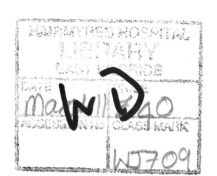

Infertility in the Male

Fourth Edition

Infertility in the Male

Fourth Edition

Edited by

Larry I. Lipshultz, Stuart S. Howards and Craig S. Niederberger

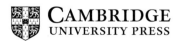
CAMBRIDGE
UNIVERSITY PRESS

CAMBRIDGE UNIVERSITY PRESS
Cambridge, New York, Melbourne, Madrid, Cape Town, Singapore,
São Paulo, Delhi, Dubai, Tokyo

Cambridge University Press
The Edinburgh Building, Cambridge CB2 8RU, UK

Published in the United States of America by Cambridge University Press, New York

www.cambridge.org
Information on this title: www.cambridge.org/9780521872898

First edition published by Churchill Livingstone 1983
Second and third edition published by Mosby Year Book 1991, 1997
Fourth edition published by Cambridge University Press 2009

Printed in the United Kingdom at the University Press, Cambridge

A catalogue record for this publication is available from the British Library

Library of Congress Cataloguing in Publication data
Infertility in the male / [edited by] Larry I. Lipshultz, Stuart S.
    Howards, Craig S. Niederberger. – 4th ed.
        p. ; cm.
    Includes bibliographical references and index.
    ISBN 978-0-521-87289-8 (hardback)
    1. Infertility, Male. I. Lipshultz, Larry I., 1942– II. Howards,
    Stuart S., 1937– III. Niederberger, Craig S.
    [DNLM: 1. Infertility, Male. WJ 709 I43 2009]
    RC889.I563 2009
    616.6'92–dc22   2009027850

ISBN 978-0-521-87289-8 Hardback

Contents

Color plate section appears between pages 276 and 277.

Contributors

Ashok Agarwal PhD HCLD
Glickman Urological and Kidney Institute, Cleveland Clinic, Cleveland, OH, USA

Joseph P. Alukal MD
Department of Urology, NYU School of Medicine, New York, NY, USA

Deborah J. Anderson PhD
Department of Obstetrics & Gynecology, Boston University School of Medicine, Boston, MA, USA

Linda D. Applegarth EdD
The Ronald O. Perelman and Claudia Cohen Center for Reproductive Medicine & Infertility, Weill Medical College of Cornell University, New York, NY, USA

Saleh Binsaleh MD FRCSC
Division of Urology, Department of Surgery, Faculty of Medicine, King Saud University, Riyadh, Saudi Arabia

Elizabeth M. Bloom JD
New England School of Law, Boston, MA, USA

Karen E. Boyle MD
Shady Grove Fertility Reproductive Science Center, Rockville, MD, & Greater Baltimore Medical Center (GBMC), Baltimore, MD, USA

Nancy L. Brackett PhD HCLD
The Miami Project to Cure Paralysis, University of Miami Miller School of Medicine, Miami, FL, USA

Robert E. Brannigan MD
Department of Urology, Northwestern University Feinberg School of Medicine, Chicago, IL, USA

James V. Bruckner PhD
Department of Pharmaceutical & Biomedical Sciences, College of Pharmacy, University of Georgia, Athens, GA, USA

Victor M. Brugh III MD
Department of Urology, Eastern Virginia Medical School, Norfolk, VA, USA

Ettore Caroppo MD
ASL BARI, Reproductive Unit, Conversano, Bari, Italy

Grace M. Centola PhD
LifeCell Dx, Inc., Buffalo, NY; New England Cryogenic Center, Newton, MA, USA

Aleksander Chudnovsky MD
Division of Urology, University of Massachusetts, Worcester, MA, USA

Susan L. Crockin JD
The Crockin Law & Policy Group LLC, Newton, MA, USA

Fnu Deepinder MD
Glickman Urological and Kidney Institute, Cleveland Clinic, Cleveland, OH, USA

David M. Fenig
Department of Pharmaceutical & Biomedical Sciences, College of Pharmacy, University of Georgia, Athens, GA, USA

Aaron B. Grotas MD
Sol & Margaret Berger Department of Urology, Beth Israel Medical Center, New York, NY, USA

Matthew P. Hardy (deceased)
Population Council, New York, NY, USA

Wayne J. G. Hellstrom MD
Department of Urology, Tulane University Health Sciences Center, New Orleans, LA, USA

Stanton C. Honig MD
Urology Center, New Haven, CT, & Division of Urology, University of Connecticut, Farmington, CT, USA

Stuart S. Howards MD
Department of Urology, University of Virginia
School of Medicine, Charlottesville, VA, USA

Keith Jarvi MD FRCSC
Division of Urology, Mount Sinai Hospital,
University of Toronto, Toronto, Ontario, Canada

Rajasingam S. Jeyendran PhD
Andrology Laboratory Services, Inc., Chicago, IL,
USA

William E. Kaplan MD
Division of Pediatric Urology, Children's
Memorial Hospital, Chicago, IL, USA

Edward Karpman MD
El Camino Urology, Mountain View, CA, USA

Sanjay S. Kasturi MD
Department of Urology, University of Pennsylvania
School of Medicine, Philadelphia, PA, USA

Mohit Khera MD MBA MPH
Scott Department of Urology, Baylor College of
Medicine, Houston, TX, USA

Nancy A. Klein MD
Seattle Reproductive Medicine, Seattle, WA, USA

Dolores J. Lamb PhD HCLD
Scott Department of Urology and Department of
Molecular and Cellular Biology, Baylor College of
Medicine, Houston, TX, USA

Jane M. Lewis MD
Department of Urologic Surgery, University of
Minnesota, Minneapolis, MN, USA

Larry I. Lipshultz MD
Scott Department of Urology, Baylor College of
Medicine, Houston, TX, USA

Kirk C. Lo MD CM FRCSC
Division of Urology, Mount Sinai Hospital,
University of Toronto, Toronto, Ontario, Canada

Charles M. Lynne MD
Department of Urology, University of Miami
Miller School of Medicine, Miami, FL, USA

R. Dale McClure MD FACS FRCSC
Department of Urology, Virginia Mason Medical
Center, Seattle, WA, USA

Antoine A. Makhlouf MD PhD
Department of Urologic Surgery, University of
Minnesota, Minneapolis, MN, USA

Myles Margolis MD FRCPC
Department of Medical Imaging, Mount Sinai
Hospital, University of Toronto, Toronto, Ontario,
Canada

Clara I. Marín-Briggiler PhD
Laboratory of Molecular Studies of the Gamete
Interaction Process, Instituto de Biología y
Medicina Experimental, CONICET, Buenos
Aires, Argentina

Randall B. Meacham MD
Division of Urology, University of Colorado
School of Medicine, Denver, CO, USA

Jesse N. Mills MD
The Urology Center of Colorado, Denver, CO,
USA

John P. Mulhall MD
Urology Service, Memorial Sloan–Kettering
Cancer Center, New York, NY, USA

Alexander Müller MD
Urology Service, Memorial Sloan–Kettering
Cancer Center, New York, NY, USA

Christine Mullin MD
Rockville Centre, NY, USA

Harris M. Nagler MD FACS
Sol and Margaret Berger Department of
Urology, Beth Israel Medical Center & Albert
Einstein College of Medicine, Yeshiva University,
NY, USA

Craig S. Niederberger MD FACS
Department of Urology, UIC College of
Medicine, & Department of Bioengineering,
UIC College of Engineering, University of
Illinois at Chicago, Chicago, IL, USA

Robert D. Oates MD
Department of Urology, Boston University School
of Medicine, Boston, MA, USA

Dana A. Ohl MD
Department of Urology, University of Michigan,
Ann Arbor, MI, USA

E. Charles Osterberg BS
Department of Urology, Northwestern
University Feinberg School of Medicine,
Chicago, IL, USA

Rodrigo L. Pagani MD
Department of Urology, University of São Paulo
School of Medicine, São Paulo, Brazil

Vassilios Papadopoulos DPharm PhD
The Research Institute of the McGill University
Health Center and Department of Medicine,
McGill University, Montreal, Quebec, Canada

Joseph A. Politch PhD
Department of Obstetrics & Gynecology,
Boston University School of Medicine, Boston,
MA, USA

Gail S. Prins PhD
Department of Urology, UIC College of
Medicine, University of Illinois at Chicago,
Chicago, IL, USA

Angela A. Reese BS
Fertility Solutions Inc, Cleveland, OH, USA

Susan A. Rothmann PhD HCLD
Fertility Solutions Inc, Cleveland, OH, USA

Edmund S. Sabanegh Jr. MD
Glickman Urological and Kidney Institute,
Cleveland Clinic, Cleveland, OH, USA

Denny Sakkas PhD
Department of Obstetrics, Gynecology &
Reproductive Sciences, Yale University School of
Medicine, New Haven, CT, USA

Jay I. Sandlow MD
Department of Urology, Medical College of
Wisconsin, Milwaukee, WI, USA

Richard A. Schoor MD FACS
Private Practice Urology, Smithtown, NY, USA

Paulo C. Serafini MD
Department of Gynecology, University of São
Paulo School of Medicine, São Paulo, Brazil

Mark Sigman MD
Division of Urology (Department of
Surgery), Brown University,
Providence, RI, USA

Suresh C. Sikka PhD HCLD
Andrology Clinical Laboratories,
Department of Urology, Tulane University
Health Sciences Center,
New Orleans, LA, USA

Rebecca Z. Sokol MD MPH
Keck School of Medicine, University of Southern
California, Los Angeles, CA, USA

Jens Sønksen MD DMSci PhD
Department of Urology, Herlev Hospital, Herlev,
Denmark

Miguel Srougi MD
Department of Urology, University of São Paulo
School of Medicine, São Paulo, Brazil

James Stelling MD
Reproductive Specialists of New York, Stony
Brook, NY, USA

Justin Tannir MD
Department of Ophthalmology, Kresge Eye
Institute, Detroit Medical Center, Detroit, MI,
USA

Anthony J. Thomas Jr. MD
Glickman Urological and Kidney Institute,
Cleveland Clinic, Cleveland, OH, USA

Paul J. Turek MD
The Turek Clinic, San Francisco, CA, USA

Terry T. Turner PhD
Department of Urology, University of
Virginia School of Medicine, Charlottesville,
VA, USA

Mónica H. Vazquez-Levin PhD
Laboratory of Molecular Studies of the Gamete
Interaction Process, Instituto de Biología y
Medicina Experimental, CONICET, Buenos
Aires, Argentina

Moshe Wald MD
Department of Urology, University of Iowa, Iowa
City, IA, USA

Thomas J. Walsh MD MS
Department of Urology, University of
Washington School of Medicine, Seattle,
WA, USA

Thomas M. Wheeler MD
Department of Pathology, Baylor College of
Medicine, Houston, TX, USA

Daniel H. Williams IV MD
Department of Urology, University of
Wisconsin School of Medicine and Public Health,
Madison, WI, USA

Armand Zini MD
Division of Urology, McGill University, Montreal,
Quebec, Canada

Barry R. Zirkin PhD
Division of Reproductive Biology, Department
of Biochemistry & Molecular Biology, Johns
Hopkins Bloomberg School of Public Health,
Baltimore, MD, USA

Foreword

Alan H. DeCherney

This fourth edition of *Infertility in the Male* certainly disproves the call to arms of the reproductive medicine community: when, in 1992, ICSI (intracytoplasmic sperm injection) appeared in the armamentarium of the infertility physicians it was claimed that urologists no longer had a role in the management of infertile men, except for obtaining sperm. This concept is certainly refuted and defeated by this exquisite revision of a book whose first edition was published in 1983.

The editors have assembled all of the leaders in the field to contribute on their individual areas of expertise, yet the text has editorial consistency. All of the chapters are extremely well written, providing a basic foundation for practice and for the understanding of male factors in infertility. The contributions are critical and crucial, with exciting new information combining modern insights on topics such as the determination of seminal oxidants, the measurement of DNA fragmentation and its role in infertility, and the genetic and epidemiologic impact on infertility, to cite just a few, along with historically documented concepts.

The book is well organized, and it is fascinating to follow the course of the field through its development and enhancement by rigorous scientific research. Of special interest is the in-depth chapter on analyzing male fertility data: as the authors put it, "our knowledge of male infertility, its causes and treatments, ultimately derives from raw observational and experimental data. Transforming those data into information depends on statistical analysis." This chapter provides a basic understanding of statistical analysis, which, although brief, is thorough.

The chapter on adverse effects of environmental chemicals and drugs illustrates how current this text is, as does the material on microdeletions found in the Y chromosome. It is clear that male factor infertility is a viable and exciting subspecialty of urology with a bright, sanguine, and important future. This is further illustrated by the stimulating chapter on genetic aspects of infertility, which includes a discussion of apoptotic

changes – research which will be applied in the clinic setting in the future.

The book provides comprehensive descriptions of normal and abnormal male reproductive physiology and pathophysiology, while also supplying great insights into diagnosis and treatment of the range of conditions underlying infertility in the male. It is therefore the "bible" for urologists, urologists in training, and individuals having a profound interest in male reproduction (i.e. reproductive endocrinologists).

This beautifully illustrated and well-edited text also provides an exciting forum for what the future holds. The book not only provides academic material, but also serves as a manual for carrying out procedures. This is a required read for anyone interested in male infertility.

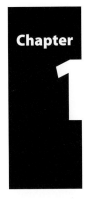

Chapter

1

Anatomy and embryology of the male reproductive tract and gonadal development

Jane M. Lewis and William E. Kaplan

Introduction

The understanding of embryology provides a foundation for the mastery of anatomy. In the treatment of men with infertility, it is only appropriate that one return to the basics of fetal development of the male reproductive tract. This chapter will review the germ layers from which all tissues organize themselves and develop. It will also review the ductal system and its critical role in reproduction. The cloacal development, with its eventual division of the urogenital sinus, will be reviewed, including the various roles the urogenital sinus plays in male reproductive tract anatomy. Testis growth and descent will be discussed. And finally the events involved in the development of external male genitalia will be reviewed.

The germ layers

After fertilization of the ovum by sperm, prenatal development happens quite rapidly. By day two, the first cell division creates a zygote. On day three, with ongoing rapid cell division known as cleavage, the morula (from the Latin word for mulberry) forms and travels down the fallopian tube into the uterus. On day four, the morula develops a fluid-filled cavity, the yolk sac. With the development of tightly packed cells along the periphery, it becomes a blastocyst. **At day six, implantation into the uterus has begun**.

During the second week of development, the inner cell mass also develops a fluid-filled space called the amniotic cavity, and once again the most central or anterior cells organize themselves into a bilaminar disc. The blastocyst becomes completely implanted in the wall of the uterus and the placenta begins to form (Fig. 1.1). **By the third week, the blastocyst develops a primitive streak, a notochord, and turns the bilaminar disc into three germ layers – ectoderm, mesoderm, and endoderm** (Fig. 1.2).

After the fourth week of development, the primitive streak stops producing mesoderm and the widely dispersed mesenchyme, and the streak essentially disappears. The intraembryonic mesoderm in the trilaminar disc further differentiates into paraxial mesoderm on either side of the notochord, followed laterally by the intermediate mesoderm and most laterally by the lateral mesoderm. **Both the urinary and genital systems develop from this intermediate mesoderm** (Fig. 1.3) [1,2].

Normal development of the urinary ductal system

The urogenital system consists of two distinct systems (urinary and genital/reproductive) which are developmentally very interrelated. In the adult male they remain interrelated, but in the adult female these systems are separate, although still very close neighbors. **Before expression of gonadal genotype, all embryos undergo the same development of three urinary excretory systems, the second of which will be significant for the male reproductive system**.

First, the pronephroi (singular – pronephros) appear and disappear in developing embryos during the fourth week. In humans, the pronephros itself has no function but the longitudinal ducts, known as pronephric or nephric ducts, empty into the cloaca. This lays the groundwork for the development of the more permanent structures.

Second, the mesonephroi (singular – mesonephros) are paired organs that appear as the pronephroi are disintegrating. They have glomeruli as well as tubules that empty into the mesonephric ducts, which were originally the paranephric ducts. Hence, sometime during the fifth week of development the mesonephroi function as a primitive filtering system and empty waste into the cloaca (Fig. 1.4).

Infertility in the Male, 4th edition, ed. Larry I. Lipshultz, Stuart S. Howards, and Craig S. Niederberger. Published by Cambridge University Press. © Cambridge University Press 2009.

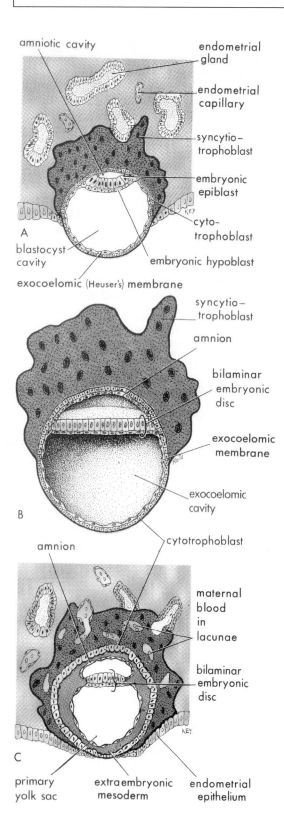

amniotic cavity

endometrial gland

endometrial capillary

syncytio-trophoblast

embryonic epiblast

cyto-trophoblast

KEY

A

blastocyst cavity

embryonic hypoblast

exocoelomic (Heuser's) membrane

syncytio-trophoblast

amnion

bilaminar embryonic disc

exocoelomic membrane

exocoelomic cavity

B

cytotrophoblast

amnion

maternal blood in lacunae

bilaminar embryonic disc

C

KEY

primary yolk sac

extraembryonic mesoderm

endometrial epithelium

Fig. 1.1. Blastocyst in the endometrium, showing the bilaminar disc formation. (A) Partially implanted in the endometrium at around 8 days. (B) Enlarged, three-dimensional representation of blastocyst. (C) A blastocyst that has completely embedded in the endometrium; the lacunae seen in the syncytiotrophoblast will eventually communicate with the endometrial vessels, establishing the primitive ureteroplacental circulation. (Reproduced with permission from Moore KL, Persaud TVN. *The Developing Human: Clinically Oriented Embryology*, 5th edn. Philadelphia, PA: Saunders, 1993.)

Third, the metanephroi (singular – metanephros), or the permanent kidneys, develop in the fifth week and begin to function in the ninth week, corresponding to when the mesonephroi degenerate. **There are two distinct parts that contribute to the creation of the metanephroi: the ureteric bud and the metanephric blastema.** A diverticulum from the (meso)nephric duct, known as the ureteric bud, grows out into some neighboring metanephric mesoderm, which is the blastema for the future kidney. The contact of the ureteric bud induces the metanephric mesoderm to grow and differentiate. Nephrons grow through a process of branching and ongoing cell induction. The developing tubules are eventually invaginated by glomeruli from the developing aorta [3].

Finally, during the seventh to eighth week post-fertilization, the effects of the gonads start to play a role. If testes are present and testosterone is being secreted, and the body's cells are receptive to it, the (meso)nephric ducts will become what are known as the Wolffian ducts and will shift their function from the urinary system to the reproductive system. They are paired, run longitudinally on either side of the midline, and empty into the cloaca. The proximal, most cranial, portion of them will become the epididymis and the remainder will form the ductus (vas) deferens and the ejaculatory duct. If testosterone is not present or is not being sensed, these ducts will disappear and leave only a few vestigial remnants. Another duct that is unique to the genital system instead of coopted from the urinary system will develop parallel to the mesonephric ducts. These are the paramesonephric ducts, to be discussed in more detail later.

The cloaca

During the rapid cell growth in the third week of the trilaminar embryo, the head and tail fold ventrally. During this folding, a part of the yolk sac is incorporated into the embryo as the hindgut, and the distal portion of this dilates into a region known as the cloaca, from the Latin word for sewer. Within this piece of incorporated yolk sac exists a diverticulum called the allantois, from

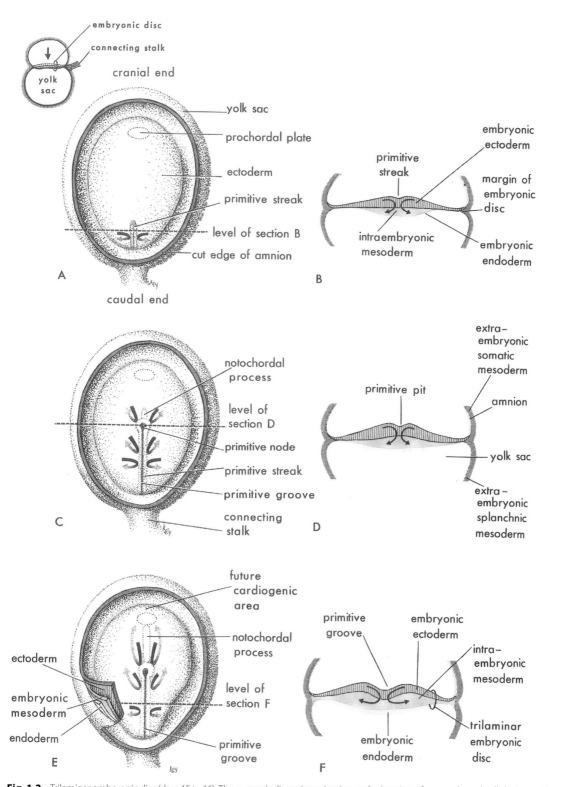

Fig. 1.2. Trilaminar embryonic disc (days 15 to 16). The arrows indicate invagination and migration of mesenchymal cells between the ectoderm and endoderm. (A, C & E) Dorsal views, with the amnion removed; (B, D, & F) corresponding cross-section views. (Reproduced with permission from Moore KL, Persaud TVN. *The Developing Human: Clinically Oriented Embryology*, 5th edn. Philadelphia, PA: Saunders, 1993.)

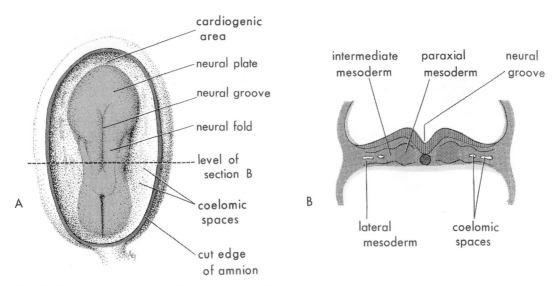

Fig. 1.3. Embryo at 18 days, showing differentiation of mesoderm: (A) dorsal view, with the amnion removed; (B) cross section indicated in image A. (Reproduced with permission from Moore KL, Persaud TVN. *The Developing Human: Clinically Oriented Embryology*, 5th edn. Philadelphia, PA: Saunders, 1993.)

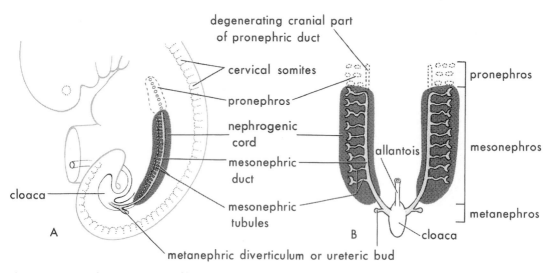

Fig. 1.4. Junction of excretory organs in fifth week. (A) lateral view; (B) ventral view with the mesonephric tubules rotated laterally for ease of viewing. (From Moore KL, Persaud TVN. *The Developing Human: Clinically Oriented Embryology*, 5th edn. Philadelphia, PA: Saunders, 1993.)

the Greek word *allas* meaning sausage. It extends up into the connecting stalk of the embryo and, although much more important in other animals' developing respiratory function, in humans it is associated with the developing bladder, and its blood vessels become the umbilical arteries and vein. The vestigial remnants are the urachus and the median umbilical ligament.

The cloaca, as incorporated yolk sac, is an endoderm-lined cavity, anchored at the caudal end by the cloacal membrane. **Currently, there are two leading theories as to the separation of the cloacal membrane.** The classic view was that mesenchyme continues to grow rapidly, extending caudally and dorsally, between the more ventral allantois and the relatively dorsal hindgut. This mesenchyme is known as the urorectal septum. As it grows caudally, it eventually fuses with the cloacal membrane, and this point of fusion in adults is known as the perineal body. The migration and fusion

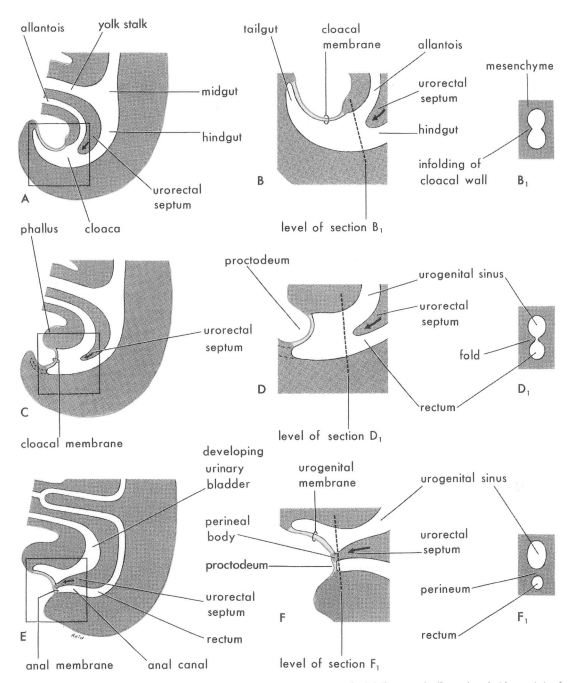

Fig. 1.5. Cloaca and urogenital sinus division: (A & B) at 4 weeks; (C & D) at 6 weeks; (E & F) at 7 weeks. (Reproduced with permission from Moore KL, Persaud TVN. *The Developing Human: Clinically Oriented Embryology*, 5th edn. Philadelphia, PA: Saunders, 1993.)

of the urorectal septum effectively divides the cloaca into a ventral urogenital sinus (which is contiguous with the allantois cranially) and a dorsal area including the rectum and anal canal during the seventh week of development. The cloacal membrane associated with the ventral urogenital sinus is now referred to as the urogenital membrane, and the dorsal portion is the anal membrane. By the end of the eighth week, the anal membrane usually ruptures and the urogenital membrane is degenerating (Fig. 1.5) [4].

This theory was challenged by more recent studies utilizing three-dimensional magnetic resonance imaging. These observations led to the theory that the descending urorectal septum never fuses with the cloacal membrane [5]. Rather, the cloaca undergoes preprogrammed cell death during the eighth week of development, and the urorectal septum, which is immediately posterior to the cloacal membrane, still defines the boundary between the urogenital sinus on the ventral side, and the rectum/anal canal on the dorsal side. The tip of the urorectal septum then becomes the perineal body.

The trigone and excretory ducts

During the fifth week of development, as the final kidney is beginning to form as described above, the portion of the urogenital sinus that will become bladder is beginning to take shape. As discussed above, the mesonephric ducts, which are mesodermal structures, are connected to the urogenital sinus (ventral portion of the cloaca, and therefore endodermally lined) bilaterally. **The portions of the mesonephric ducts distal to where the ureteric buds have sprouted become known as the common excretory ducts.** The common excretory ducts then fuse in the midline and become known as the primitive trigone. With ongoing growth of the urogenital sinus, the trigone migrates more and more caudal, which causes the ureteric buds eventually to become individually invaginated into the developing trigone as well (Fig. 1.6). It is assumed that the rapid growth of the bladder, along with the relative ascent of the kidneys, exerts a force on the ureteric orifices to move superolaterally after incorporation into the bladder.

The common excretory ducts eventually move into the prostatic part of the urethra and become known as the verumontanum. Anomalies in development can occur depending on the distance between the orifice of the mesonephric duct within the urogenital sinus and the ureteric bud. If it is too short, the resultant ureteral orifice may develop distally in the bladder neck or urethra; if it is too long, it may never become incorporated into the bladder. Also, the migration of the excretory ducts, as well as the appearance of the paramesonephric ducts, all occur before testosterone and anti-Müllerian hormone (AMH), also known as Müllerian-inhibiting substance (MIS), are present [3].

The urogenital sinus: male

The urogenital sinus has three distinct regions, all lined with the same endodermal cells. The most cranial is the vesical part, which is contiguous with the allantois, which will become the bladder. There is a middle pelvic part, which in males will become the prostate and bulbourethral glands. And finally there is a caudal, phallic part, which is in contact with the urogenital membrane. This is the region that will become the spongy urethra. The distal part of the urethra originates from ectodermal cells along the glandular plate at the tip of the glans penis. This plate is evident at eleven weeks of development. By the twelfth week, the plate becomes canalized and starts growing down to meet the spongy urethra coming from the urogenital sinus by the fourteenth week. Connective tissue and smooth muscle of the urethra derive from neighboring splanchnic mesenchyme (Fig. 1.7) [6].

The growing circulation of androgens from the developing testes promotes the start of prostate development. As the urethra is growing distally from the most caudal part of the urogenital sinus, the prostate develops from the middle pelvic part of the urogenital sinus during the tenth week of gestation. This starts with various outpouchings of endoderm into the neighboring mesenchyme, which will then differentiate into stroma and smooth muscle. The endodermal or epithelial cords eventually canalize, and the lining develops into two distinct cell types, luminal and basal.

The bulbourethral glands develop as paired outgrowths from the spongy part of the urethra, just distal to the prostate [6]. As with the prostate, the epithelial portion of these glands comes from the endoderm of the urogenital sinus. The outpouchings of endoderm then induce the local mesenchyme to form the smooth-muscle fibers and stroma of the glands. These glands will produce secretions that contribute to semen (Fig. 1.8).

The urogenital sinus: female

The urogenital sinus, in its undifferentiated state, is composed of three sections: a cranial (vesical) part, a middle (pelvic) part, and a caudal (phallic) part. The fate of the vesical part is the same for females and males – it becomes the bladder. This is the area into which the distal mesonephric ducts invaginate, fuse, migrate caudally, then receive the invagination of the ureteric buds, all forming the trigone. The middle (pelvic) and the caudal (phallic) portions have slightly different fates in the developing female. **As there is no testosterone or anti-Müllerian hormone (AMH) present in the eighth week, the phallus does not grow but the urethra undergoes the same transformation,**

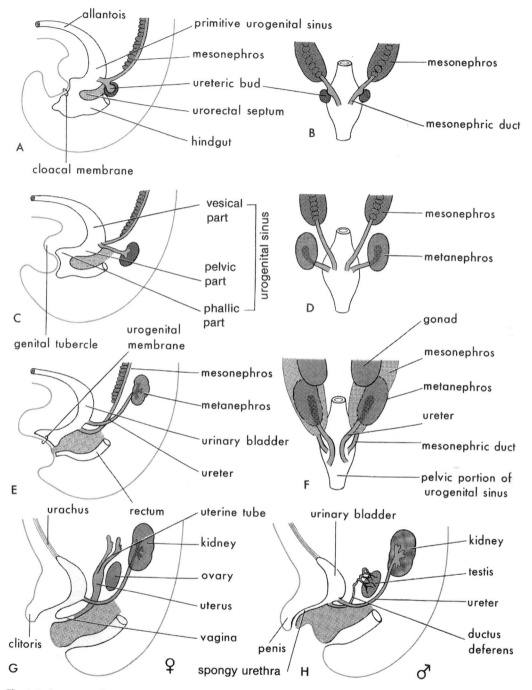

Fig. 1.6. Formation of urogenital sinus and rectum; movement of the mesonephric ducts and ureters; formation of bladder, urethra, and urachus. Shown in stages from 5 weeks to 12 weeks. (Reproduced with permission from Moore KL, Persaud TVN. *The Developing Human: Clinically Oriented Embryology*, 5th edn. Philadelphia, PA: Saunders, 1993.)

albeit much shorter, from the caudal portion of the urogenital sinus (Fig. 1.6).

In the hormonal female, the mesonephric (Wolffian) ducts degenerate, but the paramesonephric ducts persist. The ends of these ducts fuse together and then fuse into the posterior wall of the middle (pelvic) urogenital sinus – that point of fusion becomes known as the sinusal tubercle. The ducts continue to fuse with

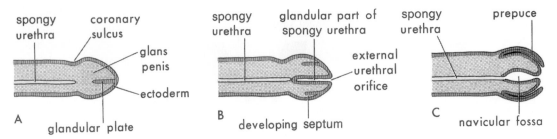

Fig. 1.7. Developing penis from 11 to 14 weeks. (Reproduced with permission from Moore KL, Persaud TVN. *The Developing Human: Clinically Oriented Embryology*, 5th edn. Philadelphia, PA: Saunders, 1993.)

the urogenital sinus and open up into a common, single-lumen chamber, known as the ureterovaginal canal. This becomes the uterus as well as the proximal portion of the vagina.

The sinusal tubercle eventually contributes to the vaginal plate, which elongates and becomes canalized. The final barrier to the outside world is a thin endodermal layer of urogenital sinus, which normally dissolves by the fifth month, but a remnant will be left as the vaginal hymen. The epithelial layer of the entire vagina and cervix may extend in from this endodermal urogenital sinus connection (Fig. 1.8) [3].

The genital ducts

To review, there are a series of ducts that develop in the genitourinary systems. Some are primarily for the rudimentary urinary system (pronephric), some start in the urinary system but are coopted by the genital system (mesonephric), and some are proprietary of the genital system (paramesonephric). **While the fate of the pronephric duct is the same for both males and females, the development of the other two ducts is dependent on gonadal differentiation.**

Regardless of chromosomal gender, during the fifth week of development, gonadal development begins. It is undifferentiated for the first two weeks. Both gonads, the testis and the ovary, arise from a mix of mesothelium (mesodermal epithelium) from the posterior abdominal wall, mesenchyme, and primordial germ cells. The process starts with the appearance of a thickened area of epithelium, the gonadal ridge. The primordial germ cells are first identified in the developing embryo during the fourth week. They eventually migrate towards the gonadal ridge. Additional epithelial tissue of the gonadal ridge thickens, becoming known as the primary sex cords. The sex cords incorporate the primordial germ cells which are now present. **At this point, the gonadal ridge is identified as having**

two distinct regions: the epithelial layer (cortex) and the mesenchymal area (medulla) (Fig. 1.9) [4].

Still in an undifferentiated gonadal state, the paramesonephric ducts appear. The cranial ends of these ducts are funnel-shaped and open into the future peritoneal cavity. These ducts become known as the Müllerian ducts.

By the sixth week of development, if the embryo is chromosomally XY, cells in the sex cords in the medulla will grow and become Sertoli cells, under the influence of SRY (sex-determining region of the Y sex chromosome), and the cortex will disappear. The Sertoli cells will start to produce AMH, which will halt the development of the paramesonephric ducts and eventually cause rapid regression during the eighth to tenth week of development [7]. Remnants in the males include a small piece of tissue on the superior pole of the testis called the appendix testis. Also, extra tissue along the posterior urethra can remain, becoming known as the prostatic utricle. Rarely, a genetic male due to an AMH malfunction will have persistence of the Müllerian ducts (and thus a uterus and fallopian tubes will develop), a condition called hernia uteri inguinale. The Sertoli cells, along with the primordial germ cells, will become seminiferous tubules at puberty.

The seminiferous or testis cords are separated by mesenchyme that is stimulated to become Leydig cells by the SRY protein. This occurs from the eighth to the tenth week of development, at which point these cells start producing testosterone. Initially, the production is regulated by placental chorionic gonadotropin, but eventually the developing embryo's own hypothalamus–pituitary axis takes over control with the pituitary secretion of human chorionic gonadotropin (hCG).

Testosterone stimulates numerous changes in the existing ductal system. Specifically, the mesonephric duct definitively becomes the Wolffian duct. The most

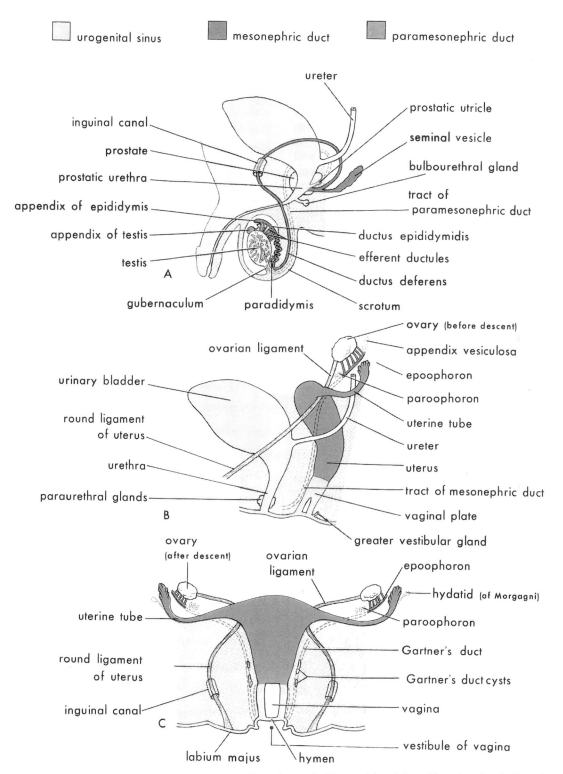

Fig. 1.8. Urogenital sinus and genital duct integration: (A) newborn male; (B) 12-week female fetus; (C) newborn female. (Reproduced with permission from Moore KL, Persaud TVN. *The Developing Human: Clinically Oriented Embryology*, 5th edn. Philadelphia, PA: Saunders, 1993.)

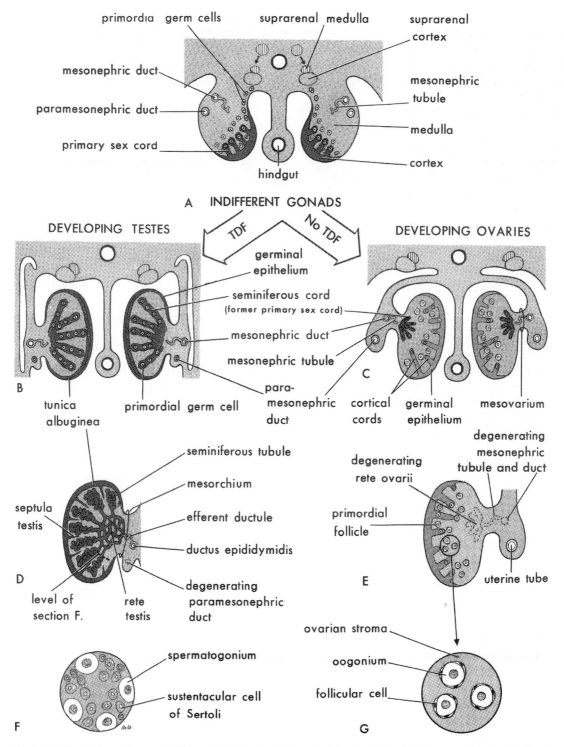

Fig. 1.9. Differentiation of the gonads: (A) 6 weeks; (B) 7 weeks; (C) 12 weeks; (D) testis at 20 weeks; (E) ovary at 20 weeks; (F & G) sections of testis and ovary at 20 weeks. TDF, testis-determining factor. (Reproduced with permission from Moore KL, Persaud TVN. *The Developing Human: Clinically Oriented Embryology*, 5th edn. Philadelphia, PA: Saunders, 1993.)

distal portion of the Wolffian duct becomes invested with more smooth muscle and becomes the ductus (vas) deferens. Near the urogenital sinus/developing prostate, during the tenth week, a pair of lateral buds develops from the duct and become the seminal vesicles. The most cranial portion of the duct will disintegrate, and the remnant tissue is called the appendix epididymis. The mesonephric tubules (not ducts) that grew near the developing testes will become incorporated into the testis–epididymis structure as efferent ductules. **As already structured, these former tubules (now efferent ductules) empty into the Wolffian duct, which in proximity to the developing testis, are transforming into part of the ductus epididymis.** The more distal ends of the testis cords will form the tubuli recti and the rete testis. But the communications between rete testis and efferent ductules of the epididymis will not be established until after the twelfth week of development [8].

Testis development continues. In addition to the sex cords forming with germ cells and Sertoli cells, and Leydig cells in the interstices, the development of the tunica albuginea is a characteristic and diagnostic feature of testicular development. This is a thick, fibrous capsule of connective tissue that causes the separation of the sex cords from the epithelial layer. The testis then becomes suspended in a developing mesentery of its own called the mesorchium, along with two major attachments: the cranial suspensory ligament and the gubernaculum. During the fourth month of development, as the abdominal cavity is enlarging, the cranial suspensory ligament, stimulated by the presence of testosterone, regresses. The gubernaculum, however, thickens regardless of androgen, and holds the testis in the inguinal region. Increasing intra-abdominal pressure up to this point is likely unimportant in testis travel, but for its migration through the inguinal canal and down into the scrotum it becomes more important [3].

The descent of the testis into the scrotum is complicated. During the seventh month of development, the peritoneal cavity evaginates through each inguinal canal down into the scrotum. This outpouching is called the processus vaginalis. While this is happening, the gubernaculum continues to thicken and shorten its hold on the testis [9]. **Testosterone appears to be important in the dissolution of the cranial suspensory ligament as well as in the migration of the testis from the inguinal canal into the scrotum. The androgenic mechanism of action is poorly understood.** Researchers have also looked at the role of

AMH from Sertoli cells [10], *Hoxa10* gene expressed in the gubernaculum, as well a Leydig cell gene product called INSL3 [11,12], with promising research but no definitive conclusions. It was observed that if the genitofemoral nerve is transected, cryptorchidism occurs [13]. Over years of study, this has implicated androgen action via this nerve [14] and denervation of the gubernaculum as well as resultant lack of the neurotransmitter calcitonin gene-related peptide [15]. Once again, no consensus has been reached.

Phenotypic sex development

The external genitalia begin their development in an undifferentiated state. As with the internal ductal system, the presence or absence of a Y sex chromosome with the *Sry* gene and the production of testosterone will drive the differentiation to a male or female phenotype [16]. There are, however, many other gene loci implicated in successful male differentiation, some for the formation of the urogenital ridge – *Wt1* (Wilms' tumor 1), *Sf1* (steroidogenic factor 1), and *Dax1* (dosage-sensitive sex reversal, adrenal hypoplasia congenital, X chromosome) [17]; others for Sertoli cell functions – *Sox9*, *FGF9*, *Sry* [18,19]; and still others for transcription of the AMH gene – *Fog2*, *Igf1* [20,21]. Actual phenotypic male expression involves testosterone production from Leydig cells, but several genes have been identified as producers of essential enzymes – *StAR*, *Cyp11a1*, *Cyp17*, and *3βHSD* [22].

Before these gene products come into play, during the fourth week of development in the undifferentiated state, the embryo's growing mesenchyme gathers together at the cranial end of the cloacal membrane forming the genital tubercle. Additional proliferating tissue is noted on either side of the cloacal membrane; this becomes what is known as the labioscrotal swellings and the urogenital folds. The genital tubercle elongates and becomes what is known as a phallus. As previously discussed, the cloacal membrane is divided into the ventral urogenital membrane and the dorsal anal membrane. The urogenital membrane becomes the urethral groove, which is bordered on either side by the urogenital folds. This membrane, along with the anal membrane, ruptures in the eighth week, which coincides with the presence or absence of testosterone, resulting in the urethral groove that will extend along the ventrum of the phallus in males, and a common vestibule of the vagina in females [7].

In the presence of testosterone, the phallus lengthens and enlarges to form the penis. The urethral groove grows as well, with the lateral walls made

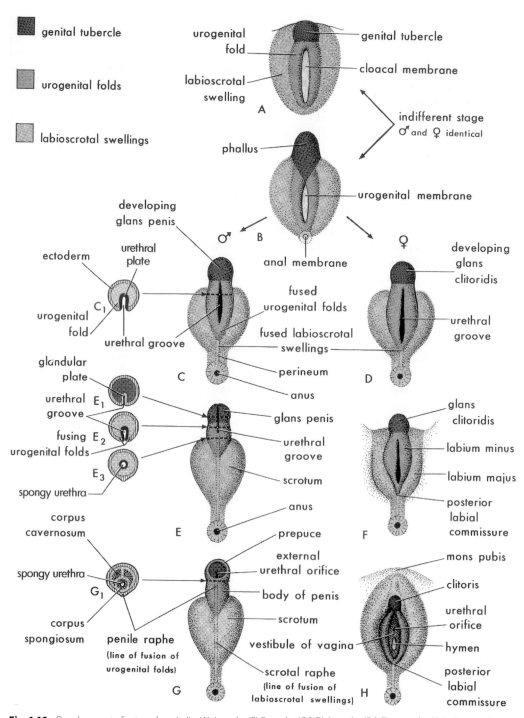

Fig. 1.10. Development of external genitalia: (A) 4 weeks; (B) 7 weeks; (C & D) 9 weeks; (E & F) 11 weeks; (G & H) 12 weeks. (Reproduced with permission from Moore KL, Persaud TVN. *The Developing Human: Clinically Oriented Embryology*, 5th edn. Philadelphia, PA: Saunders, 1993.)

up of urogenital folds, and the inner lining made up of endodermal cells from the phallic portion of the urogenital sinus called the urethral plate. The urogenital folds fuse in the midline, enclosing the spongy urethra

with the penis, and the result is the externally visible median raphe. This is an extension of the fusion that has occurred with the labioscrotal swellings, forming the median raphe of the scrotum. As mentioned previously in the section on urethral development, the ectoderm from the glandular plate at the tip of the glans penis forms a cellular cord that grows down into the penis to meet the spongy urethra (Fig. 1.10).

During the twelfth week, there is a proliferation of ectoderm around the glans, forming the prepuce. Eventually, there is a breakdown of the preputial tissue from the glans, but this may not happen until the child reaches infancy [8].

Conclusion

The embryology of the genitourinary tract is quite complicated, involves many pieces being in the exact place at the correct time, and requires that the underlying genome provide all the appropriate gene products in the right sequence. Many errors can and do occur. Fortunately for the developing embryo, these errors of the genitourinary tract are rarely fatal, but certainly can cause problems for the individual born into the world. An understanding of how things are formed can greatly aid in diagnosis and treatment of these patients.

References

[1] Moore KL, Persaud TVN. The beginning of human development. *The Developing Human: Clinically Oriented Embryology*, 5th edn. Chapter 2. Philadelphia, PA: Saunders, 1993: 15–41.

[2] Moore KL, Persaud TVN. Formation of the bilaminar embryonic disc. *The Developing Human: Clinically Oriented Embryology*, 5th edn. Chapter 3. Philadelphia, PA: Saunders, 1993: 43–53.

[3] Park JM. Normal development of the urogenital system. In: Wein AJ, Kavoussi LR, Novick AC, Partin AW, Peters CA, eds. *Campbell–Walsh Urology*, 9th edn. Philadelphia, PA: Saunders Elsevier, 2007: 3121–48.

[4] Cuckow PM, Nyirady P. Embryology of the urogenital tract. In: Gearhart JP, Rink RC, Mouriquand PDE, eds. *Pediatric Urology*. Philadelphia, PA: Saunders, 2001: 3–13.

[5] Nievelstein RA, van der Werff JF, Verbeek FJ, Valk J, Vermeij-Keers C. Normal and abnormal embryonic development of the anorectum in human embryos. *Teratology* 1998; 57: 70–8.

[6] Moore KL. The pelvis and perineum. *Clinically Oriented Anatomy*, 3rd edn. Chapter 3. Baltimore, MD: Williams & Wilkins, 1992: 277–312.

[7] Moore KL, Persaud Tvn. The urogenital system. *The Developing Human: Clinically Oriented Embryology*, 5th edn. Chapter 12. Philadelphia, PA: Saunders, 1993: 265–303.

[8] Lerman SE, McAleer IM, Kaplan GW. Embryology of the genitourinary tract. In: Belman AB, King LR, Kramer SA, eds. *Clinical Pediatric Urology*, 4th edn. London: Martin Dunitz, 2002: 1–23.

[9] Heyns CF. The gubernaculum during testicular descent in the human fetus. *J Anat* 1987; 153: 93–112.

[10] Josso N, Picard JY, Imbeaud S, et al. The persistent mullerian duct syndrome: a rare cause of cryptorchidism. *Eur J Pediatr* 1993; 152 (Suppl 2): S76–8.

[11] Adham IM, Brukhardt E, Benahmed M, Engel W. Cloning of a cDNA for a novel insulin-like peptide of the testicular Leydig cells. *J Biol Chem* 1993; 268: 26668–72.

[12] Nef S, Parada LF. Cryptorchidism in mice mutant for Insl3. *Nat Genet* 1999; 22: 295–9.

[13] Beasley SW, Hutson JM. Effect of division of genitofemoral nerve on testicular descent in the rat. *Aust N Z J Surg* 1987; 57: 49–51.

[14] Hutson JM, Beasley SW, Bryan AD. Cryptorchidism in spina bifida and spinal cord transection: a clue to the mechanism of transinguinal descent of the testis. *J Pediatr Surg* 1988; 23: 275–7.

[15] Park WH, Hutson JM. The gubernaculum shows rhythmic contractility and active movement during testicular descent. *J Pediatr Surg* 1991; 26: 615–7.

[16] Greenfield A, Koopman P. SRY and mammalian sex determination. *Curr Top Dev Biol* 1996; 34: 1–23.

[17] Nachtigal MW, Hirokawa Y, Enyeart-VanHouten DL, et al. Wilms' tumor 1 and Dax-1 modulate the orphan nuclear receptor SF-1 in sex-specific gene expression. *Cell* 1998; 93: 445–54.

[18] Sekido R, Bar I, Narvaez V, Penny G, Lovell-Badge R. SOX9 is up-regulated by the transient expression of SRY specifically in Sertoli cell precursors. *Dev Biol* 2004; 274: 271–9.

[19] Colvin JS, Green RP, Schmahl J, Capel B, Ornitz DM. Male-to-female sex reversal in mice lacking fibroblast growth factor 9. *Cell* 2001; 104: 875–89.

[20] Tevosian SG, Albrecht KH, Crispino JD, et al. Gonadal differentiation, sex determination and normal Sry expression in mice require direct interaction between transcription partners GATA4 and FOG2. *Development* 2002; 129: 4627–34.

[21] Nef S, Verma-Kurvari S, Merenmies J, et al. Testis determination requires insulin receptor family function in mice. *Nature* 2003; 426: 291–5.

[22] Brennan J, Tilmann C, Capel B. Pdgfr-α mediates testis cord organization and fetal Leydig cell development in the XY gonad. *Genes Dev* 2003; 17: 800–10.

Male hypothalamic–pituitary–gonadal axis

Ettore Caroppo

Introduction

The male hypothalamic–pituitary–gonadal (HPG) axis is a finely controlled system whose role is to promote spermatogenesis and androgen biosynthesis. Hypothalamus, pituitary, and testes secrete hormones and peptides that feed back at multiple levels of the reproductive axis to control their own synthesis and secretion, resulting in a tightly regulated system (Fig. 2.1). Specific neurons in the hypothalamus secrete the decapeptide gonadotropin-releasing hormone (GnRH) in an episodic pattern of pulses. GnRH is transported through the hypophyseal portal circulation to the anterior pituitary gland, where it binds to its own receptors on a specific pituitary cell type, the gonadotrope, to modulate the synthesis and secretion of the gonadotropins, luteinizing hormone (LH) and follicle-stimulating hormone (FSH). Gonadotropins, in turn, are secreted into the systemic circulation and act on the testes to regulate spermatogenesis and androgen biosynthesis. Gonadal steroids and peptides are finally secreted into the systemic circulation and act to modulate hypothalamic and pituitary function in both positive and negative feedback loops. Such a dynamic system achieves homeostasis via axis-specific, time-delayed, and dose-responsive feedback and feedforward linkages.

GnRH

GnRH is a decapeptide produced in the GnRH neurons located in the preoptic area and projected to the median eminence of hypothalamus. It is released in the portal blood in discrete pulses, and the frequency and amplitudes of such pulses determine the pattern of FSH and LH release from the pituitary. GnRH secretion is regulated by autocrine, paracrine, and endocrine mechanisms as follows (Table 2.1).

Regulation of GnRH secretion

Autocrine regulation

GnRH is thought to regulate its own release by means of an ultrashort loop feedback mechanism. GnRH agonists have been shown to reduce GnRH release both in vivo [1] and in vitro [2], as a result of the interaction with the GnRH receptor (GnRHR), which is expressed within the hypothalamus.

Synchronization of GnRH neuron activity is critical for episodic hormone release, but the mechanisms for GnRH neuron coordination remain unclear. One possible mechanism involves synaptic interactions among these cells [3,4], with GnRH itself being implicated in the mediation of such communication. To understand this mechanism, acutely prepared brain slices from castrate adult male mice were chosen to examine GnRH and non-GnRH (control) neurons (Fig. 2.2) for both type 1 GnRHR (GnRHR-1) expression and electrophysiological responses to GnRH [5]. It was found that a substantial subpopulation of adult GnRH neurons expressed GnRHR-I, and that the response to activation of this receptor was dose-dependent, with low doses inhibiting and high doses stimulating firing rate (Fig. 2.3). The reduction in firing rate induced by a low-dose GnRH signal supported the hypothesis that GnRH exerts an ultrashort negative feedback loop upon its own release. On the other hand, the increased firing rate seen with high doses suggested that autoregulation of GnRH neurons would vary depending on the level of GnRH near the receptor. **GnRH neurons could, therefore, activate and suppress their own activity using GnRH itself as an intra-GnRH neural network signal, a strategy that could have important implications for generation of the GnRH surge in addition to the regulation of pulsatile release.**

Infertility in the Male, 4th edition, ed. Larry I. Lipshultz, Stuart S. Howards, and Craig S. Niederberger. Published by Cambridge University Press. © Cambridge University Press 2009.

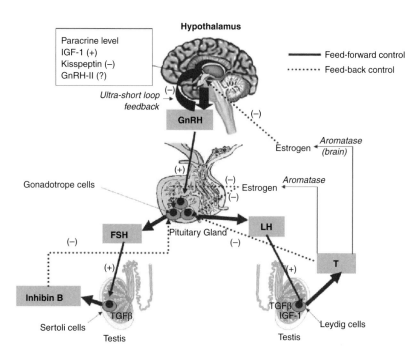

Fig. 2.1. Schematic overview of feed-forward and feedback controls within the male hypothalamic–pituitary–gonadal axis.

Table 2.1. Regulation of GnRH release

Modulators	Autocrine regulation	Paracrine regulation	Endocrine regulation
GnRH-I	Ultrashort loop feedback	–	–
Endocannabinoids	Ultrashort feedback	–	–
GnRH-II	–	(Stimulatory) role in GnRH-I secretion	–
IGF-1	–	Enhances GnRH gene transcription	–
Kisspeptin	–	Stimulates GnRH release through GPR54	–
Testosterone	–	–	Restrains activity of the GnRH-LH unit
Oestrogens	–	–	Reduces the frequency of GnRH secretion
Neurotensin	–	–	Activates GnRH electrical activity
Norepinephrine	–	–	Activates GnRH electrical activity

This hypothesis has been corroborated by evaluation of the behavior of immortalized GnRH neural GT1 cell line in primary culture. Treatment of these cells with GnRH agonists altered their pattern of GnRH secretion, increasing amplitude and decreasing frequency, with a net effect of increasing the amount of GnRH release [6–8], while GnRH antagonists eliminated pulsatile release and caused an increase in basal release, likely due to suppression of GnRH neuron activity. GT1 cells have been also found to exhibit episodic GnRH release in the absence of other cell types, a finding that strengthens the hypothesis of an autocrine regulation of pulsatile GnRH release. The finding that GT1 cells express GnRH receptors, the activation of which influences the pattern of pulsatile GnRH release by changing pulse frequency and amplitude [6], is consistent with this proposal. In addition, a study performed on hypothalamic tissue removed from fetuses of 17-day pregnant Sprague Dawley rats demonstrated that pulsatile GnRH secretion can be re-established even when all neuronal pathways and interconnections within the hypothalamus are disrupted by dispersion and culture of the hypothalamic cell population. The resulting pattern of GnRH secretion resembled the profile of GnRH release from intact hypothalamic explants and that observed in pituitary portal blood vessels. Dispersed hypothalamic cells were able to retain the ability to form interconnections,

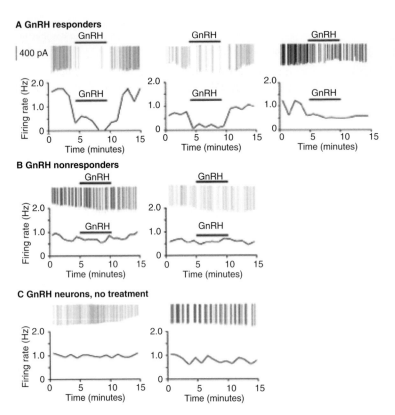

A GnRH responders

B GnRH nonresponders

C GnRH neurons, no treatment

Fig. 2.2. GnRH inhibits firing rate of a sub-population of GnRH neurons. Representative examples of firing rate of GnRH neurons that responded to GnRH treatment (bar) with (A, left and center) reversible inhibition or (A, right) inhibition that did not reverse, (B) that did not respond with inhibition, and (C) that were not treated. Vertical lines at the top of each plot are individual action currents detected, with corresponding scale bar. Graph beneath plots represent firing rate in 1-minute bins. (Reproduced with permission from: Xu C *et al.* Dose-dependent switch in response of gonadotropin-releasing hormone (GnRH) neurons to GnRH mediated through the type I GnRH receptor. *Endocrinology* 2004; **145**: 728–35. Copyright 2004 The Endocrine Society.)

and continued to generate a neuropeptide secretory pattern similar to that observed in vivo. The persistence of such a pattern, with changes in pulse frequency and amplitude, indicated that neuropeptide release from a reconstituted neuronal network can occur in the absence of inputs from extrahypothalamic neurons and peripheral endocrine glands [7].

Interestingly, it has been found that GnRH neurons could modulate their own GnRH secretion through the synthesis of factors other than GnRH itself. GnRH neurons, in fact, are able to synthesize two different endocannabinoids, anandamide and 2-arachidonyl monoacylglycerol, as demonstrated in immortalized GnRH neurons [9]. Cannabinoids have been demonstrated to reduce sperm counts, depress serum testosterone level, and suppress serum LH level. On the other hand, treatment with the opioid antagonist naloxone increases, and morphine decreases, LH secretion in castrated rams [10,11]. The highest levels of expression of cannabinoid receptors in the hypothalamus are in the medial preoptic area and arcuate nucleus [12]; taken together, these data suggest that endocannabinoids may play a role in the ultrashort feedback system of GnRH regulation by autocrine or juxtacrine interactions with cells in close apposition to GnRH neurons.

Paracrine regulation

In addition to GnRH-I, a second GnRH subtype (GnRH-II), originally identified in the chicken hypothalamus, has been found in humans [13]. This GnRH form differs from GnRH-I by three amino acid residues at position 5, 7 and 8 (His^5-Trp^7-Tyr^8-GnRH-I). Cell bodies of GnRH-II neurons are concentrated in the preoptic area and basal hypothalamus, but they can also be found in the septal region and anterior olfactory area as well as the cortical and medial amygdaloid nuclei. GnRH-II signals have been localized mainly in the periaqueductal region of the midbrain, in the caudate nucleus and, to a lesser extent, in the hippocampus and amygdala [14].

The role of GnRH-II has not yet been established. A role in reproductive behavior has been suggested by several studies, due to peptide localization in brain areas associated with this function. GnRH-II was found, indeed, to be a potent stimulator of reproductive behavior in ring doves, song sparrows, and musk shrews [15]. Moreover, recent evidence suggests that

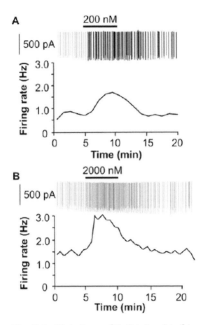

Fig. 2.3. High doses of GnRH stimulate firing activity in GnRH neurons. Representative examples of firing rate of GnRH neurons that responded to GnRH treatment (bar) at (A) 200 nM and (B) 2000 nM. Vertical lines at the top of each plot are individual action currents detected. Graph beneath plots represent firing rate in 1-minute bins. (Reproduced with permission from: Xu C *et al*. Dose-dependent switch in response of gonadotropin-releasing hormone (GnRH) neurons to GnRH mediated through the type I GnRH receptor. *Endocrinology* 2004; **145**: 728–35. Copyright 2004 The Endocrine Society.)

GnRH-II may function similarly in other mammals, including humans, to fine-tune reproductive efforts with periods of sufficient energy resources [16].

GnRH-II was found to be as effective as GnRH-I in stimulating LH release both in vivo and in vitro, as well as in stimulating FSH release in vitro [17]. The physiological relevance of this finding is yet to be ascertained. Because it seems that GnRH-II most likely exerts its physiological action via the established GnRH-I pathway, its involvement in the paracrine control of GnRH-I secretion has been hypothesized.

It has been suggested that insulin-like growth factor 1 (IGF-1) is involved in the paracrine control of GnRH secretion. Indeed, IGF-1 receptors were found to be expressed on GnRH-expressing neuronal cell line (NLT), where IGF-1 promotes DNA synthesis by stimulating hGnRH promoter activities, enhances mGnRH mRNA expression, and promotes NLT cells proliferation. IGF-1 has been shown to regulate GnRH neuronal activities under in-vivo conditions and is believed to play an important role in the regulation of

pubertal development. Moreover, IGF-1 signal is transmitted to the nucleus to regulate GnRH gene expression [references reviewed in 18]. IGF-1 could, therefore, directly act on GnRH neurons in the hypothalamus to enhance GnRH gene transcription and play a crucial role in controlling the onset of puberty.

Recently it has been proposed that kisspeptin, an RF-amide peptide ligand for G-protein-coupled receptor 54 (GPR54), may have a role in regulating GnRH secretion [19]. Direct measurements showed that kisspeptin administration provoked rapid GnRH release, with a sharp rise in both GnRH and LH within minutes of kisspeptin infusion. Kisspeptin may act directly at the level of GnRH neurons, as GPR54 was found to be localized in GnRH neurons. Moreover, peripheral and central administration of this peptide can provoke a robust gonadotropin release.

Endocrine regulation

Testosterone is thought to feed back to restrain activity of the GnRH–gonadotrope secretory unit. Pharmacological amounts of testosterone suppress LH release in healthy men, and excessive estrogen delivery represses gonadotropin secretion in the human. Conversely, selective nonsteroidal antagonists of the estrogen or androgen receptor moderately augment LH and FSH secretion.

Studies in rams and in male rhesus monkeys suggest that testosterone's predominant site of action is within the central nervous system; the employment of hypophysiotropic clamp models has confirmed that testicular steroids do not act at the pituitary gland to suppress the secretion of gonadotropins in male rhesus monkeys [20].

In rams, testosterone is capable of decreasing the secretion of GnRH. Following castration of rams, a clear and progressive increase was observed in the frequency of GnRH pulses [21], and treatment of castrated rams with testosterone decreased the frequency of GnRH pulses [22,23]. Castration of adult male rhesus monkeys resulted in increased secretion of LH and GnRH messenger RNA (mRNA) levels in the mediobasal hypothalamus, and the testes may exert an action at the hypothalamus to inhibit GnRH gene expression [24].

Studies with aromatase inhibitors suggest that aromatization of testosterone to estradiol within the brain is an important step in the feedback regulation of GnRH secretion. It has been postulated that estrogen modulates activity of GnRH neuron activity by using a variety of different mechanisms to regulate the biosynthetic and secretory activity of the GnRH neurons. In terms of estrogen's stimulatory actions on GnRH neurons, there is good evidence for at least five different neurotransmitter pathways being involved in stimulating GnRH secretion at the time of the surge [25].

It seems that estrogen orchestrates the activity patterns of several neurotransmitter systems within the GnRH network to bring about the GnRH surge. It uses the excitatory amino acids, neurotensin and norepinephrine, to activate GnRH electrical activity at the level of the GnRH cell body, while neuropeptide Y and norepinephrine have a similar role within the median eminence, presumably on GnRH terminals. Estrogen also utilizes the β-endorphin neurons but reduces their level of activity to disinhibit GnRH neurons. The neurotensin input, however, is the only component that could be regarded as originating from the anteroventral periventricular nucleus, the principal site at which estrogen is thought to act to initiate the GnRH surge in the rat. It is suggested that the very substantial projections from the anteroventral periventricular nucleus to the arcuate nucleus may represent an important pathway through which estrogen coordinates neuropeptide Y and β-endorphin neurons to help induce the surge. The norepinephrine component of the network should be regarded as a permissive neuromodulatory element. Each of these interconnected components must be functional for the GnRH surge to occur; the acute pharmacological disruption of any one will prevent its occurrence. The prolonged period of estrogen exposure required for the GnRH surge to occur is entirely consistent with the generation by estrogen of a coordinated cascade of events mediated by estrogen receptor-dependent alterations in gene transcription [25].

Estrogen seems to be able to influence GnRH pulse generator function. Experiments on brain slice preparations demonstrated that estradiol reduces the frequency of GnRH secretion and, consequently, LH release through a pathway involving GABAergic and glutamatergic neurons [26]. Indeed, GABA itself has been found to inhibit GnRH secretion in rams [20].

Pattern of GnRH secretion

GnRH is released from the hypothalamus in a pulsatile pattern, and the stimulation of gonadotropin biosynthesis and secretion by GnRH is dependent on the pulsatile nature of GnRH delivery to the anterior pituitary. Administration of exogenous GnRH in a continuous fashion results, in effect, in the downregulation of gonadotropin subunit mRNA levels and

of LH and FSH secretion, whereas pulsatile GnRH stimulates mRNA levels and secretion [27–29]. In particular, LH-β subunit mRNA levels seem to be stimulated to a greater extent by a GnRH pulse frequency of every 30 minutes, while FSH-β subunit mRNA levels are stimulated to a greater extent by a lower GnRH pulse frequency, every 120 minutes [30]. This variability in GnRH responsiveness seems to correlate, at least partially, with the concentration of GnRH receptors on the cell surface [31,32]. This may suggest that the differential effects of varying GnRH pulse frequencies on gonadotropin subunit gene expression occur directly at the level of the pituitary, not involving extrapituitary steroid or neuroendocrine factors.

The frequency and amplitude of GnRH pulses secreted by the hypothalamus vary under different physiological conditions. **It has been postulated that the frequency and amplitude of GnRH stimulation provide signals for the differential regulation of LH and FSH secretion. At higher GnRH pulse frequencies, LH secretion increases disproportionately more than FSH secretion, whereas at lower GnRH pulse frequencies, FSH secretion is favored** [33,34].

The pattern of GnRH pulsatile secretion seems to be intrinsic to GnRH neurons. GnRH neurons have been found to display rhythmic activity in multiple time domains, ranging from burst firing on the order of seconds to episodes of increased firing rate that occur on the order of many minutes. Analysis of burst-firing characteristics revealed a relationship between the high-frequency rhythms (bursts) and the low-frequency rhythms (clusters and episodes). These findings suggest a working model in which distinct rhythm generators in GnRH neurons interact to produce secretion at intervals relevant to reproductive function [35].

Burst firing has been observed in acutely isolated GnRH neurons, indicating that this mode of firing is intrinsic. Furthermore, in other neuroendocrine systems, burst firing has been positively correlated with hormone release. A burst can thus be considered the fundamental unit of activity of a GnRH neuron.

Estradiol has been found to produce the increase in episode interval by reducing the frequency with which interburst interval is altered [35]. Estradiol may alter the low-frequency rhythm, which in turn affects patterning but not the other characteristics of the high-frequency rhythm. Such a differential sensitivity to estradiol supports the notion that multiple distinct rhythm generators exist in GnRH neurons. In addition to influences such as steroids arising external to the GnRH neurosecretory network, rhythms intrinsic to individual GnRH neurons could also be modulated by interactions among GnRH neurons. In this regard, rhythms emerging from networked cells have been shown to differ from those of isolated component cells.

Gonadotropins

Gonadotropins FSH and LH are glycoproteins consisting of a common α subunit and a hormone-specific β subunit that are associated through noncovalent interactions. While the β subunits determine the functional specificity of gonadotropins, their intrinsic bioactivity is to a great extent determined by their degree of glycosylation. Weakly glycosylated forms of the hormones have a short circulatory half-time, and although totally deglycosylated gonadotropins are able to interact with their cognate receptor, they are unable to evoke generation of the second messenger signal [36]. Since gonadotropins are secreted from the pituitary as a mixture of differently glycosylated isoforms, with composition varying according to the physiological state, it is reasonable to hypothesize that the intrinsic bioactivity of gonadotropins is one variable determining their overall function.

Gonadotropins are essential for spermatogenesis and secretion of testicular androgens. Lack of gonadotropins results in suppression of spermatogenesis, as demonstrated by hypophysectomy, by GnRH immunization, and by GnRH analog treatment. Both FSH and LH play an important role in regulating spermatogenesis. FSH seems to be essential to promote spermatogenesis in men, as four men identified with inactivating FSH-β mutation were found to be azoospermic [37–39]. The integrity of FSH receptors is also a prerequisite for intact spermatogenesis, as inactivation of FSH receptor genes was found to lead to a variable degree of spermatogenic failure and infertility [40], while targeted disruption of FSH receptor genes has clearly demonstrated that FSH signaling is required for maintaining normal testicular size, seminiferous tubular diameter, sperm number, and sperm motility [41].

FSH increases spermatogonial number and maturation of spermatocytes, including meiosis, but it is unable to complete spermatogenesis. LH participates in regulating spermatogenesis by stimulating the synthesis of testosterone, which plays an essential role in spermatid maturation. It has been found, indeed, that total functional inactivation of LH caused arrest of spermatogenesis and absence of Leydig cells in men with mutation of the LH-β gene, while treatment with human chorionic gonadotropin (hCG) resulted in onset of spermatogenesis [42].

LH is essential for testosterone secretion by Leydig cells. A permissive role of FSH is postulated, as FSH-stimulated Sertoli cells secrete IGF-1, which acts in an autocrine and paracrine fashion to induce LH receptors and enhance proliferation and steroidogenesis in mouse Leydig cells [43,44]. As a matter of fact, in mice with targeted deletion of IGF-1, Leydig cells remain functionally immature with a decline in steroidogenic capacity [45], and neutralization of FSH in the EDS-treated rat model results in a reduction of serum testosterone and in-vitro testosterone production, as well as in a significant reduction in steady mRNA concentration of steroidogenic acute regulatory protein (StAR), LH receptor, and IGF-1 [46].

An episode of LH secretion induced by GnRH results in stimulation of the side-chain cleavage enzyme with the subsequent release of testosterone within 30–60 minutes of LH stimulation [47]. This testosterone response lasts approximately 24–48 hours [48]. It has been observed that between 24 and 48 hours after an LH or hCG injection, Leydig cells are refractory to further stimulation by either hormone. This phenomenon is thought to be mediated by the inhibition of C_{17-20} liase and 17α hydroxilase activity.

Regulation of gonadotropin secretion

Regulation of gonadotropin secretion in the human involves a complex interplay between feed-forward stimulation by GnRH from the hypothalamus, feedback control by sex steroids and inhibin from the testes, and, probably, autocrine/paracrine modulation by other factors within the pituitary.

Feed-forward regulation

GnRH stimulates in vitro the synthesis of gonadotropin subunits and increases α, LH-β, and FSH-β subunit mRNA levels as well as the transcriptional activity of corresponding gene promoters. Individual gonadotropin genes respond differentially to the frequency of GnRH pulses: low frequencies (one stimulus every two or four hours) appear to preferentially increase FSH-β mRNA levels whereas higher frequencies preferentially stimulate LH-β mRNA, but permanent exposure to GnRH leads to a more or less rapid depletion of both FSH-β and LH-β mRNA in a manner that suggests a rapid transcription arrest followed by RNA degradation [49]. It seems that specific mechanisms differentially regulate the expression of three genes within a single cell. These may involve not only GnRH receptor signaling but also an indirect modulation by steroids or members of the transforming growth factor β

19

superfamily, activin and inhibin. Indeed, these substances, as well as follistatin, a polypeptide that binds and functionally incapacitates activins, are produced in the anterior pituitary and seem to be involved in the paracrine/autocrine regulation of FSH secretion. It is unclear, however, if their action could explain the existing divergence between FSH and LH secretion under GnRH stimuli.

Feedback regulation

Testicular steroids play a crucial role in the feedback control of gonadotropin secretion. It has been established that testosterone's action at the pituitary level can be direct (mediated by its binding to the androgen receptor) as well as indirect, mediated by aromatization to estrogens and binding to pituitary estrogen receptors.

Testosterone seems to exert a direct feedback control of LH secretion, while its action on FSH secretion is mostly indirect. Selective suppression of estradiol secretion with an aromatase inhibitor results in a significant increase in both gonadotropins, with the increase in LH approximating that in FSH (Fig. 2.4). On the other hand, suppression of both testosterone and estradiol to castrate levels using ketoconazole (Fig. 2.5) causes an increase in LH three times greater than FSH [50]. Men with estradiol receptor mutations and congenital aromatase deficiency have a two- to threefold increase in FSH despite elevated testosterone levels,

similar to increases observed in studies employing aromatase inhibitors. Similarly, adult male mice with targeted disruption of the aromatase *Cyp19* gene exhibit elevated levels of gonadotropins despite high circulating testosterone concentrations. Patients with congenital androgen insensitivity syndrome (AIS) have normal or minimally elevated FSH despite markedly elevated LH levels, and treatment with clomiphene has been shown to exert similar effects on FSH secretion in these men compared with normal men. Finally, administration of nonaromatizable androgens, such as DHT or fluoxymesterone, has been shown to have no impact on FSH secretion except at very high doses [references reviewed in 50].

A number of studies have demonstrated the pituitary site of estrogen feedback action. Patients with isolated GnRH deficit were shown to have increased gonadotropin levels after aromatase treatment [51], and in men with estrogen resistance or aromatase deficiency, serum gonadotropins were found elevated or at the upper limit of the normal range despite normal or elevated serum testosterone levels, indicating that aromatization of testosterone to estradiol is required for normal functioning of gonadotropin feedback [52–54].

Estradiol inhibits LH secretion by decreasing LH pulse amplitude and LH responsiveness to GnRH, consistent with a pituitary site of action. Administration

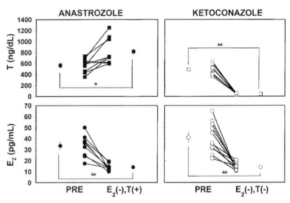

Fig. 2.5. Changes in T and E_2 in normal men in response to anastrozole (left panels) and ketoconazole (right panels). Individual and mean 6 SEM data are depicted for subjects before and after selective E_2 suppression by aromatase blockade [E_2(2), T(1)] and after biochemical castration [E_2(2), T(2)]. Asterisks represent a significant change from baseline: *, $P < 0.05$; **, $P < 0.0005$. To convert the values for T to nanomoles per L, multiply by 0.03467. To convert the values for E_2 to picomoles per L, multiply by 3.671. (Reproduced with permission from Hayes FJ *et al.* Differential regulation of gonadotropin secretion by testosterone in the human male: absence of a negative feedback effect of testosterone on follicle-stimulating hormone secretion. *J Clin Endocrinol Metab* 2001; **86**: 53–8. Copyright 2001 The Endocrine Society.)

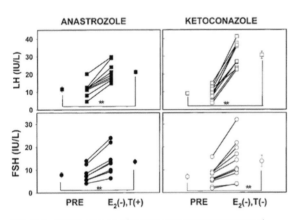

Fig. 2.4. Changes in gonadotropin concentrations in normal men in response to anastrozole (left panels) and ketoconazole (right panels). Individual and mean 6 SEM data are depicted for subjects before and after selective E_2 suppression by aromatase blockade [E_2(2), T(1)] and after biochemical castration [E_2(2), T(2)]. Asterisks represent a significant change from baseline: **, $P < 0.0005$. (Reproduced with permission from Hayes FJ *et al.* Differential regulation of gonadotropin secretion by testosterone in the human male: absence of a negative feedback effect of testosterone on follicle-stimulating hormone secretion. *J Clin Endocrinol Metab* 2001; **86**: 53–8. Copyright 2001 The Endocrine Society.)

of antiestrogens to normal men results in an increase in LH pulse frequency [51]. In men, pharmacological infusions of estradiol and pathological hyperestrogenism tend to blunt spontaneous LH pulse amplitude and bolus GnRH-stimulated LH release without repressing LH pulse frequency, while administration of nonsteroidal estrogen-receptor antagonists does augment LH pulse frequency [55].

Estrogen does not fully account for the negative feedback regulation of FSH secretion. The existence of a testicular, nonsteroidal, endocrine factor controlling FSH secretion was first postulated in 1932, when the inhibin family was discovered and characterized. At least two forms of inhibin, inhibin A and inhibin B, exist, and they share a common α subunit linked by disulfide bonds to different β subunits, which are termed βA and βB. Inhibin A is a dimeric protein consisting of αβA, whereas inhibin B consists of αβB. The testes are the principal source of circulating inhibin, and within the testes, Sertoli cells are generally agreed to be the predominant site of inhibin production. The principal form of circulating inhibin in men is inhibin B, and the inverse relationship between circulating inhibin B and FSH suggests that this is the physiologically relevant form involved in the testicular regulation of FSH secretion.

The importance of inhibin B in feedback regulation of FSH regulation in males has been clearly demonstrated in animal studies. Treatment of castrated rams with a physiological dose of testosterone decreased FSH plasma concentrations by approximately only 15%. Moreover, in castrated rams infused for 12 hours with a dose of human recombinant (hr) inhibin that resulted in the plasma inhibin concentrations found in intact rams, FSH plasma concentrations were reduced to values similar to those found in intact rams. This result was achieved without any effect on LH secretion. Furthermore, administration of hr-inhibin to castrated hypothalamo-pituitary disconnected rams treated with GnRH pulses suppressed FSH plasma concentrations, demonstrating that the negative feedback actions exerted on FSH occur at pituitary gland level. Administration of testosterone and charcoal-extracted porcine follicular fluid as a source of inhibin to hypophysiotropically clamped adult male rhesus monkeys maintained circulating FSH concentrations at the intact level following castration. Passive immunization against the α subunit of human inhibin resulted in increased FSH secretion, with no effect on LH or testosterone, in hypophysiotropically clamped juvenile rhesus monkeys infused intermittently with GnRH and in normal intact male rhesus monkeys. Finally, in hypophysiotropically clamped juvenile rhesus monkeys, treatment with hr-inhibin A alone (and in combination with testosterone) held circulating FSH and FSH-β mRNA at control levels following castration, whereas testosterone alone did not restrain the post-castration rise in FSH synthesis and secretion [references reviewed in 20].

Similar results have been obtained in human males. Selective ablation of sex steroids in men resulted in a modest increase in FSH levels, which remained within the normal adult male range [56]. In subjects with primary gonadal failure, sex steroid administration alone failed to reduce FSH levels to the normal range, and in normal men treated with ketoconazole no significant change was observed in FSH levels, whereas LH levels were elevated [56]. Finally, chemotherapy-induced testicular damage produces a decrease in inhibin B level with a consequent rapid increase in FSH level [57].

Pattern of gonadotropin secretion

Direct monitoring of hypothalamic–pituitary portal blood in the rat, sheep, and monkey has demonstrated that secretory bursts of GnRH are followed uniformly by a slightly time-delayed pulse of LH secretion. GnRH release from the hypothalamus into the portal circulation is episodic rather than continuous, which in turn causes LH to be released in a series of secretory bursts, resulting in intermittently elevated LH concentrations in the blood (Fig. 2.6). The amplitude of such serum LH concentration peaks in healthy men ranges from 35% to 270% (increase from nadir to peak). Although LH pulses do not exhibit strictly regular periodicity, they typically occur in an ultradian fashion, with a mean frequency in men of approximately one event per hour or one every 90–120 minutes [58].

Pulsatile LH concentrations bathing Leydig cells in the testes in turn stimulate testosterone secretion in a dose-dependent manner. Some evidence suggests that LH and testosterone levels show circadian variations, with maximal hormone concentrations occurring during the later portion of nighttime sleep. In general, the amplitude of LH pulses tends to vary inversely with event frequency and to be maximal at night, but mean daily serum LH and testosterone concentrations remain within a relatively narrow physiological range, probably reflecting homeostatic feedback control. In young men, serum LH and testosterone concentrations are cross-correlated, reflecting LH's dose-dependent

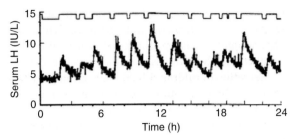

Fig. 2.6. Serum luteinizing hormone (LH) concentrations (mean of duplicates) measured by radioimmunoassay in blood collected at 1-minute intervals over 24 hours in a healthy young adult male. Deflections above the data are cluster-identified LH pulses. (Reproduced with permission from Bergendahl M *et al*. Current concepts on ultradian rhythms of luteinizing hormone secretion in the human. *Hum Reprod Update* 1996; **2**: 507–18.)

feed-forward action on Leydig cell testosterone biosynthesis as well as testosterone's negative feedback on GnRH–LH secretion. Reduction or removal of testosterone's negative-feedback signal via an androgen-receptor antagonist or an inhibitor of Leydig cell steroidogenesis increases the frequency and amplitude of pulsatile LH release. Conversely, continuous intravenous infusion of testosterone in steroidogenesis-inhibited men suppresses pulsatile LH release by reduced LH (and presumptively GnRH) pulse frequency with escape of occasional higher-amplitude LH pulses [references reviewed in 59].

Evaluations performed on blood samples collected from the peripheral and hypophyseal portal circulation of ovariectomized ewes have shown that FSH is secreted in two modes: tonic (basal secretion) and episodic. The episodic mode of secretion included both GnRH-associated and non-GnRH-associated episodes of FSH secretion [60]. **Unlike LH, which is secreted primarily in pulses, the predominant mode of FSH secretion is basal.** Previous findings demonstrated that circulating FSH concentrations remain detectable for several days in sheep after interruption of hypothalamic inputs to the pituitary and in hypophysectomized rats [61], and continues to be secreted in long-term pituitary cultures while LH secretion declines [62]. Almost all of the GnRH pulses in this study were associated with FSH pulses. Such a close relationship was, however, not evident when FSH pulses were identified in the peripheral circulation. The very discrete nature of the GnRH-associated bursts of FSH in the hypophyseal portal blood and the close time-lag relationship between GnRH and FSH suggest that the primary factor responsible for induction of the GnRH-associated pulses of FSH is GnRH. It is interesting to note that

secretory excursions of FSH were also identified in the absence of detectable GnRH pulses. Furthermore, many of the GnRH-associated pulses of FSH themselves appeared to develop on top of a previously elicited episode of FSH release .

Testicular factors

Testes participate in the feedback regulation of the HPG axis through the synthesis and secretion of steroids and peptides, chiefly testosterone and inhibin B, whose role and action have been spelled out in the previous sections of this chapter. Recently other factors have been evaluated and their contribution to the feedback regulation of the HPG axis has been postulated.

Testosterone

Testosterone is synthesized from cholesterol through a series of enzymatic transformations that occur in the Leydig cell mitochondria and microsomes through the activation of cholesterol ester hydrolase by LH. The rate-limiting step in steroidogenesis is the transfer of cholesterol to the inner mitochondrial membrane for bioconversion to pregnenolone by the cytochrome P450 side-chain cleavage enzyme. LH feed-forward activity is crucial for spermatogenesis, as the gonadotropin stimulates the labile regulatory protein StAR, which in turn activates cytochrome P450. Moreover, LH increases the association between cholesterol and cytochrome P450. Pregnenolone is converted to testosterone through the $\Delta 4$ pathway (pregnenolone → progesterone → 17a-hydroxyprogesterone → androstenedione) or through the $\Delta 5$ pathway (pregnenolone → 17a-hydroxypregnenolone → dehydroepiandrosterone → 5-androstenediol), $\Delta 5$ being the predominant pathway in men.

Testosterone is the main secretory product of the testis, the daily production rate being 5–7 mg in men. As the testicular content of testosterone in adult men is approximately 50 mg/testis, it is assumed that testosterone is continuously produced and released into the circulation. Testosterone is transported in plasma bound to albumin or to sex hormone-binding globulin, and approximately only 2% of total testosterone circulates freely in blood.

Testosterone plasma levels are strictly correlated to LH levels. Individual LH pulses in peripheral blood were found to precede testosterone pulses in the spermatic vein by 80 minutes, with a consequent strongly positive correlation among their levels in the spermatic vein. This correlation suggests the existence of a feed-forward relationship between LH and testosterone, which in turn reflects pituitary LH drive of testosterone secretion by gonadal Leydig cells [63]. On the other hand, the increase in testosterone level leads to a quite prompt (60-minute delay) decrease in LH level, due to the feedback interplay within the GnRH–LH–testosterone axis.

These findings have been validated by the employment of a specific GnRH-receptor antagonist peptide, which reduced LH and testosterone concentrations during the subsequent 8–10 hours, with values greater than 65% suppressed for an additional 15 hours. Repeated LH injections increased total testosterone concentrations from the suppressed nadir of less than 120 ng/dL to a predicted asymptotic plateau of 611 ng/dL at a half-time of 97 minutes [64].

Inhibin B

Inhibin is a glycoprotein hormone secreted by the Sertoli cells composed of an α subunit disulfide-linked to one of two β subunits, the βA subunit to form inhibin A or the βB subunit to form inhibin B. Its testicular origin was demonstrated when its levels were found to be undetectable in agonadal men and to be significantly lower than normal in men with other testicular disorders [65].

Immunocytochemical investigation demonstrated the presence of inhibin α subunit in both Sertoli cells and Leydig cells but not in the germ cells of adult human testes with normal or altered spermatogenesis. βB subunit was immunolocalized in pachytene spermatocytes to round spermatids as well as in Leydig cells but not in Sertoli cells in testes with normal spermatogenesis and with spermatogenic arrest. In testes with Sertoli cells only, βB subunit was localized only in Leydig cells [66]. These findings suggest that germ cells could directly contribute to inhibin B production. As a matter of fact it was observed that inhibin B concentrations fall to undetectable levels following loss of all germ cells in men after chemotherapy or radiotherapy, and similar results were obtained in the irradiated nonhuman primate model. Moreover, a direct positive correlation between inhibin B and sperm concentration in normal men is noted, and studies in which serum inhibin B levels were related to the histologic pattern of testicular biopsies have confirmed that inhibin B levels are reduced in men with severe spermatogenetic defects [references reviewed in 66].

The localization of α and βB subunits in the Leydig cells could suggest that Leydig cells could contribute to inhibin B production. However, it has been demonstrated that LH (or hCG) does not stimulate inhibin B production in hypogonadal as well as in normal men [67,68]. It is reasonable to think, therefore, that Leydig cells simply participate in the regulation of inhibin production by Sertoli cells.

Secretion of inhibin B is controlled by many factors including gonadotropins and intrinsic factors involving Sertoli, Leydig, and germ cells. It is recognized that there is a reciprocal relationship between plasma FSH and inhibin B levels. This relationship is not modified in infertile men as it is in fertile men, as demonstrated by the evaluation of plasma levels of inhibin B and its bio-inactive precursors [69]. That FSH stimuli are required for inhibin B secretion has been confirmed by studies evaluating men with acquired hypogonadotropic hypogonadism, whose inhibin B levels were markedly below those of normal men but were promptly restored by recombinant FSH administration. In contrast, recombinant LH treatment was found to be ineffective [67].

There are two discrete developmental periods in which there is a rise in FSH secretion leading to an increase in inhibin B levels [70]. The first period of increased circulating levels of inhibin B occurs following the rise in gonadotropins seen during the first year of infancy. The further decline in gonadotropin levels accompanied by an increase in inhibin B suggests that maturation of a feedback inhibitory system occurs. Once inhibin B secretion is initiated and brought within the normal range, the maintenance of inhibin B until the onset of puberty seems to be independent of further gonadotropin stimulation. Inhibin B decreases gradually to a nadir at 6–10 years of age, then increases rapidly in early adolescence to reach a new plateau at 12–17 years [71]. The second cycle of FSH secretion, followed by inhibin B secretion and suppression of FSH production, occurs with the onset of puberty in males [70,71]. Inhibin B increases progressively from pubertal stages G1 to G3 but then decreases slightly at stages G4 to G5 [71]. At puberty there is active mitotic division with spermatogonial maturation and accumulation of germ cells undergoing spermatogenesis leading to an increase in testicular size. During this period there is also a dramatic rise in FSH and LH and a sharp increase in the circulating levels of inhibin B. Before the initiation of puberty, the Sertoli cell is the predominant cell type within the seminiferous tubules, while germ cells prevail over the Sertoli cells in adult testis. This scenario may be required for maintenance of inhibin B secretion and FSH suppression before puberty. The integrity of Sertoli cells but not of germ cells, indeed, is required for inhibin B secretion, as demonstrated by lack of modification of acute inhibin B response to FSH during spermatogenesis suppression by combined testosterone and depot medroxyprogesterone acetate administration for hormonal contraceptive purposes [72].

Insulin-like growth factor 1 (IGF-1)

The testis is a site of IGF-1 biosynthesis and action. IGF-1 mRNA, protein, and specific IGF-1 receptors are present in the testis and have been identified in Leydig cells, peritubular cells, and spermatocytes. LH and hCG stimulate IGF-1 secretion and up-regulate type I IGF-1 receptor gene expression in rodent Leydig cells. IGF-1 stimulates the proliferation of Leydig cell precursors, and pretreatment of these cells with LH augments the mitogenic effect. As a matter of fact, IGF-1 null mutant mice have fewer and smaller Leydig cells than normal, and lower serum T levels in adulthood [73], and mice with a targeted gene deletion of IGF-1 had an abnormal pattern of Leydig cell proliferation and differentiation and attenuated testosterone production in response to LH stimulation [74]. These data suggest that IGF-1 is required for establishment of normal numbers of adult Leydig cells and steroidogenic function.

Evidence in IGF-1 null male mice suggests that LH is unable to produce a sufficient signal for adequate testosterone production in the absence of IGF-1. IGF-1 null male mice show, indeed, unaltered basal and LH-stimulated testosterone levels. However, while LH increases testosterone production in wild-type testes, neither IGF-1 nor LH treatment can stimulate testosterone production beyond basal levels in mutant mice. The lack of response to LH probably is related to the decrease in testicular LH receptors observed in these mice. Only the combination of LH plus IGF-1 is able to increase testosterone production in mutant testes, but the response is significantly attenuated relative to wild-type animals [75].

The proliferative effects of IGF-1 on Leydig cells are potentiated by LH at low concentrations. Taken together, the evidence supports the conclusion that IGF-1 and LH act in concert to facilitate Leydig cell proliferation and differentiation.

Transforming growth factor β (TGF-β)

TGF-β family peptides have been shown to be present in the testis. TGF-β1 has been reported to be a modulator of hormone formation in both cultured Leydig and Sertoli cells, and of contractility, shape, and organization of peritubular myoid cells. In TGF-β2-deficient mice, testis hypoplasia, cryptorchidism, and ectoplasia were observed. Overproduction of TGF-β1 may also affect the testis with atrophy of the gonad and thickened tubular basement membranes [76].

The positive regulatory action of LH/hCG on TGF-β receptor expression in Leydig cells has been demonstrated using porcine Leydig cells [76]. Other evidence suggests that TGF-β antagonizes LH/hCG steroidogenic action in Leydig cells [77,78]. These data, together with the demonstration that LH increases the expression of functional TGF-β receptors, and thus potentially TGF-β action, may suggest the existence of a short loop between the hormone and the growth factor at the Leydig cell level. LH may use the TGF-β system to end or reduce its own steroidogenic action or that of other growth factors that enhance LH-stimulated steroid hormone production in Leydig cells, such as epidermal growth factor/TGF-α and IGF-1. In fact, it has been shown that TGF-β antagonizes the stimulatory action of epidermal growth factor/TGF-α [79] and IGF-1 [80] on LH-induced testosterone formation. Such interactions between the growth factors and the gonadotropin may occur to modulate the intratesticular levels of testosterone required for correct spermatogenesis.

Other factors

It has been hypothesized that corticotropin-releasing hormone (CRH) may have direct inhibitory effects on steroidogenesis. In-vitro studies showed that CRH acts rapidly in the fetal and adult rat Leydig cell to exert highly effective negative autoregulation of the Leydig cell steroidogenic response to the LH stimulus [81].

Interleukin 1α (IL-1α) has been demonstrated to exert both inhibitory and stimulatory effects on steroidogenesis by Leydig cells. Recent studies have revealed that the effect exerted by IL-1α in this context depends on the stage of maturation of the Leydig cells, and that it is mediated by stimulation of StAR. Stimulation of the expression of StAR in immature Leydig cells by IL-1α is dose- and time-dependent. The proposed sources of constitutive production of IL-1α in the testis are the Sertoli cells [82].

Growth hormone (GH) plays a role in gonadal steroidogenesis and gametogenesis, exerting endocrine action either directly at gonadal sites or indirectly via IGF-1. In male subjects, congenital GH deficiency may result in a delay in the onset of puberty, and it has also been associated with decreased sperm counts and motility and reduced testicular size. In addition, GH influences Leydig cell steroidogenesis by increasing the expression of several genes that code for steroidogenic enzymes, including 3β-hydroxysteroid dehydrogenase, and by regulating the secretion of IGF-1 [82].

Conclusions

The male hypothalamic–pituitary–gonadal axis is a complex, dynamic, finely controlled, and tightly regulated system operating at multiple levels (endocrine, paracrine, and autocrine).

GnRH secretion is modulated by several factors, including GnRH itself by means of an ultrashort loop feedback, and with the important contribution of testosterone through its aromatization to estrogens. The fine control of GnRH secretion is required for the appropriate feed-forward regulation of FSH and LH, which respond differently to different frequencies and amplitudes of GnRH release.

LH is released in a pulsatile manner; its interaction with Leydig cells, most likely mediated by IGF-1 and TGF-β, is followed by a prompt rise in testosterone level, which in turn, together with its aromatase-derived products, decreases the release of LH itself.

FSH secretion is predominantly tonic (basal), but GnRH-associated and non-GnRH-associated episodes of FSH secretion are observed. A stable FSH level is achieved through the feedback control of estrogens and inhibin B; the latter peptide is secreted by germ cells, and its secretion is controlled by FSH and by intrinsic factors involving Sertoli, Leydig, and germ cells.

Understanding of such dynamics represents the correct approach to the diagnosis and treatment of disorders of the male reproductive system.

References

[1] Padmanabhan V, Evans NP, Dahl GE, *et al*. Evidence for short or ultrashort loop negative feedback of gonadotropin-releasing hormone secretion. *Neuroendocrinology* 1995; **62**: 248–58.

[2] DePaolo LV, King RA, Carrillo AJ. In vivo and in vitro examination of an autoregulatory mechanism for luteinizing hormone-releasing hormone. *Endocrinology* 1987; **120**: 272–9.

[3] Witkin JW, Silverman AJ. Synaptology of luteinizing hormone-releasing hormone neurons in rat preoptic area. *Peptides* 1985; **6**: 263–71.

[4] Pompolo S, Rawson JA, Clarke IJ. Projections from the arcuate/ventromedial region of the hypothalamus to the preoptic area and bed nucleus of stria terminalis in the brain of the ewe: lack of direct input to gonadotropin-releasing hormone neurons. *Brain Res* 2001; **904**: 1–12.

[5] Xu C, Xu XZ, Nunemaker CS, Moenter SM. Dose-dependent switch in response of gonadotropin-releasing hormone (GnRH) neurons to GnRH mediated through the type I GnRH receptor. *Endocrinology* 2004; **145**: 728–35.

[6] Krsmanovic LZ, Stojilkovic SS, Mertz LM, Tomic M, Catt KJ. Expression of gonadotropin-releasing hormone receptors and autocrine regulation of neuropeptide release in immortalized hypothalamic neurons. *Proc Natl Acad Sci U S A* 1993; **90**: 3908–12.

[7] Krsmanovic LZ, Martinez-Fuentes AJ, Arora KK, *et al*. Autocrine regulation of gonadotropin-releasing hormone secretion in cultured hypothalamic neurons. *Endocrinology* 1999; **140**: 1423–31.

[8] Krsmanovic LZ, Mores N, Navarro CE, Arora KK, Catt KJ. An agonist-induced switch in G protein coupling of the gonadotropin-releasing hormone receptor regulates pulsatile neuropeptide secretion. *Proc Natl Acad Sci U S A* 2003; **100**: 2969–74.

[9] Gammon CM, Freeman GM, Xie W, Petersen SL, Wetsel WC. Regulation of gonadotropin-releasing hormone secretion by cannabinoids. *Endocrinology* 2005; **146**: 4491–9.

[10] Ebling FJP, Lincoln GA. Endogenous opioids and the control of seasonal LH secretion in Soay rams. *J Endocrinol* 1985; **107**: 341–53.

[11] Schanbacher BD. Effects of intermittent pulsatile infusion of luteinizing hormone-releasing hormone on dihydrotestosterone-suppressed gonadotropin secretion in castrate rams. *Biol Reprod* 1985; **33**: 603–11.

[12] Moldrich G, Wenger T. Localization of the CB1 cannabinoid receptor in the rat brain: an immunohistochemical study. *Peptides* 2000; **21**: 1735–42.

[13] White RB, Eisen JA, Kasten TL, Fernald RD. Second gene for gonadotropin-releasing hormone in humans. *Proc Natl Acad Sci U S A* 1998; **95**: 305–9.

[14] Cheng CK, Leung Pck. Molecular biology of gonadotropin-releasing hormone (GnRH)-I, GnRH-II and their receptors in humans. *Endocr Rev* 2005; **26**: 283–306.

[15] Millar RP, Lu ZL, Pawson AJ, *et al*. Gonadotropin-releasing hormone receptors. *Endocr Rev* 2004; **25**: 235–75.

[16] Kauffman AS, Bojkowska K, Wills A, Rissman EF. Gonadotropin-releasing hormone-II messenger ribonucleic acid and protein content in the mammalian brain are modulated by food intake. *Endocrinology* 2006; **147**: 5069–77.

[17] Densmore VS, Urbanski HF. Relative effect of gonadotropin-releasing hormone (GnRH)-I and GnRH-II on gonadotropin release. *J Clin Endocrinol Metab* 2003; **88**: 2126–34.

[18] Zhen S, Zakaria M, Wolfe A, Radovick S. Regulation of gonadotropin-releasing hormone (GnRH) gene expression by insulin-like growth factor I in a cultured GnRH-expressing neuronal cell line. *Mol Endocrinol* 1997; **11**: 1145–55.

[19] Messager S, Chatzidaki EE, Ma D, *et al*. Kisspeptin directly stimulates gonadotropin-releasing hormone release via G protein-coupled receptor 54. *Proc Natl Acad Sci U S A* 2005; **102**: 1761–6.

[20] Tilbrook AJ, Clarke IJ. Negative feedback regulation of the secretion and actions of gonadotropin-releasing hormone in males. *Biol Reprod* 2001; **64**: 735–42.

[21] Caraty A, Locatelli A. Effect of time after castration on secretion of LHRH and LH in the ram. *J Reprod Fertil* 1988; **82**: 263–9.

[22] Jackson GL, Kuehl D, Rhim TJ. Testosterone inhibits gonadotropin-releasing hormone pulse frequency in the male sheep. *Biol Reprod* 1991; **45**: 188–94.

[23] Tilbrook AJ, de Kretser DM, Cummins JT, Clarke IJ. The negative feedback effects of testicular steroids are predominantly at the hypothalamus in the ram. *Endocrinology* 1991; **129**: 3080–92.

[24] El Majdoubi M, Ramaswamy S, Sahu A, Plant TM. Effects of orchidectomy on levels of the mRNAs encoding gonadotropin-releasing hormone and other hypothalamic peptides in the adult male rhesus monkey (Macaca mulatta). *J Neuroendocrinol* 2000; **12**: 167–76.

[25] Herbison AE. Multimodal influence of estrogen upon gonadotropin-releasing hormone neurons. *Endocr Rev* 1998; **19**: 302–30.

[26] Nunemaker CS, Defazio RA, Moenter SM. Estradiol-sensitive afferents modulate long-term episodic firing patterns of GnRH neurons. *Endocrinology* 2002; **143**: 2284–92.

[27] Belchetz PE, Plant TM, Nakai Y, Keogh EJ, Knobil E. Hypophysial responses to continuous and intermittent delivery of hypothalamic gonadotropin-releasing hormone. *Science* 1978; **202**: 631–3.

[28] Weiss J, Jameson JL, Burrin JM, Crowley WF. Divergent responses of gonadotropin subunit messenger RNAs to continuous vs. pulsatile gonadotropin-releasing hormone in vitro. *Molecular Endocrinology* 1990; **4**: 557–64.

[29] Wierman ME, Rivier JE, >Wang C. Gonadotropin-releasing hormone-dependent regulation of gonadotropin subunit messenger ribonucleic acid levels in the rat. *Endocrinology* 1989; **124**: 272–8.

[30] Kaiser UB, Jakubowiak A, Steinberger A, Chin WW. Differential effects of gonadotropin-releasing hormone (GnRH) pulse frequency on gonadotropin subunit and GnRH receptor messenger ribonucleic acid levels in vitro. *Endocrinology* 1997; **138**: 1224–31.

[31] Loumaye E, Catt KJ. Homologous regulation of gonadotropin-releasing hormone receptors in cultured pituitary cells. *Science* 1982; **215**: 983–5.

[32] Savoy-Moore RT, Schwartz NB, Duncan JA, Marshall JC. Pituitary gonadotropin-releasing hormone receptors during the rat estrous cycle. *Science* 1985; **209**: 942–4.

[33] Savoy-Moore RT, Swartz KH. Several GnRH stimulation frequencies differentially release FSH and LH from isolated, perfused rat anterior pituitary cells. *Adv Exp Med Biol* 1987; **219**: 641–5.

[34] Wildt L, Hausler A, Marshall G, *et al*. Frequency and amplitude of gonadotropin-releasing hormone stimulation and gonadotropin secretion in the rhesus monkey. *Endocrinology* 1981; **109**: 376–85.

[35] Nunemaker CS, Straume M, Defazio RA, Moenter S. Gonadotropin-releasing hormone neurons generate interacting rhythms in multiple time domains. *Endocrinology* 2003; **144**: 823–31.

[36] Sairam MR, Fleshner P. Inhibition of hormone-induced cyclic AMP production and steroidogenesis in interstitial cells by deglycosylated lutropin. *Mol Cell Endocrinol* 1981; **22**: 41–54.

[37] Themmen AP, Huhtaniemi I. Mutations of gonadotropins and gonadotropin receptors: elucidating the physiology and pathophysiology of pituitary-gonadal function. *Endocr Rev* 2000; **21**: 551–83.

[38] Layman LC, Porto AL, Xie J, *et al*. FSHβ gene mutations in a female with partial breast development and a male sibling with normal puberty and azoospermia. *J Clin Endocrinol Metab* 2002; **87**: 3702–7.

[39] Clark AD, Layman LC. Analysis of the Cys82Arg mutation in follicle-stimulating hormone beta (FSHβ) using a novel FSH expression vector. *Fertil Steril* 2003; **79**: 379–85.

[40] Tapanainen JS, Aittomäki K, Min J, Vaskivuo T, Huhtaniemi IT. Men homozygous for an inactivating mutation of the follicle-stimulating hormone (FSH) receptor gene present variable suppression of spermatogenesis and fertility. *Nat Genet* 1997; **15**: 205–6.

[41] Dierich A, Sairam MR, Monaco L, *et al*. Impairing follicle-stimulating hormone (FSH) signaling in vivo: targeted disruption of the FSH receptor leads to aberrant gametogenesis and hormonal imbalance. *Proc Natl Acad Sci U S A* 1998; **95**: 13612–17.

[42] Weiss J, Axelrod L, Whitcomb RW, *et al*. Hypogonadism caused by a single amino acid substitution in the β subunit of luteinizing hormone. *N Engl J Med* 1992; **326**: 179–83.

[43] Wang GM, O'Shaughnessy PS, Chubb C, *et al*. Effects of insulin-like growth factor I on steroidogenic enzyme expression levels in mouse Leydig cells. *Endocrinology* 2003; **144**: 5058–64.

[44] Wang GM, Hardy MP. Development of Leydig cells in the insulin-like growth factor I (IGF-1) knockout mouse: effects of IGF-1 replacement and gonadotropic stimulation. *Biol Reprod* 2004; **70**: 632–9.

[45] Baker J, Hardy MP, Zhow J, *et al*. Effects of an IGF-1 gene null mutation on mouse reproduction. *Mol Endocrinol* 1996; **10**: 903–18.

[46] Sriraman V, Sairam MR, Rao AJ. Evaluation of relative roles of LH and FSH in regulation of differentiation of Leydig cells using an ethane 1,2-dimethylsulfonate-treated adult rat model. *J Endocrinol* 2003; **176**: 151–61.

[47] Payne AH, Hardy MP, Russell LD, eds. *The Leydig Cell.* Vienna, IL: Cache River Press, 1996.

[48] Hodgson YM, de Kretser DM. Serum testosterone response to single injection of hCG ovine-LH and LHRH in male rats. *Int J Androl* 1982; **5**: 81–91.

[49] Counis R, Laverrière JN, Garrel G, *et al.* Gonadotropin-releasing hormone and the control of gonadotrope function. *Reprod Nutr Dev* 2005; **45**: 243–54.

[50] Hayes FJ, DeCruz S, Seminara SB, Boepple PA, Crowley WF. Differential regulation of gonadotropin secretion by testosterone in the human male: absence of a negative feedback effect of testosterone on follicle-stimulating hormone secretion. *J Clin Endocrinol Metab* 2001; **86**: 53–8.

[51] Hayes FJ, Seminara SB, Decruz S, Boepple PA, Crowley WJ. Aromatase inhibition in the human male reveals a hypothalamic site of estrogen feedback. *J Clin Endocrinol Metab* 2000; **85**: 3027–35.

[52] Smith EP, Boyd J, Frank GR, *et al.* Estrogen resistance caused by a mutation in the estrogen-receptor gene in a man. *N Engl J Med* 1994; **331**: 1056–61.

[53] Morishima A, Grumbach MM, Simpson ER, Fisher C, Qin K. Aromatase deficiency in male and female sibling caused by a novel mutation and the physiological role of estrogens. *J Clin Endocrinol Metab* 1995; **80**: 3689–99.

[54] Carani C, Qin K, Simoni M, *et al.* Effect of testosterone and estradiol in a man with aromatase deficiency. *N Engl J Med* 1997; **337**: 91–5.

[55] Schnorr JA, Bray MJ, Veldhuis JD. Aromatization mediates testosterone's short-term feedback restraint of 24-hour endogenously driven and acute exogenous gonadotropin-releasing hormone-stimulated luteinizing hormone and follicle-stimulating hormone secretion in young men. *J Clin Endocrinol Metab* 2001; **86**: 2600–6.

[56] Hayes FJ, Pitteloud N, DeCruz S, Crowley WF, Boepple PA. Importance of inhibin B in the regulation of FSH secretion in the human male. *J Clin Endocrinol Metab* 2001; **86**: 5541–6.

[57] Wallace EM, Groome NP, Riley SC, Parker AC, Wu FCW. Effects of chemotherapy-induced testicular damage on inhibin, gonadotropin, and testosterone secretion: a prospective longitudinal study. *J Clin Endocrinol Metab* 1997; **82**: 3111–15.

[58] Bergendahl M, Evans WS, Veldhuis JD. Current concepts on ultradian rhythms of luteinizing hormone secretion in the human. *Hum Reprod Update* 1996; **2**: 507–18.

[59] Keenan D, Veldhuis JD. A biomathematical model of time-delayed feedback in the human male hypothalamic–pituitary–Leydig cell axis. *Am J Physiol* 1998; **275**: E157–76.

[60] Padmanabhan V, McFadden C, Mauger DT, Karsch FJ, Midgley AR. Neuroendocrine control of follicle-stimulating hormone (FSH) secretion. I. Direct evidence for separate episodic and basal components of FSH secretion. *Endocrinology* 1997; **138**: 424–32.

[61] Hamernik DL, Nett TM. Gonadotropin-releasing hormone increases the amount of messenger ribonucleic acid for gonadotropins in ovariectomized ewes after hypothalamic–pituitary disconnection. *Endocrinology* 1988; **122**: 959–66.

[62] Sheridan R, Loras B, Surardt L, Ectors F, Pasteels JL. Autonomous secretion of follicle-stimulating hormone by long term organ cultures of rat pituitaries. *Endocrinology* 1979; **104**: 198–204.

[63] Foresta C, Bordon P, Rossato M, Mioni R, Veldhuis JD. Specific linkages among luteinizing hormone, follicle-stimulating hormone, and testosterone release in the peripheral blood and human spermatic vein: evidence for both positive (feed-forward) and negative (feedback) within-axis regulation. *J Clin Endocrinol Metab* 1997; **82**: 3040–6.

[64] Veldhuis JD, Iranmanesh A. Pulsatile intravenous infusion of recombinant human luteinizing hormone under acute gonadotropin-releasing hormone receptor blockade reconstitutes testosterone secretion in young men. *J Clin Endocrinol Metab* 2004; **89**: 4474–9.

[65] Anawalt BD, Bebb RA, Matsumoto AM, *et al.* Serum inhibin B levels reflect Sertoli cell function in normal men and men with testicular dysfunction. *J Clin Endocrinol Metab* 1996; **81**: 3341–5.

[66] Marchetti C, Hamdane M, Mitchell V, *et al.* Immunolocalization of inhibin and activin α and βB subunits and expression of corresponding messenger RNAs in the human adult testis. *Biol Reprod* 2003; **68**: 230–5.

[67] Young J, Couzinet B, Chanson P, *et al.* Effects of human recombinant luteinizing hormone and follicle-stimulating hormone in patients with acquired hypogonadotropic hypogonadism: study of Sertoli and Leydig cell secretions and interactions. *J Clin Endocrinol Metab* 2000; **85**: 3239–44.

[68] Kinniburgh D, Anderson RA. Differential patterns of inhibin secretion in response to gonadotropin stimulation in normal men. *Int J Androl* 2001; **24**: 95–101.

[69] Robertson DM, Stephenson T, McLachlan RI. Characterization of plasma inhibin forms in fertile and infertile men. *Hum Reprod* 2003; **18**: 1047–54.

[70] Byrd W, Bennett MJ, Carr BR, *et al.* Regulation of biologically active dimeric inhibin A and B from infancy to adulthood in the male. *J Clin Endocrinol Metab* 1998; **83**: 2849–54.

27

[71] Crofton PM, Evans AE, Groome NP, *et al.* Inhibin B in boys from birth to adulthood: relationship with age, pubertal stage, FSH and testosterone. *Clin Endocrinol (Oxf)* 2002; **56**: 215–21.

[72] Matthiesson KL, Robertson DM, Burger HG, McLachlan RI. Response of serum inhibin B and pro-αC levels to gonadotrophic stimulation in normal men before and after steroidal contraceptive treatment. *Hum Reprod* 2003; **18**: 734–43.

[73] Baker J, Hardy MP, Zhou J, *et al.* Effects of an IGF1 gene null mutation on mouse reproduction. *Mol Endocrinol* 1996; **10**: 903–18.

[74] Wang G, Hardy MP. Development of Leydig cells in the insulin-like growth factor-I (IGF-1) knockout mouse: effects of IGF-1 replacement and gonadotropic stimulation. *Biol Reprod* 204; **70**: 632–9.

[75] Chatelain PG, Sanchez P, Saez JM. Growth hormone and insulin-like growth factor I treatment increase testicular luteinizing hormone receptors and steroidogenic responsiveness of growth hormone deficient dwarf mice. *Endocrinology* 1991; **128**: 1857–62.

[76] Goddard I, Bouras M, Keramidas M, *et al.* Transforming growth factor-β receptor types I and II in cultured porcine Leydig cells: expression and hormonal regulation. *Endocrinology* 2000; **141**: 2068–74.

[77] Benahmed M. Growth factors and cytokines in the testis. In: Comhaire FH, ed. *Male Infertility.* London: Chapman and Hall, 1996: 55–97.

[78] Gnessi L, Fabbri A, Spera G. Gonadal peptides as mediators of development and functional control of the testis: an integrated system with hormones and local environment. *Endocr Rev* 1997; **18**: 541–609.

[79] Sordoillet C, Chauvin MA, Hendrick JC, *et al.* Sites of interaction between epidermal growth factor and transforming growth factor-β1 in the control of steroidogenesis in cultured porcine Leydig cells. *Endocrinology* 1992; **130**: 1352–8.

[80] Besset V, Collette J, Chauvin MA, Franchimont P, Benahmed M. Effect of transforming growth factor-β1 on the insulin-like growth factor system in cultured porcine Leydig cells. *Mol Cell Endocrinol* 1994; **99**: 251–7.

[81] Fabbri A, Tinajero JC, Dufau ML. Corticotropin releasing factor is produced by rat Leydig cells and has major local antireproductive role. *Endocrinology* 1990; **127**: 1541–3.

[82] Colon E, Svechnikov KV, Carlsson-Skwirut C, Bang P, Soder O. Stimulation of steroidogenesis in immature rat leydig cells evoked by interleukin-1α is potentiated by growth hormone and insulin-like growth factors. *Endocrinology* 2005; **146**: 221–30.

Chapter 3

Leydig cell development and function

Barry R. Zirkin, Vassilios Papadopoulos, and Matthew P. Hardy (deceased)

Introduction

Androgens are the predominant reproductive hormones in the male; testosterone is the primary androgen in the circulation. **In all mammalian species studied to date, testosterone is by far the predominant bioactive androgen within the testis.** In the rat, for example, the concentration of 5α-dihydrotestosterone is only 5% that of testosterone [1]. Testosterone also has been shown to be the major androgenic steroid in the human testis [2]. **It is well established that testosterone is essential for normal spermatogenesis; reduced intratesticular levels can result in oligospermia or azoospermia** [2]. Among the known causes of male infertility, about 50% might be correctable with therapy, perhaps including the administration of testosterone so as to increase intratesticular concentrations [2]. However, the introduction of in-vitro fertilization by intracytoplasmic sperm injection has made it possible for couples who previously were labeled "sterile" due to male-factor infertility to have offspring without therapy. In some ways this is unfortunate, because there are disadvantages to this method of management, including its high cost and incidence of multiple gestations. Moreover, the use of assisted reproductive technologies for treatment of male-factor infertility transfers all of the risks of intervention from the partner with an abnormality to his spouse. The importance of testosterone also is apparent from studies showing that its perturbation by chemicals in the environment may be involved in developmental anomalies in the male reproductive tract in wildlife and declining sperm counts in humans [3,4].

Leydig cells, located in the interstitial compartment of the mammalian testis, are the primary testosterone-producing cells in males. Adult Leydig cells emerge at puberty, and most persist thereafter without turning over [5]. **Recently, the origin of Leydig cells has been clarified by the identification of stem Leydig**

cells from the testes of postnatal day 7 Sprague Dawley rats that were shown to self-renew under specific conditions or to differentiate into Leydig cells under other conditions [6]. In rodents, the differentiation of progenitor Leydig cells from the stem Leydig cells, which occurs between postnatal days 10 and 14 [6–9], signals the beginning of the Leydig cell lineage. By approximately day 28 postpartum, the progenitor Leydig cells begin to transition into immature Leydig cells [8–11], and these cells then divide once or twice and differentiate into testosterone-secreting adult Leydig cells. **With aging, progressive decreases in serum concentrations of testosterone occur** in both men [12] and rodents [13–18]. **In men, these decreases are associated with significant health consequences, including reduced sexual function, energy, muscle function, and bone density, and increased frailty and cognitive impairment** [12,19,20]. Figure 3.1 illustrates this sequence of events in the human male.

In this chapter, we first will discuss the development of the adult population of Leydig cells from the stem cell precursor through the progenitor and immature Leydig cell stages. We then will address what currently is understood about the regulation of adult Leydig cell steroidogenic function. Finally, we will discuss our understanding of the mechanisms that account for the reduced steroidogenesis that occurs with Leydig cell aging.

Development of the adult population of Leydig cells
Fetal Leydig cells

Leydig cells are the primary source of testosterone in the male. There are two separate Leydig cell generations that develop successively in the testis between embryogenesis and puberty. In rats, the first generation, the fetal Leydig cells, differentiate from stromal

Infertility in the Male, 4th edition, ed. Larry I. Lipshultz, Stuart S. Howards, and Craig S. Niederberger. Published by Cambridge University Press. © Cambridge University Press 2009.

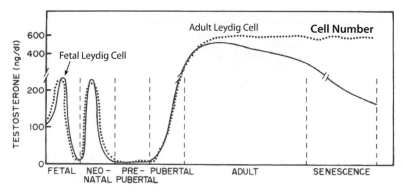

Fig. 3.1. Relative numbers of Leydig cells (dotted line) and levels of serum testosterone (solid line) in the human male throughout life. There are three peaks in serum testosterone: the fetal peak induces male sexual differentiation; the neonatal peak at 2–3 months of life hormonally imprints the hypothalamus, liver, and prostate so that they respond appropriately to androgen later in life; and the pubertal rise at the beginning of the second decade elicits the development of secondary sexual characteristics and supports spermatogenesis during adulthood. Serum testosterone levels are maintained at 6 ng/mL during adulthood and decline with aging. (Modified from Adashi EY, *et al. Reproductive Endocrinology, Surgery, and Technology*. Philadelphia, PA: Lippincott-Raven, 1996, Chapter 25. Used with permission.)

cells between the nascent testis cords during gestation. Once formed, fetal Leydig cells are terminally differentiated and fully competent to produce testosterone. The majority of fetal Leydig cells dedifferentiate or undergo apoptosis after birth [10,21], and therefore are unlikely to contribute significantly to postnatal steroidogenesis.

The morphogenetic events of early testis differentiation are controlled by the *Sry* **(sex-determining region on the Y chromosome) gene**. The *Sry* gene product, a nuclear transcription factor, acts in concert with other transcription factors, including WT-1, SOX-9, and DAX-1, to initiate male sexual differentiation [22,23]. Differentiation of fetal Leydig cells is one of the downstream events of *Sry* signaling. Fibroblastic cells in the testis interstitium become identifiable as fetal Leydig cells by day 12.5. Recent studies by Capel and others have shown that the morphogen DHH (Desert Hedgehog) and platelet-derived growth factor α (PDGFα) induce the fibroblastic cells to express P450 side-chain cleavage enzyme (CYP11A1) on day 12.5 [24–26].

The origin of the fetal Leydig cells is a subject of ongoing debate. The most widely held view has been that mesenchymal cells of the mesonephros, originally derived from embryonic mesoderm, migrate into the testis and furnish a source of fetal Leydig stem cells [27]. Capel and colleagues, however, have reported that interference with the mesonephric migratory process does not perturb the eventual differentiation of fetal Leydig cells [24], and have proposed that their stem cells move in from the coelomic epithelium overlying

the developing gonad [25]. Neural crest cells provide another potential source of fetal Leydig stem cells [28]. The neural crest is an ephemeral body that extends along the rostrocaudal axis of the developing vertebrate embryo. Formed during neurulation, the migratory neural crest cells give rise to most of the peripheral nervous system, facial skeleton, and numerous other derivatives throughout the embryo, including neuroendocrine cells and possibly fetal Leydig cells.

Fetal Leydig cell function appears to be independent of luteinizing hormone (LH). For example, these cells function normally in hypogonadal mice that lack endogenous circulating gonadotropins, and also in LH receptor knockout (LHRKO) males that do not have functional LH receptors [29–33]. Steroidogenic factor 1 (SF-1), a nuclear transcription factor that is produced under the direction of SRY, is reported to direct fetal Leydig stem cells towards the steroidogenic lineage by inducing the expression of the cytochrome P450 steroidogenic enzymes [26,34,35]. SF-1 also promotes the differentiation of Sertoli cells [36]. Among the consequences of the actions of SF-1 in embryonic Sertoli cells are the secretion of Desert Hedgehog, PDGFα, and other paracrine regulatory factors such as IGF-1 [26,37] and vasoactive intestinal peptide [38] that promote the differentiation and function of fetal Leydig cells. Negative regulatory factors, such as transforming growth factor β1 (TGF-β1) [39] and anti-Müllerian hormone (AMH, also known as Müllerian-inhibiting substance) [40] partially inhibit fetal Leydig cell steroidogenesis. Fetal Leydig cells maintain high rates of steroidogenic activity, secreting primarily

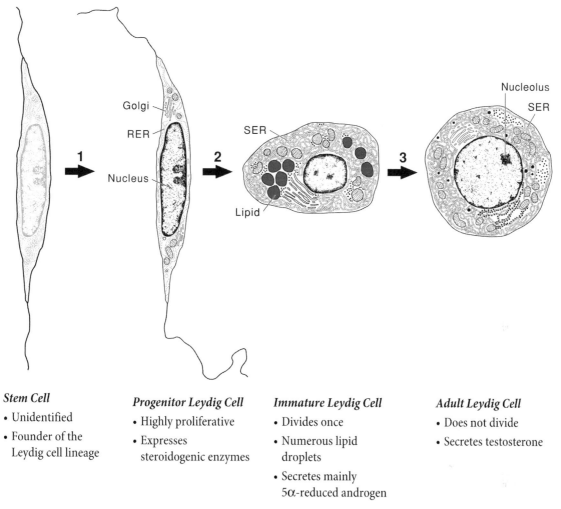

Stem Cell
- Unidentified
- Founder of the Leydig cell lineage

Progenitor Leydig Cell
- Highly proliferative
- Expresses steroidogenic enzymes

Immature Leydig Cell
- Divides once
- Numerous lipid droplets
- Secretes mainly 5α-reduced androgen

Adult Leydig Cell
- Does not divide
- Secretes testosterone

Fig. 3.2. Rat Leydig cells at successive stages of their development. RER, rough endoplasmic reticulum; SER, smooth endoplasmic reticulum. (Modified from Adashi EY, *et al. Reproductive Endocrinology, Surgery, and Technology*. Philadelphia, PA: Lippincott-Raven, 1996, Chapter 25. Used with permission.)

testosterone, during the last week of gestation leading up through birth [41]. The testosterone that is secreted is critical for male secondary sexual differentiation, including the development of the penis and sex accessory glands.

Adult Leydig cell ontogeny

As illustrated in Figure 3.2, **three separate transitions of cells have been shown to be involved in the development and differentiation of adult Leydig cells**. These transitions have been described most fully for the rat [42], but similar transitions are thought to occur in other species as well, including humans [43]. The first recognized cell type in the Leydig cell lineage in the rat, referred to as progenitor Leydig cells (PLCs), is first

seen in the testis between postnatal days 10 and 14. The PLCs are small, spindle-shaped cells that are similar in appearance to the undifferentiated fibroblastic cells seen in the early postnatal testis, but express markers of Leydig cell differentiated function including P450 side-chain cleavage enzyme (CYP11A1), 3β-hydroxysteroid dehydrogenase (3β-HSD) [44], cytochrome P450 17α-hydroxylase/C_{17-20}-lyase (CYP17), and a truncated form of the luteinizing hormone receptor (LHR) [45,46]. The PLCs contain negligible amounts of smooth endoplasmic reticulum, the organelle that houses several steroidogenic enzymes, but nonetheless are competent to produce steroids, secreting mainly androsterone (AO) [47]. PLCs gradually enlarge and become round, and their proliferative capacity is reduced.

The second transition results in another intermediate, the immature Leydig cells (ILCs). ILCs are seen most commonly in the testis during days 28–56 postpartum. These cells have more smooth endoplasmic reticulum (SER) than PLCs and are able to produce high levels of 5α-reduced androgens, primarily 3α, 5α-androstanediol [23]. ILCs undergo a final division before the third transition, the development of the adult Leydig cell (ALC) by day 56 [47]. ALCs are relatively large cells with an abundance of SER, few lipid droplets, and high levels of steroidogenic enzyme activities. Testosterone is the predominant androgen secreted by these cells. ALCs comprise the predominant population of Leydig cells in the sexually mature testis. After puberty, there is little or no further proliferation (or death) of the ALCs [21]; renewal occurs very slowly under physiological conditions [48].

Differences in steroidogenic and metabolizing enzymes lead to different androgen end products in PLCs, ILCs, and ALCs [47]. Due to high levels of 5α–reductase and 3α-HSD activity, and low levels of 17β-HSD, androsterone is the major steroid produced by rat PLCs. In ILCs, more 5α–reduced androgens are produced as a result of high levels of 5α-reductase and 3αHSD activities that convert testosterone into 5α–androstane–3α,17β–diol (3α–DIOL), the major end product secreted by ILCs. Testosterone secretion prevails in ALCs due to increased 17β-HSD activity together with sharply decreased 5α–reductase activity. In addition to the regulators already discussed, a balance between testosterone biosynthetic and degradative enzyme activities determines the amount of testosterone secreted by Leydig cells [10].

In the adult, LH binding to its Leydig cell receptor triggers the cAMP signaling pathway and a cascade of intercellular events, including increased gene transcription, steroidogenic enzyme activity, and testosterone production [49,50]. **Lack of LH stimulation results in reduced steroidogenic enzyme activities and in Leydig cell atrophy** [51]. **However, LH stimulation is unlikely to be the initial stimulus for cells to enter the Leydig cell lineage, or to trigger the initial expression of Leydig cell-specific genes.** Evidence for this conclusion comes from the fact that the LH receptor protein is truncated in PLCs, resulting in an attenuated response to gonadotropin stimulation [52]. That LH plays a critical role in the further development of Leydig cells, however, is apparent from studies of GnRH[hpg] mice, which are deficient in circulating LH. In these mice, Leydig cell numbers are about 10% of control [53]. Moreover, Leydig cells are severely hypoplastic

in LHRKO mice; these cells may not progress beyond a mesenchymal-like stage that has attenuated expression of steroidogenic enzymes, with 3β-HSD the only enzyme present [30,54,55]. Increased Leydig cell proliferation occurs following LH/hCG administration in vivo [56]. In adult Snell dwarf mice, a deficiency in plasma gonadotropin prevents full differentiation of Leydig cells without affecting their numbers [57]. Although LH stimulates DNA synthesis in immature rat Leydig cells in vitro, significant enhancement of the LH effect is achieved by coadministration of growth factors such as IGF-1 [58,59], raising the possibility that the action of LH on Leydig cell proliferation may be preceded by the action of other factors.

Stem Leydig cells

The first identified cell type in the sequence leading to adult Leydig cells, the PLCs, are LH receptor-positive/3β-HSD-positive cells that divide a limited number of times in vivo and then give rise to immature Leydig cells (ILCs) and ultimately to ALCs [42]. **Until recently, a fundamental unanswered question was whether the ultimate source of the PLCs and thus of ALCs might be a pool of undifferentiated, self-renewing stem Leydig cells (SLCs)** (Fig. 3.2).

In general, stem cells are defined by their capacity for self-renewal and by their ability to give rise to one or more differentiated lines of cells without depleting the stem cell pool. Thus, based on well-characterized stem cells from other systems [60–63], the features that would be expected of stem Leydig cells (SLCs) are (1) self-renewal, (2) commitment, (3) amplification, and (4) differentiation. SLCs would be expected to be present in the testis in small numbers that are maintained by renewal cell divisions during postnatal life through adulthood; one or both of the progeny of an SLC division would be expected to undergo commitment to the Leydig cell lineage; and the numbers of committed SLCs would be expected to increase through amplification cell divisions, creating a pool of cells that undergo differentiation into androgen-secreting progenitor Leydig cells (PLCs).

There have been attempts to identify stem Leydig cells (SLCs). In one study, putative testicular stem Leydig cells from cryptorchid mice were isolated and transplanted into mice with a targeted deletion of the LH receptor gene (LHRKO) [64]. Serial serum testosterone assays revealed significant increases in circulating testosterone levels, suggesting that the transplanted cells or their progeny differentiated to produce at least some Leydig cells. This study showed the promise of

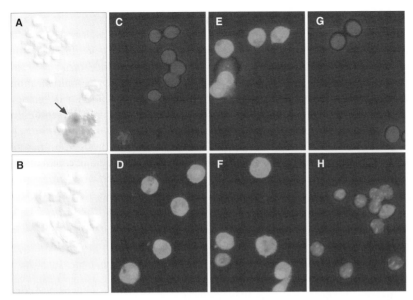

Fig. 3.3. Characteristics of stem Leydig cells (SLCs). Freshly isolated SLCs contaminated by fetal Leydig cells (FLCs) are shown in panel A with a cluster of FLCs stained strongly for 3β-HSD (arrow). After negative immunoselection to eliminate LHR-positive cells and positive selection of PDGFRα-expressing cells, none of the cells stained for 3β-HSD (Panel B). LHR^{neg} PDGFRα^{pos} SLCs did not stain for 3β-HSD (C) or LHR (G). They were, however, positively stained for PDGFRα (D), c-kit (E), LIFR (F), and GATA4 (H). DAPI staining (blue) was used to provide nuclear contrast. (From Ge RS, *et al.* In search of rat stem Leydig cells: identification, isolation, and lineage-specific development. *Proc Natl Acad Sci U S A* 2006; **103**: 2719–24, with permission of the publisher.) *See color plate section.*

the LHRKO mouse to furnish Leydig cell-depleted host testes for further analysis of transplanted stem cells. A second study reported the presence of nestin-positive cells in the interstitial compartment of testes, and suggested that there were stem cells that ultimately gave rise to ALCs [65]. The observation that SLCs express nestin may provide important clues to the ontogeny of these cells in the embryo. For example, one might infer that they are of neural or neural-crest origin.

In a recently reported study, spindle-shaped cells were seen in the interstitium of the testis at one week postpartum, prior to the differentiation of the PLCs, that were 3β-HSD-negative and platelet-derived growth factor receptor α (PDGFRα)-positive [6]. Enriched populations of these cells were harvested from rat testes and purified following immunoselection for cells that lacked LH receptor (LHR^{neg}) and contained PDGFRα (PDGFRα^{pos}). The cells obtained in this way also were 3β-HSD^{neg} and contained proteins known to be involved in Leydig cell development, including the GATA4 transcription factor, c-kit receptor, and leukemia inhibitory factor receptor (LIFR), the latter a well-known stem cell marker (Fig. 3.3). Culture of these cells in media containing PDGF-BB, LIF, and kit ligand stimulated the proliferation of the putative SLCs over the course of six months while the

cells maintained spindle-shaped morphology and did not differentiate. However, when the putative SLCs cells were placed for seven days in a differentiation-inducing medium that contained a combination of thyroid hormone (T3), insulin-like growth factor 1 (IGF-1), and luteinizing hormone (LH), about 40% of the cells expressed 3β-HSD, and the cells synthesized testosterone (Fig. 3.4). Based on these characteristics, the isolated cells seemed likely to be the sought-after stem Leydig cells (SLCs).

The ability to colonize its niche is an essential feature of the stem cell. Thus, it was essential to determine whether the cells that were identified as putative SLCs were able to colonize the interstitial compartment of the testis and to differentiate. The Leydig cell cytotoxin ethane dimethanesulfonate (EDS) was administered to adult rats to eliminate ALCs in the host testes, and fluorescently labeled LHR^{neg}, PDGFRα^{pos}, 3β-HSD^{neg} cells were injected into the parenchyma at the cranial pole of the testis. On day 10 thereafter, all of the fluorescent labeling in the testis was confined to the interstitium, and significant numbers of the labeled cells were positively stained for 3β-HSD activity. In contrast, EDS-treated rats that received saline control injections without cells lacked fluorescence on day 10, and there were no cells that stained for 3β-HSD, indicating that

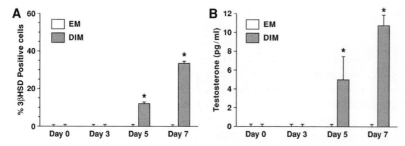

Fig. 3.4. Differentiation of stem Leydig cells (SLCs) into Leydig cells in vitro. SLCs were cultured in expansion medium (EM) or in differentiation-inducing medium (DIM). Testosterone production (right) progressively increased with culture DIM, with its rate correlated with increases in 3β-HSD-positive cells (left). *Denotes a significant change compared to control. (From Ge RS, *et al.* In search of rat stem Leydig cells: identification, isolation, and lineage-specific development. *Proc Natl Acad Sci U S A* 2006; **103**: 2719–24, with permission of the publisher.)

regeneration of Leydig cells from host cells had not yet occurred. This study, which demonstrated that the putative SLCs were able to colonize the testicular interstitium and subsequently differentiate in vivo, made it clear that the cells indeed were SLCs.

Do stem Leydig cells age?

There is growing evidence that stem and progenitor cells age, and that this contributes at least in part to age-related alteration in tissue maintenance and repair. For example, hematopoietic stem cells in older mice have been shown to have decreased ability to self-renew and proliferate [66]. Similarly, the proliferation and self-renewal potential of stem (or progenitor) cells have been shown to decline with age in the mouse forebrain, and there is age-related reduced pancreatic islet proliferation and regeneration [67–69]. Age-related decline in stem cell function might result from intrinsic stem cell aging, and/or from changes in the environment of the stem cell niche. Changes within the niche could include alterations in its content of proteins and lipids, factors released from damaged cells, and/or paracrine and endocrine factors.

Previous studies have shown that a single injection of the alkylating agent EDS specifically destroys all Leydig cells in both the young adult and aged rat testis, and that thereafter new populations of Leydig cells are restored to the testes at both ages [70]. The earliest restored cells were found to produce high amounts of 5α-reduced androgens. Later, the restored cells produced testosterone as the predominant androgen. By 10 weeks after EDS, the ability of the cells restored to the testes of young adult and aged rats to produce testosterone was equivalent. Thus, although situated in an aged testis and in the environment of an aged hypothalamic–pituitary axis, the steroidogenic

function of the Leydig cells restored to aged rat testes was equivalent to that of young rat Leydig cells rather than reduced as in controls. The sequence of events following EDS, from the appearance of cells producing 5α-reduced androgens to the maturation of these cells to produce testosterone, resembled Leydig cell maturation during puberty. These observations suggest that **although there is little turnover of adult Leydig cells, there may be stem cells that reside in the testicular interstitium that are capable of giving rise to adult, well-functioning Leydig cells**.

Adult Leydig cell steroidogenic function

Adult Leydig cell testosterone production depends upon LH, secreted in pulses into the peripheral circulation by the pituitary gland [71,72]. Acting through a cAMP-dependent pathway, LH has both rapid (acute) and long-term (trophic) effects on Leydig cell testosterone production [73–75]. In its acute actions, LH binds to specific high-affinity receptors on the Leydig cell plasma membrane, initiating a cascade of events that include coupling of the LH receptor (LHR) with G proteins, activation of adenylate cyclase, increased intracellular cAMP formation, cAMP-dependent phosphorylation of proteins, and translocation of cholesterol to the inner mitochondrial membrane [50,76]. The conversion of cholesterol to pregnenolone is catalyzed by CYP11A1, located on the inner mitochondrial membrane. Following its production in the mitochondria, pregnenolone moves out of the mitochondria to the smooth endoplasmic reticulum, where it binds to the 3β-HSD enzyme and is converted to progesterone. Progesterone is then acted upon by CYP17 to produce 17α-hydroxyprogesterone and then androstenedione.

Finally, androstenedione is converted to testosterone by 17β-ketosteroid reductase [73].

Although the aforementioned enzymatic steps are well recognized (i.e., traditional) [77], there is evidence that the steroidogenic enzymes may have catalytic functions in addition to or different from their traditional ones. For example, CYP17, in addition to its 17α-hydroxylase/C17–20 lyase activity, is a potent oxidant that recently was shown to be associated with squalene monoxygenase (epoxidase) activity, which is critical in cholesterol biosynthesis by MA-10 Leydig cells [78]. Moreover, CYP17-independent steroid synthesis has been shown in brain and testis [79,80], suggesting the existence of other, not yet understood, mechanisms of steroid biosynthesis.

Numerous studies have shown that the expressions of the mRNAs for the steroidogenic enzymes are regulated by LH via cAMP [17,74,77,81,82]. Intracellular cAMP concentration derives from a balance between the rates of cAMP synthesis and degradation, which are regulated by adenylate cyclases and cyclic nucleotide phosphodiesterases, respectively [50,83–85]. A great deal is known about the mechanism by which the binding of LH to its receptor ultimately produces cAMP [84–89]. In brief, binding of LH to the LHR induces the binding of the cytosolic domain of the receptor to a guanine nucleotide-binding (G) protein. In its resting state, the α subunit of the trimeric G protein is bound to GDP. LHR binding to the G protein stimulates the exchange of bound GDP for GTP. This activates the α subunit, which then dissociates from the β and γ subunits of the G protein, and the active GTP-bound α subunit then interacts with adenylate cyclase to convert ATP to cAMP. The activity of the α subunit is terminated by hydrolysis of the bound GTP by the action of the intrinsic GTPase activity of the α subunit. The inactive α subunit, now with GDP bound, reassociates with the βγ complex, restarting the cycle. GTPase activating proteins (GAPs), termed RGS (regulators of G protein signaling), are able to increase GTP hydrolysis and thus return the α subunit to its inactive state. To date, about 20 distinct α subunits have been cloned. These can be divided into four major subfamilies: Gsα, Giα, Gq/IIα, and G12α. There are G proteins (Gs) that are activators of adenylate cyclase, and those (Gi) that are involved in adenylate cyclase inhibition. At least nine closely related isoforms of adenylate cyclases have been identified, and some 40 phosphodiesterases. The receptor and effector proteins involved in cAMP production are thought to be mobile within the plane of the membrane, and so are influenced by the state of membrane fluidity. Consequently, changes in membrane fluidity could have significant consequences for cAMP production [50,84,88–90].

The primary point of control in the acute stimulation of steroidogenesis by LH is the conversion of cholesterol to pregnenolone on the inner mitochondrial membrane by CYP11A1 [91–93]. **The rate-determining step in the cholesterol transport pathway is the transport of cholesterol from intracellular sources into the mitochondria** [91–93]. Cyclic AMP is integrally involved in this process. Cyclic AMP binds to PKA, an enzymatically inactive tetramer consisting of two catalytic and two regulatory subunits, and the tetramer then dissociates into the regulatory dimer and two free active catalytic subunits that phosphorylate and activate serine and threonine residues on specific protein substrates [94]. Protein phosphorylation is a key regulatory step in hormone-stimulated steroid formation [92,95]. Maximal stimulation of cholesterol transport and steroid formation can occur at lower cAMP levels than are normally present in the Leydig cells; the concentration of hCG needed to induce maximal cAMP synthesis is about 15 times higher than that needed for maximal testosterone production [91]. However, the exact mechanism by which cAMP is able to induce cholesterol transport from the cytosol to the inner mitochondrial membrane remains uncertain.

A number of molecules have been proposed to mediate cholesterol transfer into mitochondria [92,93,95]. During the last 15 years, **two cholesterol transport molecules in particular, TSPO (translocator protein) and StAR (steroidogenic acute regulatory protein), have emerged as playing critical roles** (Fig. 3.5).

TSPO: a mitochondrial high-affinity cholesterol-binding protein

Translocator protein (18 kDa), previously known as the peripheral-type benzodiazepine receptor (PBR) [96], was originally discovered because it binds the benzodiazepine diazepam with relatively high affinity [97]. Although present in all tissues examined, TSPO was found to be particularly high in steroid-producing tissues, where it was localized primarily in the outer mitochondrial membrane (OMM) [97–99]. It has been observed in various cell systems and in isolated mitochondria [97,100] that TSPO drug ligands stimulate the formation of steroids. To identify the step activated

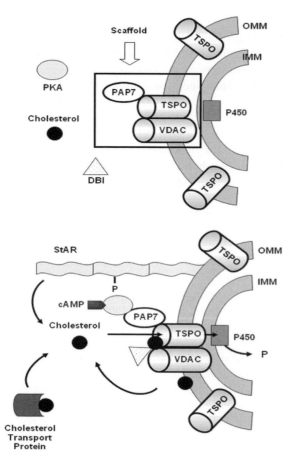

Fig. 3.5. Schematic representation of the putative mitochondrial signaling complex mediating the acute hormonal regulation of cholesterol transport into mitochondria. Top: shows the basal state in which PAP7–TSPO–VDAC interactions are thought to recruit PKA to mitochondria. The box delineates the mitochondrial scaffold formed by these three proteins. This scaffold allows the anchoring of PKARIα to the mitochondria and the recruitment of hormone-induced StAR protein to this complex (bottom). According to this proposed mechanism, StAR phosphorylation and activation initiates cholesterol movement into TSPO and through TSPO into the mitochondria via outer mitochondrial membrane (OMM)–inner mitochondrial membrane (IMM) contact sites. Cholesterol then can be converted by CYP11A1 (P450 side-chain cleavage enzyme) into pregnenolone (P).

by TSPO ligands, the amounts of cholesterol present in the OMM and inner mitochondrial membrane (IMM) were quantified before and after treatment with TSPO ligands. These experiments demonstrated that TSPO ligands induced TSPO-mediated translocation of cholesterol from OMM to IMM [101]. Targeted disruption of the TSPO gene in Leydig cells resulted in the arrest of cholesterol transport into mitochondria as well as the arrest of steroid formation, while transfection of the TSPO-disrupted cells with a TSPO

cDNA rescued steroidogenesis [102]. Moreover, a TSPO 7-mer peptide antagonist was found to inhibit the benzodiazepine-stimulated steroid formation by directly inhibiting drug binding, as well as hormone-stimulated Leydig cell steroidogenesis [103]. The role of TSPO in cholesterol transport was further clarified by site-directed mutagenesis and in-vitro expression studies [104] which showed that a region of the cytosolic carboxyl-terminus of the receptor was the cholesterol-binding site that is critical for cholesterol-binding activity [104,105]. In-vitro reconstitution experiments revealed that TSPO binds cholesterol with low nanomolar affinity [105,106]. In-vivo studies, in which adrenal and ovarian TSPO levels were pharmacologically [107–109] or developmentally [110, 111] modulated, further demonstrated a correlation between TSPO levels and steroidogenesis. In addition, knocking out TSPO by gene targeting resulted in early embryonic lethality [98], indicating its important role during development.

Analysis of the cDNA sequences from different mammals indicated that the 18 kDa TSPO protein contains 169 amino acids, and that there is a high degree of identity and homology among species [97–99]. Hydropathy profile analysis of the amino acid sequence suggested a putative five-transmembrane structure that has been experimentally confirmed [112]. Three-dimensional models of human and mouse TSPO were developed that showed the five transmembrane segments as α helices spanning the OMM [113,114], suggesting that TSPO functions as a channel that accommodates cholesterol molecules in the space delineated by the five helices and thus allows cholesterol molecules to cross the OMM to the IMM. The mitochondrial 18 kDa TSPO protein is organized in clusters of 4–6 molecules that redistribute upon addition of hCG to Leydig cells, inducing a rapid increase in TSPO ligand binding [115,116]. Studies with recombinant TSPO and radiolabeled ligands collectively demonstrated that TSPO is a high-affinity cholesterol-binding protein [106].

A search for endogenous TSPO ligands identified a 10 kDa polypeptide, the diazepam-binding inhibitor (DBI) [97], which was originally purified from brain [117]. It is highly expressed in steroidogenic cells, displaces radiolabeled benzodiazepines in competition studies [118], can be cross-linked to TSPO [119], and stimulates mitochondrial pregnenolone formation [120,121]. Taken together, these observations suggest that DBI plays a crucial role in steroidogenesis.

TSPO-associated mitochondrial proteins have been described, including the voltage-dependent anion channel (VDAC) and the adenine nucleotide transporter (ANT) [122] (Fig. 3.5). The 18 kDa TSPO is the isoquinoline-binding component of the complex [106], whereas the presence of VDAC, a large conductance ion channel referred to as a "mitochondrial porin," increases the ability of the 18 kDa protein to bind benzodiazepines [123]. As yet, the role of ANT in this complex remains unclear. Although it is clear that these proteins are involved in the formation of TSPO-containing contact sites, their roles seem to be constitutive rather than regulatory. Thus, there must exist certain cytosolic proteins that interact with and regulate these mitochondrial membrane elements. A TSPO-associated protein, PAP7, was identified which binds the regulatory subunit RIα of cAMP-dependent protein kinase (PKA; [124,125]). PAP7 is targeted to mitochondria in response to hormone treatment [125], thus allowing for local (mitochondrial) catalytic activation of PKA and phosphorylation of protein substrates, such as StAR [126].

StAR: a unique hormone-induced mitochondrial cholesterol transporter

StAR is a 37 kDa protein that contains an N-terminal mitochondrial signal sequence [93,127]. It has been known for some time that StAR is integrally involved in regulating cholesterol transport. For example, the transfection of StAR protein, CYP11A1, and adreno-doxin into COS-1 cells led to a sixfold increase in the formation of 3β-hydroxy-5-cholestenoic acid [128]. In gonadal and adrenal cells, StAR de novo synthesis was shown to parallel the maximal steroid synthesis in response to trophic hormones [129,130], and expression of the 37 kDa StAR precursor in the absence of hormones induced a two- to threefold increase in progesterone production by MA-10 cells and by isolated mitochondria. The 37 kDA StAR preprotein was shown to be cleaved in mitochondrial membrane contact sites to produce the 30 kDa "mature" StAR protein, an event initially believed to be responsible for cholesterol transport across the mitochondrial membranes [93,131,132]. However, the hormonal stimulation of steroidogenesis, both in vitro and in vivo, was observed within 5–15 minutes of hormone addition [91,92,133], whereas StAR mRNA and protein expression has been shown to begin 30–60 minutes after hormone stimulation [129].

StAR does not need to enter into mitochondria to stimulate steroidogenesis [93,131]. Indeed, mitochondrial import and proteolysis of StAR may terminate its action [134]. Moreover, the issue of how effectively StAR can bind cholesterol has been raised. For example, evidence based on fluorescence energy transfer experiments has shown that cholesterol can bind to StAR with an affinity of 32 nM and a stoichiometry of two molecules per molecule of StAR [135]. Other studies, too, have indicated that StAR is a low-affinity (high-micromolar) cholesterol-binding protein [136]. These observations are consistent with the idea of a transporter/transfer activator role for StAR that does not require high-affinity cholesterol binding and that does not require StAR to enter into mitochondria to stimulate steroidogenesis [134,137]. In this model, there is no requirement for StAR to bind cholesterol. An alternative model suggesting that StAR acts as an intermembrane shuttle [138] has been now dismissed, since it does not account for the strong evidence that StAR acts at the OMM [134]. In a more recent study it was shown that the cholesterol binding and transfer activities of StAR are distinct [139].

There is no question that StAR initiates cholesterol transfer from OMM to IMM [134]. However, the fact that a "receptor" for StAR in the OMM has not been identified [134] suggests that there may be few high-affinity binding sites for StAR, that there are transient interactions of StAR with components of OMM, or that the recognition may be done through a mediator molecule (protein or cholesterol). Evidence for the requirement for additional components involved in the regulation of gonadal steroidogenesis stems from studies of StAR knockout mice. Disruption of the StAR gene in StAR$^{-/-}$ mice did not suppress steroidogenesis completely [140]. In addition, hormone-stimulated steroidogenesis was maintained in the presence of nigericin, a K$^+$/H$^+$ exchanger that abolishes the hormone-induced accumulation of StAR [141].

Taken together, **the studies of TSPO and StAR suggest that the two are indispensable elements of the steroidogenic machinery.** One possibility is that TSPO and StAR function in a coordinated manner to transfer cholesterol into mitochondria [133]. Thus, treatment with oligodeoxynucleotides (ODNs) antisense for each of the proteins inhibited the respective protein expression and the ability of the cells to synthesize steroids in response to hCG [133]. Treatment of the cells with ODNs antisense to TSPO or with a peptide antagonist to TSPO resulted in inhibition of the accumulation of the mature mitochondrial 30 kDa StAR protein, suggesting that the presence of TSPO is required for StAR import into mitochondria. Pregnenolone formation by mitochondria from control cells was increased by the addition of 37 kDa StAR or a fusion protein of Tom20 (translocase of outer membrane) to StAR (Tom/StAR). In contrast, mitochondria isolated from cells treated with ODNs antisense to TSPO failed to form pregnenolone and to respond to either StAR or Tom/StAR proteins. These studies clearly demonstrated that there is a functional interaction between StAR and TSPO required for cholesterol delivery into mitochondria and subsequent steroid formation, with TSPO the mitochondrial site of import of StAR-mobilized cholesterol. StAR and TSPO may interact at the level of a mitochondrial multivalent scaffold in the outer mitochondrial membrane that mediates the effect of hormones on mitochondrial cholesterol transport and steroidogenesis [142]. This would be consistent with the idea that StAR is recruited to the outside of the mitochondria to induce cholesterol transfer [131,132], and that TSPO interacts with or mediates the action of StAR [133] to transfer cholesterol to the inner mitochondrial membrane.

Leydig cell aging

As men age, progressive decreases in serum concentrations of testosterone occur [12] (Fig. 3.6). Associated with these decreases are significant health consequences, including reduced sexual function, energy, muscle function, and bone density, and increased frailty and cognitive impairment [12,19,20]. Circulating LH concentrations do not decline as men age [143–147], suggesting that reduced testosterone results from a primary gonadal deficit rather than from changes at the hypothalamic–pituitary level. Consistent with this, the administration of hCG has been shown to stimulate testosterone production to a lesser extent in older than in younger men [148–151], suggesting reduced responsiveness of Leydig cells to LH. As yet, however, the mechanism by which testosterone levels decline in aging men is unknown.

Decreases in serum levels of testosterone also occur with aging in rodents [13–18]. In most rat strains, declines in serum LH accompany reduced testosterone [13,16,152]. This suggests that in such strains, and in contrast to humans, age-related decline in serum testosterone is secondary to hypothalamic–pituitary changes. In the Brown Norway rat strain, however, serum testosterone levels decline but LH levels do not, and serum FSH levels rise [70,153]. These similarities to the human, as well as the long life span and relative absence of disease, are among the reasons that Brown Norway rats have become widely used for studies of Leydig cell aging.

Reduced serum testosterone levels might be caused by reduced numbers of Leydig cells or by reduced steroidogenic activity of the cells. The number of Leydig cells per testis has been shown to remain unchanged with Brown Norway rat aging [70,153], suggesting that changes in the steroidogenic function of individual Leydig cells, not their reduced numbers, are responsible for reduced serum testosterone levels. In fact, Leydig cells from aged Brown Norway rats have been shown to produce less cAMP and testosterone in response to LH than those from young rats [154], and the cells to have reduced levels of StAR and PBR protein and mRNA [81,111,155], and reduced activities of CYP11A1, 3β-HSD, CYP17, and 17β-KSD [81,82].

Such changes in the steroidogenic machinery of aging Leydig cells might result from extrinsic factors (i.e., changes outside the Leydig cells that impinge upon them) or from intrinsic factors (i.e., changes within the Leydig cells themselves). **Although serum LH levels do not change significantly with age [70,153], age-related changes in LH pulse amplitude and frequency have been reported [156,157], and such changes could affect Leydig cell testosterone production.** In fact, studies have shown that neither the in-vivo administration of exogenous LH to old rats [158,159] nor the in-vitro culture of old cells with LH [159] resulted in the increased ability of old Brown Norway Leydig cells to produce testosterone at the high levels of young rats. Such observations strongly support the idea that LH deficits are not the major cause of reduced testosterone production by aging Leydig cells, and indeed may not

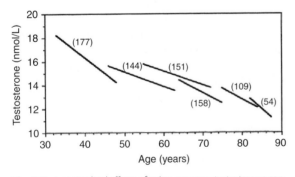

Fig. 3.6. Longitudinal effects of aging on serum testosterone concentrations in cohorts (parentheses) of men. (Redrawn with permission from Harman SM, *et al.* Longitudinal effects of aging on serum total and free testosterone levels in healthy men. *J Clin Endocrinol Metab* 2001; **86**: 724–31. Copyright 2001, The Endocrine Society)

be involved. Rather, the responsiveness of aged Leydig cells to LH is reduced relative to young cells.

Culturing aged cells for three days with dibutyryl cAMP (dbcAMP), a membrane-permeable cAMP agonist that bypasses the LH receptor–adenylate cyclase cascade, has been shown to restore testosterone production by old Leydig cells to levels approximating those of young cells [83]. StAR and CYP11A1 also were restored to young levels by culturing aged cells with dbcAMP. The observation that bypassing signal transduction by culturing cells with dbcAMP largely reversed the steroidogenic decline by the aged cells suggests that the reduced ability of old cells to transduce the signal between LH and cAMP production may play a major role in the reduced steroidogenesis by aged Leydig cells.

Free radicals and redox environment of aging Leydig cells

A number of hypotheses have been put forward over the years to explain changes that occur in aging cells, including late-onset gene expression, telomere shortening, gene modifications, changes in the immune system, and accumulated reactive oxygen-induced damage to DNA, lipids, and/or proteins [160–167]. Among these, **there is evidence that alterations in the Leydig cell reactive oxygen environment, leading to increased oxidative stress, might be involved in Leydig cell age-related functional changes** [168,169].

The basis of the free-radical or oxidative-stress theory of aging is that cells exist in a chronic state of oxidative stress resulting from an imbalance between pro-oxidants and antioxidants, and that because of this imbalance there is an accumulation of oxidative damage to a variety of macromolecules. The steady-state accumulation of oxidative damage is thought to be an important mechanism underlying longevity, age-related pathology, and progressive decline in the functional efficiency of various cellular processes [168,170–172]. Over the last several years, data have accumulated indicating the involvement of reactive oxygen species (ROS) in normal cell-signaling processes as well [173]. To date, most of the evidence in support of the free-radical theory for any cell type has been correlative. Numerous studies have shown age-related increase in oxidative damage to a variety of molecules, including lipid, protein, and DNA, in organisms ranging from invertebrates to humans [168,170–172,174,175]. The physiological importance

of oxidative damage to protein was recognized 20 years ago when it was shown that the oxidative modification of one of the histidine residues of glutamine synthetase to a carbonyl group inactivated the enzyme [175]. More recently, age-related increases in protein oxidation have been shown in various rodent and nonhuman primate tissues and cells, as well as in fibroblasts from patients with Werner syndrome or progeria [175–180]. Manipulations that increase life span have been shown to reduce the expected age-related increases in oxidatively damaged biomolecules. Thus, caloric restriction (CR), which delays aging, has been shown to be associated with reduced levels of oxidative damage in a variety of tissues of rats and mice, and with decreases in lipid peroxidation [181]. CR also has been shown to reduce age-related increases in global protein carbonyl content [182, 183], and to decrease oxidative damage to DNA [184].

Steroidogenic cells produce ROS via the P450 enzymes as well as via the mitochondrial electron transport chain [185,186]. There is compelling evidence in the literature for a central role for oxidative stress in steroidogenic function in the ovary [187–189] and adrenal gland [190]. With respect to the ovary, rat luteal cells have been shown to respond to hydrogen peroxide by reduced progesterone synthesis. The acute blockage of steroidogenesis by hydrogen peroxide has been shown to be due to uncoupling of the LHR and adenylate cyclase, and to impaired cholesterol utilization by mitochondrial CYP11A1. Similarly, studies of rat luteal cells demonstrated that the in-vitro generation of superoxide radicals by xanthine oxidase disrupted LH-stimulated cAMP production and progesterone secretion [191].

With respect to Leydig cells, mitochondrial-derived ROS content of aged cells, measured by lucigenin-derived chemiluminescence, has been shown to be greater than that of young cells [169], suggesting increased production of ROS by the aging cells. Alteration of the antioxidant defense system also occurs in aging Leydig cells. Thus, SOD1, SOD2, glutathione peroxidase 1 (GPX-1), catalase (CAT), and reduced glutathione, major enzymatic and nonenzymatic antioxidants, all have been shown to decrease with age in Leydig cells [192,193]. The hypothesis that increased ROS and reduced antioxidants may affect cell function is supported by the observation that the extent of lipid peroxidation in isolated Leydig cell membrane fractions has been shown to be significantly elevated with age [186]. This is significant because lipid peroxidation can affect membrane structure and/or fluidity, and virtually every event associated with steroidogenesis is dependent on the integrity of cell membranes. In particular, it has been shown that perturbation of membrane composition and/or fluidity can affect cAMP production [191,194]. Additionally, the inclusion of high levels of the antioxidant vitamin E in the feed has been shown to delay age-related decreases in steroidogenesis in Brown Norway rats [195]. None of these observations, by itself, proves that oxidative stress plays a significant role in the reduced ability of old Leydig cells to produce testosterone; but the results, taken together, are consistent with the hypothesis that oxidative stress, resulting from an altered redox environment of the aging Leydig cells, in some way results in the reduced LH signaling that characterizes aging Leydig cells; and that reduced LH signaling, in turn, affects cAMP production, cholesterol transport via StAR and/PBR, and the steroidogenic enzymes, and ultimately testosterone production.

Summary

Testosterone-secreting adult Leydig cells, which first appear around the time of puberty, ultimately derive from a pool of stem Leydig cells that are negative for Leydig lineage-specific markers 3β-HSD and LHR, and positive for the stem cell marker PDGFRα. The differentiated progeny of the stem Leydig cells, the progenitor Leydig cells, are characterized by Leydig cell lineage-specific markers including 3β-HSD, CYP11A1, and CYP17, and by their ability to produce steroids (mainly androsterone). After a number of divisions, the progenitor Leydig cells give rise to immature Leydig cells that are characterized by increases in CYP11A1, CYP17, and 3β-HSD, increased androgen metabolism by 5α-reductase and 3α-HSD, and ultimately the production of high levels of 5α-reduced androgens (primarily 3α, 5α-androstanediol). The mature Leydig cells, which derive from the immature cells, are characterized by their high levels of testosterone production and low turnover.

The primary point of control in the acute stimulation of steroidogenesis in adult Leydig cells is the conversion of cholesterol to pregnenolone on the inner mitochondrial membrane by CYP11A1. The rate-determining step in the cholesterol transport pathway is the transport of cholesterol from intracellular sources into the mitochondria. Two cholesterol transport molecules, TSPO (translocator protein) and StAR (steroidogenic acute regulatory protein), have emerged as playing critical roles in mediating cholesterol transfer into the mitochondria, the rate-limiting step in steroidogenesis. Although still far from established, current evidence is consistent with the idea that StAR is recruited to the outside of the mitochondria to induce cholesterol transfer, and that TSPO interacts with or mediates the action of StAR to transfer cholesterol to the inner mitochondrial membrane. Finally, with aging, decreases in serum levels of testosterone occur, which, in men and in Brown Norway rats, are not secondary to declines in serum LH. In the rat, changes in the steroidogenic machinery of individual Leydig cells, not their reduced numbers, are responsible for reduced serum testosterone levels. Such changes might result from extrinsic factors (i.e., changes outside the Leydig cells that impinge upon them) or from intrinsic factors (i.e., changes within the Leydig cells themselves). From studies in which the steroidogenic decline by the aged Leydig cells was reversed with dbcAMP, it appears that the reduced ability of old cells to transduce the signal between LH and cAMP production may play a major role in the reduced steroidogenesis by aged Leydig cells. Among the many hypotheses that have been put forward over the years to explain changes that occur in aging cells, there is evidence that alterations in the Leydig cell reactive oxygen environment, leading to increased oxidative stress (i.e., imbalance between the intracellular antioxidant and pro-oxidant environment of aging Leydig cells) might be involved in Leydig cell age-related functional changes.

Acknowledgments

Supported by NIH grants AG021092 (BZ), HD055740 (BZ), HD37031 (VP), ES07747 (VP), HD32588 (MPH), and ES10233 (MPH).

References

[1] Turner TT, Jones CE, Howards SS, et al. On the androgen microenvironment of maturing spermatozoa. *Endocrinology* 1984; **115**: 1925–32.

[2] Jarow JP, Zirkin BR. The androgen microenvironment of the human testis and hormonal control of spermatogenesis. *Ann N Y Acad Sci* 2005; **1061**: 208–20.

[3] Moline JM, Golden AL, Bar-Chama N, et al. Exposure to hazardous substances and male reproductive health: a research framework. *Environ Health Perspect* 2000; **108**: 803–13.

[4] Adami HO, Bergstrom R, Mohner M, et al. Testicular cancer in nine northern European countries. *Int J Cancer* 1994; **59**: 33–8.

[5] Teerds KJ, de Rooij DG, Rommerts FF, Wensing CJ. Development of a new Leydig cell population after the destruction of existing Leydig cells by ethane

dimethane sulphonate in rats: an autoradiographic study. *J Endocrinol* 1990; **126**: 229–36.

[6] Ge RS, Dong Q, Sottas CM, *et al.* In search of rat stem Leydig cells: identification, isolation, and lineage-specific development. *Proc Natl Acad Sci U S A* 2006; **103**: 2719–24.

[7] Hardy MP, Kelce WR, Klinefelter GR, Ewing LL. Differentiation of Leydig cell precursors in vitro: a role for androgen. *Endocrinology* 1990; **127**: 488–90.

[8] Mendis-Handagama SM, Ariyaratne HB. Differentiation of the adult Leydig cell population in the postnatal testis. *Biol Reprod* 2001; **65**: 660–71.

[9] Ge RS, Dong Q, Sottas CM, *et al.* Gene expression in rat Leydig cells during development from the progenitor to adult stage: a cluster analysis. *Biol Reprod* 2005; **72**: 1405–15.

[10] Ge RS, Hardy MP. Variation in the end products of androgen biosynthesis and metabolism during postnatal differentiation of rat Leydig cells. *Endocrinology* 1998; **139**: 3787–95.

[11] Haider SG. Cell biology of Leydig cells in the testis. In: Jeon K, ed. *International Review of Cytology*. New York, NY: Academic Press, 2004: 181–241.

[12] Harman SM, Metter EJ, Tobin JD, Pearson J, Blackman MR. Longitudinal effects of aging on serum total and free testosterone levels in healthy men. Baltimore Longitudinal Study of Aging. *J Clin Endocrinol Metab* 2001; **86**: 724–31.

[13] Steiner RA, Bremner WJ, Clifton DK, Dorsa DM. Reduced pulsatile luteinizing hormone and testosterone secretion with aging in the male rat. *Biol Reprod* 1984; **31**: 251–8.

[14] Wang C, Leung A, Sinha-Hikim AP. Reproductive aging in the male brown-Norway rat: a model for the human. *Endocrinology* 1993; **133**: 2773–81.

[15] Zirkin BR, Santulli R, Strandberg JD, Wright WW, Ewing LL. Testicular steroidogenesis in the aging Brown Norway rat. *J Androl* 1993; **14**: 118–23.

[16] Gruenewald DA, Naai MA, Hess DL, Matsumoto AM. The Brown Norway rat as a model of male reproductive aging: evidence for both primary and secondary testicular failure. *J Gerontol* 1994; **49**: B42–50.

[17] Chen H, Luo L, Zirkin BR. Leydig cell structure and function during aging. In: Payne AH, Hardy MP, Russell LD, eds. *The Leydig Cell*. Vienna, IL: Cache River Press, 1996: 221–30.

[18] Zirkin BR, Chen H. Regulation of Leydig cell steroidogenic function during aging. *Biol Reprod* 2000; **63**(4): 977–81.

[19] Swerdloff RS, Wang C. Androgens and the ageing male. *Best Pract Res Clin Endocrinol Metab* 2004; **18**: 349–62.

[20] Matsumoto AM. Andropause: Clinical implications of the decline in serum testosterone levels with aging in men. *J Gerontol A Biol Sci Med Sci* 2002; **57**: M76–99.

[21] Hardy MP, Zirkin BR, Ewing LL. Kinetic studies on the development of the adult population of Leydig cells in testes of the pubertal rat. *Endocrinology* 1989; **124**: 762–70.

[22] Parker KL, Schimmer BP, Schedl A. Genes essential for early events in gonadal development. *Cell Mol Life Sci* 1999; **55**: 831–8.

[23] de Santa Barbara P, Moniot B, Poulat F, Berta . Expression and subcellular localization of SF-1, SOX9, WT1, and AMH proteins during early human testicular development. *Dev Dyn* 2000; **217**: 293–8.

[24] Yao HH, Whoriskey W, Capel B. Desert Hedgehog/Patched 1 signaling specifies fetal Leydig cell fate in testis organogenesis. *Genes Dev* 2002; **16**: 1433–40.

[25] Brennan J, Tilmann C, Capel B. Pdgfr-α mediates testis cord organization and fetal Leydig cell development in the XY gonad. *Genes Dev* 2003; **17**: 800–10.

[26] Park SY, Tong M, Jameson JL. Distinct roles for Steroidogenic Factor 1 and Desert Hedgehog pathways in fetal and adult Leydig cell development. *Endocrinology* 2007; **148**: 3704–10.

[27] De Kretser DM, Kerr JB. The cytology of the testis. In: Knobil E, Neill JD, eds. *The Physiology of Reproduction*. New York, NY: Raven Press, 1988: 837–932.

[28] Ortega HH, Lorente JA, Salvetti NR. Immunohistochemical study of intermediate filaments and neuroendocrine marker expression in Leydig cells of laboratory rodents. *Anat Histol Embryol* 2004; **33**: 309–15.

[29] El-Gehani F, Tena-Sempere M, Huhtaniemi I. Vasoactive intestinal peptide is an important endocrine regulatory factor of fetal rat testicular steroidogenesis. *Endocrinology* 1998; **139**: 1474–80.

[30] Lei ZM, Mishra S, Zou W, *et al.* Targeted disruption of luteinizing hormone/human chorionic gonadotropin receptor gene. *Mol Endocrinol* 2001; **15**: 184–200.

[31] Zhang FP, Poutanen M, Wilbertz J, Huhtaniemi I. Normal prenatal but arrested postnatal sexual development of luteinizing hormone receptor knockout (LHRKO) mice. *Mol Endocrinol* 2001; **15**: 172–83.

[32] O'Shaughnessy PJ, Baker P, Sohnius U, *et al.* Fetal development of Leydig cell activity in the mouse is independent of pituitary gonadotroph function. *Endocrinology* 1998; **139**: 1141–6.

[33] Majdic G, Saunders PT, Teerds KJ. Immunoexpression of the steroidogenic enzymes 3-beta hydroxysteroid dehydrogenase and 17 α-hydroxylase, c17,20 lyase and the receptor for luteinizing hormone (LH) in the fetal rat testis suggests that the onset of Leydig cell steroid production is independent of LH action. *Biol Reprod* 1998; **58**: 520–5.

[34] Crawford PA, Sadovsky Y, Milbrandt J. Nuclear receptor steroidogenic factor 1 directs embryonic stem cells toward the steroidogenic lineage. *Mol Cell Biol* 1997; **17**: 3997–4006.

41

[35] Ikeda Y. SF-1: a key regulator of development and function in the mammalian reproductive system. *Acta Paediatr Jpn* 1996; **38**: 412–19.

[36] Ikeda Y, Swain A, Weber TJ, *et al.* Steroidogenic factor 1 and Dax-1 colocalize in multiple cell lineages: potential links in endocrine development. *Mol Endocrinol* 1996; **10**: 1261–72.

[37] Rouiller-Fabre V, Lecref L, Gautier C, Saez JM, Habert R. Expression and effect of insulin-like growth factor I on rat fetal Leydig cell function and differentiation. *Endocrinology* 1998; **139**: 2926–34.

[38] El-Gehani F, Tena-Sempere M, Ruskoaho H, Huhtaniemi I. Natriuretic peptides stimulate steroidogenesis in the fetal rat testis. *Biol Reprod* 2001; **65**: 595–600.

[39] Olaso R, Pairault C, Saez JM, Habert R. Transforming growth factor β3 in the fetal and neonatal rat testis: immunolocalization and effect on fetal Leydig cell function. *Histochem Cell Biol* 1999; **112**: 247–54.

[40] Rouiller-Fabre V, Carmona S, Merhi RA, *et al.* Effect of anti-Müllerian hormone on Sertoli and Leydig cell functions in fetal and immature rats. *Endocrinology* 1998; **139**: 1213–20.

[41] Habert R, Brignaschi P. Developmental changes in in vitro testosterone production by dispersed Leydig cells during fetal life in rats. *Arch Androl* 1991; **27**: 65–71.

[42] Benton L, Shan LX, Hardy MP. Differentiation of adult Leydig cells. *J Steroid Biochem Mol Biol* 1995; **53**: 61–8.

[43] Prince FP. The Triphasic Nature of Leydig cell development in humans, and comments on nomenclature. *J Endocrinol* 2001; **168**: 213–16.

[44] Warren DW, Huhtaniemi IT, Tapanainen J, Dufau ML, Catt KJ. Ontogeny of gonadotropin receptors in the fetal and neonatal rat testis. *Endocrinology* 1984; **114**: 470–6.

[45] Eskola V, Rannikko A, Huhtaniemi I, Warren DW. Ontogeny of the inhibitory guanine nucleotide-binding regulatory protein in the rat testis: MRNA expression and modulation of LH and FSH action. *Mol Cell Endocrinol* 1994; **102**: 63–8.

[46] Tena-Sempere M, Rannikko A, Kero J, Zhang FP, Huhtaniemi IT. Molecular mechanisms of reappearance of luteinizing hormone receptor expression and function in rat testis after selective Leydig cell destruction by ethylene dimethane sulfonate. *Endocrinology* 1997; **138**: 3340–8.

[47] Hardy MP, Sprando RL, Ewing LL. Leydig cell renewal in testes of seasonally breeding animals. *J Exp Zool* 1992; **261**: 161–72.

[48] Teerds KJ, de Rooij DG, Rommerts FF, van der Tweel I, Wensing CJ. Turnover time of Leydig cells and other interstitial cells in testes of adult rats. *Arch Androl* 1989; **23**: 105–11.

[49] Hakola K, Pierroz DD, Aebi A, *et al.* Dose and time relationships of intravenously injected rat recombinant luteinizing hormone and testicular testosterone secretion in the male rat. *Biol Reprod* 1998; **59**: 338–43.

[50] Dufau ML. The luteinizing hormone receptor. *Annu Rev Physiol* 1998; **60**: 461–96.

[51] Manova K, Nocka K, Besmer P, Bachvarova RF. Gonadal expression of C-kit encoded at the W locus of the mouse. *Development* 1990; **110**: 1057–69.

[52] Abney TO, Zhai J. Gene expression of luteinizing hormone receptor and steroidogenic enzymes during Leydig cell development. *J Mol Endocrinol* 1998; **20**: 119–27.

[53] Baker PJ, Johnston H, Abel M, Charlton HM, O'Shaughnessy PJ. Differentiation of adult-type Leydig cells occurs in gonadotrophin-deficient mice. *Reprod Biol Endo* 2003; **1**: (online publication).

[54] Zhang FP, Poutanen M, Wilbertz J, Huhtaniemi I. Normal prenatal but arrested postnatal sexual development of luteinizing hormone receptor knockout (LuRKO) mice. *Mol Endocrinol* 2001; **15**: 172–83.

[55] Zhang FP, Pakarainen T, Zhu F, Poutanen M, Huhtaniemi I. Molecular characterization of postnatal development of testicular steroidogenesis in luteinizing hormone receptor knockout mice. *Endocrinology* 2004; **145**: 1453–63.

[56] Christensen AK, Peacock KC. Increase in Leydig cell number in testes of adult rats treated chronically with an excess of human chorionic gonadotropin. *Biol Reprod* 1980; **22**: 383–91.

[57] Hochereau-de Reviers MT, de Reviers MM, Monet-Kuntz C, *et al.* Testicular growth and hormonal parameters in the male snell dwarf mouse. *Acta Endocrinol (Copenh)* 1987; **115**: 399–405.

[58] Khan S, Teerds K, Dorrington J. Growth factor requirements for DNA synthesis by Leydig cells from the immature rat. *Biol Reprod* 1992; **46**: 335–41.

[59] Wang GM, O'Shaughnessy PJ, Chubb C, Robaire B, Hardy MP. Effects of insulin-like growth factor I on steroidogenic enzyme expression levels in mouse Leydig cells. *Endocrinology* 2003; **144**: 5058–64.

[60] Yazawa T, Mizutani T, Yamada K, *et al.* Differentiation of adult stem cells derived from bone marrow stroma into Leydig or adrenocortical cells. *Endocrinology* 2006; **147**: 4104–11.

[61] Galli D, Innocenzi A, Staszewsky L, *et al.* Mesoangioblasts, vessel-associated multipotent stem cells, repair the infarcted heart by multiple cellular mechanisms: a comparison with bone marrow progenitors, fibroblasts, and endothelial cells. *Arterioscler Thromb Vasc Biol* 2005; **25**: 692–7.

[62] Leri A, Kajstura J, Anversa P. Cardiac stem cells and mechanisms of myocardial regeneration. *Physiol Rev* 2005; **85**: 1373–416.

[63] Zhong JF, Zhao Y, Sutton S, *et al.* Gene expression profile of murine long-term reconstituting vs. short-term reconstituting hematopoietic stem cells. *Proc Natl Acad Sci U S A* 2005; **102**: 2448–53.

[64] Lo KC, Lei Z, Rao ChV, Beck J, Lamb DJ. De novo testosterone production in luteinizing hormone receptor knockout mice after transplantation of Leydig stem cells. *Endocrinology* 2004; **145**: 4011–15.

[65] Davidoff MS, Middendorff R, Enikolopov G, *et al.* Progenitor cells of the testosterone-producing Leydig cells revealed. *J Cell Biol* 2004; **167**: 935–44.

[66] Ito K, Hirao A, Arai F, *et al.* Reactive oxygen species act through P38 MAPK to limit the lifespan of hematopoietic stem cells. *Nat Med* 2006; **12**: 446–51.

[67] Janzen V, Forkert R, Fleming HE, *et al.* Stem-cell ageing modified by the cyclin-dependent kinase inhibitor P16INK4a. *Nature* 2006; **443**: 421–6.

[68] Molofsky AV, Slutsky SG, Joseph NM, *et al.* Increasing P16INK4a expression decreases forebrain progenitors and neurogenesis during ageing. *Nature* 2006; **443**: 448–52.

[69] Krishnamurthy J, Ramsey MR, Ligon KL, *et al.* P16INK4a induces an age-dependent decline in islet regenerative potential. *Nature* 2006; **443**: 453–7.

[70] Chen H, Huhtaniemi I, Zirkin BR. Depletion and repopulation of Leydig cells in the testes of aging Brown Norway rats. *Endocrinology* 1996; **137**: 3447–52.

[71] Bremner WJ, Bagatell CJ, Christensen RB, Matsumoto AM. Neuroendocrine aspects of the control of gonadotropin secretion in men. In: Whitcomb RW, Zirkin BR, eds. *Understanding Male Infertility: Basic and Clinical Aspects.* New York, NY: Raven Press, 1993: 29–41.

[72] Ellis GB, Desjardins C, Fraser HM. Control of pulsatile LH Release in male rats. *Neuroendocrinology* 1983; **37**: 177–83.

[73] Ewing LL, Zirkin BR. Leydig cell structure and steroidogenic function. *Recent Prog Horm Res* 1983; **39**: 599–635.

[74] Ewing LL, Keeney DS. Leydig cells: structure and function. In: Desjardins C, Ewing LL, eds. *Cell and Molecular Biology of the Testis.* New York, NY: Oxford University Press; 1993: 137–65.

[75] Browne ES, Bhalla VK. Does gonadotropin receptor complex have an amplifying role in CAMP/testosterone production in Leydig cells? *J Androl* 1991; **12**: 132–9.

[76] Dufau ML, Baukal AJ, Catt KJ. Hormone-induced guanyl nucleotide binding and activation of adenylate cyclase in the Leydig cell. *Proc Natl Acad Sci U S A* 1980; **77**: 5837–41.

[77] Payne AH, Hales DB. Overview of steroidogenic enzymes in the pathway from cholesterol to active steroid hormones. *Endocr Rev* 2004; **25**: 947–70.

[78] Liu Y, Yao ZX, Papadopoulos V. Cytochrome P450 17α hydroxylase/17,20 lyase (CYP17) Function in cholesterol biosynthesis: identification of squalene monooxygenase (epoxidase) activity associated with CYP17 in Leydig cells. *Mol Endocrinol* 2005; **19**: 1918–31.

[79] Lieberman S, Warne PA. 17-Hydroxylase: an evaluation of the present view of its catalytic role in steroidogenesis. *J Steroid Biochem Mol Biol* 2001; **78**: 299–312.

[80] Prasad VV, Vegesna SR, Welch M, Lieberman S. Precursors of the neurosteroids. *Proc Natl Acad Sci U S A* 1994; **91**: 3220–3.

[81] Luo L, Chen H, Zirkin BR. Leydig cell aging: steroidogenic acute regulatory protein (StAR) and cholesterol side-chain cleavage enzyme. *J Androl* 2001; **22**: 149–56.

[82] Luo L, Chen H, Zirkin BR. Are Leydig cell steroidogenic enzymes differentially regulated with aging? *J Androl* 1996; **17**: 509–15.

[83] Chen H, Liu J, Luo L, Zirkin BR. Dibutyryl cyclic adenosine monophosphate restores the ability of aged Leydig cells to produce testosterone at the high levels characteristic of young cells. *Endocrinology* 2004; **145**: 4441–6.

[84] Conti M. Phosphodiesterases and cyclic nucleotide signaling in endocrine cells. *Mol Endocrinol* 2000; **14**: 1317–27.

[85] Conti M, Jin SL. The molecular biology of cyclic nucleotide phosphodiesterases. *Prog Nucleic Acid Res Mol Biol* 1999; **63**: 1–38.

[86] Kishi M, Liu X, Hirakawa T, *et al.* Identification of two distinct structural motifs that, when added to the C-terminal tail of the rat LH receptor, redirect the internalized hormone-receptor complex from a degradation to a recycling pathway. *Mol Endocrinol* 2001; **15**: 1624–35.

[87] Richard FJ, Tsafriri A, Conti M. Role of phosphodiesterase type 3A in rat oocyte maturation. *Biol Reprod* 2001; **65**: 1444–51.

[88] Weinstein LS, Yu S, Warner DR, Liu J. Endocrine manifestations of stimulatory G protein α-subunit mutations and the role of genomic imprinting. *Endocr Rev* 2001; **22**: 675–705.

[89] Spiegel AM. Signal transduction by guanine nucleotide binding proteins. *Mol Cell Endocrinol* 1987; **49**: 1–16.

[90] Marinero MJ, Ropero S, Colas B, Prieto JC, Lopez-Ruiz MP. Modulation of guanosine triphosphatase activity of g proteins by arachidonic acid in rat Leydig cell membranes. *Endocrinology* 2000; **141**: 1093–9.

[91] Catt KJ, Harwood JP, Clayton RN, *et al.* Regulation of peptide hormone receptors and gonadal steroidogenesis. *Recent Prog Horm Res* 1980; **36**: 557–662.

[92] Simpson ER, Waterman MR. Regulation by ACTH of steroid hormone biosynthesis in the adrenal cortex. *Can J Biochem Cell Biol* 1983; **61**: 692–707.

[93] Jefcoate CR. High-flux mitochondrial cholesterol trafficking, a specialized function of the adrenal cortex. *J Clin Invest* 2002; **110**: 881–90.

[94] Hansson V, Skalhegg BS, Tasken K. Cyclic-AMP-dependent protein kinase (PKA) in testicular cells: cell specific expression, differential regulation and targeting of subunits of PKA. *J Steroid Biochem Mol Biol* 1999; **69**: 367–78.

[95] Kimura T. Transduction of ACTH signal from plasma membrane to mitochondria in adrenocortical steroidogenesis: effects of peptide, phospholipid, and calcium. *J Steroid Biochem* 1986; **25**: 711–6.

[96] Papadopoulos V, Baraldi M, Guilarte TR, *et al.* Translocator protein (18kDa): new nomenclature for the peripheral-type benzodiazepine receptor based on its structure and molecular function. *Trends Pharmacol Sci* 2006; **27**: 402–9.

[97] Papadopoulos V. Peripheral-type benzodiazepine/diazepam binding inhibitor receptor: biological role in steroidogenic cell function. *Endocr Rev* 1993; **14**: 222–40.

[98] Lacapere JJ, Papadopoulos V. Peripheral-type benzodiazepine receptor: structure and function of a cholesterol-binding protein in steroid and bile acid biosynthesis. *Steroids* 2003; **68**: 569–85.

[99] Gavish M, Bachman I, Shoukrun R, *et al.* Enigma of the peripheral benzodiazepine receptor. *Pharmacol Rev* 1999; **51**: 629–50.

[100] Papadopoulos V, Nowzari FB, Krueger KE. Hormone-stimulated steroidogenesis is coupled to mitochondrial benzodiazepine receptors. Tropic hormone action on steroid biosynthesis is inhibited by flunitrazepam. *J Biol Chem* 1991; **266**: 3682–7.

[101] Papadopoulos V, Mukhin AG, Costa E, Krueger KE. The peripheral-type benzodiazepine receptor is functionally linked to Leydig cell steroidogenesis. *J Biol Chem* 1990; **265**: 3772–9.

[102] Papadopoulos V, Amri H, Li H, *et al.* Targeted disruption of the peripheral-type benzodiazepine receptor gene inhibits steroidogenesis in the R2C Leydig tumor cell line. *J Biol Chem* 1997; **272**: 32129–35.

[103] Gazouli M, Han Z, Papadopoulos V. Identification of a peptide antagonist to the peripheral-type benzodiazepine receptor that inhibits hormone-stimulated Leydig cell steroid formation. *J Pharmacol Exp Ther* 2002; **303**: 627–32.

[104] Li H, Papadopoulos V. Peripheral-type benzodiazepine receptor function in cholesterol transport: identification of a putative cholesterol recognition/interaction amino acid sequence and consensus Pattern. *Endocrinology* 1998; **139**: 4991–7.

[105] Li H, Yao Z, Degenhardt B, Teper G, Papadopoulos V. Cholesterol binding at the cholesterol recognition/interaction amino acid consensus (CRAC) of the peripheral-type benzodiazepine receptor and inhibition of steroidogenesis by an HIV TAT-CRAC peptide. *Proc Natl Acad Sci U S A* 2001; **98**: 1267–72.

[106] Lacapere JJ, Delavoie F, Li H, *et al.* Structural and functional study of reconstituted peripheral benzodiazepine receptor. *Biochem Biophys Res Commun* 2001; **284**: 536–41.

[107] Amri H, Ogwuegbu SO, Boujrad N, Drieu K, Papadopoulos V. In vivo regulation of peripheral-type benzodiazepine receptor and glucocorticoid synthesis by ginkgo biloba extract EGb 761 and isolated ginkgolides. *Endocrinology* 1996; **137**: 5707–18.

[108] Amri H, Drieu K, Papadopoulos V. Ex vivo regulation of adrenal cortical cell steroid and protein synthesis, in response to adrenocorticotropic hormone stimulation, by the ginkgo biloba extract EGb 761 and isolated ginkgolide B. *Endocrinology* 1997; **138**: 5415–26.

[109] Amri H, Drieu K, Papadopoulos V. Transcriptional suppression of the adrenal cortical peripheral-type benzodiazepine receptor gene and inhibition of steroid synthesis by ginkgolide B. *Biochem Pharmacol* 2003; **65**: 717–29.

[110] Zilz A, Li H, Castello R, Papadopoulos V, Widmaier EP. Developmental expression of the peripheral-type benzodiazepine receptor and the advent of steroidogenesis in rat adrenal glands. *Endocrinology* 1999; **140**: 859–64.

[111] Culty M, Luo L, Yao ZX, *et al.* Cholesterol transport, peripheral benzodiazepine receptor, and steroidogenesis in aging Leydig cells. *J Androl* 2002; **23**: 439–47.

[112] Joseph-Liauzun E, Delmas P, Shire D, Ferrara P. Topological analysis of the peripheral benzodiazepine receptor in yeast mitochondrial membranes supports a five-transmembrane structure. *J Biol Chem* 1998; **273**: 2146–52.

[113] Culty M, Li H, Boujrad N, *et al.* In vitro studies on the role of the peripheral-type benzodiazepine receptor in steroidogenesis. *J Steroid Biochem Mol Biol* 1999; **69**: 123–30.

[114] Bernassau JM, Reversat JL, Ferrara P, Caput D, Lefur G. A 3D model of the peripheral benzodiazepine receptor and its implication in intra mitochondrial cholesterol transport. *J Mol Graph* 1993; **11**: 236–44, 235.

[115] Boujrad N, Gaillard JL, Garnier M, Papadopoulos V. Acute action of choriogonadotropin on Leydig tumor cells: induction of a higher affinity benzodiazepine-binding site related to steroid biosynthesis. *Endocrinology* 1994; **135**: 1576–83.

[116] Boujrad N, Vidic B, Papadopoulos V. Acute action of choriogonadotropin on leydig tumor cells: changes in the topography of the mitochondrial peripheral-type benzodiazepine receptor. *Endocrinology* 1996; **137**: 5727–30.

[117] Costa E, Guidotti A. Diazepam binding inhibitor (DBI): a peptide with multiple biological actions. *Life Sci* 1991; **49**: 325–44.

[118] Papadopoulos V, Guarneri P, Kreuger KE, Guidotti A, Costa E. Pregnenolone biosynthesis in C6–2B glioma cell mitochondria: regulation by a mitochondrial diazepam binding inhibitor receptor. *Proc Natl Acad Sci U S A* 1992; **89**: 5113–17.

[119] Garnier M, Boujrad N, Ogwuegbu SO, Hudson JR, Papadopoulos V. The polypeptide diazepam-binding inhibitor and a higher affinity mitochondrial peripheral-type benzodiazepine receptor sustain constitutive steroidogenesis in the R2C Leydig tumor cell line. *J Biol Chem* 1994; **269**: 22105–12.

[120] Besman MJ, Yanagibashi K, Lee TD, *et al*. Identification of des-(Gly-Ile)-endozepine as an effector of corticotropin-dependent adrenal steroidogenesis: stimulation of cholesterol delivery is mediated by the peripheral benzodiazepine receptor. *Proc Natl Acad Sci U S A* 1989; **86**: 4897–901.

[121] Papadopoulos V, Berkovich A, Krueger KE, Costa E, Guidotti A. Diazepam binding inhibitor and its processing products stimulate mitochondrial steroid biosynthesis via an interaction with mitochondrial benzodiazepine receptors. *Endocrinology* 1991; **129**: 1481–8.

[122] McEnery MW, Snowman AM, Trifiletti RR, Snyder SH. Isolation of the mitochondrial benzodiazepine receptor: association with the voltage-dependent anion channel and the adenine nucleotide carrier. *Proc Natl Acad Sci U S A* 1992; **89**: 3170–4.

[123] Garnier M, Dimchev AB, Boujrad N, *et al*. In vitro reconstitution of a functional peripheral-type benzodiazepine receptor from mouse Leydig tumor cells. *Mol Pharmacol* 1994; **45**: 201–11.

[124] Li H, Degenhardt B, Tobin D, *et al*. Identification, localization, and function in steroidogenesis of PAP7: a peripheral-type benzodiazepine receptor- and PKA (RIα)-associated protein. *Mol Endocrinol* 2001; **15**: 2211–28.

[125] Liu J, Cavalli LR, Haddad BR, Papadopoulos V. Molecular cloning, genomic organization, chromosomal mapping and subcellular localization of mouse PAP7: a PBR and PKA-RIα associated protein. *Gene* 2003; **308**: 1–10.

[126] Liu J, Li H, Papadopoulos V. PAP7, a PBR/PKA-RIα-associated protein: a new element in the relay of the hormonal induction of steroidogenesis. *J Steroid Biochem Mol Biol* 2003; **85**: 275–83.

[127] Stocco DM. Tracking the role of a StAR in the sky of the new millennium. *Mol Endocrinol* 2001; **15**: 1245–54.

[128] Sugawara T, Lin D, Holt JA, *et al*. Structure of the human steroidogenic acute regulatory protein (StAR) gene: StAR stimulates mitochondrial cholesterol 27-hydroxylase activity. *Biochemistry* 1995; **34**: 12506–12.

[129] Stocco DM, Clark BJ. Regulation of the acute production of steroids in steroidogenic cells. *Endocr Rev* 1996; **17**: 221–44.

[130] Strauss JF, Kallen CB, Christenson LK, *et al*. The steroidogenic acute regulatory protein (StAR): a window into the complexities of intracellular cholesterol trafficking. *Recent Prog Horm Res* 1999; **54**: 369–94.

[131] Arakane F, Sugawara T, Nishino H, *et al*. Steroidogenic acute regulatory protein (StAR) retains activity in the absence of its mitochondrial import sequence: implications for the mechanism of StAR action. *Proc Natl Acad Sci U S A* 1996; **93**: 13731–6.

[132] Bose HS, Lingappa VR, Miller WL. The steroidogenic acute regulatory protein, StAR, works only at the outer mitochondrial membrane. *Endocr Res* 2002; **28**: 295–308.

[133] Hauet T, Yao ZX, Bose HS, *et al*. Peripheral-type benzodiazepine receptor-mediated action of steroidogenic acute regulatory protein on cholesterol entry into Leydig cell mitochondria. *Mol Endocrinol* 2005; **19**: 540–54.

[134] Strauss JF, Kishida T, Christenson LK, Fujimoto T, Hiroi H. START domain proteins and the intracellular trafficking of cholesterol in steroidogenic cells. *Mol Cell Endocrinol* 2003; **202**: 59–65.

[135] Petrescu AD, Gallegos AM, Okamura Y, Strauss JF, Schroeder F. Steroidogenic acute regulatory protein binds cholesterol and modulates mitochondrial membrane sterol domain dynamics. *J Biol Chem* 2001; **276**: 36970–82.

[136] Mathieu AP, Fleury A, Ducharme L, Lavigne P, LeHoux JG. Insights into steroidogenic acute regulatory protein (StAR)-dependent cholesterol transfer in mitochondria: evidence from molecular modeling and structure-based thermodynamics supporting the existence of partially unfolded states of StAR. *J Mol Endocrinol* 2002; **29**: 327–45.

[137] Kallen CB, Billheimer JT, Summers SA, *et al*. Steroidogenic acute regulatory protein (StAR) is a sterol transfer protein. *J Biol Chem* 1998; **273**: 26285–8.

[138] Tsujishita Y, Hurley JH. Structure and lipid transport mechanism of a StAR-related domain. *Nat Struct Biol* 2000; **7**: 408–14.

[139] Baker BY, Epand RF, Epand RM, Miller WL. Cholesterol binding does not predict activity of the

steroidogenic acute regulatory protein, StAR. *J Biol Chem* 2007; **282**: 10223–32.

[140] Caron KM, Clark BJ, Keda Y, Parker KL. Steroidogenic factor-1 acts at all levels of the reproductive axis. *Steroids* 1997; **62**: 53–6.

[141] King SR, Walsh LP, Stocco DM. Nigericin inhibits accumulation of the steroidogenic acute regulatory protein but not steroidogenesis. *Mol Cell Endocrinol* 2000; **166**: 147–53.

[142] Liu PY, Swerdloff RS, Christenson PD, Handelsman DJ, Wang C. Rate, extent, and modifiers of spermatogenic recovery after hormonal male contraception: an integrated analysis. *Lancet* 2006; **367**: 1412–20.

[143] Harman SM, Tsitouras PD. Reproductive hormones in aging men. I. Measurement of sex steroids, basal luteinizing hormone, and leydig cell response to human chorionic gonadotropin. *J Clin Endocrinol Metab* 1980; **51**: 35–40.

[144] Winters SJ, Troen P. Episodic luteinizing hormone (LH) secretion and the response of LH and follicle-stimulating hormone to LH-releasing hormone in aged men: evidence for coexistent primary testicular insufficiency and an impairment in gonadotropin secretion. *J Clin Endocrinol Metab* 1982; **55**: 560–5.

[145] Neaves WB, Johnson L, Porter JC, Parker CR, Petty CS. Leydig cell numbers, daily sperm production, and serum gonadotropin levels in aging men. *J Clin Endocrinol Metab* 1984; **59**: 756–63.

[146] Tenover JS, Matsumoto AM, Plymate SR, Bremner WJ. The effects of aging in normal men on bioavailable testosterone and luteinizing hormone secretion: response to clomiphene citrate. *J Clin Endocrinol Metab* 1987; **65**: 1118–26.

[147] Kaufman JM, Giri M, Deslypere JM, Thomas G, Vermeulen A. Influence of age on the responsiveness of the gonadotrophs to luteinizing hormone-releasing hormone in Males. *J Clin Endocrinol Metab* 1991; **72**: 1255–60.

[148] Nankin HR, Lin T, Murono EP, Osterman J. The aging Leydig Cell: III. Gonadotropin stimulation in men. *J Androl* 1981; **2**: 181–9.

[149] Liu PY, Takahashi PY, Roebuck PD, Iranmanesh A, Veldhuis JD. Aging in healthy men impairs recombinant human luteinizing hormone (LH)-stimulated testosterone secretion monitored under a two-day intravenous pulsatile LH clamp. *J Clin Endocrinol Metab* 2005; **90**: 5544–50.

[150] Veldhuis JD, Veldhuis NJ, Keenan DM, Iranmanesh A. Age diminishes the testicular steroidogenic response to repeated intravenous pulses of recombinant human LH during acute GnRH-receptor blockade in healthy men. *Am J Physiol Endocrinol Metab* 2005; **288**: E775–81.

[151] Liu PY, Takahashi PY, Roebuck PD, Iranmanesh A, Veldhuis JD. Age-specific changes in the regulation of LH-dependent testosterone secretion: assessing responsiveness to varying endogenous gonadotropin output in normal men. *Am J Physiol Regul Integr Comp Physiol* 2005; **289**: R721–8.

[152] Harman SM, Danner RL, Roth GS. Testosterone secretion in the rat in response to chorionic gonadotrophin: alterations with age. *Endocrinology* 1978; **102**: 540–4.

[153] Chen H, Hardy MP, Huhtaniemi I, Zirkin BR. Age-related decreased Leydig cell testosterone production in the Brown Norway rat. *J Androl* 1994; **15**: 551–7.

[154] Chen H, Hardy MP, Zirkin BR. Age-related decreases in Leydig cell testosterone production are not restored by exposure to LH in vitro. *Endocrinology* 2002; **143**: 1637–42.

[155] Leers-Sucheta S, Stocco DM, Azhar S. Down-regulation of steroidogenic acute regulatory (StAR) protein in rat Leydig cells: implications for regulation of testosterone production during aging. *Mech Ageing Dev* 1999; **107**: 197–203.

[156] Bonavera JJ, Swerdloff RS, Leung A, *et al.* In the male brown-Norway (BN) male rat, reproductive aging is associated with decreased LH-pulse amplitude and area. *J Androl* 1997; **18**: 359–65.

[157] Bonavera JJ, Swerdloff RS, Sinha Hakim AP, Lue YH, Wang C. Aging results in attenuated gonadotropin releasing hormone-luteinizing hormone axis responsiveness to glutamate receptor agonist N-methyl-D-aspartate. *J Neuroendocrinol* 1998; **10**: 93–9.

[158] Grzywacz FW, Chen H, Allegretti J, Zirkin BR. Does age-associated reduced Leydig cell testosterone production in Brown Norway rats result from under-stimulation by luteinizing hormone? *J Androl* 1998; **19**: 625–30.

[159] Wang C, Sinha Hikim AP, Lue YH, *et al.* Reproductive aging in the Brown Norway rat is characterized by accelerated germ cell apoptosis and is not altered by luteinizing hormone replacement. *J Androl* 1999; **20**: 509–18.

[160] Guarente L, Kenyon C. Genetic pathways that regulate ageing in model organisms. *Nature* 2000; **408**: 255–62.

[161] Ohyama Y, Kurabayashi M, Masuda H, *et al.* Molecular cloning of rat klotho CDNA: markedly decreased expression of klotho by acute inflammatory stress. *Biochem Biophys Res Commun* 1998; **251**: 920–5.

[162] Klapper W, Parwaresch R, Krupp G. Telomere biology in human aging and aging syndromes. *Mech Ageing Dev* 2001; **122**: 695–712.

[163] Tollefsbol TO, Andrews LG. Mechanisms for methylation-mediated gene silencing and aging. *Med Hypotheses* 1993; **41**: 83–92.

[164] Franceschi C, Valensin S, Bonafe M, *et al*. The network and the remodeling theories of aging: historical background and new perspectives. *Exp Gerontol* 2000; **35**: 879–96.

[165] Finkel T,.Holbrook NJ. Oxidants, oxidative stress and the biology of ageing. *Nature* 2000; **408**: 239–47.

[166] Beckman KB, Ames BN. The free radical theory of aging matures. *Physiol Rev* 1998; **78**: 547–81.

[167] Floyd RA, West M, Hensley K. Oxidative biochemical markers: clues to understanding aging in long-lived species. *Exp Gerontol* 2001; **36**: 619–40.

[168] Sohal RS. The free radical hypothesis of aging: an appraisal of the current status. *Aging (Milano)* 1993; **5**: 3–17.

[169] Chen H, Cangello D, Benson S, *et al*. Age-related increase in mitochondrial superoxide generation in the testosterone-producing cells of Brown Norway rat testes: relationship to reduced steroidogenic function? *Exp Gerontol* 2001; **36**: 1361–73.

[170] Warner HR. Superoxide dismutase, aging, and degenerative disease. *Free Radic Biol Med* 1994; **17**: 249–58.

[171] Sohal RS, Weindruch R. Oxidative stress, caloric restriction, and aging. *Science* 1996; **273**: 59–63.

[172] Martin GM, Austad SN, Johnson TE. Genetic analysis of ageing: role of oxidative damage and environmental stresses. *Nat Genet* 1996; **13**: 25–34.

[173] Usatyuk PV, Vepa S, Watkins T, *et al*. Redox regulation of reactive oxygen species-induced P38 MAP kinase activation and barrier dysfunction in lung microvascular endothelial cells. *Antioxid Redox Signal* 2003; **5**: 723–30.

[174] Bohr VA, Anson RM. DNA Damage, mutation and fine structure DNA repair in aging. *Mutat Res* 1995; **338**: 25–34.

[175] Levine RL. Oxidative modification of glutamine synthetase. I. Inactivation is due to loss of one histidine residue. *J Biol Chem* 1983; **258**: 11823–7.

[176] Stadtman ER. Protein oxidation and aging. *Science* 1992; **257**: 1220–4.

[177] Oliver CN, Ahn BW, Moerman EJ, Goldstein S, Stadtman ER. Age-related changes in oxidized proteins. *J Biol Chem* 1987; **262**: 5488–91.

[178] Smith MA, Perry G, Richey PL, *et al*. Oxidative damage in Alzheimer's. *Nature* 1996; **382**: 120–1.

[179] Zainal TA, Oberley TD, Allison DB, Szweda LI, Weindruch R. Caloric restriction of rhesus monkeys lowers oxidative damage in skeletal muscle. *Faseb J* 2000; **14**: 1825–36.

[180] Moskovitz J, Yim MB, Chock PB. Free radicals and disease. *Arch Biochem Biophys* 2002; **397**: 354–9.

[181] Weindruch R, Walford RL, *The Retardation of Aging and Disease by Dietary Restriction*. Springfield, IL: C. C. Thomas, 1988.

[182] Sohal RS, Ku HH, Agarwal S, Forster MJ, Lal H. Oxidative damage, mitochondrial oxidant generation and antioxidant defenses during aging and in response to food restriction in the mouse. *Mech Ageing Dev* 1994; **74**: 121–33.

[183] Forster MJ, Sohal BH, Sohal RS. Reversible effects of long-term caloric restriction on protein oxidative damage. *J Gerontol A Biol Sci Med Sci* 2000; **55**: B522–9.

[184] Sohal RS, Agarwal S, Candas M, Forster MJ, Lal H. Effect of age and caloric restriction on DNA oxidative damage in different tissues of C57BL/6 mice. *Mech Ageing Dev* 1994; **76**: 215–24.

[185] Hall PF. Testicular steroid synthesis: organization and regulation. In: Knobil E, Neill JD, eds. *Physiology of Reproduction*, 2nd edn. New York, NY: Raven Press, 1994: 1335–62.

[186] Peltola V, Huhtaniemi I, Metsa-Ketela T, Ahotupa M. Induction of lipid peroxidation during steroidogenesis in the rat testis. *Endocrinology* 1996; **137**: 105–12.

[187] Carlson JC, Wu XM, Sawada M. Oxygen radicals and the control of ovarian corpus luteum function. *Free Radic Biol Med* 1993; **14**: 79–84.

[188] Behrman HR, Kodaman PH, Preston SL, Gao S. Oxidative stress and the ovary. *J Soc Gynecol Investig* 2001; **8** (1 Suppl): S40–2.

[189] Behrman HR, Aten RF. Evidence that hydrogen peroxide blocks hormone-sensitive cholesterol transport into mitochondria of rat luteal cells. *Endocrinology* 1991; **128**: 2958–66.

[190] Azhar S, Cao L, Reaven E. Alteration of the adrenal antioxidant defense system during aging in rats. *J Clin Invest* 1995; **96**: 1414–24.

[191] Wu X, Yao K, Carlson JC. Plasma membrane changes in the rat corpus luteum induced by oxygen radical generation. *Endocrinology* 1993; **133**: 491–5.

[192] Cao L, Leers-Sucheta S, Azhar S. Aging alters the functional expression of enzymatic and non-enzymatic anti-oxidant defense systems in testicular rat Leydig cells. *J Steroid Biochem Mol Biol* 2004; **88**: 61–7.

[193] Luo L, Chen H, Trush MA, *et al*. aging and the Brown Norway rat Leydig cell antioxidant defense system. *J Androl* 2006; **27**: 240–7.

[194] Kolena J, Blazicek P, Horkovics-Kovats S, Ondrias K, Sebokova E. Modulation of rat testicular LH/HCG receptors by membrane lipid fluidity. *Mol Cell Endocrinol* 1986; **44**: 69–76.

[195] Chen H, Liu J, Luo L, Baig MU, Kim JM, Zirkin BR. Vitamin E, aging and Leydig cell steroidogenesis. *Exp Gerontol* 2005; **40**: 728–36.

The Sertoli cell: morphology, function, and regulation

Joseph P. Alukal and Dolores J. Lamb

Introduction

Since its discovery by Enrico Sertoli in 1865 [1], the Sertoli cell has proved a fascinating subject for physiologists, histologists, and clinicians alike. **The Sertoli cell is implicated centrally in spermatogenesis, organogenesis, male phenotypic development, and the hypothalamic–pituitary–gonadal axis [2–4]. Its role in phenotypic maleness is absolutely crucial.**

On the other hand, many questions about the specifics of Sertoli cell function remain unanswered. Since the last edition of this textbook, numerous experiments have further delineated the pathways by which the Sertoli cell performs these important functions. These include such projects as simple knockouts of follicle-stimulating hormone receptor (FSHR) and the resultant downstream effects [5]. Recent research into interference with Sertoli cell–germ cell adhesion offers a potentially fruitful future model for male contraception [6,7]. But despite this rapidly growing body of knowledge, many simple questions about the Sertoli cell remain unanswered. How does the Sertoli cell regulate the balance between spermatogenesis and germ cell apoptosis? What is the intracellular mechanism by which the Sertoli cell modulates and maintains the blood–testis barrier (BTB)? What is the trigger within the primordial Sertoli cell that initiates testis differention in the embryo? These and many other questions remain unanswered.

This chapter summarizes the existing body of knowledge regarding the human Sertoli cell. In addition, it offers an extensive consideration of the murine and rat Sertoli cell, as they are studied in many of the experiments that have proved most enlightening with regard to Sertoli cell function. This summary includes a brief overview of cellular structure, basic physiology, the role in spermatogenesis, the role in organogenesis, feedback through the hypothalamic–pituitary–gonadal axis, and future directions for inquiry.

Cell structure

Sertoli cell morphology has been well described by others [1,8,9]. **The cells form an epithelial layer on a monolayer basement membrane. They have a characteristic tripartite nucleolus. They are nondividing, columnar cells with interdigitations projecting into the lumen of the seminiferous tubule; these interdigitations provide for spaces within which spermatid elongation occurs** (Figs. 4.1–4.4).

Basement membrane

The basement membrane upon which Sertoli cells rest is an acellular matrix consisting primarily of laminin and type IV collagen [10]. This layer is produced in part by Sertoli cells and in part by peritubular myoid cells, although the major portion of laminin and collagen deposition is due to Sertoli cell action [11]. Peritubular myoid cell produced mesenchymal factor, or PModS, is in large part responsible for regulation and coordination of function between the two cells [12,13] (Fig. 4.5). A more detailed discussion of PModS follows later in this chapter.

Ultrastructural features

Sertoli cells are responsible for both the maintenance of the blood–testis barrier and the development of germ cells; it is not surprising that they secrete a vast number of proteins [2]. As is consistent with a highly transcriptionally active cell, the Sertoli cell has an extensive Golgi apparatus extending from the basal aspect of the cell all the way to the cell's apex [14,15]. **Somewhat paradoxically, Sertoli cells demonstrate little rough endoplasmic reticulum [16].** This is not completely consistent with constant and active protein secretion. Smooth endoplasmic reticulum, with associated lipid inclusions, is seen in significant amounts, correlating with active steroid synthesis (Fig. 4.6).

Infertility in the Male, 4th edition, ed. Larry I. Lipshultz, Stuart S. Howards, and Craig S. Niederberger. Published by Cambridge University Press. © Cambridge University Press 2009.

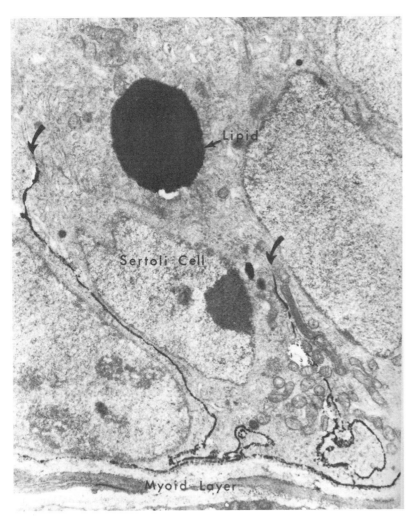

Fig. 4.1. Electron micrograph from an irradiated 30-day-old testis perfused with peroxidase. The tracer passes through the myoid layer and into the intercellular spaces between Sertoli cells. It is stopped there from deeper penetration by tight junctions (× 7200). (From Tindall DJ *et al.* Androgen binding protein as a biochemical marker of formation of the blood–testis barrier. *Endocrinology* 1975; **97**: 636–48, with permission. Copyright 1975, The Endocrine Society.)

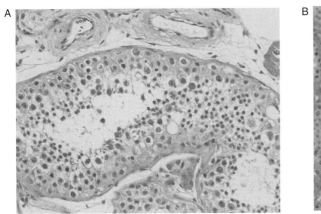

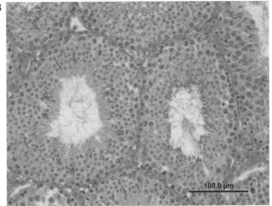

Fig. 4.2. Light microscope images of sections of the (A) human and (B) rodent testis. Hematoxylin and eosin staining (× 40). *See color plate section.*

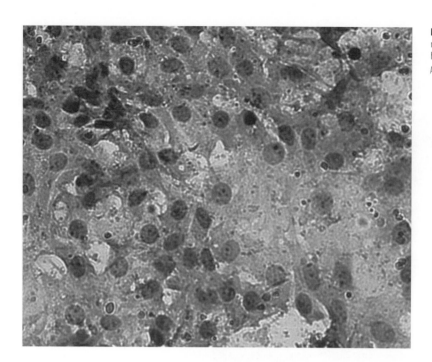

Fig. 4.3. Light microscope images of mouse Sertoli cells in culture 5 days post harvest. DAPI staining (× 40). *See color plate section.*

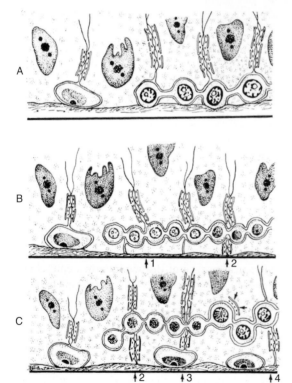

Fig. 4.4. Schematic representation of passage of spermatocytes across blood–testis barrier, composed of tight junctions, ectoplasmic specializations, and other junctional components. (A) Types A and B spermatogonia lie in the basal compartment, and adjacent Sertoli cells meet in tight junctional complexes. The B spermatogonia divide to form preleptotene spermatocytes. (B1) Slips of Sertoli cell cytoplasm extend beneath these cells. Later in time (B2 and C2), new tight junctions develop between basal slips of Sertoli cell cytoplasm, sequestering what are now leptotene spermatocytes in an intermediate compartment. Soon therafter the original tight junctions begin to disassemble (C3) and disappear (C4). The fate of these components is not clear. Midway in pachytene spermatocyte development, ectoplasmic specializations appear (arrows); these resemble one half of a tight junction. Further information regarding their processing is found later in the chapter.

other cells, however, this cytoskeletal architecture is tasked with constant change as spermatogenesis proceeds. Actin filaments, as structural components of ectoplasmic specializations, move spermatogonia. Tight junctions, also attached to actin filaments, disassemble and reform around migrating germ cells. **Thus the cytoskeletal architecture of the Sertoli cell is as crucially important to its function as any other aspect of the cell.** This chapter provides a discussion of actin filaments, intermediate filaments, and microtubules, and a brief consideration of other structures within the Sertoli cell that relate to each of these three structural elements.

Cytoskeletal architecture

The cytoskeletal architecture of the Sertoli cell, as in many other cells, consists of actin filaments, intermediate filaments, and microtubules. Different from

Actin filaments

Actin filaments are composed of actin monomers that polymerize within cells to filamentous structures

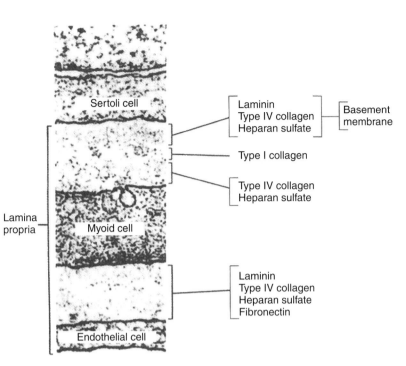

Sertoli cell

Laminin
Type IV collagen
Heparan sulfate

Basement
membrane

Type I collagen

Type IV collagen
Heparan sulfate

Lamina
propria

Myoid cell

Laminin
Type IV collagen
Heparan sulfate
Fibronectin

Endothelial cell

Fig. 4.5. Electron micrograph of the testicular lamina propria and basement membrane. (From Hadley MA, Dym M. Immunocytochemistry of extracellular matrix in the lamina propria of the rat testis: electron microscopic localization. *Biol Reprod* 1987; **37**: 1283–9, with permission.)

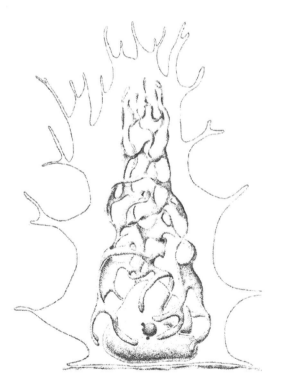

Fig. 4.6. Schematic representation of the Golgi apparatus (trans-Golgi network, TGN) of the Sertoli cell. TGN extends through the entire length of the cell. (From Rambourg A *et al*. Three-dimensional architecture of the Golgi apparatus in Sertoli cells of the rat. *Am J Anat* 1979; **154**: 455–76, with permission from John Wiley & Sons, Inc. Copyright 1979.)

5–8 nm in size. Actin filaments allow for motorized movement within cells through their attachment to myosin, another globular protein [17,18]. Functionally, actin filaments are therefore central to cell movement, attachment, polarity, and intracellular transport.

Specifically within Sertoli cells, actin filaments are predominantly found as components of tubulobulbar complexes and ectoplasmic specializations. Both structures are unique to Sertoli cells and crucially important to spermatogenesis.

Tubulobulbar complexes

Tubulobulbar complexes are identified in two places within the Sertoli cell: first, attached to spermatids at the apical surface of the seminiferous epithelium, and second, along the basolateral membrane between adjoining Sertoli cells [19,20] (Figs. 4.7, 4.8). The complexes are elongated in shape with a bulbous flared tip, and they are composed of approximated plasma membrane from both adjoining cells (Sertoli cell/spermatid and Sertoli cell/Sertoli cell). Encircling the plasma membrane interface, a tubule of actin filaments extends the length of the structure. Finally, rough endoplasmic reticulum and vesicles are located in close proximity to the flared tip of the structure [19].

The function of tubulobulbar complexes within the Sertoli cell is not completely understood. **With regard**

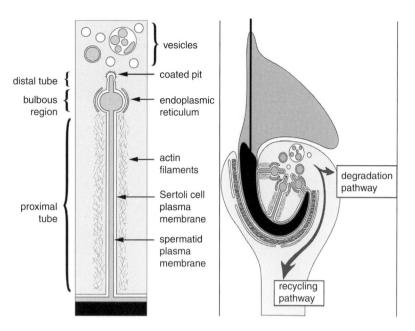

Fig. 4.7. Schematic representation of the tubulobulbar complex. The complex is associated with elongating spermatid and ectoplasmic specializations. The image on the right demonstrates internalization of vesicles by the tubulobulbar complex, which are then either recycled or degraded. (Reprinted with permission from Guttman JA *et al.* Evidence that tubulobulbar complexes in the seminiferous epithelium are involved with internalization of adhesion junctions. *Biol Reprod* 2004; **71**: 548–59.)

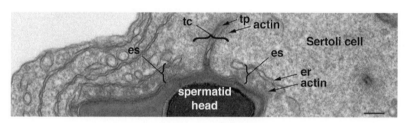

Fig. 4.8. Electron micrograph of the tubulobulbar complex (tc) and associated elongated spermatid. The complex is flanked by ectoplasmic specializations (es). Also identified are tubulobulbar process (tp) and endoplasmic reticulum (er). Bar = 200 nm. (Reprinted with permission from Guttman JA *et al.* Evidence that tubulobulbar complexes in the seminiferous epithelium are involved with internalization of adhesion junctions. *Biol Reprod* 2004; **71**: 548–59.)

to spermatids, it is thought that the tubulobulbar complex may play a role in modeling the spermatid head by removing and processing spermatid cytoplasm [21]. They are known to be the last structure to disengage from mature spermatids before their spermiation – the release of the spermatid into the lumen of the seminiferous tubule [19,22,23].

Tubulobulbar complexes between adjacent Sertoli cells may play a different role; they are identified consistently in association with both ectoplasmic specializations and tight junction/adherens junction complexes. It is hypothesized that they are involved in junction disassembly and turnover. This process may be mediated by clathrin-coated vesicles [24]. The role of actin filaments in the function of tubulobulbar complexes is not yet firmly defined. However, as these complexes are required to be highly mobile, actin

filaments could represent the means for both transport and assembly of tubulobulbar complexes. This process may be regulated through the protein kinase C pathway [25]; additionally, other kinases, including protein kinase G and carboxyl-terminal Src kinase, may be involved [26–28].

Ectoplasmic specializations

Similar to tubulobulbar complexes, ectoplasmic specializations are also located along the apical seminiferous epithelium in association with spermatids. In addition, they, too, are found along the basolateral membrane between adjoining Sertoli cells and the basement membrane [21] (Fig. 4.9).

Ectoplasmic specializations are unique to Sertoli cells. **Functionally, they are thought to be predominantly responsible for adherence of Sertoli cells to**

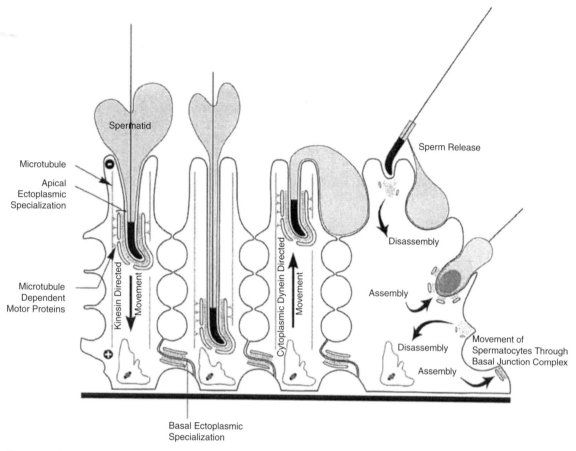

Fig. 4.9. Schematic representation of ectoplasmic specializations (ES) and their role in spermatid translocation. ES are also found between adjacent Sertoli cells. (Reprinted with permission from Vogl AW *et al*. Unique and multifunctional adhesion junctions in the testis: ectoplasmic specializations. *Arch Histol Cytol* 2000; **63**: 1–15.)

each other and to maturing spermatocytes and spermatids. They comprise three layers: plasma membrane most superficially, an intermediate layer of actin filaments, and a deep layer of endoplasmic reticulum. Associated adhesion molecules that are known to be functionally relevant to ectoplasmic specialization function include integrin α6β1, nectin 2, N-cadherin and junctional adhesion molecules (JAMs) [22,29–31]. Interestingly, nectin 2 knockout mice have been successfully engineered. Confirming the importance of ectoplasmic specializations in spermatogenesis, these animals are infertile [32–34].

Regulation of ectoplasmic specialization function is thought to be mediated through TGF-β, possibly through the ERK signaling pathway [35,36]. TGF-β is also implicated in regulation of tight junctions and thereby of the blood–testis barrier [37,38].

Intermediate filaments

Intermediate filaments are filamentous polymers that occur in almost all cell types. They are thought to perform a scaffolding function within the cell, protecting the cell from mechanical forces. They are classified into four types (I–IV) [39,40].

Within Sertoli cells, the predominant type of intermediate filament identified is vimentin (type III) [40]. In addition, keratins (type I and II) and nestin (type IV) are present in smaller amounts. Intermediate filaments radiate outward from the area surrounding the nucleus towards the periphery of the cell. Specifically, they are associated peripherally with Sertoli cell surface complexes including desmosome-like junctions, hemidesmosome-like junctions, and ectoplasmic specializations [41]. Neither desmosome-like junctions nor hemidesmosome-like junctions are completely understood with regard to their function or structural composition. Desmosome-like junctions are found both between adjoining Sertoli cells and between Sertoli cells and spermatogenic cells. They are presumed to be involved also in cell–cell attachment. Cadherins and catenins, components of desmosomes in other cells, have not as yet been conclusively identified in desmosome-like junctions of Sertoli cells [41].

A vimentin knockout mouse has been engineered; it has no defect in fertility and a normal-appearing seminiferous epithelium despite absence of evidence of intermediate filaments within Sertoli cells of the animal [42]. Further work to gain understanding of the complete role of intermediate filaments, desmosome-like junctions, and hemidesmosome-like junctions is under way.

Microtubules

Microtubules are long tubular polymers composed of dimerized α and β tubulin. They are identified in numerous types of cells and are predominantly responsible for directionalized transport within cells; polarity of the heterodimeric units comprising each microtubule allows for this. Microtubules are typically arrayed in cells in outward spokes from a microtubule organizing center (MTOC). They have both a plus (fast-growing) and minus (slow-growing) orientation in relation to this MTOC [17,39] (Fig. 4.10).

Microtubules within Sertoli cells differ from those in other cells in that they are not organized around centrally located MTOCs [43]. **Instead, they originate from the peripheral aspect of the cell, organizing towards the center of the cell; this is confirmed by reversible disruption of the microtubular architecture with fungicides (such as carbendazim and nocodozole) and subsequent observation of microtubular reorganization** [44–46]. These and other experiments in which the microtubular architecture of the Sertoli cell is disrupted via treatment with colchicine or vinblastine confirm a second function of microtubules in the Sertoli cell; the characteristic columnar morphology is lost in treated Sertoli cells, implying that microtubules provide assistance in maintaining the architecture of the Sertoli cell [47–49].

Amongst other functions within the Sertoli cell, microtubules also appear to be involved in the entrenchment and then release of elongating spermatids. Molecules including dynein and kinesin are responsible for this movement, along with movement of other substances within the cell [17]. **Again,**

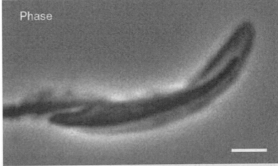
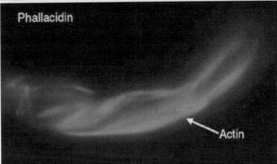
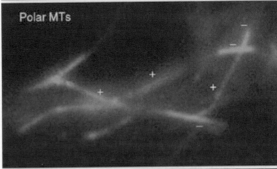
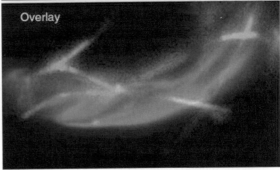

Fig. 4.10. Phase-contrast image of polarity-marked microtubules bound to ectoplasmic specializations. Overlay images of actin (to show the presence of the ectoplasmic specialization) and the polarity-marked microtubules attached to the junction plaque as well as an overlay of the polar microtubules on the ectoplasmic specialization. Actin = red, polar microtubules = green. Bar = 2.5 μm. (Reprinted with permission from Guttman JA *et al.* Dynein and plus-end microtubule-dependent motors are associated with specialized Sertoli cell junction plaques (ectoplasmic specializations). *J Cell Sci* 2000; **113**: 2167–76.) *See color plate section.*

the polarity of microtubules allows for this organized movement of spermatids and substances towards either the apical or basal surface of the cell; microtubules are consistently arranged with the minus end situated apically [17].

The blood–testis barrier

The interaction of adjoining Sertoli cells with each other and with the basement membrane is crucially important to the function of the Sertoli cell: tight junctions and adherens junctions between Sertoli cells allow for the creation of an immunologically privileged space within the seminiferous tubule. This barrier, created by Sertoli cells and the basement membrane, is known as the blood–testis barrier [50].

Interestingly, the blood–testis barrier represents the only barrier of immunologic privilege in the human that is composed of both tight junctions and adhesion junctions in contiguous locations and functioning together. This is in contradistinction to the blood–brain barrier and the blood–retina barrier, where tight junctions and adhesion junctions are separate and have unique functions [51–53]. **Moreover, the blood–testis barrier is uniquely tasked to perform several unique and complex functions of its own: namely, anchoring of Sertoli cells to each other, coordinated disassembly to allow the migration of developing spermatogenic cells into the tubule lumen, and coordinated reassembly in order to maintain the blood–testis barrier throughout this process** [41] (Fig. 4.11).

Extensive research into both the regulation of the blood–testis barrier and the structure and function of

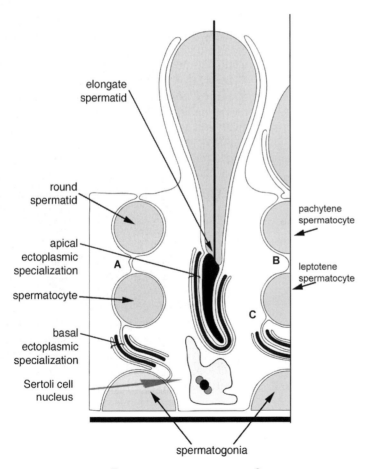

Fig. 4.11. Schematic representation of the blood–testis barrier. Tight-junction components are listed in the key. Locations of adherens junctions, hemidesmosomes, and tight junctions are as noted in the key. (Adapted with permission from Guttman JA *et al.* Evidence that tubulobulbar complexes in the seminiferous epithelium are involved. *Biol Reprod* 2004; **71**: 548–59.)

elongate spermatid

round spermatid

apical ectoplasmic specialization

spermatocyte

basal ectoplasmic specialization

Sertoli cell nucleus

pachytene spermatocyte

leptotene spermatocyte

A

B

C

spermatogonia

A
adherens junctions
desmosome-like junctions

B
tight junctions
(junctional adhering molecule, zonula occludens, claudin, nectin, testin)

C
adherens junctions
desmosome-like junctions

tight junctions and adhesion junctions has been undertaken. TGF-β signaling has been implicated in regulation of the blood–testis barrier [for review see 54]. Discussion of this topic in greater scope is found later in this chapter; however, it is important to understand that the function of the blood–testis barrier changes greatly in the course of the life of the animal. The developing fetus, the prepubertal animal, and the adult animal all differ in terms of number of germ cells, presence or absence of dividing germ cells, and presence or absence of active spermatogenesis [55]. **Therefore, regulation of blood–testis barrier function is crucially important to normal mammalian fertility**.

Structural analysis of Sertoli cell tight junctions and adherens junctions demonstrates many of the components that make up these junctions. These include membrane proteins such as occludins, claudins, zonula occludens (ZO), and junctional adhesion molecules (JAMs) [41]. Somewhat less well understood is the regulation of these components and their interactions with each other. A brief summary of this regulatory pathway will follow.

Occludins

Occludins are 65 kDa proteins found in Sertoli cell tight junctions of rats and mice, although not in human Sertoli cells [56]. They have four transmembrane domains, two extracellular loops, and one intracellular loop (Fig. 4.11). They are crucially important to spermatogenesis, as is evidenced by two sets of experiments conducted in rodents. First, occludin knockout mice become infertile by 40 weeks of age with atrophy of the testis [57]. Second, a 22 amino acid synthetic peptide that corresponds to the second extracellular loop of the occludin protein causes reversible impairment of spermatogenesis through detachment of germ cells in both mice and rats [58].

Claudins and other proteins

Claudins are a family of proteins with more than 20 members [59,60]. **Claudin 11 is also a transmembrane protein identified in tight junctions of Sertoli cells** [61]. **Claudin 11 knockout mice are infertile throughout life**. They do not show evidence of tight junctions in Sertoli cells examined on EM [62].

Also involved in the tight junction of Sertoli cells is junctional adhesion molecule 1, another transmembrane protein. **Together, occludin, claudin 11, and JAM-1 interact together with identical peptides on the surface of adjoining cells** [41,63]. The intracellular

portions of these proteins are associated with zonula occludens 1 and 2 (ZO-1, ZO-2). In turn, ZO-1 and ZO-2 link the tight junction to intracellular actin [41]. Interestingly, another junctional adhesion molecule, JAM-3, is implicated in proper polar elongation of the maturing spermatid [64].

Together, the interaction between the two adjoining multiprotein complexes that constitute each tight junction results in a significant portion of the barrier function of the blood–testis barrier. **This barrier function is measured experimentally by determining transepithelial electrical resistance. Interestingly, Sertoli cells in Matrigel culture organize functionally into a confluent layer similar to an epithelium; these cells have a weak barrier function in culture (100 ohm/cm²). Treatment of cultures with testosterone or testosterone and FSH increases the transepithelial resistance (TER) by as much as a factor of 10** [65–67]. It is hypothesized that testosterone has a direct effect on tight junction and therefore on blood–testis barrier function. Confirming this further are experiments with Sertoli-cell-specific knockouts of androgen receptor (SCARKO) mice that demonstrate intact, but weakened, blood–testis barrier function [68]. Other regulation of blood–testis barrier function appears to involve TGF-β3 through the p38 MAP–kinase pathway [69]. Further regulatory input may derive from TNF-α [70].

Spermiogenesis and spermiation

A brief discussion of spermiogenesis and spermiation follows here within the context of the functional aspects of the Sertoli cell necessary for spermiation. For more detail please refer to Chapter 5.

Spermiogenesis is the process by which the haploid round spermatid is remodeled into a functionally mature elongate spermatid; spermiation is the detachment of the mature elongated spermatid from the Sertoli cell in a coordinated fashion. As discussed above, all of the cytoskeletal architecture of the Sertoli cell contributes to this effort: ectoplasmic specializations attach the round spermatid to the Sertoli cell membrane, and microtubular movement drags the spermatid towards the basolateral membrane of the Sertoli cell, deepening the membrane crypt where the spermatid rests and elongating the cell. The now elongated spermatid is returned to the apical membrane via microtubular movement again. Finally, tubulobulbar complexes form, the ectoplasmic specializations dissolve, and the elongate spermatid is released into the lumen of the seminiferous tubule. The remaining ecto-plasmic specialization is phagocytosed [71,72].

Many theories exist as to regulation of this process. **The cyclic-AMP response element (CRE) is a likely candidate; activation of CRE located within the promoter for nectin 2 results in increased transcription of nectin 2, an intracellular protein found in ecto-plasmic specializations [73]. As mentioned previously, nectin 2 knockout mice are infertile [32–34]. CRE is known to be bound and therefore activated by, amongst other proteins, cAMP response binding protein, or CREB**. CREB is a member of the basic-domain leucine-zipper family of transcription factors. CREB is thought to unbind from CRE in the presence of increased cAMP, thereby resulting in decreased tran-scription of nectin 2 [73,74]. This contributes to the ability of the elongated spermatid to detach from now weakened ectoplasmic specializations. This obviously represents only one pathway on which spermiation might depend; research continues with the goal of fur-ther elaborating this complex process.

Sertoli cell differentiation

Sertoli cells in adult mammals exist as a terminally differentiated, postmitotic population. Sertoli cell number becomes fixed during puberty in all mam-mals [75–78]. After this point, spermatogenesis is maximally limited by the fixed number of Sertoli cells that exist in a testis. Prepubertal regulation of Sertoli cell number and division is therefore vitally important to future fertility.

Peritubular myoid cell secreted mesenchymal factor (PModS)

PModS was first described by Norton and Skinner in 1989 [12]; at the time, preliminary evidence indicated that peritubular myoid cells might play a central role in regulation of Sertoli cell differentiation. PModS was thought to act through c-Fos, a nuclear transcription factor within the Sertoli cell, to cause up-regulation of Sertoli-cell-specific factors that enabled germ cell dif-ferentiation [79,80]; these factors included transfer-rin (transferrin levels and transcription of transferrin mRNA were quantified in this study) and androgen-binding protein. At this time, investigators were just beginning to appreciate the nature of the complex intercellular interactions in the testis regulating sper-matogenesis through endocrine, paracrine, and auto-crine pathways that are discussed below.

Basic helix-loop-helix transcription factors

Continued investigation into the regulation of Sertoli cell differentiation focused on up-regulation of trans-ferrin as a downstream effect of PModS; Chadhuary and colleagues demonstrated the existence of an E-box response element within the promoter region for trans-ferrin known as SE2 [81]. E-box response elements are known targets for basic helix-loop-helix (bHLH) tran-scription factors; bHLH transcription factors dimer-ize at a conserved helix-loop-helix region and then bind E-box response elements at their conserved basic region, thereby initiating transcription of the E-box response element in question [82]. Through examin-ation of Sertoli cell cultures, a ubiquitously expressed bHLH, E12, was identified in Sertoli cells. Levels of E12 were shown to correlate with transferrin expression [83]. Also identified was a bHLH inhibitory factor, Id, which, when expressed, blocked bHLH activation of the E-box response element within SE2, again through a conserved helix-loop-helix region [84]. Transferrin levels dropped in the presence of increased levels of Id. Examination of mitotic, actively dividing Sertoli cells (prepubertal) demonstrated increased levels of Id protein.

Id proteins as regulators of Sertoli cell proliferation

Further investigation of the Id family of proteins yielded a total of four molecules, Id1, Id2, Id3, and Id4 [85]. Levels of Id proteins were found to be low in postmi-totic populations of Sertoli cells, again consistent with a terminally differentiated population of cells. Through integration and overexpression of human Id1 and Id2 into an adult population of rat Sertoli cells, Chaudhary and colleagues were able to cause postmitotic Sertoli cells to begin to proliferate [86]; correspondingly, lev-els of transferrin, androgen-binding protein, and FSH receptor dropped in treated populations of cells.

Taken together, these findings are consistent with the hypothesis that prepubertal populations of Sertoli cells divide in the testis under the influence of Id proteins, thereby populating the seminiferous tubules with adequate Sertoli cells for spermato-genesis later in life. Upon entering puberty, PModS is secreted by peritubular myoid cells in response to some other signal. In addition to the action of FSH on the Sertoli cell, this results in an increase in bHLH E12 within Sertoli cells. This overwhelms the effect of Id proteins, resulting in a halt in mitosis and an

up-regulation of Sertoli cell gene targets whose products are necessary for spermatogenesis, such as transferrin. Many questions remain. What causes the increase in PModS secretion at puberty? Is it simply a rise in intratesticular testosterone? By what intracellular pathway are Id levels changed within the cell? Chaudhary and Skinner hypothesize protein kinase A acting downstream of an activated FSH receptor; as yet this remains to be confirmed [86]. Contrary to this hypothesis, Johnston and colleagues demonstrated that Sertoli cell number in mice was regulated through testosterone and not FSH through analysis of FSH and FSH receptor knockout animals [87].

Finally, what other terminally differentiated cells within the body can be induced to proliferate through overexpression of Id family proteins? Could this be a potential future treatment for other injuries in the human body involving terminally differentiated cells such as nerve transection? Does this represent a possible future treatment for male infertility? Further research into these questions is obviously needed .

Regulation of spermatogenesis

Regulation of the Sertoli cell in its function as "nurse cell" for developing spermatogenic cells is obviously multifaceted and complex. Autocrine, paracrine, and endocrine regulatory pathways all exist simultaneously; many are well defined. As this regulation basically equates to regulation of spermatogenic function, it is vital to have a thorough understanding of these pathways in order to begin to understand the molecular basis of male infertility.

Spermatogenesis: overview

A brief overview of spermatogenesis in the rodent follows here; for further detail please see Chapter 5. **Put simply, spermatogenesis is the process by which diploid spermatogonial stem cells are turned into mature haploid spermatozoa.** Obviously, the process is far more complex than this understatement – meiotic reduction division must occur properly, the characteristic and functionally important shape of the mature sperm must be molded somehow, and the process needs to be coordinated for all germ cells arising at the same time. This is an incredibly complex process, and it is not yet fully understood in either the human or the rodent. However, a tremendous amount of knowledge can be gleaned from studying spermatogenesis as it proceeds with the help of the Sertoli cell.

Spermatogonial stem cells exist in the seminiferous tubules; as yet, these cells have not been conclusively identified in humans, but their existence is both safely assumed and functionally confirmed [88,89]. **These haploid cells must be capable of both self-renewal – thereby maintaining the stem cell population – and differentiation**. Differentiation, occurring as a result of some unknown signal, potentially arising from the Sertoli cell, starts the spermatogonial stem cell along the pathway to becoming a mature elongated spermatid. **Along this pathway, the cell passes through the following stages: spermatogonia, spermatocyte, spermatid, spermatozoon** [76,77,90–92]. The basic processes vary during these stages as well, encompassing mitosis, meiosis, and differentiation, to lead ultimately to the release of the mature spermatozoa into the lumen of the seminiferous epithelium.

Within the rodent [78,93,94], type A, intermediate, and type B spermatogonia are recognized as spermatogonial subtypes. Type A0, or undifferentiated spermatogonia, appear to be the first stage in this process (different from type As spermatogonia – the presumed spermatogonial stem cell). Type A spermatogonia are further subdivided into type A1–4 spermatogonia (differentiating). Cells then proceed through stages as intermediate and type B spermatogonia. **It is cohorts of connected type B spermatogonia that undergo mitotic division in order to become primary spermatocytes.** Spermatocytic differentiation then proceeds through several meiotic stages: preleptotene primary, leptotene primary, zygotene primary, pachytene primary, and secondary.

An alternative scheme of classification exists, outlined by Huckins [93,94]. In this system, spermatogonial stem cells, or As cells (for type A stem) are identified by the fact that they lack intercellular bridging. They divide to form either two daughter stem cells, or two paired spermatogonia (Apr) connected by a cytoplasmic bridge due to incomplete cytokinesis. The Apr cells continue division to form chains of 4, 8, and 16 A-aligned (Aal) spermatogonia. These in turn differentiate into A1 spermatogonia, which undergo another series of six divisions, still with incomplete cytokinesis. The result of this is a clonal syncitium of up to 4000 primary spermatocytes.

Taken broadly, spermatocytic differentiation can be thought of simply as primary spermatocytes undergoing meiotic reduction division followed by equatorial divisions. The result of this process is a haploid round spermatid (Fig. 4.12). As has been previously described in this chapter, the round spermatid undergoes extensive modification with regard to its cellular architecture; the result is an elongated

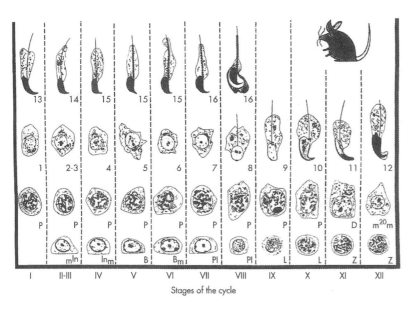

Fig. 4.12. Map of spermatogenesis in the mouse. Vertical columns, designated by Roman numerals, depict cell associations (stages). A cycle is a complete series of cell associations that are placed in logical order. The developmental progression of a cell is followed horizontally until the right-hand border of the map is reached; the cell progression then continues at the left of the map one row up. The map (cycle) ends with the completion of spermiation. The symbols designate specific phases of cell development. (Reproduced with permission from Russell LD, *et al*. Stages, cycle, and wave. In: Russell LD, *et al*, eds. *Histological and Histopathological Evaluation of the Testis*. Clearwater, FL: Cache River Press, 1990.)

Stages of the cycle

spermatid that is ready for release into the seminiferous tubule. **The process by which the mature spermatozoon is made from a round spermatid is termed spermiogenesis; the process by which the mature spermatid is released into the tubular lumen is called spermiation**.

Questions about the regulation of this process are many. They include the means by which the Sertoli cell communicates with developing cohorts of germ cells, while coordinating their individual efforts with other cells along the seminiferous tubule. In addition, the entire process needs to be subject to endocrine control, depending on the state of the organism in question. The most obvious and simplest example of this is the need for a coordinated onset to spermatogenesis when an animal enters puberty. We will first examine this endocrine regulation by specifically considering the hypothalamic–pituitary–gonadal axis.

Hypothalamic–pituitary–gonadal axis

Spermatogenesis is essentially controlled by the gonadotropic hormones, follicle-stimulating hormone (FSH) and luteinizing hormone (LH). FSH and LH are secreted by the anterior pituitary in response to secretion of gonadotropin-releasing hormone (GnRH) by the hypothalamus. LH, in turn, acts upon the Leydig cell to produce testosterone. FSH from the pituitary and testosterone from the Leydig cells then act upon the Sertoli cell to promote maturation of spermatogenic cells [95] (Fig. 4.13). Ultimately, both high levels of intratesticular testosterone and FSH are

necessary for spermatogenesis to occur in an efficient manner [96].

Negative feedback in this pathway occurs on several levels. First, inhibin, a heterodimeric protein that belongs to the TGF-β family of glycoproteins, feeds back at the level of both the hypothalamus and the pituitary to decrease secretion of gonadotropins [97,98]. Inhibin B, secreted by Sertoli cells in response to stimulation by FSH, feeds back directly on the pituitary to inhibit transcription of the gene encoding the β subunit of FSH [96,99]. Second, testosterone itself feeds back to decrease secretion of GnRH and LH together [95]. Tight internal control of FSH and testosterone secretion is necessary for normal spermatogenesis in the fertile male.

Investigation into the specific role of each of these hormones with regard to spermatogenesis has taken several forms. Knockout experiments in rodents have demonstrated the specific effects of loss of function at various points along this pathway. A brief description of these experiments follows; for an excellent review consult Kumar [100].

FSH-β knockout mice

Kumar and colleagues engineered knockout mice for the β subunit of FSH in 1997 [101]. Phenotypically, male mice were smaller on average, and they had smaller testes. Despite decreased numbers of epididymal and testis sperm, these animals were fertile. This was in part explained by the discovery that FSH receptor demonstrates some low

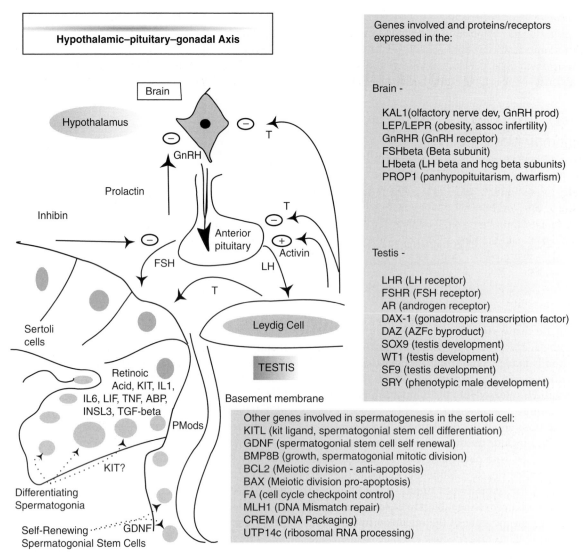

Fig. 4.13. Schematic representation of the hypothalamic–pituitary–gonadal axis. Specific attention is paid to downstream interactions within the testis at the cellular level.

level of constitutive activity even in the absence of circulating FSH [102].

This finding in mice did confirm work in humans with an isolated point mutation in the FSH receptor; of three males identified who were homozygous for the mutation, two were fertile [103]. At the same time, other mutations in the human FSH receptor in the setting of complete male infertility have been identified [104]. Female animals with this mutation were completely infertile; this also paralleled what was observed in human females with mutation of the FSH receptor [105].

FSH receptor knockout mice (FORKO)

FSH receptor is a G-protein-coupled receptor with seven transmembrane spanning regions. **To further elucidate the question of the role of FSH in spermatogenesis, Diermice for FSH receptor in 1998 [106]. The phenotypiich and colleagues successfully generated knockout c appearance of these animals was animals and dec also consistent with FSH-β KO animals, with small reased testis size observed. FORKO males were observed to enter puberty at a later stage than wild-type animals and did have impaired fertility [107].** Interestingly, male animals were found to have low levels of testosterone and did not demonstrate a normal increase in testosterone production with administration of exogenous LH; this indicates derangement in Leydig cell–Sertoli cell interaction due to absence of FSH signaling in the Sertoli cell [108].

LH-β knockout mice and LH receptor knockout mice (LHRKO)

Ma and colleagues generated knockout mice for LH-β subunit in 2004 [109]. Males were phenotypically hypogonadal; both serum and intratesticular testosterone levels were extremely low. Both male and female animals were completely infertile. On histological examination of the testes, knockout animals demonstrated few Leydig cells and no elongated spermatids.

With regard to the Sertoli cell, these animals offered an opportunity to examine how the absence of testosterone would affect Sertoli cell function despite the presence of FSH. Interestingly, expression of FSH receptor did not change in knockout animals, although up-regulation of inhibin B and anti-Müllerian hormone (AMH) was observed [109].

LH receptor knockout mice (LHRKO) were generated by Lei et al. in 2001 [110]. Male knockout animals were again found to be infertile; in addition, however, males demonstrated varying degrees of ambiguity, with undescended testes and accessory sex organs. Treatment with testosterone did not completely reverse this phenotype and did not restore fertility. Females were also completely infertile. Importantly, Lo and colleagues used this model to demonstrate the feasibility of Leydig stem cell transplantation with de novo testosterone production in these animals [111].

Androgen receptor knockout mice (ARKO, SCARKO)

The above experiments clearly demonstrated the fact that LH and/or LH receptor, and therefore testosterone, are necessary for spermatogenesis in these animals; this is as opposed to FSH, which when knocked out resulted in impaired, but not absent, fertility. Confirmatory experiments using total knockout of androgen receptor and Sertoli-cell-specific knockout of androgen receptor (SCARKO) were undertaken by De Gendt et al. in 2004 [68,112]. ARKO mice were found to have a completely ambiguous phenotype; this parallels the phenotype of testicular feminization in the human (complete androgen insensitivity syndrome). Obviously, these animals were completely infertile [112].

SCARKO animals instead demonstrated a normal male genitourinary tract and normal testicular descent. Testis size was small on average, and histological examination of the testis demonstrated no evidence of elongated spermatids; this was despite normal numbers of Sertoli cells and apparently normal numbers of early spermatogenic cells [68]. Quantitative reverse transcriptase polymerase chain reaction (RT-PCR) experiments considering a number of testis function genes demonstrated qualitative defects in the ability of ARKO/SCARKO animals to create and maintain a functional blood–testis barrier [113]. The ARKO/SCARKO experiments demonstrated that while androgen action is crucially important to spermatogenesis, it may act through some mechanism other than the Sertoli cell androgen receptor itself. Further investigation in this area will obviously prove to be important.

Other local regulators of spermatogenesis

Endocrine control of the spermatogenic process is well understood; the above experiments represent an effort to further elaborate the specifics of how LH, FSH, and testosterone contribute to spermatogenesis and phenotypic maleness through the hypothalamic–pituitary–gonadal axis. Regulation of spermatogenesis and Sertoli cell function is affected on many other levels, however. In recent years, tremendous advances have been made regarding autocrine and paracrine regulation of the Sertoli cell.

Paracrine regulators of Sertoli cell and testis function include testicular cytokines and growth factors; many of these are listed in Figure 4.13. Some of these that are of particular interest are interleukins 1 and 6, leukemic inhibitory factor (LIF), stem cell factor or KIT ligand (SCF or KIT), tumor necrosis factor (TNF), and interferon gamma (IFN-γ). The interplay of these factors between Sertoli cells and adjacent Leydig cells, peritubular myoid cells, testicular macrophages, and germ cells is one of the means by which local communication in the testis occurs. This communication is vitally important to the coordination of Sertoli cells and germ cells as spermatogenesis proceeds.

Interleukin 1

Interleukin 1 (IL-1) is actually a family of molecules consisting of IL-1α, IL-1β, and IL-1RA, a naturally occurring receptor antagonist [114–116]. In addition, IL-1 has two predominate receptor types, IL-1R1 and IL-1R2 [117]. IL-1 in general is a pro-inflammatory cytokine; its effects are mediated by the fact that IL1-R2 is a scavenging receptor type that binds circulating IL-1 and blocks its effects. In addition, IL-1R1 can exist both as a membrane-bound receptor and as a soluble, nonsignaling receptor, in essence also acting as an IL-1 block. Taken together, IL-1R2, soluble IL-1R1, and IL-1RA act together to down-regulate the pro-inflammatory effects of IL-1 [118–120].

In varying degrees, IL-1α, IL1-β, IL-1RA, and both receptor types are expressed throughout the testis. **Specifically, experiments demonstrate IL-1 receptor in Sertoli cells, Leydig cells, and germ cells [117]. FSH, TNF-α, and lipopolysaccharides (LPS) all increase expression of IL-1 by the Sertoli cell [121,122]. Finally, remains of degenerating germ cells (i.e., residual bodies from elongate spermatids) also increase expression of IL-1 [121,123].**

What emerges is a complex picture. Does IL-1 mediate something akin to the inflammatory response within the seminiferous tubule? Is IL-1 responsible for coordinated germ cell apoptosis?

Interleukin 6 and leukemic inhibitory factor

Interleukin 6 is a well-known pro-inflammatory cytokine. Specifically, it is implicated in the differentiation of both B cells and T cells [124]. It complexes with a transmembrane protein, IL-6Rα, which then associates with a receptor subunit, gp130, which then causes a downstream intracellular cascade through Map kinase [125].

LIF is a subtype of this family. **LIF, which halts germ cell apoptosis and encourages proliferation, is a murine model. It is expressed within the testis by peritubular myoid cells and acts through IL-6Rα expressed on Sertoli cells. Expression of LIF increases with administration of hCG; IL-6 increases with administration of FSH [126–128].** LIF appears to promote both Sertoli cell and germ cell survival in addition to promoting germ cell differentiation [129,130].

Again, a complex and incompletely understood picture emerges. As IL-6 secretion is stimulated by IL-1, it appears that a mechanism for tight, self-regulated control of apoptosis and germ cell proliferation exists within the testis. Elaboration of this pathway and its implications for germ cell development are of paramount importance.

TGF-β signaling as a regulator of spermatogenesis

The transforming growth factor β superfamily of proteins is a group of ligands involved in cell signaling that share a common mechanism of action. When active, these proteins dimerize through conserved cysteine residues in each subunit that attach via disulfide bonds. **Members of this family of proteins include TGF-β1–3, inhibin, activin, bone morphogenic protein (BMP), anti-Müllerian hormone (AMH), growth and differentiation factors (GDF), and the glial-cell-line-derived neurotropic factor (GDNF)** [131–136] (Table 4.1).

TGF superfamily ligands bind common receptors with shared downstream signaling pathways within the cell. Type I and type II receptors both have either serine or threonine kinase activity; type II receptors are constitutively active, whereas type I receptors are not [137]. One of the downstream signaling pathways that is well understood is that of Smad [138]. **Knockout mice for several different BMPs and Smads were generated; the results varied tremendously as a result of the critical importance of TGF-β signaling to proper development and morphogenesis. Through analysis of these results, the role of BMPs, inhibin, activin, and TGF-β in spermatogonial differentiation has become clearer.**

Sertoli cell protein secretion

All of the uniqueness of the Sertoli cell derives from its role as the "nurse" cell for developing spermatogenic cells. The blood–testis barrier protects differentiating germ cells from exposure to the immune system of the host organism in question. **On the other hand, by isolating germ cells from circulating nutrients and other factors, the blood–testis barrier necessitates active delivery of these factors to germ cells on the part of the Sertoli cell. Amongst other compounds that perform this function in some part, androgen-binding protein, transferrin, and SPARC are considered here.**

Androgen-binding protein (ABP)

A testicular analog to serum sex hormone-binding globulin, androgen-binding protein was initially isolated from the rat epididymis [139]; secretion of this protein was then localized to the Sertoli cell [140]. ABP binds both testosterone and dihydrotestosterone with high affinity [141].

Table 4.1. Selected TGF-β superfamily growth factors and receptors

Protein	Receptor	Human disease?	Human phenotype	Animal knockout model	Testis function
TGF-β1	ALK1, ALK2, ALK5 (type I), TβRII (type II)	Yes	Camurati–Engelmann disease; hypertension, osteoporosis, atherosclerosis (other diseases associated with altered receptor function including pre-eclampsia)	Yolk sac defects, inflammatory disorders, lethal	Steroidogenesis; possible paracrine regulator of spermatogenesis
TGF-β2	ALK2, ALK5 (type I), TβRII (type II)	Yes	Amyloidosis, Alzheimer's disease, oculopathy/retinopathy, cleft palate	Lethal in utero; skeletal, craniofacial, cardiac, renal defects	Early gonadal development
TGF-β3	ALK1, ALK2, ALK5 (type I), TβRII (type II)	Yes	Cleft palate	Lethal in utero; cleft palate	Early gonadal development, adult tight junction/adherens junction regulation
Inhibin	ActRII, ActRIIb (type II)			Gonadal and adrenal tumors	Autocrine/paracrine regulation of spermatogenesis
Activin	ALK1, ALK2, ALK4 (type I), ActRIB, ActRII, ActRIIb (type II)	Yes	Huntington's disease, Parkinson's disease	Variable presentation depending on subunit lost	Autocrine/paracrine regulation of spermatogenesis
BMP2	ALK3, ALK6 (type I), ActRII, ActRIIb, BMPRII (type II)	Yes	Osteoporosis, myeloproliferative disease, myelofibrosis	Lethal in utero; cardiac defects	Primordial germ cell development
BMP4	ALK3, ALK6 (type I), BMPRII (type II)	Yes	Fibrodysplasia Ossificans Progressiva	Lethal in utero; abnormal mesodermal differentiation	Primordial germ cell development
BMP8a	ALK3, ALK6 (type I), BMPRII (type II)	Yes	Myeloproliferative disease, myelofibrosis	Viable; males subfertile, degeneration of epididymal epithelium	Adult spermatogenesis
BMP8b	ALK3, ALK6 (type I) BMPRII (type II)	Yes	Myeloproliferative disease, myelofibrosis	Viable; males subfertile	Primordial germ cell development; adult spermatogenesis
BMP15	ALK3, ALK6 (type I), BMPRII (type II)	Yes	Ovarian dysgenesis	Viable, females subfertile	
GDF-9	ALK6 (type I), ActRII, BMPRII (type II)	Yes	Brachydactyly, chondroplasia	Viable; females infertile	
GDNF	c-RET	Yes	Hirschsprung disease	Lethal in utero; abnormal renal development	
AMH/MIS	ALK2 (type I), MISRII (type II)	Yes	Persistent Müllerian duct syndrome	Viable; males develop uteri, infertile	Proper male differentiation through initiation of Müllerian duct structure regression

Table 4.1. continued

Protein	Receptor	Human disease?	Human phenotype	Animal knockout model	Testis function
SMAD2	n/a	Yes	Colorectal cancer, lung cancer, hepatocellular cancer	Lethal in utero; no mesodermal formation	Downstream mediation of above listed effects
SMAD4	n/a	Yes	Multiple cancers; juvenile polyposis	Lethal; defective endodermal formation, gastrulation defect	Downstream mediation of above listed effects
SMAD5	n/a			Lethal in utero; abnormal primordial germ cell development	Downstream mediation of above listed effects

Secretion of ABP by the Sertoli cell is stimulated by both FSH and testosterone independently [142]. The majority of ABP produced in the cell is secreted apically into the lumen of the seminiferous tubule; some lesser amount (approx 20%) is secreted basally into the interstitium of the testis [143]. In addition, germ cells have been demonstrated to internalize ABP complexed to testosterone via endocytosis [144].

Therefore, it has been theorized that ABP represents a crucial "reservoir" of circulating testosterone in the testis that might be utilized by differentiating germ cells. Recent evidence argues against this, however. First, Joseph and colleagues (1997) engineered ABP-transgenic mice that constitutively overexpressed ABP. Phenotypically, animals demonstrated deranged spermatogenesis which progressed ultimately to complete infertility [145]. The authors concluded that this was due to decreased bioavailability of circulating androgens within the testis; this contradicts the idea that ABP-bound testosterone represents the fraction of intratesticular androgen that germ cells rely upon for differentiation.

Second, Jarow and colleagues (2005) demonstrated in both mice and humans a significant discrepancy between serum free testosterone, intratesticular free testosterone, intratesticular ABP-bound testosterone, and ABP levels [146,147]. They concluded that some other, as yet unidentified, molecule must account for the majority of bound testosterone in the testis – total testosterone levels in the testis being far higher than in serum. Obviously, continued research into the regulation of intratesticular androgen levels is necessary.

Transferrin

Unlike glucose, which is transported across the blood–testis barrier and then converted to lactate for germ cells to metabolize [148–152], shuttling iron into germ cells requires a complex series of steps including receptor-mediated endocytosis of transferrin, which is centrally important [153,154]. A serum glycoprotein, transferrin must be complexed to iron at both the Sertoli cell membrane and the germ cell membrane in order for iron to cross the cell membrane. Iron is vitally important to cell division, and therefore it is needed by germ cells and spermatocytes. As is mentioned elsewhere in this chapter, this rationale has been the basis for using transferrin levels as a marker of Sertoli cell differentiation.

Transferrin mediates iron transport throughout the body; most transferrin is synthesized in the liver and secreted into the circulation. Transferrin represents a major component of total body iron metabolism [155]. Skinner and Griswold first demonstrated synthesis of transferrin in the Sertoli cell in 1980 [156]. Since then, considerable research has been undertaken into the function and regulation of transferrin in the testis.

As in many other tissues in the body, serum transferrin bound to two Fe^{3+} molecules is internalized into the Sertoli cell via receptor-mediated endocytosis. A pH-driven reaction within the CURL (compartment of uncoupling and recycling of ligand) frees transferrin to allow it to return to the basolateral membrane and thereby to be recycled. Meanwhile, free Fe^{3+} within the intracellular space is bound by testicular transferrin and then secreted into the adluminal compartment. Free iron is again bound by transferrin, this time on the germ cell surface, and then the complex is internalized by the germ cell, again via receptor-mediated endocytosis [153,154].

Much effort has gone into identifying the regulation of transferrin production within the Sertoli cell; theoretically, regulation of transferrin should offer insight into overall regulation of spermatogenesis.

Lecureuil and colleagues engineered a transgenic mouse that expressed human transferrin in Sertoli cell cultures isolated from the testis. They ultimately identified FSH, vitamin A, insulin, and TNF-α as independent factors that increased transferrin expression. Interestingly, testosterone alone had no effect on transferrin levels [157].

Seminal transferrin levels correlate with basic semen parameters including sperm density; this finding is consistent with the central importance of iron metabolism to successful spermatogenesis [158].

SPARC (secreted protein, acidic and rich in cystein)

A divalent ion transporter that is presumably involved in calcium transport, SPARC was first demonstrated in the gonad by Howe and colleagues in 1988 [159]. Although it is unclear exactly what function SPARC provides in the Sertoli cell, several important pieces of information are known. First, SPARC is known to regulate other signaling molecules, including TGF-β, that are responsible for differentiation of the Sertoli cell [160,161]. Second, SPARC is known to regulate the expression of molecules such as matrix metalloproteases (MMPs) that are involved in cell adhesion, another crucially important function of the Sertoli cell [162]. Third, SPARC is expressed in germ cells. In testing the hypothesis that SPARC may be important in the differentiating embryonic testis, Wilson and colleagues demonstrated a significant increase in level of SPARC identified in the fetal testis of rats when compared with levels in adult males and in fetal ovaries [163]. The conclusion that SPARC is necessary for fetal development of the testis is contradicted by the finding that SPARC knockout animals are fertile [164].

Matrix metalloproteases (MMP)

MMP secretion is vitally important to the fluidity of the BTB and its role in spermatogenesis. Metalloproteases, such as MMP-2 (gelatinase A), MMP-4 (type IV collagenase), MMP-9 (gelatinase B), degrade the collagen network and thereby disrupt tight junction function and the blood–testis barrier [165,166].

Interestingly, MMP secretion (in addition to secretion of tissue inhibitor of metalloproteases 1, TIMP-1) is directly affected by both TNF-α and TGF-β in vitro [167–169]. This is consistent with the hypothesis that TNF-α secreted by the basement membrane of the seminiferous tubule can regulate assembly and disassembly of the BTB depending on the presence of conditions suitable for spermatogenesis; also, this evidence is consistent with models that allow for TGF-β as a central regulator.

Cellular retinol-binding protein (CRBP) and cellular retinoic acid-binding protein (CRABP)

Retinol (vitamin A) is centrally important to spermatogenesis; it helps to maintain the blood–testis barrier, enhances the effects of testosterone on the Sertoli cell, and helps enable both adhesion of spermatogonia and proper spermiation [170–172]. This effect is dependent upon retinoic acid (RA), which is transcriptionally active through two nuclear receptors (RAR α and β) [173,174].

The major portion of retinoic acid used for this process is synthesized in the testis from circulating retinol bound to retinol-binding protein (RBP) [175]. Within the Sertoli cell, retinol is bound to one of two proteins (CRBP-1 and CRBP-2) [176–178], while retinoic acid is bound to CRABP-2 [179]. CRABP-1 is expressed predominantly in spermatogonia [180]. The crucial effects of retinoic acid on spermatogenesis were experimentally delineated in vitamin A deficient (VAD) rats [170], and in retinoic acid receptor mutated mice. Spermatogenesis is absent in these animals at baseline, but it can be rescued with administration of retinoic acid. Interestingly, these animals do not demonstrate uniform absence of fertility at a prepubertal age [181,182].

Sertoli cell regulation of testis development

A more comprehensive discussion of testis development is found in Chapter 1; however, for the purposes of this chapter, a brief consideration of the Sertoli cell's role in sexual differentiation is necessary. Brennan and Capel have published an excellent review of this topic [183].

In the mouse embryo, expression of Sry, the Y-chromosomal testis-determining factor, causes differentiation of Sertoli cells as early as 10.5 days postcoitum [184–186]. This single event represents the earliest recognizable step in male differentiation; subsequent to this, Sertoli cells act to organize the primordial gonad into testis cords with segregated germ cells that will eventually differentiate into seminiferous tubules [187]. Between the cords, peritubular myoid cells and Leydig cell precursors begin to fill what will become the interstitium of the testis.

By 12.5 days, the primordial gonad is organized into what is recognizably an early precursor to the testis. **Numerous downstream genes in the Sertoli cell are implicated in this differentiation; these genes include *Dax1*, *Fgf9*, *Sox9*, and *Gata4* amongst many others** [188–191]. Selective knockouts of these genes resulted in phenotypes ranging from sex reversal, to infertility, to fetal demise [192–195].

Oddsex mutation, for example, first described by Bishop and colleagues in 2000, has provided tremendous insight into *Sry*-driven sexual differentiation [196]. **Infertile, sex-reversed XX mice were initially found to have an upstream deletion that was thought to result in overexpression of *Sox9* despite the absence of *Sry*.** Further research into this animal instead determined that insertion of a tyrosinase minigene upstream of *Sox9* was responsible for *Sox9* overexpression [197]. This autosomal dominant gene, *Ods*, contains a dopamine tautomerase promoter region (Dct) that specifically causes *Sox9* overexpression [198]. Interestingly, in order to determine the role of this mutation in nonXX animals, Qin and Bishop generated SRY-XY *Ods*/+ male mice [199]. These mice were subfertile, with initially normal male differentiation and progressive loss of fertility with age. In order to answer the question whether quantitative expression of *Sox9* could completely reverse the infertility phenotype, SRY-XY *Ods*/*Ods* homozygous mutants were generated; these animals exhibited a normal male phenotype and intact fertility.

Future directions

Continued research into the Sertoli cell is ongoing. Microarray techniques, including proteomic and genomic analysis, have begun to yield huge volumes of information about this complex and transcriptionally very active cell. Many of the answers to long-standing questions regarding stage-specific function of the cell may be found in the proteosome of Sertoli cells at various stages of development.

Further understanding of Sertoli cell physiology opens the door for continued research in male infertility; successful transplantation of germ cells has been demonstrated as a technique for restoration of fertility in animals [88,89]. The future potential for human germ cell co-culture remains an area with huge possible yields as a treatment option for male infertility.

Finally, the Sertoli cell's unique physiologic properties have attracted researchers from other fields to its study. For example, ongoing research in animal transplantation demonstrates the immunoprotective value of co-transplantation of Sertoli cells. The possible future application of this to human transplantation could also be very fruitful.

Conclusions

The Sertoli cell has fascinated researchers for years. Its complex physiology, its unique and central role in reproductive function, and its cornerstone status in phenotypic maleness have made it a favorite target of investigators. However, as so much has been gained in terms of understanding of the Sertoli cell, each new piece of information illuminates much more that warrants further research. A greater understanding of the Sertoli cell, its physiology, and its function, will be absolutely central to treating male infertility in the twenty-first century.

Acknowledgments

Supported in part by Grants No. 2P01 HD 36289, AUAF, and the National Institutes of Health Cooperative Centers Program in Reproductive Research (U54 HD07495) from the National Institutes of Health.

References

[1] Sertoli E. Dell'esistencia di particolari cellule remificati nei canalicoli seminiferi del testicolo umano. *Morgagni* 1865; 7 (31).

[2] Russell LD, Griswold MD. *The Sertoli Cell*. Clearwater, FL: Cache River Press, 1993.

[3] Fawcett DW. The mammalian spermatozoon. *Dev Biol* 1975; **44**: 394–436.

[4] Skinner MK, Griswold MD. *Sertoli Cell Biology*. Amsterdam/Boston: Elsevier Academic Press, 2005.

[5] Kumar TR, Low MJ, Matzuk MM. Genetic rescue of follicle-stimulating hormone beta-deficient mice. *Endocrinology* 1998; **139**: 3289–95.

[6] Wolski KM, Mruk DD, Cameron DF. The Sertoli-spermatid junctional complex adhesion strength is affected in vitro by adjudin. *J Androl* 2006; **27**: 790–4.

[7] Xia W, Mruk DD, Lee WM, Cheng CY. Unraveling the molecular targets pertinent to junction restructuring events during spermatogenesis using the Adjudin-induced germ cell depletion model. *J Endocrinol* 2007; **192**: 563–83.

[8] Fawcett DW, Leak LV, Heidger PM. Electron microscopic observations on the structural components of the blood–testis barrier. *J Reprod Fertil* (Suppl) 1970; **10**: 105–22.

[9] Dym M, Fawcett DW. The blood–testis barrier in the rat and the physiological compartmentation of the seminiferous epithelium. *Biol Reprod* 1970; **3**: 308–26.

[10] Hadley MA, Dym M. Immunocytochemistry of extracellular matrix in the lamina propria of the rat testis: electron microscopic localization. *Biol Reprod* 1987; **37**: 1283–9.

[11] Tung PS, Skinner MK, Fritz IB. Cooperativity between Sertoli cells and peritubular myoid cells in the formation of the basal lamina in the seminiferous tubule. *Ann N Y Acad Sci* 1984; **438**: 435–46.

[12] Norton JN, Skinner MK. Regulation of Sertoli cell function and differentiation through the actions of a testicular paracrine factor P-Mod-S. *Endocrinology* 1989; **124**: 2711–19.

[13] Skinner MK, Norton JN, Mullaney BP, *et al.* Cell–cell interactions and the regulation of testis function. *Ann N Y Acad Sci* 1991; **637**: 354–63.

[14] Rambourg A, Clermont Y, Hermo L. Three-dimensional architecture of the Golgi apparatus in Sertoli cells of the rat. *Am J Anat* 1979; **154**: 455–76.

[15] Clermont Y, Rambourg A, Hermo L. Trans-Golgi network (TGN) of different cell types: three-dimensional structural characteristics and variability. *Anat Rec* 1995; **242**: 289–301.

[16] Schulze C. On the morphology of the human Sertoli cell. *Cell Tissue Res* 1974; **153**: 339–55.

[17] Guttman JA, Kimel GH, Vogl AW. Dynein and plus-end microtubule-dependent motors are associated with specialized Sertoli cell junction plaques (ectoplasmic specializations). *J Cell Sci* 2000; **113**: 2167–76.

[18] Guttman JA, Janmey P, Vogl AW. Gelsolin: evidence for a role in turnover of junction-related actin filaments in Sertoli cells. *J Cell Sci* 2002; **115**: 499–505.

[19] Guttman JA, Takai Y, Vogl AW. Evidence that tubulobulbar complexes in the seminiferous epithelium are involved with internalization of adhesion junctions. *Biol Reprod* 2004; **71**: 548–59.

[20] Guttman JA, Obinata T, Shima J, Griswold M, Vogl AW. Non-muscle cofilin is a component of tubulobulbar complexes in the testis. *Biol Reprod* 2004; **70**: 805–12.

[21] Mruk DD, Cheng CY. Cell–cell interactions at the ectoplasmic specialization in the testis. *Trends Endocrinol Metab* 2004; **15**: 439–47.

[22] Mruk DD, Cheng CY. Sertoli–Sertoli and Sertoli–germ cell interactions and their significance in germ cell movement in the seminiferous epithelium during spermatogenesis. *Endocr Rev* 2004; **25**: 747–806.

[23] Lee NP, Cheng CY. Ectoplasmic specialization, a testis-specific cell–cell actin-based adherens junction type: is this a potential target for male contraceptive development? *Hum Reprod Update* 2004; **10**: 349–69.

[24] Segretain D. Endocytosis in spermatids during spermiogenesis of the mouse. *Biol Cell* 1989; **67**: 289–98.

[25] Le TL, Joseph SR, Yap AS, Stow JL. Protein kinase C regulates endocytosis and recycling of E-cadherin. *Am J Physiol Cell Physiol* 2002; **283**: C489–99.

[26] Zhang J, Wong CH, Xia W, *et al.* Regulation of Sertoli–germ cell adherens junction dynamics via changes in protein-protein interactions of the N-cadherin-beta-catenin protein complex which are possibly mediated by c-Src and myotubularin-related protein 2: an in vivo study using an androgen suppression model. *Endocrinology* 2005; **146**: 1268–84.

[27] Lee NP, Cheng CY. Protein kinases and adherens junction dynamics in the seminiferous epithelium of the rat testis. *J Cell Physiol* 2005; **202**: 344–60.

[28] Cheng J, Watkins SC, Walker WH. Testosterone activates mitogen-activated protein kinase via Src kinase and the epidermal growth factor receptor in sertoli cells. *Endocrinology* 2007; **148**: 2066–74.

[29] Tachibana K, Nakanishi H, Mandai K, *et al.* Two cell adhesion molecules, nectin and cadherin, interact through their cytoplasmic domain-associated proteins. *J Cell Biol* 2000; **150**: 1161–76.

[30] Sakamoto Y, Ogita H, Hirota T, *et al.* Interaction of integrin αvβ3 with nectin: implication in cross-talk between cell–matrix and cell–cell junctions. *J Biol Chem* 2006; **281**: 19631–44.

[31] Fukuhara A, Irie K, Nakanishi H, *et al.* Involvement of nectin in the localization of junctional adhesion molecule at tight junctions. *Oncogene* 2002; **21**: 7642–55.

[32] Mueller S, Rosenquist TA, Takai Y, Bronson RA, Wimmer E. Loss of nectin-2 at Sertoli–spermatid junctions leads to male infertility and correlates with severe spermatozoan head and midpiece malformation, impaired binding to the zona pellucida, and oocyte penetration. *Biol Reprod* 2003; **69**: 1330–40.

[33] Ozaki-Kuroda K, Nakanishi H, Ohta H, *et al.* Nectin couples cell–cell adhesion and the actin scaffold at heterotypic testicular junctions. *Curr Biol* 2002; **12**: 1145–50.

[34] Bouchard MJ, Dong Y, McDermott BM, *et al.* Defects in nuclear and cytoskeletal morphology and mitochondrial localization in spermatozoa of mice lacking nectin-2, a component of cell–cell adherens junctions. *Mol Cell Biol* 2000; **20**: 2865–73.

[35] Crepieux P, Marion S, Martinat N, *et al.* The ERK-dependent signalling is stage-specifically modulated by FSH, during primary Sertoli cell maturation. *Oncogene* 2001; **20**: 4696–709.

[36] Martinat N, Crepieux P, Reiter E, Guillou F. Extracellular signal-regulated kinases (ERK) 1, 2 are required for luteinizing hormone (LH)-induced steroidogenesis in primary Leydig cells and control steroidogenic acute regulatory (StAR) expression. *Reprod Nutr Dev* 2005; **45**: 101–8.

[37] Siu MK, Cheng CY. Dynamic cross-talk between cells and the extracellular matrix in the testis. *Bioessays* 2004; **26**: 978–92.

[38] Xia W, Mruk DD, Lee WM, Cheng CY. Differential interactions between transforming growth factor-β3/TβR1, TAB1, and CD2AP disrupt blood–testis barrier and Sertoli–germ cell adhesion. *J Biol Chem* 2006; **281**: 16799–813.

[39] Amlani S, Vogl AW. Changes in the distribution of microtubules and intermediate filaments in mammalian Sertoli cells during spermatogenesis. *Anat Rec* 1988; **220**: 143–60.

[40] Aumuller G, Steinbruck M, Krause W, Wagner HJ. Distribution of vimentin-type intermediate filaments in Sertoli cells of the human testis, normal and pathologic. *Anat Embryol (Berl)* 1988; **178**: 129–36.

[41] Yan HH, Cheng CY. Blood–testis barrier dynamics are regulated by an engagement/disengagement mechanism between tight and adherens junctions via peripheral adaptors. *Proc Natl Acad Sci U S A* 2005; **102**: 11722–7.

[42] Colucci-Guyon E, Portier MM, Dunia I, *et al*. Mice lacking vimentin develop and reproduce without an obvious phenotype. *Cell* 1994; **79**: 679–94.

[43] Vogl AW, Weis M, Pfeiffer DC. The perinuclear centriole-containing centrosome is not the major microtubule organizing center in Sertoli cells. *Eur J Cell Biol* 1995; **66**: 165–79.

[44] Carter SD, Hess RA, Laskey JW. The fungicide methyl 2-benzimidazole carbamate causes infertility in male Sprague-Dawley rats. *Biol Reprod* 1987; **37**: 709–17.

[45] Parvinen M, Kormano M. Early effects of antispermatogenic benzimidazole derivatives U 32.422 E and U 32.104 on the seminiferous epithelium of the rat. *Andrologia* 1974; **6**: 245–53.

[46] Russell LD, Lee IP, Ettlin R, Malone JP. Morphological pattern of response after administration of procarbazine: Alteration of specific cell associations during the cycle of the seminiferous epithelium of the rat. *Tissue Cell* 1983; **15**: 391–404.

[47] Nakai M, Hess RA, Netsu J, Nasu T. Deformation of the rat Sertoli cell by oral administration of carbendazim (methyl 2-benzimidazole carbamate). *J Androl* 1995; **16**: 410–16.

[48] Russell LD, Malone JP, MacCurdy DS. Effect of the microtubule disrupting agents, colchicine and vinblastine, on seminiferous tubule structure in the rat. *Tissue Cell* 1981; **13**: 349–67.

[49] Vogl AW, Linck RW, Dym M. Colchicine-induced changes in the cytoskeleton of the golden-mantled ground squirrel (Spermophilus lateralis) Sertoli cells. *Am J Anat* 1983; **168**: 99–108.

[50] Russell L. Desmosome-like junctions between Sertoli and germ cells in the rat testis. *Am J Anat* 1977; **148**: 301–12.

[51] Denker BM, Nigam SK. Molecular structure and assembly of the tight junction. *Am J Physiol* 1998; **274**: F1–9.

[52] Tsukita S, Furuse M, Itoh M. Structural and signalling molecules come together at tight junctions. *Curr Opin Cell Biol* 1999; **11**: 628–33.

[53] Tsukita S, Furuse M, Itoh M. Multifunctional strands in tight junctions. *Nat Rev Mol Cell Biol* 2001; **2**: 285–93.

[54] Itman C, Mendis S, Barakat B, Loveland KL. All in the family: TGF-β family action in testis development. *Reproduction* 2006; **132**: 233–46.

[55] Zhao GQ, Garbers DL. Male germ cell specification and differentiation. *Dev Cell* 2002; **2**: 537–47.

[56] Moroi S, Saitou M, Fujimoto K, *et al*. Occludin is concentrated at tight junctions of mouse/rat but not human/guinea pig Sertoli cells in testes. *Am J Physiol* 1998; **274**: C1708–17.

[57] Saitou M, Furuse M, Sasaki H, *et al*. Complex phenotype of mice lacking occludin, a component of tight junction strands. *Mol Biol Cell* 2000; **11**: 4131–42.

[58] Chung NP, Mruk D, Mo MY, Lee WM, Cheng CY. A 22-amino acid synthetic peptide corresponding to the second extracellular loop of rat occludin perturbs the blood–testis barrier and disrupts spermatogenesis reversibly in vivo. *Biol Reprod* 2001; **65**: 1340–51.

[59] Furuse M, Fujita K, Hiiragi T, Fujimoto K, Tsukita S. Claudin-1 and -2: novel integral membrane proteins localizing at tight junctions with no sequence similarity to occludin. *J Cell Biol* 1998; **141**: 1539–50.

[60] Morita K, Furuse M, Fujimoto K, Tsukita S. Claudin multigene family encoding four-transmembrane domain protein components of tight junction strands. *Proc Natl Acad Sci U S A* 1999; **96**: 511–16.

[61] Morita K, Sasaki H, Fujimoto K, Furuse M, Tsukita S. Claudin-11/OSP-based tight junctions of myelin sheaths in brain and Sertoli cells in testis. *J Cell Biol* 1999; **145**: 579–88.

[62] Gow A, Southwood CM, Li JS, *et al*. CNS myelin and Sertoli cell tight junction strands are absent in Osp/claudin-11 null mice. *Cell* 1999; **99**: 649–59.

[63] Sluka P, O'Donnell L, Bartles JR, Stanton PG. FSH regulates the formation of adherens junctions and ectoplasmic specialisations between rat Sertoli cells in vitro and in vivo. *J Endocrinol* 2006; **189**: 381–95.

[64] Gliki G, Ebnet K, Aurrand-Lions M, Imhof BA, Adams RH. Spermatid differentiation requires the assembly of a cell polarity complex downstream of junctional adhesion molecule-C. *Nature* 2004; **431**: 320–4.

[65] Wong CC, Chung SS, Grima J, *et al*. Changes in the expression of junctional and nonjunctional complex component genes when inter-sertoli tight junctions are formed in vitro. *J Androl* 2000; **21**: 227–37.

[66] Lui WY, Lee WM, Cheng CY. Transforming growth factor-β3 perturbs the inter-Sertoli tight junction permeability barrier in vitro possibly mediated via its effects on occludin, zonula occludens-1, and claudin-11. *Endocrinology* 2001; **142**: 1865–77.

[67] Grima J, Wong CC, Zhu LJ, Zong SD, Cheng CY. Testin secreted by Sertoli cells is associated with the cell surface, and its expression correlates with the disruption of Sertoli–germ cell junctions but not the inter-Sertoli tight junction. *J Biol Chem* 1998; **273**: 21040–53.

[68] De Gendt K, Swinnen JV, Saunders PT, *et al.* A Sertoli cell-selective knockout of the androgen receptor causes spermatogenic arrest in meiosis. *Proc Natl Acad Sci U S A* 2004; **101**: 1327–32.

[69] Wong CH, Mruk DD, Lui WY, Cheng CY. Regulation of blood–testis barrier dynamics: An in vivo study. *J Cell Sci* 2004; **117**: 783–98.

[70] Hellani A, Ji J, Mauduit C, *et al.* Developmental and hormonal regulation of the expression of oligodendrocyte-specific protein/claudin 11 in mouse testis. *Endocrinology* 2000; **141**: 3012–19.

[71] Vogl AW, Pfeiffer DC, Mulholland D, Kimel G, Guttman J. Unique and multifunctional adhesion junctions in the testis: ectoplasmic specializations. *Arch Histol Cytol* 2000; **63**: 1–15.

[72] Mulholland DJ, Dedhar S, Vogl AW. Rat seminiferous epithelium contains a unique junction (ectoplasmic specialization) with signaling properties both of cell/cell and cell/matrix junctions. *Biol Reprod* 2001; **64**: 396–407.

[73] Lui WY, Sze KL, Lee WM. Nectin-2 expression in testicular cells is controlled via the functional cooperation between transcription factors of the Sp1, CREB, and AP-1 families. *J Cell Physiol* 2006; **207**: 144–57.

[74] Don J, Stelzer G. The expanding family of CREB/CREM transcription factors that are involved with spermatogenesis. *Mol Cell Endocrinol* 2002; **187**: 115–24.

[75] Clermont Y. Kinetics of spermatogenesis in mammals: seminiferous epithelium cycle and spermatogonial renewal. *Physiol Rev* 1972; **52**: 198–236.

[76] Heller CG, Clermont Y. Spermatogenesis in man: an estimate of its duration. *Science* 1963; **140**: 184–6.

[77] Clermont Y. The cycle of the seminiferous epithelium in man. *Am J Anat* 1963; **112**: 35–51.

[78] Leblond CP, Clermont Y. Definition of the stages of the cycle of the seminiferous epithelium in the rat. *Ann N Y Acad Sci* 1952; **55**: 548–73.

[79] Skinner MK, Schlitz SM, Anthony CT. Regulation of Sertoli cell differentiated function: Testicular transferrin and androgen-binding protein expression. *Endocrinology* 1989; **124**: 3015–24.

[80] Norton JN, Skinner MK. Regulation of Sertoli cell differentiation by the testicular paracrine factor PModS: potential role of immediate-early genes. *Mol Endocrinol* 1992; **6**: 2018–26.

[81] Chaudhary J, Cupp AS, Skinner MK. Role of basic-helix-loop-helix transcription factors in Sertoli cell differentiation: identification of an E-box response element in the transferrin promoter. *Endocrinology* 1997; **138**: 667–75.

[82] Johnson JE, Birren SJ, Saito T, Anderson DJ. DNA binding and transcriptional regulatory activity of mammalian achaete-scute homologous (MASH) proteins revealed by interaction with a muscle-specific enhancer. *Proc Natl Acad Sci U S A* 1992; **89**: 3596–600.

[83] Chaudhary J, Skinner MK. Comparative sequence analysis of the mouse and human transferrin promoters: hormonal regulation of the transferrin promoter in Sertoli cells. *Mol Reprod Dev* 1998; **50**: 273–83.

[84] Chaudhary J, Skinner MK. Basic helix-loop-helix proteins can act at the E-box within the serum response element of the c-fos promoter to influence hormone-induced promoter activation in Sertoli cells. *Mol Endocrinol* 1999; **13**: 774–86.

[85] Chaudhary J, Johnson J, Kim G, Skinner MK. Hormonal regulation and differential actions of the helix-loop-helix transcriptional inhibitors of differentiation (Id1, Id2, Id3, and Id4) in Sertoli cells. *Endocrinology* 2001; **142**: 1727–36.

[86] Chaudhary J, Sadler-Riggleman I, Ague JM, Skinner MK. The helix-loop-helix inhibitor of differentiation (ID) proteins induce post-mitotic terminally differentiated Sertoli cells to re-enter the cell cycle and proliferate. *Biol Reprod* 2005; **72**: 1205–17.

[87] Johnston H, Baker PJ, Abel M, *et al.* Regulation of Sertoli cell number and activity by follicle-stimulating hormone and androgen during postnatal development in the mouse. *Endocrinology* 2004; **145**: 318–29.

[88] Brinster RL, Avarbock MR. Germline transmission of donor haplotype following spermatogonial transplantation. *Proc Natl Acad Sci U S A* 1994; **91**: 11303–7.

[89] Brinster RL, Zimmermann JW. Spermatogenesis following male germ-cell transplantation. *Proc Natl Acad Sci U S A* 1994; **91**: 11298–302.

[90] Heller CH, Clermont Y. Kinetics of the germinal epithelium in man. *Recent Prog Horm Res* 1964; **20**: 545–75.

[91] Clermont Y. Spermatogenesis in man. A study of the spermatogonial population. *Fertil Steril* 1966; **17**: 705–21.

[92] Clermont Y. Renewal of spermatogonia in man. *Am J Anat* 1966; **118**: 509–24.

[93] Huckins C. The spermatogonial stem cell population in adult rats. 1. Their morphology, proliferation and maturation. *Anat Rec* 1971; **169**: 533–57.

[94]   Huckins C. The spermatogonial stem cell population in adult rats. 3. Evidence for a long-cycling population. *Cell Tissue Kinet* 1971; **4**: 335–49.

[95]   Steinberger E, Root A, Ficher M, Smith KD. The role of androgens in the initiation of spermatogenesis in man. *J Clin Endocrinol Metab* 1973; **37**: 746–51.

[96]   Anawalt BD, Bebb RA, Matsumoto AM, *et al.* Serum inhibin B levels reflect Sertoli cell function in normal men and men with testicular dysfunction. *J Clin Endocrinol Metab* 1996; **81**: 3341–5.

[97]   Burger HG, Igarashi M. Inhibin: Definition and nomenclature, including related substances. *J Clin Endocrinol Metab* 1988; **66**: 885–6.

[98]   de Kretser DM, McLachlan RI, Robertson DM, Burger HG. Serum inhibin levels in normal men and men with testicular disorders. *J Endocrinol* 1989; **120**: 517–23.

[99]   Illingworth PJ, Groome NP, Byrd W, *et al.* Inhibin-B: A likely candidate for the physiologically important form of inhibin in men. *J Clin Endocrinol Metab* 1996; **81**: 1321–5.

[100] Kumar TR. What have we learned about gonadotropin function from gonadotropin subunit and receptor knockout mice? *Reproduction* 2005; **130**: 293–302.

[101] Kumar TR, Wang Y, Lu N, Matzuk MM. Follicle stimulating hormone is required for ovarian follicle maturation but not male fertility. *Nat Genet* 1997; **15**: 201–4.

[102] Baker PJ, Pakarinen P, Huhtaniemi IT, *et al.* Failure of normal Leydig cell development in follicle-stimulating hormone (FSH) receptor-deficient mice, but not FSHβ-deficient mice: Role for constitutive FSH receptor activity. *Endocrinology* 2003; **144**: 138–45.

[103] Tapanainen JS, Aittomaki K, Min J, Vaskivuo T, Huhtaniemi IT. Men homozygous for an inactivating mutation of the follicle-stimulating hormone (FSH) receptor gene present variable suppression of spermatogenesis and fertility. *Nat Genet* 1997; **15**: 205–6.

[104] Levallet J, Pakarinen P, Huhtaniemi IT. Follicle-stimulating hormone ligand and receptor mutations, and gonadal dysfunction. *Arch Med Res* 1999; **30**: 486–94.

[105] Aittomaki K, Herva R, Stenman UH, *et al.* Clinical features of primary ovarian failure caused by a point mutation in the follicle-stimulating hormone receptor gene. *J Clin Endocrinol Metab* 1996; **81**: 3722–6.

[106] Dierich A, Sairam MR, Monaco L, *et al.* Impairing follicle-stimulating hormone (FSH) signaling in vivo: targeted disruption of the FSH receptor leads to aberrant gametogenesis and hormonal imbalance. *Proc Natl Acad Sci U S A* 1998; **95**: 13612–17.

[107] Krishnamurthy H, Babu PS, Morales CR, Sairam MR. Delay in sexual maturity of the follicle-stimulating hormone receptor knockout male mouse. *Biol Reprod* 2001; **65**: 522–31.

[108] Krishnamurthy H, Kats R, Danilovich N, Javeshghani D, Sairam MR. Intercellular communication between Sertoli cells and Leydig cells in the absence of follicle-stimulating hormone-receptor signaling. *Biol Reprod* 2001; **65**: 1201–7.

[109] Ma X, Dong Y, Matzuk MM, Kumar TR. Targeted disruption of luteinizing hormone beta-subunit leads to hypogonadism, defects in gonadal steroidogenesis, and infertility. *Proc Natl Acad Sci U S A* 2004; **101**: 17294–9.

[110] Lei ZM, Mishra S, Zou W, *et al.* Targeted disruption of luteinizing hormone/human chorionic gonadotropin receptor gene. *Mol Endocrinol* 2001; **15**: 184–200.

[111] Lo KC, Lei Z, Rao Ch V, Beck J, Lamb DJ. De novo testosterone production in luteinizing hormone receptor knockout mice after transplantation of Leydig stem cells. *Endocrinology* 2004; **145**: 4011–15.

[112] De Gendt K, Atanassova N, Tan KA, *et al.* Development and function of the adult generation of Leydig cells in mice with Sertoli cell-selective or total ablation of the androgen receptor. *Endocrinology* 2005; **146**: 4117–26.

[113] Wang RS, Yeh S, Chen LM, *et al.* Androgen receptor in sertoli cell is essential for germ cell nursery and junctional complex formation in mouse testes. *Endocrinology* 2006; **147**: 5624–33.

[114] March CJ, Mosley B, Larsen A, *et al.* Cloning, sequence and expression of two distinct human interleukin-1 complementary DNAs. *Nature* 1985; **315**: 641–7.

[115] Arend WP. Interleukin-1 receptor antagonist. *Adv Immunol* 1993; **54**: 167–227.

[116] Roux-Lombard P. The interleukin-1 family. *Eur Cytokine Netw* 1998; **9**: 565–76.

[117] Gomez E, Morel G, Cavalier A, *et al.* Type I and type II interleukin-1 receptor expression in rat, mouse, and human testes. *Biol Reprod* 1997; **56**: 1513–26.

[118] Arend WP. Cytokine imbalance in the pathogenesis of rheumatoid arthritis: the role of interleukin-1 receptor antagonist. *Semin Arthritis Rheum* 2001; **30** (5 Suppl 2): 1–6.

[119] Arend WP, Malyak M, Smith MF Jr, *et al.* Binding of IL-1 alpha, IL-1 beta, and IL-1 receptor antagonist by soluble IL-1 receptors and levels of soluble IL-1 receptors in synovial fluids. *J Immunol* 1994; **153**: 4766–74.

[120] Mantovani A, Locati M, Vecchi A, Sozzani S, Allavena P. Decoy receptors: a strategy to regulate inflammatory cytokines and chemokines. *Trends Immunol* 2001; **22**: 328–36.

[121] Gerard N, Syed V, Jegou B. Lipopolysaccharide, latex beads and residual bodies are potent activators of Sertoli cell interleukin-1 alpha production. *Biochem Biophys Res Commun* 1992; **185**: 154–61.

[122] Okuma Y, Saito K, O'Connor AE, Phillips DJ, de Kretser DM, Hedger MP. Reciprocal regulation of activin A and inhibin B by interleukin-1 (IL-1) and follicle-stimulating hormone (FSH) in rat Sertoli cells in vitro. *J Endocrinol* 2005; **185**: 99–110.

[123] Wang JE, Josefsen GM, Hansson V, Haugen TB. Residual bodies and IL-1α stimulate expression of mRNA for IL-1α and IL-1 receptor type I in cultured rat Sertoli cells. *Mol Cell Endocrinol* 1998; **137**: 139–44.

[124] Heinrich PC, Castell JV, Andus T. Interleukin-6 and the acute phase response. *Biochem J* 1990; **265**: 621–36.

[125] Kishimoto T, Akira S, Narazaki M, Taga T. Interleukin-6 family of cytokines and gp130. *Blood* 1995; **86**: 1243–54.

[126] Boockfor FR, Schwarz LK. Effects of interleukin-6, interleukin-2, and tumor necrosis factor alpha on transferrin release from Sertoli cells in culture. *Endocrinology* 1991; 129(1): 256–62.

[127] Boockfor FR, Wang D, Lin T, Nagpal ML, Spangelo BL. Interleukin-6 secretion from rat Leydig cells in culture. *Endocrinology* 1994; **134**: 2150–5.

[128] Cudicini C, Lejeune H, Gomez E, *et al.* Human Leydig cells and Sertoli cells are producers of interleukins-1 and -6. *J Clin Endocrinol Metab* 1997; **82**: 1426–33.

[129] Pesce M, Farrace MG, Piacentini M, Dolci S, De Felici M. Stem cell factor and leukemia inhibitory factor promote primordial germ cell survival by suppressing programmed cell death (apoptosis). *Development* 1993; **118**: 1089–94.

[130] De Miguel MP, De Boer-Brouwer M, Paniagua R, *et al.* Leukemia inhibitory factor and ciliary neurotropic factor promote the survival of Sertoli cells and gonocytes in coculture system. *Endocrinology* 1996; **137**: 1885–93.

[131] Hogan BL. Bone morphogenetic proteins in development. *Curr Opin Genet Dev* 1996; **6**: 432–8.

[132] Massague J. The transforming growth factor-beta family. *Annu Rev Cell Biol* 1990; **6**: 597–641.

[133] Matzuk MM, Finegold MJ, Su JG, Hsueh AJ, Bradley A. Alpha-inhibin is a tumour-suppressor gene with gonadal specificity in mice. *Nature* 1992; **360**: 313–19.

[134] Lee MM, Donahoe PK. Mullerian inhibiting substance: a gonadal hormone with multiple functions. *Endocr Rev* 1993; **14**: 152–64.

[135] Lin LF, Doherty DH, Lile JD, Bektesh S, Collins F. GDNF: A glial cell line-derived neurotrophic factor for midbrain dopaminergic neurons. *Science* 1993; **260**: 1130–2.

[136] Ying SY. Inhibins, activins and follistatins. *J Steroid Biochem* 1989; **33**: 705–13.

[137] Kingsley DM. The TGF-beta superfamily: New members, new receptors, and new genetic tests of function in different organisms. *Genes Dev* 1994; **8**: 133–46.

[138] Heldin CH, Miyazono K, ten Dijke P. TGF-beta signalling from cell membrane to nucleus through SMAD proteins. *Nature* 1997; **390**: 465–71.

[139] French FS, Ritzen EM. A high-affinity androgen-binding protein (ABP) in rat testis: evidence for secretion into efferent duct fluid and absorption by epididymis. *Endocrinology* 1973; **93**: 88–95.

[140] Hagenas L, Ritzen EM, Plooen L, *et al.* Sertoli cell origin of testicular androgen-binding protein (ABP). *Mol Cell Endocrinol* 1975; **2**: 339–50.

[141] Joseph DR. Structure, function, and regulation of androgen-binding protein/sex hormone-binding globulin. *Vitam Horm* 1994; **49**: 197–280.

[142] Sharpe RM, Maddocks S, Millar M, Kerr JB, Saunders PT, McKinnell C. Testosterone and spermatogenesis: identification of stage-specific, androgen-regulated proteins secreted by adult rat seminiferous tubules. *J Androl* 1992; **13**: 172–84.

[143] Reventos J, Sullivan PM, Joseph DR, Gordon JW. Tissue-specific expression of the rat androgen-binding protein/sex hormone-binding globulin gene in transgenic mice. *Mol Cell Endocrinol* 1993; **96**: 69–73.

[144] Gerard H, Gerard A, En Nya A, Felden F, Gueant JL. Spermatogenic cells do internalize Sertoli androgen-binding protein: a transmission electron microscopy autoradiographic study in the rat. *Endocrinology* 1994; **134**: 1515–27.

[145] Joseph DR, O'Brien DA, Sullivan PM, Becchis M, Tsuruta JK, Petrusz P. Overexpression of androgen-binding protein/sex hormone-binding globulin in male transgenic mice: tissue distribution and phenotypic disorders. *Biol Reprod* 1997; **56**: 21–32.

[146] Jarow JP, Zirkin BR. The androgen microenvironment of the human testis and hormonal control of spermatogenesis. *Ann N Y Acad Sci* 2005; **1061**: 208–20.

[147] Jarow JP, Wright WW, Brown TR, Yan X, Zirkin BR. Bioactivity of androgens within the testes and serum of normal men. *J Androl* 2005; **26**(3): 343–8.

[148] Robinson R, Fritz IB. Metabolism of glucose by Sertoli cells in culture. *Biol Reprod* 1981; **24**: 1032–41.

[149] Grootegoed JA, Jansen R, Van der Molen HJ. The role of glucose, pyruvate and lactate in ATP production by rat spermatocytes and spermatids. *Biochim Biophys Acta* 1984; **767**: 248–56.

[150] Grootegoed JA, Jansen R, van der Molen HJ. Spermatogenic cells in the germinal epithelium utilize alpha-ketoisocaproate and lactate, produced by Sertoli cells from leucine and glucose. *Ann N Y Acad Sci* 1984; **438**: 557–60.

[151] Mita M, Hall PF. Metabolism of round spermatids from rats: Lactate as the preferred substrate. *Biol Reprod* 1982; **26**: 445–55.

[152] Mita M, Price JM, Hall PF. Stimulation by follicle-stimulating hormone of synthesis of lactate by Sertoli cells from rat testis. *Endocrinology* 1982; **110**: 1535–41.

[153] Morales C, Clermont Y. Receptor-mediated endocytosis of transferrin by Sertoli cells of the rat. *Biol Reprod* 1986; **35**: 393–405.

[154] Dautry-Varsat A, Ciechanover A, Lodish HF. pH and the recycling of transferrin during receptor-mediated endocytosis. *Proc Natl Acad Sci U S A* 1983; **80**: 2258–62.

[155] Aisen P, Listowsky I. Iron transport and storage proteins. *Annu Rev Biochem* 1980; **49**: 357–93.

[156] Skinner MK, Griswold MD. Sertoli cells synthesize and secrete transferrin-like protein. *J Biol Chem* 1980; **255**: 9523–5.

[157] Lecureuil C, Saleh MC, Fontaine I, Baron B, Zakin MM, Guillou F. Transgenic mice as a model to study the regulation of human transferrin expression in Sertoli cells. *Hum Reprod* 2004; **19**: 1300–7.

[158] Holmes SD, Lipshultz LI, Smith RG. Transferrin and gonadal dysfunction in man. *Fertil Steril* 1982; **38**: 600–4.

[159] Howe CC, Overton GC, Sawicki J, Solter D, Stein P, Strickland S. Expression of SPARC/osteonectin transcript in murine embryos and gonads. *Differentiation* 1988; **37**: 20–5.

[160] Schiemann BJ, Neil JR, Schiemann WP. SPARC inhibits epithelial cell proliferation in part through stimulation of the transforming growth factor-beta-signaling system. *Mol Biol Cell* 2003; **14**: 3977–88.

[161] Francki A, McClure TD, Brekken RA, *et al.* SPARC regulates TGF-beta1-dependent signaling in primary glomerular mesangial cells. *J Cell Biochem* 2004; **91**: 915–25.

[162] Murphy-Ullrich JE. The de-adhesive activity of matricellular proteins: Is intermediate cell adhesion an adaptive state? *J Clin Invest* 2001; **107**: 785–90.

[163] Wilson MJ, Bowles J, Koopman P. The matricellular protein SPARC is internalized in Sertoli, Leydig, and germ cells during testis differentiation. *Mol Reprod Dev* 2006; **73**: 531–9.

[164] Gilmour DT, Lyon GJ, Carlton MB, *et al.* Mice deficient for the secreted glycoprotein SPARC/osteonectin/BM40 develop normally but show severe age-onset cataract formation and disruption of the lens. *Embo J* 1998; **17**: 1860–70.

[165] Siu MK, Lee WM, Cheng CY. The interplay of collagen IV, tumor necrosis factor-alpha, gelatinase B (matrix metalloprotease-9), and tissue inhibitor of metalloproteases-1 in the basal lamina regulates Sertoli cell-tight junction dynamics in the rat testis. *Endocrinology* 2003; **144**: 371–87.

[166] Siu MK, Cheng CY. Interactions of proteases, protease inhibitors, and the beta1 integrin/laminin gamma3 protein complex in the regulation of ectoplasmic specialization dynamics in the rat testis. *Biol Reprod* 2004; **70**: 945–64.

[167] Poncelet AC, Schnaper HW. Regulation of human mesangial cell collagen expression by transforming growth factor-beta1. *Am J Physiol* 1998; **275**: F458–66.

[168] Li YY, Feng YQ, Kadokami T, *et al.* Myocardial extracellular matrix remodeling in transgenic mice overexpressing tumor necrosis factor alpha can be modulated by anti-tumor necrosis factor alpha therapy. *Proc Natl Acad Sci U S A* 2000; **97**: 12746–51.

[169] Siwik DA, Chang DL, Colucci WS. Interleukin-1beta and tumor necrosis factor-alpha decrease collagen synthesis and increase matrix metalloproteinase activity in cardiac fibroblasts in vitro. *Circ Res* 2000; **86**: 1259–65.

[170] Morales C, Griswold MD. Retinol-induced stage synchronization in seminiferous tubules of the rat. *Endocrinology* 1987; **121**: 432–4.

[171] Huang HF, Marshall GR. Failure of spermatid release under various vitamin A states: an indication of delayed spermiation. *Biol Reprod* 1983; **28**: 1163–72.

[172] Appling DR, Chytil F. Evidence of a role for retinoic acid (vitamin A-acid) in the maintenance of testosterone production in male rats. *Endocrinology* 1981; **108**: 2120–4.

[173] Petkovich M, Brand NJ, Krust A, Chambon P. A human retinoic acid receptor which belongs to the family of nuclear receptors. *Nature* 1987; **330**: 444–50.

[174] Brand N, Petkovich M, Krust A, *et al.* Identification of a second human retinoic acid receptor. *Nature* 1988; **332**: 850–3.

[175] Soprano D, Blaner W. *Plasma Retinol-Binding Protein*, 2nd edn. New York, NY: Raven Press, 1994.

[176] Ghyselinck NB, Bavik C, Sapin V, *et al.* Cellular retinol-binding protein I is essential for vitamin A homeostasis. *Embo J* 1999; **18**: 4903–14.

[177] E X Zhang L, Lu J, *et al.* Increased neonatal mortality in mice lacking cellular retinol-binding protein II. *J Biol Chem* 2002; **277**: 36617–23.

[178] Rajan N, Sung WK, Goodman DS. Localization of cellular retinol-binding protein mRNA in rat testis and epididymis and its stage-dependent expression during the cycle of the seminiferous epithelium. *Biol Reprod* 1990; **43**: 835–42.

[179] Li E, Demmer LA, Sweetser DA, Ong DE, Gordon JI. Rat cellular retinol-binding protein II: use of a cloned cDNA to define its primary structure, tissue-specific expression, and developmental regulation. *Proc Natl Acad Sci U S A* 1986; **83**: 5779–83.

[180] Zheng WL, Bucco RA, Schmitt MC, Wardlaw SA, Ong DE. Localization of cellular retinoic acid-binding protein (CRABP) II and CRABP in developing rat testis. *Endocrinology* 1996; **137**: 5028–35.

[181] Kastner P, Mark M, Leid M, *et al.* Abnormal spermatogenesis in RXR beta mutant mice. *Genes Dev* 1996; **10**: 80–92.

[182] Lufkin T, Lohnes D, Mark M, *et al.* High postnatal lethality and testis degeneration in retinoic acid receptor alpha mutant mice. *Proc Natl Acad Sci U S A* 1993; **90**: 7225–9.

[183] Brennan J, Capel B. One tissue, two fates: Molecular genetic events that underlie testis versus ovary development. *Nat Rev Genet* 2004; **5**: 509–21.

[184] Lovell-Badge R, Robertson E. XY female mice resulting from a heritable mutation in the primary testis-determining gene, Tdy. *Development* 1990; **109**: 635–46.

[185] Koopman P, Gubbay J, Vivian N, Goodfellow P, Lovell-Badge R. Male development of chromosomally female mice transgenic for Sry. *Nature* 1991; **351**: 117–21.

[186] Miyamoto N, Yoshida M, Kuratani S, Matsuo I, Aizawa S. Defects of urogenital development in mice lacking Emx2. *Development* 1997; **124**: 1653–64.

[187] Bullejos M, Koopman P. Spatially dynamic expression of Sry in mouse genital ridges. *Dev Dyn* 2001; **221**: 201–5.

[188] Tevosian SG, Albrecht KH, Crispino JD, Fujiwara Y, Eicher EM, Orkin SH. Gonadal differentiation, sex determination and normal Sry expression in mice require direct interaction between transcription partners GATA4 and FOG2. *Development* 2002; **129**: 4627–34.

[189] Meeks JJ, Crawford SE, Russell TA, Morohashi K, Weiss J, Jameson JL. Dax1 regulates testis cord organization during gonadal differentiation. *Development* 2003; **130**: 1029–36.

[190] Meeks JJ, Weiss J, Jameson JL. Dax1 is required for testis determination. *Nat Genet* 2003; **34**: 32–3.

[191] Colvin JS, Green RP, Schmahl J, Capel B, Ornitz DM. Male-to-female sex reversal in mice lacking fibroblast growth factor 9. *Cell 23* 2001; **104**: 875–89.

[192] Arango NA, Lovell-Badge R, Behringer RR. Targeted mutagenesis of the endogenous mouse Mis gene promoter: In vivo definition of genetic pathways of vertebrate sexual development. *Cell* 1999; **99**: 409–19.

[193] Palmer SJ, Burgoyne PS. In situ analysis of fetal, prepuberal and adult XX – -XY chimaeric mouse testes: Sertoli cells are predominantly, but not exclusively, XY. *Development* 1991; **112**: 265–8.

[194] Schmahl J, Kim Y, Colvin JS, Ornitz DM, Capel B. Fgf9 induces proliferation and nuclear localization of FGFR2 in Sertoli precursors during male sex determination. *Development* 2004; **131**: 3627–36.

[195] De Santa Barbara P, Bonneaud N, Boizet B, *et al.* Direct interaction of SRY-related protein SOX9 and steroidogenic factor 1 regulates transcription of the human anti-Mullerian hormone gene. *Mol Cell Biol* 1998; **18**: 6653–65.

[196] Bishop CE, Whitworth DJ, Qin Y, *et al.* A transgenic insertion upstream of sox9 is associated with dominant XX sex reversal in the mouse. *Nat Genet* 2000; **26**: 490–4.

[197] Qin Y, Poirier C, Truong C, Schumacher A, Agoulnik AI, Bishop CE. A major locus on mouse chromosome 18 controls XX sex reversal in Odd Sex (Ods) mice. *Hum Mol Genet* 2003; **12**: 509–15.

[198] Qin Y, Kong LK, Poirier C, Truong C, Overbeek PA, Bishop CE. Long-range activation of Sox9 in Odd Sex (Ods) mice. *Hum Mol Genet* 2004; **13**: 1213–18.

[199] Qin Y, Bishop CE. Sox9 is sufficient for functional testis development producing fertile male mice in the absence of Sry. *Hum Mol Genet* 2005; **14**: 1221–9.

Spermatogenesis in the adult

Joseph P. Alukal, Dolores J. Lamb, Craig S. Niederberger, and Antoine A. Makhlouf

Introduction

Spermatogenesis refers to the production and development of spermatozoa, the mature male gametes of most sexually reproducing species. **In mammals, spermatogenesis begins with diploid stem cells that resemble other somatic cells; it ends with highly specialized motile haploid cells that are remarkably unique in appearance and function.** While somewhat lengthy, taking about 64 days in humans [1,2], spermatogenesis is a highly efficient procedure leading to the production of an estimated 70 million spermatozoa daily [3]. **This coordinated development proceeds through sequential stages that have been well characterized in classic morphological studies and whose molecular mechanisms are currently under intensive investigation** [4–7]. The stages of spermatogenesis are summarized in Table 5.1. These will be examined later in the chapter; first, we will describe the end product – the mature spermatozoon – and the theater of production – the seminiferous tubule of the testis.

Structure of the mature spermatozoon

Spermatozoa exhibit a wide variation in shape between species. Rodent spermatozoa have a falciform head shape, while the spermatozoa of humans and other mammals have a spatulated head [8]. Electron microscopy has given us detailed images of the mature spermatozoon; simply, it is divided into a head and flagellum with a small connecting neck in between.

The head is further subdivided into the acrosomal and postacrosomal regions. The acrosomal cap forms the more rostral part of the acrosome, and it is followed by the equatorial segment (or posterior acrosome). The largest part of the sperm head volume is occupied by an ovoid nucleus, which is surrounded by a perinuclear theca. The nucleus lies deep to the posterior acrosome and extends into the postacrosomal region all the way

to the basal plate; this forms the boundary with the neck region.

The connecting piece consists of a truncated cone, with its base lodged in a small fossa of the nuclear envelope and its tip connecting to the flagellum [4]. It contains the proximal centriole, arranged perpendicularly to the axis of the spermatozoon. At its tip, the distal or longitudinal centriole is modified to give rise to the axoneme of the flagellum [4,8,9].

The flagellum itself consists of a central axoneme surrounded by periaxonemal structures. The axoneme consists of two central microtubules surrounded by a circle of nine microtubule doublets (9 + 2 configuration). Two dynein arms extend from each microtubule pair and are responsible for flagellar motion. Mutations in the left-to-right dynein gene (*Lrd*) cause immotile cilia syndrome with associated infertility in males. The flagellum can be subdivided into "pieces" based on the type of periaxonemal structure present. The most rostral part is the midpiece, where the axoneme is surrounded by nine outer dense fibers (ODF) and a mitochondrial sheath. This is followed by the principal piece, where the number of outer dense fibers drops to seven, and the mitochondria are replaced by a fibrous sheath [9]. The fibrous sheath consists of semicircular transverse ribs extending from two anchoring columns associated with axonemal doublets 3 and 8. **This arrangement of the sheath poses a limit on the plane of motion of the flagellum, presumably enhancing sperm motility** [9,10]. The flagellum terminates in the endpiece, which consists of remnants of the axoneme [9, 11].

Histology of seminiferous tubules

The adult human testis measures 15–25 cm^3 in volume [12]. It is surrounded by a fibrous capsule, the tunica albuginea. It is divided into 200–300 lobules

---

Infertility in the Male, 4th edition, ed. Larry I. Lipshultz, Stuart S. Howards, and Craig S. Niederberger. Published by Cambridge University Press. © Cambridge University Press 2009.

Table 5.1. Cell types and steps of spermatogenesis

Starting cell type	Ploidy	Process	Ending cell type
A spermatogonium	Diploid (2n)	Spermatocytogenesis (renewal)	A spermatogonium B spermatogonium
B spermatogonium	Diploid (2n)	Spermatocytogenesis (differentiation)	Primary spermatocyte
Primary spermatocyte	Diploid (4n)	Meiosis I	Secondary spermatocyte
Secondary spermatocyte	Haploid (2n)	Meiosis II	Spermatid
Spermatid	Haploid (1n)	Spermiogenesis	Spermatozoa
Spermatozoon	Haploid (1n)	Spermiation	Free spermatozoa

by septations that extend from the tunica albuginea towards the testicular mediastinum (or hilum) [4]. Each of these lobules contains several seminiferous tubules, where spermatogenesis occurs. Each seminiferous tubule arises and ends at the rete testis, an anastomosing network of tubules that empties into the efferent ductules. Seminiferous tubules are highly convoluted, averaging 70–80 cm in length [4,13]. **This arrangement results in a large surface of germinal epithelium that occupies a small compact space, thereby allowing the production of a large number of spermatozoa daily** [3].

Each seminiferous tubule consists of a basement membrane lined by Sertoli cells interspersed with germ cells at various stages of maturation. Maturation of the germ cells occurs in a centripetal fashion, with immature cells starting out at the periphery in apposition to the basement membrane, and migrating towards the lumen as they go through the various stages of spermatogenesis. Using light microscopy, Heller and Clermont initially identified 13 types of germ cells in humans [5,14]. **In ascending order of maturity these are: dark type A spermatogonia (Ad); pale type A spermatogonia (Ap); type B spermatogonia (B); preleptotene primary spermatocytes (R); leptotene primary spermatocytes (L); zygotene primary spermatocytes (z); pachytene primary spermatocytes (p); diplotene primary spermatocytes (d); secondary spermatocytes (II); and Sa, Sb1, Sb2, Sc, Sd1, and Sd2 spermatids.**

Spermatogenic cycles and waves

Histological analysis of seminiferous tubules shows that neighboring germ cells differentiate in a synchronous manner. **Thus, each section of tubule exhibits a specific pattern of cell types and cell–cell associations, and this allows classification of the epithelial sections into distinct stages.** The number of stages is highly variable per species; there are six in humans and

12–14 in rodents [6,14,15]. Stages are conventionally denoted by roman numerals, and follow a specific progression (i.e., in humans stage I is followed by II, then III, and so on, with the sequence repeating after stage VI). The number of stages depends on the duration of the spermatogenic cycle, the number of generations between spermatogonia and mature sperm, and the frequency of divisions of spermatogonia. Interestingly, in rodents, stages that follow each other temporally are also spatially adjacent, and thus the entire sequence can be described as a "spermatogenic wave" along the tubules. In rodents, any particular stage occupies the entire circumference of the tubule, making detection of the spermatogenic wave fairly straightforward. Humans, however, can exhibit more than one stage per cross section [6,14]. Careful mapping and three-dimensional reconstruction of the various stages in human biopsies has shown that this is due to a spiral arrangement of the spermatogenic wave in humans, rather than a random patchwork of various stages [16]. **In humans, the entire cycle of six stages takes approximately 64 days** [1]. Because differentiating spermatogonia divide approximately every 16 days, there are usually four cohorts of maturing germ cells seen in any particular stage.

Spermatogenesis
Spermatogonia: renewal, proliferation, and death

Spermatogonia are specialized diploid cells located on the basement membrane of the seminiferous tubule; these cells are the ancestors of all the other germ cell types [4,17]. Because spermatogonia are the only germ cells that undergo meiosis, the final product of spermatogenesis is ultimately dependent on their function. To ensure a steady supply of mature spermatozoa throughout life, spermatogonia must perform three functions: (1) differentiation into spermatozoa, (2) self-renewal, and (3) control of the ratio of germ cells to Sertoli cells by apoptosis [18].

Embryonic development of spermatogonia

The embryonic development of germ cells has been described in Chapter 1. **Briefly, primordial germ cells of the gonadal ridge associate with Sertoli cells and then become gonocytes.** Between birth and 6 months of age, gonocytes differentiate into spermatogonia [19]. Although generally considered to be quiescent before puberty, **are observed to increase in number of spermatogonia between ages 7 and 13 years**, according to stereological studies of autopsy specimens from accidental deaths [20,21]. The increase in spermatogonial cell numbers, in absolute counts as well as relative to Sertoli cell numbers, accounts for most of the increase in testicular size seen in this period [21]. This period of mitotic activity has been confirmed in other primates [22]. **Following the onset of puberty, spermatogonia begin the parallel processes of proliferation and differentiation towards spermatozoa.**

Stem cells and self-renewal

Continuous production of spermatozoa throughout life requires that spermatogonia replenish themselves. This self-renewal depends on a subgroup of spermatogonia, known as stem cells; these stem cells can undergo either mitosis, leading to daughter stem cells, or differentiation. Identification of these stem cells is of obvious importance, because preservation and expansion of this group can theoretically restart spermatogenesis after exposure to gonadotoxic insults such as radiation or chemotherapy.

Spermatogonia can be broadly divided into type A and type B subpopulations based on their heterochromatin contents, with type B cells having more heterochromatin than type A. Since heterochromatin consists predominantly of transcriptionally silent DNA, an increase in heterochromatin is a sign of differentiation in many cell lineages [18]. Thus it has always been theorized that type A spermatogonia are precursors of the type B subpopulation, and that spermatogonial stem cells (SSCs) must be a subgroup of A spermatogonia [23]. The exact identity of SSCs and their proliferation schema have been extensively studied in many species. Because much greater progress has been made in rodents than in primates, we will describe the former first.

In rodents, spermatogonial stem cells (as described by Huckins) are referred to as As cells (for type A single or type A stem) [7], and they are characterized by the fact that they are the only germ cells that lack intercellular bridges [24]. They divide to form either two daughter stem cells or two paired spermatogonia (Apr) connected by a cytoplasmic bridge due to incomplete cytokinesis. The Apr cells are then committed to continue division to form chains of 4, 8 and 16 A-aligned (Aal) spermatogonia. These in turn differentiate into A1 spermatogonia, which undergo another series of six divisions, still with incomplete cytokinesis, to form a clonal syncitium of up to 4000 primary spermatocytes [25,26]. There is a debate as to whether As stem cells continuously divide to give rise to Apr and subsequent progeny during normal spermatogenesis or merely act as a reserve population that is activated only after depletion of more differentiated spermatogonia due to a toxic insult [18]. In the latter model, A4 spermatogonia are believed to give rise to A1 spermatogonia to ensure self-renewal under normal circumstances [5]. Most investigators, however, hold to the former (As) model [27].

The picture is less clear in primates. In his classic morphological studies, Clermont classified spermatogonia based on their nuclear chromatin staining pattern when treated with Zenker-formol [23]. He identified three subtypes: type A dark spermatogonia (denoted as Ad), type A pale spermatogonia (Ap), and type B spermatogonia (B). Type B spermatogonia were designated as the immediate precursors of spermatocytes, on the basis of the similarity of their nuclear volume to that of spermatocytes, and the fact that type B cells were most abundant in spermatogenic stages VI, I, and II, just before the peak numbers of preleptotene spermatocytes in stages III and IV. In addition, quantitative studies found that Ad, Ap, and B spermatogonia and preleptotene primary spermatocytes were found in the approximate ratio of $1:1:2:4$, suggesting that division of B cells led to development of spermatocytes [23]. Assignment of Ap cells as the precursors of B cells was more tenuous, being based solely on the closer nuclear morphology. He thus proposed a model in which Ad cells were the stem cell that divided to give rise to more Ad cells for purposes of self-renewal, or to Ap cells that go on to produce B cells and spermatocytes. **While Clermont's Ap → B → spermatocyte progression has generally been accepted, his identification of Ad cells as the SSCs has been disputed** [18,26,27].

In testicular biopsies of men treated with chemotherapy or radiation, Schulze found that Ad cells were totally absent, while some Ap cells survived. Arguing that stem cells ought to be more resistant to gonadotoxic insults, it was proposed that Ap cells functioned as the SSCs [28]. In irradiated rhesus monkey testes, repopulation of the seminiferous tubules began with clonal patches of both dark and pale spermatogonia found as single, paired, or chained cells [29]. This suggested that Ap and Ad cells formed parallel populations that could both function as SSCs. More recently, Ehmcke *et al.* used the fact that stem cells in many lineages can be identified by their ability to retain BrdU labeling longer than other more frequently dividing cells. They thus identified single (i.e., not paired or chained) Ap cells as the self-renewing stem cells in macaque testis. In other words, the earliest indicator of spermatogonial commitment along the path of differentiation is incomplete cytokinesis after mitotic division, and only single spermatogonial cells function as true stem cells. They further confirmed that primate spermatogonia proliferate into synchronized clones that enter meiosis in lockstep, just as in rodents [30]. Compared to rodents, however, the number of mitotic divisions leading from SSCs to spermatocytes is much lower in primates, particularly humans. This leads to a lower efficiency of spermatozoa production, but a higher fidelity of DNA copying in the longer-lived primates [26]. With Ap cells now known to function as self-renewing SSCs, single Ad cells are currently believed to act as reserve stem cells that only activate when Ap cells are depleted [27,31]. This belief is supported by the fact that acutely radiated testes show extensive depletion of Ap cells with preservation of Ad cells. After longer intervals, however, Ad cells decrease as Ap cells transiently increase, suggesting a conversion from the former to the latter [29]. In addition, involution of Ap cells as a result of aging in humans is seen in the sixth decade, while Ad spermatogonia persist in large numbers until the eighth decade, a finding consistent with Ad spermatogonia being precursors of Ap cells [32].

Stem cell transplantation

Spermatogonial stem cells are believed to be fairly rare, with an estimated frequency of less than 0.1% in rodents [33]. This has made the isolation and study of an enriched population of SSCs fairly difficult. One breakthrough came in 1994, when Brinster and colleagues reported the successful re-establishment of spermatogenesis and production of offspring after transplantation of SSCs into sterile recipient mice testes [34,35]. This provided a functional assay to measure enrichment of stem cells via various approaches. These approaches have combined the use of cryptorchid mouse testes (which have lower differentiated and haploid germ cell numbers), with fluorescent cell sorting based on surface markers of stem cells, extrusion of vital dyes, or expression of stem-cell-specific marker transgenes [27,36–38].

Crucially important to the goal of achieving successful culture and differentiation of SSCs is the expression of the c-kit tyrosine kinase receptor. Expression of this receptor allows for binding of the kit ligand in vivo; this ligand (also known as mast cell growth factor [MGF], stem cell factor [SCF], and Steel factor) is produced by Sertoli cells, and **binding of this ligand is thought to represent an initial event in the differentiation of SSCs to spermatids.** Successful co-culture experiments with Sertoli cells and early undifferentiated spermatogonia demonstrate both the presence of kit ligand and spermatogonial expression of the c-kit receptor [39, 40].

Another benefit of the transplantation experiments has been the ability to generate transgenic animals through the male germline [41]. Successful transplantation across related species has also been reported [42, 43]. **Still, technical difficulties and safety concerns have so far kept the ultimate benefit, transplantation of human SSC to treat infertility, from being realized** [27].

Regulation of spermatogonial fate

Spermatogonial stem cells (SSCs) maintain a tight balance between differentiation and self-renewal. One of the earliest models proposed for this was invariant asymmetric division, in which an SSC divides into one daughter SSC and one Ap spermatogonium that undergoes differentiation [23]. Most evidence, however, points to a symmetric model in which the daughter cells of SSC divisions are identical. Whether the division leads to two single cells, or to paired A spermatogonia that undergo proliferation and differentiation, depends on the microenvironment of the parent cell [18]. **Only when present within the so-called "stem cell niche" would a stem cell avoid differentiation and remain uncommitted.**

The stem cell niche concept has been developed in studies of other cell lineages, particularly epithelial and hematopoetic lines [44]. The factors that characterize the niche include secreted factors, extracellular matrix proteins, and cell–cell adhesion molecules [44]. In the case of SSCs, only a few of these factors have been identified so far [45]. Not surprisingly, these factors, and therefore the presence and maintenance of the niche, are controlled by Sertoli cells.

The first factor to be implicated in SSC niche maintenance is Glial-derived neurotrophic factor (GDNF), a member of the TGF-β superfamily that is secreted by Sertoli cells [46]. Mice knockouts of GDNF die in the neonatal period, but single GDNF-null allele males survive with significantly diminished spermatogenesis and Sertoli-cell-only tubules increasingly found with advancing age [47]. In contrast, overexpression of GDNF leads to spermatogonial accumulation and failure of differentiation [47]. Neonatal GDNF$^{-/-}$ testes transplanted into nude mice (to bypass the lethality of the GDNF$^{-/-}$ phenotype) exhibit severe loss of SSCs with the first wave of spermatogenesis on day 7 [48]. GDNF acts on the SSC through both the Ret receptor and GDNF-family receptor α1 (GFRα1). Both of these molecules are surface antigens expressed by SSCs; antibodies to these molecules have been utilized in isolation protocols for SSCs, albeit with variable degrees of success. Thus, GDNF seems to be necessary for maintenance of the SSC cell niche, at least in the prepubertal period; it is not, however, sufficient by itself to cause this process to occur [45].

ERM (Ets-related molecule) is a member of the Ets family of transcription factors. ERM$^{-/-}$ mice complete the first wave of spermatogenesis, but exhibit a severe germ cell loss thereafter, with adult testes progressively exhibiting a Sertoli-cell-only picture [49]. This is due to failure of SSCs to undergo self-renewal [49]. ERM expression has been localized to Sertoli cells, where it appears to regulate a number of secreted cytokines that could transmit the self-renewal signal to SSCs [49]. GDNF expression, however, is normal in ERM$^{-/-}$ mice, indicating that other factors are necessary for maintenance of the stem cell niche in adult mice [45] .

Meiosis
Overview of meiosis

Type B spermatogonia undergo mitosis to give rise to diploid primary spermatocytes [4]. This marks the end of the proliferative portion of spermatogenesis, which has so far taken place in the nutrient-rich basal compartment of the tubule. **The spermatocytes then cross the blood–testis barrier formed by the Sertoli tight junctions to the adluminal compartment. It is there, shielded from the immune system, that the differentiation phase of spermatogenesis occurs** [6].

Meiosis is the process through which diploid germ cells give rise to haploid progeny. Briefly summarized, it consists of a single round of DNA

replication followed by two rounds of division. The DNA replication step results in having two chromatids per chromosome. This is followed by the first division (meiosis I or reduction division), when homologous chromosomes are paired and held together by the synaptonemal complex. The DNA strands of the paired chromosomes (also known as bivalent) then undergo reciprocal recombination at crossover sites or chiasmata. Following that, the homologs line up at the equatorial plate during metaphase, and each homolog migrates to a separate pole during anaphase. **This results in secondary spermatocytes containing a haploid number of chromosomes, with each chromosome containing two chromatids.** A second division follows (meiosis II or equational division), which resembles the equational division of mitosis in that the two chromatids of each chromosome segregate to either pole. **The end result is a total of four spermatids, each containing a haploid number of chromosomes with a single chromatid each.**

Prophase I and homologous recombination

Prophase I is the first stage of meiosis I and is the stage at which most of the events unique to meiosis (as opposed to mitosis) are observed. On the basis of the microscopic appearance of the chromosomal material, it is subdivided into leptonema (from greek "thin threads"), zygonema ("paired threads"), pachynema ("thick threads"), diplonema ("double threads"), and diakinesis ("through motion").

Following DNA synthesis in interphase, the chromosomes start to condense during leptonema, and can be seen by electron microscopy as fine threads attached to the nuclear membrane [4]. Each consists of two sister chromatids held together by a complex of cohesin proteins [50]. This association will continue until the metaphase of the second division, due in part to the presence of meiosis-specific cohesins [51]. Pairing of homologous chromosomes commences in the zygotene stage, and is mediated by the formation of the synaptonemal complex [52]. Pairing begins with the association of chromatids to specific synaptonemal complex proteins (SCP) that form an axial structure along the length of the chromosome, with loops of DNA extending out at a perpendicular angle to the protein core. The importance of these proteins is underscored by the finding that knockout of one such protein, SCP3, leads to maturation arrest at the level of spermatocytes in male mice [53].

Completion of synapsis marks the beginning of the pachytene stage, the longest of all prophase stages.

Pachytene spermatocytes are readily visible in microscopic sections, and are the largest germ cells in terms of size. During pachynema, the synaptonemal complex acts as a docking site for the assembly of proteins responsible for the process of DNA recombination at crossover sites known as chiasmata [54]. Recombination starts with double strand breaks in chromatid DNA mediated by Spo11, a topoisomerase first identified in yeast and found to be conserved across many species [55,56].

Spermatocytes of male Spo11$^{-/-}$ mice exhibit massive apoptosis in prophase I, confirming the essential role of this protein in mammals [57]. Following double strand breakage, a 3' DNA overhang is generated and used to invade the DNA strands of the homologous chromosome, where a homology search is initiated leading to formation of hetero-duplex DNA complexes [58]. Homologous recombination occurs when resolution of the four-strand complexes leads to the DNA strands from one chromatid continuing on a chromatid of the homologous chromosome. A detailed description of this process is beyond the scope of the present chapter (see also Chapter 8). Suffice it to say that many of the proteins involved have been identified in lower eukaryotes such as yeast, and some have had their role confirmed in mice through knockout studies [59]. The frequency of homologous recombination in humans can be estimated by counting the foci of recombination in pachytene spermatocytes immunostained for MLH1, a DNA mismatch-repair protein that is part of the meiotic recombination apparatus [60]. In normal males, this was found to be around 50 foci per cell [60,61]. Clinical studies found that the number of recombination sites is much lower in about 10% of men with nonobstructive azoospermia, and in up to 50% of men with maturation arrest [62].

Desynapsis starts in the diplotene stage, where the bivalents are held together only at sites of chiasmata. This is followed by diakinesis, during which the chromosomes condense further, and detach from the dissolving nuclear membrane in preparation for their alignment in metaphase.

Remainder of meiosis I

The remainder of the first meiotic division consists of metaphase I, anaphase I, and telophase I. During metaphase, the two chromosomes of each bivalent attach through their centromeres to the equatorial plane of the microtubule spindle. The orientation of each bivalent at the equator is random and independent of other bivalents, leading to independent assortment of the chromosomes in the resulting gametes. During anaphase, the two chromosomes of each pair are pulled toward opposite poles by shortening microtubules, leading to the final disappearance of recombination sites. This is followed by reformation of the nuclear membrane and disappearance of the spindle in telophase. Incomplete cytokinesis leads to the formation of secondary spermatocytes connected to each other by inter-cytoplasmic bridges.

Meiosis II and secondary spermatocytes

Secondary spermatocytes contain a haploid number of chromosomes but with a 2n content of DNA due to duplication of each chromosome into two chromatids during interphase. Secondary spermatocytes therefore undergo a single equational division to yield spermatids. Their size and location are intermediate between that of primary spermatocytes and spermatids, hinting at their transitional nature. The equational division, dubbed meiosis II, is mechanistically very similar to mitosis of somatic cells: the chromosomes align at the equatorial plate during metaphase, and then the two chromatids segregate to each pole during anaphase. This process occurs fairly rapidly, as evidenced by the sparse number of secondary spermatocytes identified in microscopic sections [14]. This correlates with the relative infrequency of maturation arrest at the secondary spermatocyte stage in men with nonobstructive azoospermia [63]. Reports of successful completion of the second meiotic division in secondary spermatocytes injected into oocytes in both mice and humans suggest that it is preprogrammed once the reductional division has occurred [63–65].

Spermiogenesis and spermiation

The metamorphosis of round spermatids into compact highly motile cells capable of traversing the reproductive tracts of two organisms and fertilizing an oocyte is a remarkable phenomenon. This transformation is traditionally divided into the processes of spermiogenesis and spermiation. **Spermiogenesis refers to the acquisition by the germ cell of several organelles and accessory structures such as the acrosome and the flagellum. Spermiation involves shedding of the germ cell into the tubule lumen and removal of the last vestiges of the cytoplasm (the cytoplasmic droplet) as it transits to the rete testis and caput epididymidis.** Teratozoospermia, a common clinical finding on semen analyses, presumably is due to disturbances in these processes [66].

Early studies have subdivided spermiogenesis into a series of steps based on organellar changes and nuclear condensation, with a different number of steps recognized in each species (14 in humans) [6,15]. However, it is easiest to describe the various changes to the sperm cell in a functional, rather than chronological, manner.

Acrosome formation

It has long been recognized that the acrosome arises from the Golgi apparatus [15,67]. The first visible step (in pachytene spermatocytes) is the fusion of proacrosomal granules originating in the Golgi to form a single acrosomal vesicle [68]. In spermatids, this acrosomal vesicle flattens and spreads around the nuclear membrane. It enlarges by incorporating newer vesicles supplied by the Golgi, so that, eventually, the mature human acrosome covers approximately 60% of the nuclear membrane [4,69]. The Golgi itself, meanwhile, migrates towards the opposite pole, to be later removed with the residual body [70].

The contents of the acrosome have been reviewed elsewhere [71,72]. They consist mostly of hydrolytic enzymes including proteases, hydroglycolases, and esterases. Many, such as hyalouronidase and cathepsins, are found in somatic lysosomes, while some, like acrosin, are specific to acrosomes [68,73]. The targeting of specific products to the acrosome is believed to follow the same pathways of vesicular trafficking of somatic cells, sharing a close similarity with lysosomal transport [68].

Nuclear changes and DNA compaction

In round spermatids, the nucleus is found in a central position. As spermatids elongate, it moves to an eccentric position and undergoes significant condensation, reaching a final size one-tenth of its starting volume [4,74]. At the molecular level, this is paralleled by changes in the compaction of chromatin and composition of nucleoproteins. In round spermatids, as in somatic cells, nuclear DNA is arranged around nucleosomes composed of an octamer of histone proteins. The DNA strand is wrapped around the nucleosome like a spool, giving the classical form of "beads on a string." **In contrast, mature spermatozoal DNA is arranged in compact toroidal loops (doughnut-shaped) with protamines replacing the histones as nucleoproteins.** This transformation is responsible for the much higher condensation of sperm DNA and its superior resistance to denaturation [75,76]. In mammals, this switch goes through an intermediate phase where the histones are replaced by aptly named transition proteins, which are later replaced by protamines [75,77].

Protamines are small arginine-rich proteins. The level of protamines in human sperm has been clinically measured using chromomycin A_3 and aniline blue staining of smears, and this has been proposed as a measure of DNA sperm quality [78,79]. Humans have two protamine classes, denoted protamine 1 and protamine 2, which are expressed in an approximately one-to-one ratio [80]. **Alterations of this ratio, through the absence or underexpression of one of the two forms, have been associated with male subfertility** [81–83]. Mouse knockouts of protamine 1 or protamine 2 are infertile and exhibit abnormal embryonic development [84]. However, men with abnormal sperm protamine content have successfully completed ICSI with viable pregnancies [81,82]. A possible explanation for this discrepancy was proposed by Aoki *et al.*, who found a high degree of variability of protamine expression between the spermatozoa of a single individual [81].

The purpose of this transition in nucleoproteins remains a matter of intense study. Beyond giving sperm a more hydrodynamic shape through higher compaction, protection of DNA integrity and genetic imprinting have also been proposed as goals of this transformation [85]. Another effect is the suppression of transcription, making spermatids beyond the round nucleus stage increasingly dependent on stored mRNA and post-transcriptional regulation of gene expression [86].

Growing evidence points to DNA compaction or packaging as a crucial marker of intact spermatogenesis. The clinical implication of DNA fragmentation indices (DFI) is well documented [87], and tests measuring DFI are increasingly utilized in clinical infertility practices. Further information on DNA fragmentation index and sperm chromatin structural assay (SCSA) is found in Chapter 40.

As stated previously, during DNA condensation, nuclear DNA in round spermatids is loosely associated with histones, similar to the association of compacted DNA in somatic cells. As the spermatid nucleus is remodeled, histones are replaced by transition proteins, which are then replaced with protamines, around which sperm DNA is now tightly wound. **Poor DNA packaging results in loosely wound DNA that can be demonstrably disrupted using tests such as a comet assay.** This poor packaging is thought to be caused by, amongst other etiologies, elevated levels of reactive oxygen species and deficiencies in protamine [84,88,89].

Germ cell nuclear factor (GCNF), a member of the nuclear receptor factory, is an orphan receptor expressed in both Sertoli cells and germ cells. It is implicated in early embryologic development and female fertility. In the male, GCNF mRNA is expressed preferentially during the spermatid stages of development, declining as the spermatid enters the elongate stage. Hummelke and Cooney demonstrated that expression of the protamine genes *Prm1* and *Prm2* is mediated by interference between GCNF and cAMP-responsive transcription factor (CREM-tau) [90–92]. This implicates GCNF centrally in the process of DNA condensation.

Loss of cytoplasm

Spermatid cytoplasm is removed as a residual body containing remnants of the Golgi apparatus, the chromatoid body, ribosomes, some mitochondria, and lipid droplets [93]. The residual body appears as a distinct bulge formed by caudal movement of cytoplasmic material in the spermatid [4,70]. Most residual bodies are phagocytosed by the Sertoli cells, but some are shed into the lumen of the tubule [93]. The residual body should not be confused with the cytoplasmic droplet that consists of leftover cytoplasm present in mature spermatozoa. The cytoplasmic droplet, in turn, is released into the lumen of the corpus epididymidis by the transiting spermatozoa, so that ejaculated spermatozoa have virtually no cytoplasm left, presumably in order to maximize their motility [94].

Formation of the tail

The early spermatid contains two centrioles arranged at right angles to each other. The distal longitudinal centriole, which orients parallel to the long axis of the sperm cell, gives rise to the axial filament of the flagellum, or axoneme. **The axoneme consists of microtubules arranged in the classical 2 + 9 formation of cilia (two central microtubules, surrounded by a circular arrangement of nine microtubule doublets)** [4,11,95]. The axoneme forms early in spermiogenesis, and can be seen as a protrusion from elongating spermatids, surrounded by a rim of cytoplasm [4]. This is then followed by lodging of the budding axoneme at the caudal pole of the nuclear membrane (i.e., opposite the emerging acrosomal cap), leading to the formation of the neck or connecting piece. In the meantime, outer dense fibers (ODF) are assembled from small anlagen associated with the doublets of the axoneme [96]. Thickening of the ODF continues throughout the remainder of spermiogenesis, with accretion of newly synthesized protein material, mainly Odf1, Odf2, and Spag4 (sperm-associated antigen 4) [97–99]. The fibrous sheath becomes visible slightly later, at the Sc

spermatid stage [4,96]. Its assembly proceeds from distal to proximal, taking place through most of the stages of spermiogenesis [8]. Its main components are ~80 kDa proteins known as AKAPs (cAMP-dependent kinase anchoring proteins) that are associated with sperm-specific isoforms of glycolytic enzymes [8]. The structure and composition of the fibrous sheath confirm its role in regulating flagellar motion, and its assembly requires both protein synthesis and protein degradation via the ubiquitin system [100]. Improper assembly of the periaxonemal components has been proposed as the etiology of some forms of male asthenospermia, and it is linked to abnormalities in ubiquitin-mediated degradation [95]. **Associations between abnormalities of axonemal structure and the immotile cilia syndromes, such as Kartagener and Young syndromes, are well described.**

Spermiation

Spermiation refers to the release of fully developed spermatids into the tubule lumen as mature spermatozoa. When spermatids are first formed, they are surrounded by processes of the Sertoli cell without a specific orientation, and reside close to the lumen of the tubule. As they elongate, their heads orient basally and become deeply embedded within the Sertoli cells using desmosome-like cell junctions [101]. Contact is lost caudally first, and then progressively towards the head until spermatids are attached by only a small area of the head just before spermiation. Attachment to the Sertoli cells at that point is maintained by small tubulobulbar processes of the spermatid cell membrane that project into the Sertoli cell cytoplasm [102]. At spermiation, all these attachments are lost and the spermatid is released as a free spermatozoon. While many of the cell adhesion molecules involved in the attachment of spermatids to Sertoli cells have been identified [103], the detailed mechanism of spermiation remains under investigation [104]. The facts that spermiation fails as a result of FSH and testosterone withdrawal [105], and that it is sensitive to various toxins such as cadmium [106], indicate that it is an active and complex process. Thus the yet-to-be-identified "spermiation signal" or its downstream effector is a potential target for male contraception [31].

Aspects of spermatogenesis regulation
Hormonal influences

Testosterone and FSH are the two major regulatory hormones of spermatogenesis. Both are necessary for initiation and maintenance of spermatogenesis in humans at quantitative levels [107]. Testosterone alone is capable of initiating qualitative spermatogenesis only, as evidenced by the occurrence of some spermatogenesis in a prepubertal boy with a testosterone-producing Leydig cell tumor and normal FSH levels [108].

Quantitative spermatogenesis requires high levels of testicular testosterone, which in humans are ~100-fold higher than in serum, due to the local production by Leydig cells [109]. Thus, exogenous administration of testosterone in humans leads to azoospermia or profound oligospermia even with normal circulating testosterone levels [110]. **Testosterone acts presumably via stimulation of Sertoli cells, as germ cells lack the androgen receptor** [107]. Stereological studies in male hormonal contraception trials show that exogenous testosterone administration in humans causes severe reduction in the number of B spermatogonia, followed by Ap spermatogonia [111]. In addition, spermiation is affected, with a resulting further drop in ejaculated sperm numbers. Meiosis and spermiogenesis, however, appear to proceed in humans despite lack of testosterone; this is contrary to findings in rodents, where meiosis is considered exquisitely sensitive to androgen effects and to the stage at which Sertoli cells express the highest numbers of androgen receptors [107].

A brief consideration of the regulatory mechanisms of spermatogenesis is necessary for completeness; for further information on this topic the reader is referred to Chapter 2 (on the hypothalamic–pituitary–gonadal axis) and Chapter 27 (on male contraception). This discussion will review endocrine, paracrine, and autocrine regulatory mechanisms; this topic is covered in greater detail in Chapter 4.

Endocrine regulation of spermatogenesis

Central control of spermatogenesis is mediated by the gonadotropic hormones, FSH and LH; these hormones are secreted by the anterior pituitary. This process is under the control of gonadotropin-releasing hormone (GnRH) secreted by the hypothalamus. Downstream, LH is bound by receptors on the Leydig cell and causes the production of testosterone. FSH is bound by receptors on the Sertoli cell and acts to promote maturation of spermatogenic cells [107,108] (see Fig. 4.13 in Chapter 4: specific attention is paid to downstream interactions within the testis at the cellular level). Efficient spermatogenesis depends upon the intact nature of this entire pathway.

Negative feedback in the HPG axis is mediated by inhibin and testosterone. Inhibin, a heterodimeric protein that belongs to the TGF-β family of glycoproteins, acts to decrease secretion of gonadotropins. **Secreted by Sertoli cells in response to stimulation by FSH, inhibin feeds back directly on the pituitary to inhibit transcription of the gene encoding the B subunit of FSH.** Meanwhile, testosterone feeds back directly upon both the hypothalamus and anterior pituitary to decreased secretion of both GnRH and LH together [107]. A cartoon representation of this feedback loop and the genes that influence its function is found in Figure 4.13.

A significant portion of our understanding of these molecules and their effects derives from knockout experiments performed in animals over the past several years. A brief summary of these experiments and their findings follows here.

FSH-β and FSH-receptor knockout (FORKO) mice

Initial attempts at transgenic knockout of HPG hormones targeted FSH. In 1997, **Kumar et al. successfully knocked out the β subunit of FSH in mice. Males were smaller on average, and they had smaller testes, but despite decreased numbers of epididymal and testis sperm, these animals were fertile** [112,113].

FSH receptor (FSHR) is a G-protein-coupled receptor with seven transmembrane spanning regions; Dierich et al. successfully generated knockout mice for FSHR in 1998 [114]. The phenotypic appearance of these animals was consistent with FSH-β KO animals. FORKO males were observed to enter puberty at a later stage than wild-type animals, and they did have impaired fertility.

LH-β knockout mice and LH receptor knockout mice (LHRKO)

LH receptor knockout mice (LHRKO) were generated by Lei et al. in 2001. Male knockout animals were infertile; in addition, males demonstrated varying degrees of ambiguity, with undescended testes and accessory sex organs. Treatment with testosterone did not completely reverse this phenotype and did not restore fertility. Females were also completely infertile [115].

Ma and colleagues generated knockout mice for LH-β subunit in 2004. Males were phenotypically hypogonadal; both serum and intratesticular testosterone levels were extremely low. Both male and female animals were completely infertile. On histological examination of the testes, knockout animals demonstrated few Leydig cells and no elongated spermatids. However, the ambiguous genitalia phenotype observed in LHRKO animals was not present in LH knockout animals [116].

Androgen receptor knockout mice (ARKO, SCARKO)

The above experiments clearly demonstrated the role of LH, LH receptor, and testosterone in the fertility of these animals. Confirmatory experiments using total knockout of androgen receptor and Sertoli-cell-specific knockout of androgen receptor (SCARKO) were undertaken by De Gendt in 2004 [117,118]. **ARKO mice were found to have a completely ambiguous phenotype; this parallels the phenotype of testicular feminization in the human** (complete androgen insensitivity syndrome). These animals were completely infertile [119].

SCARKO animals instead demonstrated a normal male genitourinary tract and normal testicular descent. Testis size was small, and histological examination of the testis demonstrated no evidence of late spermatids; this was despite normal numbers of Sertoli cells and apparently normal numbers of early spermatogenic cells [119].

Gene expression control

The transformation from diploid to haploid chromosomal complement and the tight packaging of DNA during spermiogenesis pose some unique constraints on gene transcription in differentiating male germ cells. Therefore **it is not surprising that germ cells possess several unique gene-expression control mechanisms**, at both the transcriptional and the translational levels. A detailed discussion of the molecular mechanisms is beyond the scope of this chapter, and we will only briefly touch upon some of the unique gene-expression features of cells of the spermatogenic cycle (for excellent reviews see [120] and [121]). A representation of the genes expressed at each level of spermatogenesis appears in Figure 5.1.

Germ-cell-specific gene isoforms

To maintain balanced gene expression, **germ cells must somehow "make up" for the loss of half of the chromosomal content during meiosis.** One mechanism to accomplish this is sharing of mRNA between sibling cells through intercellular bridges that persist due to incomplete cytokinesis after division. Another mechanism is activation of testis-specific isoforms [120]. This is particularly true of X-linked genes because the sex-chromosomes – unlike the

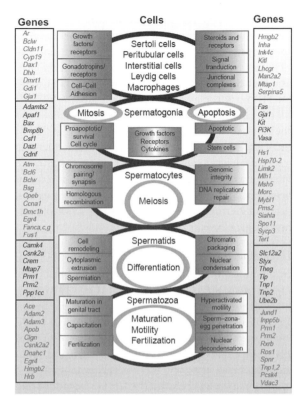

Fig. 5.1. Genes crucially involved in spermatogenesis, organized by function and location. (From Matzuk MM, Lamb DJ. Genetic dissection of mammalian fertility pathways. *Nat Cell Biol* 2002; **4**: s41–9. With permission from Macmillan Publishers Ltd. Copyright 2002.)

autosomes – are completely transcriptionally silent during the long pachytene phase, when they are heterochromatized as the XY body [122,123]. The X chromosome in mammals carries many highly conserved genes (such as enzymes of the glycolytic pathways [124,125]), which were found to be duplicated onto autosomes as retrogenes, and whose expression is restricted to testis [126].

Germ-cell-specific promoter function

The gene promoters of germ-cell-specific genes are generally shorter and more guanine-cytosine-rich than somatic promoters [120]. In addition, several of the transcription factors involved in RNA–polymerase II binding and transcription initiation have germ-cell-specific isoforms. For example, TLF (TBP-like factor) is a highly conserved protein that shares homology with TATA-binding protein (TBP). While present in all tissues, TLF is significantly overexpressed in germ cells through a separate testis-specific promoter [127]. Male TLF[-/-] mice were viable but completely sterile due to apoptosis of round spermatids [128]. These variants of core-transcription machinery give germ cells a mechanism for directing specific gene expression. Of course, more conventional signaling pathways are also operational in germ cells. **The best characterized system is arguably the CREM (cAMP response element modulator) pathway. FSH binding to its receptor activates adenylate cyclase, and the resultant rise in cAMP triggers binding of CREM to ACT (activator of CREM).** The complex then acts as a molecular master-switch for a number of genes involved in spermatogenesis [129,130]. This important role has been confirmed in CREM knockout mice, which exhibit deficient spermiogenesis, with severe restriction of post-meiotic gene expression [131].

Chromatoid body

Another fascinating element in spermatogenic gene regulation is the chromatoid body (CB). This structure, identified over 100 years ago, **consists of cloudy electron-dense material that first appears in pachytene spermatocytes, and moves around the cytoplasm in a nonrandom fashion,** associating at times with the Golgi complex, the nuclear membrane, and mitochondria [86,132,133]. The CB has been found to be devoid of DNA, instead consisting mostly of RNA and associated proteins [134]. Recently, these have been found to include the ribonuclease dicer, which cleaves double-stranded RNA to produce small interfering RNAs (siRNA) that promote the degradation of complementary mRNA in the RNA silencing pathway [135,136]. **Thus the chromatoid body appears to function in the storage and processing of RNA** [133]. Its prominence in germ cells points to the significance of the post-transcriptional control mechanisms of gene expression in spermatogenesis.

Conclusions

Spermatogenesis is one of the most fascinating biological processes observed in the animal kingdom. Billions of sperm are produced over the lifetime of one animal. A majority of them are made with an extraordinarily high degree of fidelity. Reproduction depends upon this process.

At the same time, spermatogenesis exists only in a terribly fragile balance, easily deranged by changes in hormonal milieu, genetic errors, or physiologic insults. Further investigation of spermatogenesis can help us to understand how we might prevent this derangement to the benefit of our patients. In addition, a thorough understanding of this process may lead us to discoveries such as a male contraceptive pill – a drug that would prove itself a real boon to world and public health.

This investigation, which began with the light-microscope experiments of van Leeuwenhoek, and continues today with successful experiments describing the isolation and transplantation of spermatogonial stem cells, must be grown even further. This research presents us the opportunity to identify new treatments for patients with infertility and to gain a better understanding of hormonal control of spermatogenesis. Spermatogenesis itself is a fertile ground for furthering our understanding of stem cell biology. Meaningful research in spermatogenesis must continue.

Acknowledgments

Supported in part by Grants No. 2P01 HD 36289, AUAF, and the National Institutes of Health Cooperative Centers Program in Reproductive Research (U54 HD07495) from the National Institutes of Health.

References

[1] Clermont Y. Kinetics of spermatogenesis in mammals: seminiferous epithelium cycle and spermatogonial renewal. *Physiol Rev* 1972; **52**: 198–236.

[2] Heller CG, Clermont Y. Spermatogenesis in man: an estimate of its duration. *Science* 1963; **140**: 184–6.

[3] Amann RP, Howards SS. Daily spermatozoal production and epididymal spermatozoal reserves of the human male. *J Urol* 1980; **124**: 211–15.

[4] Kerr JB, *et al.* Cytology of the testis and intrinsic control mechanisms. In: Neill JD, ed. *Knobil and Neill's Physiology of Reproduction*, 3rd edn. New York, NY: Academic Press, 1994: 827–947.

[5] Clermont Y. The cycle of the seminiferous epithelium in man. *Am J Anat* 1963; **112**: 35–51.

[6] Sutovsky P, Manandhar G. Mammalian spermatogenesis and sperm structure: anatomical and compartmental analysis. In: Jonge CJD, Barratt CLR, eds. *The Sperm Cell: Production, Maturation, Fertilization, Regeneration*. Cambridge: Cambridge University Press, 2006: 1–30.

[7] Huckins C. The spermatogonial stem cell population in adult rats. I. Their morphology, proliferation and maturation. *Anat Rec* 1971; **169**: 533–57.

[8] Eddy E. The spermatozoon. In: Neill JD, ed. *Knobil and Neill's Physiology of Reproduction*, 3rd edn. New York, NY: Academic Press, 1994: 3–54.

[9] Toshimori K. Biology of spermatozoa maturation: an overview with an introduction to this issue. *Microsc Res Tech* 2003; **61**: 1–6.

[10] Eddy EM, Toshimori K, O'Brien DA. Fibrous sheath of mammalian spermatozoa. *Microsc Res Tech* 2003; **61**: 103–15.

[11] Fawcett DW. The mammalian spermatozoon. *Dev Biol* 1975; **44**: 394–436.

[12] Prader A. Testicular size: assessment and clinical importance. *Triangle* 1966; **7**: 240–3.

[13] Lennox B, Ahmad KN. The total length of tubules in the human testis. *J Anat* 1970; **107**: 191.

[14] Heller CH, Clermont Y. Kinetics of the germinal epithelium in man. *Recent Prog Horm Res* 1964; **20**: 545–75.

[15] Leblond CP, Clermont Y. Definition of the stages of the cycle of the seminiferous epithelium in the rat. *Ann N Y Acad Sci* 1952; **55**: 548–73.

[16] Schulze W. Evidence of a wave of spermatogenesis in human testis. *Andrologia* 1982; **14**: 200–7.

[17] Clermont Y. Spermatogenesis in man: a study of the spermatogonial population. *Fertil Steril* 1966; **17**: 705–21.

[18] de Rooij DG, Russell LD. All you wanted to know about spermatogonia but were afraid to ask. *J Androl* 2000; **21**: 776–98.

[19] Print CG, Loveland KL. Germ cell suicide: new insights into apoptosis during spermatogenesis. *Bioessays* 2000; **22**: 423–30.

[20] Muller J, Skakkebaek NE. Quantification of germ cells and seminiferous tubules by stereological examination of testicles from 50 boys who suffered from sudden death. *Int J Androl* 1983; **6**: 143–56.

[21] Paniagua R, Nistal M. Morphological and histometric study of human spermatogonia from birth to the onset of puberty. *J Anat* 1984; **139**: 535–52.

[22] Rey RA, Campo SM, Bedecarrás P, Nagle CA, Chemes HE. Is infancy a quiescent period of testicular development? Histological, morphometric, and functional study of the seminiferous tubules of the cebus monkey from birth to the end of puberty. *J Clin Endocrinol Metab* 1993; **76**: 1325–31.

[23] Clermont Y. Renewal of spermatogonia in man. *Am J Anat* 1966; **118**: 509–24.

[24] Weber JE, Russell LD. A study of intercellular bridges during spermatogenesis in the rat. *Am J Anat* 1987; **180**: 1–24.

[25] Chiarini-Garcia H, Russell LD. High-resolution light microscopic characterization of mouse spermatogonia. *Biol Reprod* 2001; **65**: 1170–8.

[26] Aponte PM, van Bragt MP, de Rooij DG, van Pelt AM. Spermatogonial stem cells: characteristics and experimental possibilities. *APMIS* 2005; **113**: 727–42.

[27] Khaira H, McLean D, Ohl DA, Smith GD. Spermatogonial stem cell isolation, storage, and transplantation. *J Androl* 2005; **26**: 442–50.

[28] Schulze C. Morphological characteristics of the spermatogonial stem cells in man. *Cell Tissue Res* 1979; **198**: 191–9.

[29] van Alphen MM, van de Kant HJ, de Rooij DG. Repopulation of the seminiferous epithelium of the rhesus monkey after X irradiation. *Radiat Res* 1988; **113**: 487–500.

[30] Ehmcke J, Simorangkir DR, Schlatt S. Identification of the starting point for spermatogenesis and characterization of the testicular stem cell in adult male rhesus monkeys. *Hum Reprod* 2005; **20**: 1185–93.

[31] McLachlan RI, O'Donnell L, Meachem SJ, et al. Identification of specific sites of hormonal regulation in spermatogenesis in rats, monkeys, and man. *Recent Prog Horm Res* 2002; **57**: 149–79.

[32] Nistal M, Codesal J, Paniagua R, Santamaria L. Decrease in the number of human Ap and Ad spermatogonia and in the Ap/ Ad ratio with advancing age: new data on the spermatogonial stem cell. *J Androl* 1987; **8**: 64–8.

[33] Tegelenbosch RA, de Rooij DG. A quantitative study of spermatogonial multiplication and stem cell renewal in the C3H/101 F1 hybrid mouse. *Mutat Res* 1993; **290**: 193–200.

[34] Brinster RL, Avarbock MR. Germline transmission of donor haplotype following spermatogonial transplantation. *Proc Natl Acad Sci U S A* 1994; **91**: 11303–7.

[35] Brinster RL, Zimmermann JW. Spermatogenesis following male germ-cell transplantation. *Proc Natl Acad Sci U S A* 1994; **91**: 11298–302.

[36] Shinohara T, Orwig KE, Avarbock MR, Brinster RL. Spermatogonial stem cell enrichment by multiparameter selection of mouse testis cells. *Proc Natl Acad Sci U S A* 2000; **97**: 8346–51.

[37] Lo KC, Brugh VM, Parker M, Lamb DJ. Isolation and enrichment of murine spermatogonial stem cells using rhodamine 123 mitochondrial dye. *Biol Reprod* 2005; **72**: 767–71.

[38] Shimizu Y, Motohashi N, Iseki H, et al. A novel subpopulation lacking Oct4 expression in the testicular side population. *Int J Mol Med* 2006; **17**: 21–8.

[39] Ohta H, Yomogida K, Dohmae K, Nishimune Y. Regulation of proliferation and differentiation in spermatogonial stem cells: The role of c-kit and its ligand SCF. *Development* 2000; **127**: 2125–31.

[40] Schrans-Stassen BH, van de Kant HJ, de Rooij DG, van Pelt AM. Differential expression of c-kit in mouse undifferentiated and differentiating type A spermatogonia. *Endocrinology* 1999; **140**: 5894–900.

[41] Nagano M, Brinster CJ, Orwig KE, et al. Transgenic mice produced by retroviral transduction of male germ-line stem cells. *Proc Natl Acad Sci U S A* 2001; **98**: 13090–5.

[42] Dobrinski I. Germ cell transplantation and testis tissue xenografting in domestic animals. *Anim Reprod Sci* 2005; **89**: 137–45.

[43] Nagano M, McCarrey JR, Brinster RL. Primate spermatogonial stem cells colonize mouse testes. *Biol Reprod* 2001; **64**: 1409–16.

[44] Watt FM, Hogan BL. Out of Eden: stem cells and their niches. *Science* 2000; **287**: 1427–30.

[45] Hess RA, Cooke PS, Hofmann MC, Murphy KM. Mechanistic insights into the regulation of the spermatogonial stem cell niche. *Cell Cycle* 2006; **5**: 1164–70.

[46] Hu J, Shima H, Nakagawa H. Glial cell line-derived neurotropic factor stimulates sertoli cell proliferation in the early postnatal period of rat testis development. *Endocrinology* 1999; **140**: 3416–21.

[47] Meng X, Lindahl M, Hyvönen ME, *et al*. Regulation of cell fate decision of undifferentiated spermatogonia by GDNF. *Science*, 2000. **287**: 1489–93.

[48] Naughton CK, Jain S, Strickland AM, Gupta A, Milbrandt J. Glial cell-line derived neurotrophic factor-mediated RET signaling regulates spermatogonial stem cell fate. *Biol Reprod* 2006; **74**: 314–21.

[49] Chen C, Ouyang W, Grigura V, *et al*. ERM is required for transcriptional control of the spermatogonial stem cell niche. *Nature* 2005; **436**: 1030–4.

[50] Michaelis C, Ciosk R, Nasmyth K. Cohesins: chromosomal proteins that prevent premature separation of sister chromatids. *Cell* 1997; **91**: 35–45.

[51] Eijpe M, Offenberg H, Jessberger R, Revenkova E, Heyting C. Meiotic cohesin REC8 marks the axial elements of rat synaptonemal complexes before cohesins SMC1beta and SMC3. *J Cell Biol* 2003; **160**: 657–70.

[52] Haering CH, Nasmyth K. Building and breaking bridges between sister chromatids. *Bioessays* 2003; **25**: 1178–91.

[53] Yuan L, Liu JG, Zhao J, Brundell E, Daneholt B, Höög C. The murine SCP3 gene is required for synaptonemal complex assembly, chromosome synapsis, and male fertility. *Mol Cell* 2000; **5**: 73–83.

[54] Kleckner N, Storlazzi A, Zickler D. Coordinate variation in meiotic pachytene SC length and total crossover/chiasma frequency under conditions of constant DNA length. *Trends Genet* 2003; **19**: 623–8.

[55] Esposito MS, Esposito RE. The genetic control of sporulation in Saccharomyces. I. The isolation of temperature-sensitive sporulation-deficient mutants. *Genetics* 1969; **61**: 79–89.

[56] Keeney S, Giroux CN, Kleckner N. Meiosis-specific DNA double-strand breaks are catalyzed by Spo11, a member of a widely conserved protein family. *Cell* 1997; **88**: 375–84.

[57] Baudat F, Manova K, Yuen JP, Jasin M, Keeney S. Chromosome synapsis defects and sexually dimorphic meiotic progression in mice lacking Spo11. *Mol Cell* 2000; **6**: 989–98.

[58] Hays FA, Watson J, Ho PS. Caution! DNA crossing: crystal structures of Holliday junctions. *J Biol Chem* 2003; **278**: 49663–6.

[59] Pittman DL, Cobb J, Schimenti KJ, *et al*. Meiotic prophase arrest with failure of chromosome synapsis in mice deficient for Dmc1, a germline-specific RecA homolog. *Mol Cell* 1998; **1**: 697–705.

[60] Lynn A, Koehler KE, Judis L, *et al*. Covariation of synaptonemal complex length and mammalian meiotic exchange rates. *Science* 2002; **296**: 2222–5.

[61] Barlow AL, Hulten MA. Crossing over analysis at pachytene in man. *Eur J Hum Genet* 1998; **6**: 350–8.

[62] Gonsalves J, Sun F, Schlegel PN, *et al*. Defective recombination in infertile men. *Hum Mol Genet* 2004; **13**: 2875–83.

[63] Tesarik J, Balaban B, Isiklar A, *et al*. In-vitro spermatogenesis resumption in men with maturation arrest: Relationship with in-vivo blocking stage and serum FSH. *Hum Reprod* 2000; **15**: 1350–4.

[64] Sofikitis N, Mantzavinos T, Loutradis D, *et al*. Ooplasmic injections of secondary spermatocytes for non-obstructive azoospermia. *Lancet* 1998; **351**: 1177–8.

[65] Kimura Y, Yanagimachi R. Development of normal mice from oocytes injected with secondary spermatocyte nuclei. *Biol Reprod* 1995; **53**: 855–62.

[66] Toshimori K, Ito C. Formation and organization of the mammalian sperm head. *Arch Histol Cytol* 2003; **66**: 383–96.

[67] Bowen RH. On the idiosome, Golgi apparatus and acrosome in the male germ cells. *The Anatomical Record* 1922; **24**: 158–160.

[68] Moreno RD, Alvarado CP. The mammalian acrosome as a secretory lysosome: new and old evidence. *Mol Reprod Dev* 2006; **73**: 1430–4.

[69] Hermo L, Rambourg A, Clermont Y. Three-dimensional architecture of the cortical region of the Golgi apparatus in rat spermatids. *Am J Anat* 1980; **157**: 357–73.

[70] Sakai Y, Yamashina S. Mechanism for the removal of residual cytoplasm from spermatids during mouse spermiogenesis. *Anat Rec* 1989; **223**: 43–8.

[71] Tulsiani DR, NagDas SK, Skudlarek MD, Orgebin-Crist MC. Rat sperm plasma membrane mannosidase: localization and evidence for proteolytic processing during epididymal maturation. *Dev Biol* 1995; **167**: 584–95.

[72] Abou-Haila A, Tulsiani DR. Mammalian sperm acrosome: formation, contents, and function. *Arch Biochem Biophys* 2000; **379**: 173–82.

[73] Klemm U, Muller-Esterl W, Engel W. Acrosin, the peculiar sperm-specific serine protease. *Hum Genet* 1991; **87**: 635–41.

[74] Holstein AF, Schulze W, Davidoff M. Understanding spermatogenesis is a prerequisite for treatment. *Reprod Biol Endocrinol* 2003; **1**: 107.

[75] Dadoune JP. Expression of mammalian spermatozoal nucleoproteins. *Microsc Res Tech* 2003; **61**: 56–75.

[76] D'Occhio MJ, Hengstberger KJ, Johnston SD. Biology of sperm chromatin structure and relationship to male fertility and embryonic survival. *Anim Reprod Sci* 2007; **101**: 1–17.

[77] Meistrich ML, Mohapatra B, Shirley CR, Zhao M. Roles of transition nuclear proteins in spermiogenesis. *Chromosoma* 2003; **111**: 483–8.

[78] Hammadeh ME, Zeginiadov T, Rosenbaum P, *et al.* Predictive value of sperm chromatin condensation (aniline blue staining) in the assessment of male fertility. *Arch Androl* 2001; **46**: 99–104.

[79] Sakkas D, Urner F, Bianchi PG, *et al.* Sperm chromatin anomalies can influence decondensation after intracytoplasmic sperm injection. *Hum Reprod* 1996; **11**: 837–43.

[80] Corzett M, Mazrimas J, Balhorn R. Protamine 1: protamine 2 stoichiometry in the sperm of eutherian mammals. *Mol Reprod Dev* 2002; **61**: 519–27.

[81] Aoki VW, Emery BR, Liu L, Carrell DT. Protamine levels vary between individual sperm cells of infertile human males and correlate with viability and DNA integrity. *J Androl* 2006; **27**: 890–8.

[82] Carrell DT, Liu L. Altered protamine 2 expression is uncommon in donors of known fertility, but common among men with poor fertilizing capacity, and may reflect other abnormalities of spermiogenesis. *J Androl* 2001; **22**: 604–10.

[83] Balhorn R, Reed S, Tanphaichitr N. Aberrant protamine 1/protamine 2 ratios in sperm of infertile human males. *Experientia* 1988; **44**: 52–5.

[84] Cho C, Willis WD, Goulding EH, *et al.* Haploinsufficiency of protamine-1 or -2 causes infertility in mice. *Nat Genet* 2001; **28**: 82–6.

[85] Oliva R. Protamines and male infertility. *Hum Reprod Update* 2006; **12**: 417–35.

[86] Kotaja N, Sassone-Corsi P. The chromatoid body: a germ-cell-specific RNA-processing centre. *Nat Rev Mol Cell Biol* 2007; **8**: 85–90.

[87] Carrell DT, Liu L, Peterson CM, *et al.* Sperm DNA fragmentation is increased in couples with unexplained recurrent pregnancy loss. *Arch Androl* 2003; **49**: 49–55.

[88] Kodama H, Yamaguchi R, Fukuda J, Kasai H, Tanaka T. Increased oxidative deoxyribonucleic acid damage in the spermatozoa of infertile male patients. *Fertil Steril* 1997; **68**: 519–24.

[89] Sun JG, Jurisicova A, Casper RF. Detection of deoxyribonucleic acid fragmentation in human sperm: Correlation with fertilization in vitro. *Biol Reprod* 1997; **56**: 602–7.

[90] Hummelke GC, Meistrich ML, Cooney AJ. Mouse protamine genes are candidate targets for the novel orphan nuclear receptor, germ cell nuclear factor. *Mol Reprod Dev* 1998; **50**: 396–405.

[91] Hummelke GC, Cooney AJ. Germ cell nuclear factor is a transcriptional repressor essential for embryonic development. *Front Biosci* 2001; **6**: D1186–91.

[92] Hummelke GC, Cooney AJ. Reciprocal regulation of the mouse protamine genes by the orphan nuclear receptor germ cell nuclear factor and CREMtau. *Mol Reprod Dev* 2004; **68**: 394–407.

[93] Breucker H, Schafer E, Holstein AF. Morphogenesis and fate of the residual body in human spermiogenesis. *Cell Tissue Res* 1985; **240**: 303–9.

[94] Akbarsha MA, Latha PN, Murugaian P. Retention of cytoplasmic droplet by rat cauda epididymal spermatozoa after treatment with cytotoxic and xenobiotic agents. *J Reprod Fertil* 2000; **120**: 385–90.

[95] Escalier D. New insights into the assembly of the periaxonemal structures in mammalian spermatozoa. *Biol Reprod* 2003; **69**: 373–8.

[96] Irons MJ, Clermont Y. Formation of the outer dense fibers during spermiogenesis in the rat. *Anat Rec* 1982; **202**: 463–71.

[97] Morales CR, Oko R, Clermont Y. Molecular cloning and developmental expression of an mRNA encoding the 27 kDa outer dense fiber protein of rat spermatozoa. *Mol Reprod Dev* 1994; **37**: 229–40.

[98] Shao X, van der Hoorn FA. Self-interaction of the major 27-kilodalton outer dense fiber protein is in part mediated by a leucine zipper domain in the rat. *Biol Reprod* 1996; **55**: 1343–50.

[99] Shao X, Tarnasky HA, Lee JP, Oko R, van der Hoorn FA. Spag4, a novel sperm protein, binds outer dense-fiber protein Odf1 and localizes to microtubules of manchette and axoneme. *Dev Biol* 1999; **211**: 109–23.

[100] Sutovsky P. Ubiquitin-dependent proteolysis in mammalian spermatogenesis, fertilization, and sperm quality control: Killing three birds with one stone. *Microsc Res Tech* 2003; **61**: 88–102.

[101] Russell L. Desmosome-like junctions between Sertoli and germ cells in the rat testis. *Am J Anat* 1977; **148**: 301–12.

[102] Russell LD. Further observations on tubulobulbar complexes formed by late spermatids and Sertoli cells in the rat testis. *Anat Rec* 1979; **194**: 213–32.

[103] Wine RN, Chapin RE. Adhesion and signaling proteins spatiotemporally associated with spermiation in the rat. *J Androl* 1999; **20**: 198–213.

[104] Chung SS, Wang X, Wolgemuth DJ. Male sterility in mice lacking retinoic acid receptor alpha

involves specific abnormalities in spermiogenesis. *Differentiation* 2005; **73**: 188–98.

[105] Saito K, O'Donnell L, McLachlan RI, Robertson DM. Spermiation failure is a major contributor to early spermatogenic suppression caused by hormone withdrawal in adult rats. *Endocrinology* 2000; **141**: 2779–85.

[106] Hew KW, Ericson WA, Welsh MJ. A single low cadmium dose causes failure of spermiation in the rat. *Toxicol Appl Pharmacol* 1993; **121**: 15–21.

[107] O'Donnell L, *et al*. Endocrine regulation of spermatogenesis. In: Neill JD, ed. *Knobil and Neill's Physiology of Reproduction*, 3rd edn. New York, NY: Academic Press, 1994: 1017–69.

[108] Steinberger E, Root A, Ficher M, Smith KD. The role of androgens in the initiation of spermatogenesis in man. *J Clin Endocrinol Metab* 1973; **37**: 746–51.

[109] Jarow JP, Zirkin BR. The androgen microenvironment of the human testis and hormonal control of spermatogenesis. *Ann N Y Acad Sci* 2005; **1061**: 208–20.

[110] Coviello AD, Bremner WJ, Matsumoto AM, *et al*. Intratesticular testosterone concentrations comparable with serum levels are not sufficient to maintain normal sperm production in men receiving a hormonal contraceptive regimen. *J Androl* 2004; **25**: 931–8.

[111] Zhengwei Y, Wreford NG, Royce P, de Kretser DM, McLachlan RI. Stereological evaluation of human spermatogenesis after suppression by testosterone treatment: Heterogeneous pattern of spermatogenic impairment. *J Clin Endocrinol Metab* 1998; **83**: 1284–91.

[112] Kumar TR, Low MJ, Matzuk MM. Genetic rescue of follicle-stimulating hormone beta-deficient mice. *Endocrinology* 1998; **139**: 3289–95.

[113] Kumar TR, Wang Y, Lu N, Matzuk MM. Follicle stimulating hormone is required for ovarian follicle maturation but not male fertility. *Nat Genet* 1997; **15**: 201–4.

[114] Dierich A, Sairam MR, Monaco L, *et al*. Impairing follicle-stimulating hormone (FSH) signaling in vivo: targeted disruption of the FSH receptor leads to aberrant gametogenesis and hormonal imbalance. *Proc Natl Acad Sci U S A* 1998; **95**: 13612–17.

[115] Lei ZM, Mishra S, Zou W, *et al*. Targeted disruption of luteinizing hormone/human chorionic gonadotropin receptor gene. *Mol Endocrinol* 2001; **15**: 184–200.

[116] Ma X, Dong Y, Matzuk MM, Kumar TR. Targeted disruption of luteinizing hormone beta-subunit leads to hypogonadism, defects in gonadal steroidogenesis, and infertility. *Proc Natl Acad Sci U S A* 2004; **101**: 17294–9.

[117] De Gendt K, Atanassova N, Tan KA, *et al*. Development and function of the adult generation of Leydig cells in mice with Sertoli cell-selective or total ablation of the androgen receptor. *Endocrinology* 2005; **146**: 4117–26.

[118] De Gendt K, Swinnen JV, Saunders PT, *et al*. A Sertoli cell-selective knockout of the androgen receptor causes spermatogenic arrest in meiosis. *Proc Natl Acad Sci U S A* 2004; **101**: 1327–32.

[119] Denolet E, De Gendt K, Allemeersch J, *et al*. The effect of a sertoli cell-selective knockout of the androgen receptor on testicular gene expression in prepubertal mice. *Mol Endocrinol* 2006; **20**: 321–34.

[120] DeJong J. Basic mechanisms for the control of germ cell gene expression. *Gene* 2006; **366**: 39–50.

[121] Eddy EM. Male germ cell gene expression. *Recent Prog Horm Res* 2002; **57**: 103–28.

[122] Solari AJ. The behavior of the XY pair in mammals. *Int Rev Cytol* 1974; **38**: 273–317.

[123] Richler C, Ast G, Goitein R, *et al*. Splicing components are excluded from the transcriptionally inactive XY body in male meiotic nuclei. *Mol Biol Cell* 1994; **5**: 1341–52.

[124] Hendriksen PJ, Hoogerbrugge JW, Baarends WM, *et al*. Testis-specific expression of a functional retroposon encoding glucose-6-phosphate dehydrogenase in the mouse. *Genomics* 1997; **41**: 350–9.

[125] McCarrey JR, Thomas K. Human testis-specific PGK gene lacks introns and possesses characteristics of a processed gene. *Nature* 1987; **326**: 501–5.

[126] Wang PJ. X chromosomes, retrogenes and their role in male reproduction. *Trends Endocrinol Metab* 2004; **15**: 79–83.

[127] Sugiura S, Kashiwabara S, Iwase S, Baba T. Expression of a testis-specific form of TBP-related factor 2 (TRF2) mRNA during mouse spermatogenesis. *J Reprod Dev* 2003; **49**: 107–11.

[128] Martianov I, Fimia GM, Dierich A, *et al*. Late arrest of spermiogenesis and germ cell apoptosis in mice lacking the TBP-like TLF/TRF2 gene. *Mol Cell* 2001; **7**: 509–15.

[129] Foulkes NS, Mellström B, Benusiglio E, Sassone-Corsi P. Developmental switch of CREM function during spermatogenesis: from antagonist to activator. *Nature* 1992; **355**: 80–4.

[130] Monaco L, Kotaja N, Fienga G, *et al*. Specialized rules of gene transcription in male germ cells: the CREM paradigm. *Int J Androl* 2004; **27**: 322–7.

[131] Blendy JA, Kaestner KH, Weinbauer GF, Nieschlag E, Schütz G. Severe impairment of spermatogenesis in mice lacking the CREM gene. *Nature* 1996; **380**: 162–5.

[132] Parvinen M, Parvinen LM. Active movements of the chromatoid body: a possible transport mechanism for haploid gene products. *J Cell Biol* 1979; **80**: 621–8.

[133] Parvinen M. The chromatoid body in spermatogenesis. *Int J Androl* 2005; **28**: 189–201.

[134] Biggiogera M, Fakan S, Leser G, Martin TE, Gordon J. Immunoelectron microscopical visualization of ribonucleoproteins in the chromatoid body of mouse spermatids. *Mol Reprod Dev* 1990; **26**: 150–8.

[135] Kotaja N, Bhattacharyya SN, Jaskiewicz L, *et al*. The chromatoid body of male germ cells: similarity with processing bodies and presence of Dicer and microRNA pathway components. *Proc Natl Acad Sci U S A* 2006; **103**: 2647–52.

[136] Zamore PD, Haley B. Ribo-gnome: the big world of small RNAs. *Science* 2005; **309**: 1519–24.

Chapter 6

The epididymis and accessory sex organs

Terry T. Turner

Urogenital embryology

The urogenital tract of males and females is identical prior to the seventh week of human development [1]. Before the seventh week, genetic males and females have both Müllerian and Wolffian duct systems, but at the end of this indifferent phase of sexual differentiation, the dual duct systems form the primordia of the internal, accessory organs of reproduction (Fig. 6.1). **Two secretory substances of the testes, anti-Müllerian hormone (AMH), also called Müllerian-inhibiting substance (MIS), and testosterone, induce masculine extragonadal differentiation.** Genetic males and females are both responsive to the masculinizing effects of the testis; thus, in some circumstances, the karyotype of extragonadal cells may not be consistent with the differentiation of the internal reproductive structures.

If the fetus is a genetic male, the *Sry* gene on the Y chromosome encodes the testis-determining factor (TDF), and in the seventh week of gestation primitive sex cords penetrate the formerly indifferent gonad. Clearly, other gene expressions are required for testis development, among whose products are SOX-9, DAX-1, GATA-4, and DHH [2]. Some of these genes may be direct targets of TDF. The sex cords become the seminiferous tubules containing primitive germ cells and Sertoli cells, and the initial endocrine function of those Sertoli cells is the secretion of AMH, a 70 kDa glycoprotein that causes regression of the Müllerian ducts [3]. Although AMH has been purified and much is known about the structure of the protein and the genes that encode the protein, the mechanism of its action remains incompletely understood [4].

In the presence of a normal testis producing AMH, the Müllerian system regresses. Development of the Müllerian system does not require secretions from the fetal ovaries since the female phenotype occurs in the absence of the gonads. **Müllerian regression** is followed by transformation of the Wolffian ducts into the male excurrent duct system (Fig. 6.1). The upper segment becomes the epididymis; the middle portion, the vas deferens; and the terminal area, the ejaculatory duct and seminal vesicles. This differentiation of the Wolffian duct is completed in humans by day 84 of gestation [5].

The intimately associated urinary and reproductive tracts both develop from the mesodermal ridge, a mass of intermediate mesoderm along the posterior wall of the abdominal cavity. The nephrogenic cords and the urogenital ridges appear by 25 days in the human embryo, long before the primordial germ cells begin their migration from the yolk sac. During subsequent development of the kidneys a series of intermediate renal structures appears, which are the pronephros, mesonephros, and metanephros. The pronephros is nonfunctioning and is replaced by the mesonephros by the fifth week of life. In some species, possibly including the human, the mesonephros becomes a transiently functioning primitive kidney, but the permanent kidney arises later from the metanephros, which is also beginning to appear in the fifth week. Over the next few weeks the mesonephros degenerates as the metanephros develops, but in the male embryo the distal regions of the mesonephros persist to become the excurrent ducts of the male reproductive tract [3].

The mesonephric duct becomes the epididymis and vas deferens, and the residual mesonephric tubules form the efferent ducts. The efferent ducts unite with the rete testis, thus making the connection between the separately developing testis and the excurrent duct system. Mesonephric tubules failing to connect with the rete testis typically atrophy, but a few may persist as paraepididymides or appendices of the epididymis. Gene expressions necessary for epididymal development at these early stages include members

Infertility in the Male, 4th edition, ed. Larry I. Lipshultz, Stuart S. Howards, and Craig S. Niederberger. Published by Cambridge University Press. © Cambridge University Press 2009.

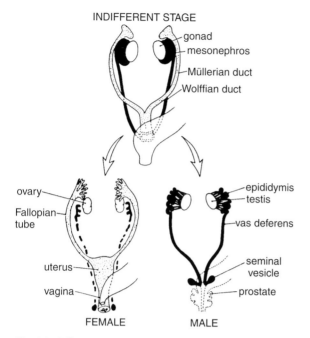

INDIFFERENT STAGE

gonad
mesonephros
Müllerian duct
Wolffian duct

ovary
Fallopian tube
uterus
vagina
FEMALE

epididymis
testis
vas deferens
seminal vesicle
prostate
MALE

Fig. 6.1. Differentiation of female and male internal genitalia from the indifferent stage. (From Wilson JD *et al*. The hormonal control of sexual development. *Science* 1981; **211**: 1278–80. Copyright 1981 by American Association for the Advancement of Science. Used with permission.)

of the Wnt family, e.g., *Wnt4*, *Wnt7α*, a number of homeobox genes, e.g., *Hoxa10*, *Hoxa11*, *Hoxd13*, and so-called paired-box genes, e.g., *Pax2* and *Pax8* [2]. Since the adult efferent ducts and epididymis share a common origin with the primitive kidney, it is not surprising that congenital absence of the vas deferens or epididymis is occasionally associated with concurrent, ipsilateral renal agenesis [6].

Any genetic defect that inhibits testosterone biosynthesis can result in abnormal development of the epididymis, although very early development of the accessory sex organs may well be independent of the hypothalamic–pituitary–gonadal axis. It seems that testosterone–androgen receptor complexes clearly mediate later fetal Wolffian duct virilization and 5α-dihydrotestosterone (DHT)–androgen receptor complexes mediate differentiation of the male external genitalia [5]. This could explain why patients with 5α-reductase deficiency and the inability to convert testosterone to DHT have normally virilized internal genitalia (epididymis, vas deferens, prostate, seminal vesicle, and ejaculatory duct), but predominately female external genitalia. On the other hand, patients with a disorder of the androgen receptors, such as those

with testicular feminization, fail to develop Wolffian structures and appear as phenotypic females [7].

Additionally, Cunha *et al.* have established the significance of epithelial–mesenchymal interactions in the prenatal development of urogenital sinus (prostate) and Wolffian duct (epididymis, vas deferens, seminal vesicles) structures [8]. The mesenchyme of these tissues also likely plays an important role in postnatal development and maintenance of adult accessory sex organs. The adult structure and function of these organs will be discussed below with a primary emphasis on the epididymis, since its contribution to the ejaculate is required for natural-mating fertility. That does not appear to be the case with the other organs, individually.

The epididymis

Direct studies of the human epididymis are uncommon. **Nonpathological specimens of men within their reproductive years are understandably difficult to obtain, and even when such epididymides are made available, they often lack the proper preservation for good biological studies**; nevertheless, some attributes of the tissue can be evaluated directly.

As the human epididymis appears upon surgical exposure, the distal portion disappears into the epididymal fat (Fig. 6.2a). This makes it appear that the epididymis has almost no cauda. In fact, the human epididymis is 10–12 cm long before becoming the convoluted vas (Fig. 6.2b), and the coiled, convoluted vas extends for another 7–8 cm (these estimates refer to the length of the epididymal organ, not to the length of the uncoiled epididymal tubule). So, while it does not appear that the human epididymis has a bulbous cauda for sperm storage, as occurs in most nonprimate species [9], the "tail" of the human epididymis contains at least 50% of the sperm present in the epididymis [10,11], a percentage similar to that in other species with bulbous caudae [12]. Since the demarcation of the tail or the cauda of the epididymis has been unclear in most human studies, it seems likely that much of this sperm storage capacity is in what some would call the proximal convoluted vas (Fig. 6.2). It seems, then, that the bulbous cauda seen in most species is simply extended into what is called the proximal convoluted vas in the human, and the high proportion of epididymal sperm stored in the distal tubule implies that a relatively large, functional cauda still exists in the human.

Histology of the epididymis reflects the fact that the bulk of the caput epididymidis consists of efferent

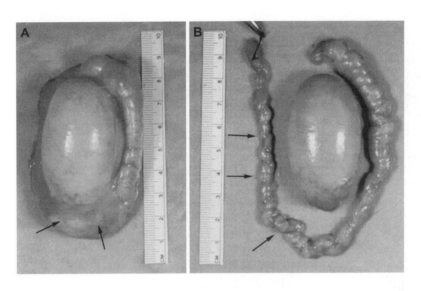

Fig. 6.2. The human testis and epididymis. (A) The testis and epididymis as taken from the scrotum; the distal part of the organ disappears into the epididymal fat pad (arrows). (B) The testis and epididymis after dissection, illustrating the absence of enlarged cauda epididymidis but an extensive convoluted vas deferens (arrows).

duct tubules and the cauda is the site of sperm storage (Fig. 6.3). Of the six types of efferent duct epithelium [13], Figure 6.3 illustrates only one (type 2), with the tissues taken from the regions illustrated by the arrows. By the midcorpus, the epithelium has taken on the appearance of a tall, relatively uniform, stereociliated, columnar epithelium, and in the cauda, the epithelium surrounding the enlarged tubule lumen, has become very short, allowing room for maximum sperm storage and reflecting the lower metabolic activity of this epithelium relative to that of the more proximal duct.

Anatomy texts typically report the uncoiled epididymal tubule to be 6–7 m long, though the origin of this estimate is uncertain. **Epididymal transit time for human sperm has been estimated to require 2–6 days** [10,11], in contrast to transit times estimated for most other species, which are consistently greater than 10 days regardless of the presumed or measured length of the epididymal tubule [14]. In the rat, for example, epididymal transit time has been estimated to be approximately 13 days in a tubule measuring 3.2 m from initial segment through cauda [15]. **An important consequence of rapid epididymal transit in the human is that sperm maturation in the caput and corpus epididymidis must happen very quickly relative to other species.** This, in turn, may be related to results from clinical cases in which at least some sperm experiencing very little epididymal transit are said to be fertile.

The epididymis contributes to a fertile ejaculate through four classical functions: sperm maturation, sperm transport, sperm concentration, and sperm storage. Each of these is considered below.

Sperm maturation

Silber reported two cases in which human males with patent efferent duct–vas deferens anastomoses (efferentiovasostomy) achieved natural-mating pregnancies with their partners [16]. He subsequently reported that 16 of 37 patients (43%) with patent caput vasoepididymostomies were eventually able to achieve a pregnancy with their partners using natural methods [17]. Schoysman and Bedford had also previously reported pregnancies after caput vasoepididymostomies [18]. The implication of these reports was that functional maturity of at least some human sperm has been gained with either no or relatively little epididymal transit. These reports raised the issue of whether or not the human epididymis is truly necessary for human sperm maturation.

It is well established that mammalian sperm, in general, mature in the epididymis, and the changes that occur in sperm during maturation have been recently reviewed [19]. Gene and protein expressions vary along the duct [20,21], leading to a changing intraluminal microenvironment for the maturing spermatozoa [22,23]. This sperm maturation process can be compared across species if sperm development characteristics are scaled on a common model as in Figure 6.4. This illustration scales data from mice, boars, and humans along an abscissa reflecting a common proportionate length of tubule in the initial segment, caput, corpus, and cauda epididymidis. The scale used in this model is that of the rat, the only species in which segment lengths have been reported [15].

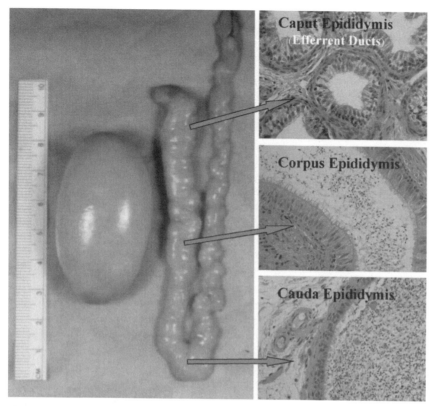

Fig. 6.3. The histology of the adult human epididymis. Much of the caput epididymidis is actually efferent duct tubule, of which there are several leading to the single true epididymal tubule. Based on histological appearance, there are six types of ciliated efferent duct tubule [13], of which only type 2 is illustrated. In the midcorpus region there is a single, highly coiled epididymal tubule with a tall, columnar, stereociliated epithelium. Sperm concentration is increasing in the epididymal lumen. In the cauda epididymidis, a short, stereociliated epithelium surrounds the large tubule lumen full of densely packed spermatozoa. *See color plate section.*

Different measurements of sperm maturation are illustrated in Figure 6.4 (e.g., percent progressive motility, percent ova fertilized with intrauterine insemination, percent ova fertilized with in-vitro fertilization (IVF), and percent ova-binding spermatozoa after subzonal injection). **The overall data reflect the obvious trends that sperm motility and fertilizing potential increase dramatically from caput to cauda epididymidis.** In the mouse and boar, as well as other species, the most striking increases in maturation occur between distal caput epididymidis and the proximal cauda. Thus, sperm maturation is essentially complete when sperm arrive in the proximal cauda epididymidis. In the human epididymis, the increasing sperm maturation parameters between proximal and distal epididymis appear to be less dramatic than in the other species (Fig. 6.4), but the function of mature human sperm in these epididymides could be limited by natural consequences; i.e., unobstructed human epididymides are typically acquired from patients well

beyond their reproductive years, and the function of even normally ejaculated cells could be compromised in those patients.

It is important to note that the data in Figure 6.4 are all from sperm obtained from unobstructed epididymides, and regardless of the species studied, sperm from the caput epididymidis are essentially immotile and infertile. They gain the capacity for motility and fertility during epididymal transit [24].

Schoysman and Bedford [18] first reported that fertile ejaculates could occur in the human, even though the ejaculated sperm had bypassed most of the epididymis. Silber subsequently reported pregnancies following bilateral caput vasoepididymostomies and even bilateral efferentiovasostomies [16,17], and in more recent years others have reported pregnancies following caput vasoepididymostomies and natural mating (as opposed to additional assistance from advanced reproductive technologies, such as IVF and intracytoplasmic sperm injection

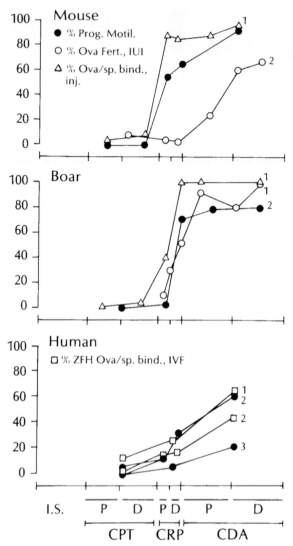

Fig. 6.4. Evidence of sperm maturation in the epididymides of mouse, boar, and human. The data extracted are percent progressive motility, percent ova fertilized after intrauterine insemination, percent ova binding spermatozoa after subzonal injection, or percent zona-free hamster (ZFH) ova binding human sperm after in vitro insemination. I.S., initial segment; P, proximal; D, distal; CPT, caput; CRP, corpus; CDA, cauda. The references noted by numbers in each panel are as follows: **Mouse**: (1) Lacham O, Trounson A. *Mol Reprod Dev* 1991; **29**: 85; (2) Pavlok A. *J Reprod Fertil* 1974; **35**: 303. **Boar**: (1) Hunter AG, *et al. J Reprod Fertil* 1976; **46**: 463; (2) Dacheux JL, Paquignon M. *Reprod Nutr Dev* 1980; **20**: 1085. **Human**: (1) Hinrichsen MJ, Blaquier JA. *J Reprod Fertil* 1980; **60**: 291; (2) Moore HDM, *et al. Int J Androl* 1983; **6**: 310; (3) Turner TT. Unpublished data from micropuncture of epididymides from men > 50 years of age immediately after orchiectomy for prostatic cancer, 1993.

[ICSI], which make fewer demands for sperm maturation).

The consensus is that after vasoepididymostomy, the chances for development of a fertile ejaculate

increases with the length of the epididymis the sperm were able to transit [16,17,25,26]. The only paradox is that 20–40% of patients whose sperm are exposed to only the initial part of the caput eventually become fertile, even if the time to pregnancy exceeds the conventional one year of most fertility trials. Silber, for example, noted that some of his fertile patients required up to four years of attempting pregnancy before success was achieved [17]. That caveat aside, reports do indicate that a significant minority of patients with severely abbreviated epididymides can eventually acquire a fertile ejaculate even if, overall, the motility and fertility of those sperm remain quite low.

Since some sperm that have been exposed to only a short portion of the epididymis can fertilize an egg in vivo, it is not surprising that sperm in epididymal aspirates from the obstructed proximal epididymis can fertilize an egg in vitro. **It is now well established that the proximal regions of an obstructed epididymis can yield sperm with a relatively high fertility potential when used with ICSI or even conventional IVF.** In fact, due to the increasing experience with pairing surgical aspiration techniques with ICSI, current inquiries are no longer about the in-vitro fertility of sperm from the different regions of the epididymis, but about the in-vitro fertility of sperm collected directly from the testis [27].

The use of aspirated sperm in ICSI bypasses the requirement that sperm be motile and be able to acrosome react, penetrate the zona, bind to the egg plasma membrane, fuse with the membrane, and complete fertilization on their own. Even in IVF, there is no requirement for survival in seminal plasma, then in cervical mucus, in the uterine environment, and finally in the oviductal fluids. Neither is there a need for the kind of motility capable of propelling the sperm through the cervical mucus into the uterus and through the uterotubal junction where it must still propel itself into the oviduct en route to the site of fertilization; thus, in either ICSI or IVF it is not surprising that the epididymis can be bypassed either in part (IVF) or in toto (ICSI). It is surprising, however, that spermatozoa can acquire the necessary characteristics for fertilization in vivo without having to pass through a substantial length of epididymal tubule. At first glance, this would not be expected, and it is reasonable to question how such a thing can occur.

Caput vasoepididymostomy and efferentiovasostomy allow for either brief or no exposure of sperm to the epididymal microenvironment. In both cases, however, sperm cells are exposed to the vas deferens microenvironment. One possible explanation for sperm maturation in these situations is that long-term obstruction causes remodeling of the caput or efferent duct epithelium, and the changes there make the proximal microenvironment more conducive to sperm maturation. A positive indication of this is that changes in caput protein secretion induced by vasectomy have been shown not to return to normal after vasovasostomy in the rat model [28]. A second possibility is that the microenvironment of the vas deferens may be more suitable for sperm maturation than is commonly appreciated.

In the rare reported cases of natural-mating fertility after efferentiovasostomy, sperm have been exposed to no epididymal microenvironment at all and have only the vas exposure to assist in maturation. While this would seem to make a fertile ejaculate even more improbable, there is an explanation of how even this could occur. **Sperm cell maturation presumably follows a Gaussian distribution; i.e., a few cells will mature much more easily than the average and a few cells will mature much less easily than the average.** A small minority of sperm cells, those tending toward very early maturation, may find sufficient stimulation in the microenvironment of the efferent ducts and vas deferens to reach functional maturity. This could lead to an occasional, perhaps even rare, fertile ejaculate. In the case of Silber's two patients with efferentiovasostomy [29], for example, it took longer than a year for a pregnancy to be achieved, but it may be fair to assume that the vigor of the attempt was substantial. The fertile sperm might have been rare, indeed.

The situation with sperm aspiration is different than with proximal tubule reconstruction. Sperm from caput epididymidal or even testicular aspirations are exposed to little or no epididymal secretion and to no vas deferens secretion. These sperm cells have considerable fertility potential in the assisted reproductive technology (ART) setting, because the requirements put upon them are quite different than in the cases of vasoepididymostomy and natural mating. As already mentioned, aspirated sperm used in ART procedures are not required to possess all the motility and survival capacities of sperm cells attempting natural fertilization. For such sperm there is no exposure to seminal plasma, no deposition in the vagina, no movement required through the viscous cervical fluids, and no exposure to potentially damaging uterine or oviductal environments. With these impediments removed,

sperm with an even less complete maturation than those found in an ejaculate after caput vasoepididymostomy might reasonably be expected to fertilize an ovum in vitro.

There is also the apparent paradox that sperm aspirated more proximally in the obstructed epididymis appear to have greater motility and fertility than do sperm collected more distally [29–31], which seems counter to the idea that the greater the length of tubule traversed, the greater the fertility potential the sperm should have. In fact, this paradox arises only because the more distally one moves along the patent tubule, the closer one becomes to the obstruction site. The "sperm pack" at the obstruction site is also the site of sperm degeneration and the filling of the lumen with cell debris. Moving upstream from the obstruction site, i.e., toward the more proximal caput and the efferent ducts, allows the operator to access tubules with a higher proportion of intact, grossly normal cells. This helps explain the improved motility and fertility characteristics found in cells collected more proximally than distally when approaching the site of obstruction. It remains true that the longer the unobstructed portion of epididymis above the obstruction, the better the chance of achieving fertility with sperm aspiration [30,31], even if the sperm aspiration is performed at a site relatively proximal to the site of obstruction.

It is also the case that some degree of sperm mixing between proximal and distal sites can occur, especially in the obstructed epididymis. **Sperm movement through the epididymis is positive and pendular; that is, the fluid moves back and forth in the tubule even as it makes net progress down the tubule** [15]. This back and forth movement of lumen content establishes a potential for sperm mixing as the cells make their way down the epididymal tubule, and it has been our general observation in acute, in-vivo experiments in laboratory animals that the vigor of the back and forth surges tends to increase with epididymal obstruction. In the case of chronically obstructed human epididymides, it seems likely that this type of movement of luminal content over several days could result in the eventual mixing of sperm from a more distal part of the patent duct with sperm from a more proximal portion; thus, sperm which have been exposed to the secretion of some more distal parts of the obstructed tubule could be found in the more proximal region, where sperm aspiration might occur. Such a phenomenon would explain why greater epididymal length is associated with increased likelihood of sperm fertility, even though sperm aspiration occurs much more proximally than the actual end of the patent tubule.

Sperm maturation occurs as sperm are exposed to the specialized intraluminal microenvironment within the epididymal lumen. This microenvironment is made up of the secretory products of the seminiferous and epididymal epithelia, and the list of proteins and small organic molecules secreted into the epididymis is long [14,20,23]. **Multiple reports have demonstrated that epididymal proteins are acquired by epididymal sperm cell membranes and that they affect such characteristics as sperm–zona binding, sperm binding to the egg membrane, membrane fusion, and fertility** [32,33]. Because of this protein–sperm interaction, a number of laboratories are currently investigating the molecular regulation of epithelial gene expression and protein synthesis and secretion in hopes of identifying the specific mechanisms underlying sperm maturation. Such mechanisms can potentially be useful in further understanding of male infertility as well as in male contraceptive development.

For example, microarray analysis of all 10 segments of the mouse epididymis has revealed the gene expression patterns of over 30 000 gene transcripts [34]. Many of these gene expressions are highly regulated along the length of the epididymis (Fig. 6.5). Electronic data mining of human genome datasets can find homologous genes expressed in the human epididymis and determine which expressions in the human are unique to the epididymis. Further studies of the products (proteins) of these highly selected, epididymal-specific genes can detect which may be subject to interference by specifically designed drugs, thus making them potentially useful in male contraceptive strategies [35,36].

Sperm transport

The propelling forces for sperm transport through the epididymis are (1) hydrostatic pressure from fluid secretion in the testis, and (2) peristaltic contractions of the tubule [15]. There has been little development in this area in recent years, but empirical observation during in-vivo micropuncture experiments indicates that

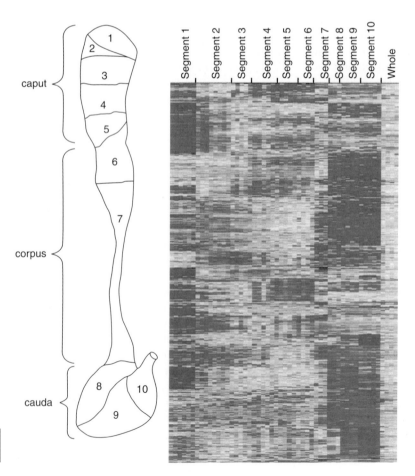

Fig. 6.5. Illustration of the segments of the mouse epididymis and gene expression patterns in each segment. Left: schematic of segmentation; segments consist of lobules of coiled tubule separated by connective tissue septa. Right: heat map of the 1100 most highly regulated genes in the different epididymal segments as determined by microarray analysis of gene expression in each segment [34]. Colors indicate relative expression level: red, high; white, moderate; blue, low. Results from multiple microarray analyses (3–6) of each segment are displayed. These results indicate that individual segments or groups of contiguous segments can be unique in their gene expression profiles, which implies a functional difference between those segments. *See color plate section.*

the contractile activity, and the subsequent back and forth agitation of the luminal contents, increases with increasing intraluminal pressure. How such neurogenic activity is stimulated, and the role of intraluminal pressure in the regulation of normal intraluminal fluid movement, remains unknown.

Net fluid transport rates are rapid in the proximal epididymis, where fluid is nonviscous and water is being rapidly absorbed from the lumen, but transport rates slow considerably in the distal tubule, where the lumen content can be quite viscous and little water absorption is occurring. As stated previously, the time required for sperm to transit the epididymis has been assessed in a variety of ways and is notable for its relative consistency between species (10–13 days) except for humans (2–6 days) [14]. The amount of time the human sperm spends in the proximal epididymis is consequently relatively short, and this may relate to the relative rapidity with which human sperm are matured.

Regulation of fluid movement along the epididymal lumen might be more important than generally recognized, since the concentration of secreted or absorbed molecules present in luminal fluid at any point along a duct is a function of proluminal and antiluminal epithelial transport activities and the time the intraluminal fluid is exposed to the ductal epithelium. In the case of the epididymal lumen fluid, the concentrations of ions, organic molecules, or specific proteins are likely important for sperm maturation or for later, downstream activities of the epididymal epithelium. For example, the relatively high sodium ion and chloride ion concentrations in the efferent ducts and proximal epididymis allow for antiluminal sodium ion and chloride ion pumping, which leads to vigorous reabsorption of water from the lumen [23,37] and subsequent concentration of spermatozoa. Radically altered rates of movement of luminal content down the epididymal tubule could alter the amount of fluid reabsorbed at any one point, and this could affect the final concentration of sperm awaiting ejaculation.

Sperm concentration

The sperm-concentrating ability of the epididymis has been established for many years [38,39], and this concentrating effect is due to fluid reabsorption subsequent to antiluminal electrolyte transport [37,40]. In rats and mice, 90–95% of fluid leaving the rete testis has been reabsorbed by the time the remaining fluid reaches the caput epididymidis (Fig. 6.6). Previous investigators have suggested that catecholamines [41],

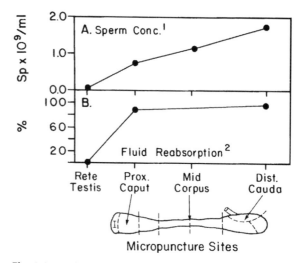

Fig. 6.6. Intraluminal sperm concentrations in the rat epididymis and the percentage of fluid coming over from the rete testis that has been reabsorbed by the time the sperm cells reach the proximal caput or distal cauda epididymidis. The references referred to by numbers are: (1) Turner TT, Cesarini DM. *J Androl* 1983; **3**: 197 [42]; (2) Turner TT. *Ann NY Acad Sci* 1991; **637**: 364 [22].

aldosterone [42,43], and the renin–angiotensin system [44] play a regulatory role in this fluid reabsorption, making the mechanism of lumen volume regulation in vivo very complex. Ion transport channels such as the cystic fibrosis transmembrane conductance regulator (a cAMP-activated chloride channel) and antiluminal sodium transporters cause osmotic shifts that draw water through aquaporin channels in the cell membranes [45]. The regulators mentioned previously can influence these transporters and either stimulate or repress the regulation of net water movement out of the epididymal lumen.

Understanding the regulation of water reabsorption, and thus the regulation of sperm concentration, in the epididymal lumen could be important to a more general understanding of how intraluminal molecules, especially those other than androgens, play a role in the regulation of the epididymis.

Sperm storage

Approximately 55–65% of total epididymal sperm are stored in the human cauda epididymidis [46]. While sperm can pass through this portion of the tubule within 3–13 days, depending on species [14], fertile sperm can be stored for longer periods [47]. Little is understood about the characteristics of the luminal environment that are pertinent to sperm storage because this aspect of epididymal function, including the cell and tissue

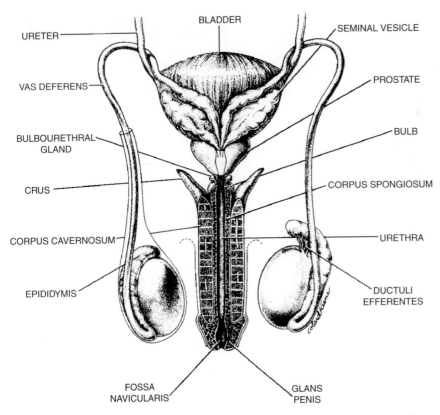

Fig. 6.7. Schematic illustration of the male reproductive tract depicting the major structures and accessory sex glands. (From Dym M. The male reproductive system. In: Weiss L, Greep RO, eds. *Histology*. New York, NY: McGraw-Hill, 1977: 980. Used with permission.)

biology of the cauda epididymal epithelium, has been largely ignored. **Specific proteins secreted into the lumen by the more proximal epithelium, as well as intraluminal ionic concentrations and osmolality, have been shown to play a role in maintaining sperm in a quiescent state in the cauda of several species [48], and, doubtless, providing protection against xenobiotics and oxidative stress is also important to the storage of viable sperm [14,49].**

Caudal sperm in aged men exhibit significantly less progressive motility than do cells from their corpus epididymidis [50]. This may seem to stand convention on its ear, but it was speculated to be due to the fact that the epididymides studied were obtained from sexually inactive, older men with extended periods of sperm storage. This explanation makes intuitive sense, but the observation illustrates the necessity for developing new information on the biology of the cauda epididymidis and its role in maintaining fertile spermatozoa.

In conclusion, it is clear that the epididymis makes a significant contribution to the development of a fertile ejaculate. Most investigations of the last quarter-century have focused on the role of the epididymis in sperm maturation, and have provided information on various aspects of epididymal sperm biology, on the characteristics of the luminal microenvironment, and on the cell and molecular biology of the epididymal epithelium. These studies have largely focused on the mechanisms supporting sperm maturation, with much less investment in understanding the other epididymal functions of sperm transport, sperm concentration, and sperm storage.

The prostate

The prostate develops embryologically from the genitourinary sinus [51,52] during the third month of fetal life, and develops postnatally under the influence of testosterone, dihydrotestosterone, and a variety of growth factors in a complex cross-talk between mesenchymal cells and the prostatic epithelium [53]. In the adult human the prostate is made up of 30–50 tubuloalveolar glands all opening to the prostatic urethra [52,54]. The gland is inferior to the bladder and surrounds the proximal portion of the urethra

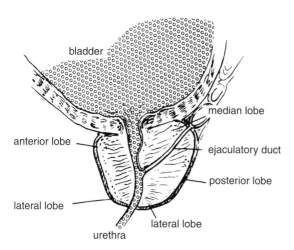

Fig. 6.8. Schematic illustration of a transverse section of the prostate identifying the anterior, lateral, and posterior "lobes" of the prostate. (From Kovi J. *Surgical Pathology of the Prostate and Seminal Vesicles*. Boca Raton, FL: CRC Press, 1989: 5. Used with permission.)

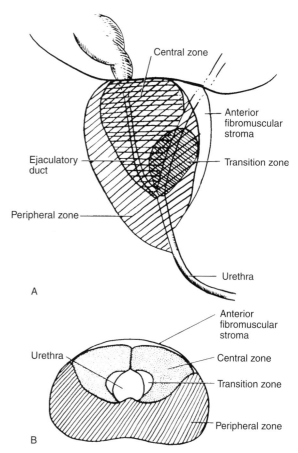

Fig. 6.9. Illustration of the zones of the prostate as suggested by McNeal [54,55]. The peripheral zone is the site of origin for most prostatic cancers, and the transition zone is the site of origin of benign prostatic hypertrophy. (From Lepor H, Lawson RK. *Prostatic Diseases*. Philadelphia, PA: Saunders, 1993: 19. Used with permission.)

where it emerges from the bladder (Fig. 6.7). The prostate averages 3.4 cm in length, 4.4 cm in width, and 2.6 cm in depth [54,55], and is often described as approximately the size of a walnut. The glands of the prostate are made up of a tall columnar epithelium embedded in a fibromuscular stroma.

The urethra and ejaculatory ducts divide the prostate into ventral, dorsal, and median portions, giving rise to an old nomenclature referring to anterior, posterior, lateral, and median lobes (Fig. 6.8), with the anterior and posterior lobes being thought of as largely fibromuscular and glandular, respectively [52,54,55]. Also, the urethra undergoes a 35° angulation approximately midway between the apex of the gland and its base (Figs. 6.8, 6.9). This point of angulation divides the urethra into the proximal and distal segments, and the opening of the ejaculatory ducts at the verumontanum are within the distal segment. **With the ejaculatory ducts and the urethra as geographical borders, the glandular prostate can actually be divided into three major zones: the peripheral zone, the central zone, and the transition zone** (Fig. 6.9) [52,54].

The peripheral zone comprises about 70% of the glandular prostate, and the ducts of the glands enter the urethra along its distal portion (Fig. 6.9) [52]. Prostatic cancer most commonly arises in the peripheral zone. The central zone accounts for approximately 20% of the glandular prostate, and the ducts of this region run with the ejaculatory ducts toward the urethra (Fig. 6.9). The transition zone makes up approximately 4–5% of the prostatic tissue, and consists of two small lobules of

glandular prostate lateral to a collar of smooth muscle which envelopes the posterior aspect of the proximal urethra. **The transition zone is the site of origin of benign prostatic hypertrophy.** The periurethral gland zone (not illustrated) contains less than 1% of total glandular prostate tissue. These small glands empty into the proximal urethra and seem to be an extension of the peripheral and transition zones. The ventral or anterior fibromuscular stroma can make up as much as 30% of the total tissue within the prostatic capsule (Fig. 6.9). This tissue contains smooth-muscle fibers, many of which are continuous proximally with the detrusor muscle fibers of the bladder neck [52,54,55].

In an average 3.0–3.5 mL ejaculate, the prostatic contribution is approximately 0.5 mL [53]; it is rich in citrate, zinc, polyamines, cholesterol, acid phosphatases, prostaglandins, and various proteases

important in the liquefaction of semen [55,56]. The functions of many of these constituents are unclear, but there are suggestions of their potential uses. For example, citrate is an important contributor to osmotic balance and may also be important as a metal ion chelator. Zinc is a constituent of many metalloenzymes, and free zinc has been claimed to be bacteriostatic in seminal plasma [57]. Others have highlighted the potential role of zinc in the regulation of citrate metabolism [58]. While the general function of acid phosphatases is known (hydrolysis of organic monophosphate esters), the specific biological role of acid phosphatase in semen is uncertain. Nevertheless, the enzyme is clinically important, since metastasizing prostatic cancer cells secrete the enzyme into serum. For this reason, acid phosphatase has served as an important marker for prostatic adenocarcinoma. More recently, prostate-specific antigen (PSA) has become widely used as a marker for prostatic cancer [59,60]. PSA is a 33 kD protein, a serine protease, secreted by the prostatic epithelium, but its function in nature remains uncertain. The molecule potentially plays a role in epithelial cell regulation, but it also acts as a protease degrading a major galactosaminoglycan (GAG) secreted into the ejaculate by the seminal vesicles, suggesting a role of the molecule in the liquefaction of semen [53,61].

The seminal vesicles

The seminal vesicles are two large lobulated glands, 5–10 cm in length, which lie inferiorly and dorsally to the bladder wall (Fig. 6.7). The paired organs lie almost horizontally when the bladder is empty and are pulled vertically when the bladder is distended. The glands consist of blind-coiled alveoli with several diverticula. The epithelial cells range from cuboidal to columnar but contain numerous organelles associated with secretory processes [62]. The name of the glands arose from early beliefs that they stored spermatozoa, but this is not the case. The ducts of the seminal vesicles join with the ampulla of the vasa and enter the urethra at the verumontanum.

Secretions of the seminal vesicles make up approximately 1.5–2.0 mL of the average 3 mL ejaculate [53,56]. The most important products of the seminal vesicles are fructose, prostaglandins, and coagulating proteins. Fructose concentrations in secretions of seminal vesicles are approximately 3 mg/mL, while a total concentration of other sugars is only 0.1 mg/mL. Fructose is thus the major energy substrate of sperm metabolism [56,63], and is important for the maintenance of sperm motility.

Prostaglandin concentrations in seminal plasma range from 100 to 300 µg/mL, and this is sufficient to produce pharmacological effects [64,65]. Von Euler proposed the name "prostaglandin" because he believed the active agent found in seminal plasma came from the prostate [64]. It is now known that prostaglandin arises primarily from the seminal vesicles [66], and that the prostaglandins appear in many molecular variants. There are approximately 15 types of prostaglandins, and these are conventionally divided into four major groups (A, B, C, and D) according to their structure. The E group of prostaglandins is the major form in the male reproductive tract, and has been associated with the induction of muscular contractions, changes in cervical mucus, and improvement in sperm transport.

Seminal vesicle proteins are thought to play a role in forming the viscous coagulum evident after ejaculation [53,56], and various proteases from the prostate, e.g., PSA, and perhaps from the seminal vesicles themselves, then digest these proteins and cause liquefaction. There is also a potential role for seminal vesicle secretions in protecting sperm from reactive oxygen species present in the semen [67], whether produced by leukocytes or generated by the spermatozoa themselves.

The bulbourethral glands and the glands of Littré

The bulbourethral glands are encased in the urogenital diaphragm. Embryologically, they arise from epithelia projecting from the urogenital sinus, and in the adult, the ducts of the glands penetrate the inferior layer of the diaphragm to enter the penile urethra (Fig. 6.7). Comparative biochemical and histochemical studies demonstrate the primarily GAG nature of the bulbourethral gland secretion [68,69]. **This secretion forms the first part of the ejaculate, or the "preejaculate," and serves to flush the tract with a buffered lubricant prior to the transport of sperm.** The glands of Littré are small, simple glands emptying into the penile urethra. These glands have little secretory capacity, and their function is unknown.

References

[1] Sadler TW. *Langman's Medical Embryology*, 7th edn. Baltimore, MD: Williams and Wilkins, 2003: 281.

[2] Parker KL, Schimmer BP. Embryology and genetics of the mammalian gonads and ducts. In: Neill JD, ed. *Knobil and Neill's Physiology of Reproduction*, 3rd edn. New York, NY: Elsevier, 2006: 313–36.

[3] Larsen WJ. *Human Embryology*, 2nd edn. New York, NY: Churchill Livingstone, 1997: 261–79.

[4] di Clemente N, Josso N, Gouédard L, Belville C. Components of anti-Müllerian hormone signaling pathways in the gonads. *Mol Cell Endocrinol* 2003; **211**: 9–14.

[5] Wilson JD, George FW, Griffin JE. The hormonal control of sexual development. *Science* 1981; **211**: 1278–80.

[6] van Wingerden JJ, Franz A. The presence of a caput epididymidis in congenital absence of the vas deferens. *J Urol* 1984; **131**: 764–6.

[7] George FW, Wilson JD. Sex determination and differentiation. In: Knobil E, Neill JD, eds. *The Physiology of Reproduction*. New York, NY: Raven Press, 1988: 3–26.

[8] Cunha GR, Cooke PS, Kurita T. Role of stromal-epithelial interactions in hormonal responses. *Arch Histol Cytol* 2004; **67**: 417–34.

[9] Hinton BT, Snoswell AM, Setchell BP. The concentration of carnitine in the luminal fluid of the testis and epididymis of the rat and some other mammals. *J Reprod Fertil* 1979; **56**: 105–11.

[10] Amann RP, Howards SS. Daily spermatozoal production and epididymal spermatozoal reserves of the human male. *J Urol* 1980; **124**: 211–15.

[11] Johnson L, Varner DD. Effect of daily spermatozoan production but not age on transit time of spermatozoa through the human epididymis. *Biol Reprod* 1988; **39**: 812–17.

[12] Robb GW, Amann RP, Killian GJ. Daily sperm production and epididymal sperm reserves of pubertal and adult rats. *J Reprod Fertil* 1978; **59**: 103–7.

[13] Yeung CH, Cooper TG, Bergmann M, Schulze H. Organization of tubules in the human caput epididymidis and the ultrastructure of their epithelia. *Am J Anat* 1991; **191**: 261–79.

[14] Robaire B, Hinton BT, Orgebin-Crist MC. The epididymis. In: Neill JD, ed. *Knobil and Neill's Physiology of Reproduction*, 3rd edn. New York, NY: Elsevier, 2006: 1071–148.

[15] Turner TT, Gleavy JL, Harris JM. Fluid movement in the lumen of the rat epididymis: effect of vasectomy and subsequent vasovasostomy. *J Androl* 1990; **11**: 422–8.

[16] Silber SJ. Pregnancy caused by sperm from vasa efferentia. *Fertil Steril* 1988; **49**: 373–5.

[17] Silber SJ. Apparent fertility of human spermatozoa from the caput epididymidis. *J Androl* 1989; **10**: 263–9.

[18] Schoysman RJ, Bedford JM. The role of the human epididymis in sperm maturation and sperm storage as reflected in the consequences of epididymovasostomy. *Fertil Steril* 1986; **46**: 293–9.

[19] Toshimori K. Biology of spermatozoa maturation: an overview with an introduction to this issue. *Microsc Res Tech* 2003; **61**: 1–6.

[20] Dacheux JL, Gatti JL, Castella S, *et al.* The epididymal proteome. In: Hinton BT, Turner TT, eds. *The Third International Conference on the Epididymis*. Charlottesville, VA: Van Doren, 2003: 115–22.

[21] Kirchhoff C, Derr P, von Horsten HH, *et al.* Gene expression in the human epididymis. In: Hinton BT, Turner TT, eds. *The Third International Conference on the Epididymis*. Charlottesville, VA: Van Doren, 2003: 192–201.

[22] Turner TT. Spermatozoa are exposed to a complex microenvironment as they traverse the epididymis. *Ann N Y Acad Sci* 1991; **637**: 364–83.

[23] Turner TT. Necessity's potion: inorganic ions and small organic molecules in the epididymal lumen. In: Robaire B, Hinton BT, eds. *The Epididymis: From Molecules to Clinical Practice*. New York, NY: Kluwer/Plenum, 2002: 131–49.

[24] Yeung CH, Cooper TG. Acquisition and development of sperm motility upon maturation in the epididymis. In: Robaire B, Hinton BT, eds. *The Epididymis: From Molecules to Clinical Practice*. New York, NY: Kluwer/Plenum, 2002: 417–34.

[25] Schlegel PH, Goldstein M. Microsurgical vasoepididymostomy: refinements and results. *J Urol* 1993; **150**: 1165–8.

[26] Belker AM. Predictors of success in microsurgical correction of vasal and epididymal obstruction. *Curr Urol Rep* 2001; **2**: 443–7.

[27] Buffat C, Patrat C, Merlet F, *et al.* ICSI outcomes in obstructive azoospermia: influence of the origin of surgically retrieved spermatozoa and the cause of obstruction. *Hum Reprod* 2006; **21**: 1018–24.

[28] Turner TT, Riley TA, Vagnetti M, *et al.* Postvasectomy alterations in protein synthesis and secretion in the rat caput epididymidis are not repaired after vasovasostomy. *J Androl* 2000; **21**: 276–90.

[29] Silber SJ, Ord T, Balmaceda J, Patrizio P, Asch RH. Congential absence of the vas deferens: the fertilizing capacity of human epididymal sperm. *N Engl J Med* 1990; **323**: 1788–92.

[30] Schlegel PN, Berkley AS, Goldstein M, *et al.* Epididymal micropuncture with in vitro fertilization and oocyte manipulation for treatment of surgically unreconstructable vasal obstruction. *Fertil Steril* 1994; **61**: 895–901.

[31] Marmar JL, Corson SL, Batzer FR, Gocial B, Go K. Microsurgical aspiration of sperm from the epididymis: a mobile program. *J Urol* 1993; **249**: 1368–73.

[32] Cooper TG. In defense of the human epididymis. *Fertil Steril* 1990; **54**: 965–73.

[33] Cuasnicu PS, Cohen DJ, Ellerman DA, *et al.* Changes in sperm proteins during epididymal maturation. In: Robaire B, Hinton BT, eds. *The Epididymis: From Molecules to Clinical Practice*. New York, NY: Kluwer/Plenum, 2002: 389–404.

[34] Johnston DS, Jelinsky SA, Bang HJ, *et al.* The mouse epididymal transcriptome: transcriptional profiling

of segmented gene expression in the epididymis. *Biol Reprod* 2005; **73**: 404–13.

[35] Johnston DS, Bai Y, Kopf G. Utilization of human genome databases in strategies for contraceptive development. In: Hinton BT, Turner TT, eds. *The Third International Conference on the Epididymis.* Charlottesville, VA: Van Doren, 2003; 256–70.

[36] Turner TT, Johnston DS, Jelinsky SA. Epididymal genomics and the search for a male contraceptive. *Mol Cell Endocrinol* 2006; **250**: 178–83.

[37] Wong PYD, Gong XD, Leung GPH, Cheuk BLY. Formation of the epididymal fluid microenvironment. In: Robaire B, Hinton BT, eds. *The Epididymis: From Molecules to Clinical Practice.* New York, NY: Kluwer/Plenum, 2002: 119–30.

[38] Crabo B. Studies on the composition of epididymal content in bulls and boars. *Acta Vet Scand* 1965; **6** (Suppl 5): 1–94.

[39] Levine N, Marsh DJ. Micropuncture studies of the electrochemical aspects of fluid and electrolyte transport in individual seminiferous tubules, the epididymis, and vas deferens. *J Physiol* 1971; **215**: 557–70.

[40] Wong PYD, Au CL, Ngai HK. Electrolyte and water transport in rat epididymis: its possible role in sperm maturation. *Int J Androl* 1978; **1**: 608–28.

[41] Wong PYD, Yeung CH. Hormonal control of fluid reabsorption in isolated rat cauda epididymidis. *Endocrinology* 1977; **101**: 1391–7.

[42] Turner TT, Cesarini DM. The ability of the rat epididymis to concentrate spermatozoa: responsiveness to aldosterone. *J Androl* 1983; **3**: 197–202.

[43] Hinton BT, Keefer DA. Binding of 3H-aldosterone to a single population of cells within the rat epididymis. *J Steroid Biochem* 1985; **23**: 231–7.

[44] Leung PS, Wong TP, Lam SY, Chan HC, Wong PYD. Testicular hormonal regulation of the rennin–angiotensin system in the rat epididymis. *Life Sci* 2000; **66**: 1317–24.

[45] Cheung KH, Leung CT, Leung GPH, Wong PYD. Synergistic effects of cystic fibrosis transmembrane conductance regulator and aquaporin-9 in the rat epididymis. *Biol Reprod* 2003; **68**: 1505–10.

[46] Amann RP. A critical review of methods for evaluation of spermatogenesis from seminal characteristics. *J Androl* 1981; **2**: 37–58.

[47] Setchell BP, Sanchez-Partida LG, Chairussyuhur A. Epididymal constituents and related substances in the storage of spermatozoa: a review. *Reprod Fertil Dev* 1993; **5**: 601–12.

[48] Jones RC, Murdoch RN. Regulation of the motility and metabolism of spermatozoa for storage in the epididymis of eutherian and marsupial mammals. *Reprod Fertil Dev* 1996; **8**: 553–68.

[49] Hinton BT, Palladino MA, Rudolph D, Labus JC. The epididymis as protector of maturing spermatozoa. *Reprod Fertil Dev* 1995; **7**: 731–45.

[50] Yeung CH, Cooper TG, Oberpenning F, Shulze H, Nieschlag E. Changes in movement characteristics of human sperm along the length of the epididymis. *Biol Reprod* 1993; **49**: 274–80.

[51] Cunha GR. Role of mesenchymal–epithelial interactions in normal and abnormal development of the mammary gland and prostate. *Cancer* 1994; **74**: 1030–44.

[52] Janulis L, Lee C. The prostate gland. In: Knobil E, Neill JD, eds. *Encyclopedia of Reproduction.* New York, NY: Academic Press, 1998: 77–85.

[53] Partin AW, Rodriguez R. The molecular biology, endocrinology, and physiology of the prostate and seminal vesicles. In: Walsh PC, Retik AB, Vaughan ED, Wein AJ, eds. *Campbell's Urology,* 8th edn. Philadelphia, PA: Saunders, 2002: 1381–428.

[54] McNeal JE. The zonal anatomy of the prostate. *Prostate* 1983; **2**: 35–49.

[55] McNeal JE. The anatomic heterogeneity of the prostate. *Prog Clin Biol Res* 1980; **37**: 149–60.

[56] Risbridger GP, Taylor RA. Physiology of the male accessory sex structures: the prostate gland, seminal vesicles, and bulbourethral glands. In: Neill JD, ed. *Knobil and Neill's Physiology of Reproduction,* 3rd edn. New York, NY: Elsevier, 2006; 1149–72.

[57] Fair WR, Wehner N. The prostatic antibacterial factor: identity and significance. *Prog Clin Biol Res* 1976; **6**: 383–403.

[58] Costello LC, Franklin RB. Novel role of zinc in the regulation of prostatic citrate metabolism and its implications in prostate cancer. *Prostate* 1998; **35**: 285–96.

[59] Catalona WJ, Smith DS, Ratliff TL, Basler JW. Detection of organ-confined prostate cancer is increased through prostate-specific antigen-based screening. *JAMA* 1993; **270**: 948–54.

[60] McCormack RT, Rittenhouse HG, Finlay JA, *et al.* Molecular forms of prostate-specific antigen and the human kallikrein gene family: a new era. *Urology* 1995; **45**: 729–44.

[61] Lilja H. A kallikrien-like serum protease in prostatic fluid cleaves the predominant seminal vesicle protein. *J Clin Invest* 1985; **76**: 1899–903.

[62] Brandes D. Hormonal regulation of fine structures. In: Brandes D, ed. *Male Accessory Sex Organs.* New York, NY: Academic Press, 1974; 17.

[63] Mann T, Lutwak-Mann CL. *Male Reproductive Function.* New York, Springer-Verlag, 1991; 107.

[64] von Euler US. Zur kenntnis der pharmakologischen wirkungen von natirsekreten un extrackten

mammlicher accessorischer geschlechtsdrusen. *Arch Pathol Pharmacol* 1934; **175**: 78–87.

[65] Goldblatt MW. Properties of human seminal plasma. *J Physiol* 1935; **84**: 208–18.

[66] Eliasson R. Studies on prostaglandins, occurrence, formation, and biological actions. *Acta Physiol Scand* 1959; **158** (Suppl 46): 1–12.

[67] Zubkova EV, Robaire B. Effect of glutathione depletion on antioxidant enzymes on the epididymis, seminal vesicles and liver and on sperm metabolism in the aging Brown Norway rat. *Biol Reprod* 2004; **71**: 1002–8.

[68] Cavazos LF. Fine structure and functional correlates of male accessory sex glands of rodents. In: Hamilton DW, Greep RO, eds. *Handbook of Physiology: Endocrinology*, Vol. 5. Baltimore, MD: American Physiological Society, 1975: 353.

[69] Setchell BP, Brooks DE. Anatomy, vasculature, innervation and fluids of the male reproductive tract. In: Knobil E, Neill JD, eds. *The Physiology of Reproduction*. New York, NY: Raven Press, 1988; 753.

An overview of the molecular mechanisms involved in human fertilization

Mónica H. Vazquez-Levin and Clara I. Marín-Briggiler

Introduction

Fertilization is a fundamental process that involves a highly coordinated sequence of interactions between the female and male gametes, giving rise to a diploid zygote. During this process, spermatozoa that have successfully completed spermatogenesis, epididymal maturation, and transport through the female reproductive tract first bind to the extracellular matrix that surrounds the egg, called the zona pellucida (ZP). Sperm binding to ZP glycoproteins triggers sperm acrosomal exocytosis (AE), involving fusion of the sperm plasma and outer acrosomal membranes and the release of the content from the acrosomal granule; these components, in conjunction with the hyperactivated vigorous motility, help sperm penetration through the ZP. The spermatozoon reaches the perivitelline space, binds and fuses to the egg plasma membrane (oolemma); the sperm head enters the egg cytoplasm (ooplasm), and the sperm nucleus undergoes decondensation. Ultimately, sperm entrance triggers mechanisms to block polyspermia. Each of these steps is schematically represented in Figure 7.1.

Although in the last 30 years some of the mechanisms involved in mammalian fertilization have been elucidated, the molecular basis of human sperm–egg interaction is still not completely known. Defective sperm–ZP interaction and disordered ZP-induced AE have been identified as major causes of fertilization failure in standard in-vitro fertilization (IVF) procedures performed in couples under infertility treatment, and a major contribution to this outcome has been attributed to abnormalities in the male gamete [1,2]. **An understanding of the molecular mechanisms underlying the processes by which spermatozoa reach, recognize, bind to, and fuse with the egg will provide new tools for the improvement of current methods of treatment and diagnosis of male infertility, as well as methods for regulation of male fertility.**

This chapter aims to present an overview of the current knowledge regarding the molecular mechanisms involved in human fertilization and the components participating in this process. Due to space limitations, most of the original publications on each topic could not be listed. Cited literature is mainly a selection of review and individual articles on recent advances in human reproduction. Reports from studies in animal models are mentioned when strictly needed. For supplementary information, readers should refer to a number of review articles from highly recognized professionals in the field [3–10].

Sperm transport in the female tract

Human semen is ejaculated into the anterior vagina and, within minutes, spermatozoa enter the cervix by traversing the cervical mucus. The mucus acts as a sperm filter, and only cells with good motility and morphology can enter the uterine cavity; in the uterus, spermatozoa are subjected to muscular contractions, and a few thousand cells are able to reach the Fallopian tubes. During their transport and storage in the female genital tract, spermatozoa undergo several metabolic and structural changes, collectively known as capacitation, and develop a distinct pattern of motility named hyperactivation. These changes prepare sperm cells to be guided to the egg by thermotaxis and chemotaxis, and are required for the occurrence of AE and for sperm penetration through the egg vestments (see below). The close relationship and dynamic interactions between spermatozoa and secretions and/or cells of the female genital tract are essential for the regulation and development of in-vivo sperm fertilizing ability. While sperm storage in the

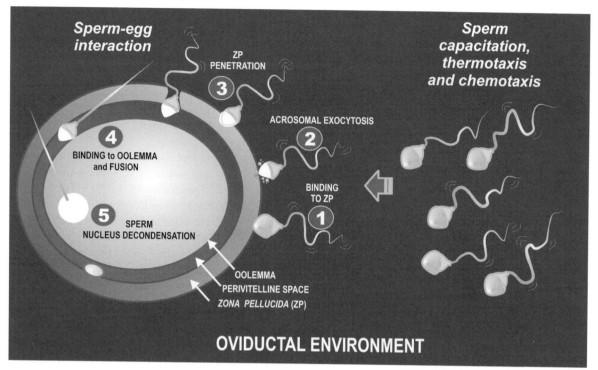

Fig. 7.1. Schematic representation of mammalian sperm–egg interaction. Once deposited in the female reproductive tract, spermatozoa undergo a series of biochemical and functional changes known as sperm capacitation, and are able to follow guidance mechanisms towards the egg known as sperm thermotaxis and chemotaxis. In the vicinity of the egg, the fertilizing spermatozoon undergoes the following interaction steps: (1) after penetrating the cumulus oophorus cells that surround the egg, the spermatozoon reaches the zona pellucida (ZP) and binds to it; (2) sperm binding to the ZP triggers sperm acrosomal exocytosis (AE), allowing the release of acrosomal content; (3) the spermatozoon penetrates the ZP; (4) the spermatozoon reaches the perivitelline space, binds to and fuses with the egg plasma membrane (oolemma); (5) the sperm head enters the egg cytoplasm (ooplasm) and the sperm nucleus undergoes decondensation [3].

oviduct mediated by binding to oviductal epithelial cells has been described in several animal species, the existence of a sperm reservoir in human Fallopian tubes remains to be proven [11,12].

Sperm capacitation

The need for sperm capacitation to achieve fertilization in mammals was independently described nearly 60 years ago by Austin [13] and Chang [14]; however, the molecular mechanisms underlying this process are only beginning to be clarified. Because of ethical and technical limitations, most studies leading to an understanding of the basis of in-vivo sperm capacitation, and most of the knowledge gained, have resulted from in-vitro evidence.

Human sperm capacitation is initiated when the male gamete traverses the cervical mucus, with the removal of inhibitory factors from the seminal plasma. Several capacitation-related events take place during sperm passage through the uterus

and Fallopian tubes or penetration of the cumulus oophorus, and **capacitation is completed on the surface of the ZP, with AE [11]. Evidence indicates that sperm capacitation is an asynchronous event, and that only a small proportion of the cells from an ejaculate (approximately 10% in humans [15]) are capacitated at a given time;** the continuous replacement of the capacitated sperm population would ensure the availability of "egg-responsive" spermatozoa for a relatively extended period of time.

Capacitation has been associated mainly with (1) modifications in the sperm plasma membrane composition and fluidity, (2) changes in intracellular ion concentrations, (3) generation of low and controlled levels of reactive oxygen species, and (4) an increase in protein phosphorylation. A brief outline of each event in human spermatozoa is presented here; a detailed description of this process in mammalian spermatozoa has been reviewed elsewhere [3,7,11,16,17].

Sperm plasma membrane modifications

Sperm capacitation has been associated with the removal, alteration, and acquisition of sperm plasma membrane components during migration into cervical mucus or during passage through the uterus and oviduct [11].

An important modification related to sperm capacitation is the cholesterol efflux. Cholesterol provided by the seminal plasma is the principal inhibitor of sperm capacitation; as a result of cholesterol removal, there is a decrease in the cholesterol/phospholipid ratio and an increase in membrane fluidity. Loss of sperm sterols also leads to a decrease of lipid order; such changes are associated with an increase in ion permeability and protein tyrosine phosphorylation, and with a redistribution of cell surface proteins [7,17,18]. In particular, cholesterol efflux has been connected with the exposure of mannose receptors on the sperm surface [19] that may interact with sugar residues of ZP glycoproteins (see below).

Proteins of epididymal and/or seminal plasma origin, which act by stabilizing the plasma membrane and by preventing a premature AE, are removed from the sperm surface during capacitation [20]. Other proteins can be unmasked after sperm incubation under capacitating conditions, as shown for the epididymal protein P34H [21]. Moreover, protein redistribution may occur during capacitation; for example, the human testicular protein TPX1 is localized in the acrosomal region of ejaculated spermatozoa, but in the equatorial segment of capacitated cells [22].

Some seminal plasma components can bind to specific sperm receptors and regulate the expression of sperm fertilizing ability. It has been reported that fertilization-promoting peptide (FPP), adenosine, calcitonin, and angiotensin II stimulate the initiation of capacitation, by modulation of membrane-associated adenylate cyclase (AC) activity, and hence intracellular levels of cyclic adenosine monophosphate (cAMP) [23]. The incorporation by the sperm plasma membrane of some uterine and oviductal proteins has also been reported. As an example, sialic acid-binding protein (SABP) is secreted by human endometrial cells and would bind to the sperm head, facilitating calcium (Ca^{2+}) influx into sperm [24].

Changes in intracellular ion concentrations

An increase in intracellular Ca^{2+} ion concentration during human sperm capacitation has been reported. It is suggested that binding of this cation to some proteins (calmodulin) may affect the activity of several enzymes, such as soluble AC or phosphodiesterase, modulating the intracellular levels of cAMP; moreover, Ca^{2+} ions may directly interact with membrane phospholipids, modifying their fluidity [16,17,25]. Ca^{2+} signaling in human spermatozoa would be regulated by the release of this cation from intracellular stores, as well as by activation of several transporters and channels in the sperm plasma membrane [26].

Capacitation has also been linked with bicarbonate (HCO_3^-) and sodium (Na^+) influx into spermatozoa and with potassium (K^+) efflux. As a result of HCO_3^- influx, there is a rise in intracellular pH; HCO_3^- may also activate soluble AC and then be involved in cAMP metabolism. Enhanced K^+ permeability and decreased Na^+ permeability may lead to sperm plasma membrane hyperpolarization; hyperpolarization would be essential to revert to inactivation of Ca^{2+} channels, leaving them with the ability to be activated by the ZP during AE (see below) [16,17,25,27].

Reactive oxygen species

Spermatozoa incubated under aerobic conditions generate reactive oxygen species (ROS), such as superoxide anion (O_2^-), which spontaneously dismutates to hydrogen peroxide (H_2O_2). Although high ROS concentrations are harmful to the cell, low concentrations are beneficial for the development of sperm capacitation and AE. ROS are produced in high quantities by leukocytes, but O_2^- production by spermatozoa has also been reported as an early capacitation-related event [28]. ROS would regulate enzymes involved in cAMP synthesis and in protein phosphorylation (see below) [29].

Increase in protein phosphorylation

The occurrence of sperm capacitation has been associated with an increase in protein phosphorylation on tyrosine residues; a large number of studies have been performed in several mammalian species, including humans [17]. Most tyrosine-phosphorylated proteins have been localized to the sperm flagellum, although tyrosine phosphorylation of head proteins has also been reported [30]. In particular, A-kinase anchor proteins (AKAP82, pro-AKAP82, AKAP3, and FSP95) and calcium-binding and tyrosine phosphorylation-regulated protein (CABYR) localized on the human sperm tail undergo phosphorylation on tyrosine residues during capacitation; these proteins are involved in the maintenance of sperm motility, and probably in the development of hyperactivation (see below) [31–34].

Recent evidence has shown that human **sperm capacitation is also related to protein phosphorylation on serine and threonine residues** [35–37], although the identity of the target proteins and their function are still unknown. Phosphorylation on tyrosine, serine, and threonine residues has been associated with cholesterol efflux and is modulated by ROS. However, the relationship between these phosphorylation pathways remains obscure [17,29,37].

Altogether, the findings summarized above show that multiple changes at the sperm plasma membrane level and the activation of several intracellular pathways must occur on the sperm cell as a prerequisite for acrosomal responsiveness.

Development of hyperactivated motility

At ejaculation, spermatozoa display activated progressive motility that allows them to be propelled through the female genital tract. While residing in the oviduct, or following incubation under capacitating conditions, **mammalian spermatozoa are able to change their motility pattern and show a less progressive, vigorous movement, characterized by a high-amplitude and asymmetrical flagellar beating; this phenomenon has been termed hyperactivation** [38]. **Hyperactivation is associated with sperm capacitation; however, the development of hyperactivated motility may be regulated by a separate or divergent pathway from that modulating the acquisition of acrosomal responsiveness** [39]. Although ATP and cAMP are necessary for sperm hyperactivation, there is evidence showing that an increase in intracellular Ca^{2+} concentrations is essential for the development of this type of motility, which may be linked with the phosphorylation of specific flagellar proteins [40]. Concomitant with the ability to undergo in-vitro capacitation, a small proportion of the human spermatozoa synchronously develops hyperactivation (approximately 20% of the cells [41]), and hyperactivation is a reversible process since it can be "switched on and off" in individual cells [40].

Hyperactivated motility may be required for sperm release from the oviductal epithelium, for reaching the fertilization site, and for penetrating the cumulus oophorus and ZP [3]. A detailed description of the characteristics and regulation of mammalian sperm hyperactivation has been reviewed elsewhere [3,40,42–44].

Conditions to achieve in-vitro human sperm capacitation

Capacitation-related events can be accomplished in vitro by incubating spermatozoa for a certain period of time, under specific environmental conditions, and using defined culture media. Considering that seminal plasma contains decapacitating factors, its removal is mandatory to achieve capacitation. Semen samples are subjected to dilution or to sperm separation techniques; immotile spermatozoa and round cells are removed, and a population of high-quality sperm cells is obtained [45].

Capacitation is a temperature-dependent process [3]. Human sperm incubation at body temperature has proven to be essential for the occurrence of protein tyrosine phosphorylation, for displaying hyperactivated motility, and for undergoing AE in response to a physiological stimulus, since none of these events occurs in cells incubated at room temperature [46].

Sperm culture media have been formulated to mimic the complex composition of the oviductal fluid. They consist of balanced salt solutions supplemented with appropriate concentrations of electrolytes, metabolic energy sources (glucose, lactate, and pyruvate), and a protein supply (albumin). **The ionic composition of culture media is fundamental to maintain sperm function. While most media contain millimolar concentrations of Ca^{2+} ions, results from our studies have shown that 0.22 mM of this cation are sufficient to support the development of some capacitation-related events** [47], and that Ca^{2+} in the incubation medium can be replaced by strontium (Sr^{2+}) ions [48]. **The presence of HCO_3^- and albumin in the culture medium is essential to promote capacitation.** HCO_3^- activates soluble AC, which would result in the activation of protein kinase A (PKA), while albumin assists in membrane cholesterol removal. All of these events are associated with protein phosphorylation on tyrosine residues [17].

The in-vitro conditions described above provide the minimum requirements that allow the occurrence of sperm capacitation-related events. It is obvious, however, that they are unable to completely mimic the complexity of the natural environment where capacitation takes place. In IVF conditions, the egg, its surrounding cells, and their secretions may contribute additional as-yet unidentified factors that may be required for spermatozoa to develop their full fertilizing ability.

Sperm thermotaxis and chemotaxis

Evidence has indicated that mammalian spermatozoa do not reach the egg by random encounter and that, instead, capacitated cells follow guidance mechanisms towards the female gamete. In addition to passive sperm drag by muscle contraction in the oviduct, the existence of two active mechanisms of sperm guidance, named thermotaxis and chemotaxis, has been reported in mammals. **Thermotaxis is the movement of cells in the direction of a temperature gradient, and chemotaxis is the directed movement of cells along a chemical concentration gradient** [49,50].

Capacitated human and rabbit spermatozoa have been demonstrated to display thermotaxis, as in vitro they are able to sense a temperature difference of 2 °C and to swim from a cooler to a warmer temperature [51]. In rabbits, different temperatures have been found between the sperm storage site (cooler) and fertilization site (warmer), and there is evidence of a higher temperature difference after ovulation [52]. Neither the molecular mechanisms underlying sperm thermotaxis nor the identity of the sperm thermosensors is currently known.

Chemotaxis was first reported in marine species with external fertilization [53], **and later this phenomenon was described in amphibians and animals with internal fertilization, including mice, rabbits, and humans** [50]. Many substances present in the oviductal and follicular fluids have been proposed as sperm chemoattractants [50]. Moreover, recent studies have suggested that the odorant bourgeonal is a chemoattractant for human sperm; this compound would cause the activation of signal transduction pathways leading to an increase in intracellular cAMP and Ca^{2+} concentrations [54]. These events would result in an asymmetrical beating of the flagellum, with a change in the swimming direction. Some chemoattractants can also increase the flagellar beat frequency, reflected in an increment in swimming speed, a phenomenon that has been called chemokinesis [55].

The relevance of thermotaxis and chemotaxis in vivo remains to be determined; these phenomena would have the function of recruiting a selective sperm population with the ability to fertilize the egg [15,51]. **It has been proposed that while thermotaxis may be a sperm guidance mechanism from the reservoir to the fertilization site, chemotaxis could be the way by which spermatozoa are directed through the cumulus cells to the egg** [49].

Sperm–egg interaction

Sperm–egg interaction is a specialized process that leads to fertilization and activation of development. **Studies performed in several mammalian species**

have shown that sperm cells that have completed capacitation first bind to the ZP and undergo AE; acrosome-reacted spermatozoa penetrate the ZP, reach the perivitelline space, and bind and fuse to the egg plasma membrane.** A general description of the molecular basis of sperm–ZP and sperm–oolemma interactions is presented in the following paragraphs. In addition, information about the composition of the ZP, the sperm proteins involved in these interaction events, and some of the molecular aspects of AE are summarized. Finally, a brief description is presented of the in-vitro tests available to assess sperm–egg interaction and their relevance in the diagnosis of male infertility.

Sperm binding to the zona pellucida

Sperm binding to the ZP is a highly relevant step in the interaction events leading to fertilization since it **provides species-specificity to the recognition between the two gametes, and it evokes the AE, an event that is required for sperm penetration of the ZP and fusion to the oolemma. Sperm–ZP binding involves the interaction of ZP components with sperm surface proteins of capacitated cells, known as primary binding. In addition, gamete binding involves participation of intra-acrosomal proteins exposed once spermatozoa undergo AE; this interaction, called secondary binding, helps sperm cells to remain associated with the egg extracellular matrix.** Numerous findings favor the notion that several ZP and sperm proteins participate in these events. Irrespective of the specific receptors involved, there is a general consensus that sperm interaction with ZP ligands stimulates profound changes in the sperm cell, which include activation of several signaling cascades and ion channels (see *Acrosomal exocytosis*, below). For detailed information on the mechanism of sperm–ZP interaction, the reader may refer to the review articles mentioned at the beginning of this chapter.

The zona pellucida (ZP)

The ZP surrounds all mammalian eggs, and lies between the innermost layer of follicle cells and the egg's plasma membrane. **It is the last physical barrier that the spermatozoon must traverse to achieve fertilization; in addition, it protects the egg from physical damage, provides species-specificity to gamete interaction, and contributes to the blocking of polyspermia after sperm–egg fusion. The ZP also provides a defined environment for the preimplantation embryo and protects it from any injury.**

The elucidation of molecular aspects related to the composition, structure, and function(s) of the ZP has come mainly from investigations in the murine model. Biochemical studies showed that the mouse ZP is composed mainly of three glycoproteins, named mZP1, mZP2, and mZP3, and assembled into a network of cross-linked filaments. Further work extensively characterized these proteins at a molecular level, and experimental models combining targeted mutagenesis and transgenesis have been developed. It was demonstrated that mZP3 is the ligand for sperm primary binding and triggers and/or accelerates the AE (see below). mZP2 would be involved in sperm secondary binding to the ZP (see below), and mZP1 would maintain the integrity of the ZP structure. In addition to this evidence, a recent study has proposed that mZP2 may regulate the supramolecular structure of the ZP required to support sperm binding [5,6,56,57].

Similarly to the murine model, three ZP glycoproteins were initially identified in the human ZP [58], **their primary structure was deduced from the cDNA, and they were named hZPA,[1] hZPB, hZPC** [59].[2] **Later, a transcript of an additional ZP gene (hZP1) was found, and preliminary results have described the presence of the encoded protein in the human ZP** [60]. Sequence analysis revealed that hZPA is the homolog of mZP2, hZPC is the homolog of mZP3, and hZP1 is the ortholog of mZP1 and the paralog of hZPB. ZPB would not be expressed in the mouse eggs, but recent studies identified a novel ligand that facilitates sperm adhesion to the ZP [61].

The human ZP has been found to have a selective role against morphologically and functionally abnormal spermatozoa. Sperm cells bound to the ZP show normal morphology [62], and normal nuclear chromatin [63]; in addition, a positive correlation was observed between the number of sperm bound to the ZP and sperm protein tyrosine phosphorylation patterns [64].

Human ZP glycoproteins may also participate in primary and secondary binding; accumulated evidence shows the involvement of fucose, galactose, N-acetylglucosamine and mannose residues as well

as sulfated glycans of the ZP in these events [65–71]. More recently, the interaction of these sugars with the sperm acrosomal proacrosin/acrosin system has been described [72] (see below). Nevertheless, participation of the ZP polypeptide backbone in gamete interaction should not be disregarded.

Biochemical and functional studies with isolated native human ZP glycoproteins have been hampered by the scarcity of this biological material. To overcome such limitations, several groups developed in-vitro systems to produce recombinant human ZP proteins in prokaryotic and eukaryotic cells, and evaluated their function [73–80]. Recombinant hZPC was found to be associated with the head of capacitated motile human spermatozoa [81–83] and to interfere with ZP interaction [77,83]. Human ZPB produced in bacteria or insect cells binds mainly to the equatorial segment and acrosome of capacitated spermatozoa [82]. With regard to hZPA, the recombinant protein produced in bacteria or insect cells was reported to bind only to acrosome-reacted spermatozoa [82,84], and specific antibodies were capable of blocking sperm binding and penetration of homologous ZP [84]. Our group described the binding activity of recombinant human ZP glycoproteins produced in mammalian cells to human proacrosin/acrosin proteins generated in bacteria; the molecular aspects of the interaction between the acrosomal protease system and hZPA were analyzed [85] (see below). Studies aimed at assessing the ability of recombinant human ZP proteins to induce the acrosomal loss of human spermatozoa will be discussed under *Acrosomal exocytosis* (below). The use of recombinant human ZP glycoproteins with biological activity will help us to understand the basis of sperm–ZP interaction, as well as to develop alternative tools for male infertility diagnosis. Moreover, these proteins may be used as immunocontraceptive antigens, as reported [86–88].

Sperm receptors involved in sperm–ZP interaction

A large number of sperm proteins have been proposed to participate in ZP binding, and there is an extensive literature on this subject. Studies have involved the use of experimental models in rodents as well as in other mammals; numerous methodologies have been applied to their study, from classical cell biology and biochemistry to the most sophisticated molecular biology technologies and experimental genetics, including gene knockout models. Protein candidates include a variety of enzymes (β1,4-galactosyltransferase/ GalTase; α-fucosyltransferases; α-mannosidases;

---

[1] Also named ZP2 (Symbol report: ZP2. Human Genome Organization (HUGO). Gene Nomenclature Committee, April 25, 2005. www.gene.ucl.ac.uk/nomenclature/data/get_data. php?hgnc_id=13188.

[2] Also named ZP3 (Symbol report: ZP3. Human Genome Organization (HUGO). Gene Nomenclature Committee, April 25, 2005. www.gene.ucl.ac.uk/nomenclature/data/get_data. php?hgnc_id=13189.

N-acetylglucosaminidase/Hex; phospholypase A2), and carbohydrate-binding proteins (mannose, galactose, and fucose receptors; p47/SED1 and other spermadhesins; zonadhesin; selectin-like molecules), as well as other proteins (FA-1, P34H/P26h/P25b, SLIP-1, p66, epithelial cadherin). In humans, presence of some of these proteins has been described: FA-1 and P34H (see below), GalTase [89], Hex [90], selectin [91], SLIP-1 [92], p66 [93], epithelial cadherin [94]. In addition to these surface proteins, acrosomal components have been found to display ZP binding activity, and would most likely be involved in secondary binding. Among them are proacrosin/acrosin, PH-20, Sp 56, acrin2/MC41, Sp 38/IAM38, and Sp 17; evidence supporting the expression in the human of proacrosin/acrosin (see below), PH-20 [95], Sp 17 [96], and SOB3 [97] has been reported. In the following paragraphs, a brief description of sperm proteins FA-1, P34H, and proacrosin/acrosin is presented; selection of these entities was based on the abundant data available in the literature and on reports on their relationship to human fertility.

FA-1 is a 51 kDa glycoprotein present on the postacrosomal, midpiece, and tail sperm regions first described in mice [98]; characterization of the DNA sequence encoding human protein has been published [99]. Its participation in human gamete interaction has been suggested by reports describing the ability of specific antibodies and the purified protein to block sperm–ZP binding [100]. Moreover, antibodies towards FA-1 were detected in sera from subfertile men and women [101]; their presence may be deleterious for human fertilization, as proven in animal models, in which a contraceptive effect of immunization with recombinant FA-1 or the DNA encoding the protein was described [102,103].

P34H is a 34 kDa human sperm surface protein of epididymal origin localized on the acrosomal cap of intact ejaculated and capacitated cells [21]. The involvement of P34H in human fertilization was first evidenced by the inhibitory effect of a specific antiserum upon sperm–ZP binding [104]. Further research has revealed a significantly low concentration of P34H in a group of men with idiopathic infertility [105]; a recent study also demonstrated a positive correlation between the proportion of cases with P34H and successful IVF [106]. P34H has been proposed as a "fertility marker" in the assessment of the subfertile men.

Acrosin is a sperm acrosomal protease extensively studied in numerous species. In addition to its proteolytic activity (see below), biochemical studies have shown that human acrosin and its zymogen, proacrosin, bind to either native or recombinant human ZP glycoproteins [85,107]. Proacrosin/acrosin proteins were found to bind to recombinant hZPA, hZPB, and hZPC, showing the highest binding activity in proacrosin and towards hZPA; the interaction appears to involve hZPA sugar residues [72,85], and can be blocked by antiacrosin antibodies from subfertile women [108]. Our group has proposed a model combining human proacrosin/acrosin binding ability with the proteolytic properties of the mature enzyme during gamete interaction (see below). Whether alterations in proacrosin–ZP binding are associated with infertility still has not been reported.

In conclusion, despite great effort and much research, a consensus has yet not been reached on the sperm proteins that participate in sperm–ZP interaction in any mammalian species, particularly in humans. The reader may refer to the review articles on fertilization listed earlier, for reference to some of the proteins mentioned above.

Acrosomal exocytosis (AE)

After binding to the ZP, capacitated spermatozoa are able to undergo AE. The acrosome is a lysosome-like organelle that covers the anterior portion of the sperm nucleus. The membrane that overlies the nucleus has been called inner acrosomal membrane, and the portion that underlies the plasma membrane is known as outer acrosomal membrane. The acrosome contains soluble and particulate compartments (the latter known as acrosomal matrix), constituted by many proteins with hydrolytic properties [109]. **AE is an irreversible process that involves a complex series of intracellular events, which result in the fusion of the outer acrosomal membrane and the overlying plasma membrane, with the subsequent release of the acrosomal content and the exposure of the inner acrosomal membrane. The occurrence of AE facilitates sperm penetration through the ZP, and exposure of certain molecules on the sperm equatorial segment that participate in the fusion with the oolemma** (see below) [3].

Studies performed in several species have demonstrated that most of the spermatozoa that reach the oviduct have an intact acrosome. Some cells may initiate the AE while traversing the cumulus oophorus, but the fertilizing spermatozoon completes the AE upon interaction with ZP glycoproteins [3]. Reports on the mouse model have demonstrated that binding of mZP3 to specific sperm receptors may cause their aggregation and activation [110–112]. Activated receptors trigger a cascade of events that culminates with membrane fusion and the release of the acrosomal components. Briefly, mZP3-induced AE involves the activation of G proteins, intracellular alkalinization, plasma membrane depolarization, transient Ca^{2+} elevation by activation of voltage-sensitive T-type channels, generation of inositol 1,4,5-triphosphate (IP_3), sustained rise in intracellular Ca^{2+} concentrations by depletion of IP_3-sensitive Ca^{2+} stores and opening of store-operated Ca^{2+} channels in plasma membrane, and production of fusogenic compounds [7,27,113,114].

In humans, it has been reported that native or solubilized ZP proteins induce the acrosomal loss in capacitated cells [115]; however, due to the restricted availability of biological material, the identity of ZP components responsible for triggering AE has not been determined. Studies using human recombinant proteins have shown that **recombinant hZPC produced in eukaryotic cells is able to provoke AE**, involving the activation of glycine and nicotinic acetylcholine receptors, the participation of G_i protein, and an influx of Ca^{2+} [73,74,77,79,80,116,117]. **In addition, recent findings indicate that hZPB produced in insect cells also induces AE in capacitated human spermatozoa**, by activating a G_i-independent sperm receptor [79,80].

The molecular mechanisms controlling membrane fusion during human sperm AE have been extensively studied in recent years. **The participation in the AE of the SNARE** (soluble N-ethylmaleimide-sensitive attachment protein receptors) and other associated proteins, known to regulate membrane fusion during somatic cell exocytosis, has been reported [118–120]. **Moreover, it has been shown that tyrosine kinase and phosphatase activities are required for human sperm AE**, indicating the involvement of protein tyrosine phosphorylation in this process [30,121].

In capacitated human spermatozoa, **AE can also be achieved by exposure to cumulus oophorus secretions, oviductal and follicular fluids** [122–125]. It has been demonstrated that the AE-inducing activity of human follicular fluid (hFF) resides in its progesterone content [126], and our studies indicate that antibodies present in the fluid of infertile patients are also able to provoke the acrosomal loss [127]. Although the relevance of these factors in physiological AE is still unknown, it is possible that different agonist molecules present in the vicinity of the egg trigger additive or synergistic mechanisms leading to maximization of the exocytotic response. **Progesterone and follicular fluid have shown a priming effect on ZP-induced AE in mouse and human spermatozoa** [128,129]. The exposure of human spermatozoa to a gradient of progesterone, simulating the conditions found at the fertilization site, leads to a low rise and oscillations in intracellular Ca^{2+} concentrations; such stimulus is insufficient to provoke AE, but stimulates sperm movement [130].

Since only capacitated cells are able to undergo AE in response to a physiological stimulus, the occurrence of AE indicates the completion of the capacitation process. Both phenomena are intimately related, and trying to dissociate the molecular mechanisms governing each of them has been a difficult task. Results from our studies have revealed that **while 0.22 mM of Ca^{2+} in the incubation medium is sufficient to allow the occurrence of several capacitation-related events, 0.58 mM of this cation are required to support AE in response to hFF** [47]; moreover, sperm capacitation can be accomplished in a medium in which Ca^{2+} ions have been replaced by Sr^{2+}, but this ion is unable to sustain hFF-induced AE [48]. **Incubation of spermatozoa under specific ionic conditions would allow the temporal separation of capacitation and AE, and the implementation of these models will improve the knowledge of the molecular basis of these processes.**

For further information about acrosomal exocytosis, the authors suggest that the reader refer to a number of reviews [3,16,131–135].

Sperm penetration through the ZP

Spermatozoa that have completed AE are able to penetrate the ZP and fuse with the egg plasma membrane. Studies in animal models have shown that spermatozoa about to enter the ZP have the acrosomal "ghost" around the head, or have left it on the outer ZP surface. The time that spermatozoa need to complete ZP penetration is variable (mouse spermatozoa need 15–26 minutes), and it mainly depends on the capacitation status of the spermatozoa cell at the time of insemination. **During penetration, spermatozoa beat their tails vigorously and, in most cases, take curved paths, leaving behind a thin sharply defined penetration slit** [3].

The mechanism by which mammalian spermatozoa penetrate the ZP has still not been completely elucidated. Several scenarios have been proposed, within them a "**mechanical hypothesis**" in which sperm would complete ZP penetration solely by physical thrust and independently of the acrosomal enzymatic activity, and an "**enzymatic hypothesis,**" in which sperm penetration would require enzymatic activity, and motility would not be very relevant. **A mechanism combining sperm enzymatic hydrolysis with vigorous flagellar motility as a mechanical force has also been considered** [3,6,10].

The involvement of human sperm trypsin-like hydrolases in penetration of the ZP was suggested from studies showing the blocking effect of trypsin inhibitors upon this event [136]. Among the acrosomal sperm components studied so far, the proacrosin/acrosin protein system has been the best characterized [137,138]. Acrosin (EC 3.4.21.10) is a trypsin-like endoprotease synthesized and stored in the acrosome in its zymogen form, proacrosin [139,140]; the activated mature enzyme, β-acrosin, is released during AE [141], and evidence suggests that its activation is accelerated by ZP components [142]. The classical concept that sperm penetration of ZP glycoproteins is aided by proteolysis mediated by acrosin has been under revision since knockout animals lacking this protease were found to be fertile [143,144]. However, spermatozoa from acrosin-deficient mice exhibited a delayed fertilization [143], they did not fertilize eggs if challenged with wild-type spermatozoa [144], and they performed poorly when exposed to eggs with hardened ZP [145]. Altogether, this evidence suggested a disadvantage of the spermatozoa lacking acrosin in their ability to penetrate the ZP. Other proteases found in mice may overcome the absence of acrosin, but their human homologs were not identified [146]. Further studies indicated that acrosin enzymatic activity may participate during AE in the dissolution of the acrosomal matrix and in the release of the acrosomal content [147].

In humans, an abnormal acrosin enzymatic activity has been associated with fertility failure. In particular, a group of men diagnosed with unexplained infertility showed decreased acrosin activity [148,149]; the low enzymatic activity was related to a diminished IVF outcome, and abnormalities in proacrosin activation were identified, but no changes in the DNA sequence of proacrosin were found [148].

The results summarized above show that the mechanisms underlying the sperm–ZP penetration remain to be established; future studies may help in unraveling the molecular basis of this event.

Sperm fusion to the oolemma

Spermatozoa that have completed AE and ZP penetration reach the perivitelline space, and bind and fuse to the oolemma. The interaction between the fertilizing spermatozoon and the egg plasma membrane would initially involve the contact and binding between sperm receptors located in the inner acrosomal membrane from the apical region of the head and oolemma microvilli. After this interaction is dissociated by proteases, the spermatozoon might turn parallel, attach to the oolemma, and fuse by its equatorial segment. Apparently, the anterior sperm region is engulfed by egg phagocytosis, and the postacrosomal region and tail are subsequently incorporated via membrane fusion. A visible indication of gamete fusion is the reduction of sperm tail movement that occurs seconds after the fusion event. Under physiological conditions, only one spermatozoon fuses with the oolemma [3,7,150–153].

Acrosome-intact sperm cells are unable to fuse, regardless of their capacitation status. As a result of or concomitant with AE, the sperm plasma membrane at the equatorial segment undergoes major physiological changes rendering a cell capable of fusing with the egg, making the AE an absolute prerequisite for gamete fusion. In contrast, strong sperm motility is not essential for sperm–egg fusion [3].

Several sperm proteins have been proposed to participate in mammalian gamete fusion. For many years, studies in the mouse pointed at members of the MDC (metaloprotease-like domain, desintegrin-like domain, cystein-rich domain) or ADAM (a disintegrin and metalloprotease) proteins present on spermatozoa, in particular, fertilin-β (also known as ADAM2) and cyritestin (ADAM3). However, gene deletion studies showed that fusion occurred in the absence of these proteins [154,155]. In humans, the genes encoding proteins fertilin-α (ADAM1), tMCDII, and cyritestins are nonfunctional [156], but sperm cells express other members of this protein family (ADAM18) that may be relevant to oolemma binding [157].

Recent studies have identified a novel immunoglobulin superfamily type I transmembrane protein, named IZUMO. This protein is exposed after AE, and seems to be essential for mouse sperm–egg fusion, since IZUMO$^{-/-}$ males are sterile and spermatozoa from these animals were not capable of fertilizing in vitro. In humans, an anti-IZUMO antibody can inhibit sperm performance in the ZP-free hamster egg sperm penetration assay (SPA, see below) without affecting sperm transport and interaction with the egg vestments [158]. However, a normal expression of IZUMO was observed in patients with severe oligospermia and/or asthenospermia, as well as in patients with fertilization failure in previous conventional IVF procedures [159].

The involvement of other sperm proteins in gamete fusion has been suggested by studies showing the ability of specific antibodies to inhibit sperm performance in the SPA: FLB1 [160], SOB2 [161], gp20 [162], Sp 10 [163], ARP [164], SAMP32 [165], SAMP14 [166], TPX1 [22], and epithelial as well as neural cadherins [94, Marín-Briggiler et al., unpublished data].

With regard to the egg receptor, integrins were initially thought to act as the counterpart of ADAM proteins [167], but later were found to be dispensable for sperm–egg fusion in animal models [168] and humans [169]. However, their potential accessory role in sperm–egg fusion remains to be determined, especially considering the evidence of the presence of $\alpha6\beta1$ integrin clusters at the site of sperm contact [170].

Studies done in the murine model demonstrated that CD9 has a crucial role in sperm–egg fusion. CD9$^{-/-}$ female mice showed severely reduced fertility, but the deficiency could be overcome by sperm microinjection into the egg cytoplasm [171]. In human eggs, antibodies towards CD9 inhibited clustering of other associated proteins that would be directly involved in gamete fusion [170].

Currently, there are two best-characterized examples of membrane fusion events: fusion between membranes of enveloped viruses and host cells, and fusion between cytoplasm transport vesicles and target membranes [152]. Much still needs to be studied to determine whether similar mechanisms or a novel one underlies mammalian sperm–egg fusion.

Once the fertilizing spermatozoon has entered the ooplasm, the block of polyspermia is achieved by changes in the oolemma that prevent the entry of additional sperm cells (cortical reaction); in addition, enzymatic modifications of the ZP glycoproteins alter the structure and penetrability of the ZP matrix (i.e., hardening of the ZP, ZP reaction). Ultimately, the fertilizing spermatozoon activates zygote formation, and zygote development begins by receptor-mediated signal transduction cascades and/or provision of sperm components [3].

In-vitro assays to evaluate sperm–egg interaction

Several in-vitro bioassays have been developed to test sperm–egg interaction. Some of them have also been used in experiments aimed at evaluating the molecular basis of fertilization. A brief description is presented in the following paragraphs.

The ability of human spermatozoa to recognize and bind to the homologous ZP can be tested by the hemizona and intact-ZP assays, using oocytes that have failed to fertilize in IVF cycles, or have been retrieved from surgically removed ovaries or postmortem tissue. In the hemizona assay, oocytes are microbisected in equal halves; hemizonae are exposed to two different sperm populations (spermatozoa from patient and fertile control), and the numbers of tightly bound cells in each hemizona are compared [172]. The intact-ZP assay, known as the "sperm–ZP binding ratio test," evaluates competitive binding of two differentially labeled sperm populations to human oocytes [173]. The ability of spermatozoa to bind to the ZP has been associated with sperm concentration, motility, normal morphology, and acrosomal integrity; moreover, the results of both ZP binding assays have been positively and significantly correlated with IVF outcome [174–176].

Evaluation of the acrosomal status of human spermatozoa recovered after binding to native ZP has been proposed as a test to determine sperm ability to undergo physiological AE [177]; the acrosomal loss can also be induced by sperm exposure to solubilized ZP [178]. Other physiological (hFF [179] and progesterone [180]) and pharmacological (calcium ionophore A23187 [181]) agents have been widely utilized to determine human sperm ability to undergo in-vitro AE. Different responses to these inducers have been obtained in spermatozoa from fertile men compared to those from subjects with abnormal semen parameters, and results have been highly correlated with fertilization rates in standard IVF [174,175,182,183]. In over 25% of the patients with idiopathic male infertility, disordered ZP-induced AE has been identified. Interestingly, in some cases this pathology was not related to abnormal sperm–ZP binding, **indicating that the evaluation of both sperm–ZP binding and ZP-induced AE would be required to assess human sperm function [174,176].**

Assays to evaluate the ability of human spermatozoa to penetrate the ZP and to bind to the oolemma have been developed using homologous oocytes [174]; however, these tests are rather complex to carry out and are performed with fresh oocytes, making the protocols difficult to implement. Alternatively, **the heterologous gamete assay using ZP-free hamster eggs (SPA) has been extensively used to assess**

human sperm ability to fuse with the oolemma and to undergo chromatin decondensation [184]. In the standard SPA [185], eggs are inseminated with overnight-capacitated spermatozoa; optimized protocols involve the use of spermatozoa subjected to treatments that increase the population of acrosome-reacted cells (exposure to A23187 or hFF; incubation with TEST-yolk buffer [185,186]). These modified assays have a higher power to predict natural pregnancy than conventional semen parameters [187,188], and their results have been related to normal sperm morphology [189] and IVF rates [186].

The validity of the aforementioned sperm functional assays to predict fertilization outcome under in-vitro conditions has been compared in a meta-analysis finding that, while sperm–ZP binding and induced-AE assays have a high predictive power in IVF, the standard SPA has poor clinical value as predictor of fertilization [190].

Further assessments related to sperm–egg interaction in vitro may include evaluation of the expression levels of sperm proteins involved in fertilization, such as mannose receptors [191] and P34H [106], in addition to the detection of the presence and protease activity of proacrosin/acrosin [192].

The evaluation of the subfertile male should include a basic semen analysis, followed by bioassays aimed at assessing sperm functional competence. In men without noticeable defects in routine semen parameters, assessment of sperm–egg interaction may help in the diagnosis of infertility. Moreover, the results of these tests may allow the selection of the most appropriate therapeutic procedure for each patient. As an example, spermatozoa from patients with disordered ZP-induced AE have shown a poor performance in standard IVF, but they were able to reach high fertilization and pregnancy rates after intracytoplasmic sperm injection (ICSI), demonstrating the effectiveness of the ICSI procedure as the optimal treatment in these cases [2,193].

Conclusions

This chapter has described the molecular mechanisms involved in human fertilization, focusing on the male gamete. The mechanisms underlying fertilization have been shown to be extremely complex, and many of them are triggered/regulated by the interaction between the gametes themselves and between the gametes and other cells, acellular structures, or secretions present in the male and female reproductive tracts.

The literature has accumulated evidence mainly derived from in-vitro studies, but results and conclusions are limited by the experimental approaches used. Trying to reproduce such a complex scenario in vitro is nearly impossible, and this serious technical limitation is restricting our complete knowledge of the fertilization process. Despite their deficiencies, in-vitro studies have allowed the development of several diagnostic methods and many therapeutic protocols, the human IVF procedure being the best example of their validity.

Many of the molecular mechanisms underlying mammalian sperm capacitation, AE, and fusion with the egg have been found to modulate somatic cell functions. In addition, much of what we presently know about fertilization in humans was first described in animal models. However, several differences have been identified in the components and regulatory mechanisms of animal and human gametes, suggesting that many answers to our questions about human fertilization will finally be found in the human cells.

In recent years, efforts have been made to produce genetically modified animals to study the role of certain proteins in fertilization; many of these animals remain fertile, most likely because they carry redundant mechanisms to ensure fertilization success. These experimental models, although very elegant, probably are far from reality. Working closely, researchers and clinicians may be able to capture the invaluable information that can be obtained from a comprehensive evaluation of the infertile male.

Acknowledgments

Preparation of this manuscript was carried out with grant support from the World Health Organization (LID grant 97175), and the Agencia Nacional de Promoción Científica y Tecnológica (PICT2004 05–26110) to MHVL. CMB and MHVL are career members from the National Research Council of Argentina (CONICET).

References

[1] Liu DY, Baker HW. Defective sperm–zona pellucida interaction: a major cause of failure of fertilization in clinical in-vitro fertilization. *Hum Reprod* 2000; **15**: 702–8.

[2] Liu DY, Baker HW. Disordered zona pellucida-induced acrosome reaction and failure of in vitro fertilization in patients with unexplained infertility. *Fertil Steril* 2003; **79**: 74–80.

[3] Yanagimachi R. Mammalian fertilization. In: Knobil E, Neill JD, eds. *Physiology of Reproduction*, 2nd edn. New York, NY: Raven Press, 1994: 189–317.

[4] McLeskey SB, Dowds C, Carballada R, White RR, Saling PM. Molecules involved in mammalian sperm–egg interaction. *Int Rev Cytol* 1998; **177**: 57–113.

[5] Wassarman PM. Mammalian fertilization: molecular aspects of gamete adhesion, exocytosis, and fusion. *Cell* 1999; **96**: 175–83.

[6] Wassarman PM, Jovine L, Litscher ES. A profile of fertilization in mammals. *Nat Cell Biol* 2001; **3**: E59–64.

[7] Flesch FM, Gadella BM. Dynamics of the mammalian sperm plasma membrane in the process of fertilization. *Biochim Biophys Acta* 2000; **1469**: 197–235.

[8] Primakoff P, Myles DG. Penetration, adhesion, and fusion in mammalian sperm–egg interaction. *Science* 2002; **296**: 2183–5.

[9] Talbot P, Shur BD, Myles DG. Cell adhesion and fertilization: steps in oocyte transport, sperm–zona pellucida interactions, and sperm–egg fusion. *Biol Reprod* 2003; **68**: 1–9.

[10] Bedford JM. Enigmas of mammalian gamete form and function. *Biol Rev Camb Philos Soc* 2004; **79**: 429–60.

[11] De Jonge C. Biological basis for human capacitation. *Hum Reprod Update* 2005; **11**: 205–14.

[12] Suarez SS, Pacey AA. Sperm transport in the female reproductive tract. *Hum Reprod Update* 2006; **12**: 23–37.

[13] Austin CR. Observations on the penetration of the sperm in the mammalian egg. *Aust J Sci Res (B)* 1951; **4**: 581–96.

[14] Chang MC. Fertilizing capacity of spermatozoa deposited into the fallopian tubes. *Nature* 1951; **168**: 697–8.

[15] Cohen-Dayag A, Tur-Kaspa I, Dor J, Mashiach S, Eisenbach M. Sperm capacitation in humans is transient and correlates with chemotactic responsiveness to follicular factors. *Proc Natl Acad Sci U S A* 1995; **92**: 11039–43.

[16] Baldi E, Luconi M, Bonaccorsi L, Forti G. Signal transduction pathways in human spermatozoa. *J Reprod Immunol* 2002; **53**: 121–31.

[17] Visconti PE, Westbrook VA, Chertihin O, *et al.* Novel signaling pathways involved in sperm acquisition of fertilizing capacity. *J Reprod Immunol* 2002; **53**: 133–50.

[18] Cross NL. Role of cholesterol in sperm capacitation. *Biol Reprod* 1998; **59**: 7–11.

[19] Benoff S, Hurley I, Cooper GW, *et al.* Head-specific mannose-ligand receptor expression in human spermatozoa is dependent on capacitation-associated membrane cholesterol loss. *Hum Reprod* 1993; **8**: 2141–54.

[20] Fraser LR. Sperm capacitation and the acrosome reaction. *Hum Reprod* 1998; **13** (Suppl 1): 9–19.

[21] Boué F, Blais J, Sullivan R. Surface localization of P34H, an epididymal protein, during maturation,

[22] Busso D, Cohen DJ, Hayashi M, Kasahara M, Cuasnicu PS. Human testicular protein TPX1/CRISP-2: localization in spermatozoa, fate after capacitation and relevance for gamete interaction. *Mol Hum Reprod* 2005; **11**: 299–305.

[23] Fraser LR, Adeoya-Osiguwa SA, Baxendale RW, Gibbons R. Regulation of mammalian sperm capacitation by endogenous molecules. *Front Biosci* 2006; **11**: 1636–45.

[24] Banerjee M, Chowdhury M. Induction of capacitation in human spermatozoa in vitro by an endometrial sialic acid-binding protein. *Hum Reprod* 1995; **10**: 3147–53.

[25] Fraser LR. Ionic control of sperm function. *Reprod Fertil Dev* 1995; **7**: 905–25.

[26] Jimenez-Gonzalez C, Michelangeli F, Harper CV, Barratt CL, Publicover SJ. Calcium signalling in human spermatozoa: a specialized 'toolkit' of channels, transporters and stores. *Hum Reprod Update* 2006; **12**: 253–67.

[27] Darszon A, Acevedo JJ, Galindo BE, *et al.* Sperm channel diversity and functional multiplicity. *Reproduction* 2006; **131**: 977–88.

[28] de Lamirande E, Jiang H, Zini A, Kodama H, Gagnon C. Reactive oxygen species and sperm physiology. *Rev Reprod* 1997; **2**: 48–54.

[29] O'Flaherty C, de Lamirande E, Gagnon C. Positive role of reactive oxygen species in mammalian sperm capacitation: triggering and modulation of phosphorylation events. *Free Radic Biol Med* 2006; **41**: 528–40.

[30] Naz RK, Rajesh PB. Role of tyrosine phosphorylation in sperm capacitation/acrosome reaction. *Reprod Biol Endocrinol* 2004; **2**: 75.

[31] Carrera A, Moos J, Ning XP, *et al.* Regulation of protein tyrosine phosphorylation in human sperm by a calcium/calmodulin-dependent mechanism: identification of A kinase anchor proteins as major substrates for tyrosine phosphorylation. *Dev Biol* 1996; **180**: 284–96.

[32] Mandal A, Naaby-Hansen S, Wolkowicz MJ, *et al.* FSP95, a testis-specific 95-kilodalton fibrous sheath antigen that undergoes tyrosine phosphorylation in capacitated human spermatozoa. *Biol Reprod* 1999; **61**: 1184–97.

[33] Naaby-Hansen S, Mandal A, Wolkowicz MJ, et al. CABYR, a novel calcium-binding tyrosine phosphorylation-regulated fibrous sheath protein involved in capacitation. *Dev Biol* 2002; **242**: 236–54.

[34] Luconi M, Carloni V, Marra F, *et al.* Increased phosphorylation of AKAP by inhibition of phosphatidylinositol 3-kinase enhances human sperm

motility through tail recruitment of protein kinase A. *J Cell Sci* 2004; **117**: 1235–46.

[35] Naz RK. Involvement of protein serine and threonine phosphorylation in human sperm capacitation. *Biol Reprod* 1999; **60**: 1402–9.

[36] O'Flaherty C, de Lamirande E, Gagnon C. Phosphorylation of the Arginine-X-X-(Serine/Threonine) motif in human sperm proteins during capacitation: modulation and protein kinase A dependency. *Mol Hum Reprod* 2004; **10**: 355–63.

[37] Jha KN, Salicioni AM, Arcelay E, *et al.* Evidence for the involvement of proline-directed serine/threonine phosphorylation in sperm capacitation. *Mol Hum Reprod* 2006; **12**: 781–9.

[38] Yanagimachi R. Mechanisms of fertilization in mammals. In: Mastroianni L, Biggers JD, eds. *Fertilization and Embryonic Development In Vitro*. New York, NY: Plenum Press, 1981: 81–187.

[39] Marquez B, Suarez SS. Different signaling pathways in bovine sperm regulate capacitation and hyperactivation. *Biol Reprod* 2004; **70**: 1626–33.

[40] Luconi M, Baldi E. How do sperm swim? Molecular mechanisms underlying sperm motility. *Cell Mol Biol* 2003; **49**: 357–69.

[41] Burkman LJ. Characterization of hyperactivated motility by human spermatozoa during capacitation: comparison of fertile and oligozoospermic sperm populations. *Arch Androl* 1984; **13**: 153–65.

[42] Kay VJ, Robertson L. Hyperactivated motility of human spermatozoa: a review of physiological function and application in assisted reproduction. *Hum Reprod Update* 1998; **4**: 776–86.

[43] Mortimer ST. CASA: practical aspects. *J Androl* 2000; **21**: 515–24.

[44] Ho HC, Suarez SS. Hyperactivation of mammalian spermatozoa: function and regulation. *Reproduction* 2001; **122**: 519–26.

[45] Buffone MG, Doncel GF, Marín-Briggiler CI, Vazquez-Levin MH, Calamera JC. Human sperm subpopulations: relationship between functional quality and protein tyrosine phosphorylation. *Hum Reprod* 2004; **19**: 139–46.

[46] Marín-Briggiler CI, Tezon JG, Miranda PV, Vazquez-Levin MH. Effect of incubating human sperm at room temperature on capacitation-related events. *Fertil Steril* 2002; **77**: 252–9.

[47] Marín-Briggiler CI, Gonzalez-Echeverria F, Buffone M, *et al.* Calcium requirements for human sperm function in vitro. *Fertil Steril* 2003; **79**: 1396–403.

[48] Marín-Briggiler CI, Vazquez-Levin MH, Gonzalez-Echeverria F, *et al.* Strontium supports human sperm capacitation but not follicular fluid-induced acrosome reaction. *Biol Reprod* 1999; **61**: 673–80.

[49] Bahat A, Eisenbach M. Sperm thermotaxis. *Mol Cell Endocrinol* 2006; **252**: 115–19.

[50] Eisenbach M, Giojalas LC. Sperm guidance in mammals: an unpaved road to the egg. *Nat Rev Mol Cell Biol* 2006; **7**: 276–85.

[51] Bahat A, Tur-Kaspa I, Gakamsky A, *et al.* Thermotaxis of mammalian sperm cells: a potential navigation mechanism in the female genital tract. *Nat Med* 2003; **9**: 149–50.

[52] Bahat A, Eisenbach M, Tur-Kaspa I. Periovulatory increase in temperature difference within the rabbit oviduct. *Hum Reprod* 2005; **20**: 2118–21.

[53] Kaupp UB, Hildebrand E, Weyand I. Sperm chemotaxis in marine invertebrates: molecules and mechanisms. *J Cell Physiol* 2006; **208**: 487–94.

[54] Spehr M, Schwane K, Riffell JA, Zimmer RK, Hatt H. Odorant receptors and olfactory-like signaling mechanisms in mammalian sperm. *Mol Cell Endocrinol* 2006; **250**: 128–36.

[55] Ralt D, Manor M, Cohen-Dayag A, *et al.* Chemotaxis and chemokinesis of human spermatozoa to follicular factors. *Biol Reprod* 1994; **50**: 774–85.

[56] Rankin T, Dean J. The zona pellucida: using molecular genetics to study the mammalian egg coat. *Rev Reprod* 2000; **5**: 114–21.

[57] Hoodbhoy T, Dean J. Insights into the molecular basis of sperm–egg recognition in mammals. *Reproduction* 2004; **127**: 417–22.

[58] Shabanowitz RB, O'Rand MG. Characterization of the human zona pellucida from fertilized and unfertilized eggs. *J Reprod Fertil* 1998; **82**: 151–61.

[59] Harris JD, Hibler DW, Fontenot GK, *et al.* Cloning and characterization of zona pellucida genes and cDNA from a variety of mammalian species: the ZPA, ZPB and the ZPC gene families. *DNA Seq* 1994; **4**: 361–93.

[60] Lefièvre L, Conner SJ, Salpekar A, *et al.* Four zona pellucida glycoproteins are expressed in the human. *Hum Reprod* 2004; **19**: 1580–6.

[61] Rodeheffer C, Shur BD. Characterization of a novel ZP3-independent sperm-binding ligand that facilitates sperm adhesion to the egg coat. *Development* 2004; **131**: 503–12.

[62] Menkveld R, Franken DR, Kruger TF, Oehninger S, Hodgen GD. Sperm selection capacity of the human zona pellucida. *Mol Reprod Dev* 1991; **30**: 346–52.

[63] Liu DY, Baker HW. Human sperm bound to the zona pellucida have normal nuclear chromatin as assessed by acridine orange fluorescence. *Hum Reprod* 2007; **22**: 1597–602.

[64] Liu DY, Clarke GN, Baker HW. Tyrosine phosphorylation on capacitated human sperm tail detected by immunofluorescence correlates strongly with sperm–zona pellucida (ZP) binding but not with the ZP-induced acrosome reaction. *Hum Reprod* 2006; **21**: 1002–8.

[65] Mori K, Hadito T, Kamada M, *et al.* Blocking of human fertilization by carbohydrates. *Hum Reprod* 1993; **8**: 1729–32.

[66] Lucas H, Bercegeay S, Le Pendu J, *et al.* A fucose-containing epitope potentially involved in gamete interaction on the human zona pellucida. *Hum Reprod* 1994; **9**: 1532–8.

[67] Benoff S. Carbohydrates and fertilization: an overview. *Mol Hum Reprod* 1997; **3**: 599–637.

[68] Miranda PV, Gonzalez-Echeverría F, Marín-Briggiler CI, *et al.* Glycosidic residues involved in human sperm–zona pellucida binding in vitro. *Mol Hum Reprod* 1997; **3**: 399–404.

[69] Maegawa M, Kamada M, Yamamoto S, *et al.* Involvement of carbohydrate molecules on zona pellucida in human fertilization. *J Reprod Immunol* 2002; **53**: 79–89.

[70] Oehninger S, Acosta A, Hodgen GD. Antagonistic and agonistic properties of saccharide moieties in the hemizona assay. *Fertil Steril* 1990; **53**: 143–9.

[71] Mahony MC, Oehninger S, Clark GF, Acosta AA, Hodgen GD. Fucoidin inhibits the zona pellucida-induced acrosome reaction in human spermatozoa. *Contraception* 1991; **44**: 657–65.

[72] Furlong LI, Veaute C, Vazquez-Levin MH. Binding of recombinant human proacrosin/acrosin to zona pellucida (ZP) glycoproteins. II. Participation of mannose residues in the interaction. *Fertil Steril* 2005; **83**: 1791–6.

[73] van Duin M, Polman JE, De Breet IT, *et al.* Recombinant human zona pellucida protein ZP3 produced by chinese hamster ovary cells induces the human sperm acrosome reaction and promotes sperm–egg fusion. *Biol Reprod* 1994; **51**: 607–17.

[74] Brewis IA, Clayton R, Barratt CL, Hornby DP, Moore HD. Recombinant human zona pellucida glycoprotein 3 induces calcium influx and acrosome reaction in human spermatozoa. *Mol Hum Reprod* 1996; **2**: 583–9.

[75] Chapman NR, Kessopoulou E, Andrews P, Hornby D, Barratt CLR. The polypeptide backbone of recombinant human zona pellucida glycoprotein-3 initiates acrosomal exocytosis in human spermatozoa in vitro. *Biochem J* 1998; **330**: 839–45.

[76] Harris JD, Seid CA, Fontenot GK, Liu HF. Expression and purification of recombinant human zona pellucida proteins. *Protein Expr Purif* 1999; **16**: 298–307.

[77] Dong KW, Chi TF, Juan YW, *et al.* Characterization of the biologic activities of a recombinant human zona pellucida protein 3 expressed in human ovarian teratocarcinoma (PA-1) cells. *Am J Obstet Gynecol* 2001; **184**: 835–44.

[78] Martic M, Moses EK, Adams TE, *et al.* Recombinant human zona pellucida proteins ZP1, ZP2 and ZP3 co-expressed in a human cell line. *Asian J Androl* 2004; **6**: 3–13.

[79] Chakravarty S, Suraj K, Gupta SK. Baculovirus-expressed recombinant human zona pellucida glycoprotein-B induces acrosomal exocytosis in capacitated spermatozoa in addition to zona pellucida glycoprotein-C. *Mol Hum Reprod* 2005; **11**: 365–72.

[80] Caballero-Campo P, Chirinos M, Fan XJ, *et al.* Biological effects of recombinant human zona pellucida proteins on sperm function. *Biol Reprod* 2006; **74**: 760–8.

[81] Whitmarsh AJ, Woolnough MJ, Moore HDM, Hornby DP, Barratt CLR. Biological activity of recombinant human ZP3 produced in vitro: potential for a sperm function test. *Mol Hum Reprod* 1996; **2**: 911–19.

[82] Chakravarty S, Kadunganattil S, Bansal P, Sharma RK, Gupta SK. Relevance of glycosylation of human zona pellucida glycoproteins for their binding to capacitated human spermatozoa and subsequent induction of acrosomal exocytosis. *Mol Reprod Dev* 2008; **75**: 75–88.

[83] Marín-Briggiler CI, Gonzalez-Echeverría MF, Harris JD, Vazquez-Levin MH. Recombinant human zona pellucida protein C produced in Chinese hamster ovary cells binds to human spermatozoa and inhibits sperm–zona pellucida interaction. *Fertil Steril* 2008; **90**: 879–82.

[84] Tsubamoto H, Hasegawa A, Nakata Y, *et al.* Expression of recombinant human zona pellucida protein 2 and its binding capacity to spermatozoa. *Biol Reprod* 1999; **61**: 1649–54.

[85] Furlong LI, Harris JD, Vazquez-Levin MH. Binding of recombinant human proacrosin/acrosin to zona pellucida (ZP) glycoproteins. I. Studies with recombinant ZPA, ZPB, and ZPC. *Fertil Steril* 2005; **83**: 1780–90.

[86] Paterson M, Wilson MR, Morris KD, van Duin M, Aitken RJ. Evaluation of the contraceptive potential of recombinant human ZP3 and human ZP3 peptides in a primate model: their safety and efficacy. *Am J Reprod Immunol* 1998; **40**: 198–209.

[87] Martinez ML, Harris JD. Effectiveness of zona pellucida protein ZPB as an immunocontraceptive antigen. *J Reprod Fertil* 2000; **120**: 19–32.

[88] Koyama K, Hasegawa A, Gupta SK. Prospect for immunocontraception using the NH2-terminal recombinant peptide of human zona pellucida protein (hZPA). *Am J Reprod Immunol* 47: 303–10.

[89] Miller DJ, Cross NL, Vazquez-Levin M, Shur BD. The role of sperm galactosyltransferase in fertilization: presence and possible function in humans and other mammals. In: Baccetti B, ed. *Comparative Spermatology: 20 Years After.* New York, NY: Raven Press: 569–74.

[90] Miranda PV, Gonzalez-Echeverria F, Blaquier JA, Mahuran DJ, Tezon JG. Evidence for the participation

of beta-hexosaminidase in human sperm–zona pellucida interaction in vitro. *Mol Hum Reprod* 2000; **8**: 699–706.

[91] Dell A, Morris HR, Easton RL, *et al.* Structural analysis of the oligosaccharides derived from glycodelin, a human glycoprotein with potent immunosuppressive and contraceptive activities. *J Biol Chem* 1995; **270**: 24116–26.

[92] Rattanachaiyanont M, Weerachatyanukul W, Leveille MC, *et al.* Anti-SLIP1-reactive proteins exist on human spermatozoa and are involved in zona pellucida binding. *Mol Hum Reprod* 2001; **7**: 633–40.

[93] Lasserre A, Gonzalez-Echeverria F, Moules C, *et al.* Identification of human sperm proteins involved in the interaction with homologous zona pellucida. *Fertil Steril* 2003; **79** (Suppl 3): 1606–15.

[94] Marín-Briggiler CI, Veiga MF, Matos ML, *et al.* Expression of epithelial cadherin in the human male reproductive tract and gametes and evidence of its participation in fertilization. *Mol Hum Reprod* 2008; **14**: 561–71.

[95] Lin Y, Kimmel LH, Myles DG, Primakoff P. Molecular cloning of the human and monkey sperm surface protein PH-20. *Proc Natl Acad Sci U S A* 1993; **90**: 10071–5.

[96] Lea IA, Richardson RT, Widgren EE, O'Rand MG. Cloning and sequencing of cDNAs encoding the human sperm protein, Sp17. *Biochim Biophys Acta* 1996; **1307**: 263–6.

[97] Hammami-Hamza S, Doussau M, Bernard J, *et al.* Cloning and sequencing of SOB3, a human gene coding for a sperm protein homologous to an antimicrobial protein and potentially involved in zona pellucida binding. *Mol Hum Reprod* 2001; **7**: 625–32.

[98] Naz RK, Phillips TM, Rosenblum BB. Characterization of the fertilization antigen 1 for the development of a contraceptive vaccine. *Proc Natl Acad Sci U S A* 1986; **83**: 5713–17.

[99] Naz RK, Zhu X. Molecular cloning and sequencing of cDNA encoding for human FA-1 antigen. *Mol Reprod Dev* 2002; **63**: 256–68.

[100] Kadam AL, Fateh M, Naz RK. Fertilization antigen (FA-1) completely blocks human sperm binding to human zona pellucida: FA-1 antigen may be a sperm receptor for zona pellucida in humans. *J Reprod Immunol* 1995; **29**: 19–30.

[101] Bronson RA, Cooper GW, Margalioth EJ, Naz RK, Hamilton MS. The detection in human sera of antisperm antibodies reactive with FA-1, an evolutionarily conserved antigen, and with murine spermatozoa. *Fertil Steril* 1989; **52**: 457–62.

[102] Naz RK, Zhu X. Recombinant fertilization antigen-1 causes a contraceptive effect in actively immunized mice. *Biol Reprod* 1998; **59**: 1095–100.

[103] Naz RK. Effect of fertilization antigen (FA-1) DNA vaccine on fertility of female mice. *Mol Reprod Dev* 2006; **73**: 1473–9.

[104] Boué F, Bérubé B, De Lamirande E, Gagnon C, Sullivan R. Human sperm-zona pellucida interaction is inhibited by an antiserum against a hamster sperm protein. *Biol Reprod* 1994; **51**: 577–87.

[105] Boué F, Sullivan R. Cases of human infertility are associated with the absence of P34H, an epididymal sperm antigen. *Biol Reprod* 1996; **54**: 1018–24.

[106] Sullivan R, Legare C, Villeneuve M, Foliguet B, Bissonnette F. Levels of P34H, a sperm protein of epididymal origin, as a predictor of conventional in vitro fertilization outcome. *Fertil Steril* 2006; **85**: 1557–9.

[107] Furlong LI, Hellman U, Krimer A, *et al.* Expression of human proacrosin in Escherichia coli and binding to zona pellucida. *Biol Reprod* 2000; **62**: 606–15.

[108] Veaute C, Furlong LI, Bronson R, Harris JD, Vazquez-Levin MH. Acrosin antibodies and infertility. I. Detection of antibodies towards proacrosin/acrosin in women consulting for infertility and evaluation of their effects upon the sperm protease activities. *Fertil Steril* 2008; Apr 24. [Epub ahead of print]

[109] Abou-Haila A, Tulsiani DR. Mammalian sperm acrosome: formation, contents, and function. *Arch Biochem Biophys* 2000; **379**: 173–82.

[110] Bleil JD, Wassarman PM. Sperm–egg interactions in the mouse: sequence of events and induction of the acrosome reaction by a zona pellucida glycoprotein. *Dev Biol* 1983; **95**: 317–24.

[111] Macek MB, Lopez LC, Shur BD. Aggregation of β1,4-galactosyltransferase on mouse sperm induces the acrosome reaction. *Dev Biol* 1991; **147**: 440–4.

[112] Gong X, Dubois DH, Miller DJ, Shur BD. Activation of a G protein complex by aggregation of β1,4-galactosyltransferase on the surface of sperm. *Science* 1995; **269**: 1718–21.

[113] Florman HM, Arnoult C, Kazam IG, Li C, O'Toole CM. A perspective on the control of mammalian fertilization by egg-activated ion channels in sperm: a tale of two channels. *Biol Reprod* 1998; **59**: 12–16.

[114] Roldan ER. Role of phospholipases during sperm acrosomal exocytosis. *Front Biosci* 1998; **3**: D1109–19.

[115] Cross NL, Morales P, Overstreet JW, Hanson FW. Induction of acrosome reactions by the human zona pellucida. *Biol Reprod* 1988; **38**: 235–44.

[116] Bray C, Son JH, Kumar P, Harris JD, Meizel S. A role for the human sperm glycine receptor/Cl(–) channel in the acrosome reaction initiated by recombinant ZP3. *Biol Reprod* 2002; **66**: 91–7.

[117] Bray C, Son JH, Meizel S. A nicotinic acetylcholine receptor is involved in the acrosome reaction of human sperm initiated by recombinant human ZP3. *Biol Reprod* 2002; **67**: 782–8.

[118] Michaut M, Tomes CN, De Blas G, Yunes R, Mayorga LS. Calcium-triggered acrosomal exocytosis in human spermatozoa requires the coordinated activation of Rab3A and N-ethylmaleimide-sensitive factor. *Proc Natl Acad Sci U S A* 2000; **97**: 9996–10001.

[119] Ramalho-Santos J, Moreno RD, Sutovsky P, *et al.* SNAREs in mammalian sperm: possible implications for fertilization. *Dev Biol* 2000; **223**: 54–69.

[120] De Blas GA, Roggero CM, Tomes CN, Mayorga LS. Dynamics of SNARE assembly and disassembly during sperm acrosomal exocytosis. *PLoS Biol* 2005; **3**: e323.

[121] Tomes CN, Roggero CM, De Blas G, Saling PM, Mayorga LS. Requirement of protein tyrosine kinase and phosphatase activities for human sperm exocytosis. *Dev Biol* 265: 399–415.

[122] Tesarik J. Comparison of acrosome reaction-inducing activities of human cumulus oophorus, follicular fluid and ionophore A23187 in human sperm populations of proven fertilizing ability in vitro. *J Reprod Fertil* 1985; **74**: 383–8.

[123] Suarez SS, Wolf DP, Meizel S. Induction of the acrosome reaction in human spermatozoa by a fraction of human follicular fluid. *Gam Res* 1986; **14**: 107–21.

[124] Siiteri JE, Dandekar P, Meizel S. Human sperm acrosome reaction-initiating activity associated with the human cumulus oophorus and mural granulosa cells. *J Exp Zool* 1988; **246**: 71–80.

[125] De Jonge CJ, Barratt CL, Radwanska E, Cooke ID. The acrosome reaction-inducing effect of human follicular and oviductal fluid. *J Androl* 1993; **14**: 359–65.

[126] Osman RA, Andria ML, Jones AD, Meizel S. Steroid induced exocytosis: the human sperm acrosome reaction. *Biochem Biophys Res Commun* 1989; **160**: 828–33.

[127] Marín-Briggiler CI, Vazquez-Levin MH, Gonzalez-Echeverria F, *et al.* Effect of antisperm antibodies present in human follicular fluid upon the acrosome reaction and sperm–zona pellucida interaction. *Am J Reprod Immunol* 2003; **50**: 209–19.

[128] Roldan ER, Murase T, Shi QX. Exocytosis in spermatozoa in response to progesterone and zona pellucida. *Science* 1994; **266**: 1578–81.

[129] Schuffner AA, Bastiaan HS, Duran HE, *et al.* Zona pellucida-induced acrosome reaction in human sperm: dependency on activation of pertussis toxin-sensitive G(i) protein and extracellular calcium, and priming effect of progesterone and follicular fluid. *Mol Hum Reprod* 2002; **8**: 722–7.

[130] Harper CV, Barratt CL, Publicover SJ. Stimulation of human spermatozoa with progesterone gradients to simulate approach to the oocyte: induction of [Ca(2+)].(i) oscillations and cyclical transitions in flagellar beating. *J Biol Chem* 2004; **279**: 46315–25.

[131] Brucker C, Lipford GB. The human sperm acrosome reaction: physiology and regulatory mechanisms. An update. *Hum Reprod Update* 1995; **1**: 51–62.

[132] Benoff S. Modelling human sperm–egg interactions in vitro: signal transduction pathways regulating the acrosome reaction. *Mol Hum Reprod* 1998; **4**: 453–71.

[133] Patrat C, Serres C, Jouannet P. The acrosome reaction in human spermatozoa. *Biol Cell* 2000; **92**: 255–66.

[134] Kirkman-Brown JC, Punt EL, Barratt CL, Publicover SJ. Zona pellucida and progesterone-induced Ca2+ signaling and acrosome reaction in human spermatozoa. *J Androl* 2002; **23**: 306–15.

[135] Breitbart H. Signaling pathways in sperm capacitation and acrosome reaction. *Cell Mol Biol* 2003; **49**: 321–7.

[136] Liu DY, Baker HW. Inhibition of acrosin activity with a trypsin inhibitor blocks human sperm penetration of the zona pellucida. *Biol Reprod* 1993; **48**: 340–8.

[137] Urch UA. Biochemistry and function of acrosin. In: Wassarman P, ed. *Elements of Mammalian Fertilization.* Boca Raton, FL: CRC Press, 1991: 233–48.

[138] Klemm U, Muller-Esterl W, Engel W. Acrosin, the peculiar sperm-specific serine protease. *Hum Genet* 1991; **87**: 635–41.

[139] Siegel MS, Bechtold DS, Kopta CI, Polakoski KL. The rapid purification and partial characterization of human sperm proacrosin using an automated fast protein liquid chromatography (FPLC) system. *Biochim Biophys Acta* 1986; **883**: 567–73.

[140] Zahn A, Furlong LI, Biancotti JC, *et al.* Evaluation of the proacrosin/acrosin system and its mechanism of activation in human sperm extracts. *J Reprod Immunol* 2002; **54**: 43–63.

[141] Tesarik J, Drahorad J, Testart J, Mendoza C. Acrosin activation follows its surface exposure and precedes membrane fusion in human sperm acrosome reaction. *Development* 1990; **110**: 391–400.

[142] Eberspaecher U, Gerwien J, Habenicht UF, Schleuning WD, Donner P. Activation and subsequent degradation of proacrosin is mediated by zona pellucida glycoproteins, negatively charged polysaccharides, and DNA. *Mol Reprod Dev* 1991; **30**: 164–70.

[143] Baba T, Azuma S, Kashiwabara S, Toyoda Y. Sperm from mice carrying a targeted mutation of the acrosin gene can penetrate the oocyte zona pellucida and effect fertilization. *J Biol Chem* 1994; **269**: 31845–9.

[144] Adham IM, Nayernia K, Engel W. Spermatozoa lacking acrosin protein show delayed fertilization. *Mol Reprod Dev* 1997; **46**: 370–6.

[145] Nayernia K, Adham IM, Shamsadin R, *et al.* Proacrosin-deficient mice and zona pellucida modifications in an experimental model of multifactorial infertility. *Mol Hum Reprod* 2002; **8**: 434–40.

[146] Honda A, Siruntawineti J, Baba T. Role of acrosomal matrix proteases in sperm–zona pellucida interactions. *Hum Reprod Update* 2002; **8**: 405–12.

[147] Yamagata K, Murayama K, Okabe M, *et al.* Acrosin accelerates the dispersal of sperm acrosomal proteins during acrosome reaction. *J Biol Chem* 1998; **273**: 10470–4.

[148] Mari S, Rawe V, Biancotti JC, et al. Biochemical and molecular studies of the proacrosin/acrosin system in patients with unexplained infertility. *Fertil Steril* 2003; **79**: 1676–9.

[149] Chaudhury K, Das T, Chakravarty B, Bhattacharyya AK. Acrosin activity as a potential marker for sperm membrane characteristics in unexplained male infertility. *Fertil Steril* 2005; **83**: 104–9.

[150] Evans JP. The molecular basis of sperm–oocyte membrane interactions during mammalian fertilization. *Hum Reprod Update* 2002; **8**: 297–311.

[151] Kaji K, Kudo A. The mechanism of sperm–oocyte fusion in mammals. *Reproduction* 127: 423–9.

[152] Rubinstein E, Ziyyat A, Wolf JP, Le Naour F, Boucheix C. The molecular players of sperm–egg fusion in mammals. *Semin Cell Dev Biol* 2006; **17**: 254–63.

[153] Primakoff P, Myles DG. Cell–cell membrane fusion during mammalian fertilization. *FEBS Lett* 2007; **581**: 2174–80.

[154] Cho C, Bunch DO, Faure JE, et al. Fertilization defects in sperm from mice lacking fertilin beta. *Science* 1998; **281**: 1857–9.

[155] Shamsadin R, Adham IM, Nayernia K, *et al.* Male mice deficient for germ-cell cyritestin are infertile. *Biol Reprod* 1999; **61**: 1445–51.

[156] Grzmil P, Kim Y, Shamsadin R, *et al.* Human cyritestin genes (CYRN1 and CYRN2) are non-functional. *Biochem J* 2001; **357**: 551–6.

[157] Frayne J, Hurd EA, Hall L. Human tMDC III: a sperm protein with a potential role in oocyte recognition. *Mol Hum Reprod* 2002; **8**: 817–22.

[158] Inoue N, Ikawa M, Isotani A, Okabe M. The immunoglobulin superfamily protein Izumo is required for sperm to fuse with eggs. *Nature* 2005; **434**: 234–8.

[159] Hayasaka S, Terada Y, Inoue N, *et al.* Positive expression of the immunoglobulin superfamily protein IZUMO on human sperm of severely infertile male patients. *Fertil Steril* 2007; **88**: 214–16.

[160] Boué F, Duquenne C, Lassalle B, Lefèvre A, Finaz C. FLB1, a human protein of epididymal origin that is involved in the sperm-oocyte recognition process. *Biol Reprod* 1995; **52**: 267–78.

[161] Lefèvre A, Martin Ruiz C, Chokomian S, Duquenne C, Finaz C. Characterization and isolation of SOB2, a human sperm protein with a potential role in oocyte membrane binding. *Mol Hum Reprod* 1997; **3**: 507–16.

[162] Focarelli R, Giuffrida A, Capparelli S, *et al.* Specific localization in the equatorial region of gp20, a 20 kDa sialylglycoprotein of the capacitated human spermatozoon acquired during epididymal transit which is necessary to penetrate zona-free hamster eggs. *Mol Hum Reprod* 1998; **4**: 119–25.

[163] Hamatani T, Tanabe K, Kamei K, *et al.* A monoclonal antibody to human SP-10 inhibits in vitro the binding of human sperm to hamster oolemma but not to human zona pellucida. *Biol Reprod* 2000; **62**: 1201–8.

[164] Cohen DJ, Ellerman DA, Busso D, *et al.* Evidence that human epididymal protein ARP plays a role in gamete fusion through complementary sites on the surface of the human egg. *Biol Reprod* 2001; **65**: 1000–5.

[165] Hao Z, Wolkowicz MJ, Shetty J, *et al.* SAMP32, a testis-specific, isoantigenic sperm acrosomal membrane-associated protein. *Biol Reprod* 2002; **66**: 735–44.

[166] Shetty J, Wolkowicz MJ, Digilio LC, *et al.* SAMP14, a novel, acrosomal membrane-associated, glycosylphosphatidylinositol-anchored member of the Ly-6/urokinase-type plasminogen activator receptor superfamily with a role in sperm–egg interaction. *J Biol Chem* 2003; **278**: 30506–15.

[167] Fenichel P, Durand-Clement M. Role of integrins during fertilization in mammals. *Hum Reprod* 1998; **13** (Suppl 4): 31–46.

[168] He ZY, Brakebusch C, Fassler R, *et al.* None of the integrins known to be present on the mouse egg or to be ADAM receptors are essential for sperm–egg binding and fusion. *Dev Biol* 2003; **254**: 226–37.

[169] Sengoku K, Takuma N, Miyamoto T, Horikawa M, Ishikawa M. Integrins are not involved in the process of human sperm–oolemmal fusion. *Hum Reprod* 2004; **19**: 639–44.

[170] Ziyyat A, Rubinstein E, Monier-Gavelle F, *et al.* CD9 controls the formation of clusters that contain tetraspanins and the integrin α6β1, which are involved in human and mouse gamete fusion. *J Cell Sci* 2006; **119**: 416–24.

[171] Miyado K, Yamada G, Yamada S, *et al.* Requirement of CD9 on the egg plasma membrane for fertilization. *Science* 2000; **287**: 321–4.

[172] Burkman LJ, Coddington CC, Franken DR, *et al.* The hemizona assay (HZA): development of a diagnostic test for the binding of human spermatozoa to the human hemizona pellucida to predict fertilization potential. *Fertil Steril* 1988; **49**: 688–97.

[173] Liu DY, Lopata A, Johnston WI, Baker HW. A human sperm–zona pellucida binding test using oocytes that failed to fertilize in vitro. *Fertil Steril* 1988; **50**: 782–8.

[174] Liu DY, Garrett C, Baker HW. Clinical application of sperm–oocyte interaction tests in vitro fertilization: embryo transfer and intracytoplasmic sperm

injection programs. *Fertil Steril* 2004; **82**: 1251–63, 2004.

[175] Franken DR, Oehninger S. The clinical significance of sperm–zona pellucida binding: 17 years later. *Front Biosci* 2006; **11**: 1227–33.

[176] Liu DY, Liu ML, Garrett C, Baker HW. Comparison of the frequency of defective sperm–zona pellucida (ZP) binding and the ZP-induced acrosome reaction between subfertile men with normal and abnormal semen. *Hum Reprod* 2007; **22**: 1878–84.

[177] Liu DY, Baker HW. Disordered acrosome reaction of spermatozoa bound to the zona pellucida: a newly discovered sperm defect causing infertility with reduced sperm–zona pellucida penetration and reduced fertilization in vitro. *Hum Reprod* 1994; **9**: 1694–700.

[178] Franken DR, Bastiaan HS, Oehninger SC. Physiological induction of the acrosome reaction in human sperm: validation of a microassay using minimal volumes of solubilized, homologous zona pellucida. *J Assist Reprod Genet* 2000; **17**: 374–8.

[179] Calvo L, Vantman D, Banks SM, et al. Follicular fluid-induced acrosome reaction distinguishes a subgroup of men with unexplained infertility not identified by semen analysis. *Fertil Steril* 1989; **52**: 1048–54.

[180] Krausz C, Bonaccorsi L, Luconi M, et al. Intracellular calcium increase and acrosome reaction in response to progesterone in human spermatozoa are correlated with in-vitro fertilization. *Hum Reprod* 1995; **10**: 120–4.

[181] Cummins JM, Pember SM, Jequier AM, Yovich JL, Hartmann PE. A test of the human sperm acrosome reaction following ionophore: relationship to fertility and other seminal parameters. *J Androl* 1991; **12**: 98–103.

[182] Calvo L, Dennison-Lagos L, Banks SM, et al. Acrosome reaction inducibility predicts fertilization success at in-vitro fertilization. *Hum Reprod* 1994; **9**: 1880–6.

[183] Yovich JM, Edirisinghe WR, Yovich JL. Use of the acrosome reaction to ionophore challenge test in managing patients in an assisted reproduction program: a prospective, double-blind, randomized controlled study. *Fertil Steril* 1994; **61**: 902–10.

[184] Yanagimachi R, Yanagimachi H, Rogers BJ. The use of zona-free animal ova as a test-system for the assessment of the fertilizing capacity of human spermatozoa. *Biol Reprod* 1976; **15**: 471–6.

[185] World Health Organization. *WHO Laboratory Manual for the Examination of Human Semen and Sperm–Cervical Mucus Interaction*, 4th edn. Cambridge: Cambridge University Press, 1999.

[186] Johnson A, Bassham B, Lipshultz LI, Lamb DJ. Methodology for the optimized sperm penetration assay. In: Keel BA, Webster BW, eds. *Handbook of the Laboratory Diagnosis and Treatment of Infertility*. Boca Raton, FL: CRC Press, 1990: 135–47.

[187] Aitken RJ, Irvine DS, Wu FC. Prospective analysis of sperm–oocyte fusion and reactive oxygen species generation as criteria for the diagnosis of infertility. *Am J Obstet Gynecol* 1991; **164**: 542–51.

[188] Romano R, Santucci R, Marrone V, et al. A prospective analysis of the accuracy of the TEST-yolk buffer enhanced hamster egg penetration test and acrosin activity in discriminating fertile from infertile males. *Hum Reprod* 1998; **13**: 2115–21.

[189] Vazquez-Levin MH, Chue J, Goldberg S, Medley NE, Nagler HM. The relationship between critical evaluation of sperm morphology and the TYB-optimized zona free hamster oocyte sperm penetration assay. *Int J Androl* 1999; **22**: 329–35.

[190] Oehninger S, Franken DR, Sayed E, Barroso G, Kolm P. Sperm function assays and their predictive value for fertilization outcome in IVF therapy: A meta-analysis. *Hum Reprod Update* 2000; **6**: 160–8.

[191] Benoff S, Cooper GW, Hurley I, et al. Human sperm fertilizing potential in vitro is correlated with differential expression of a head-specific mannose-ligand receptor. *Fertil Steril* 1993; **59**: 854–62.

[192] Kennedy WP, Kaminski JM, Van der Ven HH, et al. A simple clinical assay to evaluate the acrosin activity of human spermatozoa. *J Androl* 1989; **10**: 221–31.

[193] Liu DY, Bourne H, Baker HW. High fertilization and pregnancy rates after intracytoplasmic sperm injection in patients with disordered zona pellucida-induced acrosome reaction. *Fertil Steril* 1997; **67**: 955–8.

New concepts in the genetics of male reproduction and infertility

Paul J. Turek

Introduction

Our understanding of genomic medicine has vastly improved with recent developments in molecular genetics, stem cell technology, and the description of the DNA content of the human genome. Indeed, advances in these fields have had an impact on research that is focused on genetic causes of male infertility. The goal of this chapter is to show how developments in genomic medicine will likely explain much of what we currently view as unexplained male infertility. The increasing importance of the human X chromosome as a source of spermatogenesis genes, the fact that faulty recombination occurs in male infertility, and the growing knowledge of the close relationship between germ cells and stem cells will be discussed. Taken together, these developments in genetic causes of male infertility have tremendous implications for the diagnosis and treatment of this condition.

The X chromosome and male infertility

Although abnormalities of the Y chromosome have been associated with male infertility since 1976 [1], only in the last decade was the Y chromosome shown to have genes that govern spermatogenesis. More recently, it has become clear that **the X chromosome may be as important as the Y in determining male fertility potential**. Although its role as a sex-determining chromosome is well recognized, one suggestion that the X chromosome harbored male infertility genes arose from case reports of X-chromosome translocations, partial deletions, and inversions that resulted in severe infertility and azoospermia [2–6]. **Infertility from structural abnormalities may occur through direct interruption of a gene at breakpoint regions, or as a consequence of "position effect," in which**

an uninterrupted gene does not function normally because of its changed chromosomal environment. As a consequence, the X chromosome garnered suspicion as an important chromosome for male fertility.

Studies on the mouse X chromosome

Recently, Wang and colleagues began a systematic search for the genes expressed exclusively in mouse spermatogonia [7]. Of 25 genes identified by cDNA subtraction, 3 localized to the Y chromosome, 12 to autosomes, and 10 (9 novel) to the X chromosome. Verifying the value of the cDNA subtraction, these experiments recovered the mouse homologs of three well-described human Y-chromosome genes: *USP9Y*, *RBMY*, and *DAZ*. The strong and unexpected predilection of genes expressed in spermatogonia to the X chromosome, indicating 15-fold enrichment relative to chance, led the investigators to conclude that the X chromosome has a predominant role in premeiotic stages of mammalian spermatogenesis. Interestingly, many protein products of these genes were found to have a role in transcriptional or post-transcriptional gene regulation. In addition, human homologs to six of the nine novel mouse X-chromosome genes were identified and mapped to chromosomal regions of known conserved synteny between mouse and human genomes (Table 8.1) [7]. Thus, **similar to genes on the Y chromosome, X-chromosome genes may also prove to be sites of mutation in human spermatogenic failure**.

Clinical studies of human X-linked genes and infertility

Few studies have examined mutations in X-linked genes in male infertility patients (Table 8.2) [8,9]. In a study of 56 infertile men with low or no sperm counts, Raverot *et al.* observed mutations in the *SOX3* (sex determining region Y box 3) gene [8]. The mouse

Infertility in the Male, 4th edition, ed. Larry I. Lipshultz, Stuart S. Howards, and Craig S. Niederberger. Published by Cambridge University Press. © Cambridge University Press 2009.

Table 8.1. Human germ-cell-specific X-linked genes expressed in spermatogonia [7] (reproduced with permission)

Mouse gene	Mouse chromosome	Human ortholog	Comments
Fthl17	X	FTHL17	Ferritin, iron metabolism
Usp26	X	USP26	Ubiquitin specific protease 26
Tex11	X	TEX11	Testis expressed gene 11
Tafq2	X	TAFQ2	TBP-associated factor; RNA polymerase II
Nxf2	X	NXF2	Nuclear RNA export factor
Tex13	X	TEX13A, 13B	Testis expressed gene 13
mUtp14b	X	UTP14	Juvenile spermatogonia depletion (jsd) phenotype

Table 8.2. Clinical studies of X-linked genes in male infertility

Human gene	Study patients	Mutations detected	Clinical phenotype	Ref.
SOX3	56	3 nucleotide substitutions, no mutations	Oligoazoospermia	[8]
FATE	144	4 polymorphisms 2 mutations (1.4%)	Random, infertile men	[9]

homolog of this gene is found in the developing gonad and brain and, when disrupted, causes hypogonadism with loss of germ cells. Mutations in the human *FATE* gene (Xp28) have also been studied in infertile men [9]. This gene encodes a polypeptide of 21 kDa that is not related to any known proteins. The *FATE* message is testis-specific in fetal life soon after sex determination and is co-expressed with *SRY* in the 7-week-old testis. Among 144 randomly chosen infertile men and 100 proven fertile men, a study of the *FATE* gene revealed two mutations. Each mutation was found only once, and neither was found in the controls. Neither affected patient had a karyotype abnormality or a Y-chromosome microdeletion. However, in one affected patient, a maternal uncle also carried the mutation and was fertile. The authors concluded that **FATE gene mutations may contribute to but are not common or important causes of male infertility**.

There is also speculation that the *ZFX* gene in humans, a zinc finger protein on the X chromosome that appears to be a transcriptional activator, may function in sex differentiation or spermatogenesis. To study this, Luoh *et al.* used a reverse genetic strategy, mutagenized the mouse homolog *Zfx*, and noted organismal effects that might suggest a role of this gene in reproduction [10]. **The Zfx mutant had an impressive decrease in primordial germ cell number during the embryonic period before testicular differentiation**. After birth, the mutant mice were smaller, had smaller testes and epididymides, and had sperm counts reduced by one-half compared to wild-type mice.

Why does the X chromosome have a role in male fertility?

It is interesting that, at least in mice, a disproportionate number of male-specific genes are found on the X chromosome. Two theories have been offered to explain this phenomenon: meiotic drive and sexually antagonistic genes [7]. Compared to autosomes, sex chromosomes may be more susceptible to **meiotic drive**, in which there is preferential transmission of certain alleles to gametes and offspring rather than their homolog, in contrast to more random Mendelian patterns. This process could skew transmission of X over Y chromosomes, perhaps driven by X-linked genes critical for spermatogenesis. Alternatively, the theory of **sexually antagonistic genes**, often invoked to explain why the Y chromosome is laden with spermatogenesis genes, may also account for an abundance of X-chromosome genes. Sexually antagonistic genes might enhance the reproductive strength in one sex and diminish it in the other, and there is reason to believe that such genes might accumulate on the sex chromosomes. If recessive mutations exist that enhance male reproductive fitness, they would be more likely to have immediate benefit for males if located on the X chromosome rather than an autosome, thus increasing the chance that the allele would permeate the population. Once permeated, female "fitness" might decrease and adaptive pressures would serve to limit the gene expression to males, thus augmenting the number of critical spermatogenesis genes on the X chromosome [7].

This scenario is even more complicated when we consider that spermatogenesis genes also exist on autosomes. **One theory presupposes that autosomal fertility genes arose as "retrogenes" transposed from the X chromosome [11]. Silencing of the X chromosome during male meiosis could create a driving force for the shift of X-linked genes to autosomes to preserve expression of critical genes required for developing germ cells.** Interestingly, it appears that many such **"retrogenes" (genes that lack introns in contrast with their progenitors)** originated from X-linked progenitor genes and are specifically expressed in the testis [11]. The evolution of autosomal, testis-specific retrogenes, by the compensation hypothesis, is important in that they compensate for the transcriptionally silenced X-chromosome genes that participate in spermatogenesis. Corroborating this hypothesis, several retrogenes have recently been identified that are autosomally located and testis-specific, with an origin from intron-containing X-chromosome progenitor genes. The X-derived retrogene *Jsd* is an excellent example. This gene causes spermatogonial depletion in mice following a single postnatal wave of spermatogenesis. The homolog retrogene in humans is expressed only in the testis [12]. Both as "rescue" genes that explain the widely variable phenotype observed in men with AZF deletions, and as primary effectors of unexplained genetic infertility, X-derived retrogenes are likely to be important for normal human spermatogenesis.

Errors in DNA repair and recombination as causes of male infertility

Remarkably little is known about the genetic basis for human recombination, a series of events that governs proper chromosomal segregation during meiosis on one hand, but also allows for genetic variation and evolution on the other. What is clear is that human recombination occurs at genomic "hotspots," and that large variations in recombination rates occur within humans and between species [13]. This section will review our evolving knowledge of recombination and male infertility.

The mice papers and DNA mismatch repair

Defective DNA repair has been associated classically with certain hereditary forms of colon cancer, retinoblastoma, and skin cancer. For a decade, it has been clear that mutations in genes needed for DNA repair

(*PMS2, Mlh1*) in mice also lead to infertility characterized by meiotic arrest [14]. We selected a cohort of infertile human testes with a histologic "look" (a global maturation arrest pattern) similar to that of the mutant mouse model and asked whether there is evidence of defective DNA mismatch repair similar to that found in mice [15]. We analyzed the sequence of a polymorphic marker, D19S49, in both testis and blood DNA from men with normal spermatogenesis and those with maturation arrest. With defective DNA repair, we expected to see an increased number of mutations in DNA sequences from the testes of infertile men compared to those from controls. After PCR of this marker, products were cloned and sequenced. Indeed, three out of the six patients with maturation arrest had significantly more mutations in testis DNA with dinucleotide (microsatellite) repeats than the men with obstruction. In addition, the percentage error in the sequences (10–25%) was similar to that found in *Mlh1$^{-/-}$* mice compared to wild-type mice (14%) [16]. Interestingly, no mutations were observed in the blood DNA of either group. **This provides evidence that certain forms of male infertility could involve the inability to properly repair the germline DNA, and this has since been confirmed by others** [17]. Future research on the involvement of specific human DNA repair genes in this process will greatly augment our understanding of this genetic pathway in spermatogenesis. In addition, **the relationship between defective DNA repair in infertile men and the risk of cancer among their biological offspring certainly merits further research.**

Chromosomal recombination in spermatogenesis

Since an obvious source of errors in DNA mismatch repair results from the complex events of chromosomal crossing over and synapsis that occur during meiosis, we and others have investigated whether there are defects in the fidelity of meiotic recombination within the germ cells of infertile men. **Recombination is required both to introduce genetic variation and to insure proper chromosome separation during meiosis.** During meiosis prophase I there is formation of a synaptonemal complex (SC, a proteinaceous structure), pairing of homologous (maternal and paternal) chromosomes, and physical interaction of DNA molecules through reciprocal recombination at sites of crossing over (chiasmata) between homologs [18]. The SC consists of two axial elements that form

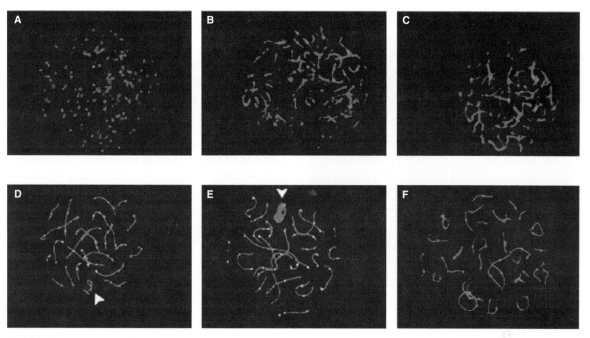

Fig. 8.1. The developmental stages of meiotic prophase I demonstrated by antibody immunofluorescence. Within these spermatocytes, antisera were directed against SCP3 (synaptonemal complex protein 3; SCs, red), MLH1 (Mut-L homolog 1; MLH1 foci, yellow), and CREST antigens (centromeres, blue). Cells are in the following stages of meiotic prophase: (A) leptotene; (B) early zygotene; (C) late zygotene; (D) early pachytene, with arrowhead indicating the sex chromosomes (X and Y); (E) late pachytene, with arrowhead indicating the desynapsed sex chromosomes; and (F) diplotene. Magnification × 1000. (From Gonsalves J *et al. Defective recombination in infertile men. Hum Mol Genet* 2004, **13**: 2875–83, by permission of Oxford University Press.) *See color plate section.*

between sister chromatids during leptotene prophase (Fig. 8.1a). As homologs get closer, transverse filaments form between axial elements. MLH1, a DNA mismatch repair protein, is thought to be involved in recombination between homologs [16,19]; the number and distribution of MLH1 foci on the SC in male and female mice correspond to the number and distribution of crossovers observed genetically and cytologically [16,20].

Chromosomal recombination in azoospermic men

The failure to form the synaptonemal complex in an infertile man with meiotic arrest and azoospermia was an important clue that defective recombination may underlie male infertility [21]. We also reported an association between reduced recombination frequencies and infertility in a cohort of 40 infertile men [22]. Newer, sophisticated immunofluorescence techniques now allow for the accurate study of proteins during meiosis [23] (Fig. 8.1). The assessment of the synaptonemal complex proteins SCP1 and SCP3, and other proteins found in late

recombination nodules such as MLH1, now allows simultaneous analysis of synapsis and meiotic recombination. Antibodies to SCP3/SCP1 allow visualization of the axial and lateral elements (as the axial elements are called after homolog synapsis) and transverse filaments, from the beginning of their assembly in early meiosis until their disassembly in diplotene prophase. Antibodies to MLH1 allow us to identify recombination foci on the synaptonemal complex. In our first study using antibody immunofluoresence, we performed the first comparison of recombination parameters within populations of spermatocytes from infertile ($n = 49$) and fertile ($n = 17$) men who reported for assisted reproduction [22]. **We observed that 10% of nonobstructive azoospermic men had significantly lower recombination frequencies than men with normal spermatogenesis, a proportion that has since been confirmed by other investigators in similar studies [24] (Fig. 8.2). Furthermore, when we focused on men who had a pathological diagnosis of "maturation arrest" on biopsy, about half had detectable defects in recombination, consistent with our previous findings on microsatellite instability in these men. In contrast, none of the men with normal spermatogenesis had**

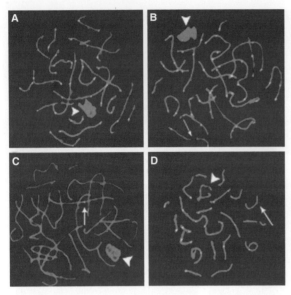

Fig. 8.2. Pachytene spermatocytes from men in (A) control, (B) obstructive and (C & D) nonobstructive azoospermia groups. (SCs, red; MLH1 foci, yellow; centromeres, blue). The sex chromosomes are indicated (arrowheads in A–D). There are several areas of faulty recombination noted: the arrow in (B) indicates a chromosomal bivalent with incomplete synapsis; the arrow in (C) indicates one of only a few SCs in this spermatocyte with any MLH1 foci; the arrow in (D) indicates a bivalent with no MLH1 foci in the SC. Magnification × 1000. (From Gonsalves J *et al.* Defective recombination in infertile men. *Hum Mol Genet* 2004, **13**: 2875–83, by permission of Oxford University Press.) *See color plate section.*

defects in recombination. This was considered **direct evidence that defects in recombination are linked to poor sperm production in some infertile men**. In addition, it suggested that severe defects in recombination in men are compatible with sperm production; moreover, sperm from men with defective recombination are likely to be used routinely (without such testing) in assisted reproductive clinics.

Characteristics of abnormal recombination in male infertility

Subsequent work with antibody immunofluorescence has shed light on other features of the recombination pathway in normal and infertile men. In testicular biopsies from azoospermic men (obstructive and nonobstructive) and controls (non-infertility-related), Sun *et al.* more accurately characterized the recombination abnormalities and divided them into two groups: (1) abnormalities in the quality of chromosomal pairing and (2) variations in recombination frequencies [25]. The quality of chromosome pairing was assessed by observing gaps (discontinuities) and splits (unpaired

chromosome regions) in the SCs. Variations in recombination were assessed by estimating the number of nonexchange SCs (complexes showing no MLH1 foci) and recombination frequencies (the mean number of MLH1 foci per cell at the pachytene stage). Among measures of chromosomal pairing quality, there were no significant differences among the three groups of men. In fact, SC gaps (35–45% of SCs) and splits (7.5% in controls) were detected in all groups. Splits or unpaired chromosomal areas tended to occur more often in obstructive and nonobstructive azoospermic men than in controls. Non-exchange SCs were rare in all groups. In the second category, they observed highly significant differences in recombination frequency between controls (mean 48 ± 4.7 MLH1 foci per pachytene spermatocyte) and men with both obstructive (46.3 ± 6.3 MLH1 foci) and nonobstructive azoospermia (40.4 ± 6.1 MLH1 foci). Finally, regarding SCs that completely lack any MLH1 foci, there was a significant difference between controls and men with nonobstructive azoospermia. **Thus, by refining the analysis of the particular recombination abnormalities in infertile men, this study confirmed that there may be decreased chromosomal pairing quality as well as recombination frequencies in men with nonobstructive azoospermia.**

Variations in recombination in normal spermatogenesis

Variations in recombination have implications for sperm aneuploidy, since reduced recombination frequency and alterations in crossover position are risk factors for human nondisjunction. **Documentation of the normal variability in recombination, therefore, is a prerequisite for the understanding of changes observed in abnormal situations, such as nondisjunction or a chromosome rearrangement.** To further define the distribution of recombination foci in normal germ cells, we investigated the variability in recombination foci across all chromosomes in men with normal spermatogenesis [26]. Recombination maps for individual chromosomes were examined with antibody immunofluorescence, and individual chromosomes were identified with centromere-specific multicolor FISH (cenM-FISH) (Fig. 8.3). **Significant heterogeneity in MLH1 focus frequency across donors was observed for larger chromosome arms. Moreover, significant inter-individual variation in overall recombination frequency per cell was also found.** Interestingly, a significant inverse correlation was also observed between mean autosomal cell MLH1 focus

A closer look at the phenomenon of non-exchange SCs, or chromosomes without any recombination nodules, has been undertaken in men with normal spermatogenesis [27]. This work has also revealed important clinical implications. Using FISH with immunofluorescence in 10 normal men showed that chromosomes 21 (2.1%) and 22 (1.7%) had a significantly higher proportion of non-exchange SCs than chromosomes 11–20. However, the sex chromosomes were affected with a much higher frequency (27%) than any autosome. **Thus it appears that G-group, as well as sex chromosomes, are most susceptible to having no recombination foci and thus are more susceptible to nondisjunction during spermatogenesis. This observation is consistent with the findings from sperm karyotyping and FISH analyses that show that chromosomes 21, 22, and the sex chromosomes have significantly increased frequencies of aneuploidy compared to other autosomes.**

Proteins involved with recombination

Our understanding of recombination and male infertility has been further broadened by the study of specific meiotic proteins involved in this process. The temporal progression and localization of five meiotic proteins in human recombination (RAD51, RPA, MSH4, MLH1, and MLH3) have recently been reported [28]. The observation of precise protein colocalization patterns within recombination foci at different times in normal germ cells implies that specific interactions exist during meiosis. In addition, **the marked persistence of MSH4 protein within recombination foci, unlike the temporal waxing and waning of other proteins, shows that it not only may initialize, but also may remain active to stabilize and maintain critical foci of recombination** throughout this critical time in prophase of human germ cells. In summary, recent research on DNA mismatch repair and recombination has been extremely fruitful in defining specific abnormalities associated with testis failure in a significant proportion of men with previously unexplained infertility.

The sperm transcriptome and male infertility

Routine semen parameters exhibit notoriously wide variability and, in general, correlate poorly with fertility. **This has suggested to researchers that oligogenic and polygenic modifiers (rather than single gene mutations) may describe the bulk of genetic male**

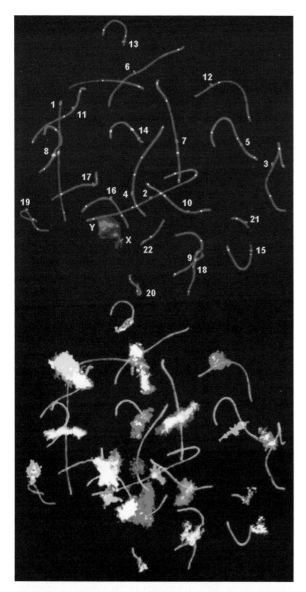

Fig. 8.3. (Upper) Human pachytene spermatocyte with SCs shown in red, centromeres in blue, and MLH1 foci in yellow. (Lower) Subsequent cenM-FISH analysis allows identification of individual chromosomes so that recombination (MLH1) foci can be analyzed for each SC on each chromosome. (From Sun F *et al*. Variation in MLH1 distribution in recombination maps for individual chromosomes from human males. *Hum Mol Genet* 2006; **15**: 2376–91, by permission of Oxford University Press.) *See color plate section.*

frequencies and advancing male age. This has also been shown in oocytes from mice and hamsters. Important for mapping and identifying diseases, this knowledge can also inform our exploration of the chromosomal effects of recombination in various patterns and provide clues to the sources of variation.

infertility. This has led to several interesting investigations of the sperm transcriptome. We have investigated the idea that "genetic signatures" can be developed from testis biopsies with cDNA microarrays [29]. Beginning by comparing the human gene expression patterns from normal versus Sertoli-cell-only testis with cDNA arrays (cDNA subtraction), we identified genes either up- or down-regulated significantly relative to normal. Analysis of these genes produced a subset of 689 genes that were mined for function and relevant homologs. From this pool, we identified 10 genes and constructed a "working" gene set to predict spermatogenic stage on biopsy. Testing this gene set with testis biopsies from infertile men showed a good correlation with routine histology. **Most exciting, however, is the potential for genetic diagnostics to be far more informative than histology**. Examples include the ability of genetic analysis to delineate with higher resolution than routine histology the presence of germ cells in testis biopsies and the ability to examine gene expression profiles in toxicology studies.

RNA transcription in spermatogenesis and RNA in sperm

Sperm classically have been viewed as being transcriptionally dormant. RNAs needed for spermiogenesis were thought to be made in early spermatogenesis and considered "left over" in mature sperm, playing no role during fertilization and beyond. **This theory has now been called into question since the molecular genetic "fingerprint" of normal sperm has been investigated with cDNA microarrays** [30]. In this work, the cDNAs from histologically normal testes, and pooled ($n = 9$ men) and single ejaculates from normal men with proven fertility were hybridized to a 30 K cDNA microarray to determine (1) which mRNAs are contained in sperm and (2) what association exists between testicular and ejaculated sperm genetic fingerprints.

In this study, 7157 unique ESTs (expressed sequence tags) were identified from the testes probe. When the pooled-ejaculate RNA or single-ejaculate RNAs were used as probes, 3281 and 2780 ESTs were identified, respectively. Additionally, all of the pooled- and single-ejaculate RNAs were contained within the larger population of ESTs identified in testis tissue. This high concordance between normal testis and ejaculated sperm **supports the view that sperm RNAs may be used to monitor past events of genetic expression during spermatogenesis**. Additional data mining

of the "ejaculated sperm ESTs revealed that contrary to earlier belief the detected RNAs reflected activity throughout the process of spermatogenesis."

The meaning of mRNA and sperm

Further research on complex sperm RNAs has led investigators to conclude that they are important to the overall paternal contribution to post-fertilization events in the early embyo [31]. In addition, given the wide heterogeneity of RNA in the sperm, it is conceivable that **small interfering RNAs (siRNAs)** exist among those transmitted to the oocyte at fertilization and may be responsible for a heretofore unrecognized level of genetic control as early imprints are established in the embryo [32]. Most recently, a study compared sperm RNAs from normal and infertile men in an attempt to develop a non-invasive diagnostic tool for identifying germline mutations in candidate infertility-associated genes [33]. With over 90% efficiency, germ-cell-expressed genes could be traced from men with a wide range of ejaculated sperm concentrations. Among 270 severely oligospermic men (< 1 million sperm/mL) and 394 controls, two of the oligospermic men and none of the controls exhibited *KLHL10* missense mutations that were clinically suggestive of a functional deficiency. Importantly, this study demonstrated the utility of this approach for the analysis of germ-cell-expressed genes that regulate sperm maturation, motility, and, possibly, fertilization. Diagnostic testing of sperm with these molecular genetic techniques has wide therapeutic implications for male reproductive medicine.

Insights into spermatogenesis from embryonic stem cell research

Until recently, it has not been possible to examine human germ cell development in vivo, for obvious ethical reasons. However, with the advent of human embryonic stem cell (hESC) technology, the study of early embryonic development, including the "birth" of germ cells, is now possible. Several exciting revelations from this research are described below.

Where do germ cells come from?

During human fetal development, hESCs from the inner cell mass of the embryo develop into primordial germ cells (PGCs). After migrating into the gonadal ridge, PGCs enter the fetal gonad as undifferentiated gonocytes, which replicate mitotically until puberty. At puberty, gonocytes become spermatogonia and either self-renew or differentiate into sperm. The type A

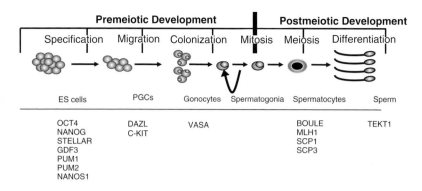

Fig. 8.4. Diagram of the different stages of human germ cell differentiation. Listed is the earliest expression of each gene at each germ cell stage. Most genes are specific to germ cells. ES, embryonic stem cells; PGCs, primordial germ cells.

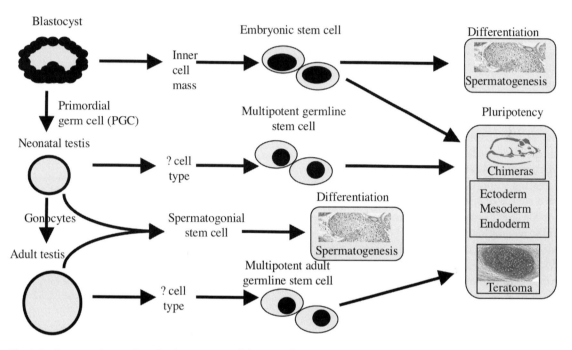

Fig. 8.5. Current understanding of embryonic stem cell derivation from animal models. Embryonic stem cells from blastocysts can differentiate into three germ layers, make chimeras and teratomas, and differentiate into sperm. Spermatogonial stem cells from neonatal and adult mouse testis can also form germline stem cells with similar properties.

spermatogonia is the adult stem cell in the testicle. Recently, human gene expression markers have been discovered that characterize these stages of development, and some of these are outlined in Figure 8.4. **Interestingly, it has been observed that undifferentiated hESC lines actually express early or premeiotic germ cell markers (in the form of both RNA and proteins), but not later postmeiotic markers [34,35]. This suggests that hESCs are very closely related to PGCs and that the germ cell lineage is one of the first lineages to form from hESCs, certainly occurring before** hESC differentiation to the intermediate precursors of ectoderm, mesoderm, or endoderm in the developing embryo.

How are germ cells similar to embryonic stem cells?

The close relationship between human hESCs and early, dedicated germ cells in the form of PGCs has major implications for our understanding of germ cell developmental potential. **Indeed, both hESC and early germ cell lines (embryonic germ cells) derived from human PGCs are pluripotent, able to self-renew, and can form all major somatic lineages [36]. This suggests that the potential of human PGCs in the developing human gonad is not strictly limited to the germ cell lineage, but may in fact have a development potential similar to hESCs. Although this has not** been convincingly demonstrated in humans, there is provocative evidence from mice models that this is true. In fact, the capacity for pluripotency has been demonstrated with germ cells derived from both the neonatal and adult mouse testis [37,38]. When cultured in vitro, under stem cell conditions, it has been observed that testis cells, likely spermatogonia, acquire properties similar to ESCs (Fig. 8.5). These cells have been differentiated into various somatic lineages, form chimeras when injected into developing blastocysts, and make teratomas when injected into nude mice. This provocative research **raises the possibility that pluripotency may exist in the germline of adult men**, and that the testis may be a valuable source of patient-specific "embryonic-like" stem cells for cell-based stem cell therapy in the future without the need for embryo manipulation.

Conclusions

The goal of this chapter was to show how developments in genomic medicine will likely explain much of what we currently view as unexplained male infertility. The increasing importance of the human X chromosome as a source of spermatogenesis genes will open the door for new diagnostic tests. The understanding that faulty recombination occurs in male infertility has wide implications not only for the explanation of the infertility but also for the use of affected gametes. Finally, our growing knowledge of the close relationship between germ cells and stem cells, and the successful manipulation of these cells in vitro, has tremendous implications not only for the treatment and cure of male infertility but also for a host of other medical diseases in the future.

References

[1] Tiepolo L, Zuffardi O. Localization of factors controlling spermatogenesis in the nonfluorescent portion of the human Y chromosome long arm. *Hum Genet* 1976; **34**: 119–24.

[2] Mattei MG, Mattei JF, Ayme S, Giraud F. X-autosome translocations: cytogenetic characteristics and their consequences. *Hum Genet* 1982; **61**: 295–309.

[3] Madan K. Balanced structural changes involving the human X: effect on sexual phenotype. *Hum Genet* 1983; **63**: 216–21.

[4] Cantu JM, Diaz M, Moller M, *et al.* Azoospermia and duplication 3qter as distinct consequences of a familial t(X; 3)(q26; q13.2). *Am J Med Genet* 1985; **20**: 677–84.

[5] Nemeth AH, Gallen IW, Crocker M, Levy E, Maher E. Klinefelter-like phenotype and primary infertility in a

[6] Lee S, Lee SH, Chung TG, *et al.* Molecular and cytogenetic characterization of two azoospermic patients with X-autosome translocation. *J Assist Reprod Genet* 2003; **20**: 385–9.

[7] Wang PJ, McCarrey JR, Yang F, Page DC. An abundance of X-linked genes expressed in spermatogonia. *Nat Genet* 2001; **27**: 422–6.

[8] Raverot G, Lejeune H, Kotlar T, Pugeat M, Jameson JL. X-linked sex-determining region Y box 3 (SOX3) gene mutations are uncommon in men with idiopathic oligoazoospermic infertility. *J Clin Endocrinol Metab* 2004; **89**: 4146–8.

[9] Olesen C, Silber J, Eiberg H, *et al.* Mutational analysis of the human FATE gene in 144 infertile men. *Hum Genet* 2003; **113**: 195–201.

[10] Luoh SW, Bain PA, Polakiewicz RD, *et al.* Zfx mutation results in small animal size and reduced germ cell number in male and female mice. *Development* 1997; **124**: 2275–84.

[11] Wang PJ. X chromosomes, retrogenes and their role in male reproduction. *Trends Endocrinol Metab* 2004; **15**: 79–83.

[12] Rohozinski J, Bishop CE. The mouse juvenile spermatogonial depletion (jsd) phenotype is due to a mutation in the X-derived retrogene, mUtp14b. *Proc Natl Acad Sci U S A* 2004; **101**: 11695–700.

[13] Coop G, Przeworski M. An evolutionary view of human recombination. *Nat Rev Genet* 2007; **8**: 23–34.

[14] Baker SM, Bronner CE, Zhang L, *et al.* Male mice defective in the DNA mismatch repair gene PMS2 exhibit abnormal chromosome synapsis in meiosis. *Cell* 1995; **82**: 309–12.

[15] Nudell DM, Castillo M, Turek PJ, Reijo Pera R. Increased frequency of mutations in DNA in infertile men with meiotic arrest. *Hum Reprod* 2000; **15**: 1289–94.

[16] Baker SM, Plug AW, Prolla TA, *et al.* Involvement of mouse Mlh1 in DNA mismatch repair and meiotic crossing over. *Nat Genet* 1996; **13**: 336–42.

[17] Maduro MR, Casella R, Kim E, *et al.* Microsatellite instability and defects in mismatch repair proteins: a new etiology for Sertoli cell-only syndrome. *Mol Hum Reprod* 2003; **9**: 61–8.

[18] Hassold T, Hunt P. To err (meiotically) is human: the genesis of human aneuploidy. *Nat Rev Genet* 2001; **2**: 280–91.

[19] Lynn A, Koehler KE, Judis L, *et al.* Covariation of synaptonemal complex length and mammalian meiotic exchange rates. *Science* 2002; **296**: 2222–5.

[20] Marcon E, Moens P. MLH1p and MLH3p localize to precociously induced chiasmata of okadaic-

male with a paracentric Xq inversion. *J Med Genet* 2002; **39**: e28.

acid-treated mouse spermatocytes. *Genetics* 2003; **165**: 2283–7.

[21] Judis L, Chan ER, Schwartz S, Seftel A, Hassold T. Meiosis I arrest and azoospermia in an infertile male explained by failure of formation of a component of the synaptonemal complex. *Fertil Steril* 2004; **81**: 205–9.

[22] Gonsalves J, Sun F, Schlegel PN, *et al.* Defective recombination in infertile men. *Hum Mol Genet* 2004; **13**: 2875–83.

[23] Peters AH, Plug AW, van Vugt MJ, de Boer P. A drying-down technique for the spreading of mammalian meiocytes from the male and female germline. *Chromosome Res* 1997; **5**: 66–8.

[24] Topping D, Brown P, Judis L, *et al.* Synaptic defects at meiosis I and non-obstructive azoospermia. *Hum Reprod* 2006; **21**: 3171–7.

[25] Sun F, Greene C, Turek PJ, *et al.* Immunofluorescent synaptonemal complex analysis in azoospermic men. *Cytogenet Genome Res* 2005; **111**: 366–70.

[26] Sun F, Oliver-Bonet M, Liehr T, *et al.* Analysis of achiasmate bivalents in pachytene cells from 10 normal men. *Hum Reprod* 2006; **21**: 2335–9.

[27] Sun F, Oliver-Bonet M, Liehr T, *et al.* Variation in MLH1 distribution in recombination maps for individual chromosomes from human males. *Hum Mol Genet* 2006; **15**: 2376–91.

[28] Oliver-Bonet M, Turek PJ, Sun F, Ko E, Martin RH. Temporal progression of recombination in human males. *Mol Hum Reprod* 2005; **11**: 517–22.

[29] Fox M, Ares XV, Turek PJ, Haqq C, Reijo Pera R. Feasibility of global gene expression analysis in testicular biopsies from infertile men. *Mol Reprod Devel* 2003; **66**: 403–21.

[30] Ostermeier GC, Dix DJ, Miller D, Khatri P, Krawetz SA. Spermatozoal RNA profiles of normal fertile men. *Lancet* 2002; **360**: 772–7.

[31] Ostermeier GC, Miller D, Huntriss JD, Diamond MP, Krawetz S. A. Reproductive biology: delivering spermatozoan RNA to the oocyte. *Nature* 2004; **429**: 154.

[32] Ostermeier GC, Goodrich RJ, Moldenhauer JS, Diamond MP, Krawetz SA. A suite of novel human spermatozoal RNAs. *J Androl* 2005; **26**: 70–4.

[33] Yatsenko AN, Roy A, Chen R, *et al.* Non-invasive genetic diagnosis of male infertility using spermatozoal RNA: KLHL10 mutations in oligozoospermic patients impair homodimerization. *Hum Mol Genet* 2006; **15**: 3411–9.

[34] Clark AT, Rodriguez RT, Bodnar MS, *et al.* Human STELLAR, NANOG, and GDF3 genes are expressed in pluripotent cells and map to chromosome 12p13, a hotspot for teratocarcinoma. *Stem Cells* 2004; **22**: 169–79.

[35] Clark AT, Bodnar MS, Fox M, *et al.* Spontaneous differentiation of germ cells from embryonic stem cells in vitro. *Hum Mol Genet* 2004; **13**: 727–39.

[36] Shamblott MJ, Axelman J, Littlefield JW, *et al.* Human embryonic germ cell derivatives express a broad range of developmentally distinct markers and proliferate extensively in vitro. *Proc Natl Acad Sci U S A* 2001; **98**: 113–18.

[37] Guan K, Nayernia K, Maier LS, *et al.* Pluripotency of spermatogonial stem cells from adult mouse testis. *Nature* 2006; **440**: 1199–203.

[38] Kanatsu-Shinohara M, Inoue K, Lee J, *et al.* Generation of pluripotent stem cells from neonatal mouse testis. *Cell* 2004; **119**: 1001–12.

Chapter 9

Erection, emission, and ejaculation: mechanisms of control

Alexander Müller and John P. Mulhall

Introduction

This chapter is dedicated to the elucidation of the current understanding of the fundamental principles involved in erection, emission, and ejaculation.

Concept of penile erection

The penis as the external genitalia in the male harbors the erectile tissue, which has the elasticity to generate tumescence by storing blood and become rigid. The achievement of a natural penile erection is the result of a complex cascade, including neurologic and hemodynamic events under psychological control, resulting in a firm enlargement of the penis. The unique anatomical particulars allow the penis to expand significantly during the erectile process.

Anatomical fundamentals of the penis

Anatomically the penis is built by paired crura forming the **corpora cavernosa** and by the bulb containing the urethra and becoming the **corpus spongiosum**, which is expanded at the tip to the glans. At the base of the penis the corpora cavernosa are covered by the ischiocavernosus muscles, and the corpus spongiosum is surrounded by the bulbocavernosus muscle. Innervated by the pudendal nerve, the contractions of the ischiocavernosus muscles enhance penile rigidity, and contractions of the bulbospongiosus muscles are involved in the expulsion of semen. Several layers wrap around the penile structures, starting with the skin from the outside followed by the Dartos fascia and **Buck's fascia** and lastly the **tunica albuginea**, which surrounds both corpora cavernosa with an outer longitudinal layer and wraps each corpus individually with an inner circular layer of tissue.

Arterial blood supply

The blood supply to the penis can be divided into a **dorsal superficial** and a **central deep (cavernosal) arterial system** that are generally derived from the internal iliac system, specifically the internal pudendal artery, which gives off a perineal branch and continues as the penile artery. Considerable variations of this most common arterial supply will be found in distinctive patients. Additional blood supply may also be found in the form of accessory pudendal arteries provided by the internal iliac, external iliac, or obturator arteries. Before dividing into the **subfascial dorsal artery** and **central cavernosal arteries**, the internal pudendal artery sends arterial branches to the posterior scrotum and to the bulbous urethra. The main **neurovascular bundle**, including the deep dorsal vein, laterally flanked by the paired dorsal penis arteries and then the dorsal nerves, runs along the dorsum of the penis. Circumflex branches of the dorsal penis arteries run around the penis. Usually there are communications between the dorsal and the deep arterial system. The deep penile arteries enter the crura cavernosa and stream on both sides centrally within the corpora cavernosa forming two sorts of terminal branches. The coiled helicine arteries directly supply the sinusoidal spaces, and the few smaller arteries travel between the trabeculae. In the flaccid state, the trabecular arteries keep the main arterial flow. During erection, the sinusoidal spaces are filled by blood supplied via the helicine arterioles.

Venous drainage

Subtunical venous plexuses collect blood from the sinusoidal spaces leading into emissary veins, which pierce the tunica albuginea. **Emissary veins** drain into spongiosal veins, circumflex veins, or directly into the deep dorsal vein and further proximally into cavernosal and crural veins ending in the **internal pudendal vein**. The retrocoronal plexus drains the glans penis into the deep dorsal vein, which also collects the blood from the bulbar veins and from the corpus spongiosum via circumflex veins from the spongiosal vein. The deep

Infertility in the Male, 4th edition, ed. Larry I. Lipshultz, Stuart S. Howards, and Craig S. Niederberger. Published by Cambridge University Press. © Cambridge University Press 2009.

dorsal vein travels along the midline between the neurovascular bundles, finally entering the periprostatic venous plexus. Via the superficial dorsal venous complex the skin and the subcutaneous tissue of the penis are drained into the saphenous vein.

Erectile function

Erectile function is the capability of the erectile tissue to store blood under expansion of the penis and to maintain the erection, allowing satisfactory sexual performance.

The erectile tissue in the corpora cavernosa surrounded by the tunica albuginea is essentially a vascular structure which appears as a spongiose tissue acting like a hydraulic device. **Trabecular structures** composed by collagen, elastin, blood vessels, and nerves contain **smooth-muscle cells** that form the sinusoidal spaces. The **sinusoids** are lined by endothelium. The endothelium is a key regulator of vascular physiology and has a fundamental role in the process of erection. In fact, this is founded in the belief that diseases in which endothelial dysfunction develops, such as in atherosclerosis, diabetes mellitus, hypertension, and hypercholesterolemia, are associated with a high prevalence of erectile dysfunction (ED). Helicine branches of the deep penile arteries are responsible for the filling. Humoral factors, neuronal transmitters, and local mediators are involved in the control of smooth-muscle tone determining arterial inflow and sinusoidal capacitance.

Terminal endings of the cavernous nerves and endothelial cells, which line the cavernosal sinusoids, release erectogenic neurotransmitters. **Nitric oxide (NO)** is believed to be the main vasoactive nonadrenergic, noncholinergic (NANC) neurotransmitter and chemical mediator of penile erection [1]. The smooth-muscle tone depends on the intracellular concentration of free calcium and the sensitivity of the contractile apparatus to calcium. With the relaxation of the intracavernosal sinusoids a rising blood inflow fills the corpora cavernosa followed by an expansion of sinusoidal spaces and volumetric augmentation. The inflatability of the corpora is limited by the surrounding tunica albuginea, which limits the growth of diameter and length under full expansion. Under the extension of the lacunar spaces following the increasing blood inflow, subtunical and emissary veins become compressed and the blood is trapped in the corpora cavernosa because of a reduced venous outflow, which is known as the **veno-occlusive mechanism**. Usually after orgasm,

there is a release of noradrenaline by adrenergic fibers mediating smooth-muscle contraction that leads to penile detumescence.

Erectile hemodynamics

The penile erection is principally a vascular event balanced by the arterial inflow and venous outflow mediated through smooth-muscle tone. Our current understanding of penile hemodynamics during erections is essentially influenced by extensive vascular studies by Lue *et al.* in the 1980s, who concluded that erection depends on increased arterial inflow, increased venous resistance, and relaxation of the cavernous smooth muscles [2]. Relaxation of the smooth muscle and the arterial inflow are actively mediated events, though the decreased venous outflow appears to be a passive process, secondary to the veno-occlusive mechanism by enlarged pressure and volume within the lacunar cavernosal sinusoids. In the flaccid state of the penis, which is dominated by the adrenergic tone of the smooth muscles under the influence of the sympathetic part of the autonomic nervous system, the arterial flow is low, based on the constricted arterioles and the contracted cavernosal smooth muscles. In this condition the arterial inflow is usually less than 15 cm/s and the blood gases taken from the sinusoids are similar to those of venous blood (20–40 mmHg PO_2) [3].

Under parasympathetic (NANC) influence, and the consequent reduction in adrenergic tone, tumescence occurs following arteriolar dilation and trabecular smooth-muscle relaxation. In the filling phase arterial inflow rises, typically reaching velocities greater than 30 cm/s, followed by the tumescent phase in which the penis expands to its maximal capacity and the compression of the subtunical venules begins. In this phase the intracavernosal pressure increases, reaching diastolic blood-pressure levels. Filling continues only during the systolic phase. At a full erection the intracavernosal pressure climbs to values of around 90% of systolic blood pressure and above. At this time the blood gas tensions are similar to those of arterial blood (90–100 mmHg PO_2) [3]. Under the contraction of the ischiocavernosus muscles the penile crura are compressed and the intracavernosal pressure raises levels above the systolic blood pressure and the penis becomes fully rigid. Contraction of the ischiocavernosus muscle may be achieved willingly but also happens under the influence of the bulbocavernosus reflex, which when activated maintains rigidity during penetration. The contraction of the bulbocavernosus muscle reinforces glans erection. The emissary veins are completely closed by the veno-occlusive mechanism and the arterial inflow concludes. Preserving circulation in the cavernosal tissue, the intracavernosal pressure falls intermittently back to those levels below the systolic pressure. Once orgasm is reached or the sexual stimulus is terminated, the erectile transmission ceases and anti-erectile neurotransmission takes over. In the detumescence phase the sympathetic stimulation leads to a fall in arterial inflow and consequently to a drop in intracavernosal pressure. The helicine arterioles constrict and the trabecular smooth muscles contract, leading to reduced compression of the subtunical veins and increased venous outflow that brings the penis back into a flaccid state dominated by a noradrenergic influence of the smooth muscles .

Neurological control of erection

The neurophysiological control of the erectile process is under the influence of central and peripheral processes. At least three kinds of erection can be distinguished in man: central, reflexogenic, and nocturnal types. The initial origin in **central erections** is located in the supraspinal centers and moves along the spinal cord and the cavernous nerves to the erectile tissue. The pathway that is responsible for **reflexogenic erections** plays an important role in maintaining an erection during stimulation by continuing neuronal activation. During mechanical stimulation of the dorsal nerve, signals in the lumbosacral cord are returned via parasympathetic fibers back to the corporeal tissue. The occurrence of **nocturnal erections** is not fully understood yet. But nocturnal penile tumescence is a robust physiologic phenomenon in all normal healthy males, and occurs several times during the night during rapid eye movement (REM) sleep [4]. Sleep-related tumescence testing has been used to differentiate psychogenic from organic impotence. Such nocturnal erections have been postulated to represent a spontaneous mechanism for repeated oxygenation of the erectile tissue during the erection at night [5].

Central control

Despite ongoing efforts, at present we know little about underlying **central control mechanisms**, and what we know is based mainly on experimental studies in animals [6]. Sexual inspirations accomplished by all human senses will be processed within central centers of the brain including the limbic system, cortical centers, and the hypothalamus, all of which seem to be involved in influencing the erectile process.

The **limbic system**, which counts as the anatomical equivalent for emotions located in the prefrontal cortex, interacts with the **hypothalamus**, which appears to be the central integration locus for erectile stimuli. Within the hypothalamus, the two most important regions involved in the erectile regulation are the **paraventricular nucleus (PVN)**, implicated in the processing of erectile stimuli, and the **medial preoptic area (MPOA)**, crucial for the display of sexual behavior, especially copulatory activities [7,8]. In addition, the **nucleus paragigantocellularis** located in the pons seems to support anti-erectile sympathetic preganglionic neurons via a serotonergic projection, which can be abolished upon sexual arousal by projections from the PVN. The central regulation of erectile function is very complex, and a number of neurotransmitters are involved in central pathways. The dopaminergic system, which appears to play a key role, currently is the focus of the pharmaceutical industry. That the PVN is under the innervation of dopaminergic neurons and includes pro-erectile neurons is supported by the report of induced penile erections in rats with dopaminergic agonists, glutamatergic agonists, or oxytocin and electrical stimulations [9]. From these areas, also including the nucleus accumbens, which is devoted to sexual motivation, pro-erectile fibers descend along the spinal cord to the sacral preganglionic neurons and increase the parasympathetic outflow. Several central transmitters and peptides shown to be involved in erectile modulation include dopamine, acetylcholine, NO, oxytocin, adrenocorticotropic/α-melanocyte-stimulating hormone in an assistant role, encephalins and noradrenaline in an inhibitory role, and serotonin in either a supportive or a preventive erectile role. Within the hypothalamus a number of neurotransmitters balance pro- and anti-erectile signals. Table 9.1 represents an overview of centrally acting neurotransmitter and peptides. Under sexual arousal an imbalance involving increased pro-erectile action and decreased anti-erectile pattern lead to a proper erectile function.

Peripheral control

The central areas are connected with centers from the autonomic nerve system located in the **spinal cord**, from which signals reach the penis and vice versa by sensitive afferences from the genitalia (Fig. 9.1). The **pro-erectile sacral parasympathetic nuclei**, which are located in the spinal cord, arise from **S2–S4 segments**, where the preganglionic parasympathetic neurons can be found in the intermediolateral cell column of the spinal cord. Along the pelvic nerve, parasympathetic

Table 9.1. Centrally acting neurotransmitters

Neurotransmitter	Receptor	Locus of action	Effects on erection	Comments
Dopamine	D_1 and D_2, D_1	PVN Spinal cord	Pro-erectile	D_2 receptors are probably predominant in the hypothalamus
NO		PVN	Pro-erectile	Involved in oxytocinergic pathway
α-MSA	Melanocortin (MC) 1–5	PVN	Pro-erectile	Involved in oxytocinergic pathway
ACTH	Unknown	PVN	Pro-erectile	Involved in oxytocinergic pathway
Opioids	Opioid μ	PVN	Anti-erectile	Mediating an oxytocinergic mechanism
GABA	GABA$_A$ GABA$_B$	MPOA Spinal cord	Anti-erectile	
Noradrenaline	$α_1$ $α_2$	Brain/spinal cord Brain	Anti-erectile	$α_2$-antagonists have improved erections
Glutamate		Hypothalamus	Pro-erectile	NO involving activation of descending oxytocinergic pathways
Serotonin (5-hydroxytryptamine, 5-HT)	5-HT$_{1A}$ 5-HT$_{2C}$	Spinal cord Spinal cord	Anti-erectile Pro-erectile	Omnipresent within the CNS, mainly anti-erectile
Oxytocin		Spinal cord	Pro-erectile	

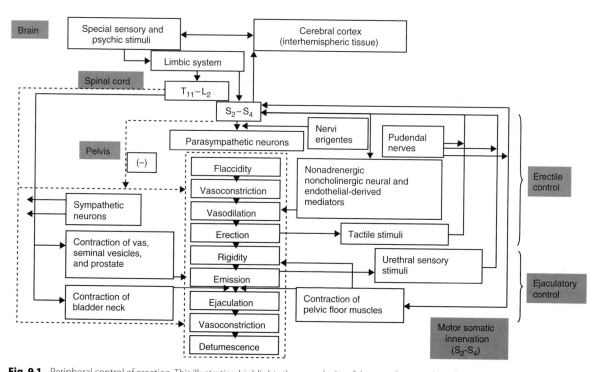

Fig. 9.1. Peripheral control of erection. This illustration highlights the complexity of the erectile control mechanisms at the peripheral level.

axons pass to the pelvic plexus, and after synaptic transfer to the postganglionic neurons, axons lead the signals along the **cavernous nerve** to the erectile tissue. That the paired cavernous nerves are essential neuronal structures embedded in the physiological erectile process is emphasized by the fact that electrical stimulation of the cavernous nerve induces penile erection, and injury of the cavernous nerve leads to changes in erectile function and structural changes in the erectile tissue [10].

The **sympathetic influence** is responsible for the basal anti-erectile tone present in the flaccid state of the penis [11]. The sympathetic nuclei are located in the intermediolateral cell column and the dorsal gray commissure at the thoracolumbar level of the spinal cord where the preganglionic sympathetic axons arise from the **thoracolumbar T11–L2 segments**. After joining the sympathetic paravertebral chain ganglia some of the axons travel along the lumbar splanchnic nerves to the inferior mesenteric and superior hypogastric plexus and reach the pelvic plexus. After synaptic communication the postganglionic neuron fibers travel in the cavernous nerves. Through the paravertebral sympathetic chain, sympathetic axons also reach sacral ganglia, and, after synaptic shifting, postganglionic axons join the pudendal nerves. The **pudendal nerves** are also collecting fibers of motoneurons arising from the dorsolateral and dorsomedial nuclei located in the ventral horn of the sacral spinal cord innervating the ischiocavernosus and bulbospongiosus muscles. Almost all sensory afferent information originating in the penis is collected by the dorsal nerve of the penis, which joins the pudendal nerves to the sacral segments S2–S4, at their origin.

Local control

Terminal nerve endings, the vascular endothelium, and smooth-muscle cells are the fundamental protagonists in the local control of the erectile process. A complex interplay of circulating humoral, neuronal, and local factors influences the arteriolar and trabecular response, both determined by the tone of the smooth muscles, which is balanced between contractile and relaxant factors. In general a principal stimulus via a membrane-bound receptor or a cytoplasmic protein translates into the production of an intracellular messenger that leads to changes in intracellular calcium (Ca) concentration and finally results in changes in the smooth-muscle tone.

Undisputedly, **smooth muscles** are a central structure in the erectile process. The smooth-muscle tone is dependent on the **intracellular Ca ion concentration**, contracting in response to a rise in intracellular Ca ion concentration and relaxing according to an intracellular Ca concentration fall. Along a concentration gradient between the extracellular environment and the smooth-muscle cell, Ca tends to get into the cell when Ca channels in the cellular membrane are open. Also the sarcoplasmic reticulum and the nucleus

can contribute to an increase in intracellular Ca concentration by Ca release. Among several different **Ca channels, the L-type** appears to be the most important in the smooth-muscle cell. Among a number of causes, the opening of the Ca channels depends on the membrane potential of the smooth-muscle cell and the phosphorylation of the channels.

Most of the time the penis is kept in a flaccid state under the influence of α-adrenergic tone through a tonic noradrenaline release from sympathetic nerves that maintain a penile arterial and corporeal smooth-muscle contraction via an α_1-receptor-mediated increase in intracellular Ca concentration [12]. This seemingly plausible explanation is supported by the findings that the density of α-adrenoceptors is 10 times higher than that of β-adrenoceptors in the human corpus cavernosum [13]. The anti-erectile influence of **noradrenaline**, tonically released from sympathetic nerve terminals, is an example of a membrane-bound adrenergic-receptor-mediated effect. The α_1-adrenoceptors appear to be most important in trabecular smooth-muscle tone, where the stimulation leads to smooth-muscle contraction, whereas both α_1- and α_2-adrenoceptors are important in the arteriolar smooth muscle. Prejunctional α_2-adrenoceptor stimulation results in an inhibition of a vasodilatory neurotransmitter release. When noradrenaline binds to the α_1-receptor of the cell, it increases the activity of the membrane-bound enzyme phospholipase C, which converts phosphatidylinositol 4,5-biphosphate to the active second messengers inositol 1,4,5-triphosphate (IP_3) and diacylglycerol (DAG). IP_3 binds on the IP_3 receptor on the endoplasmic reticulum, liberating Ca ions into the cytosol. DAG stimulates the enzyme protein kinase C and causes an opening of L-type Ca channels, leading to a rise in intracellular Ca ion concentration, and also triggers the closing of potassium channels. The rise in cytoplasmic calcium concentration initiates the contractile process of the smooth muscles and keeps the penis in a flaccid state. The increase in intracellular Ca ion concentration ($[Ca]i$) is transient and returns to near basal levels despite the fact that the constrictor activity is still present. The $[Ca]i$ leads to an activation of calcium/calmodulin-dependent myosin light chain kinase (MLCK). The activated MLCK phosphorylates the myosin light chain and initiates smooth-muscle contraction [14].

Lately, an additional pathway has been proposed that induces smooth-muscle contraction by increased Ca sensitivity via G-protein-coupled receptor activation under noradrenergic influence without changing the cytoplasmic Ca ion concentration [15]. This mechanism involves **RhoA**, a monomeric G-protein that activates **Rho-kinase**, which in turn inhibits the regulatory subunit of smooth-muscle myosin phosphatase (SMPP-1M). The inhibition of the SMPP-1M prevents the dephosphorylation of myofilaments and increases the sensitization of the myofilaments to intracellular basal Ca ion concentration in favor of smooth-muscle contraction [15]. It is believed that once the [Ca]i returns to basal levels after a transient initiation, the calcium-sensitizing pathways take over to maintain the contractile smooth-muscle tone [16].

Nitric oxide (NO) and the NO–cGMP pathway appear to be the most influential pro-erectile neurotransmitter and pathway in smooth-muscle relaxation [17]. Recent studies also documented that NO plays a role in central regions, such as the PVN, in control of penile erection and sexual activity [18]. NO is a free radical, has a half-life of only approximately 5 seconds, and is synthesized from L-arginine and molecular oxygen by the enzyme nitric oxide synthase (NOS), producing NO and L-citrulline. Three distinct isoforms of NOS have been identified. The neuronal (nNOS) is present in the cytoplasm of nerve endings, and the endothelial (eNOS) is mainly membrane-bound in endothelial cells, including penile blood vessels and trabecular tissue [19]. Both isoforms require calcium and calmodulin for activity. The third inducible isoform (iNOS) is calcium-independent, induced by inflammatory mediators, and under physiological conditions not expressed in the penis. NO is released both directly from parasympathetic nerve terminals which contain nNOS following cholinergic stimulation, and from vascular endothelium containing eNOS. Endothelium-derived-NO release can be achieved by acetylcholine via postganglionic cholinergic nerves [20], by shear stress via protein kinase Akt activation [21], and also by triggering NO production via bradykinin and oxygen. NO derived from nNOS in the nitrergic nerves appears to be responsible for the initiation and major portion of the smooth-muscle relaxation, whereas NO from eNOS contributes to the maintenance of the erection. Based on its lipophilic character, NO is able to penetrate the cellular membrane of the smooth-muscle cell and stimulate the enzyme guanylate cyclase, which converts guanosine triphosphate (GTP) to **cyclic guanosine monophosphate (cGMP)**, the active second messenger. Cyclic GMP stimulates the enzyme protein kinase G, which prompts the closure of L-type Ca channels and opening of potassium channels. Both effects result in pro-erectile smooth-muscle relaxation.

The active second messenger cGMP is converted to an inactive GMP by the enzyme **phosphodiesterase**, which will be highlighted in detail below. As mentioned before, membrane potential, which depends on the relation of ion concentration inside and outside the cell, is an important modulator of the Ca channel status. Alterations in the activity of **potassium channels, maxi-K and** K_{ATP} channels in particular as the most important in smooth-muscle cells, highly influence changes in the membrane potential. An opening of these potassium channels, which can be achieved by cGMP-dependent protein kinase, cGMP itself, and cyclic adenosine monophosphate (cAMP)-dependent protein kinase A, causes hyperpolarization and relaxation of smooth-muscle cells.

During an erection the smooth-muscle entirety works as a functional unit communicating through **gap junctions** between the smooth-muscle cells. These connexin-containing connections between individual cells allow second messengers such as cAMP and cGMP and intracellular ions such as potassium and calcium to transmit undisturbed from cell to cell and to provide the entire tissue with the same information [22]. The penile erectile tissue is able to act like a so-called **functional syncytium**.

Recent observations suggest that the interaction between the pro-erectile nitrergic pathway and the anti-erectile noradrenergic mechanism takes place on the cellular level inside the smooth muscle [23]. Cyclic GMP as the second messenger of the nitrergic pathway activates a G-kinase, which interrelates with the noradrenergic pathway by phosphorylating a regulatory protein called **IRAG** (IP$_3$-receptor-associated G-kinase substrate) associated with the IP$_3$ receptor [24]. The G-kinase-mediated IRAG phosphorylation closes the IP$_3$ receptor and thus prevents the noradrenergic- mediated increase in cytoplasmic Ca ion concentration. This may explain how the nitrergic system supersedes the noradrenergic system during erection. Furthermore, this also offers a possible explanation of a pathophysiological aspect of the development of ED. Thus an insufficient NO–cGMP pathway results in a predominance of the noradrenergic pathway [25].

In penile expansion, nitric oxide (NO) appears to be the dominant mediator of smooth-muscle relaxation [1]. But it is becoming increasingly apparent that in the complex process of erection there must be a number of mediators involving smooth-muscle contraction and relaxation that interact in a number of pathways taking place in different locations. Also important factors in smooth-muscle relaxation are acetylcholine

Table 9.2. Factors impacting on smooth-muscle tone

	Contractile	Relaxant
Neuronal	Noradrenaline Neuropeptide Y (NPY)	Nitric oxide (NO) Acetylcholine (Ach) Vasoactive intestinal polypeptide (VIP) Calcitonin gene-related peptide (CGRP)
Local	Endothelin I Prostaglandin F2α Thromboxane A2 Angiotensin II	Nitric oxide Prostaglandin E2, A2, I2 Histamine Adenosine triphosphate Bradykine Substance P Serotonin (5-hydroxytryptamine, 5-HT) Somatostatin

(ACh), vasoactive intestinal polypeptide (VIP), calcitonin gene-related peptide (CGRP), prostanoids, histamine, and adenosine triphosphate (ATP). Table 9.2 represents an overview of factors that may influence smooth-muscle tone within the penis. ACh released from the parasympathetic nerve endings stimulates NO release from the vascular endothelium and inhibits the liberation of noradrenaline from the sympathetic nerve terminals. VIP is colocalized with ACh in parasympathetic nerve endings and leads to cavernosal and arteriolar smooth-muscle relaxation. CGRP shows endothelial-dependent arteriolar dilating outcome but no effects on trabecular smooth muscles. Histamine can be found in mast cells and in walls of penile blood vessels and mediates smooth-muscle relaxation via H_2-receptors but can also lead to contraction via H_1-receptors. The mainly smooth-muscle-relaxing results of histamines are mediated by an increasing effect on endothelial NO production and an inhibition of sympathetic noradrenaline release. Other substances including bradykine, ATP, substance P, or 5-HT are able to increase endothelial NO release.

Pharmacological influence

At present the oral drugs that are commonly in use are phosphodiesterase type 5 (PDE-5) inhibitors including sildenafil, vardenafil, and tadalafil, which behave as peripheral conditioners, and dopaminergic agonists such as subinguinal apomorphine as a central initiator. The other local pharmacotherapies include intracavernosal injection therapy, intraurethral agents, and topical drugs. The introduction of intracavernosal injection therapy in the early 1980s became the foundation of ED therapy until the late 1990s with the launch of intraurethral drug application in 1997 and the orally available PDE-5 inhibitors in 1998 [26–29]. The concept of local drug absorption by the penile

skin appears very attractive and logical, but because of inadequate efficacy and local adverse events no topical agents are currently approved for use; they are therefore not discussed further in this chapter.

Phosphodiesterase inhibitors

With the introduction of sildenafil citrate (Viagra™) [30] in 1998, as a **selective type 5 phosphodiesterase inhibitor** for **oral use**, treatment options for ED have been revolutionized [29]. Vardenafil (Levitra™) [31] and tadalafil (Cialis™) [32] complete the PDE-5 inhibitor family in Europe and the USA. It is very important to recognize that such agents do not initiate an erection but act locally within the penis to facilitate and enhance the smooth-muscle response to sexual stimulation. As described above, the relaxation of the smooth muscles in the corpora cavernosa is essential in achievement of a normal penile erection. In response to sexual stimuli, NO is released by cavernous nerve endings and endothelial cells and stimulates the creation of the active second messenger cGMP by guanylate cyclase [1,33]. The extent of the nitrergic stimulus and the rate of cGMP breakdown by the enzyme phosphodiesterase control the level of the active second messenger within the smooth-muscle cell. **Sildenafil, vardenafil, and tadalafil** are selective inhibitors of cGMP-specific PDE-5, the predominant isozyme metabolizing cGMP in the corpus cavernosum [29,34,35]. Inhibiting PDE-5 and thus preventing cGMP breakdown potentiates the action of cGMP and thus facilitates erectile activity. Regarding enzyme phosphodiesterase, at least 11 different but homologous gene families (21 subfamilies) have been discovered, with each family typically having several different isoforms, and types 2, 3, 4, 5, and 11 have been identified in the human cavernosal smooth muscle [36,37]. These PDEs differ in their three-dimensional structure, kinetic properties, modes of regulation, intracellular localization, cellular expression, and inhibitor sensitivities. Overall PDE-5 appears to be the most important isozyme in the control of normal penile erectile activity. Not only cGMP but also cAMP, as another important pro-erectile second messenger in the smooth muscle, is a substrate for PDE. PDE-3 specifically hydrolyses cAMP, but is inhibited by cGMP. With an increased occurrence of cGMP by PDE-5 inhibition the cross-regulation by PDE-3 inhibition prevents cAMP breakdown in addition. Older medications with a certain specificity to inhibit PDE-5, such as dipyridamole and zaprinast, are completely replaced by the new generation of PDE-5 inhibitors, which are more potent [38].

Other remedies, including theophylline, oxpentifylline, and papaverine, inhibit PDE isozymes in a nonselective manner. **Papaverine**, as a **nonspecific PDE inhibitor**, was introduced in 1982 as a potent therapy for ED by **intracavernosal injection** and revolutionized the treatment options for ED at that time [26]. Local administration of papaverine directly into the corpora cavernosa prevents the breakdown of cGMP and cAMP by the inhibition of PDE-5 and PDE-3, respectively. The increased bioavailability of both second messengers results in lowering the cytoplasmic Ca concentration with consecutive smooth-muscle relaxation achieving an erection usually within minutes. Systemic side effects are basically abolished, because local drug levels are high, while systemic drug concentrations remain low. A single intracorporeal injection is able to induce an erection because the erectile tissue works as a so-called functional syncytium, allowing the undisturbed information transfer between the smooth-muscle cells through gap junctions [22].

Dopaminergic agonists

With the introduction of **apomorphine hydrochloride** (Uprima™, Ixense™) in Europe in 2001 (unlicensed in the USA), the brain was addressed as an organ in the treatment for ED [39]. Results from basic research by induction of penile erections via D_2 dopaminergic receptors in the paraventricular nucleus in rodents after parenteral administration of dopaminergic agonists paved the way for the use of central initiators [40].

Apomorphine is a **dopaminergic agonist** whose primary effect occurs at the brain level in the paraventricular nucleus where the D_2 **dopaminergic receptors** specifically responsible for erectile function are located [41]. Activation of these receptors triggers the processes that induce pro-erectile stimuli by neuronal

stimulation through the medullar parasympathetic route and start the penile vascular response through the pudendal nerves. Side effects including yawning, somnolence, nausea, headache, dizziness, and vasodilated syncopes are due to effects caused by co-stimulation of dopaminergic receptors D_{1-5}. In general, apomorphine is used **sublingually** and appears to be effective in patients with mild ED, with a relatively fast onset of action (30–60 minutes), but beyond this it seems to have limited application [39]. At this time there is interest in developing a transnasal delivery of this agent.

Adenylate cyclase stimulation

Prostanoids – Human corpus cavernosum tissue is able to synthesize prostanoids [42], and their production is modulated by oxygen tension and suppressed by hypoxia [43]. Prostanoids exert their effects mainly through cAMP, which is formatted after adenylate cyclase activation. This is a membrane-bound receptor-coupled enzyme, compared to guanylate cyclase, which is an intracytoplasmic enzyme. One of the prostanoid representatives is **prostaglandin E_1 (PGE_1)** (Alprostadil™), which is a potent erectogenic agent in use for direct **intracavernosal injection (ICI) therapy** and acts via specific receptors on the smooth-muscle cell membrane **stimulating the enzyme adenylate cyclase** [44]. Adenylate cyclase converts cyclic adenosine triphosphate (cATP) to cyclic adenosine monophosphate (cAMP), as the active second messenger. This again stimulates protein kinase A, which has actions similar to those of protein kinase G, leading to a fall in the intracellular Ca concentration and finally to pro-erectile smooth-muscle relaxation and increase in diameter of cavernosal arteries resulting in an erection. PGE_1 is the most widely used single drug for ICI [45,46]. However, a common side effect is the complaint of penile pain in over 30%, due to nociception of PGE_1 after ICI, causing 3–5% of patients to withdraw [47]. Nowadays PGE_1 is often used in combination with papaverine, a nonspecific PDE inhibitor, and/ or phentolamine, a nonspecific α-adrenergic receptor blocker. Among other effects, PGE_1 causes a reduction in release of noradrenaline at the presynaptic nerve endings. This has a supportive pro-erectile effect.

Another common option for PGE_1 application is the Medicated Urethral System for Erection (MUSE™), which delivers the active agent in pellet form **into the urethra**. PGE_1 reaches the smooth muscle in the corpora cavernosa after penetrating the urothelial epithelium via retrograde flow through spongiosal veins communicating with the cavernosal blood supply [48].

Vasoactive intestinal polypeptide (VIP) is also a pro-erectile compound that acts through G-protein receptor-mediated **adenylate cyclase activation** of the smooth-muscle cell [49]. In general, VIP leads only to a moderate tumescence when injected alone into the corpora cavernosa, but it shows promising rigidity results in combination with other injectable drugs such as phentolamine. Ongoing research will show whether these drugs will find a place in the clinical treatment of ED.

Melanocortin agonists – Melanocortin peptides including adrenocorticotropin and α-melanocyte-stimulating hormone, both produced in the pituitary, have been determined in different animal studies to have the ability to cause sexual excitation [50]. Two melanocortin receptor agonists, **melanotan II (MT-II)** and **PT-141** (the deaminated metabolite of MT-II), have undergone clinical trial examination for the purpose of ED treatment. Melanocortin agonists act via G-protein membrane-bound receptors and five melanocortin receptors (MC-1–5) have been identified, of which MC-3 and especially MC-4 seem to be involved in the control of penile erection. Their stimulation leads to an **adenylate cyclase activation** with initiation of the cAMP cascade finally leading to smooth-muscle relaxation. Clinical studies on **subcutaneous** MT-II administration have demonstrated a pro-erectile activity in men with ED of various origins [51]. Even more promising is the report on PT-141 in randomized, double-blind, placebo-controlled studies, especially because of the convenient **intranasal** application of PT-141 and the fact that to date no serious side effects have been reported after PT-141 administration [52].

Influence of α-adrenoceptors

Alpha-adrenoreceptors appear to play an important role in smooth-muscle tone regulation; specifically, α_1-adrenoceptor stimulation leads to smooth-muscle contraction, whereas α_2-adrenoceptor activation modulates neurotransmitter release from sympathetic and parasympathetic nerve terminals. Initiated by animal studies which demonstrated enhanced erectile response to electrical stimulation of erectogenic nerves after α-adrenoceptor blocking, clinical observations show induction of an erection after local intracavernosal injection (ICI) of a **competitive non-specific α-adrenoceptor antagonist** such as phentolamine. To improve its therapeutic effect phentolamine is often used in combination with papaverine or in a

triple combination called **trimix** that combines PGE_1, papaverine, and phentolamine, which are synergistic. The result is maximization of efficacy while at the same time minimizing side effects [53]. However, trimix itself is not licensed. Phentolamine may also have some effects on serotonin receptors, but the main location of action appears to be the arteriolar smooth muscle, and the result is an increased arterial inflow into the penis with little effect on the cavernosal smooth muscle.

Phenoxybenzamine is also a **nonspecific but irreversible α-adrenoceptor antagonist**. Because of an increased risk of prolonged erections and priapism due to its long half-life of over 24 hours, and a reported tendency to induce cavernosal fibrosis, it is not in common use for ICI.

Moxisylyte is a **nitrosylated selective inhibitor of** α_1**-adrenoceptors**, which, when injected, combines vasodilator activity as a NO donor and blockade of the tonic sympathetic neuronal action [54].

Orally administered **yohimbine** was widely used in the 1960s with the intent to improve erectile function. Yohimbine is an α_2**-adrenoceptor antagonist**, but the exact location of its action is not fully clear and it may be pharmacologically active both peripherally and centrally. The role of yohimbine has diminished, because it is much less efficacious than recently available agents such as PDE-5 inhibitors or apomorphine.

Rho-kinase pathway antagonism

The RhoA/Rho-kinase pathway supports the noradrenergic dominance of smooth-muscle contraction in the flaccid state of the penis through phosphorylated inhibition of the myosin phosphatase leading to increased sensitization of myofilaments to basal cytoplasmic Ca ion concentration [15]. Studies using Y-27632, a selective Rho-kinase inhibitor, have demonstrated prevention of vascular, bronchial, and gastrointestinal smooth-muscle contraction [25]. Rho-kinase is expressed in the penile smooth muscle as well and is expressed 17-fold in the corpus cavernosum compared to vascular smooth muscle [55]. In-vivo Rho-kinase inhibition stimulates rat penile erection independently of NO and causes relaxation in vitro [56]. Molecular studies in human corpora cavernosa have documented a high expression of RhoA contributing to the RhoA-mediated Ca sensitization in the flaccid state of the penis [57]. The finding of increased RhoA expression in human artery smooth-muscle cells in a NO/cGMP-dependent protein kinase-dependent manner suggests that the basal release of NO is necessary to maintain RhoA expression and function in vascular smooth-muscle cells [58]. The RhoA/Rho-kinase pathway plays a supportive role in the modulation of the contractile smooth-muscle tone in the flaccid penis, and it seems that this pathway might represent a promising alternative therapeutic target for ED treatment.

Angiotensin and angiotensin-converting enzyme

The renin–angiotensin system, with its active element angiotensin II, an octapeptide hormone which is involved in blood pressure and plasma volume regulation, thirst perception, sodium excretion, and sympathetic nervous activity, seems also to play a detumescent role in the erectile tissue [59]. Angiotensin II mediates its effects via AT_1 and AT_2 membrane receptors and produces and secretes it in the human corpus cavernosum causing a dose-dependent contraction of human corpus cavernosum strips [60]. Clinical studies strongly support the hypothesis that angiotensin II is involved in flaccidity and detumescence [61]. Clinical trials also clearly showed, in a prospective open design, a significant amelioration of ED documented with an improvement of the International Index of Erectile Function questionnaire score under the use of the selective angiotensin II receptor blocker valsartan in men with hypertension [62]. These findings noticeably support the belief that angiotensin II is involved in penile flaccidity and detumescence and is connected to ED.

Endothelin

Endothelins (ET), as a group of endogenous peptides primarily produced by endothelial cells, may make a contribution to the corporeal smooth-muscle tone as a potent vasoconstrictor. ETs work through ET_A and ET_B receptor stimulation and increase transmembrane Ca fluctuation due to voltage-dependent and/or receptor-operated Ca channels, and lead to smooth-muscle contraction [63]. Clinical trials do not support the effectiveness of ET_A antagonism resulting in improved erectile function found in animal studies [64]. The disconcordance between the promising results in animal studies and failure to replicate results in the clinic should raise awareness that there are differences in the transferable applicability of laboratory findings in humans, which should not be underestimated. Current opinion suggests that ETs may play only a minor role in the control of penile flaccidity [65].

Nitric oxide donors and guanylate cyclase activators

Linsidomine (SIN-1) and **nitroprusside** are NO donors which are able to **release NO** after **intracavernosal injection** stimulating the NO/cGMP pathway

[66]. Preliminary data showed potential effectiveness and safety of NO donors as intracavernosal agents, but long-term self-injection trials are needed to define their place in clinical practice recommendations [67]. NO effectiveness in smooth-muscle relaxation is coupled with the activation of guanylate cyclase. Classical NO donors tend to lose their potency due to a tachyphylactic effect, or have other side effects due to their nonspecific interaction with other biological molecules [25]. The pharmaceutical industry, including Bayer, Abbott, and Aventis, have developed NO-independent soluble guanylate cyclase activators that are at present in the animal experimental phase [68].

Serotoninergic influence (trazodone)

Serotonin, also known as 5-hydroxytryptamine (5-HT), plays a complex role in modulating sexual behavior. The 5-HT receptors appear to be able to facilitate sexual stimulation via 5-HT_{1A} receptor activation or to restrain it via 5-HT_{1B} and 5-HT_3 receptor stimulation, and therefore many drugs that influence 5-HT activity alter sexual behavior. But so far no medication which uses the serotoninergic influence is licensed for the treatment of ED.

Summary

Erection is primarily a neurovascular event combining neurotransmission and vascular biological responses under central and local control. Not surprisingly, the complexity of additional hormonal stimulation, local biochemical interactions, and biomechanical mechanisms influence the neurovascular control. Most of the time, the penis is kept in a flaccid state under the influence of α-adrenergic tone through a tonic noradrenaline release from sympathetic nerves maintaining a penile arterial and corporeal smooth-muscle contraction supported by calcium-sensitizing pathways via RhoA-kinase activation. Recent observations suggest that the interaction between the pro-erectile nitrergic cascade and the anti-erectile noradrenergic mechanism takes place on the cellular level inside the smooth muscle, where the nitrergic system supersedes the noradrenergic system during erection. An erection is inducible by various stimuli and mainly driven by the NO/cGMP pathway resulting in arterial and trabecular smooth-muscle relaxation. The balance and interaction between relaxant and contractile factors determines the final outcome of the penile smooth-muscle tone. Growing from the revolutionary introduction of an effective and safe oral treatment such as the PDE-5 inhibitors within the last decade, many advances have been made in the understanding of the physiology of penile erection. As a result, novel targets are under development, including Rho-kinase inhibition or adenylate cyclase activation, with the promise of beneficial effects in ED management in the future.

Concepts of emission and ejaculation

Alongside developments in the field of erectile physiology and function, the last decade has witnessed promising advances in the understanding of central and peripheral mechanisms of ejaculation control. Usually accompanied by orgasm, **ejaculation** constitutes the final phase of the sexual response cycle in the male and represents a reflex involving sensory stimuli processed on cerebral and spinal levels and returned on efferent pathways. Ejaculation is a reflex that requires a complex interplay between somatic, sympathetic, and parasympathetic pathways involving predominantly central dopaminergic and serotonergic neurons [69]. In an undisturbed antegrade ejaculation process three basic phases are involved: emission, ejection/expulsion, and orgasm [70]. **Emission**, as the first phase of ejaculation, is a sympathetic spinal cord reflex and is defined as the deposition of seminal fluid into the posterior urethra.

Ejaculation or **expulsion** is due to the combined action of sympathetic and somatic pathways. An antegrade ejaculation requires a synchronized interplay between periurethral muscle contractions and bladder neck closure contemporaneous with the relaxation of the external urinary sphincter.

Orgasm, generally associated with ejaculation, is a pleasurable sensation resulting from cerebral processing of the increased pressure in the posterior urethra and contraction of the urethral bulb and accessory sexual organs.

Anatomy

Several anatomical structures are involved in the ejaculation process. The ejaculate comprises secretions from the seminal vesicles (50–80% of the ejaculatory volume), the prostate (15–30%), and bulbourethral (Cowper's) glands and spermatozoa (approximately 5%).

Functional anatomy

The spermatozoa undergo final maturation in the **epididymis** and are stored there prior to ejaculation. The smooth muscles of the epididymis are innervated by adrenergic and cholinergic pathways, receiving neuronal fibers from the superior and inferior spermatic

plexus. The neurotransmitters identified in the caudal epididymis include VIP, neuropeptide Y, CGRP, substance P, and NOS [71,72].

During the emission phase, spermatozoa are transported by peristaltic contractions of the smooth muscles of the **ductus (vas) deferens**, which joins the duct of the seminal vesicles at its ampullar ending, forming the ejaculatory duct. The vasa deferentia act as conduits, carrying sperm between the epididymis and the ejaculatory ducts via the vasal ampullae. The vasal ampullae pass medially to the seminal vesicles, where they join together to form the ejaculatory duct. The ejaculatory duct travels through the prostate and enters the urethra at the level of the verumontanum. The pelvic plexus provides both adrenergic and cholinergic nerves innervating the ductus deferens. Among the neuropeptides playing a role in ductus deferens innervation, NO, VIP, and neuropeptide Y are the most abundant [73,74]. Dual innervation by sympathetic and parasympathetic fibers from the hypogastric and pelvic nerves via the pelvic plexus supply the **seminal vesicles**. These paired structures, situated lateral to the ampullary vas bilaterally, have layers of smooth muscles and are responsible for 50–80% of the ejaculatory volume. A recent microscopic study demonstrated nitrergic-mediated signal transduction in the control of human seminal vesicle function [75]. Another pelvic organ involved in the ejaculatory process is the **prostate gland**, contributing 15–30% of the ejaculatory secretion. The prostate contains simple fibromuscular tissue and alveolar epithelium. The contractile and secretory function of the prostate gland is under autonomic control, dually innervated by sympathetic and parasympathetic filaments. The adrenergic fibers traveling along the pelvic nerve are confined to innervating the blood vessels supplying the prostate. Via the hypogastric nerve the adrenergic and cholinergic influences reach the prostatic parenchyma, which is dominated by sympathic tone. Studies using radioligand binding assays and receptor autoradiography support the suggestion that prostatic muscular contraction is controlled by the sympathetic nervous system acting via α_1-adrenoceptors [76]. Muscarinic receptors and α_1-adrenoreceptors are predominant in the nonpathological prostate along with α_2- and β-adrenoreceptors. Using transneuronal mapping methods the presence of adrenergic and cholinergic endings has been documented in the outer muscle layer and inner secretory layer of the prostatic acini [77]. VIP and neuropeptide Y are the most frequent neurotransmitters in the prostate [78,79]. Enkephalin in the prostatic smooth muscles and nitrergic innervations of the epithelium, fibromuscular stroma, and blood vessels has also been described [80,81]. The bulbourethral glands or Cowper's glands are covered by the bulboglandularis muscles, and contract and expel their secretions into the urethra under cholinergic control. Interestingly, animal studies in rats have revealed only cholinergic fibers around acini in the Cowper's glands but have not shown adrenergic components [82]. The ejaculatory fluid flows via the ejaculatory ducts at the colliculus seminalis into the prostatic urethra.

As part of the ejaculatory reflex, the closure of the bladder neck sphincter prevents retrograde semen flow into the bladder during emission and ejaculation. Both the bladder neck and the **urethra** contain layers of smooth muscles receiving a dual innervation from sympathetic and parasympathetic nerves [83]. The nerve fibers pass via the hypogastric and pelvic nerves joining the pelvic plexus. Adrenergic α_1- and α_2-adrenoreceptors are found mostly in the smooth muscle but also in submucosa [84]. Cholinergic somatic efferents, via the pudendal nerve, supply the external rhabdosphincter, a striated-muscle layer at the distal segment of the urethra [85]. NOS, neuropeptide Y, VIP, enkephalin, and somatostatin have been detected in ganglion cells and/or axon endings located in the smooth-muscle layers of the bladder neck and the urethra [86,87]. Urethral afferents terminate in the lumbosacral segments of the spinal cord along pudendal, pelvic, and hypogastric nerves. CGRP and substance P have been identified in the urethra [87]. Adequate propulsion of the ejaculate requires a synchronized relaxation of the external urinary sphincter with simultaneous bladder neck closure during rhythmic contractions of the striated muscles of the pelvic floor, including the bulbocavernosus, ischiocavernosus, and levator ani muscles [69]. These muscles are innervated exclusively by motor fibers from the pudendal nerve. The ischiocavernosus muscles cover the corpora cavernosa along the crura at the base of the penis, and the bulbocavernosus muscle encircles the corpus spongiosum. The rhythmic contraction of these muscles provides the movement of the seminal fluid through the urethra and, finally, its expulsion from the urethral meatus.

Neuroanatomy

Peripheral anatomy

The pathways involved in the peripheral control of ejaculation include sensory afferents and motor efferents. The **sensory afferent** input travels along the **dorsal nerve** leading into the perineal nerve and along the **hypogastric nerve**. The majority of sensory information is gathered via free nerve terminals from the penile skin and glans. However, encapsulated receptors called Krause-Finger corpuscles have also been identified in the glans [88]. Sensory impulses trek along the dorsal nerve, which is a sensory branch of the perineal nerve, to the upper sacral and the lower lumbar segments of the spinal cord. In addition, afferents also pass via hypogastric nerve fibers, reaching the paravertebral lumbosacral sympathetic chain via thoracolumbar dorsal roots in the spinal cord [89]. The sensory afferents end in the medial dorsal horn and the dorsal gray commissure of the spinal cord [90].

The **autonomic nervous system** plays a key role in the **efferent pathway** of the ejaculatory reflex [82]. As mentioned before, the nerves primarily extend from the pelvic plexus, where sympathetic and parasympathetic nerve fibers provide a rich innervation of the male sexual organs in the pelvis. The origins of the preganglionic **sympathetic neurons** are located in the intermediolateral cell column and in the central autonomic region of the thoracolumbar segments of the spinal cord (T11–L2) [91]. The sympathetic fibers leave the spinal column bilaterally through the ventral roots and synapse in the paravertebral sympathetic chain. From there fibers proceed via the thoracic sympathetic chain to the inferior enteric plexus, the major and minor splanchnic nerves, the cranial mesenteric plexus, and the intermesenteric nerves where further descending nerves from these ganglia form the hypogastric plexus just below the aortic bifurcation. Proceeding sympathetic fibers merge into the inferior mesenteric ganglia where the paired hypogastric nerves arise. The confluence of the hypogastric nerve and the parasympathetic pelvic nerve constitutes the pelvic plexus. The outgoing branches from this plexus innervate the epididymis, vas deferens, seminal vesicle, prostate, bladder neck, and urethra [92].

The origin of the preganglionic parasympathetic neurons is located in the intermediolateral cell column of the lumbosacral segments of the spinal cord in the sacral parasympathetic nucleus (S2–S4). Neurons travel in the pelvic nerve to the pelvic plexus. Efferent somatic nerves emerge from Onuf's nuclei in the anterior horn of the sacral segments S2–S4 and travel along the motor branch of the pudendal nerve to innervate the pelvic floor striated muscles, including the bulbospongiosus and ischiocavernosus muscles.

The pudendal nerve also arises from the sacral segments S2–S4, and after leaving the pelvis through the greater sciatic foramen and re-entering via the lesser sciatic foramen it innervates the perineal striated musculature. Under the influence of both sympathetic and parasympathetic pathways the process of ejaculation can be triggered by sensory stimulation of the penis as well as influenced by various cerebral erotic stimuli integrated and processed at the spinal cord level [93].

Spinal and central anatomy

The spinal network plays a significant role in processing and directing afferent and efferent information in the ejaculatory process (Fig. 9.2). For a long time, interneurons located in the medial gray bilaterally in the lumbosacral spinal cord have been presumed to be the **spinal ejaculation generator** [94–96]. Recently, specific neurons in the central gray of lamina 7 and 10 of lumbar segments 3 and 4 (L3–4) have been discovered, and these may play a pivotal role in the control of ejaculation as a spinal ejaculation generator [97]. It has been documented that these neurons have projections to the parvocellular subparafascicular thalamic nucleus (SPFp) [98]. Based on their projection to the thalamus and their spinal location, these particular neurons are reported as **lumbar spinothalamic (LSt) cells**. The LSt cells also have projections to somatic motor neurons as well as sympathetic and parasympathetic preganglionic neurons, emphasizing their contribution to the integration of sensory afferent contributions and autonomic and motor efferent assemblies involved in the ejaculatory reflex [97,99].

The spinal centers are under descending inhibitory and excitatory influences of supraspinal regions involving cerebral sensory areas and motor centers, which are closely interrelated [100,101]. This specifically ejaculatory-related cerebral network includes the **medial preoptic area (MPOA), the paraventricular nucleus of the hypothalamus (PVN), the nucleus paragigantocellularis (nPGi), the posterodorsal medial amygdaloid nucleus (MeApd), and the SPFp**.

Physiological control of ejaculation

Thus peripheral and central sites, as well as sympathetic, parasympathetic, and somatic pathways, participate in the physiological control of the ejaculatory reflex. A normal ejaculatory response requires synchronized neurochemical interplay coordinated at different levels of the nervous system. In humans, the components of the ejaculate are released from participating organs in a particular order. The first portion of the ejaculate is provided by the bulbourethral glands, followed by fluid from the prostate that includes a few spermatozoa.

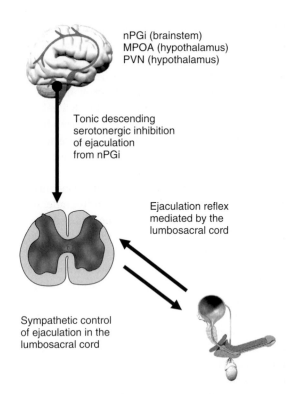

nPGi (brainstem)
MPOA (hypothalamus)
PVN (hypothalamus)

Tonic descending serotonergic inhibition of ejaculation from nPGi

Ejaculation reflex mediated by the lumbosacral cord

Sympathetic control of ejaculation in the lumbosacral cord

Fig. 9.2. Central control of ejaculation. nPGi, nucleus paragigantocellularis; MPOA, medial preoptic area; PVN, paraventricular nucleus.

Afterwards, the main fraction of the ejaculate, including the bulk of the spermatozoa, is contributed by the epididymis and vas deferens, along with prostatic and seminal vesicle fluids.

Posterior urethral distension, which is an adequate sensory stimulation of the dorsal penile nerve, appears to be sufficient to trigger an ejaculatory response. Describing a urethrogenital reflex, urethral distension in anesthetized rats induced contractions of the striated perineal muscles [102]. In other work in anesthetized rats, the electrical stimulation of the dorsal nerve of the penis and the pelvic nerve, both transmitting sensory information from the urethrogenital tract, provoked a response of somatic pathways, innervating the pelvic floor striated muscles [103]. These results have also been shown in humans, along with documentation of electromyographic activity of the bulbospongiosus muscles after sensory stimulation by distension of the posterior urethra or sacral root stimulation [104,105].

The emission of the seminal fluid is controlled by the sympathetic nervous system activating propulsive contraction of smooth muscle of the prostate, vas deferens, and seminal vesicles, as well as prostatic glandular secretion. Several studies have documented a contractile response of the vasa deferentia, seminal vesicles, prostate, and urethra as a result of sympathetic nerve system activation by stimulation of sympathetic nerve fibers within the hypogastric or splanchnic nerves or by sympathomimetic medications [86,106].

In animal species, pelvic nerve stimulation leads to a contractile response of the vasa deferentia, the prostate, and the urethra [107,108]. With the use of cholinergic drugs, contraction and secretion of prostate and seminal vesicles has been observed to be mediated by muscarinic receptors [109]. Based on these findings regarding the cholinergic activation, the sympathetic innervation of the prostate might contain both adrenergic and cholinergic elements. Clear clinical evidence for a functional role of parasympathetic innervation involved in the ejaculatory process is missing thus far [86].

Besides the adrenergic and cholinergic influence, experimental studies have revealed that VIP and neuropeptide Y are involved in the contraction and secretion of prostate and seminal vesicles [109,110]. However, the detailed process of their interaction is yet to be fully elucidated. One aspect might be the modulating influence of parasympathetic input on noradrenaline release [110].

The important role of the sympathetic pathway in the ejaculatory process in humans is emphasized by the fact that an interruption of the innervation of the bladder neck, vas deferens, or the prostate can lead to a retrograde ejaculation or failure of emission. Protection of sympathetic efferents during surgical procedures in the retroperitoneum or in the pelvis preserves normal ejaculatory function [111]. A semen sample can be acquired from patients with spinal cord injury by using electric stimulation of the hypogastric plexus, activating sympathetic efferents to achieve ejaculation [112].

The somatic nervous system represented by the pudendal nerve is exclusively responsible for the expulsion phase of the ejaculate. The synchronous activation of ischiocavernosus, bulbospongiosus, and levator ani muscles as the perineal striated muscles, and the anal and urethral external sphincters innervated by the pudendal nerve, causes the powerful thrust of seminal fluid out of the urethra [113]. Patients with sacral spinal cord injuries after trauma (the pudendal nerve arises from sacral segments S2–S4) or patients with neuropathies (e.g., diabetes) typically have a dribbling ejaculation due to the missing motor innervation of the propulsive pelvic musculature [114].

Neuropharmacology

Experimental studies in animals advocate a fundamental role for dopamine (D) and serotonin (5-hydroxytryptamine, 5-HT) in the regulation of ejaculation. Increased ejaculate volume was observed in rats after apomorphine (a nonselective D receptor agonist) administration into the MPOA [115]. And the opposite effect, showing reduced ejaculatory activity, was witnessed after the injection of flupenthixol, a nonselective D receptor antagonist. So far, five D receptors have been identified, subdivided into D_1-like (D_1 and D_5 receptors) and D_2-like (D_2, D_3, and D_4 receptors). The pharmacological stimulation of D_2 and D_3 receptors in the MPOA with quinelorane induced emission and expulsion in rats [116,117].

Cerebral serotonin (5-HT) plays an inhibitory role in ejaculation, demonstrated in several studies in rats [118]. Within the group of 14 different 5-HT receptor subtypes, some may have pro- and others anti-ejaculatory effects. The current literature supports at least the involvement of 5-HT_{1A}, 5-HT_{1B}, and 5-HT_{2C} receptors in the ejaculatory response control [119]. The stimulation of 5-HT_{1A} receptors at various places including cerebral, spinal, or peripheral autonomic ganglia has a generally positive effect on ejaculation, while stimulation of 5-HT_{2C} has the opposite effect [120]. Activation of 5-HT_{1A} autoreceptors has resulted in shortening of the ejaculatory latency time [121]. On the other hand, the stimulation of presynaptic 5-HT_{1B} autoreceptors and postsynaptic 5-HT_{2C} receptors has shown an inhibition of ejaculatory behavior in male rats [121,122].

Attention needs to be paid to patients using psychotropic agents or adrenergic α-receptor antagonists. The last drug class is frequently prescribed for the treatment of benign prostatic hyperplasia and hypertension. Ejaculatory failure described under the influence of adrenergic α-receptor antagonists appears to be related more to inhibition of seminal emission than to retrograde ejaculation. For uroselective α_1-adrenoceptor antagonists targeting the predominant α-receptor subtypes, ejaculatory dysfunction has been described from approximately 1% for alfuzosin up to 18% for tamsulosin. The drug-to-drug variability appears to be due to a different 5-HT and dopamine receptor interaction [123,124].

A well-recognized negative effect on ejaculatory function has been described for psychotropic substances including antipsychotics, anxiolytics, and antidepressants. The effects of antipsychotic drugs are usually mediated by dopaminergic receptor antagonism, especially on D_2-like subtype receptors. Among those for chlorpromazine, clozapine, and risperidone an interaction with 5-HT$_{2A}$ receptors has also been described. Based on their mechanism of action, it is not surprising that ejaculatory impairment has been shown to be caused by antipsychotic drugs. However, whether interference with the central dopaminergic or serotonergic pathways is responsible for the mediation of an ejaculatory impairment needs to be more fully elucidated. The occurrence of retrograde ejaculation has been reported in men using antipsychotics [125].

An inhibitory effect on ejaculation apparently mediated by an enhanced GABAergic effect of benzodiazepines prescribed for anxiety treatment has been reported to occur in approximately 10% [126]. Of the variety of available antidepressants, many delay or inhibit ejaculation. An increased ejaculation latency time has been reported for tricyclic antidepressants inhibiting neuronal noradrenaline transport and also 5-HT [127,128]. A consistent and frequently described finding in psychiatric patients receiving selective serotonin reuptake inhibitors (SSRIs), the youngest member of the available antidepressant family, is a lengthened ejaculation latency time, reported as 31–48% in clinical trials [129]. The impeded serotonin (5-HT) reuptake seems only one pathway involved, as it appears that dopaminergic, anticholinergic, prolactinergic, and nitrergic pathways also contribute mechanisms of SSRI-induced ejaculatory dysfunction.

On the other hand, ongoing research has tried to take advantage of the delayed ejaculation that is a side effect induced by SSRIs in developing a treatment option for premature ejaculation. Premature ejaculation, with a prevalence of 21–33%, is thought to be the most common male sexual dysfunction [130,131]. At this time, no drugs have been approved by regulatory agencies for treatment of premature ejaculation [132]. Initially, long-acting SSRIs were not made to treat premature ejaculation. However, based on their side effect of delayed ejaculation, SSRIs are used all the time off-label to treat premature ejaculation [133–135]. Other side effects of this pharmacological group include dermatological response, anticholinergic results, increasing bodyweight, psychiatric and neurological disorders, cognitive mutilation, and drug–drug interactions as well as sexual disturbances involving erectile dysfunction and loss of libido [136,137]. There are numerous definitions of premature ejaculation, but we will address only the two most common. Premature ejaculation has been defined by the

International Consultation on Urological Diseases as "persistent or recurrent ejaculation with minimal stimulation before, on, or shortly after penetration, and before the person wishes it, over which the sufferer has little or no voluntary control, or which causes the sufferer and/or his partner bother or distress" [138]. Recently the American Urological Association Guideline on the Pharmacologic Management of Premature Ejaculation defined premature ejaculation as "ejaculation that occurs sooner than desired, either before or shortly after penetration, causing distress to either one or both partners" [133]. Diagnosis and treatment are also complicated by the numerous ways of evaluating premature ejaculation. As an objective outcome measure the term "intravaginal ejaculatory latency time" (IELT) was defined and introduced in 1998 [139]. The underlying pathophysiology of premature ejaculation is not completely understood yet. In addition to a psychological aspect, basic and clinical psychopharmacological data suggest that premature ejaculation is a neurobiological phenomenon related to central serotonergic neurotransmission [140]. Lately dapoxetine, a short-acting SSRI, was developed specifically for the treatment of premature ejaculation, increasing serotonin activity by inhibition of neuronal reuptake of serotonin [141]. Taken per os, dapoxetine has a specific pharmacokinetic suitable for on-demand therapy, with only approximately 1 hour to maximum serum concentration, 1.2 hours initial half-life, and rapid elimination [142]. The first phase III trial of dapoxetine 30 mg or 60 mg on demand for the treatment of premature ejaculation, in two randomized, double-blind, placebo-controlled studies, showed a significant prolongation of IELT, roughly three- to fourfold compared to placebo ($P < 0.0001$) [143]. Dapoxetin was better than placebo on the first dose and at all subsequent time points analyzed, and also improved patients' perception of control over ejaculation, satisfaction with sexual intercourse, and overall impression of change in condition. Side effects appeared to be dose-related (30–60 mg) and affected the gastrointestinal and central nervous system the most, including nausea (8.7–20.1%), diarrhea (3.9–6.8%), headache (5.9–6.8%), dizziness (3.0–6.2%), and somnolence (3.2–3.7%). Adverse sexual events were rare and included erectile dysfunction (2.9–3.8%), abnormal ejaculation (0.7–0.8%), and decreased libido (0.7–0.3%). These data are promising for an effective and generally well-tolerated treatment option for premature ejaculation when given on demand.

Summary

The introduction of the PDE-5 inhibitors a decade ago raised a new awareness in both patients and physicians of the existence of male and female sexual dysfunction. Renewed scientific interest in the concepts of physiological control, alongside the development of new treatment options for erectile dysfunction and ejaculation disorders, has been witnessed within recent years. Additional research will be required to further expand our current knowledge of the spinal and supraspinal control mechanisms of the ejaculatory process. An improved understanding of the complex influences on ejaculation may open new therapeutic strategies for ejaculatory disorders.

References

[1] Rajfer J, Aronson WJ, Bush PA, Dorey FJ, Ignarro LJ. Nitric oxide as a mediator of relaxation of the corpus cavernosum in response to nonadrenergic, noncholinergic neurotransmission. *N Engl J Med* 1992; **326**: 90–4.

[2] Lue TF, Tanagho EA. Hemodynamics of erection. In: Tanagho EA, Lue TF, McClure RD, eds. *Contemporary Management of Impotence and Infertility*. Baltimore, MD: Williams & Wilkins, 1988: 28–38.

[3] Kim N, Vardi Y, Padma-Nathan H, *et al*. Oxygen tension regulates the nitric oxide pathway: physiological role in penile erection. *J Clon Invest* 1993; **91**: 437–42.

[4] Schmidt MH, Schmidt HS. Sleep-related erections: neural mechanisms and clinical significance. *Curr Neurol Neurosci Rep* 2004; **4**: 170–8.

[5] Gontero P, Kirby R. Proerectile pharmacological prophylaxis following nerve-sparing radical prostatectomy (NSRP). *Prostate Cancer Prostatic Dis* 2004; **7**: 223–6.

[6] Giuliano F, Rampin O. Central control of erection and its pharmacological modification. *Curr Opin Urol* 2000; **10**: 629–33.

[7] Meisel RL, Sachs BD. The physiology of male sexual behavior. In: Knobil E, Neill JD, eds. *The Physiology of Reproduction*, 2nd edn. New York, NY: Raven Press, 1994: 3–105.

[8] Zahran AR, Vachon P, Courtois F, Carrier S. Increases in intracavernous penile pressure following injections of excitatory amino acid receptor agonists in the hypothalamic para-ventricular nucleus of anesthetized rats. *J Urol* 2000; **164**: 1793–7.

[9] Melis MR, Succu S, Iannucci U, Argiolas A. Prevention by morphine of apomorphine- and oxytocin-induced penile erection and yawning: involvement of nitric oxide. *Naunyn Schmiedebergs Arch Pharmacol* 1997; **355**: 595–600.

[10] Mullerad M, Donohue JF, Li PS, *et al*. Functional sequelae of cavernous nerve injury in the rat: is there model dependency. *J Sex Med* 2006; **3**: 77–83.

[11] Giuliano F, Bernabe J, Brown K, *et al*. Erectile response to hypothalamic stimulation in rats: role of peripheral nerves. *Am J Physiol* 1997; **273**: R1990–7.

[12] Cirino G, Fusco F, Imbimbo C, Mirone V. Pharmacology of erectile dysfunction in man. *Pharmacol Ther* 2006; **111**: 400–23.

[13] Levin RM, Wein A J. Adrenergic alpha receptors outnumber beta receptors in human penile corpus cavernosum. *Invest Urol* 1980; **18**: 225–8.

[14] Berridge MJ. Inositol triphosphate and calcium signaling. *Nature* 1993; **361**: 315–25.

[15] Somlyo AP, Somlyo AV. Signal transduction by G-proteins, Rho-kinase and protein phophatase to smooth muscle and non-muscle myosin II. *J Physiol* 2000; **522**: 177–85.

[16] Saenz de Tejada I, Angulo J, Cellek S, *et al*. Physiology of erectile function. *J Sex Med* 2004; **1**: 254–65.

[17] Toda N, Ayajiki K, Okamura T. Nitric oxide and penile erection function. *Pharmacol Ther* 2005; **1006**: 233–66.

[18] Melis RM, Succu S, Mauri A, Argiolas A. Nitric oxide production is increased in the paraventricular nucleus of the hypothalamus of male rats during noncontact penile erections and copulation. *Eur J Neurosci* 1998; **10**: 1968–74.

[19] Lin CS, Lau A, Bakircioglu E, *et al*. Analysis of neuronal nitric oxide synthase isoform expression and identification of human nNOS-mu. *Biochem Biophys Res Commun* 1998; **253**: 388–94.

[20] Saenz de Tejada I, Blanco R, Goldstein I, *et al*. Cholinergic neurotransmission in human corpus cavernosum. I. Responses of isolated tissue. *Am J Physiol* 1988; **254**: H468–72.

[21] Hurt KJ, Musicki B, Pales MA, *et al*. Akt-dependent phosphorylation of endothelial nitric oxide synthase mediates penile erection. *Proc Natl Acad Sci U S A* 2002; **99**: 4061–6.

[22] Christ GJ, Richards S, Winkler A. Integrative erectile biology: the role of signal transduction and cell to cell communication in coordinating corporal smooth muscle tone and penile erection. *Int J Impot Res* 1997; **9**: 69–84.

[23] Cellek S. Nitrergic–noradrenergic interaction in penile erection: a new insight into erectile dysfunction. *Drugs Today* 2000; **36**: 135–46.

[24] Schlossmann J, Ammendola A, Ashman K, *et al*. Regulation of intracellular calcium by a signalling complex of IRAG, IP3 receptor and cGMP kinase Ibeta. *Nature* 2000; **404**: 197–201.

[25] Cellek S, Rees RW, Kalsi J. A Rho-kinase inhibitor, soluble guanylate cyclase activator and nitric oxide-releasing PDE5 inhibitor: novel approaches to

erectile dysfunction. *Expert Opin Invest Drugs* 2002; **11**: 1563–73.

[26] Virag R. Intracavernous injection of papaverine for erectile failure. *Lancet* 1982; **143**: 332–7.

[27] Brindley GS. Cavernosal alpha-blockade: a new treatment for investigating and treating erectile impotence. *Br J Psych* 1983; **143**: 332–7.

[28] Padma-Nathan H, Gellstrom W, Kaiser FE, *et al.* Treatment of men with erectile dysfunction with transurethral alprostadil. *N Engl J Med* 1997; **336**: 1–7.

[29] Goldstein I, Lue TF, Padma-Nathan H, *et al.* Oral sildenafil in the treatment of erectile dysfunction. Sildenafil Study Group. *N Engl J Med* 1998; **338**: 1397–404.

[30] Viagra® (sildenafil citrate), Pfizer Labs, Division of Pfizer, Inc, New York, NY 10017, USA.

[31] Levitra® (vardenafil HCL), Bayer HealthCare, Pharmaceuticals, Glaxo SmithKline.

[32] Cialis® (tadalafil), Eli Lilly and Company, Indianapolis, IN 46285, USA.

[33] Burnett AL. The role of nitric oxide in erectile dysfunction: implications for medical therapy. *J Clin Hypertens (Greenwich)* 2006; **8**: 53–62.

[34] Hellstrom WJG, Gittelman MC, Karlin G, *et al.* Vardenafil for treatment of men with erectile dysfunction: efficacy and safety in a randomized double-blind placebo controlled trial. *J Androl* 2002; **23**: 763–72.

[35] Brock GB, McMahon CG, Chen KK, *et al.* Efficacy and safety of tadalafil for the treatment of erectile dysfunction: results of integrated analyses. *J Urol* 2002; **168**: 1332–6.

[36] Beavo JA. Cyclic nucleotide phosphodiesterases: functional implications of multiple isoforms. *Physiol Rev* 1995; **75**: 725–48.

[37] Bender AT, Beavo JA. Cyclic nucleotide phosphodiesterases: molecular regulation to clinical use. *Pharmacol Rev* 2006; **58**: 488–520.

[38] Baxendale RW, Smith EJ, Stanley M, *et al.* Selectivity of sildenafil citrate and other phosphodiesterase type 5 inhibitors against human phosphodiesterases types 7–11. *J Clin Pharmacol* 2002; **41**: 1015.

[39] Dula E, Bukofzer S, Perdok R, George M. Apomorphine SL Study Group. Double-blind, crossover comparison of 3 mg apomorphine SL with placebo and with 4 mg apomorphine SL in male erectile dysfunction. *Eur Urol* 2001; **39**: 558–63.

[40] Melis MR, Argiolas A, Gessa GL. Apomorphine-induced penile erection and yawning: site of action in the brain. *Brain Res* 1987; **415**: 98–104.

[41] Allard J, Giuliano F. Central nervous system agents in the treatment of erectile dysfunction: how do they work? *Curr Urol Rep* 2001; **2**: 488–94.

[42] Andersson KE. Pharmacology of penile erection. *Pharm Rev* 2001; **53**: 417–50.

[43] Daley JT, Brown ML, Watkins T, *et al.* Prostanoid production in rabbit corpus cavernosum. I. Regulation by oxygen tension. *J Urol* 1996; **155**: 1482–7.

[44]. Uprima™ (apomorphine hydrochloride), Abbott Laboratories (NZ) Ltd, 227 Cambridge Terrace, Naenae, Lower Hutt.

[45] Porst H. A rational for prostaglandin E1 in erectile failure: a survey of worldwide experience. *J Urol* 1996; **155**: 802–15.

[46] Stackl W, Hasun R, Marberger M. Intracavernous injection of prostaglandin E1 in impotent men. *J Urol* 1988; **140**: 66–8.

[47] Linet OI, Ogrinc FG. Efficacy and safety of intracavernosal alprostadil in men with erectile dysfunction. The Alprostadil Study Group. *N Engl J Med* 1996; **334**: 873–7.

[48]. MUSE™ (alprostadil), MEDA Pharma GmbH & Co. KG, 61352 Bad Homburg, Germany.

[49] Iwatsubo K, Okumura S, Ishikawa Y. Drug therapy aimed at adenyl cyclase to regulate cyclic nucleotide signaling. *Endocr Metab Immune Disord Drug Targets* 2006; **6**: 239–47.

[50] Argiolas A, Melis MR, Murgia S, Schioth HB. ACTH- and alpha-MSH-induced grooming, stretching, yawning and penile erection in male rats: site of action in the brain and role of melanocortin receptors. *Brain Res Bull* 2000; **51**: 425–31.

[51] Wessells H, Gralnek D, Dorr R, *et al.* Effect of an alpha-melanocyte stimulating hormone analog on penile erection and sexual desire in men with organic erectile dysfunction. *Urology* 2000; **56**: 641–6.

[52] Molinoff PB, Shadiack AM, Earle D, Diamond LE, Quon CY. PT-141: a melanocortin agonist for the treatment of sexual dysfunction. *Ann N Y Acad Sci* 2003; **994**: 96–102.

[53] Padma-Nathan H. The efficacy and synergy of polypharmacotherapy in primary and salvage therapy of vasculogenic erectile dysfunction. *Int J Impot Res* 1990; **2**: 257–8.

[54] de Tejada IS, Garvey DS, Schroeder JD, *et al.* Design and evaluation of nitrosylated alpha-adrenergic receptor antagonists as potential agents for the treatment of impotence. *J Pharmacol Exp Ther* 1999; **290**: 121–8.

[55] Rees RW, Ziessen T, Ralph DJ, *et al.* Human and rabbit cavernosal smooth muscle cells express Rho-kinase. *Int J Impot Res* 2002; **14**: 1–7.

[56] Chitaley K, Wingard CJ, Clinton Webb R, *et al.* Antagonism of Rho-kinase stimulates rat penile erection via a nitric oxide-independent pathway. *Nat Med* 2001; **7**: 119–22.

[57] Wang H, Eto M, Steers WD, Somlyo AP, Somlyo AV. RhoA-mediated Ca2+ sensitization in erectile function. *J Biol Chem* 2002; **277**: 30614–21.

[58] Sauzeau V, Rolli-Derkinderen M, Marionneau C, Loirand G, Pacaud P. RhoA expression is controlled by nitric oxide through cGMP-dependent protein kinase activation. *J Biol Chem* 2003; **278**: 9472–80.

[59] Touyz RM, Schiffrin EL. Signal transduction mechanism mediating the physiological and pathophysiological actions of angiotensin II in vascular smooth muscle cells. *Pharm Res* 2000; **52**: 639–72.

[60] Kifor I, Williams GH, Vickers MA, *et al.* Tissue angiotensin II as modulator of erectile function. I. Angotensin peptide content, secretion and effects in the corpus cavernosum. *J Urol* 1999; **157**: 1920–5.

[61] Becker AJ, Uckert S, Stief CG, *et al.* Possible role of bradykinin and angiotensin II in the regulating of penile erection and detumescence. *Urology* 2001; **57**: 193–8.

[62] Dusing R. Effect of the angiotensin II antagonist valsartan on sexual function in hypertensive men. *Blood Press Suppl* 2003; **2**: 29–34.

[63] Christ GJ. The penis as vascular organ: the importance of corporal smooth muscle tone in erection. *Urol Clin North Am* 1995; **22**: 727–45.

[64] Kim NN, Dhir V, Azadzoi KM, *et al.* Pilot study of the endothelin-A receptor slective antagonist BMS-193884 for the treatment of erectile dysfunction. *J Androl* 2002; **23**: 76–83.

[65] Becker AJ, Uckert S, Stief CG, *et al.* Systemic and cavernosal plasma levles of endothelin (1–21) during different penile conditions in healthy males and patinets with erectile dysfunction. *World J Urol* 2001; **19**: 371–6.

[66] Stief CG, Holmquist F, Djamilian M, *et al.* Preliminary results with the nitric oxide donor linsidomine chlorhydrate in the treatment of human erectile dysfunction. *J Urol* 1992; **148**: 1437–40.

[67] Shamloul R, Atteya A, Elnashaar A, *et al.* Intracavernous sodium nitroprusside (SNP) versus papaverine/phentolamine in erectile dysfunction: a comparative study of short-term efficacy and side-effects. *J Sex Med* 2005; **2**: 117–20.

[68] Hobbs AJ. Soluble guanylate cyclase: an old therapeutic target re-visited. *Br J Pharmacol* 2002; **136**: 637–40.

[69] McMahon CG, Abdo C, Incrocci L, *et al.* Disorders of orgasm and ejaculation in men. *J Sex Med* 2004; **1**: 58–65.

[70] Lipshultz LI, Mc Connell J, Benson GS. Current concepts of the mechanisms of ejaculation: normal and abnormal states. *J Reprod Med* 1981; **26**: 499–507.

[71] Dun NJ, Dun SL, Huang RL, *et al.* Distribution and origin of nitric oxide synthase-immunoreactive nerve fibers I the rat epididimis. *Brain Res* 1996; **738**: 292–300.

[72] Torres G, Bitran M, Huidobro-Toro JP. Co-release of neuropeptide Y (NPY) and noradrenaline from the sympathetic nerve terminals supplying the rat vas deferens: influence of calcium and the stimulation intensity. *Neurosci Lett* 1992; **148**: 39–42.

[73] Giuliano F, Clement P. Neuroanatomy and physiology of ejaculation. *Annu Rev Sex Res* 2005; **16**: 190–216.

[74] Sjostrand N, Ehren I, Eldh J, Wiklund NP. NADPH-diaphorase in glandular cells and nerves and its relation to acetylcholinesterase-positive nerves in the male reproductive tract of man and guinea-pig. *Urol Res* 1998; **26**: 181–8.

[75] Uckert S, Stanarius A, Stief CG, *et al.* Immunocytochemical distribution of nitric oxide synthase in the human seminal vesicle: a light and electron microscopical study. *Urol Res* 2003; **31**: 262–6.

[76] Chapple CR, Aubry ML, James S, *et al.* Characterization of human prostatic adrenoceptors using pharmacology receptor binding and localization. *Br J Urol* 1989; **63**: 487–96.

[77] Nadelhaft I. Cholinergic axons in the rat prostate and neurons in the pelvic ganglion. *Brain Res* 2003; **989**: 52–7.

[78] Vaalasti A, Hervonen A. Nerve endings in the human prostate. *Am J Anat* 1980; **137**: 41–7.

[79] Adrian TE, Gu J, Allen JM, *et al.* Neuropeptide Y in the human male genital tract. *Life Science* 1984; **35**: 2643–8.

[80] Aumuller G, Jungblut T, Malek B, Konrad S, Weihe E. Regional distribution of opioidergic nerves in human and canine prostates. *Prostate* 1989; **14**: 279–88.

[81] Bloch W, Klotz T, Loch C, *et al.* Distribution of nitric oxide synthase implies a regulation of circulation, smooth muscle tone, and secretory function in the human prostate by nitric oxide. *Prostate* 1997; **33**: 1–8.

[82] Dail WG. Autonomic innervation of male genitalia. In: Maggi CA, ed. *Nervous Control of the Urogenital System.* Chur, Switzerland: Harwood Academic, 1993: 69–102.

[83] Lincoln J, Burnstocl G. Autonomic innervation of the urinary bladder and urethra. In: Maggi CA, ed. *Nervous Control of the Urogenital System.* Chur, Switzerland: Harwood Academic, 1993: 33–68.

[84] Monneron MC, Gillberg PG, Ohman B, Albers P. In vitro alpha-adrenoceptor autoradiography of the urethra and urinary bladder of the female pig, cat guinea-pig and rat. *Scand J Urol Nephrol* 2000; **34**: 233–8.

[85] Morrison J, Steers WD, Brading A, *et al.* Neurophysiology and neuropharmacology. In: Abrams P, Cardozo L, Khoury S, Wein A, eds. *Incontinence.* Plymouth: Health Publication, 2005: 85–164.

[86] Giuliano F, Clement P. Neuroanatomy and physiology of ejaculation. *Annu Rev Sex Res* 2005; **16**: 190–216.

[87] Crowe R, Burnstock GA. Histochemical and immunohistochemical study of the autonomic innervation of the lower urinary tract of the female pig. Is the pig a good model for the human bladder and urethra? *J Urol* 1989; **141**: 414–22.

[88] Halata Z, Munger BL. The neuroanatomical basis for the protopathic sensibility of the human glans penis. *Brain Res* 1986; **371**: 205–30.

[89] Baron R, Janig W. Afferent and sympathetic neurons projecting into lumbar visceral nerves of the male rat. *J Comp Neurol* 1991; **314**: 429–36.

[90] Ueyama T, Arakawa H, Mizuno N. Central distribution of efferent and afferent components of the pudendal nerve in rat. *Anat Embryol* 1987; **177**: 37–49.

[91] Nadelhaft I, McKenna KE. Sexual dimorphism in sympathetic preganglionic neurons of the rat hypogastric nerve. *J Comp Neurol* 1987; **256**: 308–15.

[92] Sato K, Kihara K. Spinal cord segments controlling the canine vas deference and differentiation of the primate sympathetic pathways to the vas deferens. *Microsc Res Tech* 1998; **42**: 390–7.

[93] Hellstrom W. Current and future pharmacotherapies of premature ejaculation. *J Sex Med* 2006; **3** (Suppl 4): 332–41.

[94] Marson L, Platt KB, McKenna KE. Central nervous system innervation of the penis as revealed by the transneuronal transport of pseudorabies virus. *Neuroscience* 1993; **55**: 263–80.

[95] Greco B, Edwards DA, Zumpe D, Michael RP, Clancy AN. Fos induced by mating or noncontact sociosexual interaction is colocalized with androgen receptors in neurons within the forebrain, midbrain, and lubosacral spinal cord of male rats. *Horm Behav* 1998; **33**: 125–38.

[96] Rampin O, Gougis S, Giuliano F, Rousseau JP. Spinal Fos labeling and penile erection elicited by stimulation of dorsal nerve of the rat penis. *Am J Physiol* 1997; **272**: R1425–31.

[97] Truitt WA, Coolen LM. Identification of a potential ejaculation generator in the spinal cord. *Science* 2002; **297**: 1566–9.

[98] Coolen LM, Veening JG, Wells AB, Shipley MT. Afferent connections of the parvocellular subparafascicular thalamic nucleus in the rat: evidence for functional subdivisions. *J Comp Neurol* 2003; **463**: 132–56.

[99] Xu C, Yaici ED, Conrath M, *et al.* Galanin and neurokinin-1 receptor immunoreactivity spinal neurons controlling the prostate and the bulbospongiosus muscle identified by transsynaptic labeling in the rat. *Neuroscience* 2005; **134**: 1325–41.

[100] Hamson DK, Watson NV. Regional brainstem expression of Fos associated with sexual behavior in male rats. *Brain Res* 2004; **1006**: 233–40.

[101] Heeb MM, Yahr P. Anatomical and functional connections among cell groups in the gerbil brain that are activated with ejaculation. *J Comp Neurol* 2001; **439**: 248–58.

[102] McKenna KE, Chung SK, McVary KT. A model for the study of sexual function in anesthetized male and female rats. *Am J Physiol* 1991; **261**: R1276–85.

[103] Johnson RD, Hubscher CH. Brainstem microstimulation differentially inhibits pudendal motoneuron reflex inputs. *Neuroreport* 1998; **9**: 341–5.

[104] Opsomer RJ, Caramia MD, Zarola F, Pesce F, Rossini PM. Neurophysiological evaluation of central–peripheral sensory and motor pudendal fibres. *Electroencephalogr Clin Neurophysiol* 1989; **74**: 260–70.

[105] Shafik A, El-Sibai O. Mechanism of ejection during ejaculation: identification of a urethrocavernosus reflex. *Arch Androl* 2000; **44**: 77–83.

[106] Kontani H, Shiraoya C. Method for simultaneous recording of the prostatic contractile and urethral pressure responses in anesthetized rats and the effects of tamsulosin. *Jpn J Pharmacol* 2002; **90**: 281–90.

[107] Kolbeck SC, Steers WD. Neural regulating of the vas deferens in the rat: an electrophysiological analysis. *Am J Physiol* 1992; **263**: R331–8.

[108] Watanabe H, Shima M, Kojima M, Ohe H. Dynamic study of nervous control on prostatic contraction and fluid excretion in the dog. *J Urol* 1988; **140**: 1567–70.

[109] Moss HE, Crowe R, Burnstock G. The seminal vesicle in eight and 16 week streptozotocin-induced diabetic rats: adrenergic, cholinergic and peptidergic innervation. *J Urol* 1987; **138**: 1273–8.

[110] Stjernquist M, Owman C, Sjoberg NO, Sundler F. Coexistence and cooperation between neuropeptide Y and norepinephrine in nerve fibers of guinea pig vas deferens and seminal vesicle. *Biol Reprod* 1987; **36**: 149–55.

[111] Pocard M, Zinzindohoue F, Haab F, *et al.* A prospective study of sexual and urinary function before and after total mesorectal excision with autonomic nerve preservation for rectal cancer. *Surgery* 2002; **131**: 368–72.

[112] Brindley GS, Sauerwein D, Hendry WF. Hypogastric plexus stimulators for obtaining semen from paraplegic men. *Br J Urol* 1989; **64**: 72–7.

[113] Gerstenberg TC, Levin RJ, Wagner G. Erection and ejaculation in man: assessment of the electromyographic activity of the bulbocavernosus and ischiocavernosus muscles. *Br J Urol* 1990; **65**: 395–402.

[114] Vinik AI, Maser RE, Mitchell BD, Freeman R. Diabetic autonomic neuropathy. *Diabetes Care* 2003; **26**: 1553–79.

[115] Scaletta LL, Hull EM. Systemic or intracranial apomorphine increases copulation in long-term castrated male rats. *Pharmacol Biochem Behav* 1990; **37**: 471–5.

[116] Bazzett TJ, Eaton RC, Thompson JT, *et al.* Dose dependent D2 effects on genital reflexes after MPOA injections of quinelorane and apomorphine. *Life Science* 1999; **48**: 2309–15.

[117] Ferrari F, Giulinai D. Behavioral effects induced by the dopamine D3 agonist 7-OH-DPAT in sexually-active and -inactive male rats. *Neuropharmacology* 1996; **35**: 279–84.

[118] Giuliano F, Clement P. Physiology of ejaculation: emphasis on serotonergic control. *Eur Urol* 2005; **48**: 408–17.

[119] Waldinger MD, Olivier B. Utility of selective serotonin reuptake inhibitors in premature ejaculation. *Curr Opin Investig Drugs* 2004; **5**: 743–7.

[120] Rehman J, Kaynan A, Christ G, *et al.* Modification of sexual behavior of Long-Evans male rats by drugs acting on the 5-HT1A receptor. *Brain Res* 1999; **821**: 414–25.

[121] Hillegaart V, Ahlenius S. Facilitation and inhibition of male rat ejaculatory behavior by the respective 5-HT1A and 5-HT1B receptor agonists 8-OH-DPAT and anpirtoline, as evidenced by use of the corresponding new and selective receptor antagonists NAD-2999 and NAS-181. *Br J Pharmacol* 1998; **125**: 1733–43.

[122] Foreman MM, Hall JL, Love RL. The role of the 5-HT2 receptor in the regulation of sexual performance of male rats. *Life Sci* 1989; **45**: 1263–70.

[123] Rosen RC, Giuliano F, Carson CC. Sexual dysfunction and lower urinary tract symptoms (LUTS) associated with benign prostatic hyperplasia (BPH). *Eur Urol* 2005; **47**: 824–37.

[124] Pulito VL, Li X, Varga SS, Mulcahy LS, *et al.* An investigation of the uroselective properties of four novel α1a-adrenergic receptor subtype-selective antagonists. *J Pharmacol Exp Ther* 2000; **294**: 224–9.

[125] Raja M. Risperidone-induced absence of ejaculation. *Int Clin Psychopharmacol* 1999; **14**: 317–19.

[126] Metz ME, Pryor JL. Premature ejaculation: a psychophysiological approach for assessment and management. *J Sex Marital Ther* 2000; **26**: 293–320.

[127] Hsu JH, Shen WW. Male sexual side effects associated with antidepressants: a descriptive clinical study of 32 patients. *Int J Psychiatry Med* 1995; **25**: 191–201.

[128] Harrison WM, Rabkin JG, Ehrhardt AA, *et al.* Effects of antidepressant medication on sexual function: a controlled study. *J Clin Psychopharmacol* 1986; **6**: 144–9.

[129] Montejo-Gonzalez AL, Llorca G, Izquierdo JA, *et al.* SSRI-induced sexual dysfunction: fluoxstin, paroxstine, sertraline, and fluvoxamine in a prospective, multicenter, and descriptive clinical study of 344 patients. *J Sex Marital Ther* 1997; **23**: 176–94.

[130] Laumann EO, Paik A, Rosen RC. Sexual dysfunction in the United States: prevalence and predictors. *JAMA* 1999; **281**: 537–44.

[131] Rowland DL, Perelman MA, Althof SE, *et al.* Self-reported premature ejaculation and aspects of sexual functioning and satisfaction. *J Sex Med* 2004; **1**: 225–32.

[132] Rosen RC. The premature ejaculation prevalence and attitudes (PEPA) survey: a multi-national survey. *J Sex Med* 2004; **1** (Suppl 1): 57–8.

[133] Montague DK, Jarow J, Broderick GA, *et al.* AUA guideline on the pharmacologic management of premature ejaculation. *J Urol* 2004; **172**: 290–4.

[134] McMahon CG, Touma K. Treatment of premature ejaculation with paroxetine hydrochloride as needed: 2 single-blind placebo controlled crossover studies. *J Urol* 1999; **161**: 1826–30.

[135]. Waldinger MD. Hengeveld MW, Zwinderman AH, Olieveier B. Effect of SSRI antidepressants on ejaculation: a double-blind, randomized, placebo-controlled study with fluoxetine, fluvoxamine, paroxetine, and sertraline. *J Clin Psychopharmacol* 1998; **18**: 275–81.

[136] Williams VS, Baldwin DS, Hogue SL, *et al.* Estimating the prevalence and impact of antidepressant-induced sexual dysfunction in 2 European countries: a cross-sectional patient survey. *J Clin Psychiatry* 2006; **67**: 204–10.

[137] Hu XH, Bull SA, Hunkeler EM, *et al.* Incidence and duration of side effects and those rated as bothersome with selective serotonin reuptake inhibitor treatment of depression: patient report versus physician estimate. *J Clin Psychiatry* 2004; **65**: 959–65.

[138] McMahon CG, Abdo C, Incrocci L, *et al.* Disorders of orgasm and ejaculation in men. *J Sex Med* 2004; **1**: 58–65.

[139] Waldinger MD, Hengeveld MW, Zwinderman AH, Olivier B. An empirical operationalization study of DSM IV diagnostic criteria for premature ejaculation. *Int J Psychiatry Clin Pract* 1998; **2**: 287–93.

[140] Waldinger MD, Berendesen HH, Blok BF, Olievier B, Holstege G. Premature ejaculation and serotonergic antidepressants-induced delayed ejaculation: the involvement of the serotonergic system. *Behav Brain Res* 1998; **92**: 111–18.

[141] Gengo PJ, Giuliano F, McKenna K. Monoaminergic transporter binding and inhibition profile of dapoxetine, a medication for the treatment of premature ejaculation. *J Urol* 2005; **173** (Suppl 4): 239.

[142] Modi NB, Dresser MJ, Simon M, *et al.* Single- and
multiple-dose pharmacokinetics of dapoxetine
hydrochloride, a novel agent for the treatment of
premature ejaculation. *J Clin Pharmacol* 2006; **46**:
301–9.

[143] Pryor JL, Althof SE, Steidle C, *et al.*, for the
Dapoxetine Study Group. Efficacy and tolerability of
dapoxetine in treatment of premature ejaculation: an
integrated analysis of two double-blind, randomized
controlled trials. *Lancet* 2006; **368**: 929–37.

Office evaluation of the subfertile male

Mark Sigman, Larry I. Lipshultz, and Stuart S. Howards

Introduction

Infertility is often a difficult and stressful condition for both clinicians and patients to address. The possibility of being childless often threatens both the male and female partner's self-esteem. In addition, clinicians are often unfamiliar with the plethora of diagnostic tests currently available, and the interpretation of those tests required to develop a rational management plan.

Fortunately, the last decade has seen new emphasis on practice guidelines based on evidence-based medicine when possible and on consensus opinions of experts when adequate scientific studies are lacking. The American Urological Association and the American Society for Reproductive Medicine have jointly produced guidelines covering several aspects of the evaluation and management of male infertility. The use of evidence-based medicine and outcomes research is essential to determine the appropriate role of the growing list of available diagnostic tests. In spite of the scientific community's increased emphasis on appropriately designed studies, patients are increasingly drawn to alternative medicine approaches for which, in general, there is limited or anecdotal evidence of efficacy. The wide use of the Internet has given patients rapid access to information. Unfortunately, this information is of widely varying quality, often leading the patients to have false expectations about the diagnostic utility of various tests as well as inappropriate expectations of the results of therapeutic approaches. This only emphasizes the need for the clinician to have a strong understanding of the basics of the infertility evaluation.

Pregnancy rates by intercourse in normal couples are approximately 20–25% per month, 75% by six months, and 90% by one year [1]. After one year of unprotected intercourse approximately 15% of couples of unknown fertility status are unable to conceive. In approximately 30% of these couples, infertility is due to a significant male factor alone, whereas **combined male and female factors are present in an additional 20% [2–4]. Thus, a male factor is involved in approximately 50% of infertile relationships. It is important to realize that 25–35% of infertile couples without treatment will conceive by intercourse at some point in time.** Conception rates of 23% are reported within the first two years, and an additional 10% will conceive within two more years [5,6]. **Overall, in nonazoospermic infertile couples a pregnancy rate of 1–3% per month can be expected.** While infertility is generally not considered to exist until after 12 months of attempted conception, couples often seek help prior to that period of time because they may have delayed attempts at parenthood until after career development. If conception does not occur in a timely manner, such couples face a race against the woman's biologic clock. For these reasons, a basic, simple, and cost-effective evaluation need not be postponed. The workup of the infertile male should proceed, as would the workup of any patient with a medical problem: with a thorough history and physical examination followed by an initial series of laboratory tests. The results of the history, physical examination, and laboratory tests are used to develop a differential diagnosis, which may require additional, more specific testing. Although many tests are available to evaluate different aspects of male infertility, not all patients need all tests.

The primary goals of the evaluation of the male presenting with infertility are to identify: (1) etiologic conditions that may be reversed with resultant improvement in the male's fertility status; (2) irreversible conditions that may be best managed by the use of the assisted reproductive techniques, such as intrauterine insemination (IUI) or in-vitro fertilization (IVF), using the male partner's sperm; (3) irreversible conditions not amenable to assisted reproductive techniques, such that donor insemination or adoption is more advisable; (4) medically significant

Infertility in the Male, 4th edition, ed. Larry I. Lipshultz, Stuart S. Howards, and Craig S. Niederberger. Published by Cambridge University Press. © Cambridge University Press 2009.

pathologies underlying the male's infertility; and (5) genetic etiologies that may have implications for the patient and/or his offspring. When specific etiologies are identified, treatment may be directed towards the underlying pathology. Unfortunately, in many cases, the underlying cause for the abnormal semen analysis remains unknown. In these instances, both empirical therapies and techniques such as IUI, IVF, and intracy-toplasmic sperm injection (ICSI) are often utilized. The physician should be familiar with the indications and limitations of each of these techniques, to better counsel the patient about appropriate management options.

History

A careful history should be obtained, including a detailed reproductive history and medical and surgical history, as well as a review of pertinent lifestyle factors and potential gonadal toxic exposure (Table 10.1).

Reproductive history

A notation should be made of prior conceptions for the male or the female with present or past partners, details of any prior difficulty achieving conception, as well as past evaluations and treatments for infertility and past use of contraception. The frequency and timing of intercourse should be recorded. Often neither partner understands the menstrual cycle and the fact that it is during the middle of the menstrual cycle that the female is fertile. In addition, it should be stressed that intercourse does not have to occur exactly at the time of ovulation since sperm remain viable within the cervical mucus and crypts for 48 hours or longer. **Studies of fertile couples have demonstrated that conception may occur with intercourse taking place within the five days prior to ovulation but will not occur if intercourse is performed only on the day following ovulation [7]. Most couples should be advised to have intercourse every two days near the time of ovulation.** This will ensure that viable sperm are present within the female reproductive tract during the 12–24-hour period in which the ovum is viable and in the fallopian tube, and therefore capable of being fertilized. If intercourse occurs too frequently, inadequate numbers of sperm may be deposited within the vagina. The male should be questioned about his erectile and ejaculatory function, as well as frequency of masturbation. Commonly used lubricants such as K-Y Jelly, Lubifax, SurgiLube, Keri Lotion, Astroglide, and saliva have been demonstrated to adversely affect sperm motility in vitro [8–13]. Lubricants that do not appear to affect

Table 10.1. History of the infertile male

History of infertility
Duration
Prior pregnancies
Present partner
Another partner
Previous treatments
Evaluation and treatment of partner
Sexual history
Potency
Lubricants
Timing of intercourse
Frequency of intercourse
Frequency of masturbation
Childhood and development
Cryptorchidism, orchiopexy
Herniorrhaphy
Y–V plasty of bladder neck
Testicular torsion
Onset of puberty
Medical history
Systemic illness (e.g., diabetes mellitus, multiple sclerosis)
Previous/current therapy
Surgical history
Orchiectomy (testicular cancer, torsion)
Retroperitoneal surgery
Pelvic injury
Pelvic, inguinal, or scrotal surgery
Herniorrhaphy
Y–V plasty, transurethral prostate
Infections
Viral febrile
Mumps orchitis
Venereal
Tuberculosis, smallpox (rare)
Gonadotoxins
Chemicals (pesticides)
Drugs (chemotherapeutic, cimetidine, sulfasalazine, nitrofurantoin, alcohol, marijuana, androgenic steroids, cocaine)
Thermal exposure (hot tubs, saunas)
Radiation
Smoking
Family history

Table 10.1. continued

Cystic fibrosis

Androgen receptor deficiency

Review of systems

Respiratory infections

Anosmia

Galactorrhea

Impaired visual fields

Headaches

motility include raw egg white, vegetable oil, safflower oil, peanut oil, and, recently, several commercial lubricants. While these studies were done in vitro, it is still prudent to recommend that couples use a lubricant only if needed, and use only a minimal amount of one.

Childhood illnesses and conditions

The history of specific childhood illnesses or conditions may be important in the evaluation of the infertile male. **Bilateral cryptorchidism results in a significant decrease in spermatogenesis, while the effect of unilateral cryptorchidism appears to be much milder.** Studies of formerly cryptorchid patients who have undergone orchidopexies have reported decreased sperm densities in approximately 30% of men with unilateral cryptorchidism (range 28–82%). However, some studies have reported abnormal sperm densities in only 17% of patients [14,15]. In contrast, approximately 50% of bilaterally cryptorchid patients (range 9–88%) have been reported to have decreased sperm densities. Interestingly, the majority of unilaterally cryptorchid men are able to initiate a pregnancy without difficulty. Fertility rates in couples in whom the male has unilateral cryptorchidism average 85%, which is only slightly lower than and possibly not statistically significantly different from pregnancy rates in controls [14,15]. In contrast, fertility rates in couples in whom the male had bilateral cryptorchidism are only 50–65%. Despite the trend of performing orchidopexies at an earlier age, improved fertility rates have yet to be demonstrated with this approach. On the other hand, testes that remain undescended in the postpubertal age group do not function, and fertility rates are not improved by postpubertal repair [16,17]. Testicular trauma or history of torsion of the testis should be noted, since both may result in atrophic testes. Approximately 30–40% of men with a history of testicular torsion will have abnormal results on semen analyses [18–25]. Antisperm antibodies are present in 0–11% of patients either at the time or

after the event of testicular torsion [26,27]. Interestingly, testicular biopsies of the contralateral testis at the time of torsion have demonstrated a high frequency of impaired spermatogenesis and histological abnormalities [18,28]. Thus it appears that testes susceptible to torsion may have pre-existing spermatogenic defects. Despite these findings, definitive proof demonstrating decreased fertility in adult men with a past history of torsion is lacking [22,24].

The timing of pubertal development should be noted. Significantly delayed or incomplete development may suggest an endocrinopathy. Mumps does not appear to affect the testis when experienced prepubertally. However, after the age of 11 or 12 unilateral mumps orchitis occurs in 30% of patients who contract mumps postpubertally. The orchitis is bilateral in approximately 10% of patients [29]. While this infection has been uncommon since the advent of mumps vaccine, it is still problematic in developing countries [26,30]. Importantly, the testicular damage may be quite severe, resulting in marked fibrosis and atrophy of the testis.

Systemic diseases and illnesses

Both diabetes and multiple sclerosis may affect erectile as well as ejaculatory function [31]. Myotonic dystrophy is associated with the development of testicular atrophy [30,32]. Any generalized illness resulting in fever or viremia may cause impaired testicular function, the effects of which may not appear in the ejaculate for 1–4 months. The actual time lapse between the injurious event and the appearance of abnormal cells in the ejaculate varies, depending on what stage of the spermatogenic process is affected. For this reason, if a patient gives a history of acute medical problems in the three months before his first office visit, and if laboratory analysis shows subnormal semen quality, analyses should be repeated several months later before a decision is made regarding the quality of sperm production. A history of pyospermia or prostatitis should be noted, although these are uncommon and unproven causes of infertility [33]. The history of chronic upper respiratory infections associated with severe motility defects raises the possibility of primary ciliary dyskinesia (also known as immotile cilia syndrome). When this condition is associated with situs inversus, it is known as Kartagener syndrome [34]. The association of frequent respiratory infections with azoospermia raises the possibility of Young syndrome [35]. In this condition, epididymal obstruction is due to inspissation of secretions. Any history of urinary tract infections or sexually transmitted diseases should be recorded, particularly if associated with epididymitis. Epididymal infections may result in the obstruction of the epididymis.

Past surgical history

Details of past surgeries should be obtained. Bladder neck surgery as well as prostate surgery may result in retrograde ejaculation, and patients will present with absent or low-volume ejaculates and the presence of large numbers of sperm in the postejaculate urine. Pelvic and retroperitoneal surgery may also affect ejaculatory function. Modifications of retroperitoneal lymph node dissection techniques utilizing a template method or a nerve-sparing approach preserve the sympathetic nerves and allow retention of the ejaculatory function in most patients [30,32,36–38]. Patients with ejaculatory function after retroperitoneal surgery may sometimes be effectively treated pharmacologically with sympathomimetic drugs, retrieval of sperm from a postejaculatory alkalinized urine combined with intrauterine insemination, electroejaculation, or surgical sperm retrieval combined with ICSI (see Chapter 26). The vas deferens may be injured during a herniorrhaphy itself or as a consequence of scarring from polypropylene mesh used during the repair [39].

Cancer and cancer treatments

Patients with testicular cancer may present with infertility either before or after treatment of their cancer. **Approximately 50% of testicular cancer patients have subnormal sperm densities prior to chemotherapy** [12,22,24,40]. **Of note, of those with oligo- or azoospermia, 75% normalized during surveillance** [12]. Following cisplatinum-based chemotherapy for testicular cancer, most patients will become azoospermic. However, most will recover sperm production within four years [13,41]. Radiation therapy given to patients with testicular seminoma results in impaired spermatogenesis 4–6 months after the completion of radiation. This may occur even with gonadal shielding [42]. Of those patients developing impaired spermatogenesis following retroperitoneal radiation therapy for seminoma, most will have a return to baseline semen quality within a two-year period. Three-fourths of those attempting conception will be successful within four years [41,43]. Patients with leukemia, lymphoma, and a variety of solid neoplasms often have subnormal semen parameters [44–46]. Most patients with Hodgkin's disease and leukemia become azoospermic after chemotherapy; however, some treatments may not result in permanent sterility [47]. **After bone marrow transplantation with a combination of chemotherapy and radiation therapy, permanent sterility usually results** [48].

Medication and drug use

A detailed history of medications including prescribed, over-the-counter, illicit, and neutraceuticals should be obtained. Unfortunately, for many substances, data detailing potential effects on male fertility are lacking. Online sources include databases such as Reprotox and Reprotext. Both are often available through online hospital and university databases. **Heavy marijuana use has been associated with gynecomastia, decreased serum testosterone levels, and a decrease in sperm concentration and pyospermia** [49–51]. Similarly, oligospermia and defects in morphology and motility have been reported in users of cocaine [52,53]. Antihypertensive medications are commonly associated with erectile dysfunction, but most do not directly affect fertility. Spironolactone acts as an antiandrogen and has been associated with impaired semen quality [52,54]. Calcium channel blockers have been reported to cause a reversible functional defect in sperm, impairing the ability of sperm to fertilize human eggs without affecting sperm production or standard semen analysis parameters [55,56]. However, all investigators have not reported these effects.

Diethylstilbestrol (DES) was given to pregnant women in the 1950s, and reports of epididymal cysts and cryptorchidism in males with prenatal DES exposure have raised concerns about effects on fertility [57]. However, follow-up studies on adult men with prenatal DES exposure have revealed no adverse effects on fertility [58]. **Exogenous androgens are well known to induce hypogonadotropic hypogonadism. This may be induced by testosterone directly or by synthetic anabolic steroids. The subsequent suppression of endogenous testosterone production usually results in azoospermia, which is frequently reversible over a 3–6 month period of time. Of significance, some patients do not recover normal pituitary function.** While dehydroepiandrosterone (DHEA) is commonly taken and easily available over the counter, there is no human male fertility data on this medication. Rat studies have demonstrated no effect on spermatogenesis. **Alpha-blockers may cause decreased ejaculate volume or anejaculation. This appears not to be due to retrograde ejaculation and appears to be more common with tamsulosin than with other α-blockers** [59]. Saw palmetto is another commonly used over-the-counter medication for prostate problems. Unfortunately, there are no human male fertility data on this drug.

Many antibiotics have been reported in animal studies to have potentially adverse effects on male fertility [60]. However, there are few human data regarding the majority of these medications. Very high doses of nitrofurantoin have been reported to cause early maturation arrest at the primary spermatocyte stage [61,62]. However, short-term lower-dose therapy, as is commonly used clinically, is not likely to be detrimental. While erythromycin, tetracycline, and gentamicin have been reported to have the potential to adversely affect fertility, documentation of an in-vivo effect in humans is lacking [63]. Sulfasalazine is well known to cause defects in human sperm concentration and motility [64,65]. These effects are reversible, and patients with concerns about fertility should be treated with 5-amino salicylic acid, which does not affect semen parameters [66]. Cimetidine has been reported to have antiandrogenic effects inducing gynecomastia. While a decrease in sperm count was reported, no loss of fertility has been noted [67].

Immune modulators are commonly used, but unfortunately most lack clear human data. Interferon has been used to treat mumps orchitis. However, there are no human data indicating an impairment of male fertility associated with this medication. Colchicine has been reported to induce oligospermia. However, this was reported after long-term use in patients with Behçet's disease. Short-term use in healthy males induced no effect in semen parameters [68,69]. Cyclosporine has been found to induce impaired fertility in rats. However, there are no human data [70], and there are no human or animal data on mycophenolate mofetil, a medication used commonly in transplant patients.

Cholesterol-lowering drugs such as statins (HMG-CoA reductase inhibitors) have been of concern because of potential effects on cell membranes. While there are no human data indicating adverse affects, rat data have suggested no detrimental effects on fertility [71]. Chronic opioid use, whether oral or intrathecal, may induce hypogonadotropic hypogonadism. This has commonly been noted to lead to sexual dysfunction. Effects on fertility have not been examined [72,73]. Epilepsy has been associated with decreased testosterone levels and increased estrogen levels. In addition, medications used to treat epilepsy may worsen the hormonal abnormalities and have been associated with some sperm morphologic defects [74].

Occupational and lifestyle exposures

Exposure to potential environmental toxins should be carefully noted. This includes pesticide exposure as well as occupational chemical exposure. Material safety data sheets (MSDS) may be examined for additional information [75,76]. Exposure to lead, mercury, cadmium, arsenic, hydrocarbons, particular amebicide and nematocide soil fumigants, and 2-bromopropane (a substitute for chlorofluorocarbons) has been associated with decreased spermatogenesis [75,77–82]. Serum levels of heavy metals should be obtained in patients thought to have had high exposure to these compounds. **While testicular atrophy is commonly present in alcoholics, moderate alcohol consumption does not appear to impair male fertility** [83–86]. **The effect of cigarette smoking on male fertility remains controversial. However, accumulating data suggest adverse effects.** Studies finding decreases in semen parameters and no effect on semen parameters have been reported [5,50,87–91]. Interestingly, a recent analysis reported an increase in the time to conception when the male partner of a couple smoked and the nonsmoking female partner was passively exposed to cigarette smoke [92]. Similarly, poor results during in-vitro fertilization have been reported in smokers [93], and impaired fertility in offspring of male smokers has also been reported [94]. **Caffeine consumption, while often questioned, does not appear to affect male fertility** [95]. **Exposure to excessive heat should be recorded. The use of frequent saunas and hot baths has been demonstrated to impair semen parameters** [96–98]. These habits should be discontinued if a patient undergoing evaluation has been found to have impaired semen parameters. Workers in certain occupations – such as welders; drivers of industrial machinery, taxis and trucks; bakers; ceramic oven operators; and workers in submarines – have been found to have increased rates of infertility [99]. While the use of tight underwear is commonly thought to impair spermatogenesis, a large study has not demonstrated this effect [100].

Physical examination

The physical examination of the infertile male should focus on identifying abnormalities that may affect fertility. This includes the pattern of virilization, as well as the patient's secondary sexual characteristics. Abnormalities of androgenization suggest the possibility of an endocrine disorder. Excessive estrogens or an imbalance in the estrogen-to-androgen ratio may result in gynecomastia. Kartagener syndrome is associated with immotile cilia and immotile sperm combined with situs inversus. Penile curvature or angulation should be assessed, as should the location of the urethral meatus. Anatomical abnormalities of the penis can result in improper placement of the ejaculate within the vaginal vault. The scrotal contents should be carefully palpated with the patient standing in a warm room. Testicular consistency should be noted as well as testicular size. It has been shown that a decrease in testicular size is often associated with impaired spermatogenesis [101]. This is not surprising, since 85% of the testis is involved in sperm production; consequently, when the germinal epithelium atrophies, loss of testicular mass occurs. **Testicular volume may be measured with an orchidometer, or the length and width measured with calipers.** In the normal male, the volume should be at least 20 mL and the greatest length of the testis at least 4 cm [102–104]. Of note, Asian men typically have smaller testes.

Examination of the epididymis should be carefully performed, taking note of the presence of the caput, corpus, and cauda as well as whether or not the epididymis feels indurated or full. Obstruction of the genital ductal system may be suggested by a fullness of the epididymis. While spermatoceles and epididymal cysts are commonly palpated, they usually do not indicate obstruction. **Palpation of the spermatic cords should be performed with careful notation of the presence or absence of the vas deferens as well as any areas of vasal atrophy or nodularity. The patient should be examined in a standing position for the presence of a varicocele within the spermatic cord and surrounding the testicle.** An increase in the venous diameter may be noted with the patient performing the Valsalva maneuver. Alternatively, the patient may distend his abdomen, which often increases intra-abdominal pressure without resulting in contraction of the cremasteric muscles. Varicoceles may be graded as small (grade 1) if only palpable with the patient performing the Valsalva maneuver, moderate (grade 2) when palpable with the patient in the standing position without performing the Valsalva maneuver, or large (grade 3) when the veins are visible through the scrotal skin. Varicoceles should decrease in size when the patient is in the supine position. Subclinical varicoceles are those varicoceles identifiable only with an ancillary technique and not palpable or suspected on physical exam. We do not recommend a search for subclinical varicoceles. Occasionally, because of anatomic abnormalities such as a small scrotum with high testes or very thick spermatic cords, the physical exam is indeterminate. In those cases, techniques such as ultrasonography may be employed. While a rectal examination is often recommended, the majority of abnormalities

that are detectable on transrectal ultrasonography will not be noted on digital rectal examination.

Initial laboratory testing

Following completion of the history and physical examination, appropriate laboratory testing of the male should be performed. **The cornerstone of the evaluation remains the completion of at least 2–3 semen analyses.** Nevertheless, the semen analysis is not a direct measure of fertility. While there are differences in overall semen parameters between fertile and infertile populations, there is a large amount of overlap [105]. **It is important for the clinician to understand the difference between average semen parameters and those threshold values below which fertility becomes statistically less likely.** While an average sperm density may be defined on the basis of the mean and its accompanying 95% confidence interval of a population of fertile males, samples outside of that range are not necessarily infertile. Thus, unlike the determination of normal values in other aspects of medicine, ranges used in evaluating semen parameters are based on attempts to separate fertile from infertile populations. Average sperm densities in populations of men are often reported to be in the range of 60–70 million sperm/mL. This average number is not the same as the minimal number of sperm necessary for initiating a pregnancy. In addition, it is important to realize that fertility is dependent on more than one semen parameter, as well as on the status of both partners. Thus, a patient with an average sperm count but absent motility will be infertile. **It is also important to keep in mind that semen parameters that may be adequate for pregnancy by assisted reproductive techniques, including IUI, should not be confused with those necessarily adequate for normal pregnancy rates by intercourse.** As sperm densities decrease, pregnancy rates by intercourse have also been found to decrease [106]. In addition, both sperm motility and morphology have been reported to be as important if not more important than sperm density [107,108].

In general, it is not possible on the basis of the semen analysis to separate infertile from fertile patients, since the majority of infertile men have some motile sperm in the semen. More correctly, patients may be placed in a subfertile category. In contrast, azoospermic patients are sterile. It has also become clear that equal numbers of motile sperm from different patients do not have the same fertilizing capability. Thus, men treated for hypogonadotropic hypogonadism are often fertile with sperm concentrations

Table 10.2. Common reference ranges for semen parameters [117]

Parameter	Reference range
Volume	≥ 2.0 mL
pH	≥ 7.2
Sperm concentration	≥ 20 million sperm/mL
Total sperm count per ejaculate	40 million sperm
Motility	≥ 50% with grade A + B motility or ≥ 25% with grade A motility
Morphology	≥ 15% by strict criteria
Viability	≥ 75% of sperm viable
WBC (white blood cells)	< 1 million/mL

under 5 million sperm/mL, whereas data from IVF centers indicate that even the motile sperm from oligoasthenoteratozoospermic patients do not fertilize as well as equal numbers of motile sperm from normospermic patients [109,110]. While there are no universally agreed-upon reference ranges for semen analyses, the World Health Organization reference values have been utilized increasingly (Table 10.2). While there are many additional tests of fertility, only the semen analysis is required in all patients undergoing a male fertility evaluation. The remaining tests should be utilized to narrow the differential diagnosis following the results of a history, physical examination, and semen analyses.

Semen analysis

Collection

It is important to provide patients with specific criteria for the collection of semen specimens. In general, a minimum of two semen analyses should be obtained from all patients. Consistency in the duration of sexual abstinence before collection of the specimen should be maintained, to allow accurate comparisons between the samples from the same patient. Sperm concentration has been found to increase 25% per day of abstinence for the first four days, while increases in the seminal volume, and therefore total sperm count, were also increased with increased days of abstinence; motility and morphology remained unchanged [111]. Of interest, even ejaculation within the seven days before the beginning of the abstinence period caused a lowering of sperm concentration.

When the initial semen samples have widely different parameters, additional samples should be obtained. It is useful to explain this to the patient before collection of the first specimen in case additional specimens are needed. The specimen container should be clean, although not necessarily sterile, and wide-mouthed to minimize collection error. Some plastics may contain residual spermicidal chemicals; thus, batches of containers should be checked to rule out spermatotoxic contaminating material. This may easily be performed by incubating raw semen samples in the plastic containers for several hours to assure that motility does not decrease. While in the past glass containers were commonly utilized, this is currently uncommon. **Collection of the semen may be by masturbation, coitus interruptus, or with special seminal collection condoms devoid of spermicidal agents.** Ordinary latex condoms may interfere with the viability of spermatozoa and may contain spermacides, and therefore should not be used. **Although coitus interruptus may be employed, it is not an ideal technique as the initial portion of the ejaculate may be lost.** In addition, acidic vaginal secretions and bacteria may contaminate the specimen. The specimen should be transported to the laboratory at room or body temperature. This is easily accomplished by having the patient place the container in a pocket next to his body. The laboratory should specify how long from the time of ejaculation the specimen should be brought to the laboratory; in most laboratories this is stated to be 1–2 hours. A specimen container should be labeled with the patient's name, date, and time of collection, as well as the abstinence period.

Physical characteristics

Freshly produced semen is a coagulum that liquefies 5–25 minutes after ejaculation. The seminal constituents responsible for coagulation originate in the seminal vesicles; the proteolytic enzymes that initiate liquefaction are found in the prostate. **Patients with congenital bilateral absence of the vas deferens usually have absent or hypoplastic seminal vesicles. Thus, semen from these patients has a low volume, is acidic, and does not coagulate.**

Details of the measurement of semen parameters and characteristics may be found in Chapter 33. Abnormal viscosity is commonly reported, and it is important to be able to differentiate semen with failure of liquefaction from semen that remains hyperviscous after liquefaction. Since, prior to liquefaction, semen consists of a coagulum, nonliquefied semen remains a coagulum following ejaculation. In contrast, hyperviscous semen is semen that has liquefied and becomes less of a coagulum after ejaculation. However, its consistency remains thicker than normal. Normally liquefied semen may be poured drop by drop, in contrast to hyperviscous semen, which forms thick strands instead of drops. While in the past hyperviscous and nonliquefied semen have been thought to be causes of infertility, it is unclear if this is actually the case. Normal postcoital tests have been reported in patients with nonliquefied semen, while sperm have been found in the cervical mucus before semen liquefaction [112]. Although some have ascribed hyperviscosity to genital tract infections, this is not supported by current data [113]. If hyperviscous or nonliquefying semen is reported, a postcoital test (PCT) may be obtained. The presence of normal numbers of motile sperm in the cervical mucus strongly suggests that the consistency of semen is not a factor in the couple's infertility. In those instances when the PCT demonstrates few motile sperm in association with good-quality cervical mucus, semen processing and IUI using the male partner's sperm may be employed.

Concentration

The term *sperm count* **typically refers to the sperm density reported as millions of sperm per milliliter of semen. An accompanying parameter, total sperm count, generally refers to the total number of sperm within the whole ejaculate.** This is obtained by multiplying the sperm concentration by the seminal volume. There are a variety of methods to determine sperm concentration. The majority utilize counting chambers in which sperm are counted within a grid. Recent data have demonstrated significant differences in sperm counts depending on the type of chamber used [114,115]. Samples in which no sperm are identified should be centrifuged, and the pellet examined for the presence of spermatozoa.

Motility and forward progression

Motility refers to the percentage of sperm demonstrating any motion, whereas forward progression is a qualitative assessment of the relative speed with which spermatozoa move in a forward direction. There are two common scoring systems in use. In one, a five-point scale is utilized, with a rating of 0 indicating no motility, 1 indicating sluggish or nonprogressive movement, 2 referring to sperm moving with a slow, meandering, forward progression, 3 indicating movement in a reasonably straight line with moderate speed, 4 indicating sperm movement with high speed in a straight line [116]. The report indicates the motility category of the majority of moving sperm. An alternative system categorizes all of the moving sperm into one of four categories: category A indicates rapid progressive motility, B represents sluggish or slowly progressive motility, C is motility that is nonprogressive, and D indicates lack of motility. The percentage of sperm falling into each category is reported [117].

Clumps of agglutinated sperm occasionally appear in semen specimens; significant amounts of sperm agglutination are suggestive of the presence of the antisperm antibodies. **Under wet-mount microscopy, round cells without tails are commonly identified.** These should be properly termed round cells. **Both immature germ cells, such as spermatocytes, and white blood cells may have this appearance.** The presence of excessive numbers of round cells should be recorded. Subsequent assays may be used to differentiate between immature germ cells and white blood cells. Because nonmotile sperm may be alive, the term *necrospermia* should not be used unless a sperm viability assay has demonstrated that all sperm are nonviable. In those cases in which motility is less than 5–10%, a viability stain should be used to determine if the immotile sperm are alive. A high percentage of viable nonmotile sperm suggests the presence of an ultrastructural abnormality, such as primary ciliary dyskinesia. Electron microscopy of the spermatozoa to examine the sperm cytoskeleton may be utilized to confirm the diagnosis (see Chapter 11).

Morphology

The microscopic examination of sperm shape (morphology) is a sensitive index of the state of the germinal epithelium [118]. While a rough gauge of morphology can be obtained using wet-mount microscopy with a phase-contrast microscope, detailed and accurate evaluation requires stained cytological smears. The traditional evaluation of sperm morphology classifies sperm as normal if they do not fit into one of several defined categories. A common classification scheme classifies sperm as normal (oval), amorphous (including large and small sperm), tapered, duplicated, and immature. The observation of spermatozoa recovered from postcoital cervical mucus, or from the surface of zona pellucida, has led to more strict criteria to define normal spermatozoa (see Chapter 34) [119–122]. **There are multiple morphology scoring systems currently in use with no consensus among laboratories.** Currently, lower limits of normal of 60%, 30%, 14%, and 4% are in use. **Thus interpretation of the morphology score on the semen analysis report requires that the physician be familiar with the individual laboratory's classification system.** The physician must also be aware of what clinical studies have been done to allow interpretation of various levels of normal morphologic forms. Initial studies utilizing strict morphologic criteria studied patients undergoing IVF, and reported better fertilization rates in those with greater than 14% normal forms by strict criteria than in those with less than 14% normal forms. Further studies reported that the poorest fertilization rates occurred in those with less than 4% normal forms. Thus some laboratories report a normal threshold of greater than 4% while others report its being greater than 14% [123]. Similar problems exist when morphology scores are used to predict pregnancy rates with IUI [124–126] and with intercourse [103,105,127]. **What has become clear is that pregnancies are possible when morphology scores are low, and therefore morphology scores should not be used in isolation from other parameters.**

Computer-assisted semen analysis

Efforts to improve upon the manual semen analysis have resulted in computer-assisted semen analyses (CASA). Most systems utilize video with multiple frames that are then analyzed to determine specific semen parameters. In addition to motility, sperm concentration, and in some cases sperm morphology, additional parameters that are not measurable manually are often reported. The average distance per unit time between sequential positions of individual sperm is known as the curvilinear velocity. In contrast, the straight-line velocity is the speed of the sperm in a forward direction. This correlates with manual methods of determination of the forward progression [128]. The straight-line velocity divided by curvilinear velocity yields linearity. CASA systems are often used to measure hyperactivation, which is a state sperm obtain following capacitation. Hyperactivated sperm demonstrate large-amplitude

Table 10.3. Distribution of semen abnormalities in 8758 patients

Azoospermia	4%
Predominance of a single abnormal parameter	29%
Motility	18%
Volume	2%
Morphology	7%
Density	2%
Defects in two or more parameters	37%
All parameters normal	30%

movements of the head and tail with slow or nonprogressive motility [129 130]. The clinical utility of these, as well as other CASA-derived semen parameters, remains limited. Advantages of CASA systems include the ability to obtain precise quantitative data as well as the potential for standardization of semen analysis procedures. However, these advantages have been largely overshadowed by disadvantages including a lack of standardization in procedures, which may affect the results, as well as the significant expense of acquiring the equipment [131]. While CASA remains a valuable research tool, it has not proven itself more useful in the clinical arena than the manual semen analysis [132–134].

Interpretation of the initial evaluation

Following the history, physical examination, and initial semen analysis, a differential diagnosis should be developed. **Additional laboratory studies may then be employed to further refine the diagnosis and help determine management options.** The results of the initial evaluation may be utilized in diagnostic algorithms, which direct the clinician to obtain pertinent diagnostic tests in a systematic and organized manner and with the least chance of omitting appropriate steps. When this approach is used, semen analysis results may be categorized into (1) all parameters normal; (2) azoospermia (lack of sperm in the semen); (3) diffuse abnormalities in sperm density, sperm morphology and motility; and (4) isolated problems restricted to one parameter of the semen evaluation such as seminal volume, sperm density, motility, or morphology. Utilizing our own patient population, we have calculated the frequencies of these classifications of subcategories (Table 10.3).

Normal semen parameters

The finding of normal semen parameters raises the possibility of a female factor, inappropriate coital habits, erectile dysfunction, defects in sperm function, or the presence of antisperm antibodies. The term *unexplained infertility* is used to characterize infertility in which female factors have been ruled out and the male has a normal evaluation with normal semen parameters. Consideration should be given to testing for the presence of antisperm antibodies in the male. While uncommon, some men with normal semen parameters have a functional defect interfering with the ability of sperm to fertilize eggs. This may be diagnosed with the use of sperm function testing such as the sperm penetration assay, hemizona assay, acrosome reaction testing, reactive oxygen species (ROS) determination, or DNA fragmentation analysis . If functional defects are identified, the male evaluation should be repeated to try to identify any reversible causes. If no etiologies are identified, then the couple with clear sperm functional defects should be directed towards IVF with ICSI. In those cases of unexplained infertility without sperm function defects, IUI combined with controlled ovarian hyperstimulation or IVF may be considered.

Azoospermia

The term *azoospermia* refers to the absence of sperm from the semen. This should be differentiated from a dry ejaculate in which no antegrade semen is produced. The first step in evaluating an azoospermic patient is to be certain that the semen is truly azoospermic by centrifuging the specimen [135]. It is not unusual to find sperm in the specimen of a patient initially reported to be sterile. In this instance, total ductal obstruction or complete lack of spermatogenesis has been ruled out. Azoospermia is commonly categorized into either obstructive azoospermia or nonobstructive azoospermia. The term *nonobstructive azoospermia* refers to a lack of sperm production, whereas *obstructive azoospermia* implies adequate sperm production in the presence of obstruction of the ductal system. The physician should take careful note during the physical exam of the testicular size and presence of the vas deferens, and should obtain a serum FSH. These parameters will help differentiate between the various causes of normal-volume azoospermia. Low testicular volume suggests a nonobstructive azoospermic etiology. Congenital bilateral absence of the vas deferens (CBAVD) is diagnosed by physical exam. This

defect is usually due to a mutation in the cystic fibrosis transmembrane regulator gene (*CFTR*) [136]. Semen from CBAVD patients is commonly low-volume and azoospermic with an acidic pH. A small proportion of patients may have vasal agenesis due to a non-cystic-fibrosis-mediated embryologic defect. These cases are often associated with renal anomalies, specifically unilateral absence of the kidney [137]. Thus a renal ultrasound should be obtained. Normal testicular size is generally found in these patients. Because spermatogenesis is normal, a screening FSH should be obtained. The presence of a normal testicular volume and a normal FSH is a sufficient evaluation for diagnosis. A diagnostic testicular biopsy is not required in these patients unless the history, the physical exam, or the finding of an elevated FSH suggests a spermatogenic defect.

The finding of atrophic testes suggests a spermatogenic defect. This may be primarily due to an inherent testicular dysfunction or secondarily due to a hormonal deficiency. Thus azoospermic patients with normal seminal volumes and palpable vas deferens should have FSH and testosterone levels measured. The finding of small testes in association with a low FSH and testosterone suggests hypogonadotropic hypogonadism, and the patient's LH and prolactin levels should be evaluated. Low gonadotropin levels associated with an elevated prolactin level raise the possibility of a pituitary prolactinoma, and a pituitary MRI should be obtained. The finding of atrophic testes and elevated FSH levels indicates germ cell failure. It is important to realize that the normal ranges of FSH commonly utilized in commercial laboratories may have been determined from males whose fertility status was unknown. **Thus patients with normal sperm production typically have FSH values in the lower end of the normal range (less than 5–6 mIU/mL). Levels above this should raise the suspicion of a defect in spermatogenesis.** While patients with normal spermatogenesis bilaterally usually have FSH levels in the low normal range, it should be kept in mind that an FSH above this range does not rule out intact spermatogenesis. Patients with unilateral testicular disease may have elevated FSH levels. In patients with elevated FSH levels, a diagnostic testicular biopsy should only be performed in conjunction with sperm retrieval if IVF/ICSI is being considered. **Patients with nonobstructive azoospermia due to a primary testicular defect and not due to a hormonal deficiency should be offered genetic testing consisting of a** karyotype and a Y-chromosome microdeletion analysis (see Chapter 15). **If abnormalities are found, the couples should be offered genetic counseling prior to proceeding with assisted reproductive techniques.**

The finding of normal-sized testes in the presence of a normal FSH raises the possibility of obstructive azoospermia. Genetic testing should also be offered to these patients. A testicular biopsy is required to differentiate between spermatogenic defects and obstruction. If IVF/ICSI is an option, the diagnostic biopsy should be performed in conjunction with sperm retrieval. Sperm may be cryopreserved for later use in an IVF/ICSI cycle. The presence of normal spermatogenesis on the biopsy indicates obstructive azoospermia. Scrotal exploration with microscopic vasotomy and sampling of the vas fluid with either vasal irrigation or standard contrast vasography may be performed. The absence of sperm in the vas fluid suggests a more proximal obstruction. The presence of sperm in the vas fluid in association with inability to irrigate fluid distally in the vas deferens indicates a more distal obstruction. The rare finding of sperm in the vas fluid and a normal ability to irrigate the vas deferens distally, in the presence of normal-volume azoospermia, suggests the possibility of ectopic entrance of the distal vas deferens into the genitourinary system.

When performing vasography, retrograde injection towards the epididymis should be avoided, as it may cause epididymal trauma and extravasation secondary to increased intraductal pressure. Generally, bilateral vasograms are not necessary. A unilateral patent vas is all that necessary to rule out obstruction as the cause of azoospermia. Epididymal obstruction can often be appreciated at the time of scrotal exploration when dilated epididymal tubules are identified under magnification during examination of the epididymis. Microsurgical epididymostomy of an individual epididymal tubule with inspection of the fluid in the operating room under high dry magnification ($\times$ 400) can verify the presence of sperm. If epididymal obstruction is encountered, vasoepididymostomy using the techniques described in Chapter 21 should be performed. When the vasogram results demonstrate normal patency in the absence of sperm in the vasal fluid and the presence of nondilated epididymal tubules, consideration should be given to the obstruction of the efferent ductules or rete testis.

Low-volume azoospermic semen specimens may be due to hypogonadism (low testosterone levels), ejaculatory duct obstruction, or seminal vesicle absence or hypofunction. Both patients with bilateral ejaculatory duct obstruction and patients with CBAVD (which is usually associated with absence or hyperplasia of the seminal vesicles) produce low-volume, azoospermic, and acidic semen specimens. In all patients with low-volume ejaculates (see next section) postejaculate urine should be obtained to rule out retrograde ejaculation. In patients with low-volume azoospermic semen specimens, retrograde ejaculation with sperm found only in the urine is very unusual. This is in contrast to those patients with dry ejaculates, in whom retrograde ejaculation, with sperm found in the postejaculate urine, is much more common. If retrograde ejaculation is identified, attempts may be made to initiate antegrade ejaculation with sympathomimetic agents. Alternatively, urinary alkalinization may be achieved and sperm may be retrieved from voided urine, or culture medium may be instilled into the empty bladder prior to ejaculation. The medium may then be voided and sperm retrieved for IUI or IVF (see Chapter 26). If the postejaculate urine does not contain spermatozoa the seminal vesicles and the ejaculatory ducts should be examined with transrectal ultrasonography (TRUS). Historically, obstruction of the ejaculatory ducts was evaluated through the use of seminal fructose measurements, but the advent of TRUS has made this unnecessary (Chapter 20). Dilated seminal vesicles suggestive of ejaculatory duct obstruction may be aspirated at the time of the TRUS. The presence of millions of sperm identified under wet-mount microscopy of the seminal vesicle aspirate is diagnostic of ejaculatory duct obstruction [138]. In addition, the finding of sperm in the seminal vesicle fluid indicates the presence of intact spermatogenesis. Patients with these characteristics do not need testis biopsies for diagnosis. If ejaculatory duct obstruction is identified, transurethral resection of the ejaculatory ducts may be an option (Chapter 23). In those azoospermic patients with low-volume ejaculates and in whom no ejaculatory duct obstruction is identified by TRUS, the evaluation should proceed as for normal-volume azoospermia.

In a series of 133 azoospermic patients, biopsies were performed in 101 cases and 41% demonstrated normal spermatogenesis. The remainder of the azoospermic patients had testicular failure: Sertoli-cell-only (38%), maturation arrest (20%), or focal scarring (2%) [139].

Multiple semen abnormalities

The finding of defects in sperm density, motility, and morphology are commonly referred to as

oligoasthenoteratozoospermia (OAT). **By far the most common cause of this pattern is varicocele.** The presence of a varicocele is a clinical diagnosis based on physical examination, and routine use of ancillary testing is not indicated (Chapter 18). Ancillary techniques such as ultrasonography or venography may be utilized when the physical exam is suboptimal but suggestive of the varicocele – as in those patients who are obese, have very small scrotums, or are unable to tolerate a physical exam due to a vasovagal response [140]. Transient distresses such as heat from the environment or from fevers should be considered if they have occurred within three months prior to obtaining the semen analysis. Additional causes of OAT include environmental toxins, drugs or medications, and cryptorchidism. Finally, the possibility of partial ejaculatory duct obstruction should be considered, as it may be associated with low seminal volume and defects in the majority of semen parameters [141]. While some have advocated diagnosis and treatment of these patients, the criteria for diagnosis remain unclear. Clinicians should be careful in utilizing partial ejaculatory duct obstruction to explain what is, more commonly, idiopathic male infertility.

Defects in isolated semen parameters

Approximately 30% of patients have isolated defects in seminal volume, sperm density, motility, or morphology (Table 10.3).

Defects in seminal volume

Complete ejaculatory failure, also called *aspermia*, or a dry ejaculate, exists when no fluid is produced in an antegrade fashion during the male orgasm. This should be differentiated from *azoospermia*, in which semen is produced in an antegrade fashion but there are no sperm present within the semen. **Ejaculatory failure may be due to retrograde ejaculation, in which semen flows in a retrograde fashion into the bladder, or due to failure of emission, in which there is no semen expulsed through the vas deferens and ejaculatory ducts into the urethra.** Common causes of ejaculatory failure include neurologic abnormalities such as spinal cord injury, diabetes mellitus, and multiple sclerosis, and, in addition, the use of α-blockers. Approximately 10% of patients taking tamsulosin report ejaculatory dysfunction. This appears to be much less common with the nonselective α-blockers, as well as with alfuzosin [59]. Retroperitoneal surgery, including colon surgery and retroperitoneal lymph

node dissections, may also impair ejaculation. True absence of ejaculation should be differentiated from complete inability to obtain orgasm, which may be due to medications such as serotonin reuptake inhibitors or to psychological disturbances.

Much more common than complete lack of ejaculation are low-volume ejaculate specimens. The most common cause of this finding is an incomplete collection. Multiple specimens should be obtained to be sure that low volume is a consistent finding. In addition, the patient should be questioned to be sure the specimen results from a complete collection. Finally, partial retrograde ejaculation is another common cause of low-volume ejaculates. The previously mentioned neurological disorders, medications, and bladder neck or prostatic surgery, as well as idiopathic causes, should be considered. Evaluation of low-volume azoospermia is discussed above, in the section on azoospermia. Some patients are unable to collect complete specimens by masturbation. The use of special seminal collection condoms will allow the collection of a specimen through intercourse. The abstinence period should be recorded for each specimen, since short abstinence periods will result in lower seminal volumes. **Postejaculate urine analysis should be performed in all patients with absent ejaculation and low-volume nonazoospermic semen specimens.** Specimens are most easily obtained by having the patient urinate prior to ejaculation. The patient is then instructed to ejaculate, and any antegrade specimen is collected into one container. The patient may then void into a second container. The urine is centrifuged at $\geq 300 \times g$ for 10 minutes and the pellet examined. In those patients with aspermia, the presence of any sperm in the postejaculate urine indicates either retrograde ejaculation or at least the passage of some semen into the urethra. In those patients with low-volume nonazoospermic semen specimens, the finding of greater numbers of sperm in the urine than in the antegrade specimen indicates at least a functionally important component of retrograde ejaculation. **It should also be kept in mind that the finding of any sperm in postejaculate urine in azoospermia rules out complete bilateral ductal obstruction.** In the absence of sperm in the postejaculate urine, ejaculatory duct obstruction should be suspected. Complete bilateral ejaculatory duct obstruction will result in azoospermic, low-volume, and acidic semen specimens. The workup of these patients is described in the section on azoospermia. It is important to keep in mind that both congenital bilateral absence of the vas deferens and isolated ejaculatory duct obstruction may have these findings. A careful physical examination will identify those patients with CBAVD. Transrectal ultrasonography should be obtained to rule out ejaculatory duct obstruction [142]. In the presence of low-volume nonazoospermic semen specimens, the diagnosis of partial ejaculatory duct obstruction by TRUS remains controversial and should not be made without seminal vesicle aspiration. While some would advocate the performance of resection of the ejaculatory ducts in these cases, others would utilize sperm in the antegrade ejaculate for the assisted reproductive techniques. A large ejaculate volume (>5 mL) may in theory dilute the sperm density and thereby cause subfertility. This occurrence is extremely uncommon and should only be suspected when there is an abnormal postcoital test despite adequate total sperm per ejaculate. In these instances, IUI combined with semen processing, which concentrates the sperm into a smaller volume, may be considered.

Defects in sperm concentration

In some patients, the only abnormality in the semen analysis is a decrease in the sperm density (<20 million sperm per mL). **In patients with less than 10 million sperm per mL, serum FSH and testosterone should be determined. In those patients with less than 5 million sperm per mL, a karyotype and Y-chromosome microdeletion analysis should also be considered. If** deficiencies in gonadotropins are identified, a complete endocrine evaluation should be performed (Chapter 12). The finding of an elevated FSH may indicate a primary testicular defect. Most commonly, oligospermia is idiopathic. While varicoceles are commonly associated with decreases in sperm density, decreases in other sperm parameters such as motility usually accompany these findings. If hormonal deficiencies and genetic abnormalities have been ruled out, remaining treatment options include empiric medical therapy (Chapter 25) and assisted reproductive techniques, such as IUI and IVF/ICSI.

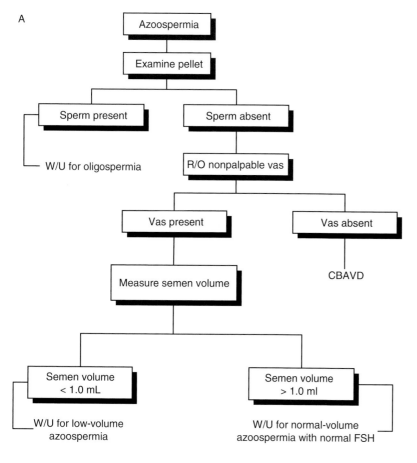

Fig. 10.1. (A–C) Algorithms for the workup of azoospermia. CBAVD, congenital bilateral absence of vas deferens; ED, ejaculatory duct; FSH, follicle-stimulating hormone; hCG, human chorionic gonadotropin; ICSI, intracytoplasmic sperm injection; LH, luteinizing hormone; MRI, magnetic resonance imaging; R/O, rule out; T, testosterone; TDI, therapeutic donor insemination; TRUS, transrectal ultrasonography; TURED, transurethral resection of ejaculatory duct; W/U, workup; YCMD, Y-chromosome microdeletion.

B

Fig. 10.1 continued

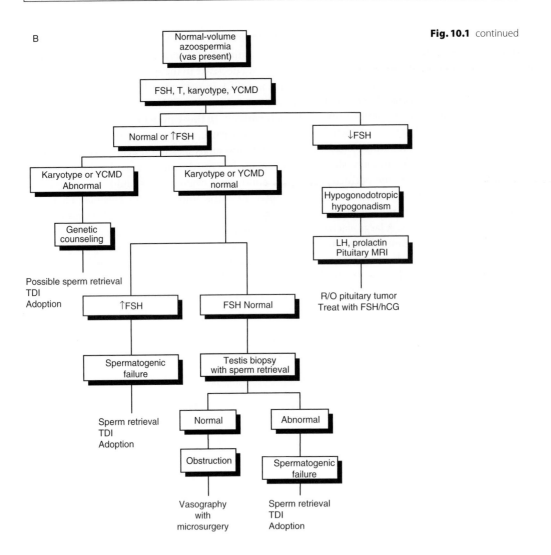

Defects in motility

The term *asthenospermia* refers to defects in sperm movement. This may be manifested by a low percentage of sperm that demonstrate any movement (motility) or by sperm that move forward slowly (poor forward progression). Prolonged abstinence periods, genital tract infections associated with pyospermia, antisperm antibodies, spermatozoal ultrastructural defects, partial ejaculatory duct obstruction, varicoceles, defective transport through the genital ductal system, and idiopathic causes may account for asthenospermia. Asthenospermia should be differentiated from sperm agglutination, which is the clumping together of individual spermatozoa identified under the microscope. Both asthenospermia and the presence of sperm agglutination suggest the presence of antisperm

antibodies. In general, it is preferable to use direct assays, since these determine the presence of sperm-bound antisperm antibodies, as compared with indirect assays that determine the presence of antisperm antibodies in a body fluid, such as serum (Chapter 16). **If antibody-positive, these patients may be treated with immunosuppressive steroids; however, the effectiveness of this medical treatment is low and there is the risk, albeit small, of serious side effects, such as aseptic necrosis of the hip. More commonly, patients are directed towards IUI or ICSI.** Patients with isolated asthenospermia will not have hormonal deficiencies; therefore, hormone assays are not indicated in this patient population.

Nonmotile sperm in the semen specimen are most commonly dead and therefore not viable. The clinician should consider the possibility of the semen specimen

C

Fig. 10.1 continued

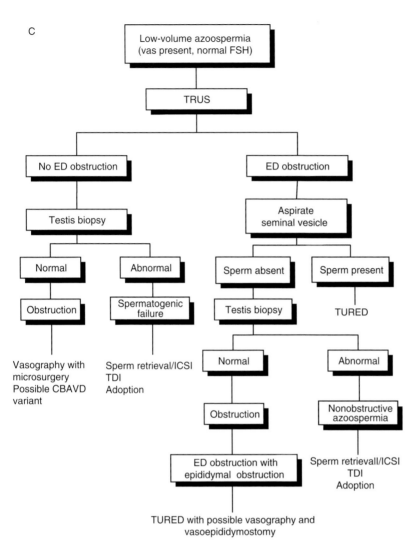

being exposed to contaminants within the container or to extremes of temperature, or extremely prolonged abstinence periods.

The complete absence of motility, or instances with less than 5–10% motility, also suggests the possible presence of ultrastructural defects in the spermatozoa. In these instances, a viability assay should be obtained. If all sperm are nonviable, *necrospermia* accurately describes the condition. In contrast, the finding of a high proportion of viable sperm with extremely low motility is consistent with the presence of an ultrastructural defect. In these instances, sperm should be evaluated by electron microscopy. The most common of such abnormalities include primary ciliary dyskinesia, also know as immotile cilia syndrome. When this is combined with situs inversus, it is known as Kartagener syndrome.

Defects in morphology

Teratozoospermia **refers to defects in sperm morphology.** This has been reported increasingly with the application of "strict" criteria. The majority of the cases are idiopathic, while varicoceles and temperature insults to spermatogenesis are also potential causes. Rare ultrastructural defects, such as the presence of round-headed sperm (globozoospermia), are characterized by an absence of acrosome [139,143]. While these cases may be treated with ICSI, pregnancy rates have been low.

Other abnormalities of semen

The presence of increased numbers of round cells in the semen suggests pyospermia. A study to differentiate between immature germ cells and white blood

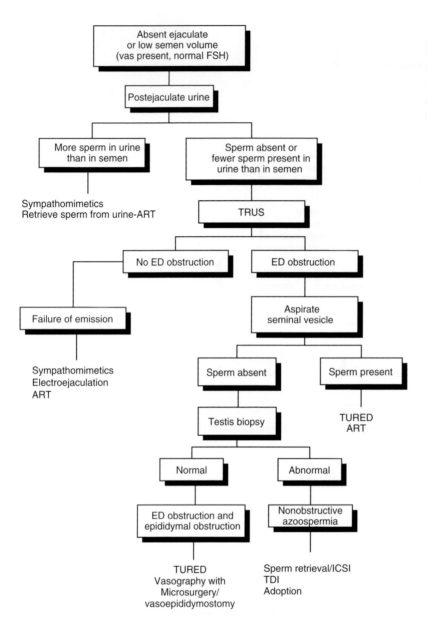

Fig. 10.2. Algorithm for the workup of absent or low-volume ejaculate. ART, assisted reproductive technologies; ED, ejaculatory duct; ICSI, intracytoplasmic sperm injection; TDI, therapeutic donor insemination; TRUS, transrectal ultrasonography; TURED, transurethral resection of ejaculatory duct.

cells should be considered. In cases of true pyospermia, the patient should be evaluated for *Mycoplasma genitalium* and *Chlamydia trachomatis*. These tests can be performed utilizing urine assays that use polymerase chain reaction (PCR) techniques. While semen cultures for bacteria have been advocated, the specimens are commonly contaminated by distal urethral organisms [144]. As previously mentioned, hyperviscosity should rarely be suspected as a cause of infertility.

Additional laboratory tests

After the history, physical examination, and initial semen analyses, the algorithms shown in Figures 10.1–10.4 are used to narrow down the differential diagnoses. Often additional testing is indicated. It should be emphasized that supplemental testing may be called for only when required to help narrow down diagnostic possibilities or to help in determining patient management. The etiologic categories of a large population of our patients are presented in Table 10.4.

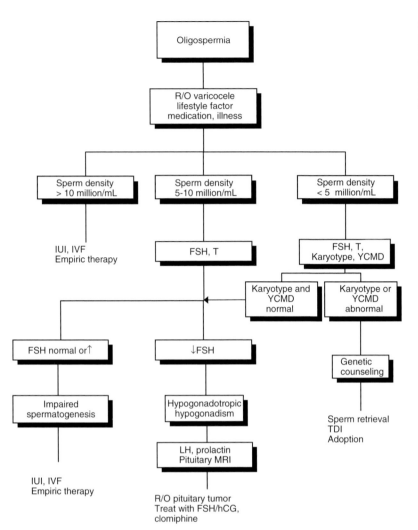

Fig. 10.3. Algorithm for the workup of oligospermia. FSH, follicle-stimulating hormone; hCG, human chorionic gonadotropin; IUI, intrauterine insemination; IVF, in-vitro fertilization; LH, luteinizing hormone; MRI, magnetic resonance imaging; R/O, rule out; T, testosterone; YCMD, Y-chromosome microdeletion.

Hormonal studies

The performance of a hormonal evaluation serves two purposes in the evaluation of the subfertile male: to identify endrocrinological abnormalities causing male infertility, or to yield prognostic information that is useful in the management of the male. Indications for hormonal testing include evidence from the patient's history suggestive of hormonal abnormalities, such as complaints of sexual dysfunction or decreased libido, or particular findings on physical examination, such as decreased androgenization or gynecomastia. However, the most common indication is oligospermia, with the vast majority of hormonal abnormalities being found in men with sperm densities of less than 10 million sperm per mL [145]. While gonadotropins are secreted episodically, pooled hormonal studies are seldom required, since a single determination performed in the morning rarely inaccurately determines a patient's true clinical endocrine status. **Morning determinations should be performed because testosterone is secreted diurnally, with higher levels in the morning. However, doing so consistently and routinely is often not feasible due to scheduling difficulties. Pooled samples should be reserved for those situations when the results of a single determination do not fit the patient's clinical evaluation** [146]. In patients with sperm densities of less than 10 million sperm per mL, determination of FSH and testosterone should be obtained. The most common abnormality identified is an elevated FSH, which generally indicates an impairment of spermatogenesis. In contrast, a normal FSH may be present with normal spermatogenesis or impaired spermatogenesis.

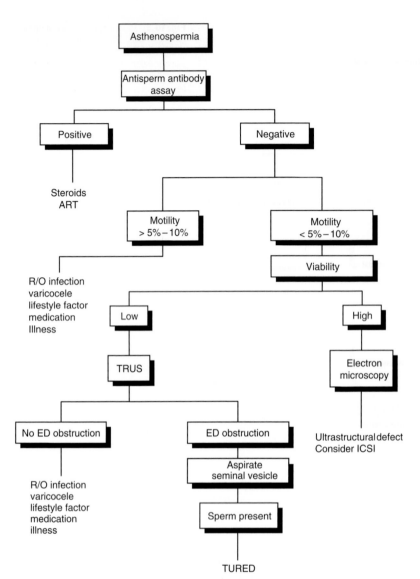

Fig. 10.4. Algorithm for the workup of asthenospermia. ART, assisted reproductive technologies; ED, ejaculatory duct; ICSI, intracytoplasmic sperm injection; R/O, rule out; TRUS, transrectal ultrasonography; TURED, transurethral resection of ejaculatory duct.

True endocrinologic causes of male infertility are uncommon, being present in less than 3% of cases [145]. **If deficiencies in FSH or testosterone are noted on the initial hormonal evaluation, repeat studies with the addition of LH and prolactin should be considered** (see Chapter 12).

Quantification of leukocytes in semen

Some infertile patients have numerous round cells in their semen. Both leukocytes and spermatocytes (immature germ cells) appear similar under wet-mount microscopy and therefore should be referred to as round cells. While many laboratories report these as white blood cells, their presence usually cannot be accurately determined without special staining techniques. The

WHO considers more than 1 million white blood cells per mL to be abnormal. Thus consideration should be given to performing white blood cell staining of semen in those patients with > 1 million round cells per mL, or more than 10–15 round cells per high-powered field (see Chapter 17). There remains controversy about the significance of true pyospermia. Many patients with pyospermia do not have documented infection, and not all studies demonstrate decreased fertility rates in couples with increased numbers of leukocytes in the semen [147]. Pyospermia is more frequent in patients with genital tract infection and in patients with infertility [148,149]. Bacterial cultures are not always positive in cases with pyospermia [150]. **Approximately one-third of patients with excess round cells in the**

Table 10.4. Distribution of final diagnostic categories found in a male infertility clinic

Category	Number	%
Immunologic	121	–
Idiopathic	1535	32.6%
Varicocele	1253	26.6%
Obstruction	720	15.3%
Normal female factor	503	10.7%
Cryptorchidism	129	2.7%
Ejaculatory failure	95	2.0%
Endocrinologic	70	1.5%
Drug/Radiation	64	1.4%
Genetic	56	1.2%
Testicular failure	52	1.1%
Sexual dysfunction	32	0.7%
Pyospermia	25	0.5%
Cancer	20	0.4%
Systemic disease	15	0.3%
Infection	10	0.2%
Torsion	5	0.1%
Ultrastructural	5	0.1%
Total	4710	100.0%

semen will be found to have true pyospermia, with the remainder having increased numbers of immature germ cells and not true pyospermia [151]. Those patients with true pyospermia should be evaluated for genital tract infection (see Chapter 17). The treatment of pyospermia in the absence of genital tract infection remains controversial. Suggested treatments have included empiric antibiotic therapy, anti-inflammatory medications, frequent ejaculations, and prostatic massage. Despite a lack of proven efficacy [152], consideration may be given to semen processing to remove the leukocytes. The processed sperm may then be utilized for IUI or IVF.

Antisperm antibodies

Despite the availability of antisperm antibody assays for many years, the indications for testing, the interpretation of the tests, and the management of immunologic infertility remain controversial. Risk factors for the development of antisperm antibodies include any process that may have potentially disrupted the blood–testis barrier, including obstruction of the genital tract. The finding of immotile sperm with a shaking motion

on a postcoital test has correlated with the presence of antisperm antibodies [153–155]. Additional indications have included asthenospermia or sperm agglutination as well as unexplained infertility. Management strategies have ranged from attempts to decrease the production of antisperm antibodies to semen processing techniques to remove the antibodies or the use of ICSI to bypass potential fertilization problems induced by the antibodies (see Chapter 16).

Functional assays

The standard semen analysis measures objective parameters of semen such as sperm count, motility, or seminal volume. Although these variables may correlate with fertilization, they do not directly measure those processes required for fertilization. For fertilization to occur in vivo, a sperm must be able to reach the site of the ovum by traversing the cervical mucus, undergo capacitation and the acrosome reaction, fuse with the oolemma, and be incorporated into the ooplasm. There are currently a variety of functional assays that measure the ability of the sperm to progress through these various stages.

The sperm–cervical mucus interaction is generally measured by the PCT. The ability of sperm to undergo capacitation and the acrosome reaction may be evaluated through acrosome reaction assays, which determine the percentage of sperm able to undergo the acrosome reaction, as well as the sperm penetration assay. The ability of sperm to bind to the zona pellucida may be evaluated by the hemizona assay. These specialized tests of sperm function are discussed in Chapter 11.

Additional tests

Additional tests, including those that measure reactive oxygen species (ROS) in semen, are being used with increasing frequency. While small amounts of ROS are normally present in semen, higher concentrations may injure sperm plasma membranes and induce DNA strand breaks [156] (see Chapters 11 and 39). Recent studies have demonstrated that sperm from subfertile males have poorer DNA integrity than sperm from fertile males. The roles of these tests remain controversial, and they are discussed in Chapters 11 and 40.

Conclusions

While there are a variety of sophisticated assays and investigations into the etiology of male infertility, the basic evaluation of the subfertile male remains founded on the performance of a proper history, physical examination, and basic semen analyses. Additional diagnostic tests are utilized in specific instances as suggested in the algorithms (Figs 10.1–10.4). The following chapters will provide details of further specialized diagnostic tests as well as specific causes of infertility. **At the conclusion of the evaluation, the physician should evaluate options for improving the male's fertility status and thus allowing the couple to conceive by intercourse. In addition, the physician should be aware of the appropriate role of assistive reproductive techniques that allow the use of spermatozoa that might be present.** In some instances both approaches may be employed so that patients with azoospermia or severely low sperm counts may be treated, with resultant improvement in the semen parameters. While the semen parameters may not normalize, they may improve to the point where other treatment options such as IUI are available. Options for both surgical and medical treatment of the subfertile male are discussed in depth in subsequent chapters. Finally, it is important to keep in mind that adoption and donor sperm insemination remain viable management choices.

References

[1] Spira A. Epidemiology of human reproduction. *Hum Reprod* 1986; **1**: 111–15.

[2] MacLeod J. Human male infertility. *Obstet Gynecol Surv* 1971; **26**: 335–51.

[3] Mosher WD. Reproductive impairments in the United States, 1965–1982. *Demography* 1985; **22**: 415–30.

[4] Simmons FA. Human infertility. *N Engl J Med* 1956; **255**: 1140–6.

[5] Vine MF, Tse CK, Hu P, Truong KY. Cigarette smoking and semen quality. *Fertil Steril* 1996; **65**: 835–42.

[6] Aafjes JH, van der Vijver JC, Schenck PE. The duration of infertility: an important datum for the fertility prognosis of men with semen abnormalities. *Fertil Steril* 1978; **30**: 423–5.

[7] Wilcox AJ, Weinberg CR, Baird DD. Timing of sexual intercourse in relation to ovulation: effects on the probability of conception, survival of the pregnancy, and sex of the baby. *N Engl J Med* 1995; **333**: 1517–21.

[8] Goldenberg RL, White R. The effect of vaginal lubricants on sperm motility in vitro. *Fertil Steril* 1975; **26**: 872–3.

[9] Kutteh WH, Chao CH, Ritter JO, Byrd W. Vaginal lubricants for the infertile couple: effect on sperm activity. *Int J Fertil Menopausal Stud* 1996; **41**: 400–4.

[10] Tagatz GE, Okagaki T, Sciarra JJ. The effect of vaginal lubricants on sperm motility and viability *in vitro*. *Am J Obstet Gynecol* 1972; **113**: 88–90.

[11] Tulandi T, Plouffe L, McInnes RA. Effect of saliva on sperm motility and activity. *Fertil Steril* 1982; **38**: 721–3.

[12] Carroll PR, Whitmore WF, Herr HW, *et al.* Endocrine and exocrine profiles of men with testicular tumors before orchiectomy. *J Urol* 1987; **137**: 420–3.

[13] Boyers SP, Corrales MD, Huszar G, DeCherney AH. The effects of Lubrin on sperm motility in vitro. *Fertil Steril* 1987; **47**: 882–4.

[14] Lee PA. Fertility after cryptorchidism: epidemiology and other outcome studies. *Urology* 2005; **66**: 427–31.

[15] Lee PA. Fertility in cryptorchidism: does treatment make a difference? *Endocrinol Metab Clin North Am* 1993; **22**: 479–90.

[16] Grasso M, Buonaguidi A, Lania C, *et al.* Postpubertal cryptorchidism: review and evaluation of the fertility. *Eur Urol* 1991; **20**: 126–8.

[17] Okuyama A, Nonomura N, Nakamura M, *et al.* Surgical management of undescended testis: retrospective study of potential fertility in 274 cases. *J Urol* 1989; **142**: 749–51.

[18] Anderson JB, Williamson RC. The fate of the human testes following unilateral torsion of the spermatic cord. *Br J Urol* 1986; **58**: 698–704.

[19] Anderson JB, Williamson RC. Fertility after torsion of the spermatic cord. *Br J Urol* 1990; **65**: 225–30.

[20] Bartsch G, Frank S, Marberger H, Mikuz G. Testicular torsion: late results with special regard to fertility and endocrine function. *J Urol* 1980; **124**: 375–8.

[21] Dondero F, Lenzi A, Picardo M, Pastore R, Valesini G. Cell-mediated antisperm immunity in selected forms of male infertility. *Andrologia* 1980; **12**: 25–9.

[22] Fraser I, Slater N, Tate C, Smart JG. Testicular torsion does not cause autoimmunization in man. *Br J Surg* 1985; **72**: 237–8.

[23] Mastrogiacomo I, Zanchetta R, Graziotti P, Betterle C, Scrufari P, Lembo A. Immunological and clinical study of patients after spermatic cord torsion. *Andrologia* 1982; **14**: 25–30.

[24] Puri P, Barton D, O'Donnell B. Prepubertal testicular torsion: subsequent fertility. *J Pediatr Surg* 1985; **20**: 598–601.

[25] Thomas WE, Cooper MJ, Crane GA, Lee G, Williamson RC. Testicular exocrine malfunction after torsion. *Lancet* 1984; **2**: 1357–60.

[26] Hagen P, Buchholz MM, Eigenmann J, Bandhauer K. Testicular dysplasia causing disturbance of spermiogenesis in patients with unilateral torsion of the testis. *Urol Int* 1992; **49**: 154–7.

[27] Anderson MJ, Dunn JK, Lipshultz LI, Coburn M. Semen quality and endocrine parameters after acute testicular torsion. *J Urol* 1992; **147**: 1545–50.

[28] Hadziselimovic F, Snyder H, Duckett J, Howards S. Testicular histology in children with unilateral testicular torsion. *J Urol* 1986; **136**: 208–10.

[29] Werner CA. Mumps orchitis and testicular atrophy: a factor in male sterility. *Ann Intern Med* 1950; **32**: 1075–86.

[30] Casella R, Leibundgut B, Lehmann K, Gasser TC. Mumps orchitis: report of a mini-epidemic. *J Urol* 1997; **158**: 2158–61.

[31] Greene LF, Kelalis PP. Retrograde ejaculation of semen due to diabetic neuropathy. *J Urol* 1967; **98**: 696.

[32] Drucker WD, Blanc WA, Rowland MM, *et al.* The testis in myotonic muscular dystrophy: a clinical and pathologic study with a comparison with Klinefelter's syndrome. *J Clin Endocrinol Metab* 1963; **23**: 59.

[33] Weidner W, Krause W, Ludwig M. Relevance of male accessory gland infection for subsequent fertility with special focus on prostatitis. *Hum Reprod Update* 1999; **5**: 421–32.

[34] Wilton LJ, Teichtahl H, Temple-Smith PD, De Kretser DM. Kartagener's syndrome with motile cilia and immotile spermatozoa: axonemal ultrastructure and function. *Am Rev Respir Dis* 1986; **134**: 1233–6.

[35] Wilton LJ, Teichtahl H, Temple-Smith PD, *et al.* Young's syndrome (obstructive azoospermia and chronic sinobronchial infection): a quantitative study of axonemal ultrastructure and function. *Fertil Steril.* 1991; **55**: 144–51.

[36] Donohue JP, Thornhill JA, Foster RS, Rowland RG, Bihrle R. Retroperitoneal lymphadenectomy for clinical stage A testis cancer (1965 to 1989): modifications of technique and impact on ejaculation. *J Urol* 1993; **149**: 237–43.

[37] Jewett MA. Nerve-sparing technique for retroperitoneal lymphadenectomy in testis cancer. *Urol Clin North Am* 1990; **17**: 449–56.

[38] Jacobsen KD, Ous S, Waehre H, *et al.* Ejaculation in testicular cancer patients after post-chemotherapy retroperitoneal lymph node dissection. *Br J Cancer* 1999; **80**: 249–55.

[39] Shin D, Lipshultz LI, Goldstein M, *et al.* Herniorrhaphy with polypropylene mesh causing inguinal vasal obstruction: a preventable cause of obstructive azoospermia. *Ann Surg* 2005; **241**: 553–8.

[40] Dubin L, Amelar RD. Sexual causes of male infertility. *Fertil Steril* 1972; **23**: 579–82.

[41] Ohl DA, Sønksen J. What are the chances of infertility and should sperm be banked? *Semin Urol Oncol* 1996; **14**: 36–44.

[42] Hahn EW, Feingold SM, Simpson L, Batata M. Recovery from aspermia induced by low-dose radiation in seminoma patients. *Cancer* 1982; **50**: 337–40.

[43] Fossa SD, Aass N, Kaalhus O. Long-term morbidity after infradiaphragmatic radiotherapy in young men with testicular cancer. *Cancer* 1989; **64**: 404–8.

[44] Hallak J, Kolettis PN, Sekhon VS, Thomas AJ, Agarwal A. Cryopreservation of sperm from patients with leukemia: is it worth the effort? *Cancer* 1999; **85**: 1973–8.

[45] Rueffer U, Breuer K, Josting A, *et al.* Male gonadal dysfunction in patients with Hodgkin's disease prior to treatment. *Ann Oncol* 2001; **12**: 1307–11.

[46] Agarwal A, Allamaneni SS. Disruption of spermatogenesis by the cancer disease process. *J Natl Cancer Inst Monogr* 2005; (34): 9–12.

[47] Meistrich ML, Wilson G, Mathur K, *et al.* Rapid recovery of spermatogenesis after mitoxantrone, vincristine, vinblastine, and prednisone chemotherapy for Hodgkin's disease. *J Clin Oncol* 1997; **15**: 3488–95.

[48] Anserini P, Chiodi S, Spinelli S, *et al.* Semen analysis following allogeneic bone marrow transplantation: additional data for evidence-based counselling. *Bone Marrow Transplant* 2002; **30**: 447–51.

[49] Harmon J, Aliapoulios MA. Gynecomastia in marihuana users. *N Engl J Med* 1972; **287**: 936.

[50] Close CE, Roberts PL, Berger RE. Cigarettes, alcohol and marijuana are related to pyospermia in infertile men. *J Urol* 1990; **144**: 900–3.

[51] Hembree WC, Zeidenbert P, Nahas G. Marijuana effects on human gonadal function. In: Nahas G, Poton WDM, Indanpaan-Heittila J, eds. *Marijuana: Chemistry, Biochemistry and Cellular Effects.* New York, NY: Springer-Verlag, 1976: 521–7.

[52] Bracken MB, Eskenazi B, Sachse K, *et al.* Association of cocaine use with sperm concentration, motility, and morphology. *Fertil Steril* 1990; **53**: 315–22.

[53] Hurd WW, Kelly MS, Ohl DA, *et al.* The effect of cocaine on sperm motility characteristics and bovine cervical mucus penetration. *Fertil Steril* 1992; **57**: 178–82.

[54] Tidd MJ, Horth CE, Ramsay LE, Shelton JR, Palmer RF. Endocrine effects of spironolactone in man. *Clin Endocrinol (Oxf)* 1978; **9**: 389–99.

[55] Benoff S, Cooper GW, Hurley I, *et al.* The effect of calcium ion channel blockers on sperm fertilization potential. *Fertil Steril* 1994; **62**: 606–17.

[56] Hershlag A, Cooper GW, Benoff S. Pregnancy following discontinuation of a calcium channel blocker in the male partner. *Hum Reprod* 1995; **10**: 599–606.

[57] Coscrove MD, Benton B, Henderson BE. Male genitourinary abnormalities and maternal diethylstilbestrol. *J Urol* 1977; **117**: 220–2.

[58] Wilcox AJ, Baird DD, Weinberg CR, Hornsby PP, Herbst AL. Fertility in men exposed prenatally to diethylstilbestrol. *N Engl J Med* 1995; **332**: 1411–16.

[59] Giuliano F. Impact of medical treatments for benign prostatic hyperplasia on sexual function. *BJU Int* 2006; **97** (Suppl 2): 34–8.

[60] Schlegel PN, Chang TS, Marshall FF. Antibiotics: potential hazards to male fertility. *Fertil Steril* 1991; **55**: 235–42.

[61] Nelson WO, Steinberger E. The effect of Furadroxyl upon the testis of the rat. *Anat Rec* 1952; **112**: 367.

[62] Nelson WO, Bunge RB. The effect of therapeutic dosages of nitrofurantoin upon spermatogenesis in man. *J Urol* 1957; **77**: 275–82.

[63] Hargreaves CA, Rogers S, Hills F, *et al.* Effects of co-trimoxazole, erythromycin, amoxycillin, tetracycline and chloroquine on sperm function in vitro. *Hum Reprod* 1998; **13**: 1878–86.

[64] Birnie GG, McLeod TI, Watkinson G. Incidence of sulphasalazine-induced male infertility. *Gut* 1981; **22**: 452–5.

[65] Toovey S, Hudson E, Hendry WF, Levi AJ. Sulphasalazine and male infertility: Reversibility and possible mechanism. *Gut* 1981; **22**: 445–51.

[66] Riley SA, Lecarpentier J, Mani V, *et al.* Sulphasalazine induced seminal abnormalities in ulcerative colitis: Results of mesalazine substitution. *Gut* 1987; **28**: 1008–12.

[67] Sawyer D, Conner CS, Scalley R. Cimetidine: adverse reactions and acute toxicity. *Am J Hosp Pharm* 1981; **38**: 188–97.

[68] Sarica K, Suzer O, Gurler A, *et al.* Urological evaluation of Behcet patients and the effect of colchicine on fertility. *Eur Urol* 1995; **27**: 39–42.

[69] Haimov-Kochman R, Ben-Chetrit E. The effect of colchicine treatment on sperm production and function: A review. *Hum Reprod* 1998; **13**: 360–2.

[70] Srinivas M, Agarwala S, Datta GS, *et al.* Effect of cyclosporine on fertility in male rats. *Pediatr Surg Int* 1998; **13**: 388–91.

[71] Niederberger C. Atorvastatin and male infertility: is there a link? *J Androl* 2005; **26**: 12.

[72] Daniell HW. Hypogonadism in men consuming sustained-action oral opioids. *J Pain* 2002; **3**: 377–84.

[73] Roberts LJ, Finch PM, Pullan PT, Bhagat CI, Price LM. Sex hormone suppression by intrathecal opioids: a prospective study. *Clin J Pain* 2002; **18**: 144–8.

[74] Gates JR. Epilepsy versus antiepileptic drugs and gonadal function in men. *Neurology* 2004; **62**: 174–5.

[75] Lipshultz LI, Ross CE, Whorton D, Milby T, Smith R, Joyner RE. Dibromochloropropane and its effect on testicular function in man. *J Urol* 1980; **124**: 464–8.

[76] Strohmer H, Boldizsar A, Plockinger B, Feldner-Busztin M, Feichtinger W. Agricultural work and male infertility. *Am J Ind Med* 1993; **24**: 587–92.

[77] De Celis R, Feria-Velasco A, Gonzalez-Unzaga M, Torres-Calleja J, Pedron-Nuevo N. Semen quality of workers occupationally exposed to hydrocarbons. *Fertil Steril.* 2000; **73**: 221–8.

[78] Kim Y, Park J, Moon Y. Hematopoietic and reproductive toxicity of 2-bromopropane, a recently introduced substitute for chlorofluorocarbons. *Toxicol Lett* 1999; **108**: 309–13.

[79] Lancranjan I, Popescu HI, Gavanescu O, Klepsch I, Serbanescu M. Reproductive ability of workmen occupationally exposed to lead. *Arch Environ Health* 1975; **30**: 396–401.

[80] Telisman S, Cvitkovic P, Jurasovic J, *et al.* Semen quality and reproductive endocrine function in relation to biomarkers of lead, cadmium, zinc, and copper in men. *Environ Health Perspect* 2000; **108**: 45–53.

[81] Toth A. Reversible toxic effect of salicylazosulfapyridine on semen quality. *Fertil Steril* 1979; **31**: 538–40.

[82] Van Thiel DH, Gavaler JS, Smith WI, Paul G. Hypothalamic–pituitary–gonadal dysfunction in men using cimetidine. *N Engl J Med* 1979; **300**: 1012–15.

[83] Curtis KM, Savitz DA, Arbuckle TE. Effects of cigarette smoking, caffeine consumption, and alcohol intake on fecundability. *Am J Epidemiol* 1997; **146**: 32–41.

[84] Dunphy BC, Barratt CL, Cooke ID. Male alcohol consumption and fecundity in couples attending an infertility clinic. *Andrologia* 1991 **23**: 219–21.

[85] Goverde HJ, Dekker HS, Janssen HJ, *et al.* Semen quality and frequency of smoking and alcohol consumption: an explorative study. *Int J Fertil Menopausal Stud* 1995; **40**: 135–8.

[86] Olsen J, Bolumar F, Boldsen J, Bisanti L. Does moderate alcohol intake reduce fecundability? A European multicenter study on infertility and subfecundity. European Study Group on Infertility and Subfecundity. *Alcohol Clin Exp Res* 1997; **21**: 206–12.

[87] Chia SE, Lim ST, Tay SK, Lim ST. Factors associated with male infertility: A case–control study of 218 infertile and 240 fertile men. *BJOG* 2000; **107**: 55–61.

[88] Dikshit RK, Buch JG, Mansuri SM. Effect of tobacco consumption on semen quality of a population of hypofertile males. *Fertil Steril* 1987; **48**: 334–6.

[89] Evans HJ, Fletcher J, Torrance M, Hargreave TB. Sperm abnormalities and cigarette smoking. *Lancet* 1981; **1**: 627–9.

[90] Marshburn PB, Sloan CS, Hammond MG. Semen quality and association with coffee drinking, cigarette smoking, and ethanol consumption. *Fertil Steril* 1989; **52**: 162–5.

[91] Osser S, Beckman-Ramirez A, Liedholm P. Semen quality of smoking and non-smoking men in infertile couples in a Swedish population. *Acta Obstet Gynecol Scand* 1992; **71**: 215–18.

[92] Hull MG, North K, Taylor H, Farrow A, Ford WC. Delayed conception and active and passive smoking. The Avon Longitudinal Study of Pregnancy and Childhood Study Team. *Fertil Steril* 2000; **74**: 725–33.

[93] Zitzmann M, Rolf C, Nordhoff V, *et al.* Male smokers have a decreased success rate for in vitro fertilization and intracytoplasmic sperm injection. *Fertil Steril* 2003; **79** (Suppl 3): 1550–4.

[94] Jensen TK, Henriksen TB, Hjollund NH, *et al.* Adult and prenatal exposures to tobacco smoke as risk indicators of fertility among 430 Danish couples. *Am J Epidemiol* 1998; **148**: 992–7.

[95] Jensen TK, Henriksen TB, Hjollund NH, *et al.* Caffeine intake and fecundability: a follow-up study among 430 Danish couples planning their first pregnancy. *Reprod Toxicol* 1998; **12**: 289–95.

[96] Brown-Woodman PD, Post EJ, Gass GC, White IG. The effect of a single sauna exposure on spermatozoa. *Arch Androl* 1984; **12**: 9–15.

[97] Lue YH, Lasley BL, Laughlin LS, *et al.* Mild testicular hyperthermia induces profound transitional spermatogenic suppression through increased germ cell apoptosis in adult cynomolgus monkeys (Macaca fascicularis). *J Androl* 2002; **23**: 799–805.

[98] Saikhun J, Kitiyanant Y, Vanadurongwan V, Pavasuthipaisit K. Effects of sauna on sperm movement characteristics of normal men measured by computer-assisted sperm analysis. *Int J Androl* 1998; **21**: 358–63.

[99] Velez de la Calle JF, Rachou E, le Martelot MT, et al. Male infertility risk factors in a French military population. *Hum Reprod* 2001; **16**: 481–6.

[100] Wang C, McDonald V, Leung A, *et al.* Effect of increased scrotal temperature on sperm production in normal men. *Fertil Steril* 1997; **68**: 334–9.

[101] Lipshultz LI, Corriere JN. Progressive testicular atrophy in the varicocele patient. *J Urol* 1977; **117**: 175–6.

[102] Charny CW. The spermatogenic potential of the undescended testis before and after treatment. *J Urol* 1960; **83**: 697–705.

[103] Gunalp S, Onculoglu C, Gurgan T, Kruger TF, Lombard CJ. A study of semen parameters with emphasis on sperm morphology in a fertile population: an attempt to develop clinical thresholds. *Hum Reprod* 2001; **16**: 110–14.

[104] Lubs HJ. Testicular size in Klinefelter's syndrome in men over fifty. *N Engl J Med* 1962; **267**: 326.

[105] Guzick DS, Overstreet JW, Factor-Litvak P, *et al.* Sperm morphology, motility, and concentration in fertile and infertile men. *N Engl J Med* 2001; **345**: 1388–93.

[106] Smith KD, Rodriguez-Rigau LJ, Steinberger E. Relation between indices of semen analysis and pregnancy rate in infertile couples. *Fertil Steril* 1977; **28**: 1314–19.

[107] Bostofte E, Bagger P, Michael A, Stakemann G. Fertility prognosis for infertile men: results of follow-up study of semen analysis in infertile men from two different populations evaluated by the Cox regression model. *Fertil Steril* 1990; **54**: 1100–6.

[108] Mayaux MJ, Schwartz D, Czyglik F, David G. Conception rate according to semen characteristics in a series of 15 364 insemination cycles: results of a multivariate analysis. *Andrologia* 1985; **17**: 9–15.

[109] Battin D, Vargyas JM, Sato F, Brown J, Marrs RP. The correlation between in vitro fertilization of human oocytes and semen profile. *Fertil Steril* 1985; **44**: 835–8.

[110] Matson PL, Turner SR, Yovich JM, Tuvik AI, Yovich JL. Oligospermic infertility treated by in-vitro fertilization. *Aust N Z J Obstet Gynaecol* 1986; **26**: 84–7.

[111] Carlsen E, Petersen JH, Andersson AM, Skakkebaek NE. Effects of ejaculatory frequency and season on variations in semen quality. *Fertil Steril* 2004; **82**: 358–66.

[112] Santomauro AG, Sciarra JJ, Varma AO. A clinical investigation of the role of the semen analysis and postcoital test in the evaluation of male infertility. *Fertil Steril* 1972; **23**: 245–51.

[113] Munuce MJ, Bregni C, Carizza C, Menduluk G. Semen culture, leukocytospermia, and the presence of sperm antibodies in seminal hyperviscosity. *Arch Androl* 1999; **42**: 21–8.

[114] Mahmoud AM, Depoorter B, Piens N, Comhaire FH. The performance of 10 different methods for the estimation of sperm concentration. *Fertil Steril* 1997; **68**: 340–5.

[115] Imade GE, Towobola OA, Sagay AS, Otubu JA. Discrepancies in sperm count using improved Neubauer, Makler, and Horwells counting chambers. *Arch Androl* 1993; **31**: 17–22.

[116] Amelar RD, Dubin L, Schoenfeld C. Semen analysis: an office technique. *Urology* 1973; **2**: 605–11.

[117] World Health Organization. *WHO Laboratory Manual for the Examination of Human Semen and Sperm–Cervical Mucus Interaction*, 4th edn. Cambridge: Cambridge University Press, 1999.

[118] MacLeod J. Human seminal cytology as a sensitive indicator of the germinal epithelium. *Int J Fertil* 1964; **9**: 281–95.

[119] Fredricsson B, Bjork G. Morphology of postcoital spermatozoa in the cervical secretion and its clinical significance. *Fertil Steril* 1977; **28**: 841–5.

[120] Liu DY, Baker HW. Morphology of spermatozoa bound to the zona pellucida of human oocytes that failed to fertilize in vitro. *J Reprod Fertil* 1992; **94**: 71–84.

[121] Menkveld R, Stander FS, Kotze TJ, Kruger TF, van Zyl JA. The evaluation of morphological characteristics of human spermatozoa according to stricter criteria. *Hum Reprod* 1990; **5**: 586–92.

[122] Mortimer D, Leslie EE, Kelly RW, Templeton AA. Morphological selection of human spermatozoa in vivo and in vitro. *J Reprod Fertil* 1982; **64**: 391–9.

[123] Coetzee K, Kruge TF, Lombard CJ. Predictive value of normal sperm morphology: a structured literature review. *Hum Reprod Update* 1998; **4**: 73–82.

[124] Van Waart J, Kruger TF, Lombard CJ, Ombelet W. Predictive value of normal sperm morphology in intrauterine insemination (IUI): a structured

literature review. *Hum Reprod Update* 2001; **7**: 495–500.

[125] Spiessens C, Vanderschueren D, Meuleman C, D'Hooghe T. Isolated teratozoospermia and intrauterine insemination. *Fertil Steril* 2003; **80**: 1185–9.

[126] Shibahara H, Obara H, Ayustawati, *et al.* Prediction of pregnancy by intrauterine insemination using CASA estimates and strict criteria in patients with male factor infertility. *Int J Androl* 2004; **27**: 63–8.

[127] Roux A, Siebert TI, Van der Merwe JP, Kruger TF. Interstitial pregnancy managed medically. *J Obstet Gynaecol* 2004; **24**: 587–9.

[128] Yeung CH, Cooper TG, Nieschlag E. A technique for standardization and quality control of subjective sperm motility assessments in semen analysis. *Fertil Steril* 1997; **67**: 1156–8.

[129] Yanagimachi R. The movement of golden hamster spermatozoa before and after capacitation. *J Reprod Fertil* 1970; **23**: 193–6.

[130] Suarez SS, Ho HC. Hyperactivation of mammalian sperm. *Cell Mol Biol* 2003; **49**: 351–6.

[131] Keel BA, Quinn P, Schmidt CF, *et al.* Results of the American Association of Bioanalysts national proficiency testing programme in andrology. *Hum Reprod* 2000; **15**: 680–6.

[132] Amann RP, Katz DF. Reflections on CASA after 25 years. *J Androl* 2004; **25**: 317–25.

[133] Davis RO, Katz DF. Computer-aided sperm analysis: technology at a crossroads. *Fertil Steril* 1993; **59**: 953–5.

[134] Krause W. Computer-assisted semen analysis systems: comparison with routine evaluation and prognostic value in male fertility and assisted reproduction. *Hum Reprod* 1995; **10** (Suppl 1): 60–6.

[135] Corea M, Campagnone J, Sigman M. The diagnosis of azoospermia depends on the force of centrifugation. *Fertil Steril* 2005; **83**: 920–2.

[136] Oates RD, Amos JA. The genetic basis of congenital bilateral absence of the vas deferens and cystic fibrosis. *J Androl* 1994; **15**: 1–8.

[137] Schlegel PN, Shin D, Goldstein M. Urogenital anomalies in men with congenital absence of the vas deferens. *J Urol* 1996; **155**: 1644–8.

[138] Jarow JP. Transrectal ultrasonography in the diagnosis and management of ejaculatory duct obstruction. *J Androl* 1996; **17**: 467–72.

[139] Jarow JP, Espeland MA, Lipshultz LI. Evaluation of the azoospermic patient. *J Urol* 1989; **142**: 62–5.

[140] Sharlip ID, Jarow JP, Belker AM, *et al.* Best practice policies for male infertility. *Fertil Steril* 2002; **77**: 873–82.

[141] Meacham RB, Hellerstein DK, Lipshultz LI. Evaluation and treatment of ejaculatory duct obstruction in the infertile male. *Fertil Steril* 1993; **59**: 393–7.

[142] Belker AM, Steinbock GS. Transrectal prostate ultrasonography as a diagnostic and therapeutic aid for ejaculatory duct obstruction. *J Urol* 1990; **144**: 356–8.

[143] Singh G. Ultrastructural features of round-headed human spermatozoa. *Int J Fertil* 1992; **37**: 99–102.

[144] Kim FY, Goldstein M. Antibacterial skin preparation decreases the incidence of false-positive semen culture results. *J Urol* 1999; **161**: 819–21.

[145] Sigman M, Jarow JP. Endocrine evaluation of infertile men. *Urology* 1997; **50**: 659–64.

[146] Bain J, Langevin R, D'Costa M, Sanders RM, Hucker S. Serum pituitary and steroid hormone levels in the adult male: one value is as good as the mean of three. *Fertil Steril* 1988; **49**: 123–6.

[147] Tomlinson MJ, Barratt CL, Cooke ID. Prospective study of leukocytes and leukocyte subpopulations in semen suggests they are not a cause of male infertility. *Fertil Steril* 1993 **60**: 1069–75.

[148] Berger RE, Karp LE, Williamson RA, *et al.* The relationship of pyospermia and seminal fluid bacteriology to sperm function as reflected in the sperm penetration assay. *Fertil Steril* 1982; **37**: 557–64.

[149] Maruyama DK, Hale RW, Rogers BJ. Effects of white blood cells on the in vitro penetration of zona-free hamster eggs by human spermatozoa. *J Androl* 1985; **6**: 127–35.

[150] Rodin DM, Larone D, Goldstein M. Relationship between semen cultures, leukospermia, and semen analysis in men undergoing fertility evaluation. *Fertil Steril* 2003; **79** (Suppl 3): 1555–8.

[151] Sigman M, Lopes L. The correlation between round cells and white blood cells in the semen. *J Urol* 1993; **149**: 1338–40.

[152] Yanushpolsky EH, Politch JA, Hill JA, Anderson DJ. Antibiotic therapy and leukocytospermia: A prospective, randomized, controlled study. *Fertil Steril* 1995; **63**: 142–7.

[153] Matson PL, Junk SM, Spittle JW, Yovich JL. Effect of antispermatozoal antibodies in seminal plasma upon spermatozoal function. *Int J Androl* 1988; **11**: 101–6.

[154] Menge AC, Beitner O. Interrelationships among semen characteristics, antisperm antibodies, and cervical mucus penetration assays in infertile human couples. *Fertil Steril* 1989; **51**: 486–92.

[155] Kremer J, Jager S. The significance of antisperm antibodies for sperm–cervical mucus interaction. *Hum Reprod* 1992; **7**: 781–4.

[156] Agarwal A, Saleh RA, Bedaiwy MA. Role of reactive oxygen species in the pathophysiology of human reproduction. *Fertil Steril* 2003; **79**: 829–43.

Chapter

11

Evaluation of sperm function

Armand Zini and Mark Sigman

Introduction

The diagnosis of male infertility has traditionally been based, to some extent, on the results of the conventional semen analysis (e.g., oligospermia, azoospermia). This has resulted in great emphasis on the individual semen parameters (sperm concentration, motility, and morphology) in our discussion and understanding of male infertility. However, a number of **studies have demonstrated that the diagnostic value of the conventional semen analysis is modest at best** [1,2]. In fact, individual semen parameters exhibit significant variability and cannot be used to reliably predict male fertility potential. **Consequently, there has been an ever-growing need to develop new tests or markers of male fertility potential that may predict reproductive outcomes and further our understanding of the pathophysiology and diagnosis of male infertility** [3].

Over the past several decades, a number of in-vitro tests have been developed to assess various functional, biochemical, and molecular markers of sperm health. These tests include measurements of sperm movement, cervical mucus penetration, the acrosome reaction, zona pellucida binding, sperm–oocyte fusion, and sperm reactive oxygen species (ROS) production. Tests of sperm DNA damage and sperm chromosome anomalies have also been developed. Taken together, these advanced sperm tests yield information on the fertilizing capacity of human spermatozoa, as well as their ability to support normal embryonic development. These tests also can be used to assess male reproductive function in the context of toxicology studies. It is unlikely that there will ever be a single sperm fertility test that alone can diagnose male infertility. One must recognize that each of the advanced sperm fertility tests can only measure a very specific aspect of sperm function, and that no single test simultaneously measures every aspect of sperm

health. It is also important to note that in the human ejaculate there are different populations of spermatozoa (e.g., motile, nonmotile, nonviable), and that a test result may reflect the functional characteristics of a subpopulation of spermatozoa (e.g., motile) from the entire ejaculate. Finally, the specific nature of these sperm tests and the generally low frequency of test-specific abnormalities in infertile men makes large-scale screening of male partners not cost-effective. Therefore, the application of advanced sperm fertility tests should be carefully tailored to the individual.

The advent of intracytoplasmic sperm injection (ICSI, a technique that overcomes many sperm function defects) has, to some extent, undermined the clinical value of sperm fertility tests because the success of this technique is largely independent of sperm function. On the other hand, ICSI has raised concerns regarding the quality of the paternal genetic material that is introduced into the oocyte. Specifically, there is some concern that utilizing ICSI and bypassing natural selection barriers may increase the risk of iatrogenic transmission of DNA-damaged and/or aneuploid spermatozoa [4]. In this chapter, we will review the biological and clinical aspects of several advanced sperm fertility tests. We will evaluate the diagnostic and prognostic value of these functional tests and provide, wherever possible, a rational, evidence-based approach to the use of these tests in the assessment of the infertile man. It is important to note that for most of these tests the prognostic value of the test was only evaluated in the context of one, or rarely two, reproductive outcomes (e.g., fertilization rate at IVF [in-vitro fertilization], IUI [intrauterine insemination] pregnancy, IVF pregnancy). To date, no advanced sperm fertility test can predict all reproductive outcomes in the context of all forms of assisted reproductive technologies (ART).

Infertility in the Male, 4th edition, ed. Larry I. Lipshultz, Stuart S. Howards, and Craig S. Niederberger. Published by Cambridge University Press. © Cambridge University Press 2009.

Motility defects

Defects in sperm movement may be due to extrinsic factors, such as collection artifacts, prolonged abstinence, genital tract infections associated with pyospermia, partial ejaculatory duct obstruction, varicoceles, defective transport through the genital ductal system, antisperm antibodies, or, less commonly, to primary sperm abnormalities such as ultrastructural sperm defects or enzyme deficiency [5]. When motility is less than 5–10% or completely absent, the possibility of ultrastructural defects in spermatozoa should be considered. In these instances, some type of testing to determine whether the nonmotile sperm are viable or dead should also be performed.

Viability assays

Dye exclusion assays

Viability assays are based on the ability of live sperm to exclude certain dyes, while dead sperm will allow the dye to penetrate and thus stain the cell. Protocols utilizing either trypan blue or eosin Y may be utilized [6] (Fig. 11.1). The absence of staining in the majority of cells indicates high viability, whereas the presence of staining indicates dead sperm. The finding of a high percentage of viable sperm in the presence of extremely low motility strongly suggests the presence of an ultrastructural (cytoskeletal) sperm defect. Since the sperm are killed in the vital staining process, they cannot be used subsequently for ART.

Hypo-osmotic sperm swelling assay

The hypo-osmotic swelling test (HOS) is based on the ability of viable sperm to maintain an osmotic gradient across the cell membrane. If live sperm are placed in hypotonic media, water will enter the cell and cause the cell to increase in volume. In sperm, this becomes evident in the tail region, where swelling of the sperm tail may be easily seen using phase-contrast microscopy (Fig. 11.2). While some have proposed that this test be performed routinely along with the semen analysis in all patients, in the majority of instances the results do not change patient management. Currently the test is utilized as a diagnostic test with the same indications as a standard dye exclusion viability assay – for samples with less than 5–10% motility to determine if the non-motile sperm are alive or dead. The finding of a high percentage of sperm with tail swelling (live sperm) in the presence of extremely low motility strongly suggests the presence of an ultrastructural defect. In contrast, the finding of no tail swelling in the majority of sperm in combination with extremely low motility suggests that the nonmotile sperm are dead. Unlike dye exclusion viability assays, the HOS assay does not kill sperm. As a result **this assay has recently been utilized in a therapeutic manner in couples undergoing ICSI when only nonmotile sperm are present in the semen specimen. An HOS test may allow the technician to pick out viable nonmotile sperm**, which then may be utilized for ICSI [7]. As expected, there is a close correlation between the results of dye viability assays and hypo-osmotic sperm swelling testing [8].

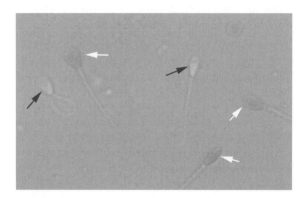

Fig. 11.1. Sperm viability stain with eosin Y. Live sperm do not take up the stain (dark arrows) while nonviable sperm stain orange-yellow (white arrows). *See color plate section.*

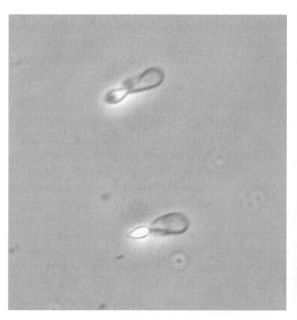

Fig. 11.2. Hypo-osmotic swelling test. Viable sperm demonstrate tail swelling, which appears as coiled tails. *See color plate section.*

Electron microscopy

Electron microscopy is indicated for those samples with less than 5–10% motility associated with high viability as measured by either a dye viability assay or hypo-osmotic sperm swelling testing. The most common abnormalities involve the structure of the sperm tail, with defects in either the axoneme or outer dense fibers. The axoneme normally contains microtubules in a 9 + 2 pattern with inner and outer dynein arms connecting the peripheral microtubules to the central doublet. The absence of both the inner and outer dynein arms is one of the most common defects identified in patients with immotile but viable sperm. Additional patterns seen in this patient population include an absence of either the inner or outer dynein arms, or abnormal positions of the microtubules or central doublet, as well as absence of the radial spokes [8–10]. Of note, identical defects are not necessarily identified in all spermatozoa of a given sample. Thus, some spermatozoa may maintain motility, indicating that the condition is heterogeneous [11,12]. The defects are commonly present in the cilia of the respiratory tract as well, and the condition is known as primary ciliary dyskinesia or immotile cilia syndrome [13]. Patients with these defects may have a history of chronic sinus infections and bronchiectasis. Fifty percent of these patients also have situs inversus, in which instance the condition is known as Kartagener syndrome. Although a variety of genetic mutations exist, only a minority of them have been identified [14]. These ciliary abnormalities generally have an autosomal recessive inheritance pattern. Sperm from patients with these patterns have been used in ICSI; although pregnancies have resulted, fertilization rates are generally quite low [15]. Okada *et al.* (1999) identified an association between the rare 9 + 0 microtubule configuration of men presenting with immotile sperm who were also found to have adult polycystic kidney disease – an important cause of end-stage renal disease, highlighting the importance of testing and counseling of couples with these rare sperm defects [16].

Defects in structures other than the axoneme have also been identified in patients with impaired motility. The fibrous sheath surrounds both the outer dense fibers and the axoneme [17]. Extremely poor or absent motility is associated with dysplasia of the fibrous sheath. Spermatozoa with this defect have short thick flagella that may have irregular shapes, leading to the term "stump tail syndrome" [18]. Complete and partial forms have been described, with 20–30% of sperm being motile in the partial variety. Disorganization and hypertrophy of the fibrous sheath are noted on electron microscopy. While defects in certain genes have been noted in some patients, the genetic abnormality in the majority of patients remains unknown [18]. Less common abnormalities in the outer dense fibers resulting in dyskinetic sperm movement has been reported [19]. *Globozoospermia* refers to the absence of the acrosome as well as the cytoskeletal protein calicin. These sperm appear as round-headed sperm under wet-mount microscopy. The classic form (type I) is characterized by a complete absence of the acrosome and the inability of sperm to fertilize human eggs. Sperm with a type II defect contain hypoplastic acrosomes and may retain some ability to fertilize ova [20]. Similar to primary ciliary dyskinesia, sperm from these patients have been utilized for ICSI, with low pregnancy rates [21]. Abnormalities of the connecting piece of the spermatozoa lead to the separation of the head from the tail, yielding headless motile flagella. These are often referred to as pinheaded sperm on a standard semen analysis report. However, electron microscopy reveals the absence of nuclear material on the tails. Defects in the junctional apparatus connecting the flagella to the sperm head have been identified. However, the genetics of this abnormality remain unknown [22]. **While ICSI is being utilized for cases of ultrastructural abnormalities, caution should be observed, since there are likely genetic bases for these conditions.**

Cervical mucus interaction

The postcoital test (PCT) assesses the ability of sperm to traverse the cervical mucus. The PCT is performed by examining the cervical mucus several hours after intercourse for the presence of sperm. This test should be scheduled just prior to ovulation in the periovulatory phase of the woman's menstrual cycle, at which point the cervical mucus becomes clear and thin. A drop of cervical mucus is examined under wet-mount microscopy for the presence of sperm [23]. While there remains some disagreement on how the test should be performed, as well as how it should be graded, a normal test result is usually defined as one in which there are more than 10–20 sperm per high-powered field (× 400), the majority of which demonstrate progressive motility. An abnormal PCT result suggests that a cervical factor or a semen deposition abnormality may be involved in the couple's infertility, but there are many other causes for an abnormal result. A frequent cause for an abnormal PCT is inappropriate timing because the test was performed on the wrong day of the cycle. In addition, a significantly abnormal semen analysis can be expected to be associated with an abnormal PCT result. Therefore, when the male has a significantly impaired semen analysis, the PCT seldom offers useful information and is not indicated. The presence of antisperm antibodies on the sperm or in the cervical mucus may result in an abnormal PCT [24]. The finding of sperm that appear to be immobilized with a shaking motion in the cervical mucus is particularly suspicious for the presence of antisperm antibodies. Additional causes of abnormal PCTs include inappropriately performed intercourse or anatomic abnormalities in either partner. While there remains some controversy as to the value of the PCT in the evaluation of the infertile couple, recent studies suggest it to be useful in approximately 50% of couples [25,26]. Because of the difficulties with variability of the PCT, in-vitro assays have been developed to try to standardize the evaluation of the interaction of the sperm and cervical mucus [27–30]. These in-vitro assays currently are not commonly used because the results generally do not change the management of the couple. However, the standard PCT should be utilized when the clinician thinks the results will affect choice of treatment [31]. **Conditions such as unexplained infertility, low-volume semen specimens with normal total sperm counts, and hyperviscous semen may benefit from the performance of postcoital testing. The finding of a persistently abnormal PCT in the presence of relatively good semen parameters suggests a defect in the quality of the cervical mucus.** The gynecologist usually performs this evaluation at the time of the PCT. The mucus is rated by its pattern of ferning and spinnbarkeit. The finding of good-quality cervical mucus indicates that timing of the PCT is likely appropriate. The finding of no sperm in cervical mucus of good quality suggests the possibility of abnormal coital technique as well as a sperm deposition abnormality, such as might be present with hypospadias.

Sperm acrosome reaction

The acrosome is a cap-like vesicle that surrounds the anterior two-thirds of the sperm head. During spermiogenesis, the Golgi apparatus progressively envelopes the spermatid nucleus. The acrosome, therefore, is originally derived from the Golgi apparatus and contains the proteolytic enzymes acrosin and hyaluronidase [26]. These acrosomal enzymes help spermatozoa penetrate the zona pellucida (ZP), the egg's glycoprotein shell [32].

The acrosome reaction (AR) is a naturally occurring exocytotic process that involves fusion of the sperm plasma membrane and outer acrosomal membrane, a process that results in the release of the acrosomal contents, e.g., proteolytic enzymes [33]. The egg's ZP is the natural stimulus for the AR, although a number of natural and artificial substances have been shown to induce the AR in vitro. Under normal circumstances, only those spermatozoa that have undergone capacitation (a maturational process that involves a series of membranous and biochemical modifications) can be acrosome-reacted [33]. One can assess the acrosomal status (acrosome-reacted or nonacrosome-reacted) of human spermatozoa using fluorescent lectins that bind to the outer acrosomal membrane (*Arachis hypogaea* agglutinin) or to the acrosomal contents (*Pisum sativum* agglutinin) [34–36]. In nonacrosome-reacted cells the probes generate a uniformly labeled acrosomal cap, and in acrosome-reacted cells only the equatorial segment of the sperm head is labeled. Simultaneous assessments of cell viability can help distinguish nonphysiological "acrosomal loss" from physiological AR [35].

Although the physiologic relevance of measuring AR in vitro is unknown, the meaningful application of the AR as a clinical test requires assessment of both baseline (spontaneous AR) and stimulated AR. As would be expected, the incidence of spontaneous AR in ejaculated human sperm populations is low, i.e., approximately 5% of ejaculated spermatozoa are acrosome-reacted [37]. The incidence of AR increases when spermatozoa are incubated with a capacitating agent to induce sperm capacitation and, subsequently, with an AR stimulant. Known AR stimulants include A23187 (a divalent cation ionophore that induces changes in intracellular calcium and pH), progesterone (P, a steroid), and the human ZP (the physiologic inducer) [38–42]. It is important to note that only a small subset (~10–25%) of spermatozoa can undergo capacitation and, subsequently, be made to acrosome-react. Moreover, it is unknown whether the subset of spermatozoa that undergo the AR in vitro ultimately have the capacity to fertilize the oocyte in vivo.

The clinical application of the AR test has revealed two types of defects associated with male infertility: AR prematurity and AR insufficiency. AR prematurity, defined as a high level of spontaneous AR (>20% of spermatozoa exhibiting spontaneous AR), has been associated with reduced capacity to fertilize at IVF [37,43]. AR insufficiency, defined as a poor responsiveness to AR stimulants (generally,

Table 11.1. Relationship between the stimulated acrosome reaction and fertilization at IVF

Study	n	r-value	TV	Sensitivity	Specificity	NPV	PPV	Stimulant[a]
Fenichel, 1991 [44]	41	–	21	92	53	77	80	A23187
Henkel, 1993 [45]	74	–	10	71	66	50	82	Cold
Pampiglione, 1993 [46]	54	–	31	50	99	85	100	A23187
Yovich, 1994 [47]	71	–	10	82	56	56	82	A23187
Calvo, 1994 [48]	232	0.37	10	55	71	75	49	FF
Parinaud, 1995 [49]	117	0.34	20	54	73	88	31	A23187
Krausz, 1996 [50]	60	0.49	7	85	77	93	59	Progesterone
Krausz, 1996 [50]	53	0.31	17	57	75	88	35	A23187
Sukcharoen, 1996 [51]	73	Negative	–	–	–	–	–	A23187
Carver-Ward, 1996 [52]	129	0.68	10	100	82	93	100	A23187
Esterhuizen, 2001 [53]	35	0.95	15	93	100	88	90	Human ZP
Liu & Baker, 2003 [42]	65	0.58	16	80	86	–	–	Human ZP
Bastiaan, 2003 [54]	30	–	8	100	63	92	100	Human ZP

[a] AR stimulant or ionophore.

n, number of treatment cycles; r, Spearman rank order or Pearson correlation between IAR and fertilization; TV, threshold value of AR; PPV, positive predictive value; NPV, negative predictive value; Human ZP, solubilized human zona pellucida; FF, follicular fluid.

<10% difference between spontaneous and induced AR), has also been associated with reduced sperm fertilizing capacity (Table 11.1).

Several independent researchers have assessed the clinical value of the stimulated AR (SAR) (Table 11.1). Several studies have shown that the SAR can help predict fertilization at conventional IVF, but the predictive value parameters (e.g., negative predictive value [NPV], positive predictive value [PPV]) vary from one study to another [42,44–54]. Overall, **the test appears to be valuable in counseling couples prior to a planned IVF: in those couples with a poor SAR score (generally, <10) ICSI rather than conventional IVF would be recommended.** The AR test may also be of value in predicting pregnancy at IUI and IVF, although there are few supporting studies in this respect [37,55]. Ultimately, each laboratory should evaluate the predictive value of the SAR with its own patient population before clinically applying the test. The SAR possesses some inherent weaknesses as a clinical test and there are some variations in test conditions that make it difficult to evaluate inter-laboratory differences in test results.

(1) The meaningful application of the test requires that it be applied to samples with normal or near-normal sperm parameters (normal motility/viability is a requisite to undergo capacitation and AR) and, as such, the test is limited to a small subset of infertile males. Indeed, Liu et al. have shown that there is a high frequency (~80% overall)

of defective sperm–ZP interaction and ZP-induced AR in oligospermic infertile men, suggesting that the test is of no clinical value in these men [56]. Overall, it has been estimated that ~10% of infertile men with normal semen parameters have a defective or low ZP-induced AR [53,57].

(2) There is no consensus amongst the laboratories as to the best stimulant or ionophore (e.g., A23187, solubilized ZP, intact ZP). This is particularly important, because there is no relationship between the intact ZP-induced AR (or sperm–ZP penetration) and A23187-induced AR [58]. The A23187-induced (as well as the P-induced) AR involves all spermatozoa in the medium. In contrast, the ZP-induced AR reflects only those spermatozoa that can bind to the ZP and, therefore, spermatozoa that possess good motility and morphology and an intact acrosome.

(3) There is no consensus amongst the laboratories as to the exact cutoff or threshold AR value that is most predictive of reproductive outcomes.

(4) The AR test requires the use of fresh semen samples, making it impossible to send samples to a distant reference laboratory for AR testing or assessment of inter-laboratory variability.

(5) A positive control sample (known fertile control with a normal response to an AR stimulant) is generally tested along with the patient sample in order to ensure that the AR test is not falsely negative.

Overall, the data suggest that the AR test can help predict fertilization at conventional IVF and, as such, may be valuable in counseling couples prior to planned IVF or ICSI. The test is particularly useful in men with normal (or near-normal) semen quality. The test may also be of value in predicting pregnancy at IUI and IVF. However, the AR possesses some weaknesses as a clinical test. The AR test requires the use of a fresh sample (with simultaneous assessment of a control sample), in-vitro induction of the AR with one of several stimulants (each with differing potency), and the establishment of a laboratory-specific threshold value, which varies from one center to another.

Sperm penetration assay

Cross-species fertilization of ova is prevented by the zona pellucida, a glycoprotein layer that surrounds the ovum [59]. **The sperm penetration assay (SPA) utilizes hamster ova, which have had the zona pellucida enzymatically removed, allowing penetration by human spermatozoa** [60]. In this assay, human sperm are processed and allowed to capacitate. The sperm are then incubated with zona-free hamster oocytes. For penetration to occur, sperm must undergo capacitation, the acrosome reaction, fusion with the oolemma, and incorporation into the ooplasm. Since the zona pellucida is removed, defects limited to binding of the sperm to the zona pellucida will not be detected by this assay. Scoring of the original assay involved determining the percentage of ova that had been fertilized. Normal samples are generally found to penetrate more than 10–30% of ova. Incubation of the sperm in more potent capacitating media allows for the majority of oocytes to be penetrated. In this modified assay, scoring is based on the number of sperm that have penetrated each ovum. Despite general agreement about the basis for the SPA, the protocols utilized for the assay have varied significantly from institution to institution. In addition, there have been several generations of revisions, which have made it difficult to compare studies [61–65]. Results of SPAs have generally correlated with semen parameters [66]. In addition, studies have reported correlations between the results of SPA and pregnancy by intercourse as well as by IVF [67–72]. However, not all studies have reported good correlations [73,74]. In general, if the test is normal, the patient's sperm will usually be able to fertilize human ova in vitro. Indeed, patients' sperm which have failed the SPA have, in some cases, been able to fertilize human ova in vitro. However, with optimized assays, semen samples that fertilize

no hamster eggs usually are unable to fertilize human ova. Because of the variable correlations between SPA results and clinical outcomes in different laboratories, the clinician utilizing this test should be familiar with the laboratory performing the test and what correlations have been documented between the results of the assay and specific clinical outcomes. The SPA should not be used as a routine test for all couples undergoing fertility evaluations. The assay may be considered in those patients who are candidates for regular IVF or IUI but have low morphology scores. Couples who fail the SPA may be better served by ICSI than by IUI or IVF. Some clinicians also recommend the test in couples with unexplained infertility to help direct couples towards IUI or ICSI. Those couples with semen samples with very poor parameters usually will be candidates only for ICSI, and therefore will not benefit from this assay. The SPA is occasionally indicated in those couples with semen samples with good parameters that have poor fertilization results in IVF. This may help determine the presence of an unexplained fertilization defect. However, most of these couples are directed toward ICSI in subsequent cycles, and therefore will not benefit from this assay.

Hemizona assay

The hemizona assay uses zona pellucida from nonfertilizable, nonliving oocytes. The zona pellucida is microscopically divided in half. Each half is then incubated with either fertile donor sperm or patient's sperm. The number of sperm bound to each zona half is determined and a ratio, called the hemizona index, is calculated by dividing the number of bound sperm from the patient by the number of bound sperm from the fertile donor [75]. **The limited availability of human oocytes has significantly limited the practical application of this test.**

Patients whose sperm have demonstrated low hemizona indices have been reported to perform poorly in IVF and IUI [75]. Most studies have considered samples abnormal if the hemizona index is less than 30–40% [2,76]. Because micromanipulation techniques are required to perform this assay, it is not frequently used. A variation allowing use of zona without micromanipulation through the use of sperm labeled with different colored fluorochromes has been described but has not gained widespread use [77]. In addition, zonae pellucidae derived from cadavers and failed IVF cycles have also been utilized [78,79]. This assay is most useful when no fertilization has occurred in IVF in the presence of a normal SPA. Since the SPA is performed without the zona pellucida, sperm that have a defect limited to zona pellucida binding have the capacity to fuse with the oolemma and therefore will not demonstrate this particular zona pellucida binding defect. Nevertheless, in the majority of cases, couples with abnormal fertilization will have broad defects not limited to abnormal zona binding that will be picked up by other sperm function assays [80]. With the availability of ICSI, most cases of failed IVF will proceed to ICSI, and therefore will not require a hemizona assay.

Semen ROS

Reactive oxygen species (ROS) are ubiquitous in aerobic biologic systems and are formed as a by-product of oxygen metabolism. ROS (also referred to as free radicals) include the superoxide anion (O_2^-), hydrogen peroxide (H_2O_2), and the highly potent oxidant, the hydroxyl radical (OH) [81]. Superoxide anion is generated as a by-product of aerobic metabolism [81]. The superoxide anion can then either spontaneously dismutate or be converted by the enzyme superoxide dismutase (SOD) to H_2O_2. The enzymes catalase or glutathione peroxidase then convert H_2O_2 to water and oxygen, eradicating the ROS. Alternatively, both superoxide anion and hydrogen peroxide can be neutralized by nonenzymatic antioxidants such as albumin, glutathione, and hypotaurine, as well as vitamins C and E [82–84].

The high ROS levels observed in some pathologic conditions, e.g., semen of some infertile men, imply an imbalance between ROS production and ROS degradation or scavenging by antioxidants in seminal plasma. These high ROS levels produce a state known as oxidative stress that can lead to biochemical or physiologic abnormalities with subsequent cellular dysfunction or cell death [85]. In contrast to the pathologic effects of excess ROS production, small amounts of ROS may be necessary for the initiation of critical sperm functions, including capacitation and the acrosome reaction [86,87]. These findings stress the importance of a balance between ROS scavenging and low physiologic levels of ROS, necessary for normal sperm function.

The detrimental effects of ROS on spermatozoa were suggested more than 60 years ago with the demonstration that exposing sperm to oxygen results in sperm toxicity [88]. Later studies confirmed that human spermatozoa and semen leukocytes have the capacity to generate ROS, and that significant levels of

ROS can be detected in the semen of 25% of infertile men [89,90]. Fertile men do not have detectable levels of semen ROS [90,91]. It has been demonstrated that activated leukocytes have a greater capacity to generate high levels of semen ROS and, consequently, increased sperm dysfunction than do spermatozoa [85,92]. The production of oxidants by semen leukocytes can be significant and can overcome the antioxidant defense afforded by seminal plasma. Human seminal plasma is a rich source of enzymatic (superoxide dismutase, catalase) and nonenzymatic (vitamins, etc.) antioxidants, and these are believed to protect spermatozoa from oxidative injury [85]. Spermatozoa also have the capacity to generate high levels of semen oxidants. In the absence of leukocyte contamination, the excessive elaboration of ROS by spermatozoa is correlated with the abnormal retention of residual sperm cytoplasm [93].

The susceptibility of human spermatozoa to oxidative stress stems from the limited capacity of these cells to protect themselves from oxidative injury and the abundance of unsaturated fatty acids in the sperm plasma membrane [89,94]. The unsaturated fatty acids provide the fluidity that is necessary for sperm motility and membrane fusion events such as the acrosome reaction and sperm–egg interaction, both required for natural fertilization. However, the unsaturated, double-bonded nature of these molecules predisposes them to lipid peroxidation. Once lipid peroxidation has been initiated, accumulation of lipid peroxides occurs on the sperm surface, with ensuing sperm dysfunction and sperm death [89,94]. Oxidative damage to DNA represents an additional mechanism for the adverse action of ROS on spermatozoa [95,96]. Semen ROS are generally measured by detection of chemiluminescence. Briefly, this is done by incubating fresh semen or sperm suspensions with a redox-sensitive, light-emitting probe, e.g., luminol, and by measuring the light emission over time with a light meter (luminometer). Sperm-specific (e.g., PMA) or leukocyte-specific (e.g., FMLP) stimulants can enhance the chemiluminescent signal [97]. Sperm ROS can also be measured by using cellular probes coupled with flow cytometry [98].

Several independent researchers have assessed the clinical value of semen ROS determination. Studies have shown that infertile men typically have higher semen ROS levels than fertile men, and that the presence of leukocytospermia (in both fertile and infertile men) is associated with high semen ROS levels [90,91]. Determination of semen ROS levels may

Table 11.2. Relationship between ROS levels in washed sperm samples and fertilization at IVF

Study	n	r-value	TV	Method	Enhancer	Stimulant
Krausz, 1994 [97]	27	NS	none	Chemiluminescence	Luminol	FMLP + PMA
Yeung, 1996 [100]	75	NS	none	Chemiluminescence	Luminol	–
Sukcharoen, 1996 [51]	73	–0.22	none	Chemiluminescence	Luminol	–
Sukcharoen, 1996 [51]	73	–0.30	none	Chemiluminescence	Luminol	FMLP
Sukcharoen, 1996 [51]	73	–0.28	none	Chemiluminescence	Luminol	PMA
Moilanen, 1998 [101]	86	NS	none	Chemiluminescence	Luminol	FMLP + PMA
Marchetti et al., 2002 [98]	45	NS	none	Flow cytometry	–	–
Zorn, 2003 [102]	41	Inverse	none	Chemiluminescence	Luminol	–
Saleh, 2003 [103]	10	–0.59	none	Chemiluminescence	Luminol	–
Hammadeh, 2006 [104]	26	–0.26	none	Colorimetric assay	–	–

PMA, 12-myristate, 13-acetate phorbol ester; FMLP, N-formyl-methionyl-leucyl-phenylalanine; n, number of treatment cycles; r, Spearman rank order or Pearson correlation between ROS levels and fertilization; TV, threshold value of ROS levels; NS, not significant ($P > 0.05$).

allow clinicians to establish a more specific diagnosis of male infertility with the potential to design more specific therapies for these men [99]. Aitken et al. observed an inverse relationship between semen ROS levels and spontaneous pregnancy outcome in a cohort of 139 untreated infertile couples [61]. However, no other studies have supported these findings.

Several studies have evaluated the relationship between semen ROS and fertilization during IVF [51,97,98,100–104]. Some of these studies have reported a significant inverse relationship between sperm ROS levels and fertilization rate at conventional IVF. However, an equal number of studies have failed to demonstrate a significant relationship between ROS levels and fertilization rates (Table 11.2). Therefore, the clinical value of semen ROS determination in predicting IVF outcome remains unproven. Semen ROS determination possesses some inherent weaknesses as a clinical test. First, there is no established cutoff or threshold semen ROS level or value that can be used to predict reproductive outcomes. Second, semen ROS determination requires the use of fresh semen samples, making it impossible to send samples to a distant reference laboratory for ROS determination or assessment of inter-laboratory variability. Finally, the protocol for ROS determination varies from laboratory to laboratory. Determination of semen ROS levels may allow clinicians to establish a more specific diagnosis of male infertility, and may be useful in predicting spontaneous pregnancy outcome, although there is only one study supporting this speculation. The value of semen ROS determination in the context of IVF is inconclusive, since only half of the reported studies support its application.

Sperm DNA damage

Mammalian fertilization involves the direct interaction of the sperm and oocyte, fusion of the cell membranes, and union of male and female gamete genomes [105]. The completion of this process, and subsequent embryo development, depends in part on the inherent integrity of the sperm DNA [106]. Indeed, there appears to be a threshold of sperm DNA damage (i.e., DNA fragmentation, abnormal chromatin packaging, protamine deficiency) beyond which embryo development and pregnancy are impaired [106,107]. There is evidence to show that the spermatozoa of infertile men possess substantially more DNA damage than spermatozoa of fertile men, and that sperm DNA damage may adversely affect reproductive outcomes [108–111]. The study of sperm DNA damage is particularly relevant in an era when advanced forms of assisted reproductive technologies (ART) are frequently utilized, and when barriers to natural selection are bypassed. However, our understanding of the etiology (or etiologies) of sperm DNA damage and the full impact of this sperm defect on reproductive outcomes in humans remains rudimentary.

This section will briefly review our current understanding of (1) the organization of sperm DNA, (2) the potential etiologies of sperm DNA damage, (3) the impact of sperm DNA damage on reproductive capacity, and (4) the clinical utility of tests of sperm DNA damage.

Human sperm DNA and chromatin structure

Sperm chromatin is tightly compacted by virtue of associations between the DNA, the nuclear matrix, and sperm nuclear proteins. During the later stages of spermatogenesis, spermatid nuclear remodeling and condensation is associated with the displacement of histones by transition proteins and then by protamines [112]. In humans, up to 15% of the nuclear DNA remains packaged by histones in sequence-specific areas [113]. Disulfide cross-links between the cysteine-rich protamines are responsible for further compaction and stabilization, and it is thought that this nuclear compaction is important in protecting the sperm genome from external stresses such as oxidation or temperature elevation in the female reproductive tract [114]. Although the bulk of the sperm DNA is nuclear, a small fraction is mitochondrial in origin. Sperm mitochondrial DNA is small (16.5 kb) circular DNA that is not bound to any proteins [115].

Etiology of sperm DNA damage

The etiology of sperm DNA damage, much like male infertility itself, is multifactorial and may be due to primary testicular or external factors. Sperm DNA damage is clearly associated with male infertility, but a small percentage of spermatozoa from fertile men also possess detectable levels of DNA damage [108–111].

Primary testicular factors

Sperm DNA damage may be the result of abnormal germ cell apoptosis. Sakkas *et al.* have proposed that some of the spermatozoa with DNA damage have initiated and then subsequently escaped apoptosis, i.e., "abortive apoptosis" [116]. Advanced paternal age and exposure to gonadotoxins have been associated with reduced levels of germ cell apoptosis and an increase in the percentage of ejaculated spermatozoa with DNA damage [117,118].

Sperm protamine deficiency has been implicated in the etiology of sperm DNA damage. Protamine deficiency (partial or complete) is frequently seen in sperm samples from infertile men but not in those of fertile men [119,120]. Studies in mice with a targeted disruption of the protamine gene [107,121] and in humans with a single nucleotide polymorphism (SNP) in the protamine gene (*PRM1*) [122] suggest a link between protamine deficiency and sperm DNA damage. This association suggests that the DNA damage is due, in part, to a defect in spermiogenesis, the period during which sperm protamines are deposited.

High levels of ROS are detected in the semen of 25% of infertile men, and have been associated with sperm DNA damage [123,124]. The DNA damage may be due to sperm- or leukocyte-derived ROS, suggesting, respectively, that DNA damage may be due to a primary testicular (i.e., spermiogenesis) or a post-testicular (e.g., genital tract inflammation) defect [125,126].

Extratesticular (external) factors

A number of extrinsic factors have also been associated with sperm DNA damage. External factors include exposure to chemotherapy, radiation, and cigarette smoke [127,128]. Genital tract inflammation, testicular hyperthermia, and varicocele are specific conditions that have also been associated with sperm DNA damage [125,126,129].

Influence of sperm DNA damage on reproductive outcomes

Sperm DNA integrity and reproductive outcomes after in-vivo fertilization

Couples in whom the man has a high percentage of spermatozoa with DNA damage (DNA fragmentation or DNA oxidation) have a reduced potential for natural fertility [108,109,130]. However, pregnancy rates by intercourse were 40% even in those couples with abnormal sperm DNA integrity testing [108]. Moreover, there is a non-statistically significant trend toward poorer sperm DNA integrity in those couples whose pregnancy resulted in miscarriage than in those who were fertile [108,109]. Investigators have also shown that sperm DNA damage is associated with poor pregnancy outcome after intrauterine insemination (IUI) [131,132]. Taken together, the data suggest that sperm DNA damage may be a predictor of lower pregnancy rates via intercourse or IUI. These studies have generally had relatively small numbers of patients with sperm DNA damage, and conclusions therefore need to be confirmed by larger studies [131,132].

Sperm DNA integrity and reproductive outcomes after in-vitro fertilization

Numerous studies have examined the possible influence of sperm DNA integrity on reproductive outcomes after both standard IVF and IVF/ICSI (Tables 11.3, 11.4). Overall, the data suggest that there is no significant relationship between sperm DNA damage and fertilization rate at IVF or IVF/ICSI [131–148].

Table 11.3. Relationships between sperm DNA damage and fertilization rate (FR), embryo quality (EQ), pregnancy rate (PR), and spontaneous abortions (SA) with IVF

Study	No. of cycles	TV	FR	EQ	PR	SA	Assay used
Sun, 1997 [134]	143	4	Inv	Inv	–	–	TUNEL
Host, 2000 [136]	50	4	Inv	–	–	–	TUNEL
Tomlinson, 2001 [137]	140	–	NS	NS	Inv	–	ISNT
Morris, 2002 [135]	20	–	NS	NS	–	–	Comet
Tomsu, 2002 [138]	40	–	NS	Inv	NS	–	Comet
Henkel, 2004 [142]	249	37	NS	–	Inv	–	TUNEL
Gandini, 2004 [143]	12	–	NS	NS	NS	–	SCSA
Huang, 2005 [144]	217	10	Inv	NS	NS	–	TUNEL
Payne, 2005 [145]	46	–	Inv	–	NS	–	SCSA
Borini, 2006 [147]	82	10	Inv	–	Inv	Pos	TUNEL
Benchaib, 2007 [148]	88	15	NS	NS	NS	Pos	TUNEL
Bungum, 2007 [132]	388	30	NS	–	NS	NS	SCSA

Comet, single cell gel electrophoresis assay; TUNEL, terminal deoxynucleotidyl transferase-mediated dUTP nick end-labeling assay; ISNT, in situ nick-translation assay; SCSA, sperm chromatin structure assay; FR, fertilization rate; EQ, embryo quality and/or development; PR, pregnancy rate; SA, spontaneous abortions; TV, threshold value of sperm DNA damage. Inv, sperm DNA damage inversely related to outcome; NS, sperm DNA damage not related to outcome; Pos, sperm DNA damage positively related to outcome; –, outcome not evaluated.

Table 11.4. Relationships between sperm DNA damage and fertilization rate (FR), embryo quality (EQ), pregnancy rate (PR), and spontaneous abortions (SA) with IVF/ICSI

Study	No. of cycles	TV	FR	EQ	PR	SA	Assay used
Lopes, 1998 [133]	150	25	Inv	NS	–	–	TUNEL
Host, 2000 [136]	61	30	NS	–	–	–	TUNEL
Morris, 2002 [135]	40	–	NS	Inv	–	–	Comet
Gandini, 2004 [143]	22	–	NS	NS	NS	–	SCSA
Huang, 2005 [144]	86	10	Inv	NS	NS	–	TUNEL
Payne, 2005 [145]	54	–	Inv	–	NS	–	SCSA
Zini, 2005 [146]	60	30	NS	Inv	NS	NS	SCSA
Borini, 2006 [147]	50	10	NS	–	Inv	Pos	TUNEL
Benchaib, 2007 [148]	234	15	Inv	Inv	NS	Pos	TUNEL
Bungum, 2007 [132]	233	30	NS	–	NS	NS	SCSA

Comet, single cell gel electrophoresis assay; TUNEL, terminal deoxynucleotidyl transferase-mediated dUTP nick end-labeling assay; SCSA, sperm chromatin structure assay; FR, fertilization rate; EQ, embryo quality and/or development; PR, pregnancy rate; SA, spontaneous abortions; TV, threshold value of sperm DNA damage. Inv, sperm DNA damage inversely related to outcome; NS, sperm DNA damage not related to outcome; Pos, sperm DNA damage positively related to outcome; –, outcome not evaluated.

Indeed, the paternal genome is not expressed until after the second cleavage division (i.e., in the four-cell embryo) so it is unlikely that sperm DNA damage would impact fertilization [149]. Similarly, the bulk of the data indicate that there is no significant relationship between sperm DNA damage and either embryo development or pregnancy outcome at IVF or IVF/ICSI. Bungum *et al.* (2007) [132] have reported that in couples with high levels of DNA damage, the ICSI pregnancy rate is higher than with IVF [132]. However, the couples that underwent IVF were not the same ones that underwent ICSI, making it difficult to draw definitive conclusions.

Adding to their observations on the relationship between sperm DNA damage and IUI pregnancy outcome, Bungum *et al.* (2007) [132] have suggested that ICSI is the treatment of choice in the setting of high levels of DNA damage (>30% DNA fragmentation by sperm chromatin structure assay [SCSA]).

These clinical observations are not consistent with animal studies, which show that DNA damage does not influence fertilization rate but is associated with both poor pregnancy outcome and poor embryo development [106]. The stringent process of sperm and embryo selection during ICSI in humans may mitigate the potential adverse effect(s) of sperm DNA damage on reproductive outcomes [143,146].

To date, the short- and long-term ramifications of successful fertilization and embryo development with DNA-damaged spermatozoa are unknown. Clearly, the understanding that sperm DNA damage is common in infertile men, together with the preliminary reports on genetic and epigenetic abnormalities in the offspring associated with ICSI, urge us to explore the subject of sperm DNA damage [150–153]. DNA that possesses measurable damage (specifically, DNA oxidation) may cause misreading errors to occur during DNA replication, and this may result in the generation of de novo mutations [154]. Although the concept has not been tested in the context of mammalian reproduction, we cannot dismiss the possibility that successful fertilization with DNA-damaged sperm may cause de novo mutations in the offspring despite the ability of the oocyte and embryo to repair sperm DNA damage [106,154].

Clinical value of tests of sperm DNA damage

Although there are insufficient data to recommend the indiscriminate application of sperm DNA testing, there are specific conditions that would benefit from further studies:

(1) Couples planning to undergo IVF or ICSI. Tests of sperm DNA damage should be performed routinely (ideally in the context of a large-scale clinical study) in order to evaluate the impact of sperm DNA damage on reproductive outcomes (fertilization, embryo development, pregnancy, miscarriage, postnatal development).

(2) Unexplained infertility. Based on evidence that tests of sperm DNA damage (specifically SCSA) may be predictors of failed natural pregnancy outcome in these couples [108,109], couples with high levels of sperm DNA damage should be studied to determine if they would be better off pursuing IVF or preferably ICSI.

(3) Couples planning to undergo ART. Based on evidence that high levels of DNA damage are associated with poor IUI pregnancy outcome, couples with high levels of sperm DNA damage should be studied to determine if they would be better off pursuing IVF or ICSI.

(4) Couples with recurrent pregnancy loss. Based on evidence that high levels of DNA damage are associated with recurrent pregnancy loss, couples with high levels of sperm DNA damage should be studied to determine if they would be better off pursuing IVF or ICSI.

The assessment of sperm DNA damage possesses some limitations as a clinical test. (1) Several tests of sperm DNA damage have been developed (e.g., DNA fragmentation, DNA denaturation, and DNA oxidation using slide- and flow-cytometry-based assays), and there is no consensus as to the most accurate test of DNA damage. (2) For each of the available tests of DNA damage, there is no consensus as to the best threshold value to predict reproductive outcomes. Moreover, there is wide variability in the threshold values from one assay to another. Therefore, each laboratory must carefully standardize the sperm DNA assay and evaluate the predictive value of the test with its own patient population before applying the test clinically. On the other hand, an advantage of these assays is that, unlike many other sperm function tests, assessment of sperm DNA damage can be performed on frozen–thawed samples with no measurable influence on test results [108,155].

Summary

Successful mammalian reproduction depends partly on the inherent integrity of the sperm DNA. Indeed, there appears to be a threshold of sperm DNA damage beyond which embryo development and subsequent pregnancy outcome are impaired. There is now clinical evidence to show that the spermatozoa of infertile men possess substantially more DNA damage than those of fertile men, and that sperm DNA damage may adversely impact reproductive outcomes. Additional studies are needed to fully define the clinical value of sperm DNA damage testing.

Sperm fluorescence in-situ hybridization (FISH) analysis for chromosomal aberrations / aneuploidy

For over a decade, FISH (fluorescence in-situ hybridization) has been used to evaluate the chromosome constitution of human spermatozoa. Studies have shown that, based on conservative estimates, the percentage of chromosomally abnormal sperm in the general population may be as high as 5–10%. In infertile male carriers of structural chromosome anomalies (e.g., Robertsonian translocations) or sex-chromosome numerical anomalies (e.g., 47,XXY) and in men with severe oligosperma, significantly higher levels of chromosomally abnormal sperm have been identified (up to 70% of spermatozoa) [156]. The clinical importance of these findings was not appreciated until the late 1990s, when studies reported an increased frequency of sex-chromosome anomalies in ICSI babies (compared to natural births) [4]. However, because of limited clinical outcome data, it remains unknown to what extent the high levels of chromosomally abnormal sperm (as is frequently seen in ICSI candidates) alone contribute to the sex-chromosome anomalies in ICSI babies. This subsection will review the risk of sperm chromosomal anomalies in different populations of men and the clinical utility of sperm FISH analysis.

Introduction

FISH is an indirect technique that has proven to be a good method to determine the chromosome content of spermatozoa. Briefly, sperm nuclei are decondensed and incubated with fluorescent, chromosome-specific probes (usually, X, Y, and one or more autosome-specific probes that hybridize to complementary DNA sequences on the target chromosomes). In order to screen for sex-chromosome abnormalities in sperm, it is necessary to look at a minimum of one autosome to distinguish disomic from diploid sperm (i.e., a sperm with two sex chromosomes and one autosome FISH signal is assumed to be disomic, whereas a sperm with two sex chromosomes and two autosome FISH signals is assumed to be diploid: Fig. 11.3) [157]. The spermatozoa are imaged microscopically, and the percentage of spermatozoa with abnormal chromosome content is recorded. The technique (FISH) is costly and labor-intensive. **The procedure requires a high-quality epifluorescence microscope, high-quality fluorescent probes, and trained personnel. The cost of an individual test is also high, due to the labor-intensive**

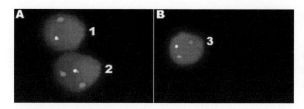

Fig. 11.3. Images of three human sperm nuclei hybridized with chromosome-specific probes (chromosome X labeled in yellow, Y in green, and 21 in red). Sperm #1 is a normal X-bearing sperm (with a single chromosome X and a single chromosome 21 signal), sperm #2 is an autosomal disomic sperm (i.e., X,21,21) and sperm #3 is a sex chromosome disomic sperm (X,Y,21). *See color plate section.*

nature of the technique (the examination of 5000–10 000 spermatozoa per sample is recommended). This latter problem may eventually be circumvented by use of automated approaches (e.g., flow cytometry) for sperm aneuploidy screens. To date, the prevalence of numerical chromosomal abnormalities in spermatozoa from a wide range of individuals and populations (fertile controls, carriers of chromosome anomalies, infertile men) has been reported. However, it is important to recognize that the majority of these studies are small, with only a handful of patients evaluated in each study.

Sperm chromosome abnormalities in fertile men

Studies in healthy donors have been used to determine the mean frequency of numerical chromosome abnormalities in sperm. A wide variability in disomy frequency for the same chromosomes has been reported by different research groups [158–160]. These results may be due to inter-individual differences or technical factors (e.g., differences in sperm decondensing protocols, scoring criteria, number of sperm analyzed, and the characteristics of the probes used). This underlines the importance of internal controls and proper methodology. An inter-chromosomal variation in the frequency of disomies has been reported, with the sex chromosomes and chromosomes 21 and 22 presenting higher rates of abnormalities than other chromosomes [159,161,162]. Although the cause of this is not known, it is suggested that the generally lower rate of meiotic recombination of these chromosomes renders them more prone to nondisjunction [163]. **Given a mean per chromosome disomy frequency of 0.13% for the autosomes and 0.37% for the sex chromosomes, and a 0.2% diploidy frequency, the overall frequency**

Table 11.5. Rate of sperm chromosome aneuploidy in infertile men with a normal karyotype

	Disomy		Diploidy	Total aneuploidy
	Autosome[a]	Sex chromosome[b]		
Fertile men	0.13% [159]	0.37% [159]	0.2% [159]	6–7% [159]
Infertile men				
Normospermic	0.11% [159]	0.44% [165]	0.3–1.0% [165]	–
Oligospermic	0.2–0.5% [159]	0.6–0.8% [161, 165]	0.3–1.0% [161, 165]	10–70% [156, 164]

[a] Per-chromosome disomy rates.
[b] Cumulative (XY + XX + YY) disomy rates.

Table 11.6. Rate of sperm chromosome aneuploidy in men with an abnormal karyotype (47,XXY, 47,XYY, Robertsonian translocation, reciprocal translocation)

	Disomy		Diploidy	Unbalanced
	Autosome[a]	Sex chromosome[b]		
Fertile men	0.1% [159]	0.37% [159]	0.2% [159]	–
47,XXY	0.2–0.7% [165]	2–20% [165, 171, 172, 189]	0.4% [172]	–
47,XYY	0.1–1.0% [173, 176]	0.6–5.2% [173]	0.8–1.5% [173]	–
Robertsonian translocation	0.1–0.8% [187]	0.2–1.3% [183, 187]	0.2–1.4% [183, 187]	5–20% [183–185]
Reciprocal translocation	0.1–2.0% [187]	0.2–0.6% [187]	0.2–5% [183, 187]	10–70% [176, 188, 190]

[a] Per-chromosome disomy rates.
[b] Cumulative (XY + XX + YY) disomy rates.

of chromosomally abnormal sperm in the general population is estimated to be ~7% (Table 11.5) [156,158–161,164,165]. The observed frequency of disomy in sperm nuclei (6–7%) is substantially higher than the estimated incidence of trisomic newborns of paternal origin. Approximately 0.3% of all newborns are trisomic and less than one-third of these are of paternal origin, with most paternal abnormalities being sex-chromosome aneuploidies [159,163]. Thus the relationship between the frequency of aneuploid spermatozoa and the paternal contribution to aneuploidy is not a simple one [163]. It is likely that natural selection barriers (aneuploid sperm exhibit a reduced capacity to bind to the oocyte [166]) and spontaneous abortions of aneuploid fetuses are both involved in reducing the incidence of paternally derived trisomic newborns [167]. Differences in sperm aneuploidy frequency among populations may be due to intrinsic and extrinsic factors. Cigarette smoke, alcohol, and chemotherapy can all cause increased sperm aneuploidy [160,168,169]. Age has also been associated with increased aneuploidy in both males and females [157,170].

Sperm chromosome abnormalities in carriers of sex chromosome numerical anomalies

Several FISH studies in sperm nuclei and germ cells from 47,XXY and 47,XYY males (both mosaic and nonmosaic) have been reported [159,171–173]. **Analysis of the spermatozoa shows a highly variable frequency of sex-chromosome disomies (range 1–20%) and of diploid sperm (range 0–1.5%)** (Table 11.6). In Klinefelter males (47,XXY), FISH analysis of the meiotic germ cells reveals that all pachytene cells are XY, although variable percentages of XXY cells are found in postmeiotic stages. These results suggest that in Klinefelter males the aneuploid cell line(s) is/are fully arrested before entering meiosis [174]. It is postulated that the high rates of sex-chromosome disomies found in the spermatozoa of some of these patients probably result from segregation errors in normal (XY) germ cells placed in a compromised testicular environment, as proposed by Mroz *et al.* [175]. **Foresta *et al.* have also reported a 2-to-1 ratio of X-bearing (23,X) to Y-bearing (23,Y)** spermatozoa in **47,XXY males** [171]. FISH analysis of testicular germ cells from 47,XYY males indicates that ~60% of pachytenes are XYY. However, the lower-than-expected sperm disomy rate in spermatozoa (0.1–1%) suggests a pachytene and/or postmeiotic arrest in this line [173,176].

Sperm chromosome abnormalities in structural reorganization carriers

The meiotic segregation of structural reorganizations depends mainly on the characteristics of the chromosome fragments involved, thus resulting in a variable percentage of chromosomally unbalanced sperm [177–182]. Sperm FISH studies (using the correct combination of probes) provide a valuable technique for assessing the percentage of abnormal sperm in translocation carriers. **In men with a Robertsonian translocation, the frequency of sperm with unbalanced chromosomes is estimated to be in the range of 5–20%** [160,183–186] (Table 11.6). These men also have a higher risk of aneuploid sperm than fertile controls (suggesting an interchromosomal effect – i.e., the reciprocal translocation impairs the meiotic segregation of noninvolved chromosomes) [186,187]. **In men with a reciprocal translocation, the frequency of sperm with unbalanced chromosomes is higher than that observed in men with a Robertsonian translocation and is estimated to be in the range of 10–70%** [160,188] (Table 11.6) [189,190]. Carriers of a reciprocal translocation also have a higher risk of aneuploid sperm than fertile controls (again suggesting an interchromosomal effect) [187]. It has been shown that the frequency of chromosomally unbalanced embryos (assessed by preimplantation genetic diagnosis with aneuploidy screen or PGD-AS) is related to the frequency of chromosomally unbalanced spermatozoa in reciprocal translocation carriers [188,191]. Depending on the nature of the reciprocal translocation, many of these abnormal embryos will likely fail to develop, and those that do develop will frequently result in abortion/stillbirth or neonatal anomalies. Therefore, it has been suggested that male structural reorganization carriers should undergo sperm FISH studies and PGD-AS, to assess the chromosomal constitution of IVF embryos [188,191,192].

Chromosomally normal infertile men

Most studies report significantly higher aneuploidy rates (mostly sex-chromosome hyperhaploidy and diploidy) in sperm nuclei of infertile compared to those of fertile men (Table 11.5). It has been suggested that meiotic disturbances, especially frequent in cases with severe oligoasthenospermia (OA), are responsible for the production of abnormal gametes [159]. **The risk of sperm chromosomal aneuploidy appears to be inversely correlated to sperm concentration and total progressive motility** [160,162,193–198]. **Severe oligospermia has been associated with aneuploidy levels of up to 70%** (total aneuploidy based on estimates) [156,164,199]. Consequently, it has been suggested that men with severe OA should undergo meiotic studies and/or sperm chromosome analyses by FISH prior to ICSI so as to undergo adequate genetic counseling. Sperm FISH analysis may also be valuable in couples with recurrent first-trimester abortions, based on studies suggesting a role for sperm chromosome abnormalities in recurrent pregnancy loss [200]. However, the parental origin of the abortions has not been determined in these studies.

Clinical utility of sperm FISH analysis

The application of sperm FISH analysis has largely been evaluated in the context of research studies. However, there may be specific clinical circumstances for which sperm FISH may be used. **Sperm FISH analysis may be useful in infertile men with sex-chromosome numerical anomalies, structural chromosome anomalies, and severe oligospermia, prior to ICSI.** Sperm FISH may also be considered in couples with a history of recurrent miscarriages and trisomic pregnancies [201]. **However, the threshold level of aneuploidy frequency (to categorize men into "high-risk" and "low-risk" groups) has not been established. Moreover, the relationship between sperm chromosome aneuploidy and chromosomally abnormal embryos is not straightforward.** Staessen et al. have shown a high frequency of chromosomally abnormal embryos (>60% abnormal embryos at IVF/ICSI) in couples with a normal chromosomal constitution (normal karyotype) and advanced maternal age [202]. Thus, counseling of couples after FISH analysis remains a challenge.

Summary

FISH analysis of sperm nuclei is a reliable technique to determine the chromosome content of spermatozoa. However, it remains a costly and labor-intensive technology. Nonetheless, the ongoing application of this technique in the context of research programs will likely provide invaluable information on the genetic risk associated with the treatment (e.g., ICSI) of severe male-factor infertility. Ultimately, the true clinical value of sperm FISH analysis can only be determined once the relationship between the frequency of aneuploid sperm and the paternal contribution to aneuploidy, particularly trisomy, has been established.

Final summary

A number of advanced sperm fertility tests have been developed and studied. Overall, the data suggest that tests of acrosome reaction and DNA damage are potentially useful clinically. Couples with an abnormal test result should consider IVF/ICSI rather than conventional IVF or IUI. However, to date, these tests cannot reliably predict pregnancy outcome after ICSI. Moreover, these clinical tests (acrosome reaction, DNA damage) exhibit some inherent weaknesses and neither has been shown to be superior to the other in the evaluation of male infertility. The data indicate that tests of sperm or semen ROS determination may help clinicians establish a more specific diagnosis and design better therapies for male infertility, although this test cannot reliably predict pregnancy outcome.

Assessment of sperm chromosome aneuploidy by FISH analysis is a labor-intensive but informative test that may be of value in specific clinical cases (e.g., men with a karyotype abnormality). However, the clinical indications for sperm FISH analysis, the threshold level of sperm aneuploidy, and the management/counseling of couples with an abnormal test result have not been fully defined.

Tests of sperm–oocyte fusion and sperm–cervical mucus penetration are of no real clinical value. Tests of zona pellucida binding are of limited clinical value owing to the difficulty in obtaining human oocytes. Therefore, these tests should not be applied in routine clinical practice.

References

[1] Guzick DS, Overstreet JW, Factor-Litvak P, *et al.* Sperm morphology, motility, and concentration in fertile and infertile men. *N Engl J Med* 2001; **345**: 1388–93.

[2] Bastiaan HS, Menkveld R, Oehninger S, Franken DR. Zona pellucida induced acrosome reaction, sperm morphology, and sperm–zona binding assessments among subfertile men. *J Assist Reprod Genet* 2002; **19**: 329–34.

[3] Consensus workshop on advanced diagnostic andrology techniques. ESHRE (European Society of Human Reproduction and Embryology) Andrology Special Interest Group. *Hum Reprod* 1996; **11**: 1463–79.

[4] Bonduelle M, Van AE, Joris H, *et al.* Prenatal testing in ICSI pregnancies: incidence of chromosomal anomalies in 1586 karyotypes and relation to sperm parameters. *Hum Reprod* 2002; **17**: 2600–14.

[5] Gagnon C, Sherins RJ, Phillips DM, Bardin CW. Deficiency of protein-carboxyl methylase in immotile spermatozoa of infertile men. *N Engl J Med* 1982; **306**: 821–5.

[6] World Health Organization. WHO Laboratory Manual for the Examination of Human Semen and Sperm–Cervical Mucus Interaction, 4th edn. Cambridge: Cambridge University Press, 1999.

[7] Sallam HN, Farrag A, Agameya AF, El-Garem Y, Ezzeldin F. The use of the modified hypo-osmotic swelling test for the selection of immotile testicular spermatozoa in patients treated with ICSI: a randomized controlled study. *Hum Reprod* 2005; **20**: 3435–40.

[8] Avery S, Bolton VN, Mason BA. An evaluation of the hypo-osmotic sperm swelling test as a predictor of fertilizing capacity in vitro. *Int J Androl* 1990; **13**: 93–9.

[9] Carbone DJ, McMahon JT, Levin HS, Thomas AJ, Agarwal A. Role of electron microscopy of sperm in the evaluation of male infertility during the era of assisted reproduction. *Urology* 1998; **52**: 301–5.

[10] Chemes EH, Rawe YV. Sperm pathology: a step beyond descriptive morphology. Origin, characterization and fertility potential of abnormal sperm phenotypes in infertile men. *Hum Reprod Update* 2003; **9**: 405–28.

[11] Jouannet P, Escaller D, Serres C, David G. Motility of human sperm without outer dynein arms. *J Submicrosc Cytol* 1983; **15**: 67–71.

[12] Sturgess JM, Chao J, Wong J, Aspin N, Turner JA. Cilia with defective radial spokes: a cause of human respiratory disease. *N Engl J Med* 1979; **300**: 53–6.

[13] Eliasson R, Mossberg B, Camner P, Afzelius BA. The immotile-cilia syndrome: a congenital ciliary abnormality as an etiologic factor in chronic airway infections and male sterility. *N Engl J Med* 1977; **297**: 1–6.

[14] Guichard C, Harricane MC, Lafitte JJ, *et al.* Axonemal dynein intermediate-chain gene (DNAI1) mutations result in situs inversus and primary ciliary dyskinesia (Kartagener syndrome). *Am J Hum Genet* 2001; **68**: 1030–5.

[15] Peeraer K, Nijs M, Raick D, Ombelet W. Pregnancy after ICSI with ejaculated immotile spermatozoa from a patient with immotile cilia syndrome: a case report and review of the literature. *Reprod Biomed Online* 2004; **9**: 659–63.

[16] Okada H, Fujioka H, Tatsumi N, *et al.* Klinefelter's syndrome in the male infertility clinic. *Hum Reprod* 1999; **14**: 946–52.

[17] Eddy EM, Toshimori K, O'Brien DA. Fibrous sheath of mammalian spermatozoa. *Microsc Res Tech* 2003; **61**: 103–15.

[18] Baccetti B, Burrini AG, Capitani S, *et al.* Notulae seminologicae. 2. The "short tail" and "stump" defect in human spermatozoa. *Andrologia* 1993; 25: 331–5.

[19] Feneux D, Serres C, Jouannet P. Sliding spermatozoa: a dyskinesia responsible for human infertility? *Fertil Steril* 1985; 44: 508–11.

[20] Singh G. Ultrastructural features of round-headed human spermatozoa. *Int J Fertil* 1992; 37: 99–102.

[21] Kilani Z, Ismail R, Ghunaim S, *et al.* Evaluation and treatment of familial globozoospermia in five brothers. *Fertil Steril* 2004; 82: 1436–9.

[22] Toyama Y, Iwamoto T, Yajima M, Baba K, Yuasa S. Decapitated and decaudated spermatozoa in man, and pathogenesis based on the ultrastructure. *Int J Androl* 2000; 23: 109–15.

[23] Moghissi KS. Postcoital test: Physiologic basis, technique, and interpretation. *Fertil Steril* 1976; 27: 117–29.

[24] Liu DY, Baker HW. Sperm nuclear chromatin normality: relationship with sperm morphology, sperm–zona pellucida binding, and fertilization rates *in vitro. Fertil Steril* 1992; 58: 1178–84.

[25] van der Steeg JW, Steures P, Eijkemans MJ, *et al.* Should the post-coital test (PCT) be part of the routine fertility work-up? *Hum Reprod* 2004; 19: 1373–9.

[26] Thorne-Tjomsland G, Clermont Y, Hermo L. Contribution of the Golgi apparatus components to the formation of the acrosomic system and chromatoid body in rat spermatids. *Anat Rec* 1988; 221: 591–8.

[27] Morgan H, Stedronska J, Hendry WF, Chamberlain GF, Dewhurst CJ. Sperm/cervical-mucus crossed hostility testing and antisperm antibodies in the husband. *Lancet* 1977; 1: 1228–30.

[28] Gaddum-Rosse P, Blandau RJ, Lee WI. Sperm penetration into cervical mucus *in vitro.* II. Human spermatozoa in bovine mucus. *Fertil Steril* 1980; 33: 644–8.

[29] Eggert-Kruse W, Gerhard I, Tilgen W, Runnebaum B. Clinical significance of crossed *in vitro* sperm–cervical mucus penetration test in infertility investigation. *Fertil Steril* 1989; 52: 1032–40.

[30] Farhi J, Valentine A, Bahadur G, *et al. In-vitro* cervical mucus–sperm penetration tests and outcome of infertility treatments in couples with repeatedly negative post-coital tests. *Hum Reprod* 1995; 10: 85–90.

[31] Practice Committee of the American Society for Reproductive Medicine. Optimal evaluation of the infertile female. *Fertil Steril* 2004; 82 (Suppl 1): S169–72.

[32] Wassarman PM. Mammalian fertilization: molecular aspects of gamete adhesion, exocytosis, and fusion. *Cell* 1999; 96: 175–83.

[33] Bedford JM. Significance of the need for sperm capacitation before fertilization in eutherian mammals. *Biol Reprod* 1983; 28: 108–20.

[34] Cummins JM, Pember SM, Jequier AM, Yovich JL, Hartmann PE. A test of the human sperm acrosome reaction following ionophore challenge: relationship to fertility and other seminal parameters. *J Androl* 1991; 12: 98–103.

[35] Aitken RJ, Brindle JP. Analysis of the ability of three probes targeting the outer acrosomal membrane or acrosomal contents to detect the acrosome reaction in human spermatozoa. *Hum Reprod* 1993; 8: 1663–79.

[36] Cross N, Morales P, Overstreet J. Two simple methods for detecting acrosome-reacted human sperm. *Gamete Res* 1986; 15: 213–26.

[37] Makkar G, Ng EH, Yeung WS, Ho PC. The significance of the ionophore-challenged acrosome reaction in the prediction of successful outcome of controlled ovarian stimulation and intrauterine insemination. *Hum Reprod* 2003; 18: 534–9.

[38] van Duin M, Polman JE, De Breet IT, *et al.* Recombinant human zona pellucida protein ZP3 produced by chinese hamster ovary cells induces the human sperm acrosome reaction and promotes sperm–egg fusion. *Biol Reprod* 1994; 51: 607–17.

[39] Franken DR, Bastiaan HS, Oehninger SC. Physiological induction of the acrosome reaction in human sperm: validation of a microassay using minimal volumes of solubilized, homologous zona pellucida. *J Assist Reprod Genet* 2000; 17: 374–8.

[40] Liu DY, Baker HW. Defective sperm–zona pellucida interaction: a major cause of failure of fertilization in clinical *in-vitro* fertilization. *Hum Reprod* 2000; 15: 702–8.

[41] Blouin JL, Meeks M, Radhakrishna U, *et al.* Primary ciliary dyskinesia: a genome-wide linkage analysis reveals extensive locus heterogeneity. *Eur J Hum Genet* 2000; 8: 109–18.

[42] Liu DY, Baker HW. Disordered zona pellucida-induced acrosome reaction and failure of *in vitro* fertilization in patients with unexplained infertility. *Fertil Steril* 2003; 79: 74–80.

[43] Takahashi K, Wetzels AM, Goverde HJ, *et al.* The kinetics of the acrosome reaction of human spermatozoa and its correlation with *in vitro* fertilization. *Fertil Steril* 1992; 57: 889–94.

[44] Fenichel P, Donzeau M, Farahifar D, *et al.* Dynamics of human sperm acrosome reaction: relation with *in vitro* fertilization. *Fertil Steril* 1991; 55: 994–9.

[45] Henkel R, Muller C, Miska W, Gips H, Schill WB. Determination of the acrosome reaction in human spermatozoa is predictive of fertilization *in vitro. Hum Reprod* 1993; 8: 2128–32.

[46] Pampiglione JS, Tan SL, Campbell S. The use of the stimulated acrosome reaction test as a test of fertilizing ability in human spermatozoa. *Fertil Steril* 1993; 59: 1280–4.

[47] Yovich JM, Edirisinghe WR, Yovich JL. Use of the acrosome reaction to ionophore challenge test in managing patients in an assisted reproduction program: a prospective, double- blind, randomized controlled study. *Fertil Steril* 1994; **61**: 902–10.

[48] Calvo L, Dennison-Lagos L, Banks SM, *et al.* Acrosome reaction inducibility predicts fertilization success at *in-vitro* fertilization. *Hum Reprod* 1994; **9**: 1880–6.

[49] Parinaud J, Vieitez G, Moutaffian H, Richoilley G, Labal B. Variations in spontaneous and induced acrosome reaction: Correlations with semen parameters and *in-vitro* fertilization results. *Hum Reprod* 1995; **10**: 2085–9.

[50] Krausz C, Bonaccorsi L, Maggio P, *et al.* Two functional assays of sperm responsiveness to progesterone and their predictive values in *in-vitro* fertilization. *Hum Reprod* 1996; **11**: 1661–7.

[51] Sukcharoen N, Keith J, Irvine DS, Aitken RJ. Prediction of the *in-vitro* fertilization (IVF) potential of human spermatozoa using sperm function tests: the effect of the delay between testing and IVF. *Hum Reprod* 1996; **11**: 1030–4.

[52] Carver-Ward JA, Jaroudi KA, Hollanders JM, Einspenner M. High fertilization prediction by flow cytometric analysis of the CD46 antigen on the inner acrosomal membrane of spermatozoa. *Hum Reprod* 1996; **11**: 1923–8.

[53] Esterhuizen AD, Franken DR, Lourens JG, Van Rooyen LH. Clinical importance of zona pellucida-induced acrosome reaction and its predictive value for IVF. *Hum Reprod* 2001; **16**: 138–44.

[54] Bastiaan HS, Windt ML, Menkveld R, *et al.* Relationship between zona pellucida-induced acrosome reaction, sperm morphology, sperm–zona pellucida binding, and *in vitro* fertilization. *Fertil Steril* 2003; **79**: 49–55.

[55] Katsuki T, Hara T, Ueda K, Tanaka J, Ohama K. Prediction of outcomes of assisted reproduction treatment using the calcium ionophore-induced acrosome reaction. *Hum Reprod* 2005; **20**: 469–75.

[56] Liu DY, Baker HW. High frequency of defective sperm–zona pellucida interaction in oligozoospermic infertile men. *Hum Reprod* 2004; **19**: 228–33.

[57] Liu DY, Clarke GN, Martic M, Garrett C, Baker HW. Frequency of disordered zona pellucida (ZP)-induced acrosome reaction in infertile men with normal semen analysis and normal spermatozoa-ZP binding. *Hum Reprod* 2001; **16**: 1185–90.

[58] Liu DY, Baker HW. A simple method for assessment of the human acrosome reaction of spermatozoa bound to the zona pellucida: lack of relationship with ionophore A23187-induced acrosome reaction. *Hum Reprod* 1996; **11**: 551–7.

[59] Barros C. *In vitro* capacitation of golden hamster spermatozoa with fallopian tube fluid of the mouse and rat. *J Reprod Fertil* 1968; **17**: 203–6.

[60] Yanagimachi R, Yanagimachi H, Rogers BJ. The use of zona-free animal ova as a test-system for the assessment of the fertilizing capacity of human spermatozoa. *Biol Reprod* 1976; **15**: 471–6.

[61] Aitken RJ, Irvine DS, Wu FC. Prospective analysis of sperm–oocyte fusion and reactive oxygen species generation as criteria for the diagnosis of infertility. *Am J Obstet Gynecol* 1991; **164**: 542–51.

[62] Muller CH. The andrology laboratory in an assisted reproductive technologies program. Quality assurance and laboratory methodology. *J Androl* 1992; **13**: 349–60.

[63] Johnson A, Smith RG, Bassham B, Lipshultz LI, Lamb DJ. The microsperm penetration assay: development of a sperm penetration assay suitable for oligospermic males. *Fertil Steril* 1991; **56**: 528–34.

[64] Lantz GD, Cunningham GR, Huckins C, Lipshultz LI. Recovery from severe oligospermia after exposure to dibromochloropropane. *Fertil Steril* 1981; **35**: 46–53.

[65] Johnson, A. Methodology for the sperm penetration assay. In: Keel BA, Webster BW, eds. *Handbook of Laboratory Diagnosis and Treatment of Infertility*. Boca Raton, FL: CRC Press, 1990.

[66] Collins JA, So Y, Wilson EH, Wrixon W, Casper RF. The postcoital test as a predictor of pregnancy among 355 infertile couples. *Fertil Steril* 1984; **41**: 703–8.

[67] Gattuccio F, D'Alia O, Pirronello S, *et al.* Varicocele and puberty: a transversal and longitudinal survey. *Acta Eur Fertil* 1988; **19**: 189–99.

[68] Shibahara H, Mitsuo M, Inoue M, *et al.* Relationship between human *in-vitro* fertilization and intracytoplasmic sperm injection and the zona-free hamster egg penetration test. *Hum Reprod* 1998; **13**: 1928–32.

[69] Corson SL, Batzer FR, Marmar J, Maislin G. The human sperm–hamster egg penetration assay: prognostic value. *Fertil Steril* 1988; **49**: 328–34.

[70] Margalioth EJ, Navot D, Laufer N, *et al.* Correlation between the zona-free hamster egg sperm penetration assay and human *in vitro* fertilization. *Fertil Steril* 1986; **45**: 665–70.

[71] Smith RG, Johnson A, Lamb D, Lipshultz LI. Functional tests of spermatozoa: sperm penetration assay. *Urol Clin North Am* 1987; **14**: 451–8.

[72] Swanson RJ, Mayer JF, Jones KH, Lanzendorf SE, McDowell J. Hamster ova/human sperm penetration: correlation with count, motility, and morphology for *in vitro* fertilization. *Arch Androl* 1984; **12** (Suppl): 69–77.

[73] Gwatkin RB, Collins JA, Jarrell JF, Kohut J, Milner RA. The value of semen analysis and sperm function assays

in predicting pregnancy among infertile couples. *Fertil Steril* 1990; **53**: 693–9.

[74] Talbert LM, Hammond MG, Halme J, *et al.* Semen parameters and fertilization of human oocytes *in vitro*: a multivariable analysis. *Fertil Steril* 1987; **48**: 270–7.

[75] Burkman LJ, Coddington CC, Franken DR, *et al.* The hemizona assay (HZA): development of a diagnostic test for the binding of human spermatozoa to the human hemizona pellucida to predict fertilization potential. *Fertil Steril* 1988; **49**: 688–97.

[76] Arslan M, Morshedi M, Arslan EO, *et al.* Predictive value of the hemizona assay for pregnancy outcome in patients undergoing controlled ovarian hyperstimulation with intrauterine insemination. *Fertil Steril* 2006; **85**: 1697–707.

[77] Liu DY, Clarke GN, Lopata A, Johnston WI, Baker HW. A sperm–zona pellucida binding test and *in vitro* fertilization. *Fertil Steril* 1989; **52**: 281–7.

[78] Franken DR. The clinical significance of sperm–zona pellucida binding. *Front Biosci* 1998; **3**: E247–53.

[79] Henkel R, Muller C, Stalf T, Schill WB, Franken DR. Use of failed-fertilized oocytes for diagnostic zona binding purposes after sperm binding improvement with a modified medium. *J Assist Reprod Genet* 1999; **16**: 24–9.

[80] Oehninger S, Acosta AA, Veeck LL, *et al.* Recurrent failure of *in vitro* fertilization: Role of the hemizona assay in the sequential diagnosis of specific sperm-oocyte defects. *Am J Obstet Gynecol* 1991; **164**: 1210–15.

[81] Grisham M. Chemistry and cytotoxicity of reactive oxygen metabolotes. In: Taylor AE, Matalon S, Ward P, eds. *Biology of Oxygen Radicals*. Bethesda, MD: American Physiological Society, 1986: 1–18.

[82] Alvarez JG, Storey BT. Taurine, hypotaurine, epinephrine and albumin inhibit lipid peroxidation in rabbit spermatozoa and protect against loss of motility. *Biol Reprod* 1983; **29**: 548–55.

[83] Chow CK. Vitamin E and *oxidative stress*. *Free Radic Biol Med* 1991; **11**: 215–32.

[84] Niki E. Action of ascorbic acid as a scavenger of active and stable oxygen radicals. *Am J Clin Nutr* 1991; **54**: 1119–24S.

[85] Aitken J, Fisher H. Reactive oxygen species generation and human spermatozoa: the balance of benefit and risk. *Bioessays* 1994; **16**: 259–67.

[86] de Lamirande E, Gagnon C. A positive role for the superoxide anion in triggering hyperactivation and capacitation of human spermatozoa. *Int J Androl* 1993; **16**: 21–5.

[87] Griveau JF, Renard P, Le LD. An *in vitro* promoting role for hydrogen peroxide in human sperm capacitation. *Int J Androl* 1994; **17**: 300–7.

[88] MacLeod J. The role of oxygen in the metabolism and motility of human spermatozoa. *Am J Physiol* 1943; **138**: 512–18.

[89] Aitken RJ, Clarkson JS, Fishel S. Generation of reactive oxygen species, lipid peroxidation, and human sperm function. *Biol Reprod* 1989; **41**: 183–97.

[90] Iwasaki A, Gagnon C. Formation of reactive oxygen species in spermatozoa of infertile patients. *Fertil Steril* 1992; **57**: 409–16.

[91] Athayde KS, Cocuzza M, Agarwal A, *et al.* Development of normal reference values for seminal reactive oxygen species and their correlation with leukocytes and semen parameters in a fertile population. *J Androl* 2007; **28**: 613–20.

[92] Kovalski NN, de Lamirande E, Gagnon C. Reactive oxygen species generated by human neutrophils inhibit sperm motility: protective effect of seminal plasma and scavengers. *Fertil Steril* 1992; **58**: 809–16.

[93] Gomez E, Buckingham DW, Brindle J, *et al.* Development of an image analysis system to monitor the retention of residual cytoplasm by human spermatozoa: correlation with biochemical markers of the cytoplasmic space, oxidative stress, and sperm function. *J Androl* 1996; **17**: 276–87.

[94] Alvarez JG, Touchstone JC, Blasco L, Storey BT. Spontaneous lipid peroxidation and production of hydrogen peroxide and superoxide in human spermatozoa: superoxide dismutase as major enzyme protectant against oxygen toxicity. *J Androl* 1987; **8**: 338–48.

[95] Aitken RJ, Gordon E, Harkiss D, *et al.* Relative impact of oxidative stress on the functional competence and genomic integrity of human spermatozoa. *Biol Reprod* 1998; **59**: 1037–46.

[96] Sawyer DE, Mercer BG, Wiklendt AM, Aitken RJ. Quantitative analysis of gene-specific DNA damage in human spermatozoa. *Mutat Res* 2003; **529**: 21–34.

[97] Krausz C, Mills C, Rogers S, Tan SL, Aitken RJ. Stimulation of oxidant generation by human sperm suspensions using phorbol esters and formyl peptides: relationships with motility and fertilization *in vitro*. *Fertil Steril* 1994; **62**: 599–605.

[98] Marchetti C, Obert G, Deffosez A, Formstecher P, Marchetti P. Study of mitochondrial membrane potential, reactive oxygen species, DNA fragmentation and cell viability by flow cytometry in human sperm. *Hum Reprod* 2002; **17**: 1257–65.

[99] Agarwal A, Sharma R, Nallella K, *et al.* Reactive oxygen species as an independent marker of male factor infertility. *Fertil Steril* 2006; **86**: 878–85.

[100] Yeung CH, De GC, De GM, Nieschlag E. Production of reactive oxygen species by and hydrogen peroxide scavenging activity of spermatozoa in an IVF program. *J Assist Reprod Genet* 1996; **13**: 495–500.

[101] Moilanen JM, Carpen O, Hovatta O. Flow cytometric light scattering analysis, acrosome reaction, reactive oxygen species production and leukocyte contamination of semen preparation in prediction

of fertilization rate *in vitro. Hum Reprod* 1998; **13**: 2568–74.

[102] Zorn B, Vidmar G, Meden-Vrtovec H. Seminal reactive oxygen species as predictors of fertilization, embryo quality and pregnancy rates after conventional *in vitro* fertilization and intracytoplasmic sperm injection. *Int J Androl* 2003; **26**: 279–85.

[103] Saleh RA, Agarwal A, Nada EA, *et al*. Negative effects of increased sperm DNA damage in relation to seminal oxidative stress in men with idiopathic and male factor infertility. *Fertil Steril* 2003; **79** (Suppl 3): 1597–605.

[104] Hammadeh ME, Radwan M, Al-Hasani S, *et al*. Comparison of reactive oxygen species concentration in seminal plasma and semen parameters in partners of pregnant and non-pregnant patients after IVF/ICSI. *Reprod Biomed Online* 2006; **13**: 696–706.

[105] Primakoff P, Myles DG. Penetration, adhesion, and fusion in mammalian sperm–egg interaction. *Science* 2002; **296**: 2183–5.

[106] Ahmadi A, Ng SC. Fertilizing ability of DNA-damaged spermatozoa. *J Exp Zool* 1999; **284**: 696–704.

[107] Cho C, Jung-Ha H, Willis WD, *et al*. Protamine 2 deficiency leads to sperm DNA damage and embryo death in mice. *Biol Reprod* 2003; **69**: 211–17.

[108] Evenson DP, Jost LK, Marshall D, *et al*. Utility of the sperm chromatin structure assay as a diagnostic and prognostic tool in the human fertility clinic. *Hum Reprod* 1999; **14**: 1039–49.

[109] Spano M, Bonde JP, Hjollund HI, *et al*. Sperm chromatin damage impairs human fertility. The Danish First Pregnancy Planner Study Team. *Fertil Steril* 2000; **73**: 43–50.

[110] Zini A, Bielecki R, Phang D, Zenzes MT. Correlations between two markers of sperm DNA integrity, DNA denaturation and DNA fragmentation, in fertile and infertile men. *Fertil Steril* 2001; **75**: 674–7.

[111] Kodama H, Yamaguchi R, Fukuda J, Kasai H, Tanaka T. Increased oxidative deoxyribonucleic acid damage in the spermatozoa of infertile male patients. *Fertil Steril* 1997; **68**: 519–24.

[112] Balhorn R. A model for the structure of chromatin in mammalian sperm. *J Cell Biol* 1982; **93**: 298–305.

[113] Gatewood JM, Cook GR, Balhorn R, Bradbury EM, Schmid CW. Sequence-specific packaging of DNA in human sperm chromatin. *Science* 1987; **236**: 962–4.

[114] Kosower NS, Katayose H, Yanagimachi R. Thiol-disulfide status and acridine orange fluorescence of mammalian sperm nuclei. *J Androl* 1992; **13**: 342–8.

[115] Anderson S, Bankier AT, Barrell BG, *et al*. Sequence and organization of the human mitochondrial genome. *Nature* 1981; **290**: 457–65.

[116] Sakkas D, Moffatt O, Manicardi GC, *et al*. Nature of DNA damage in ejaculated human spermatozoa and the possible involvement of apoptosis. *Biol Reprod* 2002; **66**: 1061–7.

[117] Singh NP, Muller CH, Berger RE. Effects of age on DNA double-strand breaks and apoptosis in human sperm. *Fertil Steril* 2003; **80**: 1420–30.

[118] Brinkworth MH, Nieschlag E. Association of cyclophosphamide-induced male-mediated, foetal abnormalities with reduced paternal germ-cell apoptosis. *Mutat Res* 2000; **447**: 149–54.

[119] Aoki VW, Moskovtsev SI, Willis J, *et al*. DNA integrity is compromised in protamine-deficient human sperm. *J Androl* 2005; **26**: 741–8.

[120] Zhang X, San GM, Zini A. Sperm nuclear histone to protamine ratio in fertile and infertile men: evidence of heterogeneous subpopulations of spermatozoa in the ejaculate. *J Androl* 2006; **27**: 414–20.

[121] Cho C, Willis WD, Goulding EH, *et al*. Haploinsufficiency of protamine-1 or -2 causes infertility in mice. *Nat Genet* 2001; **28**: 82–6.

[122] Iguchi N, Yang S, Lamb DJ, Hecht NB. An SNP in protamine 1: a possible genetic cause of male infertility? *J Med Genet* 2006; **43**: 382–4.

[123] Twigg J, Fulton N, Gomez E, Irvine DS, Aitken RJ. Analysis of the impact of intracellular reactive oxygen species generation on the structural and functional integrity of human spermatozoa: lipid peroxidation, DNA fragmentation and effectiveness of antioxidants. *Hum Reprod* 1998; **13**: 1429–36.

[124] Fischer MA, Willis J, Zini A. Human sperm DNA integrity: correlation with sperm cytoplasmic droplets. *Urology* 2003; **61**: 207–11.

[125] Pasqualotto FF, Sharma RK, Potts JM, *et al*. Seminal oxidative stress in patients with chronic prostatitis. *Urology* 2000; **55**: 881–5.

[126] Ochsendorf FR. Infections in the male genital tract and reactive oxygen species. *Hum Reprod Update* 1999; **5**: 399–420.

[127] Potts RJ, Newbury CJ, Smith G, Notarianni LJ, Jefferies TM. Sperm chromatin damage associated with male smoking. *Mutat Res* 1999; **423**: 103–11.

[128] Rubes J, Selevan SG, Evenson DP, *et al*. Episodic air pollution is associated with increased DNA fragmentation in human sperm without other changes in semen quality. *Hum Reprod* 2005; **20**: 2776–83.

[129] Smith R, Kaune H, Parodi D, *et al*. Increased sperm DNA damage in patients with varicocele: relationship with seminal oxidative stress. *Hum Reprod* 2006; **21**: 986–93.

[130] Loft S, Kold-Jensen T, Hjollund NH, *et al*. Oxidative DNA damage in human sperm influences time to pregnancy. *Hum Reprod* 2003; **18**: 1265–72.

[131] Duran EH, Morshedi M, Taylor S, Oehninger S. Sperm DNA quality predicts intrauterine

insemination outcome: A prospective cohort study. *Hum Reprod* 2002; **17**: 3122–8.

[132] Bungum M, Humaidan P, Axmon A, *et al.* Sperm DNA integrity assessment in prediction of assisted reproduction technology outcome. *Hum Reprod* 2007; **22**: 174–9.

[133] Lopes S, Sun JG, Jurisicova A, Meriano J, Casper RF. Sperm deoxyribonucleic acid fragmentation is increased in poor-quality semen samples and correlates with failed fertilization in intracytoplasmic sperm injection. *Fertil Steril* 1998; **69**: 528–32.

[134] Sun JG, Jurisicova A, Casper RF. Detection of deoxyribonucleic acid fragmentation in human sperm: correlation with fertilization *in vitro*. *Biol Reprod* 1997; **56**: 602–7.

[135] Morris ID, Ilott S, Dixon L, Brison DR. The spectrum of DNA damage in human sperm assessed by single cell gel electrophoresis (Comet assay) and its relationship to fertilization and embryo development. *Hum Reprod* 2002; **17**: 990–8.

[136] Host E, Lindenberg S, Smidt-Jensen S. The role of DNA strand breaks in human spermatozoa used for IVF and ICSI. *Acta Obstet Gynecol Scand* 2000; **79**: 559–63.

[137] Tomlinson MJ, Moffatt O, Manicardi GC, *et al.* Interrelationships between seminal parameters and sperm nuclear DNA damage before and after density gradient centrifugation: implications for assisted conception. *Hum Reprod* 2001; **16**: 2160–5.

[138] Tomsu M, Sharma V, Miller D. Embryo quality and IVF treatment outcomes may correlate with different sperm comet assay parameters. *Hum Reprod* 2002; **17**: 1856–62.

[139] Larson-Cook KL, Brannian JD, Hansen KA, *et al.* Relationship between the outcomes of assisted reproductive techniques and sperm DNA fragmentation as measured by the sperm chromatin structure assay. *Fertil Steril* 2003; **80**: 895–902.

[140] Seli E, Gardner DK, Schoolcraft WB, Moffatt O, Sakkas D. Extent of nuclear DNA damage in ejaculated spermatozoa impacts on blastocyst development after *in vitro* fertilization. *Fertil Steril* 2004; **82**: 378–83.

[141] Virro MR, Larson-Cook KL, Evenson DP. Sperm chromatin structure assay (SCSA) parameters are related to fertilization, blastocyst development, and ongoing pregnancy in *in vitro* fertilization and intracytoplasmic sperm injection cycles. *Fertil Steril* 2004; **81**: 1289–95.

[142] Henkel R, Hajimohammad M, Stalf T, *et al.* Influence of deoxyribonucleic acid damage on fertilization and pregnancy. *Fertil Steril* 2004; **81**: 965–72.

[143] Gandini L, Lombardo F, Paoli D, *et al.* Full-term pregnancies achieved with ICSI despite high levels of sperm chromatin damage. *Hum Reprod* 2004; **19**: 1409–17.

[144] Huang CC, Lin DP, Tsao HM, *et al.* Sperm DNA fragmentation negatively correlates with velocity and fertilization rates but might not affect pregnancy rates. *Fertil Steril* 2005; **84**: 130–40.

[145] Payne JF, Raburn DJ, *Couchman GM, et al.* Redefining the relationship between sperm deoxyribonucleic acid fragmentation as measured by the sperm chromatin structure assay and outcomes of assisted reproductive techniques. *Fertil Steril* 2005; **84**: 356–64.

[146] Zini A, Meriano J, Kader K, *et al.* Potential adverse effect of sperm DNA damage on embryo quality after ICSI. *Hum Reprod* 2005; **20**: 3476–80.

[147] Borini A, Tarozzi N, Bizzaro D, *et al.* Sperm DNA fragmentation: paternal effect on early post-implantation embryo development in ART. *Hum Reprod* 2006; **21**: 2876–81.

[148] Benchaib M, Lornage J, Mazoyer C, *et al.* Sperm deoxyribonucleic acid fragmentation as a prognostic indicator of assisted reproductive technology outcome. *Fertil Steril* 2007; **87**: 93–100.

[149] Braude P, Bolton V, Moore S. Human gene expression first occurs between the four- and eight-cell stages of preimplantation development. *Nature* 1988; **332**: 459–61.

[150] Hansen M, Kurinczuk JJ, Bower C, Webb S. The risk of major birth defects after intracytoplasmic sperm injection and *in vitro* fertilization. *N Engl J Med* 2002; **346**: 725–30.

[151] Ludwig M, Katalinic A, Gross S, *et al.* Increased prevalence of imprinting defects in patients with Angelman syndrome born to subfertile couples. *J Med Genet* 2005; **42**: 289–91.

[152] Cox GF, Burger J, Lip V, *et al.* Intracytoplasmic sperm injection may increase the risk of imprinting defects. *Am J Hum Genet* 2002; **71**: 162–4.

[153] Bonduelle M, Wennerholm UB, Loft A, *et al.* A multi-centre cohort study of the physical health of 5-year-old children conceived after intracytoplasmic sperm injection, *in vitro* fertilization and natural conception. *Hum Reprod* 2005; **20**: 413–19.

[154] Kuchino Y, Mori F, Kasai H, *et al.* Misreading of DNA templates containing 8-hydroxydeoxyguanosine at the modified base and at adjacent residues. *Nature* 1987; **327**: 77–9.

[155] Zini A, Fischer MA, Sharir S, *et al.* Prevalence of abnormal sperm DNA denaturation in fertile and infertile men. *Urology* 2002; **60**: 1069–72.

[156] Pang MG, Hoegerman SF, Cuticchia AJ, *et al.* Detection of aneuploidy for chromosomes 4, 6, 7, 8, 9, 10, 11, 12, 13, 17, 18, 21, X and Y by fluorescence *in-situ* hybridization in spermatozoa from nine patients with oligoasthenoteratozoospermia

undergoing intracytoplasmic sperm injection. *Hum Reprod* 1999; **14**: 1266–73.

[157] Griffin DK, Abruzzo MA, Millie EA, *et al.* Non-disjunction in human sperm: evidence for an effect of increasing paternal age. *Hum Mol Genet* 1995; **4**: 2227–32.

[158] Downie SE, Flaherty SP, Matthews CD. Detection of chromosomes and estimation of aneuploidy in human spermatozoa using fluorescence in-situ hybridization. *Mol Hum Reprod* 1997; **3**: 585–98.

[159] Egozcue S, Blanco J, Vendrell JM, *et al.* Human male infertility: chromosome anomalies, meiotic disorders, abnormal spermatozoa and recurrent abortion. *Hum Reprod Update* 2000; **6**: 93–105.

[160] Shi Q, Martin RH. Aneuploidy in human spermatozoa: FISH analysis in men with constitutional chromosomal abnormalities, and in infertile men. *Reproduction* 2001; **121**: 655–66.

[161] Martin RH, Rademaker AW, Greene C, *et al.* A comparison of the frequency of sperm chromosome abnormalities in men with mild, moderate, and severe oligozoospermia. *Biol Reprod* 2003; **69**: 535–9.

[162] Vegetti W, Van AE, Frias A, *et al.* Correlation between semen parameters and sperm aneuploidy rates investigated by fluorescence in-situ hybridization in infertile men. *Hum Reprod* 2000; **15**: 351–5.

[163] Thomas NS, Hassold TJ. Aberrant recombination and the origin of Klinefelter syndrome. *Hum Reprod Update* 2003; **9**: 309–17.

[164] Pfeffer J, Pang MG, Hoegerman SF, *et al.* Aneuploidy frequencies in semen fractions from ten oligoasthenoteratozoospermic patients donating sperm for intracytoplasmic sperm injection. *Fertil Steril* 1999; **72**: 472–8.

[165] Rives N, Saint CA, Mazurier S, *et al.* Relationship between clinical phenotype, semen parameters and aneuploidy frequency in sperm nuclei of 50 infertile males. *Hum Genet* 1999; **105**: 266–72.

[166] Van DQ, Lanzendorf S, Kolm P, Hodgen GD, Mahony MC. Incidence of aneuploid spermatozoa from subfertile men: selected with motility versus hemizona-bound. *Hum Reprod* 2000; **15**: 1529–36.

[167] Robinson WP, McFadden DE, Stephenson MD. The origin of abnormalities in recurrent aneuploidy/polyploidy. *Am J Hum Genet* 2001; **69**: 1245–54.

[168] Robbins WA, Meistrich ML, Moore D, *et al.* Chemotherapy induces transient sex chromosomal and autosomal aneuploidy in human sperm. *Nat Genet* 1997; **16**: 74–8.

[169] Rubes J, Lowe X, Moore D, *et al.* Smoking cigarettes is associated with increased sperm disomy in teenage men. *Fertil Steril* 1998; **70**: 715–23.

[170] Hassold T, Abruzzo M, Adkins K, *et al.* Human aneuploidy: incidence, origin, and etiology. *Environ Mol Mutagen* 1996; **28**: 167–75.

[171] Foresta C, Galeazzi C, Bettella A, Stella M, Scandellari C. High incidence of sperm sex chromosomes aneuploidies in two patients with Klinefelter's syndrome. *J Clin Endocrinol Metab* 1998; **83**: 203–5.

[172] Rives N, Joly G, Machy A, *et al.* Assessment of sex chromosome aneuploidy in sperm nuclei from 47,XXY and 46,XY/47,XXY males: comparison with fertile and infertile males with normal karyotype. *Mol Hum Reprod* 2000; **6**: 107–12.

[173] Rives N, Simeon N, Milazzo JP, Barthelemy C, Mace B. Meiotic segregation of sex chromosomes in mosaic and non-mosaic XYY males: case reports and review of the literature. *Int J Androl* 2003; **26**: 242–9.

[174] Luciani JM, Mattei A, Victor-Vuillet M, *et al.* Study of meiotic chromosomes in a case of Klinefelter's disease with spermatogenesis and 46,XY-47,XXY karyotype. *Ann Genet* 1970; **13**: 249–53.

[175] Mroz K, Hassold TJ, Hunt PA. Meiotic aneuploidy in the XXY mouse: evidence that a compromised testicular environment increases the incidence of meiotic errors. *Hum Reprod* 1999; **14**: 1151–6.

[176] Shi Q, Martin RH. Multicolor fluorescence *in situ* hybridization analysis of meiotic chromosome segregation in a 47,XYY male and a review of the literature. *Am J Med Genet* 2000; **93**: 40–6.

[177] Blanco J, Egozcue J, Clusellas N, Vidal F. FISH on sperm heads allows the analysis of chromosome segregation and interchromosomal effects in carriers of structural rearrangements: Results in a translocation carrier, t(5; 8)(q33; q13). *Cytogenet Cell Genet* 1998; **83**: 275–80.

[178] Martini E, von Bergh AR, Coonen E, *et al.* Detection of structural abnormalities in spermatozoa of a translocation carrier t(3; 11)(q27.3; q24.3) by triple FISH. *Hum Genet* 1998; **102**: 157–65.

[179] Van HP, Manchester D, Lowe X, Wyrobek AJ. Meiotic segregation, recombination, and gamete aneuploidy assessed in a t(1; 10)(p22.1; q22.3) reciprocal translocation carrier by three- and four-probe multicolor FISH in sperm. *Am J Hum Genet* 1997; **61**: 651–9.

[180] Cifuentes P, Navarro J, Blanco J, *et al.* Cytogenetic analysis of sperm chromosomes and sperm nuclei in a male heterozygous for a reciprocal translocation t(5; 7)(q21; q32) by *in situ* hybridisation. *Eur J Hum Genet* 1999; **7**: 231–8.

[181] Estop AM, Cieply KM, Munne S, Feingold E. Multicolor fluorescence *in situ* hybridization analysis of the spermatozoa of a male heterozygous for a reciprocal translocation t(11; 22)(q23; q11). *Hum Genet* 1999; **104**: 412–17.

[182] Giltay JC, Kastrop PM, Tiemessen CH, *et al.* Sperm analysis in a subfertile male with a Y; 16

translocation, using four-color FISH. *Cytogenet Cell Genet* 1999; **84**: 67–72.

[183] Anton E, Blanco J, Egozcue J, Vidal F. Sperm FISH studies in seven male carriers of Robertsonian translocation t(13; 14)(q10; q10). *Hum Reprod* 2004; **19**: 1345–51.

[184] Rousseaux S, Chevret E, Monteil M, *et al*. Sperm nuclei analysis of a Robertsonian t(14q21q) carrier, by FISH, using three plasmids and two YAC probes. *Hum Genet* 1995; **96**: 655–60.

[185] Ogur G, Van AE, Vegetti W, *et al*. Chromosomal segregation in spermatozoa of 14 Robertsonian translocation carriers. *Mol Hum Reprod* 2006; **12**: 209–15.

[186] Blanco J, Egozcue J, Vidal F. Interchromosomal effects for chromosome 21 in carriers of structural chromosome reorganizations determined by fluorescence *in situ* hybridization on sperm nuclei. *Hum Genet* 2000; **106**: 500–5.

[187] Douet-Guilbert N, Bris MJ, Amice V, *et al*. Interchromosomal effect in sperm of males with translocations: report of 6 cases and review of the literature. *Int J Androl* 2005; **28**: 372–9.

[188] Yakut T, Ercelen N, Acar H, Kimya Y, Egeli U. Meiotic segregation analysis of reciprocal translocations both in sperm and blastomeres. *Am J Med Genet A*. 2006; **140**: 1074–82.

[189] Guttenbach M, Michelmann HW, Hinney B, Engel W, Schmid M. Segregation of sex chromosomes into sperm nuclei in a man with 47,XXY Klinefelter's karyotype: a FISH analysis. *Hum Genet* 1997; **99**: 474–7.

[190] Martin RH, Spriggs EL. Sperm chromosome complements in a man heterozygous for a reciprocal translocation 46,XY,t(9; 13)(q21.1; q21.2) and a review of the literature. *Clin Genet* 1995; **47**: 42–6.

[191] Escudero T, Lee M, Carrel D, Blanco J, Munne S. Analysis of chromosome abnormalities in sperm and embryos from two 45,XY,t(13; 14)(q10; q10) carriers. *Prenat Diagn* 2000; **20**: 599–602.

[192] Van AE, Staessen C, Vegetti W, *et al*. Preimplantation genetic diagnosis and sperm analysis by fluorescence *in-situ* hybridization for the most common

reciprocal translocation t(11; 22). *Mol Hum Reprod* 1999; **5**: 682–90.

[193] Bernardini L, Martini E, Geraedts JP, *et al*. Comparison of gonosomal aneuploidy in spermatozoa of normal fertile men and those with severe male factor detected by *in-situ* hybridization. *Mol Hum Reprod* 1997; **3**: 431–8.

[194] Lahdetie J, Saari N, Ajosenpaa-Saari M, Mykkanen J. Incidence of aneuploid spermatozoa among infertile men studied by multicolor fluorescence *in situ* hybridization. *Am J Med Genet* 1997; **71**: 115–21.

[195] Martin RH. Genetics of human sperm. *J Assist Reprod Genet* 1998; **15**: 240–5.

[196] McInnes B, Rademaker A, Greene CA, *et al*. Abnormalities for chromosomes 13 and 21 detected in spermatozoa from infertile men. *Hum Reprod* 1998; **13**: 2787–90.

[197] Colombero LT, Hariprashad JJ, Tsai MC, Rosenwaks Z, Palermo GD. Incidence of sperm aneuploidy in relation to semen characteristics and assisted reproductive outcome. *Fertil Steril* 1999; **72**: 90–6.

[198] Nishikawa N, Murakami I, Ikuta K, Suzumori K. Sex chromosomal analysis of spermatozoa from infertile men using fluorescence *in situ* hybridization. *J Assist Reprod Genet* 2000; **17**: 97–102.

[199] Ohashi Y, Miharu N, Honda H, Samura O, Ohama K. High frequency of XY disomy in spermatozoa of severe oligozoospermic men. *Hum Reprod* 2001; **16**: 703–8.

[200] Rubio C, Simon C, Blanco J, *et al*. Implications of sperm chromosome abnormalities in recurrent miscarriage. *J Assist Reprod Genet* 1999; **16**: 253–8.

[201] Tomascik-Cheeseman LM, Lowe XR, *et al*. A father of four consecutive trisomic pregnancies with elevated frequencies of associated aneuploid sperm. *Am J Med Genet A* 2006; **140**: 1840–5.

[202] Staessen C, Platteau P, Van AE, *et al*. Comparison of blastocyst transfer with or without preimplantation genetic diagnosis for aneuploidy screening in couples with advanced maternal age: a prospective randomized controlled trial. *Hum Reprod* 2004; **19**: 2849–58.

Chapter 12

Endocrine evaluation

Rebecca Z. Sokol

Introduction

Approximately 20% of men undergoing an infertility evaluation will be diagnosed with an underlying endocrine abnormality [1–3]. Although the percentage may appear to be small, the identification of specific endocrine abnormalities allows the patient to understand if and how his infertility may be treated. Whereas some disorders can be treated with hormonal intervention leading to successful pregnancy, others cannot. **Therefore, an evaluation of the reproductive endocrine status is an essential component in the investigation of all male partners with either an abnormal physical examination suggestive of a disorder in testosterone production and action, an abnormal semen examination, or evidence of impaired sexual function.**

Reproductive axis physiology

The important hormones of the male reproductive system are gonadotropin-releasing hormone (GnRH), produced in the hypothalamus; the pituitary gonadotropins, luteinizing hormone (LH) and follicle-stimulating hormone (FSH); the testicular steroids, testosterone and estradiol; the testicular peptide, inhibin; and the peripherally produced dihydrotestosterone (DHT) (Fig. 12.1).

GnRH synthesis and pulsatile release into the hypophyseal portal veins is regulated by GnRH receptors in the pituitary gland and stimulates the synthesis and release of the gonadotropic hormones, LH and FSH [4–7]. LH and FSH are secreted by the pituitary gland into the general circulation and carried to the testes. The gonadotropins stimulate gonadal secretion of testosterone and estradiol. Testosterone is important for the maturation and maintenance of spermatogenesis [8].

Testosterone is metabolized to DHT by the enzyme 5α-reductase [9,10]. DHT is necessary for external virilization during embryogenesis and androgen action during puberty and adulthood. Only 25% of circulating estradiol is secreted by the testes. The major portion of circulating estradiol is derived from peripheral conversion of testosterone and androstenedione [11]. Estrogen plays a role in the regulation of the secretion of GnRH and LH [12,13]. The testis also produces inhibin, a nonsteroid substance secreted by the Sertoli cells [14]. Inhibin is postulated to act primarily at the pituitary level, where it selectively inhibits the secretion of FSH [15]. Inhibin, along with testosterone, exerts local regulatory effects on spermatogenesis [16–18].

Prolactin, a polypeptide hormone, is synthesized and secreted from the pituitary gland. Elevated levels of prolactin interfere with gonadotropins and suppress testosterone synthesis in men [19].

In summary, control and coordination of testicular function occur via feedback signals, both positive and negative, exerted by the hormones secreted at each level of the hypothalamic-pituitary-testicular axis. These signals include (1) inhibition of hypothalamic GnRH secretion and pituitary LH responsiveness to GnRH by testicular steroids and (2) inhibition of pituitary FSH by testicular inhibin and, possibly, by circulating estrogens. Any disruption of the delicately coordinated interaction between the components of the hypothalamic–pituitary–testicular axis may lead to hypogonadism and/or infertility [20].

History and physical examination

The history and physical examination assist the clinician in ascertaining if an endocrine disorder is causing the man's infertility. History is obtained in order to uncover any underlying medical or endocrine conditions which might alter or disrupt testosterone production. Important milestones in a patient's developmental history include normal or abnormal descent of the testes, premature or delayed puberty, gynecomastia,

Infertility in the Male, 4th edition, ed. Larry I. Lipshultz, Stuart S. Howards, and Craig S. Niederberger. Published by Cambridge University Press. © Cambridge University Press 2009.

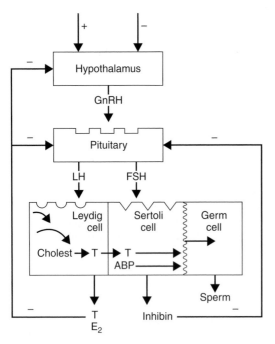

Fig 12.1. The hypothalamic–pituitary–testicular functional unit. GnRH, gonadotropin-releasing hormone; LH, luteinizing hormone; FSH, follicle-stimulating hormone; T, testosterone; ABP, androgen-binding protein; E_2, estradiol. (From Sokol RZ, Swerdloff RS. Endocrine evaluation. In: Lipshultz LI, Howards SS, eds. *Infertility in the Male*, 3rd edn. St. Louis, MO: Mosby Year Book, 1997: 210–18.)

altered libido or potency and fertility history, and urinary tract or central nervous system (CNS) abnormalities. Other important information includes past and present illnesses; surgery to the brain or the genitourinary system (e.g., orchiopexy, herniorrhaphy, vasectomy); infectious disease (e.g., venereal disease, mumps, tuberculosis, epididymitis); use of drugs, medications and alcohol; occupations and exposure to chemicals at work or at home.

Physical examination uncovers underlying general medical conditions and particularly endocrine disorders that result in hypogonadism. Assessment of cranial nerves may suggest a pituitary tumor. Midline facial defects are associated with congenital secondary hypogonadism. Thyroid disease is suspected with thyromegaly, eye changes, hyperreflexia, or hyporeflexia. Gynecomastia is associated with hypogonadism or an imbalance of the testosterone:estradiol ratio and hyperthyroidism, cirrhosis, testicular tumor, and drug use [21–23]. Hepatomegaly is associated with alcoholic liver disease and/or abnormal steroid metabolism.

Secondary sexual characteristics, which include body habitus, hair distribution pattern, body proportions, and size and anatomy of the genitalia, should be noted. Testicular examination includes assessment of shape, consistency, position, and presence of a mass. Testicular volume is measured with an orchidometer or calipers. Testicular size is primarily a reflection of the presence and activity of the seminiferous tubules. Testes smaller than 15 cm³ by Prader orchidometer are associated with an abnormally low sperm concentration and may or may not be associated with a low testosterone production. Testes larger than 25 cm³ may indicate a tumor or a hydrocele.

Determining if hypogonadism presented prior to or following puberty assists with the diagnosis. If Leydig cell function or androgen action was deficient during embryogenesis, then hypospadias, cryptorchidism, or microphallus occurs. If Leydig cell failure occurred prior to puberty, sexual maturation does not occur and features of eunuchoidism will develop. The cardinal feature of eunuchoidism is the failure of androgen-induced closure of the epiphyses of the long bones of the extremities, leading to an arm span 5 cm longer than height and a lower body segment (pubic to heel) more than 5 cm longer than the upper body segment (crown to pubic). Other findings of this condition include sparse body, pubic, and facial hair; poor skeletal muscle development; absence of male-pattern baldness; infantile genitalia with small firm testes; failure of voice to deepen; and, on occasion, gynecomastia.

Leydig cell failure following puberty is associated with more subtle physical findings. These include small, soft testes; female body habitus with female fat distribution; a decrease in skeletal muscle mass; gynecomastia; decrease in facial hair; and excessive facial wrinkling. Patients with isolated germ cell failure have normal physical findings except small testes, while patients with spermatogenic arrest or obstruction have normal-size testes.

Laboratory assessment

Initial laboratory assessment of the hypothalamic–pituitary–testicular axis includes the measurement of circulating levels of LH, FSH, and testosterone. Clinical history and the physical examination will determine if more specialized hormone testing, including free testosterone, sex hormone-binding globulin (SHBG), estradiol and prolactin, is indicated. A single sample of 10 mL of whole blood collected in the morning to minimize diurnal variation is usually adequate [24]. However, because of the pulsatile

The value for calculated free testosterone (CFT) is obtained by joining the value for TT to that for SHBG, and where the line intersects the middle curved scale is the value for CFT.

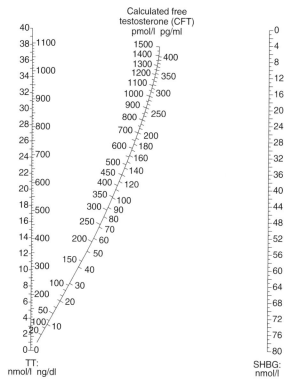

TT: nmol/l ng/dl

SHBG: nmol/l

Fig. 12.2. Nomogram for calculating free testosterone from total testosterone (TT) and sex hormone-binding globulin (SHBG). (Reprinted with permission from Carruthers M. *Androgen Deficiency in the Adult Male: Causes, Diagnosis and Treatment*. London: Taylor & Francis, 2004.)

Table 12.1. Conditions which alter sex hormone-binding globulin (SHBG) levels

Increases SHBG	Decreases SHBG
Estrogens	Androgens
Hyperthyroidism	Hypothyroidism
Aging	Growth hormone excess
Liver disease	Obesity
Anticonvulsants	Glucocorticoid excess

the amount of available SHBG alters the degree of tissue entry of testosterone [27]. Because the serum testosterone measurement includes both the bound and unbound fractions, alterations of SHBG levels may give an inaccurate estimate of the biologically active (free testosterone) concentration. Therefore, the measurement of free (unbound) testosterone is a more accurate marker of physiologically available testosterone than is the measurement of total testosterone level when conditions of altered SHBG concentrations or binding exist [28,29]. Unfortunately, free testosterone assays are often unreliable [30]. Coincident measurement of SHBG and total testosterone is an alternative to measuring free testosterone. The usefulness of the calculated free testosterone index (total testosterone level in nanomoles/L) divided by the SHBG (nanomoles/L) in lieu of a free testosterone measurement is not yet validated clinically [31,32]. A nomogram for calculating free testosterone is provided in Figure 12.2 [31].

Estradiol measurements are ordered when a patient presents with gynecomastia, a testicular mass, or a history consistent with exogenous estrogen exposure. Prolactin measurement is included in the evaluation of a patient with impotence or evidence for a CNS tumor, as well as in men with a relevant drug history. The measurement of DHT is indicated when a disorder of testosterone conversion to DHT is suggested by the clinical presentation.

Measurement of circulating LH and FSH levels allows the clinician to determine if a patient's endocrine dysfunction is the result of primary testicular failure or hypothalamic and/or pituitary deficiency. Because LH secretion is regulated by the inhibitory feedback of circulating testosterone, the measurement of serum LH reflects the adequacy of Leydig cell function in patients with testicular damage. Thus, patients with testicular failure present with elevated LH levels, and patients with hypothalamus/pituitary failure present with diminished levels.

nature of hormone secretion in men, single random measurements of serum levels may not accurately reflect the mean concentration of LH, FSH, and testosterone over a prolonged period of time [25]. Therefore, if an abnormal result is obtained, the patient should be reevaluated with a collection of multiple samples (three samples collected through an indwelling cannula at 20-minute intervals). Pooling three samples provides a more integrated measure of basal hormone secretion [25].

The measurement of free testosterone is included when clinical conditions exist that alter SHBG levels (Table 12.1). Testosterone circulates in the blood loosely bound to albumin and tightly bound to SHBG [26]. The bound testosterone is in equilibrium with the 2% of free or biologically available testosterone that enters the cells and exerts its metabolic effects. A change in

Serum FSH levels reflect the state of the seminiferous epithelium in the infertile man. In men with azoospermia due to severely damaged germ cells, serum FSH levels are usually elevated. Combined elevations of FSH and LH levels are seen in association with severe testicular damage, reflecting a decline in both the tubular (Sertoli and spermatogenic cells) and androgenic functional components of the testes. Stimulation testing of the hypothalamic–pituitary–testicular axis is rarely indicated, because it often yields unreliable results. In azoospermic or severely oligospermic men with normal-sized testes, a normal level of FSH may indicate the presence of post-testicular (epididymis and vas deferens) obstruction of the excretory duct system. Measurement of inhibin levels is not available in most laboratories, but inhibin may be a marker of testicular function [17,33].

An assessment of other pituitary hormones (adrenocorticotropic hormone [ACTH], thyroid-stimulating hormone [TSH], and growth hormone [GH]) is recommended in patients with hypogonadotropic hypogonadism in whom a pituitary tumor is suspected. Assessment of other endocrine organ functions (adrenal, thyroid, parathyroid, pancreas) is recommended in patients suspected of multiple end-organ failure.

Diagnosis and treatment

The differential diagnosis and treatment of endocrine-dependent male-factor infertility is based on the history, physical examination, and reproductive hormone levels. Based on these data, patients can be placed in four major diagnostic categories: (1) hypogonadotropic hypogonadism (secondary hypogonadism), (2) hypergonadotropic hypogonadism or testicular failure (primary hypogonadism), (3) defective androgen synthesis or response, and (4) combined primary and secondary hypogonadism (Fig. 12.3).

Hypogonadotropic hypogonadism (secondary hypogonadism)

Diagnosis

Hypogonadotropic hypogonadism, also referred to as secondary hypogonadism, can occur as the congenital condition idiopathic hypogonadotropic hypogonadism (IHH), or as an acquired condition. Men with hypogonadotropic hypogonadism are deficient in LH and FSH secretion. In the absence of LH and FSH stimulation, the testes secrete low amounts of testosterone, and spermatogenesis is disrupted (Fig. 12.4).

The original description of IHH, referred to as Kallmann syndrome, was of eunuchoidism associated with anosmia and isolated deficiency of GnRH secretion from the hypothalamus [34]. Defective migration of GnRH from the olfactory region to the hypothalamus with mutations of the *KAL1* gene is the mechanism of the impaired secretion of GnRH. This condition has a sex-linked inheritance [35]. Midline facial defects including cleft palate, color blindness, and deafness have been described. Associated renal agenesis and bimanual synkinesis may be present. IHH can also be inherited as an autosomal dominant, autosomal recessive, or GnRH receptor mutation pattern. However, the majority of cases are sporadic [36]. The incidence of the syndrome is about 1 in 10 000 males [37,38].

A variant of congenital hypogonadotropic hypogonadism, referred to as adult-onset or acquired IHH, occurs in men who have normal pubertal development and past fertility. They present with impotence and/or new-onset infertility, with inappropriately low gonadotropins in the face of lower levels of testosterone, often accompanied by oligospermia. This does not appear to be the result of aging, but rather to be a late-onset form of IHH [39].

Rarely, men will present with isolated LH deficiency, a syndrome previously referred to as the fertile eunuch syndrome. Because the absence of LH prevents normal stimulation of the Leydig cells in the testes, testosterone is not produced in adequate amounts to allow normal androgenization, but the normal secretion of FSH stimulates spermatogenesis. Rarely, men present with isolated FSH deficiency and infertility. They are normally androgenized because the LH–testosterone axis is normal [40].

Acquired causes of hypogonadotropic hypogonadism include tumor, infection, infiltrative diseases, autoimmune hypophysitis, pituitary infarction, and drug use. The most common acquired cause is a prolactin-secreting tumor. These tumors in men tend to be macroadenomas at the time of discovery and often are associated with impotence [41,42]. The tumor interferes with gonadotropin secretion by compressing the pituitary tissue and because of prolactin's inhibition of gonadotropin secretion [43]. Pituitary tumors of other cell types (GH, ACTH, FSH), nonsecreting tumors, and craniopharyngiomas act as space-occupying lesions. The associated moderately elevated prolactin is due to the inhibition of dopamine [43].

Measure serum LH, FSH, and T

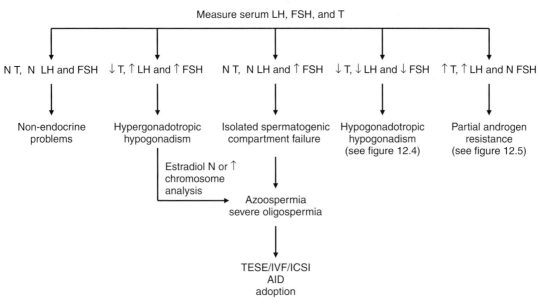

Fig. 12.3. Diagnostic evaluation of man presenting with infertility. LH, luteinizing hormone; FSH, follicle-stimulating hormone; T, testosterone; N, normal; TESE, testicular sperm extraction; IVF, in-vitro fertilization; ICSI, intracytoplasmic sperm injection; AID, artificial insemination donor. (Modified from Sokol RZ, Swerdloff RS. Endocrine evaluation. In: Lipshultz LI, Howards SS, eds. *Infertility in the Male*, 3rd edn. St. Louis, MO: Mosby Year Book, 1997: 210–18.)

Infiltrative diseases that invade the pituitary gland include sarcoidosis, histiocytosis, and infectious granulomatous diseases. Diseases that predispose the patient to increased levels of circulating levels of iron may present with hypogonadotropic hypogonadism due to iron deposition in the pituitary gland. These include hemachromatosis and those diseases that require chronic blood transfusions such as sickle cell anemia and thalassemia. Imaging studies of the hypothalamus and pituitary are necessary to determine if a tumor or infiltrative disease is present [44].

Systemic diseases with chronic malnutrition, rare neurologic disorders, estrogen-producing testicular tumors, and severe obesity may inhibit the hypothalamic–pituitary axis [45,46]. Hypogonadotropic hypogonadism has been reported in men with type 2 diabetes [47].

Patients with congenital adrenal hyperplasia secrete excess adrenal androgens, which suppress endogenous gonadotropin secretion. Thus the testes are not stimulated and spermatogenesis is suppressed. Because of the high circulating adrenal androgens, premature puberty occurs, with premature closure of the epiphyses, leading to shorter stature than genetically expected. Testes shrink, but adrenal rest tumors may be identified on testicular examination [48,49].

A number of drugs can lead to secondary hypogonadism. Drugs and medications that increase prolactin levels by interfering with the dopamine inhibition of prolactin secretion can lead to disruption of gonadotropin secretion. The use or abuse of anabolic steroids also suppresses gonadotropins. In this situation, the patient will have normal or elevated testosterone levels, variable increased estradiol levels, suppressed spermatogenesis, and normal androgenization with possible gynecomastia.

Treatment

Therapy for patients with tumors and infiltrative diseases should be dictated by the underlying pathology prior to treatment with hormone replacement therapy. Because men with hypogonadotropic hypogonadism are deficient in LH and FSH secretion, spermatogenesis can be initiated and pregnancies achieved with exogenous gonadotropins. Selection of the type of hormone therapy, as well as the ultimate success of therapy, depends on the severity of the defect. The most frequently prescribed preparations are human chorionic gonadotropin (hCG) and human menopausal gonadotropin (hMG).

HCG is biologically comparable to LH in that it stimulates Leydig cell synthesis and secretion of testosterone. Treatment with hCG alone in patients with

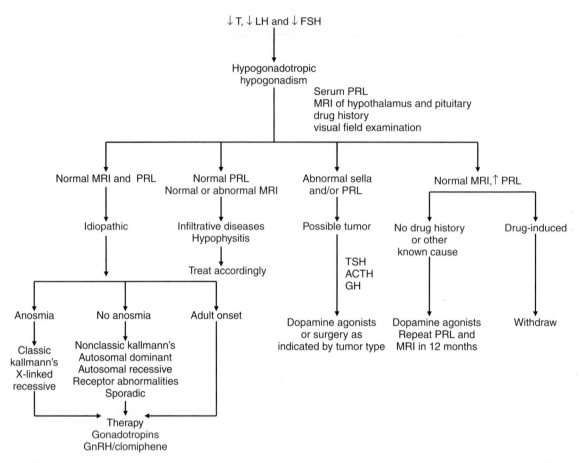

Fig. 12.4. Evaluation and treatment of patient with hypogonadotropic hypogonadism. T, testosterone; LH, luteinizing hormone; FSH, follicle-stimulating hormone; PRL, prolactin; TSH, thyroid-stimulating hormone; ACTH, adrenocorticotropic hormone; GH, growth hormone; MRI, magnetic resonance imaging examination of the sella region. (Modified from Sokol RZ, Swerdloff RS. Endocrine evaluation. In: Lipshultz LI, Howards SS, eds. *Infertility in the Male*, 3rd edn. St. Louis,MO: Mosby Year Book, 1997: 210–18.)

partial gonadotropin deficiency may increase sperm counts and result in pregnancies. HCG is administered at a dosage of 1500–2000 IU 2–3 times per week for 18–24 weeks until normal serum testosterone levels are achieved and there is no further increase in testicular growth or improvement in sperm production. Some patients with partial defects, as well as patients with complete hypogonadism, will require the addition of hMG to their regimens. HMG, which contains both LH and FSH, stimulates spermatogenesis, but only after intratesticular testosterone is brought into the normal range with hCG stimulation. HMG is administered at a dose of 75 IU 2–3 times weekly until pregnancy is achieved. After pregnancy has been achieved and maintained for three months, hMG treatment can be withdrawn and spermatogenesis usually maintained by continued administration of hCG [50].

Patients should be monitored carefully during gonadotropin therapy with monthly testicular examinations, measurement of testosterone and estradiol levels, and semen analysis. The dose is titrated to testicular size and hormone levels. Because hCG therapy stimulates estradiol production directly from the testicle as well as from conversion from testosterone, the normal ratio of testosterone to estradiol is decreased and gynecomastia as well as inhibition of spermatogenesis can occur. Other reported side effects include headaches, breast tenderness, and the development of anti-hCG and LH antibodies [51]. Selected patients may respond to treatment with clomiphene [52]. A few findings of testicular tumor have been reported [53].

If the patient has hypothalamic disease, GnRH therapy is also an option [54]. However, treatment is not user-friendly. GnRH is administered subcutaneously every two hours via continuous pump or by intranasal administration, and is not necessarily more successful in inducing spermatogenesis than is gonadotropin therapy [55–57]. Treatment with recombinant FSH may result in fertility in men with isolated FSH deficiency [40,58]. The efficacy and safety of recombinant FSH are under investigation [53,59–61]. Growth hormone therapy does not play a significant role in the treatment of hypogonadotropic hypogonadism [60,62].

Patients not interested in maintenance of spermatogenesis for fertility are often treated with testosterone replacement (see *Testosterone replacement therapy*, below). Prior chronic treatment of men with hypogonadotropic hypogonadism with testosterone does not affect the subsequent success of gonadotropic therapy [63,64].

Hypergonadotropic hypogonadism (primary hypogonadism)

Diagnosis

Men with hypergonadotropic hypogonadism can be subdivided into two major groups: (1) men with classic hypergonadotropic hypogonadism identified by elevated gonadotropin levels, low testosterone level, and severe oligospermia or azoospermia (testicular failure), and (2) men with spermatogenic failure without Leydig cell failure, who present with elevated serum FSH levels, normal LH and testosterone levels, and oligospermia or azoospermia (primary germ cell failure) (Fig. 12.3).

Klinefelter syndrome, occurring in approximately 1 in 500 men, is the most common cause of classic hypergonadotropic hypogonadism [65]. The classic chromosomal abnormality is 47,XXY. Cardiac abnormalities, cognitive and behavioral problems, and an increased incidence of breast cancer have been reported in Klinefelter patients [66–68]. Patients with karyotypes of XXY/XY or multiple X chromosome mosaicism present with a range of hypogonadal signs and symptoms [69].

Causes of primary germ cell failure include post-pubertal viral or bacterial orchitis, chemotherapeutic agents, idiopathic, and possibly secondary to exposure to environmental toxicants [70].

Treatment

At present, there is no endocrine therapy available for the treatment of infertility in these two groups of men. Artificial insemination with donor semen (AID), adoption, and, in selected cases, in-vitro fertilization (IVF)/intracytoplasmic sperm injection (ICSI) are the current options [71,72]. Recent studies suggest that these patients may benefit from recombinant FSH therapy prior to IVF/ICSI [58,73]. A subset of men with elevated FSH levels, azoospermia, and normal spermatogenesis on biopsy may be candidates for exploratory surgery to rule out an associated obstruction [74]. A small series of men with abnormal testosterone-to-estradiol ratios have been treated with aromatase inhibitors, with some improvement in spermatogenesis [75,76].

The men who present with testicular failure (both an abnormality of spermatogenesis and testosterone production) should be treated with androgens to maintain secondary sexual characteristics. If the patient has not gone through puberty, dosing should start at a lower dose than the full replacement dosage and be slowly titrated up to adult testosterone levels (see *Testosterone replacement therapy*, below).

Defective androgen synthesis or response

5α-reductase deficiency presents with a mild elevation in testosterone, decreased to absent levels of DHT, and normal LH and FSH levels. Because of the failure to convert testosterone to DHT, DHT-sensitive organs do not develop normally. Patients present with a spectrum of ambiguous genitalia, abnormal prostate development, and abnormal virilization at puberty [10,77]. These men usually have sperm production adequate to initiate a pregnancy, but, because of their genital-urinary anatomic defects, intrauterine insemination may be necessary.

Androgen resistance is associated with elevated testosterone and estradiol levels, borderline elevation of LH, and normal FSH (Fig. 12.5). This is due to insensitivity of the androgen receptor to testosterone. Androgen actions are mediated by the androgen receptor, which is encoded by the androgen receptor gene, located on the long arm of the X chromosome at Xq11–12. The androgen receptor gene contains eight axons. Axon one contains a cytosine–adenine–guanine (CAG) repeat, which varies in length in the general population and is inversely correlated with androgen receptor activity. Men with infertility are reported to have a longer CAG repeat length [78,79].

The androgen receptor defect results in a deficient cellular response to testosterone, with a secondary increase in serum LH. Because the testes are continually stimulated by an elevation of serum LH levels, the secretion rate of testosterone may be increased. Androgen receptors in the pituitary gland are also insensitive to the feedback inhibition of testosterone, and LH continues to be secreted in excess [80]. Because testosterone is normally converted to estradiol by aromatization, serum estradiol levels are usually elevated. The altered testosterone-to-estradiol ratio often produces gynecomastia.

The clinical presentation of the patient depends on the severity of the impairment in receptor function [80]. Complete androgen insensitivity (testicular feminization) is manifested as a phenotypic female with normal breast development, scant pubic and axillary hair, primary amenorrhea, and an XY karyotype. Serum testosterone and estradiol levels are markedly elevated, the latter accounting for the normal female body habitus. Patients with partial androgen resistance (Reifenstein syndrome) present with ambiguous genitalia [81]. The mildest form of androgen resistance results in a normal male phenotype, but abnormal spermatogenesis [82]. The frequency of this mildest form is not well established. Diagnosis is suggested on the basis of the hormonal pattern described, but absolute confirmation requires sequencing of the androgen receptor coding gene in specialized laboratories.

Androgen receptor abnormalities are rarely amenable to hormone therapy. No medication is currently available to overcome the defect at the receptor level. Men with partial androgen resistance have variable degrees of hypogonadism and infertility. If sperm are present either in the ejaculate or in the testes, patients may be able to father children via IVF/ICSI.

Combined primary and secondary hypogonadism

The most extensively studied category of combined primary and secondary hypogonadism is that of aging-related alterations in the hypothalamic–pituitary–testicular axis of older men. **A gradual decline in circulating testosterone levels is reported in healthy aging men** [32,83–85] (Figs 12.6, 12.7). This condition, frequently referred to as andropause, is defined as an age-related decline in circulating androgen levels below the normal range for young men, associated with signs and symptoms consistent with androgen deficiency. Although total testosterone and

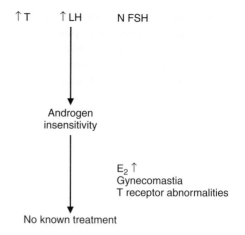

Fig. 12.5. Diagnostic evaluation of a patient with androgen resistance. T, testosterone; LH, luteinizing hormone; FSH, follicle-stimulating hormone; E₂, estradiol; N, normal. (Modified from Sokol RZ, Swerdloff RS. Endocrine evaluation. In: Lipshultz LI, Howards SS, eds. *Infertility in the Male*, 3rd edn. St. Louis, MO: Mosby Year Book, 1997: 210–18.)

bioavailable testosterone are documented to decline with aging in cross-sectional and longitudinal studies, the actual levels of these hormones tend to remain within the normal range for testosterone [84, 86–87]. Testosterone, bioavailable testosterone, and SHBG are estimated to decrease by 0.8%, 2%, and 1.6% per year, respectively [86]. Gonadotropins are reported to either increase or decrease with the testosterone levels [84,88,89]. Hypothalamic dysfunction is suggested by abnormal LH pulse frequency and reduced amplitude [90–92].

Coincident with this decline in testosterone levels is a diminution in libido and a decline in total nocturnal emissions associated with rapid-eye-movement sleep, reduced muscle mass and strength, decreased bone mass with an increased fracture rate, diminished vigor, mood changes, and possibly impaired cognition [83,93]. Chronic or acute illness, malnutrition, and a number of medications can further compromise testosterone production in the aging man.

A diagnostic workup is indicated if the patient presents with signs and symptoms of androgen deficiency. Three screening questionnaires have been developed to uncover the signs and symptoms of androgen deficiency in men: (1) the Androgen Deficiency in Aging Male questionnaire (ADAM), (2) the Massachusetts Male Aging Survey (MMAS), and (3) the Aging Male Survey (AMS) [94–96]. Unfortunately, these questionnaires have a high sensitivity but a low

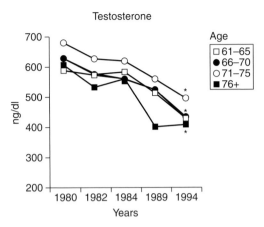

Fig. 12.6. Longitudinal changes in serum testosterone levels in four age cohorts. (From Morley JE *et al.* Longitudinal changes in testosterone, luteinizing hormone, and follicle-stimulating hormone in healthy older men. *Metabolism* 1997; **46**: 410–13. Copyright (1997), with permission from Elsevier.)

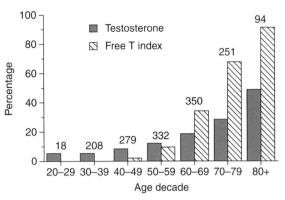

Fig. 12.7. Testosterone (T) and free T index in aging men: percentage of men in each age decade with at least one T value in the hypogonadal range. The numbers above each bar indicate the number of men studied. (From Harman SM *et al.* Longitudinal effects of aging on serum total and free testosterone levels in healthy men. *J Clin Endocrinol Metab* 2001; **86**: 724–31. With permission. Copyright 2001, The Endocrine Society.)

specificity, and correlate poorly with testosterone levels [97].

If the history and physical examination are consistent with a possible decline in circulating testosterone, then the endocrine workup should proceed as already outlined. A total testosterone below 300 µg/dL on two separate occasions is diagnostic. However, most men's testosterone values will fall in the low normal range. Preliminary results of both short-term and longer-term study trials of testosterone therapy in men more than 65 years old are inconclusive regarding the beneficial effects on muscle strength, libido and mood, and bone turnover [98]. In general, the beneficial effects of testosterone replacement are documented in those men with testosterone levels that fall below the normal range [83,99–103]. Few adverse effects have been reported, but long-term risks are uncertain [83,98,104–107].

Replacement therapy in the older man with symptoms of testosterone deficiency, but low normal circulating levels of testosterone continues to be controversial. A number of academic organizations (Endocrine Society, American Society of Andrology, International Society of Andrology, American Society for Reproductive Medicine) have published guidelines, available on their websites, regarding the diagnosis and treatment of age-related testosterone decline. Tables 12.2, 12.3, and 12.4 summarize some of those recommendations.

Testosterone replacement therapy, formulations, dosing, and potential side effects
Formulations and dosing

Testosterone replacement therapy available in the United States includes oral, intramuscular, transdermal, and buccal preparations (Table 12.5) [83]. The efficacy of oral testosterone is limited by its short half-life and potential liver toxicity. A longer-acting buccal preparation is also available.

Intramuscular preparations include both alkylated and esterified testosterone compounds. When injected intramuscularly in oil, they are absorbed more slowly, but hydrolyzed to free testosterone and metabolized the same as the free steroid. The alkylated forms are contraindicated because of their potential hepatotoxicity. Commonly prescribed esterified preparations include testosterone enanthate, testosterone cypionate, and testosterone propionate. Testosterone enanthate and cypionate esters are administered as intramuscular injections of 200 mg every two weeks. Pharmacokinetic studies of these esterified testosterones indicate that peak supraphysiologic levels are reached at 24 hours following injection, with levels falling below eugonadal levels by day 9 and returning to hypogonadal levels by day 14. Circulating estradiol levels follow a similar pattern [108,109].

Table 12.2. Contraindications to testosterone therapy

Prostate cancer
Sleep apnea
Breast cancer
Polycythemia
Significant benign prostatic hypertrophy
Unexplained PSA elevation
Undiagnosed prostate nodule
Unstable severe congestive heart failure

Table 12.3. Baseline evaluation prior to initiation of testosterone therapy

Luteinizing hormone, follicle-stimulating hormone, testosterone, estradiol, prolactin
Complete blood count
Liver function tests
Electrolytes
High-density lipoprotein cholesterol
Low-density lipoprotein cholesterol
Prostate-specific antigen
Consider bone densitometry

Table 12.4. Monitoring of testosterone therapy

Months 3, 6, 9, 12, and then yearly
Complete blood count
Liver function tests
Lipids/cholesterol
Testosterone and estradiol
Prostate-specific antigen levels and digital examination

Transdermal testosterone formulations provide a more physiologic form of androgen therapy. These include a permeation-enhanced nonscrotal testosterone patch and a topical gel. Two formulations of nonscrotal patches are available. One nonscrotal dermal system contains 12.2 mg of testosterone and delivers 2.5 mg of testosterone per 24 hours. Two patches are applied nightly to the abdomen, thighs, back, or upper arm. The 24-hour testosterone pharmacokinetic profiles mimic the normal testosterone of approximately 500 ng/dL [110]. A single large patch delivering 5 mg testosterone and applied daily to nonscrotal skin sites also mimics physiologic testosterone [111]. The testosterone : DHT ratio is normal. Testosterone : estradiol ratios are also physiologic [110].

A topical gel formulation of transdermal testosterone therapy contains 5 g of testosterone to deliver 50 mg of testosterone [112]. The gel is applied once daily to clean, dry, intact skin of the shoulders, upper arms, and/or abdomen and allowed to dry. In hypogonadal men, testosterone levels are increased to the normal range within 30 minutes and steady-state levels are reached within 24 hours. Dosage may be increased to 10 g per day to achieve normal physiologic circulating testosterone levels. A concern with this preparation is the possible transfer of the hormone through skin contact.

Potential side effects of testosterone preparations

Skin

The nonscrotal patch often causes a transient mild to moderate erythema at the application site. Approximately 17–40% of patients in published studies report severe contact dermatitis, chronic skin irritations, or local burn-like blisters [107]. Less skin irritation is reported by patients using the gel. Local pain or irritation at the site of injection is an infrequent occurrence with intramuscular injections. Acne may develop with all forms of androgen therapy.

Testis size and spermatogenesis

By suppressing endogenous gonadotropin secretion, exogenous androgens suppress spermatogenesis, resulting in a significant decrease in testicular volume and suppression of spermatogenesis.

Gynecomastia

Because testosterone is aromatized to estradiol, patients who are treated with exogenous androgens have increased circulating levels of estradiol. If the $T : E_2$ ratio is altered, this may result in gynecomastia. This side effect may be more severe in older men and is observed less often in men using transdermal forms of testosterone replacement than in men using injectable forms [106].

Prostate

Prostatic growth is primarily androgen-dependent. Therefore testosterone replacement therapy is contraindicated in patients with prostatic carcinoma. Those patients with a diagnosis of benign prostatic hypertrophy should be monitored with frequent rectal examinations. Small but significant increases in prostate size and prostate-specific antigen (PSA) are reported in hypogonadal men receiving androgen replacement [107]. To date, there is no evidence that testosterone

Table 12.5. Common testosterone (T) delivery systems

Delivery system	Route	Dose	Peak (hours)	Frequency
Testosterone enanthate/cypionate	Intramuscular	50–200 mg	48–72	2 weeks
Patch	Transdermal	5 mg	3–8	Daily
Gel	Transdermal	2.5–10 g	Flat or 3–10	Daily
Buccal	Oral	30 mg	10–12	q. 12 h

Adapted from Hijazi RA, Cunningham GR. Andropause: is androgen replacement therapy indicated for the aging male? *Ann Rev Med* 2005; **56**: 117–37.

replacement therapy causes prostate cancer; however, because the cancer is androgen-dependent, the concern is that pre-existing disease may become clinically relevant [106,112,113].

Cholesterol and lipid metabolism
An increase in low-density lipoprotein (LDL) cholesterol and a decrease in high-density lipoprotein (HDL) cholesterol are reported with intramuscular therapy. LDL and HDL may be minimally increased with patch therapy. LDL-to-HDL ratios do not change.

Behavior
The relationship between testosterone levels and aggression is controversial. Libido, potency, and depression are reported to improve in aging men taking testosterone replacement [103].

Hepatotoxicity
A number of hepatotoxic effects have been reported with the use of the 17-alkylated testosterone compounds, but not with the use of testosterone esters. These include changes in hepatic enzymes, abnormal bromsulphalein retention, and cholestatic alterations. Hepatomas and peliosis hepatitis have been reported in men with pre-existing serious medical illnesses (Fanconi anemia, aplastic anemia, hematologic malignancies) that may have predisposed them to these tumors.

Alterations in erythropoiesis
Androgens stimulate erythropoiesis, increasing the hemoglobin and hematocrit into the normal range in treated hypogonadal men [107]. Leukocyte and platelet counts may also increase. Smokers and older men appear to be more sensitive to the effects of androgens on erythropoiesis [106].

Miscellaneous
Weight gain secondary to sodium retention and protein anabolism has been reported. Patients with underlying edematous conditions such as congestive heart failure or hepatic cirrhosis may experience worsening edema. Replacement doses may reduce or exacerbate obstructive sleep apnea. These side effects are of particular concern in the older male patient.

Androgen replacement: nonprescription drugs
A number of non-FDA-approved drugs and supplements are marketed as alternative therapies for declining androgens and decreasing libido and potency in older men. These include over-the-counter testosterone or DHT-containing compounds, adrenal androgen formulations, and various herbal preparations. The former can be marketed outside the scope of the Food and Drug Administration (FDA) if the concentration in the daily dose recommended is lower than that regulated by the FDA. The exact potency of these compounds is reported to vary from manufacturer to manufacturer, and between batches produced by the same manufacturer. Minimal scientific data are available on the efficacy of over-the-counter androgen-containing supplements [114–117]. Side effects of long-term use of dehydroepiandrosterone (DHEA) and androstenedione are not known, but elevations in estradiol and DHT may potentially lead to gynecomastia and prostatic enlargement, respectively [118].

Summary
The endocrine evaluation of the male partner is an essential part of the workup of the infertile couple. A careful history, physical examination, and laboratory assessment, guided by an understanding of the physiology of the hypothalamic–pituitary–testicular axis, will allow the clinician to ascertain a diagnosis and an appropriate treatment plan.

References
[1] Baker HWG, Burger HG, de Kretser DM, Hudson B. Relative incidence of etiologic disorders in male

infertility. In: Santen RJ, Swerdloff RS, eds. *Male Reproductive Dysfunctions.* New York, NY: Marcel Dekker, 1996: 341–72.

[2] de Kretser DM. Male infertility. *Lancet* 1997; **349**: 787–90.

[3] Jequier AM, Holmes SC. Primary testicular disease presenting as azoospermia or oligozoospermia in an infertility clinic. *Br J Urol* 1993; **71**: 731–5.

[4] Barraclough CA, Wise PM. The role of catecholamines in the regulation of pituitary luteinizing hormone and follicle-stimulating hormone secretion. *Endocr Rev* 1982; **3**: 91–119.

[5] Kalra SP, Kalra PS. Neural regulation of luteinizing hormone secretion in the rat. *Endocr Rev* 1983; **4**: 311–51.

[6] Plant TM. Gonadal regulation of hypothalamic gonadotropin-releasing hormone release in primates. *Endocr Rev* 1986; **7**: 75–88.

[7] Veldhuis JD, King JC, Urban RJ, *et al.* Operating characteristics of the male hypothalamo-pituitary-gonadal axis: Pulsatile release of testosterone and follicle-stimulating hormone and their temporal coupling with luteinizing hormone. *J Clin Endocrinol Metab* 1987; **65**: 929–41.

[8] Jarow JP, Zirkin BR. The androgen microenvironment of the human testis and hormonal control of spermatogenesis. *Ann N Y Acad Sci* 2005; **1061**: 208–20.

[9] Ito T, Horton R. The source of plasma dihydrotestosterone in man. *J Clin Invest* 1971; **50**: 1621–7 .

[10] Wilson JD, Griffin JE, Russell DW. Steroid 5α-reductase 2 deficiency. *Endocr Rev* 1993; **14**: 577–93.

[11] Longcope C, Sato K, McKay C, Horton R. Aromatization by splanchnic tissue in men. *J Clin Endocrinol Metab* 1984; **58**: 1089–93.

[12] Santen RJ. Is aromatization of testosterone to estradiol required for inhibition of luteinizing hormone secretion in men? *J Clin Invest* 1975; **56**: 1555–63.

[13] Winters SJ, Troen P. Evidence for a role of endogenous estrogen in the hypothalamic control of gonadotropin secretion in men. *J Clin Endocrinol Metab* 1985; **61**: 842–5.

[14] McCullagh DR. Dual endocrine activity of the testes. *Science* 1932; **76**: 19–20.

[15] Ying SY. Inhibins, activins, and follistatins: gonadal proteins modulating the secretion of follicle-stimulating hormone. *Endocr Rev* 1988; **9**: 267–93.

[16] de Jong FH, Robertson DM. Inhibin: 1985 update on action and purification. *Mol Cell Endocrinol* 1985; **42**: 95–103.

[17] Kolb BA, Stanczyk FZ, Sokol RZ. Serum inhibin B levels in males with gonadal dysfunction. *Fertil Steril* 2000; **74**: 234–8.

[18] Tong S, Wallace EM, Burger HG. Inhibins and activins: clinical advances in reproductive medicine. *Clin Endocrinol (Oxf)* 2003; **58**: 115–27.

[19] Gillam MP, Molitch ME, Lombardi G, Colao A. Advances in the treatment of prolactinomas. *Endocr Rev* 2006; **27**: 485–534.

[20] Sokol RZ, Swerdloff RS. Endocrine evaluation. In: Lipshultz LI, Howards SS, eds. *Infertility in the Male*, 3rd edn. St. Louis, MO: Mosby Year Book, 1997: 210–18.

[21] Braunstein GD. Gynecomastia. *N Engl J Med* 1993; **328**: 490–5.

[22] Ismail AA, Barth JH. Endocrinology of gynaecomastia. *Ann Clin Biochem* 2001; **38**: 596–607.

[23] Mathur R, Braunstein GD. Gynecomastia: pathomechanisms and treatment strategies. *Horm Res* 1997; **48**: 95–102.

[24] Bain J, Langevin R, D'Costa M, Sanders RM, Hucker S. Serum pituitary and steroid hormone levels in the adult male: one value is as good as the mean of three. *Fertil Steril* 1988; **49**: 123–6.

[25] Santen RJ, Bardin CW. Episodic luteinizing hormone secretion in man: pulse analysis, clinical interpretation, physiologic mechanisms. *J Clin Invest* 1973; **52**: 2617–28.

[26] Pardridge WM. Transport of protein-bound hormones into tissues *in vivo. Endocr Rev* 1981; **2**: 103–23.

[27] Dunn JF, Nisula BC, Rodbard D. Transport of steroid hormones: binding of 21 endogenous steroids to both testosterone-binding globulin and corticosteroid-binding globulin in human plasma. *J Clin Endocrinol Metab* 1981; **53**: 58–68.

[28] Glass AR, Swerdloff RS, Bray GA, Dahms WT, Atkinson RL. Low serum testosterone and sex-hormone-binding-globulin in massively obese men. *J Clin Endocrinol Metab* 1977; **45**: 1211–19.

[29] Pugeat MM, Dunn JF, Nisula BC. Transport of steroid hormones: interaction of 70 drugs with testosterone-binding globulin and corticosteroid-binding globulin in human plasma. *J Clin Endocrinol Metab* 1981; **53**: 69–75.

[30] Vermeulen A, Verdonck L, Kaufman JM. A critical evaluation of simple methods for the estimation of free testosterone in serum. *J Clin Endocrinol Metab* 1999; **84**: 3666–72.

[31] Carruthers M. *Androgen Deficiency in the Adult Male: Causes, Diagnosis and Treatment.* London: Taylor & Francis, 2004.

[32] Harman SM, Metter EJ, Tobin JD, Pearson J, Blackman MR. Longitudinal effects of aging on serum

total and free testosterone levels in healthy men. *J Clin Endocrinol Metab* 2001; **86**: 724–31.

[33] Fernández-Arjona M, Díaz J, Cortes I, *et al.* Relationship between gonadotrophin secretion, inhibin B and spermatogenesis in oligozoospermic men treated with highly purified urinary follicle-stimulating hormone (uFSH-HP): a preliminary report. *Eur J Obstet Gynecol Reprod Biol* 2003; **107**: 47–51.

[34] Kallmann FJ, Schoenfeld WA. The genetic aspects of primary eunuchoidism. *Am J Ment Def* 1944; **158**: 203–36.

[35] Trarbach EB, Baptista MTM, Garmes HM, Hackel C. Molecular analysis of KAL-1, GnRH-R, NELF and EBF2 genes in a series of Kallmann syndrome and normosmic hypogonadotropic hypogonadism patients. *J Endocrinol* 2005; **187**: 361–8.

[36] Oliveira LMB, Seminara SB, Beranova M, *et al.* The importance of autosomal genes in Kallmann syndrome: genotype–phenotype correlations and neuroendocrine characteristics. *J Clin Endocrinol Metab* 2001; **86**: 1532–8.

[37] Bhagavath B, Podolsky RH, Ozata M, *et al.* Clinical and molecular characterization of a large sample of patients with hypogonadotropic hypogonadism. *Fertil Steril* 2006; **85**: 706–13.

[38] Santen RJ, Paulsen CA. Hypogonadotropic eunuchoidism. I. Clinical study of the mode of inheritance. *J Clin Endocrinol Metab* 1973; **36**: 47–54.

[39] Nachtigall LB, Boepple PA, Pralong FP, Crowley WF. Adult-onset idiopathic hypogonadotropic hypogonadism: a treatable form of male infertility. *N Engl J Med* 1997; **336**: 410–15.

[40] Giltay JC, Deege M, Blankenstein RA, *et al.* Apparent primary follicle-stimulating hormone deficiency is a rare cause of treatable male infertility. *Fertil Steril* 2004; **81**: 693–6.

[41] Carter JN, Tyson JE, Tolis G, *et al.* Prolactin-screening tumors and hypogonadism in 22 men. *N Engl J Med* 1978; **299**: 847–52.

[42] Franks S, Jacobs HS, Martin N, Nabarro JD. Hyperprolactinaemia and impotence. *Clin Endocrinol (Oxf)* 1978; **8**: 277–87.

[43] Ben-Jonathan N. Dopamine. a prolactin-inhibiting hormone. *Endocr Rev* 1985; **6**: 564–89.

[44] Bayrak A, Saadat P, Mor E, *et al.* Pituitary imaging is indicated for the evaluation of hyperprolactinemia. *Fertil Steril* 2005; **84**: 181–5.

[45] Hammoud AO, Gibson M, Peterson CM, Hamilton BD, Carrell DT. Obesity and male reproductive potential. *J Androl* 2006; **27**: 619–26.

[46] Plymate SR. Male hypogonadism. In: Becker KI, ed. *Principles and Practice of Endocrinology and Metabolism*. Philadelphia, PA: Lippincott, 1995: 1056–82.

[47] Dhindsa S, Prabhakar S, Sethi M, *et al.* Frequent occurrence of hypogonadotropic hypogonadism in type 2 diabetes. *J Clin Endocrinol Metab* 2004; **89**: 5462–8.

[48] Bonaccorsi AC, Adler I, Figueiredo JG. Male infertility due to congenital adrenal hyperplasia: testicular biopsy findings, hormonal evaluation, and therapeutic results in three patients. *Fertil Steril* 1987; **47**: 664–70.

[49] Stikkelbroeck NM, Otten BJ, Pasic A, *et al.* High prevalence of testicular adrenal rest tumors, impaired spermatogenesis, and Leydig cell failure in adolescent and adult males with congenital adrenal hyperplasia. *J Clin Endocrinol Metab* 2001; **86**: 5721–8.

[50] Sokol RZ. Male factor infertility. In: Lobo RA, Mishell DR, Paulson RJ, Shoupe D, eds. *Infertility, Contraception, and Reproductive Endocrinology*, 4th edn. Malden MA: Blackwell, 1997: 547–66.

[51] Sokol RZ, McClure RD, Peterson M, Swerdloff RS. Gonadotropin therapy failure secondary to human chorionic gonadotropin-induced antibodies. *J Clin Endocrinol Metab* 1981; **52**: 929–32.

[52] Whitten SJ, Nangia AK, Kolettis PN. Select patients with hypogonadotropic hypogonadism may respond to treatment with clomiphene citrate. *Fertil Steril* 2006; **86**: 1664–8.

[53] Fukagai T, Kurosawa K, Sudo N, *et al.* Bilateral testicular tumors in an infertile man previously treated with follicle-stimulating hormones. *Urology* 2005; **65**: 592.e16–18.

[54] Hoffman AR, Crowley WF. Induction of puberty in men by long-term pulsatile administration of low-dose gonadotropin-releasing hormone. *N Engl J Med* 1982; **307**: 1237–41.

[55] Kliesch S, Behre HM, Nieschlag E. High efficacy of gonadotropin or pulsatile gonadotropin-releasing hormone treatment in hypogonadotropic hypogonadal men. *Eur J Endocrinol* 1994; **131**: 347–54.

[56] Klingmuller D, Schweikert HU. Maintenance of spermatogenesis by intranasal administration of gonadotropin-releasing hormone in patients with hypothalamic hypogonadism. *J Clin Endocrinol Metab* 1985; **61**: 868–72.

[57] Skarin G, Nillius SJ, Wibell L, Wide L. Chronic pulsatile low dose GnRH therapy for induction of testosterone production and spermatogenesis in a man with secondary hypogonadotropic hypogonadism. *J Clin Endocrinol Metab* 1982; **55**: 723–6.

[58] Attia AM, Al-Inany HG, Proctor ML. Gonadotrophins for idiopathic male factor subfertility. *Cochrane Database Syst Rev* 2006; (1): CD005071.

[59] Bouloux P, Warne DW, Loumaye E, FSH Study Group in Men's Infertility. Efficacy and safety of recombinant human follicle-stimulating hormone in men with

isolated hypogonadotropic hypogonadism. *Fertil Steril* 2002; **77**: 270–3.

[60] Liu PY, Handelsman DJ. The present and future state of hormonal treatment for male infertility. *Hum Reprod Update* 2003; **9**: 9–23.

[61] Liu PY, Turner L, Rushford D, *et al.* Efficacy and safety of recombinant human follicle stimulating hormone (Gonal-F) with urinary human chorionic gonadotrophin for induction of spermatogenesis and fertility in gonadotrophin-deficient men. *Hum Reprod* 1999; **14**: 1540–5.

[62] Shoham Z, Conway CS, Ostergaard H, *et al.* Cotreatment with growth hormone for induction of spermatogenesis in patients with hypogonadotropic hypogonadism. *Fertil Steril* 1992; **57**: 1044–51.

[63] Hammar M, Berg AA. Long term androgen replacement therapy does not preclude gonadotrophin-induced improvement on spermatogenesis. *Scand J Urol Nephrol* 1990; **24**: 17–19.

[64] Ley SB, Leonard JM. Male hypogonadotropic hypogonadism: factors influencing response to human chorionic gonadotropin and human menopausal gonadotropin, including prior endogenous androgens. *J Clin Endocrinol Metab* 1985; **61**: 746–52.

[65] Bojesen A, Juul S, Gravholt CH. Prenatal and postnatal prevalence of Klinefelter syndrome: a national registry study. *J Clin Endocrinol Metab* 2003; **88**: 622–6.

[66] Bojesen A, Juul S, Birkebaek NH, Gravholt CH. Morbidity in Klinefelter syndrome: a Danish register study based on hospital discharge diagnoses. *J Clin Endocrinol Metab* 2006; **91**: 1254–60.

[67] Simm PJ, Zacharin MR. The psychosocial impact of Klinefelter syndrome: a year review. *J Pediatr Endocrinol Metab* 2006; **19**: 499–505.

[68] Weiss JR, Moysich KB, Swede H. Epidemiology of male breast cancer. *Cancer Epidemiol Biomarkers Prev* 2005; **14**: 20–6.

[69] Vernaeve V, Staessen C, Verheyen G, *et al.* Can biological or clinical parameters predict testicular sperm recovery in 47,XXY Klinefelter's syndrome patients? *Hum Reprod* 2004; **19**: 1135–9.

[70] Sokol RZ. Environmental toxins and male fertility. In: Kandeel F, ed. *Male Reproductive Dysfunction: Pathophysiology and Treatment.* New York, NY: Informa Healthcare, 2007: 203–7.

[71] Schiff JD, Palermo GD, Veeck LL, *et al.* Success of testicular sperm injection and intracytoplasmic sperm injection in men with Klinefelter syndrome. *J Clin Endocrinol Metab* 2005; **90**: 6263–7.

[72] Zitzmann M, Nordhoff V, von Schönfeld V, *et al.* Elevated follicle-stimulating hormone levels and the chances for azoospermic men to become fathers after retrieval of elongated spermatids from cryopreserved testicular tissue. *Fertil Steril* 2006; **86**: 339–47.

[73] Foresta C, Bettella A, Garolla A, Ambrosini G, Ferlin A. Treatment of male idiopathic infertility with recombinant human follicle-stimulating hormone: a prospective, controlled, randomized clinical study. *Fertil Steril* 2005; **84**: 654–61.

[74] Hauser R, Temple-Smith PD, Southwick GJ, de Kretser D. Fertility in cases of hypergonadotropic azoospermia. *Fertil Steril* 1995; **63**: 631–6.

[75] Pavlovich CP, King P, Goldstein M, Schlegel PN. Evidence of a treatable endocrinopathy in infertile men. *J Urol* 2001; **165**: 837–41.

[76] Raman JD, Schlegel PN. Aromatase inhibitors for male infertility. *J Urol* 2002; **167**: 624–9.

[77] Johnson L, George FW, Neaves WB, *et al.* Characterization of the testicular abnormality in 5α-reductase deficiency. *J Clin Endocrinol Metab* 1986; **63**: 1091–9.

[78] Dowsing AT, Yong EL, Clark M, *et al.* Linkage between male infertility and trinucleotide repeat expansion in the androgen-receptor gene. *Lancet* 1999; **354**: 640–3.

[79] Davis-Dao CA, Tuazon ED, Sokol RZ, Cortessis VK. Male infertility and variation in CAG repeat length in the androgen receptor gene: a meta-analysis. *J Clin Endocrinol Metab* 2007; **92**: 4319–26.

[80] Griffin JE. Androgen resistance: the clinical and molecular spectrum. *N Engl J Med* 1992; **326**: 611–18.

[81] Wilson JD. Roosters, Reifenstein's syndrome and hormone resistance. *N Engl J Med* 1977; **297**: 386–7.

[82] Aiman J, Griffin JE. The frequency of androgen receptor deficiency in infertile men. *J Clin Endocrinol Metab* 1982; **54**: 725–32.

[83] Hijazi RA, Cunningham GR. Andropause: is androgen replacement therapy indicated for the aging male? *Ann Rev Med* 2005; **56**: 117–37.

[84] Morley JE, Kaiser FE, Perry HM, *et al.* Longitudinal changes in testosterone, luteinzing hormone, and follicle-stimulating hormone in healthy older men. *Metabolism* 1997; **46**: 410–13.

[85] Travison TG, Araujo AB, Kupelian V, O'Donnell AB, McKinlay JB. The relative contributions of aging, health, and lifestyle factors to serum testosterone decline in men. *J Clin Endocrinol Metab* 2007; **92**: 549–55.

[86] Feldman HA, Longcope C, Derby CA, *et al.* Age trends in the level of serum testosterone and other hormones in middle-aged men: longitudinal results from the Massachusetts Male Aging Study. *J Clin Endocrinol Metab* 2002; **87**: 589–98.

[87] Gray A, Feldman HA, McKinlay JB, Longcope C. Age, disease, and changing sex hormone levels in middle-aged men: results of the Massachusetts Male Aging Study. *J Clin Endocrinol Metab* 1991; **73**: 1016–25.

[88] Harman SM, Tsitouras PD. Reproductive hormones in aging men. I. Measurement of sex steroids, basal

luteinizing hormone, and Leydig cell response to human chorionic gonadotropin. *J Clin Endocrinol Metab* 1980; **51**: 35–40.

[89] Korenman SG, Morley JE, Mooradian AD, *et al.* Secondary hypogonadism in older men: its relation to impotence. *J Clin Endocrinol Metab* 1990; **71**: 963–9.

[90] Deslypere JP, Kaufman JM, Vermeulen T, *et al.* Influence of age on pulsatile luteinizing hormone release and responsiveness of the gonadotrophs to sex hormone feedback in men. *J Clin Endocrinol Metab* 1987; **64**: 68–73.

[91] Luboshitzky R, Shen-Orr Z, Herer P. Middle-aged men secrete less testosterone at night than young healthy men. *J Clin Endocrinol Metab* 2003; **88**: 3160–6.

[92] Tenover JS, Matsumoto AM, Clifton DK, Bremner WJ. Age-related alterations in the circadian rhythms of pulsatile luteinizing hormone and testosterone secretion in healthy men. *J Gerontol* 1988; **43**: M163–9.

[93] Haren MT, Wittert GA, Chapman IM, Coates P, Morley JE. Effect of oral testosterone undecanoate on visuospatial cognition, mood and quality of life in elderly men with low-normal gonadal status. *Maturitas* 2005; **50**: 124–33.

[94] Heineman AJ, Zimmermann J, Vermeulen A, Thiel C. A new aging males' symptoms (AMS) rating scale. *Aging Male* 1998; **2**: 105–14.

[95] Morley JE, Charlton E, Patrick P, *et al.* Validation of a screening questionnaire for androgen deficiency in aging males. *Metabolism* 2000; **49**: 1239–43.

[96] Smith KW, Feldman HA, McKinlay JB. Construction and field validation of a self-administered screener for testosterone deficiency (hypogonadism) in ageing men. *Clin Endocrinol* (Oxf) 2000; **53**: 703–11.

[97] Morley JE, Perry HM, Kevorkian RT, Patrick P. Comparison of screening questionnaires for the diagnosis of hypogonadism. *Maturitas* 2006; **53**: 424–9.

[98] Bhasin S, Cunningham GR, Hayes FJ, *et al.* Clinical practice guideline: testosterone therapy in adult men with androgen deficiency syndromes: An Endocrine Soceity clinical practice guideline. *J Clin Endocrinol Metab* 2006; **91**: 1995–2010.

[99] Aminorroaya A, Kelleher S, Conway AJ, Ly LP, Handelsman DJ. Adequacy of androgen replacement influences bone density response to testosterone in androgen-deficient men. *Eur J Endocrinol* 2005; **152**: 881–6.

[100] Finas D, Bals-Pratsch M, Sandmann J, *et al.* Quality of life in elderly men with androgen deficiency. *Andrologia* 2006; **38**: 48–53.

[101] Snyder PJ, Peachey H, Hannoush P, *et al.* Effect of testosterone treatment on bone mineral density in men over 65 years of age. *J Clin Endocrinol Metab* 1999; **84**: 1966–72.

[102] Snyder PJ, Peachey H, Hannoush P, *et al.* Effect of testosterone treatment on body composition and muscle strength in men over 65 years of age. *J Clin Endocrinol Metab* 1999; **84**: 2647–53.

[103] Wang C, Cunningham G, Dobs A, *et al.* Long-term testosterone gel (AndroGel®) treatment maintains beneficial effects on sexual function and mood, lean and fat mass, and bone mineral density in hypogonadal men. *J Clin Endocrinol Metab* 2004; **89**: 2085–98.

[104] Bhasin S, Bagatell CJ, Bremner WJ, *et al.* Issues in testosterone replacement in older men. *J Clin Endocrinol Metab* 1998; **83**: 3435–45.

[105] Snyder PJ. Effects of age on testicular function and consequences of testosterone treatment. *J Clin Endocrinol Metab* 2001; **86**: 2369–72.

[106] Tenover JL. Male hormone replacement therapy including "andropause." *Endocrinol Metab Clin North Am* 1998; **27**: 969–87.

[107] Calof OM, Singh AB, Lee ML, *et al.* Adverse events associated with testosterone replacement in middle-aged and older men: a meta-analysis of randomized, placebo-controlled trials. *J Gerontol* 2005; **60A**: 1451–7.

[108] Snyder PJ, Lawrence DA. Treatment of male hypogonadism with testosterone enanthate. *J Clin Endocrinol Metab* 1980; **51**: 1335–9.

[109] Sokol RZ, Palacios A, Campfield LA, Saul C, Swerdloff RS. Comparison of the kinetics of injectable testosterone in eugonadal and hypogonadal men. *Fertil Steril* 1982; **37**: 425–30.

[110] Meikle AW, Arver S, Dobs AS, *et al.* Pharmacokinetics and metabolism of a permeation-enhanced testosterone transdermal system in hypogonadal men: influence of application site. A clinical research center study. *J Clin Endocrinol Metab* 1996; **81**: 1832–40.

[111] Yu Z, Gupta SK, Hwang SS, *et al.* Testosterone pharmacokinetics after application of an investigational transdermal system in hypogonadal men. *J Clin Pharmacol* 1997; **37**: 1139–45.

[112] Swerdloff RS, Wang C, Cunningham G, *et al.* Long-term pharmacokinetics of transdermal testosterone gel in hypogonadal men. *J Clin Endocrinol Metab* 2000; **85**: 4500–10.

[113] Morales A. Monitoring androgen replacement therapy: testosterone and prostate safety. *J Endocrinol Invest* 2005; **28** (3 Suppl): 122–7.

[114] Genazzani AR, Inglese S, Lombardi I, *et al.* Long-term low-dose dehydroepiandrosterone replacement

therapy in aging males with partial androgen deficiency. *Aging Male* 2004; **7**: 133–43.

[115] Morales AJ, Haubrich RH, Hwang JY, Asakura H, Yen SS. The effect of six months treatment with a 100 mg daily dose of dehydroepiandrosterone (DHEA) on circulating sex steroids, body composition and muscle strength in age-advanced men and women. *Clin Endocrinol (Oxf)* 1998; **49**: 421–32.

[116] Morales AJ, Nolan JJ, Nelson JC, Yen SS. Effects of replacement dose of dehydroepiandrosterone in men

and women of advancing age. *J Clin Endocrinol Metab* 1994; **78**: 1360–7.

[117] Nair KS, Rizza RA, O'Brien P, *et al*. DHEA in elderly women and DHEA or testosterone in elderly men. *N Engl J Med* 2006; **355**: 1647–59.

[118] Acacio BD, Stanczyk FZ, Mullin P, *et al*. Pharmacokinetics of dehydroepiandrosterone and its metabolites after long-term daily oral administration to healthy young men. *Fertil Steril* 2004; **81**: 595–604.

Chapter 13

Testicular biopsy in male infertility evaluation

Joseph P. Alukal, Mohit Khera, and Thomas M. Wheeler

Introduction

The testicular biopsy is one of the cornerstone surgical procedures in male reproductive surgery. It is both diagnostic and therapeutic, and while many technical modifications to the testis biopsy have been made over the past 70 years [1–3] the fundamental principles of the operation remain unchanged. **The testis biopsy offers the andrologist the opportunity to confirm the diagnosis of obstructive azoospermia, diagnose testis failure, and obtain histologic information regarding the oligospermic patient using one relatively benign operation. At the same time, the procedure allows for the extraction of any sperm identified during its course; it is this fact that has allowed for the successful treatment of millions of couples with severe male-factor infertility using intracytoplasmic sperm injection (ICSI) [4].**

As a result of the therapeutic nature of the testis biopsy when utilized as an adjunct treatment to IVF/ICSI, pressure has mounted to investigate less invasive techniques of testis biopsy. These procedures include percutaneous needle aspiration and mapping of the testis [5]. This demand is countered by efforts to increase sensitivity of biopsies with regard to the identification and extraction of any existing sperm in the severely oligospermic or virtually azoospermic patient [3,6]. The microdissection testicular sperm extraction technique (micro-TESE) is a result of this effort (Fig. 13.1); usage of an operating microscope during open testis biopsy increases the likelihood of finding sperm that can be used for IVF/ICSI.

Importantly, these two examples of modifications to the testis biopsy, with somewhat opposite goals, illustrate the continued need for a systematic approach to the histologic interpretation of testis biopsies. Application of existing technology, including flow cytometry, immunohistochemistry/immunofluorescence, and nucleic acid hybridization, to analyze and

interpret the testis biopsy continues to generate new and meaningful information regarding the pathophysiology in the infertile male. Also promising is the experimental application of *new* techniques including in-vivo near-infrared imaging and optical coherence tomography as adjuncts to the histologic assessment of the testis. These innovative techniques, although not yet ready for use in humans, represent the frontier in testis biopsy. Using these techniques, the goal of highly sensitive, noninvasive "virtual" testis biopsy with successful identification of sperm for targeted extraction can be achieved. Without a thorough understanding of the histology of the testis in normal and diseased patients, however, these future goals will remain unachievable.

This chapter will outline the relevant histologic features of both abnormal and normal testis biopsies. In addition, this chapter will include a review of the existing techniques for performing testis biopsy along with the indications for performing the procedure. As part of this review, a brief discussion of the evaluation of the infertile male and the role of testis biopsy in this evaluation is included. Finally, existing and new technologies that are being applied to testis biopsy, in addition to promising future technologies, will be reviewed.

Techniques

As previously stated, there exist numerous acceptable surgical techniques for obtaining testis tissue; moreover, there are well-understood trade-offs with regard to invasiveness and the quality of the specimen obtained, depending on the chosen technique. **Therefore, certain techniques become more or less appropriate for use, given the characteristics of the patient in question. Included here are descriptions of standard open testis biopsy (with or without the operating microscope and through use of the "window" technique when appropriate) and fine-needle aspiration/percutaneous biopsy of the testis. Also**

Infertility in the Male, 4th edition, ed. Larry I. Lipshultz, Stuart S. Howards, and Craig S. Niederberger. Published by Cambridge University Press. © Cambridge University Press 2009.

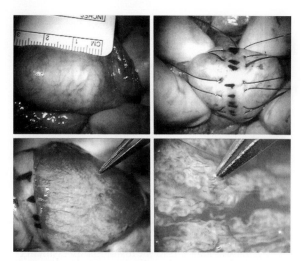

Fig. 13.1. Images from microdissection TESE (testicular sperm extraction). Top left: testis delivered into field, ruler for scale. Top right: preparation for incision in tunica albuginea; holding stitches of 5–0 chromic placed in tunica; horizontal incision marked. Bottom left: incision in tunica albuginea made, testis bivalved. Bottom right: image of same field through operative microscope (× 25), demonstrating tubules for extraction. *See color plate section.*

included is a brief description of the appropriate indications for usage of each technique.

Standard open surgical biopsy

Testis biopsy can be performed with conscious sedation, general anesthesia, or local anesthesia alone if preferred. If the procedure is performed under local anesthesia alone, a cord block in addition to a skin block at the area of the incision is typically adequate; 1% lidocaine (with or without 0.5% bupivacaine for longer-acting anesthesia) is used. **After the surgical site is properly prepared, and with the anterior scrotal skin kept on tension, a horizontal incision of 2–3 cm is made through the skin and subcutaneous tissue (dartos) to the parietal layer of the tunica vaginalis. (A vertical incision can also be used, with the potential benefit being the ability to extend the incision towards the inguinal canal if need be.) This layer is sharply divided, and the testis is delivered into the field.** A small incision (less than 1 cm) is made in the tunica albuginea using a #11 blade. Gentle pressure is then applied to the testis, and any testicular parenchyma that is extruded through the tunical opening is then excised using fine scissors (curved Iris) and set aside in an appropriate fixative or buffer, depending on the intended purpose of obtaining the biopsy. A further discussion of fixatives and buffers will follow; those typically used include Bouin's fixative for

histologic examination, and human tubal fluid for sperm extraction. If an adequate specimen has been obtained, hemostasis is achieved using electrocautery, and then the tunical opening is closed using a running fine absorbable suture (0000 chromic). The tunica vaginalis, dartos, and skin are then closed in an identical fashion. A dressing of loose gauze and a supportive garment are typically applied.

Modifications to this technique include the use of the operating microscope; this procedure is termed *microdissection testicular sperm extraction* (micro-TESE). As first described by Schlegel [3], a dual-headed operating microscope is utilized to provide magnification of 20–25×. A technique identical to that described above is used to deliver the testis into the field in a sterile fashion (care is taken to drape the microscope so that it is sterile). A larger tunical opening is made, preferably in an avascular plane, the entire testicular parenchyma exposed, and the microscope used to identify grossly normal-appearing tubules for biopsy. The opacity, color, and size of the tubules are used to decide which tubules are more likely to harbor sperm. The goals of this procedure are maximization of the likelihood of success with each procedure while minimizing unnecessarily excised testis tissue. In 684 men with nonobstructive azoospermia, Schlegel and colleagues achieved successful sperm extraction in 61% of patients.

An equally important modification to the open testis biopsy is the "window" technique. Using a smaller incision (less than 1 cm) and an eyelid retractor to provide adequate exposure, a technique like the one described above is employed to take a biopsy, with the important difference being that the testis is not delivered through the incision. The benefits of this procedure include decreased morbidity, with regard to both the size of the incision and the amount of testis tissue removed. The procedure is ideally reserved for the patient who has undergone a previous successful testis biopsy or mapping procedure; in this patient, a repeat "window" biopsy can be targeted to regions of the testis in which sperm were previously found.

Fine-needle aspiration/percutaneous testis biopsy

There are obvious trade-offs to percutaneous biopsy of the testis. Benefits of the procedure include the fact that it can be safely performed in the office and its relatively low morbidity to the patient. To its detriment is the fact that less meaningful information (primarily cyto-logical rather than histological) is returned from the procedure, simply because of the disorganized nature of the harvested tissue and the smaller amount of tissue returned. Despite this, an earlier series demonstrated that percutaneous biopsy correlated well with open biopsy [7].

Described methodologies for this procedure include use of the Tru-Cut biopsy needle, the Biopty gun, or a simple aspiration setup including a 23g butterfly needle [8–13]. All of these methodologies can be used safely with local anesthetic alone.

A by-product of the refinement of needle biopsy techniques in the testis is *fine-needle aspiration* (FNA) for systematic mapping of sites of active spermato-genesis. This technique was initially described by Turek *et al.* [5]; further refinements of this technique have also been generated from this group. A standard-ized technique of obtaining 20–30 needle aspirations is utilized. Numerous independent assessments of this technique have demonstrated that its utility is compar-able to that of open testis biopsy in terms of successful extraction of sperm from patients with azoospermia or severe oligospermia [14]. However, some disagree-ment continues to appear in the literature regarding this point. A prospective study from Scotland found increased success with extracting sperm through open biopsy as opposed to FNA mapping when the two methods were used in two comparable cohorts of patients with azoospermia [15].

Cytological assessment of biopsy or aspirate spe-cimens can be performed in several ways. The simplest, and perhaps least accurate, is a wet-prep cytologi-cal examination [16]. A wet-prep slide is prepared by placing a small sample of testis tissue on a microscope slide with a small amount of Ringer's lactate solution. A coverslip is applied and the slide is examined using a light (preferably phase) microscope. The relative ease of performing this assessment allows for its use in the operating room; ideally, a wet-prep examination can confirm that there are mature spermatozoa present in a biopsy. Unfortunately, wet-prep cytologies do not, of course, return any histologic information about the germinal epithelium, tubular architecture, or testicular interstitium.

More accurate cytological assessments can be obtained using touch-prep techniques (with H&E, Pap, or DiffQuick staining [17]) or cytocentrifugation. Both are more labor-intensive than wet-prep examinations, but they can return more meaningful histological information than wet-prep cytology.

Pathological classification of biopsy findings

Crucially important to understanding the histological appearance of a testis biopsy is an awareness of sperm-atogenesis and its progression (for further detail, refer to Chapter 5 on spermatogenesis). Cross sections of sem-iniferous tubules show samples of maturing germ cells at some point along the spermatogenic "wave." In other words, as clonal cells in a syncytium progress through spermatogenesis, they occupy adjoining spaces within tubules, and they are therefore more likely to be sam-pled together on one cross section. **In the human tes-tis, cross sections might demonstrate multiple stages in the spermatogenic "wave." In the rodent, and in other species, however, cross sections will typically demonstrate only one stage of spermatogenesis.**

Tubular architecture

The typical diameter of the seminiferous tubule in the adult human male is anywhere from 150 to 300 μm. Within the tubule, spermatogonia and Sertoli cells line the basement membrane; this basement membrane is surrounded by an interstitium that includes Leydig cells and peritubular myoid cells (Fig. 13.2). Importantly, the basement membrane is maintained by collective action of both the Sertoli cells and peritubular myoid cells. Visualization of the basement membrane is made easier by a stain such as periodic acid-Schiff.

Abnormalities of tubular architecture include such findings as tubular hypoplasia, basement membrane hyalinization, and peritubular fibrosis. Tubular hypoplasia represents a failure of the tubules

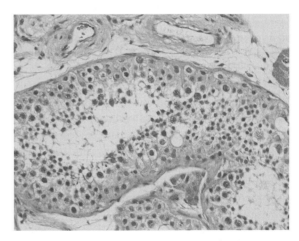

Fig. 13.2. Light-microscope image of a section of the human testis (× 200). Hematoxylin and eosin (H&E) staining. *See color plate section.*

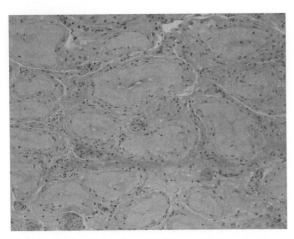

Fig. 13.3. Basement membrane hyalinization with associated peritubular fibrosis (× 200). Hematoxylin and eosin (H&E) staining. *See color plate section.*

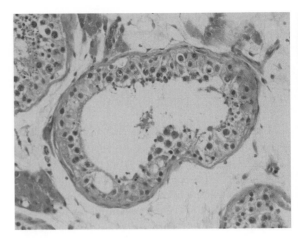

Fig. 13.4. Hypospermatogenesis. Decreased numbers of germ cells, with only some elongate spermatids noted (× 500). Hematoxylin and eosin (H&E) staining. *See color plate section.*

to enlarge during puberty; the seminiferous tubules are lined only with spermatogonia and immature Sertoli cells. This biopsy finding is potentially consistent with conditions such as hypogonadotropic hypogonadism, wherein the appropriate androgen-induced pubertal change in the testis is absent [18].

Basement membrane hyalinization (Fig. 13.3) **refers to concentric thickening of the inner basement membrane, as evidenced by deposition of hyaline (an acellular proteinaceous material that is eosinophilic on H&E staining).** This process can range from "minimal" to "complete," with complete replacement of the germinal epithelium and tubular lumen. Severe and diffused hyalinization is termed tubular sclerosis; this biopsy finding can be consistent with conditions such as hypergonadotropic hypogonadism and hyperestrogenism. Some degree of tubular sclerosis is normal in the testis of aging men, possibly as a result of arteriosclerosis [18].

Germinal epithelium

The germinal epithelium of the seminiferous tubule is composed of germ cells in various stages of development (spermatogonia, spermatocytes, spermatids) and Sertoli cells. In the infertile patient, changes in the appearance and number of these cells are characteristic. Typically defined patterns of change include hypospermatogenesis, maturation arrest, germinal cell aplasia, and end-stage changes.

Hypospermatogenesis or germ cell hypoplasia (Fig. 13.4) **is simply a reduction in the number of germ cells seen per seminiferous tubule;** it

can be characterized as mild, moderate, or severe. Hypospermatogenesis by definition implies that a consistent proportion of germ cells is observed at each stage of development. A disproportionate number of early-stage germ cells (spermatogonia or primary spermatocytes) is instead consistent with maturation arrest. There is some evidence in the literature that these two entities can be mistaken for each other [19].

Maturation arrest is simply the failure of spermatogenesis to proceed beyond a certain stage (Fig. 13.5). **Both "early" and "late" maturation arrest are well defined, with "late" maturation arrest defined as the absence of round spermatids or later stages** [20,21]. Clinically, "late" maturation arrest often correlates with normal or high-normal FSH, while "early" maturation arrest is often associated with a frankly elevated FSH.

Germinal cell aplasia, or Sertoli-cell-only syndrome, is defined by a total absence of germ cells at any stage (Fig. 13.6). **This condition can be brought about by any number of gonadotropic insults, including chemotherapy, radiation, or other toxicants.** In some patients with primary infertility, this diagnosis is made on biopsy and theoretically represents a failure of gonocytes to migrate to the gonadal ridge embryonically [22].

End-stage change implies a total absence of the germinal epithelial cells, with associated tubular sclerosis and peritubular fibrosis. This condition, clinically associated with elevated FSH and LH and testicular atrophy, can be associated with many

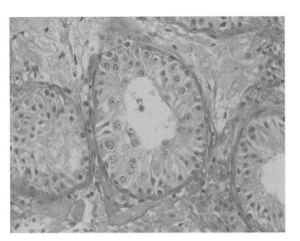

Fig. 13.5. Early maturation arrest at the level of the primary spermatocyte (× 500). Hematoxylin and eosin (H&E) staining. *See color plate section.*

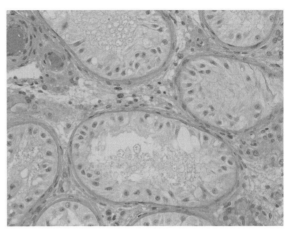

Fig. 13.6. Sertoli-cell-only or germinal cell aplasia. Empty tubules with the exception of Sertoli cells with characteristic round nucleus and tripartite nucleolus (× 500). Hematoxylin and eosin (H&E) staining. *See color plate section.*

well-known causes of male infertility, including long-term steroid abuse and Klinefelter syndrome.

Malignancy

With a lifetime incidence of approximately 0.2%, testicular cancer is rare enough to be overlooked on occasion, especially when compared to other genitourinary malignancies. Importantly, however, testicular cancer is at a peak incidence in patients aged 20–34 [23], and, as such, is more likely in patients being evaluated for infertility, who are largely drawn from the same cohort. **In fact, the adjusted incidence of testicular cancer in patients presenting for workup of infertility is reported to be as high as 1.1%, and patients with testicular cancer are known to have poorer baseline semen parameters pre-treatment [24].**

Theories regarding the relationship between testis cancer and infertility are numerous. **The most intriguing comes from the Danish literature, in which this association is termed testicular dysgenesis syndrome. In summary, this theory postulates that increasing exposure to environmental toxicants has increased the likelihood of both male infertility and testis cancer in the general population [25].** Significant debate continues regarding the testicular dysgenesis syndrome as an explanation for this phenomenon. Common risk factors for infertility and testis cancer, such as testicular atrophy, cryptorchidism, and steroid abuse may explain some of this relationship. Regardless, the potential for diagnosing an unrecognized testis cancer in the infertile patient presenting for testis biopsy is real. While a discussion of

the pathological features of testicular cancer remains outside the scope of this chapter, familiarity with the classification and treatment of testis cancer is important. Intratubular germ cell neoplasia (ITGCN) as a pre-malignant lesion is discussed here because of its unique relationship with infertility and the higher likelihood of finding it on biopsy than of finding frank testis cancer, which is more typically associated with a palpable testis mass.

ITGCN was first described by Skakkebaek in 1972 as carcinoma in situ of the testis [26]. Histologically, the tumor is defined by an intact basement membrane lined by Sertoli cells and malignant-appearing germ cells as characterized by nuclear polymorphism. ITGCN is associated with progression to invasive testis cancer; as many as 50% of patients with ITGCN progress to invasive disease within 5 years. It is commonly thought to act as a precursor lesion for all forms of testis germ cell cancer with the exception of spermatocytic seminoma [27].

Importantly, even higher incidences of ITGCN are described in patients with a history of cryptorchidism (2–8%) or contralateral testis cancer (5.5%). Given that both these conditions are associated with infertility, the likelihood of identifying ITGCN on testis biopsy is even higher in the infertile cohort than in the general population [27]. **There is no clear-cut treatment algorithm for this condition, and acceptable treatment options include observation, radiation, and orchiectomy.** Obviously, an awareness of this condition and the ability to recognize it on biopsy

219

is vitally important in the proper management of the infertile patient.

Application of novel techniques for analysis: flow cytometry, molecular biology, electron microscopy (EM)

The analysis of the testis biopsies has lent itself to the application of technologies not normally used in histopathology. This has occurred for a number of reasons. **First, the therapeutic nature of the testis biopsy depends on the ability to identify mature spermatids that might be appropriate for IVF/ICSI. In this most important regard, testis biopsy is different from any other tissue sampling in the human body.** Second, the end product of normal spermatogenesis is unique in that it is (a) haploid in chromosomal content and (b) the same cell type as that which is isolated from ejaculated semen. As a result, the application to the interpretation of testis biopsy of some techniques normally used in semen analysis has generated meaningful data. This includes the use of flow cytometry to identify haploid cells, gross assessments of DNA packaging, and fluorescence in-situ hybridization. In addition, the use of other techniques in molecular biology, including scanning electron microscopy, has provided meaningful information in the interpretation of testis biopsies.

Early data generated by flow cytometry analysis of the testis focused on the appropriate ratio of haploid, diploid, and tetraploid cells identified in the normal testis as compared to the infertile testis [28–31]. Further work in flow cytometry included efforts to identify haploid cells in the ejaculated semen of azoospermic men as a predictor of successful testis biopsy [32], and the use of flow-cytometry-enriched sorting (FACS) to identify haploid elongate spermatids in the testis biopsy of rodents [33]. These elongate spermatids were successfully used to generate embryos using IVF/ICSI. Obviously the successful use of FACS in humans to enrich testis cell populations of elongate spermatids would have tremendous clinical implications. Research in this field is ongoing.

A complete discussion of the assessment of sperm for DNA damage (or poor DNA packaging) is found in Chapter 11. **The topic is relevant to a discussion of testis biopsy in that researchers have correlated success in assisted reproductive techniques such as intrauterine insemination and in-vitro fertilization with use of sperm that have less DNA damage**

[34]. Investigations of DNA packaging in spermatids obtained from testis biopsy have followed. These studies generated contradictory conclusions: some found that DNA-damaged spermatids resulted in decreased likelihood of pregnancy after IVF/ICSI [35], and others found no difference. Additional research identified higher levels of DNA damage in testicular sperm after both in-vitro culture and freeze–thaw; the investigators concluded that fresh testis tissue should be obtained before use in assisted reproductive techniques whenever possible [36].

Finally, the application of fluorescence in-situ hybridization (FISH) techniques to analysis of the testis biopsy has also resulted in meaningful data. **FISH analysis generates data regarding defects in whole chromosome number or other large-scale chromosomal abnormalities, such as translocations.** Limitations to this technology include the ability to probe for only limited numbers of chromosomes; commonly used methodologies typically probe for chromosomes 13, 18, 21, X, and Y [37,38]. Investigators in the Netherlands considered the question of whether testis biopsies from severely oligospermic and azoospermic individuals retrieved spermatids with a higher degree of aneuploidy [39]. **Using chromosomal probes for only X, Y, and 18, they found a higher degree of aneuploidy of chromosome 18 than in results of FISH analysis of testis biopsies obtained from men with normal spermatogenesis (obstructive azoospermia secondary to vasectomy).** Results such as these illustrate the importance of continued research into the clinical implications of testicular sperm extraction from patients with severe male-factor infertility.

Scoring schema

Although the therapeutic nature of testis biopsy often dictates that biopsies be performed with the goal of identifying sperm to be used in assisted reproduction, it is still vitally important to apply a standardized schema to formal interpretation of testis biopsies. The information obtained includes valuable diagnostic data regarding the presence or absence of a contributing obstructive etiology of infertility. This is important from a therapeutic standpoint, because the recognition of a subset of patients with severe oligospermia who have an underlying obstructive etiology provides an opportunity for microsurgical reconstruction in these patients.

A standardized, reproducible, and objective grading system depends upon a number of features.

Commonly, an assessment of morphometric features (tubular diameter and basement membrane thickness) and/or cellular features (numbers of cells and types of cells seen in each field) is used to create a quantitative description of a biopsy specimen that can be communicated to other healthcare workers.

The two most widely recognized scoring schema are those of Silber and Rodriguez-Rigau [40] and Johnsen [41]. The Johnsen scoring system, which is the most commonly used method for scoring testicular biopsy, is predicated on the premise that increasing degrees of testicular damage result in successive depletion of cell types from most to least mature. Tubules are thereby scored on a scale from 1 to 10, based on the most mature cell type observed; a score of 10 represents intact spermatogenesis while a score of 1 indicates the absence of all germ cells and Sertoli cells [41]. Leydig cells are scored on the basis of presence or absence of normal numbers of cells plus hyperplasia. Importantly, Johnsen's criteria were validated in a series of 352 biopsies of patients with known diagnoses ranging from Klinefelter and Sertoli-cell-only to proven fertility (Table 13.1). Mean scores in patients with Klinefelter syndrome were 1.25, for example. This is in comparison to a mean score of 9.38 in biopsies taken from proven fertile controls.

The ultimate importance of a scoring system depends upon its ability to differentiate clinically meaningful conditions within the testis, such as maturation arrest, from hypospermatogenesis with contributing partial epididymal obstruction. No consensus regarding a particular scoring system has been reached, and the clinical utilization of scoring systems is limited in the United States at present. There is continued usage of Johnsen's scoring schema in Europe, however.

Table 13.1. Mean score counts in 352 patients reported by Johnsen

Clinical/pathologic diagnosis	Mean score
Normal testis	9.38
Eunuchoid testis	3.80
Acquired hypopituitarism	6.09
Klinefelter syndrome	1.25
Sertoli-cell-only syndrome	2.00
Severe hypospermatogenesis	5.32
Moderate hypospermatogenesis	7.80

Data from Johnsen SG. Testicular biopsy score count: a method for registration of spermatogenesis in human testes: normal values and results in 335 hypogonadal males. *Hormones* 1970; **1**: 2–25.

Indications for biopsy in the evaluation of the infertile male

Azoospermia

The azoospermic male should be evaluated in a standardized fashion to exclude the existence of a nonobstructive cause for azoospermia before a testis biopsy is undertaken. A thorough history and physical examination can yield evidence of either obstructive or nonobstructive etiologies. Findings such as dilated seminal vesicles on digital rectal examination, absent vas deferens on testis examination, or a history of prior testis surgery can point the practitioner towards a likely underlying cause for infertility.

A laboratory examination including measurement of serum gonadotropins and prolactin is important; an elevated FSH obviously points strongly toward an intrinsic cause of testis failure. Other vitally important information can be obtained from the semen analysis that indicated azoospermia in the first place. An acidic semen pH (less than 8.3), absent fructose, or an ejaculate volume less than 1.0 mL argues strongly for an obstructive cause of azoospermia. A postejaculatory urinalysis in these patients can indicate whether low-volume azoospermia is due instead to retrograde ejaculation.

Finally, a genetic evaluation including a peripheral karyotype and Y-chromosome microdeletion assay should be performed on all patients with azoospermia. These tests generate important prognostic and diagnostic information, helping to identify such conditions as Klinefelter syndrome and AZFa, b, or c deletion. These conditions carry varying likelihoods of success with regard to sperm extraction on testis biopsy, and the identification of these conditions can be useful in counseling patients regarding treatment choices (proceeding to IVF with donor sperm in the case of 46,XX male syndrome, for example).

A demonstrable cause of azoospermia is not always identified. Some patients have a normal physical examination, including normal-sized testes, a normal FSH level, and a normal 46,XY karyotype with an intact Y chromosome. These are the patients for whom a testis biopsy is most clearly indicated (with the exception of those patients in whom there is a coexisting and severe female factor that precludes IVF).

In these patients, a properly performed microdissection TESE yields the highest likelihood of recovering sperm that might then be used for IVF/ICSI. This procedure still does not, however, guarantee the recovery of sperm. Consequently, patients should be counseled as to the potential need for backup donor sperm (if they elect to proceed with IVF after a negative biopsy). No comprehensive algorithm accurately predicts the likelihood of identifying sperm on testis biopsy in these patients. In fact, the ability to determine the presence or absence of sperm in the testis noninvasively would represent a huge advance in the treatment of patients with azoospermia.

Oligospermia

The role of the testis biopsy is less clear in the patient with severe oligospermia or virtual azoospermia. In these patients, there is evidence on semen analysis of spermatogenesis, and sperm obtained from the ejaculate can theoretically be used at any time for IVF/ICSI. A complete history should be obtained and thorough physical examination should be performed in order to identify and treat any reversible causes of male infertility, such as toxin exposure or varicocele. For those patients in whom a reversible cause of infertility is not identified, the testis biopsy takes on the added role of being diagnostically important. A patient with severe oligospermia who has a normal testis biopsy should be evaluated instead for an unrecognized component of partial obstruction. Again, a proper interpretation of laboratory data, including a semen analysis and serum gonadotropins, should minimize the likelihood of this occurrence. Nevertheless, there are many patients who proceed to testis biopsy in such cases because of a normal evaluation and a need for further diagnostic information.

Malignancy/partial orchiectomy

Rarely, the testis biopsy is performed in conjunction with a partial orchiectomy for a known testis tumor; this approach can be considered in patients who have bilateral synchronous tumors, tumor in a solitary testicle, or a likely non-germ cell tumor (i.e., Leydig cell tumor). Several series have demonstrated this technique to be relatively safe when combined with adjuvant chemotherapy or radiation, depending on the pathology of the primary tumor [42,43]. Obviously, in a group of patients for whom fertility is typically important (male patients aged 20–40) and in whom a higher likelihood of subfertility is well documented, partial orchiectomy as a fertility-preserving treatment for testis malignancy is an important concept.

Typical biopsy findings in clinical states
Ductal obstruction

Some component of ductal obstruction will be identified in the workup of as many as one-third of azoospermic patients presenting to an infertility clinic. This does not include patients who have undergone vasectomy and desire reconstruction. **One might expect that the hallmark finding on testis biopsy in the setting of obstruction is quantitatively "normal" spermatogenesis. There are, however, subtle and important findings on testis biopsy that are consistent with new-onset obstruction.** These findings also potentially implicate acquired obstruction (vasectomy) as being somewhat deleterious to the testis.

Hirsch and Choi performed a retrospective review of biopsies obtained from both vasectomized men and men with a known diagnosis of congenital absence of the vas deferens. **While there was no difference in mean numbers of mature spermatids, Sertoli cells, or tubular number, significant thickening of the basement membrane was observed in the vasectomy cohort** [44].

A series of 32 testis biopsies performed by Jarow and colleagues on men who were undertaking vasectomy reversal resulted in similar findings [45]. Importantly, after vasectomy, patients had an increased likelihood of interstitial fibrosis, decreased numbers of Sertoli cells, and decreased numbers of mature spermatids. The presence of interstitial fibrosis also predicted likelihood of infertility even after a technically successful vasectomy reversal.

Other studies have all demonstrated the higher likelihood of antisperm antibody formation and change in testis weight after vasectomy [46–48]. All of these factors *may* play a role in the development of the aforementioned histological changes observed in ductal obstruction.

Varicocele

Several studies have considered testis biopsy findings in patients with a varicocele [49–52]. **Biopsy findings from the ipsilateral testis included maturation arrest, hypospermatogenesis, abnormalities in tubular number, interstitial fibrosis, and abnormalities in both Sertoli cell number and Sertoli cell junctional complexes.** Importantly, biopsies from the contralateral testis demonstrate fewer abnormalities, suggesting a greater effect of the varicocele on the ipsilateral testis.

Cryptorchidism

The hallmark finding of testis biopsy obtained from cryptorchid testes is decreased numbers of germ cells. This finding carries direct correlation to likelihood of paternity on long-term follow-up [53,54].

Andropause/hypogonadism/aging

Patients with idiopathic hypogonadism and those with hypogonadism associated with aging (andropause) show similar features on testis biopsy. These findings include a decrease in seminiferous tubular diameter and germ cell number [55,56]. Importantly, correction of the underlying condition with exogenous administration of steroids does not improve these findings. Instead, testosterone supplementation typically worsens spermatogenesis through suppression of gonadotropins.

Steroid abuse

Chronic abuse of anabolic steroids results in a far worse histological picture than replacement of testosterone in the setting of properly diagnosed hypogonadism. Severe depletion in the number of germ cells leads eventually to a decrease in gross testis size. Morphological changes in the testis typically persist for a significant period of time after discontinuation of steroid usage [57].

Future directions for pathological analysis

Ultimately, the ideal diagnostic tool for the identification of intact spermatogenesis would be noninvasive, noninjurious to the testis (minimal radiation), and highly accurate. The use of infrared confocal microscopy in several other disciplines has increased interest in the field of in-vivo imaging. The need for fluorescent markers to enable visualization in the infrared spectrum limits the potential application of this technology to patients with infertility. There are, however, other technologies that hold tremendous future potential with regard to the goal of noninvasive identification of spermatogenesis.

Near-infrared confocal imaging

Campo-Ruiz and colleagues have demonstrated the feasibility of a near-infrared confocal microscope as a tool for in-vivo renal biopsy using a rabbit model [58]. This tool, which can resolve structures to a resolution of 5 microns, potentially could be applied to the testis to assess the presence or absence of spermatogenesis and to target biopsies.

Optical coherence tomography

Kuang and colleagues presented their preliminary work using optical coherence tomography to assess the testis for spermatogenesis in patients already undergoing biopsy [59]. While their results did not show that the device is capable of determining spermatogenesis at this point, they suggest that it represents a direction for further investigation.

Conclusion

In conclusion, the testis biopsy remains a vitally important procedure in the armamentarium of the andrologist. It has a tremendous therapeutic and diagnostic utility for managing the infertile male. While there are potential directions for future inquiry with regard to improving the biopsy, it still exists unchanged in its current form as a cornerstone treatment of infertility. An understanding of the testis biopsy, including the information it yields, as well as its potential to recover sperm for treatments such as IVF/ICSI, is important for every andrologist.

References

[1] Charny CW. Testicular biopsy: Its value in male sterility. *JAMA* 1940; **115**: 1429.

[2] Hotchkiss RS. Testicular biopsy in the diagnosis and treatment of sterility in the male. *Bull N Y Acad Med* 1942; **18**: 600.

[3] Schlegel PN, Li PS. Microdissection TESE: sperm retrieval in non-obstructive azoospermia. *Hum Reprod Update* 1998; **4**: 439.

[4] Palermo G, Joris H, Derde MP, *et al.* Sperm characteristics and outcome of human assisted fertilization by subzonal insemination and intracytoplasmic sperm injection. *Fertil Steril* 1993; **59**: 826–35.

[5] Turek PJ, Cha I, Ljung BM. Systematic fine-needle aspiration of the testis: correlation to biopsy and results of organ "mapping" for mature sperm in azoospermic men. *Urology* 1997; **49**: 743–8.

[6] Schlegel PN. Testicular sperm extraction: microdissection improves sperm yield with minimal tissue excision. *Hum Reprod* 1999; **14**: 131–5.

[7] Kessaris DN, Wasserman P, Mellinger BC. Histopathological and cytopathological correlations

of percutaneous testis biopsy and open testis biopsy in infertile men. *J Urol* 1995; **153**: 1151–5.

[8] Cohen MS, Frye S, Warner RS, Leiter E. Testicular needle biopsy in diagnosis of infertility. *Urology* 1984; **24**: 439–42.

[9] Gottschalk-Sabag S, Glick T, Weiss DB. Fine needle aspiration of the testis and correlation with testicular open biopsy. *Acta Cytol* 1993; **37**: 67–72.

[10] Gottschalk-Sabag S, Glick T, Bar-On E, Weiss DB. Testicular fine needle aspiration as a diagnostic method. *Fertil Steril* 1993; **59**: 1129–31.

[11] Morey AF, Deshon GE, Rozanski TA, Dresner ML. Technique of biopty gun testis needle biopsy. *Urology* 1993; **42**: 325–6.

[12] Morey AF, Plymyer M, Rozanski TA, *et al.* Biopty gun testis needle biopsy: a preliminary clinical experience. *Br J Urol* 1994; **74**: 366–9.

[13] Rajfer J, Binder S. Use of biopty gun for transcutaneous testicular biopsies. *J Urol* 1989; **142**: 1021–2.

[14] Aridogan IA, Bayazit Y, Yaman M, Ersoz C, Doran S. Comparison of fine-needle aspiration and open biopsy of testis in sperm retrieval and histopathologic diagnosis. *Andrologia* 2003; **35**: 121–5.

[15] Ezeh UI, Moore HD, Cooke ID. A prospective study of multiple needle biopsies versus a single open biopsy for testicular sperm extraction in men with non-obstructive azoospermia. *Hum Reprod* 1998; **13**: 3075–80.

[16] Coburn M, Wheeler TM, Lipshultz LI. Cytological examination of testicular biopsy specimens. Presented at Annual Meeting of the American Fertility Society, 1986.

[17] Belker AM, Sherins RJ, Dennison-Lagos L. Improved, simple and rapid staining method for intraoperative examination of testicular biopsy touch imprints. *Fertil Steril* 1995; Abstract P-074 (October Suppl): S128.

[18] Krester DM, Burger HG. Ultrastructural studies of the human Sertoli cell in normal men and males with hypogonadotropic hypogonadism before and after gonadotropic treatment. In: Saxen BB, Berlin CG, Gandy HM, eds. *Gonadotropins*. New York, NY: Wiley-Interscience, 1972.

[19] Cooperberg MR, Chi T, Jad A, Cha I, Turek PJ. Variability in testis biopsy interpretation: implications for male infertility care in the era of intracytoplasmic sperm injection. *Fertil Steril* 2005; **84**: 672–7.

[20] Coburn M, Wheeler T, Lipshultz LI. Testicular biopsy: its use and limitations. *Urol Clin North Am* 1987; **14**: 551–61.

[21] Aumuller G, Fuhrmann W, Krause W. Spermatogenetic arrest with inhibition of acrosome and sperm tail development. *Andrologia* 1987; **19**: 9–17.

[22] del Castillo EB, Trabucco A, de la Balze FA. Syndrome produced by absence of the germinal epithelium without impairment of the Sertoli or Leydig cells. *J Clin Endocrinol* 1947; **7**: 493.

[23] Huyghe E, Matsuda T, Thonneau P. Increasing incidence of testicular cancer worldwide: A review. *J Urol* 2003; **170**: 5–11.

[24] Skakkebaek NE, Hammen R, Philip J, Rebbe H. Quantification of human seminiferous epithelium. 3. Histological studies in 44 infertile men with normal chromosome complements. *Acta Pathol Microbiol Scand [A]* 1973; **81**: 97–111.

[25] Skakkebaek NE, Rajpert-De Meyts E, Main KM. Testicular dysgenesis syndrome: an increasingly common developmental disorder with environmental aspects. *Hum Reprod* 2001; **16**: 972–8.

[26] Skakkebaek NE. Possible carcinoma-in-situ of the testis. *Lancet* 1972; **2**: 516–17.

[27] Campbell MF, Wein AJ, Kavoussi LR. In: Wein AJ, Kavoussi LR, Novick AC, Partin AW, Peters CA, eds. *Campbell–Walsh Urology*, 9th edn. Philadelphia, WB Saunders, 2007.

[28] Evenson DP. Male germ cell analysis by flow cytometry: effects of cancer, chemotherapy, and other factors on testicular function and sperm chromatin structure. *Ann N Y Acad Sci* 1986; **468**: 350–67.

[29] Hellerstein DK, *et al.* A comparison of testicular touch imprint to DNA flow cytometry in the quantitative assessment of testicular histology. Presented at 44th Annual Meeting of the American Fertility Society, October 1990, Washington, DC.

[30] Kaufman DG, Nagler HM. Aspiration flow cytometry of the testes in the evaluation of spermatogenesis in the infertile male. *Fertil Steril* 1987; **48**: 287–91.

[31] Lee SE, Choo MS. Flow-cytometric analysis of testes in infertile men: a comparison of the ploidy to routine histopathologic study. *Eur Urol* 1991; **20**: 33–8.

[32] Koscinski I, Wittemer C, Rigot JM, *et al.* Seminal haploid cell detection by flow cytometry in non-obstructive azoospermia: a good predictive parameter for testicular sperm extraction. *Hum Reprod* 2005; **20**: 1915–20.

[33] Ohta H, Sakaide Y, Wakayama T. Generation of progeny via ICSI following enrichment of elongated spermatids from mouse testis by flow-cytometric cell sorting. *Hum Reprod* 2007; **22**: 1612–16.

[34] Zini A, Meriano J, Kader K, *et al.* Potential adverse effect of sperm DNA damage on embryo quality after ICSI. *Hum Reprod* 2005; **20**: 3476–80.

[35] Greco E, Scarselli F, Iacobelli M, *et al.* Efficient treatment of infertility due to sperm DNA damage by ICSI with testicular spermatozoa. *Hum Reprod* 2005; **20**: 226–30.

[36] Dalzell LH, McVicar CM, McClure N, Lutton D, Lewis SE. Effects of short and long incubations on DNA

fragmentation of testicular sperm. *Fertil Steril* 2004; **82**: 1443–5.

[37] Egozcue J, Blanco J, Vidal F. Chromosome studies in human sperm nuclei using fluorescence in-situ hybridization (FISH). *Hum Reprod Update* 1997; **3**: 441–52.

[38] Vidal F, Blanco J, Egozcue J. Chromosomal abnormalities in sperm. *Mol Cell Endocrinol* 2001; **183** (Suppl 1): S51–4.

[39] Mateizel I, Verheyen G, Van Assche E, *et al.* FISH analysis of chromosome X, Y and 18 abnormalities in testicular sperm from azoospermic patients. *Hum Reprod* 2002; **17**: 2249–57.

[40] Silber SJ, Rodriguez-Rigau LJ. Quantitative analysis of testicle biopsy: determination of partial obstruction and prediction of sperm count after surgery for obstruction. *Fertil Steril* 1981; **36**: 480–5.

[41] Johnsen SG. Testicular biopsy score count: a method for registration of spermatogenesis in human testes: normal values and results in 335 hypogonadal males. *Hormones* 1970; **1**: 2–25.

[42] Heidenreich A, Weissbach L, Holtl W, *et al.* Organ sparing surgery for malignant germ cell tumor of the testis. *J Urol* 2001; **166**: 2161–5.

[43] Kirkali Z, Tuzel E, Canda AE, Mungan MU. Testis sparing surgery for the treatment of a sequential bilateral testicular germ cell tumor. *Int J Urol* 2001; **8**: 710–12.

[44] Hirsch IH, Choi H. Quantitative testicular biopsy in congenital and acquired genital obstruction. *J Urol* 1990; **143**: 311–12.

[45] Jarow JP, Budin RE, Dym M, *et al.* Quantitative pathologic changes in the human testis after vasectomy: a controlled study. *N Engl J Med* 1985; **313**: 1252–6.

[46] Ansbacher R, *et al.* Vas ligation: humoral sperm antibodies. *Int J Fertil* 1976; **21**: 258.

[47] Bedford JM. Adaptations of the male reproductive tract and the fate of spermatozoa following vasectomy in the rabbit, rhesus monkey, hamster and rat. *Biol Reprod* 1976; **14**: 118–42.

[48] Fawcett DW. Interpretation of the sequelae of vasectomy. In: Lepow IH, Crozier R, eds. *Immunologic and Pathophysiologic Effects in Animals and Man.* New York, NY: Academic Press, 1979: 3–23.

[49] Kass EJ, Chandra RS, Belman AB. Testicular histology in the adolescent with a varicocele. *Pediatrics* 1987; **79**: 996–8.

[50] Cameron DF, Snydle FE. The blood–testis barrier in men with varicocele: a lanthanum tracer study. *Fertil Steril* 1980; **34**: 255–8.

[51] Cameron DF, Snydle FE, Ross MH, Drylie DM. Ultrastructural alterations in the adluminal testicular compartment in men with varicocele. *Fertil Steril* 1980; **33**: 526–33.

[52] Heinz HA, Voggenthaler J, Weisbach L. Histological findings in testes with varicocele during childhood and their therapeutic consequences. *Eur J Pediatr* 1980; **133**: 139.

[53] Lipshultz LI. Cryptorchidism in the subfertile male. *Fertil Steril* 1976; **27**: 609–20.

[54] Cendron M, Keating MA, Huff DS, *et al.* Cryptorchidism, orchiopexy and infertility: a critical long-term retrospective analysis. *J Urol* 1989; **142**: 559–62.

[55] Heller CG, Moore DJ, Paulsen CA, Nelson WO, Laidlaw WM. Effects of progesterone and synthetic progestins on the reproductive physiology of normal men. *Fed Proc* 1959; **18**: 1057–65.

[56] Johnson L. Spermatogenesis and aging in the human. *J Androl* 1986; **7**: 331–54.

[57] Heller CH, Clermont Y. Kinetics of the germinal epithelium in man. *Rec Prog Horm Res* 1964; **20**: 545–75.

[58] Campo-Ruiz V, Lauwers GY, Anderson RR, Delgado-Baeza E, Gonzalez S. Novel virtual biopsy of the kidney with near infrared, reflectance confocal microscopy: a pilot study *in vivo* and *ex vivo. J Urol* 2006; **175**: 327–36.

[59] Kuang W, Davis CB, Schoenfield L, Thomas AJ. Optical coherence tomography: a novel imaging modality for testicular tissue. Abstract 1806. American Urological Association Annual Meeting, Anaheim, CA, May 2007.

Adverse effects of environmental chemicals and drugs on the male reproductive system

James V. Bruckner, David M. Fenig, and Larry I. Lipshultz

History of chemical exposures and male infertility

Despite recognition for 200 years of adverse effects of some compounds on the testes, **knowledge in the field of male reproductive toxicology is still quite limited.** Some of the first reports in the scientific literature of gonadotoxic substances in the workplace were published in the 1970s, when it was theorized in one of the initial papers that fertility was impaired in workmen exposed to lead [1]. Two years later Whorton and his colleagues reported marked reductions in sperm counts in employees who synthesized 1,2-dibromo-3-chloropropane (DBCP) at a pesticide manufacturing facility in California [2]. Subsequent monitoring studies at other DBCP production facilities across the USA yielded similar findings.

Widespread interest and concern about **a connection between the release of chemicals into the environment and human cancer incidence** resulted from Carson's 1962 book *Silent Spring* [3]. Three decades later Colborn in 1993 proposed and expounded upon the theory of **endocrine-disrupting chemicals (EDCs)**, which holds that parental exposure to EDCs has more influence on childhood development than genetics [4]. Sharpe and Skakkebaek in 1993 hypothesized that excess estrogen exposure in utero could induce reproductive abnormalities in male offspring [5]. These theories have attracted **enormous interest, controversy, debate, and research.**

There has been a parallel **explosion of interest** in the concept of **environmental estrogens (EEs)** [6]. A number of sources of EEs have been described. A variety of estrogenic growth promoters are commonly **given to livestock** in the USA and Europe. Diethylstilbestrol (DES) was widely used as a growth promoter in farm animals in Europe until the 1980s.

Zeranol, an anabolic growth promoter in meat production in the USA, is a relatively new product with estrogenic activity comparable to 17β-estradiol and DES in vitro [7]. Levels of growth promoters in meat have been found to be extremely low (i.e., in the low pg–ng per kg bodyweight per day range) [8]. Use of such substances in dairy farming has resulted in increased levels of estrogens and sulfated estrogens in milk [9]. However, current levels of EDCs in the US diet do **not** appear to be a threat to human reproductive health.

Some authorities contend that the data from epidemiological studies **in men from Western countries** demonstrate **progressive reductions in sperm density through the past century; however, this remains controversial.** Carlsen *et al.* in 1992 reported a significant global decline in sperm counts between 1938 and 1990 [10]. Swan *et al.* in 1997 expressed concerns about the data quality, model selection, and statistical designs of some published studies [11]; however, these investigators found the annual declines in sperm counts in the USA (1.5%) and Europe and Australia (3%) to be somewhat larger than described by Carlsen *et al.* in 1992 [10]. Others, however, have observed that experimental evidence for a significant decline in sperm counts in the USA is unconvincing [12]. Joffe observed that semen quality did decrease substantially in some European cities, but not in others or in five US cities. In addition, he found that data from nonWestern countries were too limited and diverse to support any conclusions [13].

Mechanisms of testicular cell injury, dysfunction, and death

For survival, all cells must: synthesize necessary endogenous molecules; assemble the molecules into macromolecular complexes, organelles, and cell membranes; produce energy; and maintain homeostasis in

Infertility in the Male, 4th edition, ed. Larry I. Lipshultz, Stuart S. Howards, and Craig S. Niederberger. Published by Cambridge University Press. © Cambridge University Press 2009.

the intracellular environment [14]. Many chemicals (parent compounds) or their metabolites may damage certain cell populations by one or a combination of mechanisms, or modes of action. Basic mechanisms of action of most chemicals are partially or poorly understood, if at all.

Necrosis and apoptosis

Apoptosis is a highly regulated form of cell death, involving a cascade-like activation of a series of catabolic processes that progressively disassemble the cell. Unlike apoptosis, necrosis predominates when ATP is depleted. Toxic substances exert their adverse effects through a variety of mechanisms which, in turn, induce apoptosis and/or necrosis.

Toxic metals such as lead, cadmium, mercury, and arsenic bind to enzymes and proteins critical to cell function, negating their role in biochemical and physiological processes. Some other gonadotoxicants (e.g., organochlorines) are **metabolically activated** to reactive, electrophilic intermediates that **bind** avidly to nucleophilic groups on enzymatic and structural proteins, as well as RNA and DNA. Free radicals interact with polyunsaturated fatty acids in lipids to form lipid peroxyradicals and lipid hydroperoxides. **Peroxidative damage** of membrane lipids leads to loss of integrity of organelles and even the cell membrane. Inhibition of thiol-containing enzymes such as calcium-transporting ATPases occurs through depletion of glutathione (GSH) by free radicals [15]. **Adduction of DNA** may **alter the expression of gene products essential for cell survival.** Production of somatic mutations through metabolite–DNA adduct formation can serve as the **initiating event in carcinogenesis.**

Several chemicals impede the process of oxidative phosphorylation, which is detrimental to cells from the depletion of ATP stores [16]. ATP deficit compromises the action of ATP-dependent sodium ion (Na^+) and calcium ion (Ca^{++}) pumps, resulting in loss of ionic and volume regulatory controls [17]. The resulting interference with processes responsible for calcium homeostasis depletes energy reserves further and activates degradative hydrolytic enzymes, including proteases, phospholipases, and endonucleases, the latter of which cause fragmentation of chromatin. These enzymes can overproduce reactive oxygen species (ROS), such as superoxide anion, and disrupt the cytoskeleton of sperm by dissociation of actin microfilaments and their attachments to the cell membrane [18]. Microfilaments are believed to play an important

role in anchoring Sertoli and germ cells and in their intercellular communications [19].

Disruption of the balance between germ cell gain via mitosis and loss by apoptosis plays a key role in mediating and modulating the action(s) of several gonadotoxicants. Germ cell survival in the seminiferous tubules is controlled by adjacent Sertoli cells via the Fas receptor–ligand system. Disruption of the Sertoli microtubules that serve to anchor and nourish germ cells results in overexpression of the Fas ligand, promoting apoptosis [20,21].

Endocrine disrupters and hormonal imbalances

"Endocrine-disrupting chemicals" (EDCs) have been defined by Younglai *et al.* [22] as a diverse group of endogenous and exogenous compounds that **mimic the effects of endogenous hormones, antagonize the effects of endogenous hormones, induce changes in the expression and/or activity of steroidogenic hormones,** and **alter circulating levels of steroid hormones.** The tremendous amount of research that has been devoted to EDCs has substantially increased our understanding of potential risks posed by these chemicals. Nevertheless, there is still a lack of scientific consensus about numerous issues, and many uncertainties remain [23–25].

The **timing** of exposure to sex hormones and exogenous substances with hormonal actions is a **critical determinant of the nature and severity of adverse effects on the male reproductive system.** The most significant **"window of susceptibility"** is undoubtedly the period of **organogenesis** during the **first trimester of pregnancy** [26–27]. The remainder of fetal development and neonatal life are somewhat less important "windows." Hormonal imbalances generally have **relatively little impact on male reproductive function during childhood and adolescence.** Induction of fertility problems in **adult** males is typically due to **high-level exposures to gonadotoxicants** [28].

Estrogens were the original substances of concern in the **"endocrine disruption hypothesis."** Estrogens are believed to act by a number of **mechanisms** to induce male reproductive disorders, including: **(1) suppression of androgen production** [27]; **(2) suppression of androgen receptor (AR) expression** [48]; **(3) reduction of Sertoli cell numbers and sperm production** [27,29]; and **(4) suppression of insulin-like factor 3 (INSL3) in fetal Leydig cells** [30]. Estrogens are also known to be involved in the negative feedback regulation of gonadotropin secretion, in masculinization of the brain, and in maintenance of sexual behavior in adult men.

A number of scientists have proposed that certain **industrial chemicals with estrogenic activity may exert such effects.** However, these xenobiotics have been noted to be 10 000–100 000-fold less potent than estradiol [6] and 100-fold less potent than phytoestrogens [31], leading some to doubt the influence of endocrine-disrupting chemicals on male reproductive tract problems [32,33]. Phytoestrogens, such as the isoflavones genistein and daidzen found in soybeans, often have mixed estrogenic and antiestrogenic effects, as they bind to, but only weakly activate, estrogen receptors (i.e., they are **partial agonists)** [34,35].

A variety of pesticides, including vinclozolin, linuron, procymidone and *p,p′*-DDT, as well as its stable metabolite *p,p′*-DDE, are included in a class of chemicals known as **antiandrogens.** These chemicals **primarily act during fetal sexual differentiation to inhibit the synthesis or actions of androgens, thereby interfering with the normal masculinization of the male fetus** [36,37].

Skakkebaek *et al.* in 2001 [38] coined the term "testicular dysgenesis syndrome" (TDS) for a **condition consisting of as many as four disorders: poor semen quality, testicular cancer, hypospadias, and cryptorchidism.** Two or more of these disorders are frequently seen together, suggesting they have a **common etiology; however, this remains speculative.** The temporal increases in incidence of the four disorders have led some researchers to propose that concurrent increases in exposures to **industrial chemicals with estrogenic or antiandrogenic activity may contribute to male reproductive dysfunction** [6,28,38]. This view, however, is not shared by all [13]. In addition, adverse effects on human growth and development, secondary sexual characteristics, the timing of puberty, and incidences of hormone-sensitive cancers are not manifest in epidemiological studies in Europe or the USA [12].

Carcinogenicity

The incidence of testicular cancer **increased by 51%** in the USA between 1975 and 1995, but **stabilized in** the first half of the 1990s [39]. There has been **considerable controversy about the relative roles of genetic and environmental factors in the etiology of testicular cancer.**

It should be recognized that **carcinogenesis is a multistage process that results from a complex interaction of multiple factors.** There is substantial evidence that factors operative during the early gestational period play an important role in the genesis of testicular cancer [40,41]. High levels of **endogenous maternal estrogens are associated with increased risks of testicular cancer and cryptorchidism** in male offspring [6,42]. In-utero exposure to DES, Premarin®, and other prescribed medications containing estrogens has been associated with increased cancer rates [41].

There likely are **a number of factors**, in addition to excessive estrogen action, that give rise to aberrant fetal germ (carcinoma in situ) cells from which **testicular cancer** develops. High exposures to antiandrogens, xenobiotics (e.g., certain pesticides) that inhibit the synthesis or actions of androgens, may play a role with some individuals [38,43]. **Epidemiology studies** have provided **some evidence** of an association between testicular cancer and **high-level environmental exposures to polyhalogenated aromatic hydrocarbons (PHAHs).** Ohlson and Hardell in 2000 found a sixfold increase in risk of testicular seminoma in polyvinyl chloride (PVC) plastic workers [44].

Factors that influence susceptibility to gonadotoxicants

Dosage, potency, exposure duration, frequency, and thresholds

There are a number of **factors** that can **significantly alter the extent of testicular injury by chemicals. Potency** and **dosage** are two of the most important factors. The inherent potency of different compounds varies dramatically. DES and ethinyl estradiol, for example, are more than 1000-fold more active disrupters of the male reproductive system than the most potent environmental estrogens [45]. It is important to recognize that the **magnitude and duration of toxic effect** are largely **a function of the amount of the toxic moiety at the site of action** and the **length of time it remains there.**

The **frequency** and **duration** of toxicant exposure are also key determinants of damage by toxic chemicals. A **chemical will accumulate** in the body if it is slowly metabolized or eliminated and repeated exposures occur frequently. DDT, dioxins, and polychlorinated biphenyls (PCBs) are examples of such agents. They are very lipid-soluble and slowly/poorly metabolized [46–48]. Thus, they readily accumulate in adipose tissue and have long half-lives (i.e., the time it takes for the internal concentration to fall by 50%). Conversely, many volatile alcohols, organic solvents, and short-chain halocarbons are rapidly eliminated by exhalation and metabolism [49].

Toxic damage can also be **cumulative**. Since spermatogonia rapidly divide throughout adulthood, complete recovery of spermatogenesis is likely after an acute, or repeated, exposure to a gonadotoxicant such as DBCP, if some viable spermatogonia remain. Should all spermatogonia be killed by intensive, prolonged DBCP exposure, azoospermia results. Epidemiological studies reveal a correlation between the duration of occupational exposure to DBCP and the severity of sperm reduction, though external exposure data are lacking [50].

The concept of **dosage threshold** is important to the understanding of both noncarcinogenic and carcinogenic effects. Considerable **controversy** exists as to the **existence of thresholds for genotoxic carcinogens**. The US Environmental Protection Agency (EPA) in 2005 published its policy that assumes that all carcinogenic chemicals have no threshold, unless there is definitive scientific evidence adequately demonstrating a nonthreshold mode of action [51]. This is rarely the case, so use of a linearized, multistage cancer risk assessment model is usually advocated. This model generates high cancer risk estimates for "vanishingly small" concentrations of chemicals [52].

The **route of exposure** can have a significant impact on the internal and target organ doses of some classes of chemicals. **Inhalation** usually results in rapid, extensive absorption of volatile organic chemicals (VOCs) into the pulmonary and arterial circulations. **GI absorption** is typically slower, less complete, and can be affected by a number of variables (such as gastric emptying time, gut motility, the presence of food, or stress). In addition, many ingested nutrients and xenobiotics undergo first-pass hepatic uptake. **First-pass elimination** is not effective in removing poorly metabolized compounds such as DDT, dioxins, and PCBs. Exhalation is an additional means of eliminating VOCs before they reach the arterial circulation [53]. DBCP, a well-metabolized VOC, is **extensively removed by first-pass, or so-called presystemic, elimination before it reaches the testes.** Thus, ingested DBCP produces less pronounced decreases in sperm count than does inhaled DBCP [54]. **Dermal absorption** of DBCP and many other chemicals is **limited** under normal circumstances.

Age, lifestyle, and personal habits

A number of lifestyle factors and personal habits have been shown to have a negative impact on general health and the capacity to reproduce. Some factors appear **not** to adversely affect fertility, while results of studies of other factors are **inconclusive**. The number of investigations of **combinations** of factors has been limited. Most of these have been binary studies, although a variety of factors unique to the individual are operative. Many factors (e.g., age, diet, exercise, smoking, stress) influence general health and well-being, which can in turn indirectly affect reproduction by altering sexual behavior.

Aging appears to have a **modest effect on male fertility**, compared with that on female fertility. The frequency of chromosomal anomalies in sperm increases somewhat with age, but there is little evidence of chromosomal abnormalities in offspring of older fathers [55]. There are modest, but progressive, decreases in Leydig cell numbers, testosterone levels, and sperm motility, as well as increases in the incidence of subfertility and time to initiate pregnancy after the age of 50. In a study of men over 50 years old, pregnancy rates were lower, even when the female partner was relatively young [56].

Obesity has been associated with a **variety of disorders** in men and women including cardiovascular disease, diabetes, certain cancers, and **delayed child bearing.** Population-based studies have supported an inverse relationship between rates of fertility and male body mass index (BMI), with odds ratios from 1.12 to 1.49 [57–59]. Obesity has been associated with decreased sperm density [60,61] and increased DNA fragmentation index [62]. Alterations of hormonal parameters likely influence spermatogenic abnormalities in obese patients. An inverse relationship between BMI and free/total testosterone levels in men has been observed [63]. Estrogen production is increased due to peripheral aromatization of androgens [64], and levels of inhibin B, a marker of Sertoli cell function and spermatogenesis, are decreased [65].

While some studies have demonstrated decreased fecundity in women with high caffeine consumption, Curtis *et al.* in 1997 saw no overall association with fecundity in female tea and cola drinkers, or male coffee, tea, and cola drinkers [66]. Most epidemiological studies have **not** shown a **strong association between low- to moderate-level alcohol consumption by men or women and fecundity, fertility, or spontaneous abortion.** Some investigations reviewed by Homan *et al.* in 2007 found no association, while others indicated that moderate alcohol ingestion or as little as one drink per week may be implicated in reduced conception [67]. Curtis *et al.* in 1997 found no association between alcohol and time to pregnancy, with the exceptions of women who drank two glasses of wine per week and men who drank more than 10 glasses of beer a week [66]. In this study group, 41% of the women and 65% of the men drank while trying to conceive. Hassan and Killick in 2004 observed a significant reduction in fecundity **only** in **men** with **heavy** alcohol ingestion [68].

Cigarette smoking by men and/or women has been associated with decreased fertility in many studies. In males, smoking negatively affects sperm production, motility, and morphology [69,70]. Zitzman *et al.* in 2003 stated that smoking by males reduced the success rate of in-vitro fertilization and intracytoplasmic sperm injection procedures in their partners [71]. Martini *et al.* in 2004, however, failed to find alterations in seminal parameters in smokers or in those who consumed alcohol [72]. These investigators did observe reductions in seminal volume, sperm count, percentage of motile spermatozoa, and nonmotile viable gametes in subjects who **smoked and consumed alcohol.** The Practice Committee of the American Society for Reproductive Medicine in 2004 concluded that **smoking does adversely affect sperm parameters, but evidence indicating its effect on male fertility is still inconclusive** [73].

There is evidence from large-scale epidemiological studies that **maternal smoking can adversely affect semen quality in male offspring**. A study by Jensen *et al.* of 1770 young men, who were undergoing compulsory military medical examinations in five European countries, found that men who were exposed to smoke constituents in utero had a smaller testis size and a 25% reduction in total sperm count in comparison with unexposed men. Percentages of motile and morphologically normal sperm were also significantly lower [74]. Storgaard *et al.* in 2003 examined semen quality and sex hormone levels in Danish men whose mothers smoked while they were pregnant [75]. Total sperm counts and levels of inhibin B were reduced, while follicle-stimulating hormone levels were somewhat elevated in sons of mothers who smoked more than 10 cigarettes daily.

Mechanisms by which cigarette smoke affects semen quality **are not fully understood.** It is estimated that the combustion of tobacco yields ~**4000 compounds**. More than 30 of these are known to be **mutagens** and/or **carcinogens** in different systems [70]. Zenzes *et al.* in 1999 found benzo(a)pyrene diol epoxide–DNA adducts in the sperm of men exposed to cigarette smoke [76]. Smoke also contains reactive oxygen species that are mutagenic. Nuclear DNA damage, as well as mitochondrial and cytoskeleton aberrations, appears to result from oxidative stress and adduct formation in gametes. Higher numbers of chemical adducts are found in embryos of smokers than in those of nonsmokers, demonstrating transmission of modified DNA by spermatozoa [77]. Benzo(a)pyrene and most other lipid-soluble chemicals should readily pass through the intact blood–testis barrier.

The blood–testis barrier inhibits passage of large, polar molecules. Nevertheless, **nicotine** and its water-soluble metabolite, **cotinine**, are detectable in the seminal fluid of smokers. Pacifici *et al.* in 1993 reported that motility of spermatozoa is negatively correlated with seminal fluid levels of nicotine and cotinine [78]. Gandini and coworkers subsequently reported that concentrations of these two compounds normally present in smokers' seminal fluid do not significantly alter in-vitro kinetic parameters of human sperm [79]. **Cadmium** levels are markedly elevated in the serum and semen of heavy smokers. Cadmium disrupts Sertoli cell tight junctions, apparently by adverse effects on actin filaments [80]. Loss of endothelial tight junctions leads to edema, increased fluid pressure, ischemia, and tissue necrosis. Most of the **mechanisms** by which cigarette smoke affects semen quality **are unknown**, due to the large numbers and possible combinations of chemicals involved.

Metabolic activation and inactivation of sex hormones

Enzymes involved in the **steroid biosynthesis pathway** are beginning to be recognized as **targets** for the action of a number of EDCs. Interference with the synthesis of steroid hormones may result in alterations in sexual differentiation and development and function of the testes [81], and 2,3,7,8-tetrachloro-*p*-dioxin (TCDD), monobutyl phthalate (MBP), Di-*n*-butyl phthalate, lindane, and azole fungicides all exert antiandrogenic effects by interfering with the steroid biosynthesis pathway.

Only ~0.3% of circulating testosterone is converted by aromatase (CYP19), a mitochondrial P450 isozyme, to estradiol in adult human males [82]. A number of xenobiotics are reported to affect **aromatase** [81]. Conversion of testosterone to estradiol appears necessary for initiation of spermatogenesis and mitosis of spermatogonia [83]. **Elevated aromatase activity in males, induced by trazines herbicides, can result in excessive estrogen exposure and hypoandrogenesis** [81,84]. Ketoconazole, an imidazole drug, inhibits steroid biosynthesis and is used as a rapid method of castration in patients with metastatic prostate cancer.

Metabolic inactivation of testosterone, which occurs primarily in the **liver**, may be induced by methyl tertiary-butyl ether (MTBE) (an oxygenated fuel additive) and endosulfan (an organochlorine insecticide) through stimulatory effects on hepatic isozymes [85].

Blood–testis barrier

The blood–testis barrier (BTB) serves to protect spermatogenesis from many potentially cytotoxic drugs and other chemicals. It is created by tight cellular junctions and bands of contractile myoid cells [86]. **The BTB is well equipped to maintain low concentrations of many xenobiotics in the proximity of the germinal epithelium.** The **efficiency of the BTB as a barrier** depends upon the **properties** of xenobiotics. Small, uncharged, lipophilic chemicals enter the seminiferous tubules much more rapidly and extensively than large, hydrophilic molecules [87]. Small lipophilic molecules, such as 1,2-dibromo-3-chloropropane (DBCP) and ethylene dibromide (EDB), readily diffuse across BTB membranes. **P-glycoprotein, an efflux transporter, and related transporters** appear to **serve as an effective protection mechanism** against other potentially gonadotoxic xenobiotics. Relatively **few chemicals** that are **directly cytotoxic** to testicular germ cells have been identified.

Assessment of risks of exposure to male reproductive toxicants

Significance and relevance of laboratory animal models/testing to humans

Male reproductive development and functions in humans are very similar to those in other mammals. Extrapolation of findings in male rodents to men is thus quite reasonable. Sexual differentiation and fetal reproductive tract development are strikingly similar in utero, although the **timing** at which maturational events occur is **different** and must be taken into account [26,27]. The complex processes of spermatogenesis and sperm maturation are **remarkably alike**, though the timing is compressed in **mice and rats** [26]. Formation of spermatozoa and maturation of sperm in adult men take ~64 and 5–10 days, respectively. These two processes in mice and rats take 34.5 and 48–52 days, respectively. The **quality** of human sperm is lower than in rodents and most other mammals. Men produce fewer spermatozoa per gram of testis. Furthermore, there are more abnormal forms, lower motility, and fewer motile sperm in human semen [26]. Experiments can also be conducted in species (e.g., monkeys) that more closely resemble humans in metabolism and systemic disposition of xenobiotics.

Retrospective studies of potential human gonadotoxicants in laboratory animals can be very informative. Experience is limited, however, in **judging the human relevance** of certain detrimental reproductive effects of chemicals in animals. This is attributable to the limited number of situations in which humans have been subjected to exposures of **endocrine-disrupting chemicals (EDCs)** high enough to cause adverse effects [88–91]. In numerous other instances, apparent reproductive problems have been reported in populations with somewhat lower or much lower EDC exposures. Vietnam veterans, for example, tended to have lower sperm counts and fewer morphologically normal sperm than controls. Relatively few of these men, however, were heavily exposed to Agent Orange, a herbicide that contained high concentrations of dioxins [92].

Multiple **confounding variables are invariably present in most environmental and occupational settings where humans are exposed.** Common factors to consider, among others, are smoking, alcohol, drugs, industrial chemicals, diet, ethnicity, socioeconomic status, age, health, and genetics [49].

Prospective studies of the gonadotoxic potential of new or previously untested chemicals in **laboratory animals** can also be very informative. A series of tests for testicular and reproductive injury is prescribed by the US EPA under the Toxic Substances Control Act. It is **important to recognize that the susceptibility of different species to hormones and gonadotoxic chemicals can vary substantially.**

Risks associated with environmental and occupational exposures

The possibility that **EDCs** are having a **substantial impact on ecological systems and human health has been a major concern to the public since the early 1990s** [25]. Progressive increases in testicular cancer, hypospadias, cryptorchidism, and lower sperm counts (i.e., testicular dysgenesis syndrome [TDS]) in the Western world, since 1900, suggest a role for environmental factors. A number of research groups have initiated experiments to **learn whether adverse reproductive effects of frequently encountered combinations of EDCs are additive, synergistic, or even antagonistic.** Epidemiological studies have shown some spatial and temporal trends associated with high exposures to one or more EDCs. Human and animal experimentation has demonstrated that most EDCs have very weak estrogenic or antiandrogenic activity. Fortunately, **tissue concentrations of DDT, PCBs, and most other organochlorines have diminished substantially in Western countries**, in which they were **banned** in the 1960s and 1970s.

On occasion, **accidental environmental releases** or **contamination of foodstuffs can result in adverse effects on the male reproductive system.** In 1976, in Seveso, Italy, a factory producing 2,4,5,-trichlorophenol exploded. Large amounts of TCDD, an extremely toxic by-product, were released into the surrounding area. A number of detrimental effects were seen in exposed women and their offspring. Mocarelli *et al.* in 2000 observed a decrease in the male : female ratio of children with increase in the fathers' serum TCDD concentrations [93]. The Yusho incident in Japan, in 1968, involved contamination of rice oil with PCBs, as well as lesser amounts of dibenzofurans and polychlorinated terphenyls. Exposure of pregnant women to these chemicals resulted in increased fetal loss and neonates of low birthweight [94]. Pubertal boys exposed in utero had a shorter penis. A study of 195 Swedish fishermen with relatively high dietary intake of PCBs and DDT, however, failed to reveal a significant association between serum 2,2′,4,4′,5,5′-hexachlorobiphenyl or *p,p′*-DDE and semen quality or reproductive hormone levels [95]. Ayotte *et al.* in 2001 did find elevated serum *p,p′*-DDE levels in men from an area in Mexico where DDT was sprayed to control malaria [96]. The levels were 350-fold higher than levels measured in Canadians by the same laboratory. The Mexicans' serum *p,p′*-DDE levels were inversely correlated with semen volume and sperm count. Garcia-Rodriquez *et al.* in 1996 described clustering of cryptorchidism in agricultural areas with intensive pesticide use [97]. **The highest chemical exposures and the greatest likelihood of injury usually occur in agricultural and occupational settings.**

Data from **animal** toxicology studies **are generally in agreement with human experience.** Animals

must be administered **high** doses of potent EDCs for extended periods, often during pregnancy, to produce abnormalities of the male reproductive tract. Animal studies clearly show **threshold doses that must be exceeded to elicit injury.** Adverse effects in animals subjected to high exposures are like those of pregnant women given unusually high doses of EDCs. **Many authorities** now **agree** that the **uniformly weak activities and normally low levels of environmentally encountered EDCs and EEs in developed countries are far from sufficient to cause testicular disorders** [12,13,27,31,33,45,98].

Gonadotoxic and endocrine-disrupting chemicals
Short-chain aliphatic hydrocarbons (halocarbons)

Methyl bromide and methyl chloride

Methyl bromide (bromomethane) (MeBr) has been widely used as a fumigant, as a methylating agent in the chemical industry, and as a solvent for extracting oils from seeds, nuts, and wool [99]. MeBr is also **highly toxic to humans and other mammals.** As MeBr vapor is colorless and nearly odorless, inhalation of toxic concentrations can occur without the victim's knowledge. Alexeeff and Kilgore in 1983 reported 1,156 known fatalities and 843 serious injuries as of 1983 [100]. Pulmonary edema, congestion, and hemorrhage were often observed in the victims. The Montreal Protocol has significantly reduced the use of MeBr, though the USA has obtained critical-use exemptions and continues to apply several million kilograms annually to farm soil and crops [101].

A series of investigations was carried out with rodents to identify and to characterize **effects of MeBr on target organs.** Damage occurs in a variety of tissues including the cerebrum, adrenal glands, nasal cavity, liver, and **testes** [102]. Adverse male reproductive effects in rodents include a decrease in plasma testosterone levels during exposure [103], testicular atrophy and degeneration [104], and decreased fertility [105]. **No studies** were located regarding reproductive effects of MeBr in **humans.**

Methyl chloride (chloromethane) (MeCl) is a colorless, nearly odorless gas at room temperature. It is used primarily in production of silicones. It is also used as a blowing agent in molding polystyrene and polyurethane foams, as an aerosol propellant, and as a chemical intermediate in methylation reactions [106]. It is estimated that a total of 2.3 million kilograms of MeCl were released into the environment in 1996, from 96 processing facilities in the USA [107]. The general population in urban areas is not expected to be exposed to air concentrations above 3 parts per billion. Occupational exposures may result in inhalation of as much as 10 parts per million. **Methanethiol and formaldehyde** are believed to be proximate **cytotoxic metabolites** of both MeCl and MeBr.

The **reproductive toxicity of MeCl** has been characterized in **laboratory animals**, as **no pertinent human data** have apparently been made available. **MeCl, like MeBr, damages a number of tissues** (e.g., cerebrum, liver, kidney, **testes**) of rodents but is much less potent. Studies have demonstrated that the exposure of rodents to MeCl causes transient decreases in serum testosterone [108], epididymal granulomas [108,109], testicular degeneration, and decreased fertility [110].

The **pharmacokinetics and mode of action of MeCl and MeBr are quite similar**. Both are small, uncharged, lipophilic molecules. Thus, they are quickly and extensively absorbed from the lungs and GI tract. Distribution to the testes and brain is similar to that to a number of other tissues, despite the blood–testis and blood–brain barriers [111]. These findings are indicative of the ability of these and other volatile organic chemicals (VOCs) to diffuse readily through membranes and tight junctions between cells. Both MeCl and MeBr are metabolically activated to the cytotoxic metabolites formaldehyde (via the P450 oxidative pathway) and methanethiol (via the glutathione conjugation pathway [112,113].

Ethylene dibromide

The primary use of ethylene dibromide (1,2-dibromoethane) (EDB) since the 1920s has been as a **lead scavenger in tetra-alkyl gasoline**. Its use began to decline in the late 1970s, with increasing restrictions by the US EPA on the sale of leaded gasoline [114]. The second largest use of EDB was as a **fumigant** for stored grains and other food products, as well as for golf courses and soil used to cultivate citrus, vegetable, and grain crops. The EPA began a review of EDB's potential health effects that led to cancellation of many of its agricultural applications in the mid-1980s [115]. It is **still used in the USA for designated pest-control situations**. The major route of human exposure to this VOC is **inhalation**. Improper disposal of EDB, and its widespread use as a soil sterilant, led to its **contamination of groundwater** in many

nations [116]. Controlled experiments in animals have confirmed that EDB is gonadotoxic [117–122].

A number of **epidemiological studies of occupationally exposed populations** have focused on spermatotoxicity and fertility. Takahashi *et al.* in 1981 reported a reduction in sperm count in a small group of pineapple farm workers in Hawaii, but concurrent marijuana use and DBCP exposure confounded the findings [123]. A group of 46 men exposed to EDB for five years in a papaya fumigation operation in Hawaii were compared to matched controls [124]. There were statistically significant reductions in the papaya workers' sperm viability, motility, and count, as well as increases in the proportion of morphological abnormalities. Schrader *et al.* in 1988 described a longitudinal study of 10 EDB-exposed forestry employees and 6 unexposed men [125]. There were substantial decreases in sperm velocity and semen volume in the EDB group. Ter Haar in 1980 evaluated 59 men exposed to EDB in a plant producing gasoline additives [126]. Employees with relatively high (500–5000 ppb) vapor exposure had lower sperm counts than those with lower (< 500 ppb) exposures. No unexposed controls were included. A reduction in male fertility of 29% was observed in one of four EDB manufacturing plants investigated by Wong *et al.* in 1979 [127]. Unfortunately, several of the aforementioned studies lacked sufficient statistical power, due to small sample sizes and other methodological weaknesses, to reliably detect an association between EDB exposure and **infertility** [114]. These studies **do** indicate that **sufficiently high doses of the VOC adversely affect human sperm**, though it is **not clear what inhaled concentration and duration of exposure** are required to have such an effect.

1,2-Dibromo-3-chloropropane (DBCP)

DBCP enjoyed **widespread use** as a nematocide in the USA and a number of other nations from the mid-1960s until its use was **restricted and then banned in the late 1970s** [54]. DBCP is a relatively volatile, lipophilic halocarbon that is well absorbed from the lungs and GI tract [128]. Although Torkelson *et al.* reported severe atrophy and degeneration of the testes of several species of laboratory animals exposed to DBCP by inhalation [129], adverse effects on **human** testicular function were not recognized until the mid 1970s. **Azoospermia** and **oligospermia** were originally discovered in 14 of 25 employees who were synthesizing and packaging DBCP at a northern California agricultural chemical plant [2]. These findings prompted epidemiological studies at other facilities that produced

233

the pesticide in the USA and Israel [130–132]. The incidence of oligospermia and azoospermia at each facility was dependent upon the **duration** of the workers' exposures to DBCP. Inhalation and dermal contact were the major exposure routes. There was a **paucity of exposure data** in these occupational exposure settings, so **dosages of the chemical required to adversely affect reproductive function in men are still unknown.**

Experiments in laboratory animals have demonstrated that the **spermatotoxic effects of DBCP are dose-, route-, and species-dependent.** Inhaled DBCP is much more toxic than ingested DBCP, as the liver removes much more of such chemicals before they reach and damage the testes [49]. Rats consuming DBCP in their drinking water are less susceptible [133] than rats given the same daily dose as an oral bolus [134], due to the animals' cytotoxicity defense and repair processes. Foote *et al.* saw testicular injury in rabbits at lower drinking water levels than in rats [135]. Rao *et al.* reported rabbits to be approximately 10 times more sensitive than rats to inhaled DBCP [136,137]. In-vitro metabolism and toxicity experiments reveal that human testicular cells activate less DBCP metabolically than rat cells and experience less pronounced adverse effects.

There have been a **limited** number of studies of possible **reproductive effects** of DBCP on **male pesticide applicators and agricultural workers.** Reduced sperm counts have been reported in some pesticide applicators [138,139] and DBCP formulators and users [140]. However, two comprehensive investigations of pineapple farm workers in Hawaii by the National Institute of Occupational Safety and Health (NIOSH) demonstrated no changes in sperm count or morphology [141,142].

Because DBCP and several structurally related halocarbons are small, uncharged, lipophilic molecules, they readily pass from the blood through the blood–testis barrier to the Sertoli and germ cells. A **very limited number of drugs and other chemicals** have the properties that allow them to **enter and act** in the immediate proximity of the Sertoli cells and gonocytes of adults. There are a number of chlorinated and brominated **propanes** that have these properties and are quite **gonadotoxic** [143].

Polyhalogenated aromatic hydrocarbons (PHAHs)

DDT and DDE

1,1,1-Trichloro-2,2′-bis(*p*-chlorophenyl)ethane (DDT) has been used widely throughout much of the world

since its introduction by Allied forces in World War II to control mosquitoes that carried typhus and malaria [144]. DDT remained **the most widely used insecticide in the world until the mid to late 1960s,** when its use was **severely restricted or banned** by most developed countries. DDT has **continued to be applied in some developing countries** for vector control [145,146].

DDT and its major metabolites are **very persistent** in the environment and in humans and animals. They accumulate in animals' **adipose tissue** because of their **lipophilicity** and **slow metabolism.** These properties result in their **accumulation in food chains**, with predatory fish, birds, and mammals at the tops of the chains exhibiting the highest body burdens [144]. **Fatty fish, dairy products** and other such foods continue to be the **primary sources** of human exposure to DDT, DDE, and other polyhalogenated aromatic hydrocarbons (PHAHs) in developed countries. It is estimated that current intakes in developing countries in Asia are up to 100-fold higher than in more advanced nations. Nevertheless, it was concluded by the World Health Organization that the public health benefits from using DDT were far greater than its potential risks [147].

In-utero and lactational exposure of **experimental animals** to DDT and its major metabolites have been shown to produce a **variety** of reproductive abnormalities in male offspring. Antiandrogenic actions affecting male sexual development have been demonstrated in rats and rabbits resulting in hypospadias, cryptorchidism, and decreased weights of androgen-dependent tissues such as seminal vesicle and prostate [148–151].

Adverse effects of DDT and certain of its stable metabolites apparently result from a **combination of estrogenic, antiandrogenic, and cytochrome P450 (CYP)-inducing actions. Early developmental stages are particularly sensitive to endocrine modulation.** Kelce *et al.* in 1995 found that *p,p′*-DDE had little ability to bind to estrogen receptors (ERs), but it inhibited androgen binding to the AR and androgen-induced transcriptional activity, as well as growth of androgen-dependent tissues, in developing and in adult rats [150]. DDT and its metabolites may also disrupt male sexual development and function through induction of aromatase [152,153] and site-specific testosterone CYP hydroxylases in the liver [154].

There have been a number of **epidemiological studies** of potential relationships between **levels** of DDT and certain of its metabolites in humans and **reproductive dysfunction.** On the basis of studies of diverse populations, including US men [155,156], Swedish fisherman [157], Inuits, and Ukrainians, **it** can be concluded that current DDT/*p,p'*-DDE levels in European populations exert minimal, if any, adverse effects on male reproductive functions [156,158–160].

Adverse reproductive effects **have** been observed in males **subjected for years to extremely high DDT exposures.** Young men in regions of Mexico where malaria was endemic and DDT routinely sprayed were found to have decreased sperm motility [161], semen volume, sperm count, and serum testosterone [96]. Dalvie *et al.* in 2004 examined 60 South African malaria control workers who had been employed for ~16 years [162]. There was an increase in abnormal sperm morphology, as well as a negative association between *p,p'*-DDE levels and sperm count. Longnecker *et al.* in 2007 found no evidence that in-utero exposure to *p,p'*-DDE in Chiapas, Mexico, reduced androgen action, as reflected by anogenital distance and penile dimensions, in 781 newly delivered male infants [163]. These research projects demonstrate that **extremely high DDT/DDE exposures can significantly impact sperm quality in adults.** The data are **inadequate,** however, **to indicate what risks in-utero exposure to such large amounts of the pesticide may pose to normal development** of the male reproductive tract.

There is concern that the weak endocrine-disrupter effects of the **numerous PHAHs, PAHs,** and **halocarbons,** to which we are **exposed environmentally,** may be **additive,** or even **synergistic.** In one study, **combined levels** of the eight most abundant pesticides, including *o,p'*-DDT and *p,p'*-DDT, were significantly higher in the breast milk ingested by boys with cryptorchidism [164]. As the **estrogenic potency** of these chemicals is **quite low** [31,33], their **combined effects** in people with **very high exposures** appear likely causes of adverse male reproductive effects.

Polychlorinated biphenyls (PCBs)

PCBs are a class of PHAHs that consist of two joined phenyl rings. PCBs are very resistant to degradation by water, acids, and alkalis and can withstand temperatures of up to 500 °C without degradation. Therefore, PCBs were widely used for moistureproofing and sealing, as a solvent for lipophilic pesticides, as flame retardants, and for heat transfer applications in auto brake systems, heating/cooling systems, power transformers, and electrical capacitors [47]. The most extensive human exposures occurred in Japan [88] and Taiwan [89] in the late 1960s and 1970s, respectively, when rice cooking oil was adulterated with PCBs containing polychlorinated dibenzofurans. As PCBs are very lipid-soluble and many isomers are resistant to metabolic clearance [165], they underwent biomagnification and accumulated in adipose tissue of wildlife and humans. PCBs remain ubiquitous environmental contaminants due to their extensive use in the past and their extreme stability. PCBs were banned in the USA in 1977 but have continued to contaminate food supplies in the USA and much of the rest of the world for years. Concentrations in human tissues have progressively decreased for 20 years since the bans in the USA [47], but have diminished more slowly during the past decade [166].

There have been a **limited** number of investigations of potential effects of PCBs on the male reproductive tract in **experimental animals.** Adverse effects on the **female reproductive system, fertility, and pregnancy outcomes were found to be much more pronounced** and were more thoroughly characterized. Fertility was impaired in male offspring of rats exposed lactationally to PCBs in their first nine days of life. **Limited information** on PCB-induced gonadotoxicity in **primates** was found in the literature. Allen and Norback in 1976 did report that one of four male rhesus monkeys ingesting 0.1 mg Aroclor 1248/kg for 17 months exhibited decreased libido [167]. Histological examination of the affected animal's seminiferous tubules revealed an absence of mature spermatozoa and a predominance of Sertoli cells.

Adverse effects on the **human** male reproductive system have been documented in the two situations involving the **highest known** exposures to PCBs. Mass exposure to PCBs through contamination of cooking oil occurred in Japan in 1968 and Taiwan in the late 1970s [168].

A study of the sperm of young men born to exposed women revealed **abnormal sperm morphology, reduced motility, and diminished capacity to penetrate hamster oocytes** [169]. In 1999–2002, Huang *et al.* assessed the sperm quality of 40 adults who had been directly exposed to PCBs and PCDFs in Taiwan [170]. **After 20 years, their sperm had more abnormal forms, lower numbers, and reduced ability to penetrate hamster oocytes.** No information about gonadal effects on Japanese victims or their offspring was located.

As **fish are a major source of dietary exposure to PCBs** and other PHAHs, there have been a number of **studies of potential effects of fish consumption on human male reproductive function.** Some studies have shown an association between high-fish diets and reduced fecundability, but others have not.

High dietary exposure to PCBs may result in a slight reduction in male fertility, most likely due to modest effects on sperm motility and ability to penetrate oocytes [171–174].

Assessments of associations between PCB levels, or body burdens, and male reproductive function in the general population have yielded mixed results. The most consistent change across studies of subfertile men was reduced sperm motility [155,175,176], which raises the possibility of the absence of a dose–response relationship for this adverse effect [43].

PCBs appear to act by different mechanisms to produce multiple effects on the reproductive system. The net effect is difficult to predict, as complex mixtures of PCB isomers, DDT and p,p'-DDE, dioxins, dibenzofurans, and other PHAHs are typically encountered environmentally [177]. Certain PCBs can produce estrogenic effects by binding to α and β estrogen receptors (ERs), while others exert antiestrogenic effects [178]. Hauser et al. in 2003 concluded that individual PCB isomers have different biological activities, depending upon the number and pattern of chlorine substitutions [176].

Men show relatively little effect unless their exposures to PCBs as adults are extremely high, as in the Yucheng incident in Taiwan [170]. It appears that high levels of exposure during gestation or early childhood are associated with increased risks. As described previously, Guo et al. in 2000 reported deficits in sperm quality in young men born to highly exposed women in Taiwan [169]. High concentrations of these compounds and their hydroxylated metabolites apparently can upset the delicate estrogen/androgen balance required for proper development of the reproductive system.

The multiple mechanisms of action of the myriad of PCB isomers and metabolites, PHAHs, and PAHs make it difficult to predict whether the sum total of current low levels of these xenobiotics may subtly influence human male reproductive tract development.

Phthalates

The potential effects of phthalates on the male reproductive system are of concern, as a large proportion of the general population is currently exposed to the compounds. Phthalates are alkyl or dialkyl aryl esters of 1,2-benzenedicarboxylic acid. Widespread exposure is reflected by the common occurrence of phthalate metabolites in the urine of persons monitored in two cross-sectional studies in the USA [179,180].

Phthalate esters have been used since the 1920s as plasticizers for PVC. Phthalates are also components of many other consumer goods such as carpet backing, paints, glues, soaps, shampoos, hairsprays, cosmetics, perfumes, insect repellants, and PVC tubing that is commonly used for medical therapies. Exposures in occupational settings can occur by skin contact and inhalation of vapors and dust. The general population is subjected to lower levels of phthalates via dermal, inhalation, and oral routes. Food used to be a major source of phthalates. The lipophilic compounds will migrate from paper and plastic wraps into fatty foods, although di(2-ethylhexyl)phthalate (DEHP), one of the more commonly utilized phthalates, apparently has not been used in food wraps in the USA for the last 25 years [181].

Investigations have shown that DEHP, di-n-butyl phthalate (DBP), and certain other phthalates disrupt reproductive tract development in the male rat in an antiandrogenic manner [148,182]. Oral administration of DEHP to rats results in multinucleated gonocytes [183], Leydig cell hyperplasia, and decreased testosterone production and levels [184]. Similarly, lower dosages of DEHP have been reported to produce adverse testicular effects including aspermatogenesis when exposures are prolonged [185].

In-utero exposure of fetal male rats to DEHP and DBP induces a constellation of reproductive tract disorders remarkably similar to human testicular dysgenesis syndrome (TDS) [186,187]. Both DBP and DEHP can inhibit production of testosterone, a factor in the occurrence of hypospadias and cryptorchidism. While intake of phthalates by the general population appears to be both decreasing and substantially lower than adverse-effect levels in rodents [180], some scientists believe it is plausible that current levels of environmental antiandrogens (e.g., phthalates) have the potential to affect male reproductive health [38].

Medications

Drugs and medications may have an adverse impact on fertility through a variety of mechanisms including direct toxicity to the testicular germ cells and supporting cells, alterations of the hypothalamic–pituitary–gonadal (HPG) axis, or effects on sexual performance by impairment of libido, erections, or ejaculation.

Gonadotoxins may cause cellular damage by disrupting the balance between germ cell gain via mitosis and loss by apoptosis. Germ cell survival in the seminiferous tubules is controlled by adjacent Sertoli cells, which are susceptible to apoptosis when their microtubular structure is altered. It should be recognized that apoptosis of cells with chemically induced damage of their DNA is an important self-defense against mutagenesis and oncogenesis. Impairments of sperm density, motility, and morphology may occur, which in some instances may be permanent in nature.

Alterations in the HPG axis may result in abnormal levels of circulating gonadotropins or testosterone. Ejaculation may be impaired by medications that cause retrograde ejaculation, impair spinal reflexes, or inhibit emission. Erectile dysfunction may be impaired through neurological or vascular-mediated effects.

Common medications

Hormonal agents

Diethylstilbestrol (DES) was widely prescribed in the USA for some 25 years to prevent miscarriage and to treat a variety of complications of pregnancy. It was given to an estimated 10–20 million women in the USA from the late 1940s until 1971, despite a randomized clinical trial in 1953 that showed DES was ineffective for the conditions for which it was being prescribed. DES has greater estrogenic potency than estradiol. In-utero exposure of female fetuses significantly increased their risk of developing vaginal clear cell adenocarcinomas [188] and future infertility [189]. **Boys born to mothers who took DES have increased incidences of cryptorchidism** [13], **hypospadias** [190], **and other congenital malformations** including epididymal cysts, hypoplastic testes, and urethral stenosis. **Impairment of spermatogenesis** may also be seen [191].

Antiandrogens and luteinizing hormone-releasing hormone (LHRH) analogs are primarily used in older men as a treatment for prostate cancer, but may be used to treat sexually aggressive behavior in adolescents. These medications cause a **decrease in libido and sperm production** [192]. **The effects are typically reversible with cessation of the medication.** Similar effects are also seen with estrogenic agents used in the past for prostate cancer resulting in decreased libido, loss of potency, and testicular atrophy. Atrophy of the seminiferous tubules accounts for the abnormal semen parameters.

Finasteride, an oral 5α-reductase enzyme inhibitor, is used to treat benign prostatic hyperplasia with a 5 mg dose and male-pattern baldness with a 1 mg dose. **Two recent publications described a total of**

five patients taking finasteride, 1 mg, with impaired semen parameters ranging from azoospermia to normal counts with severely reduced motility. Cessation of medication resulted in improvements in sperm density, motility, and morphology within six months to one year [193,194]. These reports are in contrast to the findings of a double-blind, placebo-controlled, multicenter study by Overstreet *et al.* In this study of 181 men randomized to 1 mg of finasteride or placebo for 48 weeks, no changes in sperm concentration, total sperm per ejaculate, sperm motility or morphology were seen at any point in time [195]. Standard dosing of finasteride and dutasteride for benign prostatic hyperplasia, however, has been reported to result in mild decreases in sperm motility [196].

The use of testosterone replacement therapy (TRT) is more common because there are effective, safe exogenous topical gels, intramuscular agents, transdermal patches, and oral or buccal preparations. **Exogenous testosterone impairs spermatogenesis by inhibiting the HPG axis.** Reduced gonadotropin release by the pituitary gland mediates the effects on spermatogenesis and a reduction in intratesticular testosterone. **Human chorionic gonadotropin (hCG) is an alternative to testosterone replacement therapy in hypogonadal men interested in fertility.** A homolog to luteinizing hormone (LH), hCG is administered via subcutaneous injection. Both hCG and clomiphene citrate, a weak estrogen, improve serum and intratesticular testosterone without decreasing gonadotropin levels.

The use of androgenic-anabolic steroids (AAS) by professional and amateur athletes is increasing. These agents may have devastating effects on fertility. As with testosterone replacement therapy, these agents have centrally mediated effects resulting in secondary hypogonadotropic hypogonadism, which impairs spermatogenesis. Normal recovery of hormonal function may, but does not always, occur after discontinuation of these agents [197]. Recoverability of endogenous testosterone production after cessation of AAS may be achieved using hCG administration [198]. **Complete recovery of spermatogenesis using hCG, with or without human menopausal gonadotropin (hMG), has been observed as early as three months following cessation of AAS or testosterone replacement therapy** [199,200]. Human chorionic gonadotropin administration concomitant with testosterone replacement therapy theoretically may prevent impairment of spermatogenesis; however, this has yet to be definitively proven. In a study using percutaneous testicular sperm aspiration in normal men, Coviello *et al.* demonstrated that the concomitant administration of hCG at dosages of 500 IU every other day for three weeks, with testosterone enanthate 200 mg IM weekly, maintained intratesticular testosterone within the normal range [201].

Antibiotics

Antibiotics may be prescribed for infertile patients for common systemic illnesses as well as infections of the reproductive tract. Semen parameters are often depressed in these patients, possibly because of the underlying illness or, in some cases, because of the antibiotic. Commonly used antibiotics may adversely affect fertility through effects on spermatogenesis or sperm function. Tetracycline, erythromycin, clotrimoxazole, and chloroquine impair sperm motility and viability in vitro, but whether they are present in sufficiently high concentrations in semen in vivo to adversely affect fertility is unclear. In contrast, amoxicillin has not been shown to impair semen parameters [202]. While high-dose nitrofurantoins have been demonstrated to cause maturation arrest in the testis of rats [203] and depressed motility in in-vitro human studies [204], low-dose short-term use does not appear to exert these effects.

Antihypertensives

Antihypertensives may have a variety of deleterious effects on male fertility. Although traditionally used in older populations, antihypertensives are increasingly prescribed for younger men, often without discussion of their effects on sexual function [205,206]. **Antihypertensives mainly impair fertility through effects on sexual function. Semen parameters and sperm function, however, also may be impaired by certain classes of these medications.**

Beta-blockers, in particular propranolol, have been noted to cause a decrease in both libido and erectile function [207]. Cardioselective β-blockers such as atenolol and metoprolol have fewer adverse sexual side effects [208]. Thiazide diuretics may impair erections by reducing vascular resistance, resulting in decreased penile blood flow. Spironolactone causes reduced sexual desire, erectile dysfunction, and impaired semen quality. It acts as an antiandrogen through peripheral antagonism of androgens.

Calcium channel blockers may impair fertility by inhibiting the expression of mannose-ligand receptors on the sperm head. These receptors are responsible for triggering the acrosome reaction by binding to mannosyl residues on the zona pellucida of the egg [209,210]. These changes appear to be reversible [211]. Other effects on the testis are possible, as one study demonstrated that high doses of calcium channel blockers induce maturation arrest at the elongated spermatid stage in the peripubertal mouse testis [212].

Alpha-blockers such as doxazosin, terazosin, tamsulosin, and alfuzosin are commonly prescribed for benign prostatic hyperplasia or bladder neck obstruction but may have variable effects on blood pressure. Their side-effect profile is dependent on different affinities for α_1-receptor subtypes. **Retrograde ejaculation** can occur with use of these agents and may be due to effects on the vas deferens or seminal vesicles [213]. This is most commonly associated with tamsulosin. A recent randomized, placebo-controlled study demonstrated that 35% of men taking tamsulosin 0.8 mg developed anejaculation, compared to 0% for men taking alfuzosin or placebo [214]. These effects are typically reversible with discontinuation of treatment [215].

Chemotherapy and radiation

With the improving cure rates of malignancies in young men with combination chemotherapy regimens, late gonadal toxicity remains an important issue. Treatments for Hodgkin's disease and non-Hodgkin's lymphoma, testicular cancer, bone and soft tissue sarcomas, and leukemia may result in permanent sterility. The toxicity, however, depends on the agents used, individual doses, and treatment duration and interval. **Combination chemotherapy regimens using lower doses can minimize damage to spermatogonia and the supporting Sertoli cells, increasing the possibility of eventual recovery. Radiation-induced testicular damage is similarly dose-dependent.** Speed of onset and recovery as well as testis recovery are predicted by the dosage used [216].

Type B spermatogonia are most sensitive to the effects of chemotherapy, since they proliferate most actively. If type A spermatogonia, the spermatogenic stem cells, are impaired, permanent sterility can be expected [217]. On the other hand, Leydig cells and to a lesser extent Sertoli cells, which do not proliferate in adults, are less susceptible to chemotherapeutic agents and radiation [218]. Functional damage may occur, however, resulting in decreased inhibin release and secondarily elevated follicle-stimulating hormone (FSH) and LH. While serum FSH may be used to predict recovery of spermatogenesis, van Beek *et al.* found inhibin B levels superior to FSH in correlating with sperm counts and in predicting recovery [219].

The ability to recover spermatogenesis depends on the type of chemotherapeutic agent used. **Alkylating agents such as cyclophosphamide, chlorambucil, mustine, melphalan, busulfan, carmustine, and lomustine are the most gonadotoxic** [220]. Antimetabolites such as cytarabine, vinca alkaloids (vinblastine), and various other agents including platinum-based therapies also cause severe impairment of gonadal function [220–222]. Table 14.1 describes some commonly prescribed chemotherapeutic agents categorized into good, moderate, and poor risks of recovery of spermatogenesis [220,222–226].

Studies of early Hodgkin's treatment by the European Organization for Research and Treatment of Cancer demonstrated an increased FSH in 3%, 8%, and 60% of patients undergoing radiotherapy alone, chemotherapy without alkylating agents, and alkylating chemotherapy, respectively. FSH recovery occurred in 80% of patients receiving nonalkylating chemotherapy at a median of 26 months as opposed to 30% of patients receiving alkylating chemotherapy at a mean of 27 months [227]. Other studies have supported the decreased gonadotoxicity of nonalkylating therapies for Hodgkin's and non-Hodgkin's lymphoma, with non-Hodgkin's therapy the least toxic [228–230].

All newly diagnosed cancer patients should be offered sperm cryopreservation, since testicular recovery may not occur after chemotherapy or radiation. When determining sperm recovery, it should be recognized that baseline semen parameters may be depressed, as is seen most commonly with testis cancer [231]. The patient's age, general health status, time constraints, and parental anxiety may be impediments to sperm cryopreservation. With appropriate counseling, however, sperm banking programs involving young adult and adolescent patients are quite effective [232–233].

As discussed above, patients may recover spermatogenesis to varying degrees after chemotherapy. With increasing use of assisted reproductive techniques including intrauterine insemination (IUI) and in-vitro fertilization (IVF), paternity has been possible in many more patients over the past 15 years. Even patients with persistent nonobstructive azoospermia may have foci of spermatogenesis in their testis. Testicular sperm extraction (TESE) [234–236] and microdissection TESE [217] may be used to extract sperm. In a study of 20 TESE procedures in 17 patients who received

Table 14.1. Relative potential for recovery of spermatogenesis after specific chemotherapy regimens

Good	Moderate	Poor
Adriamycin	Vincristine	Cyclophosphamide
Methotrexate	PEB	Chlorambucil
Prednisone	ABVD	Mechlorethamine
Estrogens		Procarbazine
Androgens		MOPP
Cisplatin		
Thioguanin		
Doxorubicin		
6-Mercaptopurine		

ABVD, doxorubicin, bleomycin, vinblastine, dacarbazine; MOPP, nitrogen mustard, vincristine, procarbazine, prednisone; PEB, cisplatin, etoposide, bleomycin. (Data from references [220,222–226]. From Nudell DM *et al.* Common medications and drugs: how they affect male fertility. *Urol Clin North Am* 2002; **29**: 965–73. With permission.)

chemotherapy, Chan *et al.* retrieved sperm in 45% of patients. Among the 76% of patients with Sertoli-cell-only pattern on biopsy, 23% had sperm retrieved by standard or microdissection TESE. **Patients able to conceive naturally are advised to wait a minimum of 1–2 years post-chemotherapy or radiation due to the risk of chromosomal or congenital abnormalities after treatment with cytotoxic agents.**

Since radiation and chemotherapy exert effects by injury to the spermatogonia, attempts have been made to prevent or reverse sterility. The goal has been not to protect the spermatogonia from injury, but rather to help the surviving spermatogonia differentiate after cytotoxic therapy. Rat studies have demonstrated the protective effects of pretreatment with testosterone and estradiol prior to radiation therapy [237]. Similarly, suppression of intratesticular testosterone with gonadotropin-releasing hormone (GnRH) agonists or antagonists either before or after a cytotoxic insult may restore spermatogenesis and fertility in rats [218]. Human studies, however, have yielded less impressive results. Only one study of seven clinical trials demonstrated a protective benefit of hormonal agents before and during chemotherapy or radiation [218,238].

Psychotherapeutic medications

Psychotherapeutic medications affect male fertility mainly by inhibiting sexual function; however,

impairments of semen parameters may occur with use of certain antidepressants. Tricyclic antidepressants and selective serotonin reuptake inhibitors (SSRIs) may impair erections and libido via sedative and anticholinergic effects, serotonergic effects, and effects on serum prolactin [239]. It has been estimated that 62% of men taking antidepressants will experience sexual side effects [239]. SSRIs adversely affect emission and ejaculation, and therefore are used to treat patients experiencing rapid ejaculation. In addition, there is a potential for hyperprolactinemia with phenothiazines and certain tricyclic antidepressants. Hyperprolactinemia can inhibit GnRH and LH production and impair spermatogenesis [220].

Antidepressants may also directly impair male fertility via effects on sperm. **Impairment of sperm motility has been demonstrated in in-vitro studies of tricyclic antidepressants** [240,241]. A recent case report described the recovery of sperm density and motility in two patients, one taking the SSRI citalopram and the other sertraline [242].

Antipsychotic agents block dopamine production in the central nervous system, resulting in suppression of the HPG axis and decreased libido. Vasodilatory effects can also cause erectile dysfunction [192].

Miscellaneous medications

Increased awareness and recognition of erectile dysfunction has resulted in the use of phosphodiesterase type 5 (PDE-5) inhibitors in younger patients. Studies evaluating the effects of PDE-5 inhibitors on semen characteristics yield conflicting results. Single dosing studies of sildenafil reveal no effects on semen parameters in healthy volunteers [243] and an increase in motility in infertile men [244]. Likewise, an in-vitro study of sildenafil demonstrated an improvement of sperm motility but an adverse effect on fertility by causing a premature acrosome reaction [245]. **Single dosing of tadalafil has been reported to have an inhibitory effect on motility in healthy young men** [244]. The effects of chronic dosing have also been evaluated. A randomized, double-blind, placebo-controlled trial by Jarvi et al. demonstrated no adverse effects on semen parameters in patients taking vardenafil and sildenafil daily for six months [246].

Cimetidine, a histamine type 2 receptor blocker used in the treatment of peptic ulcer disease, **impairs spermatogenesis by interrupting the normal pulsatile secretion of LH** from the pituitary gland in response to GnRH. Other side effects include increased serum

prolactin concentrations, possible direct toxicity to seminiferous tubules, and impairment of the transport of sperm through the epididymis. Other medications used to treat peptic ulcer lack these effects on fertility [220].

Sulfasalazine is commonly used to treat inflammatory bowel disease. **Impairment in sperm density, motility, and morphology** occur with its use. Pregnancy rates are similarly decreased [247,248]. If sulfasalazine is discontinued, semen parameters usually will improve [249]. Mesalazine is a substitute that is effective without these fertility-related side effects [223].

Cyclosporine is an immunosuppressant commonly used after organ transplantation. In animal studies, it has been shown to decrease semen parameters and overall fertility [250]. **Cyclosporine impairs human sperm motility and viability** as well [251,252]. Though the exact mechanism is not known, it is thought that the medication interferes with signal transduction in Leydig cells in response to LH [253].

Colchicine and allopurinol alter the metabolism of uric acid and are used for the treatment of gout. These drugs may result in a reversible impairment of sperm penetration into the oocyte [220].

Lifestyle factors

The increasing use of **cell phones** has led to growing concerns that the **electromagnetic waves** emitted have harmful effects on fertility. **Recent in-vitro and in-vivo observational studies have supported a dose-dependent decrease in sperm density** [254], **motility** [254–256], **viability** [254], **and morphology** [254,256]. Whether these effects are clinically significant, or if they occur by a heat-related or electromagnetic wave-specific mechanism, remains unclear.

Testicular hyperthermia has been shown to impair spermatogenesis and negatively impact male fertility [257,258]. **Hyperthermia as a result of endogenous stressors such as high fever or exogenous heat may impair sperm density, motility, and morphology.** Laptop computers have been inconclusively demonstrated to impair fertility [259]. Wet heat from hot-tubs, Jacuzzis, or baths may cause a decline in semen quality. In a study of the recovery of semen quality after wet hyperthermia, semen parameters recovered in about half of patients after discontinuation of the hyperthermic exposure. Recovery of total motile counts among responders was largely due to improvement in mean sperm motility from 12% to 34% [260].

Alcohol and illicit drugs

Heavy consumption of **alcohol** over time often results in erectile dysfunction, decreased libido, and gynecomastia [192]. It is thought that alcohol exerts effects on the HPG axis, resulting in testicular dysfunction [192]. In addition, peripheral aromatization of testosterone is responsible for the estrogenic effects of alcohol [261]. These **hormonal alterations lead to decreases in sperm density and motility** [192]. Alcohol reduces antioxidant levels in the body, resulting in increased oxidative stress [262]. Elevated reactive oxygen species are associated with impairments in sperm motility [263]. **There is no evidence that light consumption of alcohol affects fertility** [220].

Marijuana decreases sperm density, motility, and morphology [192]. Opiates cause decreased libido and erectile dysfunction. **Opiates suppress the secretion of GnRH**, resulting in decreased circulating LH and lower testosterone levels. **Cocaine abuse causes erectile dysfunction**, while **amphetamines can cause decreased libido** [220].

Conclusion

Endocrine-disrupting chemicals (EDC) are ubiquitous in society. They are found in small amounts in food as pesticides and fumigants; in insecticides and solvents; and in plastic containers and other common household items. Offending agents such as environmental estrogens, methyl bromide and methyl chloride, ethylene dibromide, DBCP, DDT, PCBs, and phthalates may be directly gonadotoxic or cause damage through hormonally mediated events. Mediators of cellular damage such as reactive oxygen species and hydrolytic enzymes disrupt the natural balance on the cellular level between mitosis and apoptosis. Susceptibility to EDCs depends on the dosage and potency of the agent, route of exposure, and duration and frequency of exposure. Studies of laboratory animals, accidental and occupational exposures, and long-term population exposures have contributed greatly to our understanding of the effects of EDCs.

Medications, alcohol, and substances of abuse may also have deleterious effects on the male reproductive system via alterations in the HPG axis, direct gonadotoxic damage, or changes in erectile, ejaculatory, and/or sexual function. A thorough understanding of these effects is critical for appropriate prevention and treatment, particularly for those men who want to remain fertile. Chemotherapeutic agents may induce irreversible testicular damage, and therefore all patients should

be offered sperm banking prior to treatment. Lastly, results of many studies correlating lifestyle factors and impaired fertility are conflicting, but patients should be apprised of potential risks.

References

[1] Lancranjan I, Popescu HI, Gavanescu O, Serbanescu M. Reproductive ability of workmen occupationally exposed to lead. *Arch Environ Health* 1975; **30**: 396–401.

[2] Whorton D, Krauss RM, Marshall S, Milby TH. Infertility in male pesticide workers. *Lancet* 1977; **2**: 1259–61.

[3] Carson R. *Silent Spring*. New York, NY: Fawcett Press, 1962.

[4] Colborn T, vom Saal FS, Soto AM. Developmental effects of endocrine-disrupting chemicals in wildlife and humans. *Environ Health Perspect* 1993; **101**: 378–84.

[5] Sharpe RM, Skakkebaek NE. Are estrogens involved in falling sperm counts and disorders of the male reproductive tract? *Lancet* 1993; **341**: 1392–5.

[6] Toppari J, Larsen JC, Christiansen P, *et al.* Male reproductive health and environmental estrogens. *Environ Health Perspect* 1996; **104** (Suppl 4): 741–803.

[7] Leffers H, Naesby M, Vendelbo B, Skakkebaek NE, Jorgensen M. Oestrogenic properties of Zeranol, vestradiol, diethylstilbestrol, Bisphenol-A and genistein: implications for exposure assessment of potential endocrine disrupters. *Hum Reprod* 2001; **16**: 1037–45.

[8] Stephany RW. Hormones in meat: different approaches in the EU and in the USA. *APMIS Suppl* 2001; **103**: S357–64.

[9] Ganmaa D, Li XM, Wang J, *et al.* Incidence and mortality of testicular and prostatic cancers in relation to world dietary practices. *Int J Cancer* 2002; **98**: 262–7.

[10] Carlsen E, Giwercman A, Keiding N, Skakkebaek NE. Evidence for decreasing quality of semen during past 50 years. *BMJ* 1992; **305**: 609–13.

[11] Swan SH, Elkin EP, Fenster L. Have sperm densities declined? A reanalysis of global trend data. *Environ Health Perspect* 1997; **105**: 1228–32.

[12] Joffe M. Are problems with male reproductive health caused by endocrine disruption? *Occup Environ Med* 2001; **58**: 281–8.

[13] Joffe M. Infertility and environmental pollutants. *Br Med Bull* 2003; **68**: 47–70.

[14] Seeley RR, Stephens TD, Tate P. Cell biology and genetics. In: Seeley RR, Stephens TD, Tate P, eds. *Anatomy and Physiology*, 8th edn. New York, NY: McGraw-Hill, 2008: 53–93.

[15] Gregus Z, Klaassen CD. Mechanisms of toxicity. In: Klaassen CD, ed. *Casarette and Doull's Toxicology:*

241

The Basic Science of Poisons, 6th edn. New York, NY: McGraw-Hill, 2001: 35–81.

[16] Wallace KB, Starkov AA. Mitochondrial targets of drug toxicity. *Ann Rev Pharmacol Toxicol* 2000; **40**: 353–88.

[17] Buja LM, Eigenbrodt ML, Eigenbrodt EH. Apoptosis and necrosis: basic types and mechanisms of cell death. *Arch Pathol Lab Med* 1993; **117**: 1208–14.

[18] Leist M, Nicotera B. Calcium and neuronal death. *Rev Physiol Biochem Pharmacol* 1970; **132**: 79–125.

[19] Richburg JH, Boekelheide K. Mono-(2-ethylhexyl) phthalate rapidly alters both Sertoli cell vimentin filaments and germ cell apoptosis in young rat testes. *Toxicol Appl Pharmacol* 1996; **137**: 42–50.

[20] Billig H, Chun SY, Eisenhower K, Hsueh AJW. Gonadal cell apoptosis: hormone-regulated cell demise. *Hum Reprod Update* 1996; **2**: 103–17.

[21] Lee J, Richburg JH, Younkin SC, Boekelheide K. The Fas system is a key regulator of germ cell apoptosis in the testis. *Endocrinology* 1997; **138**: 2081–8.

[22] Younglai EV, Holloway AC, Foster WG. Environmental and occupational factors affecting fertility and IVF success. *Hum Reprod Update* 2005; **11**: 43–57.

[23] Damstra T, Barlow S, Bergman A, Kavlock R, Van der Kraak G. *Global Assessment of the State-of-the Science of Endocrine Disruptors*. WHO Publication Number WHO/PCS/EDC/02.2. Geneva: World Health Organization, 2002.

[24] Damstra T. Endocrine disrupters: the need for a refocused vision. *Toxicol Sci* 2003; **74**: 231–2.

[25] Daston GP, Cook JC, Kavlock RJ. Uncertainties for endocrine disrupters: our view of progress. *Toxicol Sci* 2003; **74**: 245–52.

[26] Pryor JL, Hughes C, Foster W, Hales BF, Robaire B. Critical windows of exposure for children's health: the reproductive system in animals and humans. *Environ Health Perspect* 2000; **108** (Suppl 3): 491–503.

[27] Williams K, McKinnel C, Saunders PTK, *et al.* Neonatal exposure to potent and environmental oestrogens and abnormalities of the male reproductive system in the rat: evidence for importance of the androgen-oestrogen balance and assessment of the relevance to man. *Hum Reprod Update* 2001; **7**: 236–47.

[28] Oliva A, Spira A, Multigner L. Contribution of environmental factors to the risk of male infertility. *Hum Reprod* 2001; **16**: 1768–76.

[29] Sharpe RM, Walker M, Millar MR, *et al.* Effect of neonatal gonadotropin-releasing hormone antagonist administration on Sertoli cell number and testicular development in the marmoset: comparison with the rat. *Biol Reprod* 2000; **62**: 1685–93.

[30] Nef S, Shipman T, Parada LF. A molecular basis for estrogen-induced cryptorchidism. *Develop Biol* 2000; **224**: 354–61.

[31] Safe SH. Environmental and dietary estrogens and human health: is there a problem? *Environ Health Perspect* 1995; **103**: 346–51.

[32] Safe SH. Endocrine disruptors and human health: is there a problem? An update. *Environ Health Perspect* 2000; **108**: 487–93.

[33] Safe S. Clinical correlates of environmental endocrine disrupters. *Trends Endocrinol Metab* 2005; **16**: 139–44.

[34] Ososki AL, Kennelly EJ. Phytoestrogens: a review of the present state of research. *Phytotherapy Res* 2003; **17**: 845–69.

[35] Ross JA, Kasum CM. Dietary flavonoids: bioavailability, metabolic effects, and safety. *Annu Rev Nutr* 2002; **22**: 19–34.

[36] Wolf C, Lambright C, Mann P, *et al.* Administration of potentially antiandrogenic pesticides (procymidone, linuron, iprodione, chlozolinate, p,p'-DDE and ketoconazole) and toxic substances (dibutyl- and diethylhexyl phthalate, PCB 169, and ethane dimethane sulphonate) during sexual differentiation produces diverse profiles of reproductive malformations in the male rat. *Toxicol Ind Health* 1999; **15**: 94–118.

[37] Fisher JS. Environmental anti-androgens and male reproductive health: focus on phthalates and testicular dysgenesis syndrome. *Reproduction* 2004; **127**: 305–15.

[38] Skakkebaek NE, Rajpert-DeMeyts E, Main KM. Testicular dysgenesis syndrome: an increasingly common developmental disorder with environmental aspects. *Hum Reprod* 2001; **16**: 972–8.

[39] Pharris-Ciurej ND, Cook LS, Weiss NS. Incidence of testicular cancer in the United States: has the epidemic begun to abate? *Am J Epidemiol* 1999; **150**: 45–6.

[40] Ekbom A. Growing evidence that several human cancers may originate *in utero. Cancer Biol* 1998; **8**: 237–44.

[41] Weir HK, Marrett LD, Kreiger N, Darlington GA, Sugar L. Pre-natal and peri-natal exposures and risk of testicular germ-cell cancer. *Int J Cancer* 2000; **87**: 438–43.

[42] Henderson BE, Benton B, Jing J, Yu MC, Pike MC. Risk factors for cancer of the testes in young men. *Int J Cancer* 1979; **23**: 598–602.

[43] Hauser R. The environment and male fertility: recent research on emerging chemicals and semen quality. *Semin Reprod Med* 2006; **24**: 156–67.

[44] Ohlson CG, Hardell L. Testicular cancer and occupational exposures with a focus on xenoestrogens in polyvinyl chloride plastics. *Chemosphere* 2000; **40**: 1277–82.

[45] Sharpe RM. The "oestrogen hypothesis": where do we stand now? *Internat J Androl* 2003; **26**: 2–15.

[46] ATSDR. *Toxicological Profile for Chlorinated Dibenzo-p-Dioxins (Update)*. Atlanta, GA: US Agency for Toxic Substances and Disease Registry, 1998.

[47] ATSDR. *Toxicological Profile for Polychlorinated Biphenyls (Update)*. Atlanta, GA: US Agency for Toxic Substances and Disease Registry, 2000.

[48] ATSDR. *Toxicological Profile for DDT/DDD/DDE (Update)*. Atlanta, GA: US Agency for Toxic Substances and Disease Registry, 2002.

[49] Bruckner JV, Anand SS, Warren DA. Toxic effects of solvents and vapors. In: Klaassen CD, ed. *Casarette and Doull's Toxicology: the Basic Science of Poisons*, 7th edn. New York, NY: McGraw-Hill, 2008.

[50] Whorton D, Wong O. Reproductive effects of dibromochloropropane (DBCP) on humans: a case study in occupational medicine. *Chinese J Occup Med* 1996; 3: 191–206.

[51] EPA. *Guidelines for Cancer Risk Assessment*. EPA/630/P-03/001B, Risk Assessment Forum. Washington, DC: US Environmental Protection Agency, 2005.

[52] Federal Register. *EPA National Primary Drinking Water Regulations*. Volatile Synthetic Organic Chemicals, Proposed Rulemaking 1984; 49(114): 24338.

[53] Lee KM, Bruckner JV, Muralidhara S, Gallo JM. Characterization of presystemic elimination of trichloroethylene and its nonlinear kinetics in rats. *Toxicol Appl Pharmacol* 1996; 139: 262–71.

[54] ATSDR. *Toxicological Profile for 1,2-Dibromo-3-Chloropropane*. Atlanta, GA: US Agency for Toxic Substances and Disease Registry, 1992.

[55] ESHRE Capri Workshop Group. Fertility and aging. *Hum Reprod Update* 2005; 11: 261–76.

[56] Rolf C, Behre HM, Nieschlag E. Reproductive parameters of older compared to younger men in infertile couples. *Int J Androl* 1996; 19: 135–42.

[57] Sallmen M, Sandler DP, Hoppin JA, Blair A, Baird DD. Reduced fertility among overweight and obese men. *Epidemiology* 2006; 17: 520–3.

[58] Ramlau-Hansen CH, Thulstrup AM, Nohr EA, et al. Subfecundity in overweight and obese couples. *Hum Reprod* 2007; 22: 1634–7.

[59] Nguyen R, Wilcox A, Skjaerven R, Baird DD. Men's body mass index and infertility. *Hum Reprod* 2007; 17, 2488–93.

[60] Jensen TK, Andersson AM, Jorgensen N, et al. Body mass index in relation to semen quality and reproductive hormones among 1,558 Danish men. *Fertil Steril* 2004; 82: 863–70.

[61] Magnusdottir EV, Thorsteinsson T, Thorsteinsdottir S, Heimisdottir M, Olafsdottir K. Persistent organochlorines, sedentary occupation, obesity and human male subfertility. *Hum Reprod* 2005; 20: 208–15.

[62] Kort HI, Massey JB, Elsner CV, et al. Impact of body mass index values on sperm quantity and quality. *J Androl* 2006; 27: 450–2.

[63] Svartberg J, Midtby M, Bonaa KH, et al. The associations of age, lifestyle factors and chronic disease with testosterone in men: The Tromso study. *Eur J Endocrinol* 2003; 149: 145–52.

[64] Schneider G, Kirshner MA, Berkowitz R, Ertel NH. Increased estrogen production in obese men. *J Clin Endocrinol Metab* 1979; 48: 633–8.

[65] Globerman H, Shen-Orr Z, Karnieli E, Aloni Y, Charuzi I. Inhibin B in men with severe obesity and after weight reduction following gastroplasty. *Endocr Res* 2005; 31: 17–26.

[66] Curtis KM, Savitz DA, Arbuckle TE. Effects of cigarette smoking, caffeine consumption, and alcohol intake on fecundability. *Am J Epidemiol* 1997; 146: 32–41.

[67] Homan GF, Davies M, Norman R. The impact of lifestyle factors on reproductive performance in the general population and those undergoing infertility treatment: a review. *Hum Reprod Update* 2007; 13: 209–23.

[68] Hassan MAM, Killick SR. Negative lifestyle is associated with a significant reduction in fecundity. *Fertil Steril* 2004; 81: 384–92.

[69] Omu AE, Dashti H, Mohammed AT, Mattappallil AB. Cigarette smoking causes impairment of spermatozoal quality: Andrological and biochemical evaluation. *Med Prin Pract* 1998; 7: 47–53.

[70] Kunzle R, Mueller MD, Hanggi W, et al. Semen quality of male smokers and nonsmokers in infertile couples. *Fertil Steril* 2003; 79: 287–91.

[71] Zitmann M, Rolf C, Nordhoff V, et al. Male smokers have a decreased success rate for in vitro fertilization and intracytoplasmic sperm injection. *Fertil Steril* 2003; 79: 1550–4.

[72] Martini AC, Molina RI, Estofan D, et al. Effects of alcohol and cigarette consumption on human seminal quality. *Fertil Steril* 2004; 82: 374–7.

[73] Practice Committee of the American Society for Reproductive Medicine. Smoking and infertility. *Fertil Steril* 2004; 82: S62–7.

[74] Jensen K, Jorgensen N, Punab M, et al. Association of in utero exposure to maternal smoking with reduced semen quality and testes size in adulthood: a cross-sectional study of 1,770 young men from the general population in five European countries. *Am J Epidemiol* 2004; 159: 49–58.

[75] Storgaard L, Bonde JP, Ernst E, et al. Does smoking during pregnancy affect sons' sperm counts? *Epidemiology* 2003; 14: 278–86.

[76] Zenzes MT, Bielecki R, Reed TE. Detection of benzo(a)pyrene diol epoxide-DNA adducts in sperm of men exposed to cigarette smoke. *Fertil Steril* 1999; 72: 330–5.

[77] Zenzes MT, Puy LA, Bielecki R, Reed TE. Detection of benzo(a)pyrene diol epoxide-DNA adducts in embryos from smoking couples: evidence for transmission by spermatozoa. *Mol Hum Reprod* 1999; 5: 125–31.

[78] Pacifici R, Altieri I, Gandini L, *et al.* Nicotine, cotinine, and trans-3-hydroxycotinine levels in seminal plasma of smokers: effect on sperm parameters. *Ther Drug Monitor* 1993; **15**: 358–63.

[79] Gandini L, Lombardo F, Lenzi A, *et al.* The in-vitro effects of nicotine and cotinine on sperm mobility. *Hum Reprod* 1997; **12**: 727–33.

[80] Li LH, Heindel JJ. Sertoli cell toxicants. In: Korach KS, ed. *Reproduction and Developmental Toxicology.* New York, NY: Marcel Dekker, 1998: 655–91.

[81] Sanderson JT. The steroid hormone biosynthesis pathway as a target for endocrine-disrupting chemicals. *Toxicol Sci* 2006; **94**: 3–21.

[82] Winters SJ. Androgens and antiandrogens. In: Brody TM, Larner J, Minneman KP, eds. *Brody's Human Pharmacology: Molecular to Clincal*, 4th edn. St. Louis, MO: Mosby, 2005: 454–8.

[83] Carreau S, Lambard S, Delalande C, *et al.* Aromatase expression and role of estrogens in male gonad: a review. *Reprod Biol Endocrinol* 2003; **1**: 35–40.

[84] Gammon DW, Aldons CN, Carr WC, Sanborn JR, Pfeifer KF. A risk assessment of atrazine use in California: human health and ecological aspects. *Pest Manag Sci* 2005; **61**: 331–55.

[85] Sonderfan AJ, Arlotto MP, Parkinson A. . Identification of the cytochrome P-450 isozymes responsible for testosterone oxidation in rat lung, kidney and testis: evidence that cytochrome P-450a (P450IIA1) is the physiologically important testosterone 7 alpha-hydroxylase in rat testis. *Endocrinology* 1989; **125**: 857–66.

[86] Dym M, Fawcett DW. The blood–testis barrier in the rat and the physiological compartmentation of the seminiferous epithelium. *Biol Reprod* 1970; **3**: 308–26.

[87] Setchell BP, Main SJ. Drugs and the blood–testis barrier. *Environ Health Perspect* 1978; **24**: 61–4.

[88] Kuratsune M, Yoshimura T, Matsuzaka J, Yamaguchi A. Epidemiologic study on Yusho, a poisoning caused by ingestion of rice oil contaminated with a commercial brand of polychlorinated biphenyls. *Environ Health Perspect* 1972; **60**: 321–5.

[89] Hsu ST, Ma CI, Hsu SKH, *et al.* Discovery and epidemiology of PCB poisoning in Taiwan: a four-year followup. *Environ Health Perspect* 1985; **59**: 5–10.

[90] Mocarelli P, Marocchi A, Brambilla P, *et al.* Clinical laboratory manifestations of exposure to dioxin in children. *JAMA* 1986; **256**: 2687–95.

[91] Mocarelli P, Needham LL, Marocchi A, *et al.* Serum concentrations of 2,3,7,8-tetrachlorodibenzo-p-dioxin and test results from selected residents of Seveso, Italy. *J Toxicol Environ Health* 1991; **32**: 357–66.

[92] CDC. The Centers for Disease Control Vietnam experience study. Health status of Vietnam veterans. II. Physical health. *JAMA* 1988; **259**: 2708–14.

[93] Mocarelli P, Gerthoux PM, Ferrari E, *et al.* Paternal concentrations of dioxin and sex ratio of offspring. *Lancet* 2000; **355**: 1858–63.

[94] Lione A. Polychlorinated biphenyls and reproduction. *Reprod Toxicol* 1988; **2**: 83–9.

[95] Rignell-Hydbom A, Rylander L, Giwercman A, *et al.* Exposure to CB-153 and p,p'-DDE and male reproductive function. *Hum Reprod* 2004; **19**: 2066–75.

[96] Ayotte P, Giroux S, Dewailly E, *et al.* DDT spraying for malaria control and reproductive function in Mexican men. *Epidemiology* 2001; **12**: 366–7.

[97] Garcia-Rodriquez J, Garcia-Martin M, Nogueras-Ocana M, *et al.* Exposure to pesticides and cryptorchidism: Geographical evidence of a possible association. *Environ Health Perspect* 1996; **104**: 1090–5.

[98] Foster WG, Holloway AC. Do environmental contaminants adversely affect human reproductive physiology? *J Obstet Gynaecol Can* 2003; **25**: 33–44.

[99] ATSDR. *Toxicological Profile for Bromomethane.* Atlanta, GA: US Agency for Toxic Substances and Disease Registry, 1992.

[100] Alexeeff GV, Kilgore WW. Methyl bromide. *Residue Rev* 1983; **88**: 101–53.

[101] Wedge RM, Abt EN, Hobbs CH. Methyl bromide risk characterization in California. *J Toxicol Environ Health B* 2001; **4**: 333–9.

[102] Hurtt ME, Morgan KT, Working PK. Histopathology of acute toxic responses in selected tissues from rats exposed by inhalation to methyl bromide. *Fund Appl Toxicol* 1987; **9**: 352–65.

[103] Hurtt ME, Working PK. Evaluation of spermatogenesis and sperm quality in the rat following acute inhalation exposure to methyl bromide. *Fund Appl Toxicol* 1988; **10**: 490–8.

[104] Eustis SL, Haber SB, Drew RT, Yang RSH. Toxicology and pathology of methyl bromide in F344 rats and B6C3F1 mice following repeated inhalation exposure. *Fund Appl Toxicol* 1988; **11**: 594–610.

[105] Kaneda M, Hatakenaka N, Teramoto S, Maita K. A two-generation reproduction study in rats with methyl bromide-fumigated diets. *Food Cosmet Toxicol* 1993; **31**: 533–42.

[106] ATSDR. *Toxicological Profile for Chloromethane (Updated).* Atlanta, GA: US Agency for Toxic Substances and Disease Registry, 1998.

[107] TRI96. *Toxic Chemical Release Inventory.* National Library of Medicine, National Toxicology Program Information Program. Bethesda, MD: NLM, 1998.

[108] Chapin RE, White RD, Morgan RT, Bus JS. Studies of lesions induced in the testis and epididymis of F-344 rats by inhaled methyl chloride. *Toxicol Appl Pharmacol* 1984; **76**: 328–43.

[109] Working PK, Bus JS, Hamm TE. Reproductive effects of inhaled methyl chloride in the male Fischer 344 rat. II. Spermatogonial toxicity and sperm quality. *Toxicol Appl Pharmacol* 1985; **77**: 144–57.

[110] Hamm TE, Raynor TH, Phelps MC, *et al.* Reproduction in Fischer-344 rats exposed to methyl chloride by inhalation for two generations. *Fund Appl Toxicol* 1985; **5**: 568–77.

[111] Bond JA, Dutcher JS, Medinsky MA, Henderson RF, Birnbaum LS. Disposition of [¹⁴C]. methyl bromide in rats after inhalation. *Toxicol Appl Pharmacol* 1985; **78**: 259–67.

[112] Dekant W, Frischmann C, Speerschneider P. Sex, organ and species specific bioactivation of chloromethane by cytochrome P4502E1. *Xenobiotica* 1995; **25**: 1259–65.

[113] Chellman GJ, White RD, Norton RM, Bus JS. Inhibition of the acute toxicity of methyl chloride in male B6C3F1 mice by glutathione depletion. *Toxicol Appl Pharmacol* 1986; **86**: 93–104.

[114] ATSDR. *Toxicological Profile for 1,2-Dibromoethane.* Atlanta, GA: US Agency for Toxic Substances and Disease Registry, 1992.

[115] Alexeeff GV, Kilgore WW, Li MY. Ethylene dibromide: toxicology and risk assessment. *Rev Environ Contam Toxicol* 1990; **112**: 49–122.

[116] WHO. *1,2-Dibromoethane in Drinking-Water. Background Document for Development of WHO Guidelines for Drinking-Water Quality.* WHO/SDE/WSH/03.04/66. Geneva: World Health Organization, 2004.

[117] Williams J, Gladen BC, Turner TW, Schrader SM, Chapin RE. The effects of ethylene dibromide on semen quality and fertility in the rabbit: evaluation of a model for human seminal characteristics. *Fund Appl Toxicol* 1991; **16**: 687–700.

[118] Short RD, Winston JM, Hong CB, *et al.* Effects of ethylene dibromide on reproduction in male and female rats. *Toxicol Appl Pharmacol* 1979; **49**: 97–105.

[119] Khan S, Sood C, O'Brien PJ. Molecular mechanisms of dibromoalkane cytotoxicity in isolated rat hepatocytes. *Biochem Pharamcol* 1993; **45**: 439–47.

[120] Wong LCK, Winston JM, Hong CB, Plotnick H. Carcinogenicity and toxicity of 1,2-dibromoethane in the rat. *Toxicol Appl Pharmacol* 1982; **63**: 155–65.

[121] Chiarpotto E, Biasi F, Aragno M, *et al.* Ethanol-induced potentiation of rat hepatocyte damage due to 1,2-dibromoethane. *Alcohol Alcoholism* 1995; **30**: 37–45.

[122] NTP. *Carcinogenesis Bioassay of 1,2-Dibromoethane in F344 Rats and B6C3F1 Mice (Inhalation Study).* NIH Publication Number 82–1766. Durham, NC: National Toxicology Program, 1982.

[123] Takahashi W, Wong L, Rogers BJ, Hale RW. Depression of sperm counts among agricultural workers exposed to dibromochloropropane and ethylene dibromide. *Bull Environ Contam Toxicol* 1981; **27**: 551–8.

[124] Ratcliffe JM, Schrader SM, Steenland K, *et al.* Semen quality in papaya workers with long term exposure to ethylene dibromide. *Br J Ind Med* 1987; **44**: 317–26.

[125] Schrader SM, Turner TW, Ratcliffe JM. The effects of ethylene dibromide on semen quality: a comparison of short-term and chronic exposure. *Reprod Toxicol* 1988; **2**: 191–8.

[126] Ter Haar G. An investigation of possible sterility and health effects from exposure to ethylene dibromide. In: Ames B, Infante P, Reitz R, eds. *Banbury Report*, Volume 5. Cold Springs Harbor, NY: Cold Springs Harbor Laboratory, 1980: 167–88.

[127] Wong O, Utidjian HMD, Karten VS. Retrospective evaluation of reproductive performance of workers exposed to ethylene dibromide (EDB). *J Occup Med* 1979; **21**: 98–102.

[128] Gingell R, Beatty PW, Mitschke HR, *et al.* Toxicokinetics of 1,2-dibromo-3-chloropropane (DBCP) in the rat. *Toxicol Appl Pharmacol* 1987; **91**: 386–94.

[129] Torkelson TR, Sadek SE, Rowe VK, *et al.* Toxicologic investigations of 1,2-dibromo-3-chloropropane. *Toxicol Appl Pharmacol* 1961; **3**: 545–59.

[130] Egnatz DG, Ott MG, Townsend JC, Olson RD, Johns DB. DBCP and testicular effects in chemical workers: An epidemiological survey in Midland, Michigan. *J Occup Med* 1980; **22**: 727–32.

[131] Lipshultz LI, Ross CE, Whorton D, *et al.* Dibromochloropropane and its effect on testicular function in man. *J Urol* 1980; **124**: 464–8.

[132] Potashnik G, Yamai-Inbar I, Sacks MI, Israeli R. Effects of dibromochloropropane on human testicular function. *Israel J Med Sci* 1979; **15**: 438–42.

[133] Heindel JJ, Berkowitz AS, Kyle G, Luthra R, Bruckner JV. Assessment in rats of the gonadotoxic and hepatorenal toxic potential of dibromochloropropane (DBCP) in drinking water. *Fund Appl Toxicol* 1989; **13**: 804–15.

[134] Aman RP, Berndston WE. Assessment of procedures for screening agents for effects on male reproduction: effects of dibromochloropropane (DBCP) on the rat. *Fund Appl Toxicol* 1986; **7**: 244–55.

[135] Foote RH, Schermerhorn EC, Simkin ME. Measurement of semen quality, fertility, and reproductive hormones to assess dibromochloropropane (DBCP) effects in live rabbits. *Fund Appl Toxicol* 1986; **6**: 628–37.

[136] Rao KS, Burek JD, Murray FJ, *et al.* Toxicologic and reproductive effects of inhaled 1,2-dibromo-3-chloropropane in male rabbits. *Fund Appl Toxicol* 1982; **2**: 241–51.

[137] Rao KS, Burek JD, Murray FJ, *et al.* Toxicologic and reproductive effects of inhaled 1,2-dibromo-3-chloropropane in rats. *Fund Appl Toxicol* 1983; **3**: 104–10.

[138] Glass RI, Lyness RN, Mengle DC, Powell KE, Kahn E. Sperm count depression in pesticide applicators exposed to dibromochloropropane. *Am J Epidemiol* 1979; **109**: 346–51.

[139] NIOSH. *Health Hazard Evaluation Report Number HETA 81–040-1315.* Dole Pineapple Company, Lanai, HI. Cincinnati, OH: National Institute of Occupational Safety and Health, 1983.

[140] Sandifer SH, Wilkins RT, Loadholt CB, Lane LG, Eldridge JC. Spermatogenesis in agricultural workers exposed to dibromochloropropane (DBCP). *Bull Environ Contam Toxicol* 1979; **23**: 703–10.

[141] NIOSH. *Health Hazard Evaluation Report Number HETA 81–040-1315.* Dole Pineapple Company, Lanai, HI. Cincinnati, OH: National Institute of Occupational Safety and Health, 1983.

[142] NIOSH. *Health Hazard Evaluation Report Number HETA 81–169-1935.* Maui Land and Pineapple Company, HI. Cincinnati, OH: National Institute of Occupational Safety and Health, 1990.

[143] Lag M, Soderland EJ, Omichinski JG, *et al.* Effect of bromine and chlorine positioning in the induction of renal and testicular toxicity by halogenated propanes. *Chem Res Toxicol* 1991; **4**: 528–34.

[144] Beard J. DDT and human health. *Sci Total Environ* 2006; **355**: 78–89.

[145] Torres-Arreola L, Lopez-Carrillo L, Torres-Sanchex L, *et al.* Levels of dichloro-diphenyl-trichloroethane (DDT) metabolites in maternal milk and their determinant factors. *Arch Environ Health* 1999; **54**: 123–9.

[146] Salazar-Garcia F, Gallardo-Diaz E, Ceron-Mireles P, Loomis D, Borja-Aburto VH. Reproductive effects of occupational DDT exposure among male malaria control workers. *Environ Health Perspect* 2004; **111**: 542–7.

[147] Turusov V, Rakitsky Tomatis L. Dichlorodiphenyltrichloroethane (DDT): ubiquity, persistence, and risks. Environ *Health Perspect* 2002; **110**: 125–8.

[148] Gray LE, Ostby J, Furr J, *et al.* . Perinatal exposure to the phthalates DEHP, BBP, and DINP, but not DEP, DMP, or DOTP, alters sexual differentiation of the male rat. *Toxicol Sci* 2000; **58**: 350–65.

[149] You L, Casanova M, Archibeque-Engle S, *et al.* Impaired male sexual development in perinatal Sprague-Dawley and Long-Evans hooded rats exposed in utero and lactationally to p,p′-DDE. *Toxicol Sci* 1998; **45**: 162–73.

[150] Kelce WR, Stone CR, Laws SC, *et al.* Persistent DDT metabolite p,p′-DDE is a potent androgen receptor antagonist. *Nature* 1995; **375**: 581–5.

[151] Veeramachaneni DNR, Palmer JS, Amann, RP, Pau KYF. Sequalae in rabbits following developmental exposure to p,p'-DDT or a mixture of p,p'-DDT and vinclozolin: Cryptorchidism, germ cell aplasia, and sexual dysfunction. *Reprod Toxicol* 2007; **23**: 353–65.

[152] O'Connor JC, Frame SR, Davis LG, Cook JC. Detection of the environmental antiandrogen p,p′-DDF in CD and Long-Evans rats using a tier I screening battery and a Hershberger assay. *Toxicol Sci* 1999; **51**: 44–53.

[153] Younglai EV, Holloway AC, Lim GE, Foster WG. Synergistic effects between FSH and 1,1-dichloro-2,2-bis(p-chlorophenyl)ethylene (p,p′-DDE) on human granulosa cell aromatase activity. *Hum Reprod* 2004; **19**: 1089–93.

[154] You L, Chan SK, Bruce JM, *et al.* Modulation of testosterone-metabolizing hepatic cytochrome P-450 enzymes in developing Sprague-Dawley rats following in utero exposure to p,p′-DDE. *Toxicol Appl Pharmacol* 1999; **158**: 197–205.

[155] Bush B, Bennett AH, Snow JT. Polychlorobiphenyl congeners, p,p′-DDE, and sperm function in humans. *Arch Environ Contam Toxicol* 1986; **15**: 333–41.

[156] Hauser R, Singh NP, Chen Z, Pothier L, Altshul L. Lack of an association between environmental exposure to polychlorinated biphenyls and p,p′-DDE and DNA damage in human sperm measured using the neutral comet assay. *Hum Reprod* 2003; **18**: 2525–33.

[157] Spano M, Toft G, Hagmar L, Eleuteri P, *et al.* Exposure to PCB and p,p′-DDE in European and Inuit populations: Impact on human sperm chromatin integrity. *Hum Reprod* 2005; **20**: 3488–99.

[158] Toft G, Axmon A, Giwercman A, *et al.* Fertility in four regions spanning large contrasts in serum levels of widespread persistent organochlorines: a cross-sectional study. *Environ Health* 2005; **4**: 26–39.

[159] Toft T, Rignell-Hydbom A, Tyrkiel E, *et al.* . Semen quality and exposure to persistent organochlorine pollutants. *Epidemiology* 2006; **17**: 450–8.

[160] Rignell-Hydbom JA, Rylander L, Giwercman A, *et al.* Exposure to PCBs and p,p′-DDE and human sperm chromatin integrity. *Environ Health Perspect* 2005; **113**: 175–9.

[161] de Jager C, Farias P, Barraga-Villarreal A, *et al.* Reduced seminal parameters associated with environmental DDT exposure and p,p′-DDE concentrations in men in Chiapas, Mexico: a cross-sectional study. *J Androl* 2006; **27**: 16–27.

[162] Dalvie MA, Myers JE, Thompson ML, *et al.* The long-term effects of DDT exposure on semen, fertility, and sexual function of malaria vector-control workers in Limpopo-Province, *South Africa. Environ Res* 2004; **96**: 1–8.

[163] Longnecker MP, Gladen BC, Cupul-Uicab LA, *et al.* In utero exposure to the antiandrogen 1,1-dichloro-2,2-

bis (p-chlorophenyl) ethylene (DDE) in relation to anagenital distance in male newborns from Chiopas, *Mexico. Am J Epidemiol* 2007; **165**: 1015–22.

[164] Damgaard IN, Skakkebaek NE, Toppari J, *et al.* Persistent pesticides in human breast milk and cryptorchidism. *Environ Health Perspect* 2006; **114**: 1133–8.

[165] Safe S. Toxicology, structure–function relationship, and human, and environmental health impacts of polychlorinated biphenyls: progress and problems. *Environ Health Perspect* 1992; **100**: 259–68.

[166] IPCS. *Polychlorinated Biphenyls: Human Health Aspects.* International Programe on Chemical Safety. Geneva: World Health Organization, 2003.

[167] Allen JR, Norback DH. Pathobiological responses of primates to polychlorinated biphenyl exposure. In: *Proceedings of the National Conference on Polychlorinated Biphenyls. US EPA* 1976; **560**/6–75-004: 43–9.

[168] Masuda Y. Health status of Japanese, and Taiwanese after exposure to contaminated rice oil. *Environ Health Perspect* 1985; **60**: 321–5.

[169] Guo YL, Hsu PC, Hsu CC, Lambert GH. Semen quality after prenatal exposure to polychlorinated biphenyls, and dibenzofurans. *Lancet* 2000; **356**: 1240–1.

[170] Huang W, Yao WJ, Wu MH, Guo YL, Lambert GH. Sperm changes in men exposed to polychlorinated biphenyls, and dibenzofurans. *JAMA* 2003; **289**: 2943–4.

[171] Buck GM, Mendola P, Vena JE, *et al.* Paternal Lake Ontario fish consumption, and risk of conception delay, New York State Angler cohort. *Environ Res* 1999; **80**: S13–18.

[172] Courval JM, DeHoog JV, Stein AD, *et al.* Sport-caught fish consumption and conception delay in licensed Michigan anglers. *Environ Res* 1999; **80**: S183–8.

[173] Rozati R, Reddy PP, Reddanna P, Mujtaba R. Role of environmental estrogens in the deterioration of male factor fertility. *Fertil Steril* 2002; **78**: 1187–94.

[174] Larsen L, Scheike T, Jensen TK, *et al.* Computer-assisted semen analysis parameters as predictors for fertility of men from the general population. *Hum Reprod* 2000; **15**: 1562–7.

[175] Richthoff J, Rylander L, Jonsson BAG, *et al.* Serum levels of 2, 2′, 4, 4′, 5, 5′-hexachlorobiphenyl (CB-153) in relation to markers of reproductive function in young males from the general Swedish population. *Environ Health Perspect* 2003; **111**: 409–13.

[176] Hauser R, Chen Z, Pothier L, Ryan L, Althul L. The relationship between human semen parameters and environmental exposure to polychlorinated biphenyls and p,p′-DDE. *Environ Health Perspect* 2003; **111**: 1501–11.

[177] Toft G, Hagmar L, Giwercman A, Bonde JP. Epidemiological evidence on reproductive effects of persistent organochlorines in humans. *Reprod Toxicol* 2004; **19**: 5–26.

[178] Li MH, Hansen LG. Consideration of enzyme and endocrine interactions in the risk assessment of PCBs. *Rev Toxicol* 1997; **1**: 71–156.

[179] Blount BC, Silva MJ, Caudill SP, *et al.* Levels of seven urinary phthalate metabolites in a human reference population. *Environ Health Perspect* 2000; **108**: 979–82.

[180] Silva MJ, Barr DB, Reid JA, *et al.* Urinary levels of seven phthalate metabolites in the U.S. population from the National Health and Nutrition Examination Survey (NHANES) 1999–2000. *Environ Health Perspect* 2004; **112**: 331–8.

[181] ATSDR. *Toxicological Profile for Di(2-ethyhexyl) Phthalate (Update).* Atlanta, GA: US Agency for Toxic Substances and Disease Registry, 2002.

[182] Lamb JC, Chapin RE, Teague J, Lawton AD, Reel JR. Reproductive effects for four phthalic acid esters in the mouse. *Toxicol Appl Pharmacol* 1987; **88**: 255–69.

[183] Li LH, Jester WF, Laslette AL, Orth LM. A single dose of di-(2-ethylhexyl) phthalate in neonatal rats alters gonocytes, reduces Sertoli cell proliferation, and decreases cyclin D2 expression. *Toxicol Appl Pharmacol* 2000; **166**: 222–9.

[184] Parks LG, Ostby JS, Lambright CR, *et al.* The plasticizer diethylhexylphthalate induces malformations by decreasing fetal testosterone synthesis during sexual differentiation in the male rat. *Toxicol Sci* 2000; **58**: 339–49.

[185] David RM, Moore RM, Finney DC, Guest D. Chronic toxicity of di(2-ethylhexyl) phthalate in rats. *Toxicol Sci* 2000; **55**: 433–43.

[186] Mylchreest E, Wallace DG, Cattley RC, Foster PMD. Dose-dependent alterations in androgen-regulated male reproductive development in rats exposed to di(n-butyl phthalate) during late gestation. *Toxicol Sci* 2000; **55**: 143–51.

[187] Fisher JS, Macpherson S, Marchetti N, Sharpe RM. Human "testicular dysgenesis syndrome": a possible model using in-utero exposure of the rat to dibutyl phthalate. *Hum Reprod* 2003; **18**: 1383–94.

[188] Goldberg JM, Falcone T. Effect of diethylstilbestrol on reproductive function. *Fertil Steril* 1999; **72**: 1–7.

[189] Kaufman RH, Adam E, Hatch EE, *et al.* Continued follow-up of pregnancy outcomes in diethylstilbesterol-exposed offspring. *Obstet Gynecol* 2000; **96**: 483–9.

[190] Klip H, Verloop J, van Gool JD, *et al.* Hypospadias in sons of women exposed to diethylstilbesterol in utero: A cohort study. *Lancet* 2002; **359**: 1102–7.

[191] Kinch RA. Diethylstilbestrol in pregnancy: an update. *Can Med Assoc J* 1982; **127**: 812–13.

[192] Buffum J. Pharmacosexology: the effects of drugs on sexual function-a review. *J Psychoactive Drugs* 1982; **14**: 5.

[193] Collodel G, Scapigliati G, Moretti E. Spermatozoa and chronic treatment with finasteride: a TEM and FISH study. *Arch Androl* 2007; **53**: 229–33.

[194] Liu KE, Binsaleh S, Lo KC, Jarvi K. Propecia-induced spermatogenic failure: a report of two cases. *Fertil Steril* 2007; **88**: S394.

[195] Overstreet JW, Fuh VL, Gould J, *et al.* Chronic treatment with finasteride daily does not affect spermatogenesis or semen production in young men *J Urol* 1999; **162**; 1295–300.

[196] Amory, Jkwang C,Swerdloff RS, *et al.* The effect of 5α-reductase inhibition with dutasteride and finasteride on semen parameters and serum hormones in healthy men. *J Clin Endocrinol Metab* 2007; **92**: 1659–65.

[197] Jarow JP, Lipshultz LI. Anabolic steroid-induced hypogonadotropic hypogonadism. *Am J Sports Med* 1990; **18**: 429–31.

[198] Gill GV. Anabolic steroid induced hypgonadism treated with human chorionic gonadotropin. *Postgrad Med J* 1998; **74**: 45–6.

[199] Menon DK. Successful treatment of anabolic steroid-induced azoospermia with human chorionic gonadotropin and human menopausal gonadotropin. *Fertil Steril* 2003; **79**: 1659–61.

[200] Turek PJ, Williams RH, Gilbaugh JH, Lipshultz LI. The reversibility of anabolic steroid-induced azoospermia. *J Urol* 1995; **153**: 1628–30.

[201] Coviello AD, Matsumoto AM, Bremner WJ, *et al.* Low-dose human chorionic gonadotropin maintains intratesticular testosterone in normal men with testosterone-induced gonadotropin suppression. *J Clin Endocrinol Metab* 2005; **90**: 2595–602.

[202] Hargreaves CA, Rogers S, Hills F, *et al.* Effects of co-trimoxazole, erythromycin, amoxicillin, tetracycline and chloroquine on sperm function in vitro. *Hum Reprod* 1998; **13**: 1878–86.

[203] Nelson WO, Steinberger E. The effect of furadroxyl upon the testis of the rat. *Anat Rec* 1952; **112**: 367–8.

[204] Albert PS, Mininberg DT, Davis JE. The nitrofurans as sperm immobilizing agents: their tissue toxicity and their clinical application. *Br J Urol* 1975; **47**: 459–62.

[205] Al Khaja KA, Sequeira RP, al Damanhori AH, Mathur VS. Antihypertensive drug-associated sexual dysfunction: A prescription analysis-based study. *Pharmacoepidemiol Drug Saf* 2003; **12**: 203–12.

[206] Schmieder RE, Rockstroh JK, Messerli Fh. Antihypertensive therapy: to stop or not to stop?. *JAMA* 1991; **265**: 1566–71.

[207] Rosen RC ,Kostis JB, Jekelis AW. Beta-blocker effects on sexual function in normal males.. *Arch Sex Behav* 1988; **17**: 241–55.

[208] Wilson B. The effect of drugs on male sexual function and fertility. *Nurse Pract* 1991; **16**: 12–17.

[209] Almeida SA, Teofilo JM, Anselmo Franci JA, *et al.* Antireproductive effect of the calcium channel blocker amlodipine in male rats. *Exp Toxicol Pat* 2000; **52**: 353–6.

[210] Benoff S, Cooper GW, Hurley I, *et al.* The effect of calcium ion channel blockers on sperm fertilization potential. *Fertil Steril* 1994; **62**: 606–17.

[211] Hershlag A, Cooper GW, Benoff S. Pregnancy following discontinuation of a calcium-channel blocker in the male partner. *Hum Reprod* 1995; **10**: 599–606.

[212] Lee JH, Kim H, Kim DH, Gye MC. Effects of calcium channel blockers on the spermatogenesis and gene expression in peripubertal mouse testis. *Arch Androl* 2006; **52**: 311–18.

[213] Giuliano F . Impact of medical treatments for benign prostatic hyperplasia on sexual function. *BJU Int* 2006; **97 (Suppl 2)**: 34–8.

[214] Hellstrom WJ, Sikka SC. Effects of acute treatment with tamsulosin versus alfuzosin on ejaculatory function in normal volunteers. *J Urol* 2006; **176**: 1529–33.

[215] Goktas S, Kibar Y, Kilic S, *et al.* Recovery of abnormal ejaculation by intermittent tamsulosin treatment. *J Urol* 2006; **175**: 650–2.

[216] Rowley MJ, Leach DR, Warner GA, Heller CG. Effect of graded doses of ionizing radiation on the human testis. *Radiat Res* 1974; **59**: 665.

[217] Chan PT, Palermo GD, Veeck LL, *et al.* Testicular sperm extraction combined with intracytoplasmic sperm injection in the treatment of men with persistent azoospermia postchemotherapy. *Cancer* 2001; **92**: 1632–7.

[218] Shetty G, Meistrich ML. Hormonal approaches to preservation and restoration of male fertility after cancer treatment. *J Natl Cancer Inst Monogr* 2005; **34**: 36–9.

[219] van Beek RD, Smit M, van den Heuvel-Eibrink MM, *et al.* Inhibin B is superior to FSH as a serum marker for spermatogenesis in men treated for Hodgkin's lymphoma with chemotherapy during childhood. *Hum Reprod* 2007; **22**: 3215–22.

[220] Nudell DM, Monoski MM, Lipshultz Li. Common medications and drugs: how they affect male fertility. *Urol Clin North Am* 2002; **29**: 965–73.

[221] Howell S, Shalet S. Gonadal damage from chemotherapy and radiotherapy. *Endocrinol Metab Clin North Am* 1998; **27**: 927–43.

[222] Howell SJ, Shalet SM. Testicular function following chemotherapy. *Hum Reprod Update* 2001; **7**: 363–9.

[223] Thompson ST. Prevention of male infertility: an update. *Urol Clin North Am* 1994; **21**: 365–76.

[224] Carter MD, Hollander MB, Lipshultz LI. In the medicine cabinet, clues to infertility. *Contemp Urol* 1993; **5**: 51–63.

[225] Tal R, Botchan A, Hauser R, *et al*. Follow-up of sperm concentration and motility in patients with lymphoma. *Hum Repro*d 2000; **15**: 1985–8.

[226] Meirow D, Schenker JG. Cancer and male infertility. *Hum Reprod* 1995; **10**: 2017–22.

[227] van der Kaaij MAE, Heutte N, Le Stang NL, *et al*. Gonadal function in males after chemotherapy for early-stage Hodgkin's lymphoma treated in four subsequent trials by the European Organisation for Research and Treatment of Cancer: EORTC Lymphoma Group and the Group d'Etude des Lymphomes de l'Adulte. *J Clin Oncol* 2007; **25**: 2825–32.

[228] Kulkarni SS, Sastry PS, Saikia TK, *et al*. Gonadal function following ABVD therapy for Hodgkin's disease. *Am J Clin Oncol* 1997; **20**: 354–7.

[229] Bokemeyer C, Schmoll HG, van Rhee J, *et al*. Long-term gonadal toxicity after therapy for Hodgkin's and non-Hodgkin's lymphoma. *Ann Hematol* 1994; **68**: 105–10.

[230] Sieniawski M, Reineke T, Nogova L, *et al*. Fertility in male patients with advanced Hodgkin lymphoma treated with BEACOPP: a report of the German Hodgkin Study Group (GHSG). *Blood* 2008; **111**: 71–6.

[231] Lass A, Akagbosu F, Abusheikha N, *et al*. A programme of semen cryopreservation for patients with malignant disease in a tertiary infertility centre: lessons from 8 years' experience. *Hum Reprod* 1998; **13**: 3256–61.

[232] Ginsberg JP, Ogle SK, Tuchman LK, *et al*. Sperm banking for adolescent and young adult cancer patients: sperm quality, patient, and parent perspective. *Pediatr Blood Cancer* 2008; **50**: 594–8.

[233] Bashore L. Semen preservation in male adolescents and young adults with cancer: one institution's experience. *Clin J Oncol Nurs* 2007; **11**: 381–6.

[234] Zorn B, Virant-Klun I, Stanovnik M, Drobnic S, Meden-Vrtovec H. Intracytoplasmic sperm injection by testicular sperm in patients with aspermia or azoospermia after cancer treatment. *Int J Androl* 2006; **29**: 521–7.

[235] Hibi H, Ohori T, Yamada Y, *et al*. Testicular sperm extraction and ICSI in patients with post-chemotherapy non-obstructive azoospermia. *Arch Androl* 2007; **53**: 63–5.

[236] Meseguer M, Garrido N, Remohi J, *et al*. Testicular sperm extraction (TESE) and ICSI in patients with permanent azoospermia after chemotherapy. *Hum Reprod* 2003; **18**: 1281–5.

[237] Meistrich ML, Wilson G, Kangasniemi M, *et al*. Mechanism of protection of rate spermatogenesis by hormonal pretreatment: Stimulation of spermatogonial differentiation after irradiation. *J Androl* 2000; **21**: 464–9.

[238] Masala A, Faedda R, Alagna S, *et al*. Use of testosterone to prevent cyclophosphamide-induced azoospermia. *Ann Intern Med* 1997; **126**: 292–5.

[239] Montejo AL, Llorca G, Izquierdo JA, *et al*. Incidence of sexual dysfunction associated with antidepressant agents: a prospective multicenter study of 1022 outpatients. Spanish Working Group for the Study of Psychotropic-Related Sexual Dysfunction. *J Clin Psychiatry* 2001; **62**: 10–21.

[240] Levin RM, Amsterdam JD, Winokur A, *et al*. Effects of psychotropic drugs on human sperm motility. *Fertil Ster*il 1981; **36**: 503–6.

[241] Maier U, Koinig G. Andrological findings in young patients under long-term antidepressive therapy with clomipramine. *Psychopharmacology* 1994; **116**: 357–9.

[242] Tanrikut C, Schlegel PN. Antidepressant-associated changes in semen parameters. *Urology* 2007; **69**: 185–7.

[243] Purvis K, Muirhead GJ, Harness JA. The effects of sildenafil on human sperm function in healthy volunteers. *Br J Clin Pharmacol* 2002; **53** (Suppl 1): 53–60S.

[244] Pomara G, Morelli G, Canale D, *et al*. Alterations in sperm motility after acute oral administration of sildenafil or tadalafil in young, infertile men. *Fertil Steril* 2007; **88**: 860–5.

[245] Glenn DR, McVicar CM, McClure N, Lewis SE. Sildenafil citrate improves sperm motility but causes a premature acrosome reaction in vitro. *Fertil Steril* 2007; **87**: 1064–70.

[246] Jarvi K, Dula E, Drehobl M, *et al*. Daily vardenafil for 6 months has no detrimental effects on semen characteristics or reproductive hormones in men with normal baseline levels. *J Urol* 2008; **179**: 1060–5.

[247] Toovey S, Hudson E, Hendry WF, Levi AJ. Sulphasalazine and male infertility: Reversibility and possible mechanism. *Gut* 1981; **22**: 445–51.

[248] Cosentino MJ, Chey WY, Takihara H, Cockett AT. The effects of sulfasalazine on human male fertility potential and seminal prostaglandins. *J Urol* 1984; **132**: 682–6.

[249] Wu FC, Aitken RJ, Ferguson A. Inflammatory bowel disease and male infertility: effects of sulfasalazine and 5-aminosalicylic acid on sperm-fertilizing capacity and reactive oxygen species generation. *Fertil Steril* 1989; **52**: 842–5.

[250] Srinivas M, Agarwala S, Datta Gupta S, *et al*. Effect of cyclosporine on fertility in male rats. *Pediatr Surg Int* 1998; **13**: 388–91.

[251] Cao ZG, Liu JH, Zhu YP, *et al*. Effects of different immunodepressants on the sperm parameters of kidney transplant recipients. *Zhonghua Nan Ke Xue* 2006; **12**: 405–7.

[252] Misro MM, Chaki SP, Srinivas M, Chaube SK. Effect of cyclosporine on human sperm motility in vitro. *Arch Androl* 1999; **43**: 215–20.

249

[253] Seethalakshmi L, Flores C, Diamond DA, *et al.* Reversal of the toxic effects of cyclosporine on male reproduction and kidney function of rats by simultaneous administration of hCG + FSH. *J Urol* 1990; **144**: 1489–92.

[254] Agarwal A, Deepinder F, Sharma RK, Ranga G, Li J. Effect of cell phone usage on semen analysis in men attending infertility clinic: an observational study. *Fertil Steril* 2008; **89**: 124–8.

[255] Erogul O, Oztas E, Yildirum I, *et al.* Effects of electromagnetic radiation from a cellular phone on human sperm motility: an in vitro study. *Arch Med Res* 2006; **37**: 840–3.

[256] Wdowiak A, Wdowiak L, Wiktor H. Evaluation of the effect of using mobile phones on male fertility. *Ann Agric Environ Med* 2007; **14**: 169–72.

[257] Dada R, Gupta NP, Kucheria K. Spermatogenic arrest in men with testicular hyperthermia. *Teratog Carcinog Mutagen* 2003; **1** (Suppl): 235–43.

[258] Lue YH, Lasley BL, Laughlin LS, *et al.* Mild testicular hyperthermia induces profound transitional spermatogenic suppression through increased germ cell apoptosis in adult cynomolgus monkeys (Macaca fascicularis). *J Androl* 2002; **23**: 799–805.

[259] Sheynkin Y, Jung M, Yoo P, Schulsinger D, Komaroff E. Increase in scrotal temperature in laptop computer users. *Hum Reprod* 2005; **20**: 452–5.

[260] Shefi S, Tarapore PE, Walsh TJ, Croughan M, Turek PJ. Wet heat exposure: a potentially reversible cause of low semen quality in infertile men. *Int Braz J Urol* 2007; **33**: 50–6.

[261] Purohit V. Can alcohol promote aromatization of androgens to estrogens? A review. *Alcohol* 2000; **22**: 123–7.

[262] Nordman R. Alcohol and antioxidant systems. *Alcohol* 1994; **29**: 513–22.

[263] Aitken RJ, Irvine DS, Wu FC. Prospective analysis of sperm oocyte fusion and reactive oxygen species generation as criteria for the diagnosis of infertility. *Am J Obstet Gynecol* 1991; **164**: 542–51.

Genetic aspects of infertility

Robert D. Oates and Dolores J. Lamb

Introduction: nonobstructive azoospermia and severe oligospermia

The genetic basis of male infertility, although relatively poorly understood, may ultimately represent one of the most clinically important aspects of male infertility. Diagnoses are largely descriptive, lacking a molecular basis, and generally reflect the large gaps in our understanding of the factors regulating sperm production (including endocrine, paracrine, and autocrine factors, intrinsic and extrinsic controls), the changes that occur to sperm during transit through the male and female genital tracts, fertilization, and embryonic development. Assisted reproductive technologies overcome this infertility, but also have the potential to transmit defective genes to offspring. Largely understudied over the past decade, the diagnosis and treatment of male infertility present significant challenges because of these mysteries of male reproductive tract function. Lacking the knowledge of the control factors hinders the development of definitive diagnostic tests and medical therapies. Infertility, although once thought to be largely due to defects in the female or events beyond our control (trauma or other injury, toxic exposures, infections), may reflect nature's evolutionary adaptation, which effectively limits the transmission of undesirable traits to the offspring. In this chapter, we focus on the current state of knowledge of the genetic basis of male infertility. With the molecular revolution a virtual explosion has occurred in this area of medicine, yet the translation of this knowledge to affect clinical practice has been slow. In many assisted reproductive technology laboratories across the country the presence of any sperm, despite significant functional or genetic deficiencies, is sufficient to prompt an attempt at pregnancy with intracytoplasmic sperm injection (ICSI), a procedure that was used in clinical practice before its safety and efficacy were determined. **As can be seen in the pages that follow, genetic defects associated with male infertility exist at every level of genetic information from chromosomes to genes to nucleotides to epigenetic modifications. The closer we look, the more genetic defects causing human male infertility we identify.**

Numerical chromosomal anomalies

A peripheral karyotype may identify either numerical or structural chromosomal anomalies in approximately 14% of men with severe spermatogenic deficiency [1]. **The most common finding in non-obstructive azoospermia (NOA) patients is 47,XXY Klinefelter syndrome (KS), which occurs in 1/500 to 1/1000 live births and is the underlying genetic anomaly in 10% of those NOA men** [2–5]. Most KS cases are nonmosaic, with all cells demonstrating a 47, XXY genotype, although mosaicism does occur with variable percentages of 46,XY cells admixed with the remaining 47,XXY cells. Mosaic males have less severe phenotypic consequences, and many are fertile. Whereas Y-chromosomal microdeletions affect just the spermatogenic compartment of the testis, the extra X chromosome mutes and damages the androgenic compartment as well, precipitating the major clinical manifestations of KS. This additional X, through mechanisms unknown, sets in motion the events that lead to many disparate features of KS from androgenic and spermatogenic failure to difficulties in expressive language learning [5]. The supernumerary X may be of either paternal or maternal origin. There is a dramatic increase in the number of sex-chromosome disomic sperm (24,XY) in the fathers of boys with KS that increases steadily as paternal age increases (10% higher among fathers in their twenties to 160% higher among fathers in their fifties) [6,7]. There does not appear to be an increase in autosomal disomy rates in those fathers [8].

Infertility in the Male, 4th edition, ed. Larry I. Lipshultz, Stuart S. Howards, and Craig S. Niederberger. Published by Cambridge University Press. © Cambridge University Press 2009.

The clinical spectrum of KS is wide and mostly determined by the level of androgenic function [4]. Aksglaede *et al.* demonstrated that while testosterone output is normal in the first few months of life, there is already a hint of Sertoli cell and Leydig cell dysfunction [9]. When the androgenic compartment is totally dysfunctional (complete Leydig cell failure), virilization will not occur at the expected time of puberty, gynecomastia may be present, and a eunuchoid appearance will be noted with height taller than predicted. These boys require testosterone supplementation to mature physically. The testes will be atrophic and will show extensive fibrosis and sclerosis. It is unlikely that there will be any preserved seminiferous tubules that are capable of minimal amounts of sperm production. This is the severe end of the phenotypic spectrum. On the opposite end are those KS men who have an adequate amount of testosterone secretion at puberty to androgenize as expected and thereby escape detection until they are diagnosed at the time of an infertility investigation. Libido and erectile function are normal and their height is as would be predicted [10]. However, there are young men with adequate Tanner stage progression who are detected not for either reason mentioned above but instead as an explanation for the atrophic testes found on physical examination. Small testes are common to all 47,XXY men, no matter where on the clinical spectrum they may fall, and typically they measure about 8–10 cm^3 in volume. Follicle-stimulating hormone (FSH) and luteinizing hormone (LH) are elevated, demonstrating compensatory output in response to the damaged spermatogenic and androgenic cells and functions of the testes [11,12]. The Leydig cells have little reserve, as maximal stimulation is already present and ongoing. KS men have nongonadal manifestations as well. Learning difficulties are common. KS men may have an increased mortality from breast cancer (standardized mortality ratio [SMR] 57.8) [13]. There is a slightly increased mortality from non-Hodgkin's lymphoma (SMR 3.5) [13]. Males with mediastinal germ cell tumors should be karyotyped, since KS may be detected if the genotype is not already known [14]. There may be a decreased incidence of prostate cancer in KS men [13]. Although azoospermia is the rule, there are rare exceptions of preserved fertility [15].

Even though the patient shows no sperm in the ejaculate, testicular sperm extraction (TESE) may successfully find spermatozoa in up to 69% of KS men, which can be used in conjunction with ICSI to effect fertilization, embryo development, and term pregnancy [16-18]. **Many live births of 46,XY or 46,XX children have been reported** [19-21]. Controversy exists with regard to the need for preimplantation genetic screening of embryos to identify and eliminate those that are 47,XXX, 47,XXY, or triploid for one of the autosomes [22,23]. This debate is driven by the data on individual sperm from KS men, which show a slight increase in sex-chromosomal and autosomal disomy of 0.9% and 7.5%, respectively [7,24]. However, the human clinical data reported so far show only one case of a 47,XXY fetus that was terminated – all other children reported have had normal karyotypes [25]). Where the sperm derive from is also unclear. Is there a low level of gonosomal mosaicism, with a few 46,XY spermatogonia living and working in a few functional seminiferous tubules scattered randomly and rarely about the testis parenchyma [26,27], or is it that every so often a 47,XXY spermatogonium can complete meiosis with elimination of the extra X and production of predominantly 23,X or 23,Y spermatozoa [28]?

There are no widely agreed-upon clinical or laboratory findings that predict successful sperm retrieval, although pre-TESE testis volume and testosterone level may do so, as well as age less than 35 [29–31]. Cryopreserved sperm have been used successfully, but a combined approach of TESE coincident with an ICSI cycle (tissue harvesting either the day prior to or the morning of oocyte retrieval) is the preferred approach [32]. Testosterone levels may decline after TESE is performed, especially in the first 3–6 months, but typically they rise to 95% of pre-TESE levels within 18 months [33,34]. The strategy that should be adopted for those teenage boys who are found to have KS but who have adequate virilization is unclear. Should TESE with cryopreservation of tissue/sperm be undertaken, as reported by Damani *et al.* [35]? Should tissue extraction wait until later in life, and be performed coincident with an ICSI cycle when biological paternity is desired? Is sperm production decline ongoing and progressive, beginning in infancy and accelerating at puberty [36]? Is there a better chance of success if testis tissue extraction is attempted earlier in life? Will the need for testosterone replacement be precipitated or hastened by tissue extraction at this age, remembering that these young men do not necessarily require testosterone replacement [37,38]? What is clear, however, is that a karyotype should be performed prior to any surgical intervention in all men who present with NOA.

A 46,XX testicular disorder of sex development (also known as 46,XX male syndrome) occurs in approximately 1 in 20 000 newborn males and so is a rare cause of NOA [39]. Etiologically, an abnormal XY interchange between *PRKX* and *PRKY* translocates a small portion of distal Yp to the tip of the paired X chromosome in 90% of affected men. This displaced piece of chromosomal material contains an intact *SRY*, allowing for completion of the cascade that drives gonadal differentiation along a testicular pathway. In the remaining 10%, either translocation to an autosome has occurred or the individual is SRY-negative, some other aberrant event affecting gonadal differentiation in the opposite direction than would be normally seen in a 46,XX embryo [40,41]. Whatever the mechanism, the fetal testes begin to secrete testosterone, which induces ipsilateral mesonephric duct differentiation (vasa deferentia, seminal vesicles, distal epididymides). The testes also secrete anti-Müllerian hormone, causing regression of the paramesonephric ducts. Therefore, the internal ductal anatomy is normal for a male. In the external genitalia, 5α-reductase converts testosterone to dihydrotestosterone, and morphogenesis of the anatomy here is along male lines [42]. Although fetal development seems typical for these males, there is a higher incidence of cryptorchidism in them than in the normal 46,XY population [43]. Gynecomastia may occur at puberty, and testosterone levels may be lower than those seen in 46,XY males. Height may be less than predicted for males within the family unit. **Most importantly, there is no spermatogenesis, as nearly the entirety of the male-specific Y, including the AZFa, b, and c regions** (see below), **is not present in the genome. There is no need for testis biopsy or TESE, because a karyotype will be prognostic and definitive in this circumstance, again emphasizing the point that a karyotype should be performed in all NOA men before any surgical intervention.**

Men with a 47,XYY chromosomal constitution (0.1% of males) are generally fertile but may be tall with large teeth [44]. This may be due to gonosomal mosaicism, and the greater the ratio of 46,XY to 47,XYY, the greater the sperm count. It is believed that most XYY cells will arrest at the pachytene level of meiosis I [45]. For those that do make it through this meiotic checkpoint, apoptosis may eliminate them in the round spermatid stage, as demonstrated by Milazzo *et al.* [46]. However, a slight increase in sperm aneuploidy is still present, and this may lead to an increased risk of miscarriage and perinatal death. Thus preimplantation genetic diagnosis may be helpful if in-vitro techniques are required to achieve pregnancy [47].

Structural chromosomal anomalies

Y-chromosomal microdeletions

In order to appreciate the how and why of Y-chromosomal microdeletions, it is necessary to understand the molecular geography of the Y chromosome. The Y chromosome is comprised of 60 million base pairs with a short arm (Yp) and a long arm (Yq). The euchromatic region, which contains the relevant spermatogenic genes discussed below, and the heterochromatic region (which has no presently known function) are equally divided [48]. Pseudoautosomal regions that pair and recombine with similar chromosomal stretches on the X chromosome are located at the tips of Yp and Yq [49,50]. *SRY* is located on Yp and is an essential member of the cascade of genes that ultimately determine the fate of the bipotential gonad [51]. **The male-specific Y (MSY) is that chromosomal material that bridges the two polar pseudoautosomal regions and is unique in the human genome – there is no counterpart on any other chromosome. It comprises approximately 95% of the entirety of the Y** (Fig. 15.1) [52]. It is non-recombining and houses multiple genes dispersed along its length. Most of these gene products help drive the spermatogenic machinery, but all are poorly characterized at this point [53]. Examples include *USP9Y* and *DBY* in a stretch known as AZFa, and *DAZ*, *RBMY1*, and *BPY2* in a stretch known as AZFb and AZFc (see below). Unevenly distributed throughout the length of the euchromatic portion of Yq are eight palindromic sequences, P8 closest to the centromere and P1 the most distal (Fig. 15.1). The basic structure of all eight is the same, although each is of differing total length. Each mirror-image arm expands outwards from an anchor point, a short base pair core. Each arm's sequence is nearly identical but reads in an opposite direction.

Within these palindromes, however, are subsegments known as amplicons, which are sequences that are repeated at least twice (one on each arm of a palindrome reading in an "inverted" direction) but that may have another copy or two elsewhere, spatially separate and reading in either a direct (same direction) or inverted manner [54]. For example, there are four "blue" amplicons as colorized by Kuroda-Kawaguchi *et al.*, labeled b1, b2, b3, and b4. It is the interaction of b2 and b4 that is the proximate cause of the AZFc

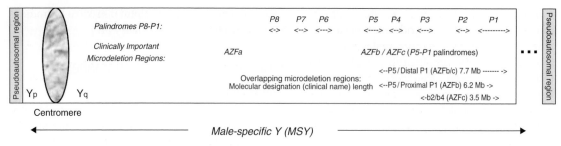

Fig. 15.1. Molecular geography of the Y chromosome.

microdeletion (see below). **Since MSY has no partner in the genome with which to pair and repair, it is believed that this unusual palindromic/ampliconic structural organization allows for self-correction to maintain the presence and fidelity of the vast majority of the Y chromosome. However, beneficial as this may be, there is a flaw in this molecular arrangement that, in rare instances, creates a circumstance of ectopic homologous recombination – an aberrant event whereby two spatially distanced amplicons fuse together as one with consequent loss of all intervening chromosomal material** [55]. As shown in Figure 15.1, these expanses may be of tremendous magnitude on the molecular scale, but they may be undetectable on the cytogenic/karyotypic scale and so are labeled as microdeletions. When a microdeletion occurs, any genes residing in this stretch are lost as well; hence the clinical consequences if these genes are requisite to optimal sperm production. In summary, Y-chromosomal organization is unique, predisposing to loss of relatively expansive segments on rare occasions that may result in male reproductive compromise.

The details of the molecular geography of the Y chromosome are indeed important to understand vis-à-vis the clinical consequences of Y-chromosomal microdeletions that eliminate genes that may be either necessary or helpful for optimal spermatogenesis. Tiepolo and Zuffardi recognized as far back as 1976 that a grossly intact Y chromosome was important for spermatogenesis to occur, and they postulated regions of necessity termed azoospermia factors (AZF) [56]. As the molecular construction of the Y was being elucidated in the mid-1990s, three specific microdeletions of significant clinical frequency were detected and described in men with sperm production deficiency. The original acronym nomenclature for these three microdeleted regions was derived from the Tiepolo and Zuffardi suggestion at a time when it was thought that each was spatially and topographically distinct.

It is now clear the AZFa region stands on its own, while the AZFb and AZFc microdeletions are just two possible microdeletions that occur within one stretch of MSY with its proximal endpoint located in P5 and its distal endpoint in P1. AZFb and AZFc are overlapping. In men with NOA or severe oligospermia, a Y-chromosomal microdeletion assay should be obtained prior to use of the ejaculated sperm or performance of tissue extraction to search for sperm. This blood test is a PCR-based assay that allows detection of clinically relevant microdeletions.

Closest to the centromere, the AZFa region is located in proximal Yq. Microdeletion of the AZFa region occurs in approximately 1% of NOA men, and the molecular anatomy of this region does not involve any of the eight palindromes mentioned above. Instead, two 10 kB endogenous retroviral elements known as HERV15yq1 and HERV15yq2 flank genomic material, which two spermatogenically important genes (*DDX3Y* and *USP9Y*) call home [57,58]. HERV15yq1 and HERV15yq2 may undergo ectopic homologous recombination, with consequent loss of all 792 kB of intervening material, including *DDX3Y* and *USP9Y* [59–61]. *DDX3Y* generates an ATP-dependent RNA helicase that may play a role in a later stage of spermatogenesis as it shuttles between cytoplasm and nucleus [62,63]. *DDX3Y* is 16.3 kB in length. *USP9Y* also plays a quantitative role, perhaps of less importance than *DDX3Y*, since mutations in *USP9Y* have been described in men with a minimal amount of spermatogenesis [64,65]. Of critical clinical importance is the fact that, as the literature suggests, if the AZFa region is microdeleted, spermatozoa will not be found on testis tissue extraction (TESE) [66,67]. **An AZFa microdeletion predicts failure of TESE. As above, a Y-chromosomal microdeletion assay will be prognostic in these circumstances if performed, as it should be, prior to TESE.**

In the chromosomal expanse from the P5 palindrome to the P1 palindrome are multiple sites of possible ectopic homologous recombination, which, when it occurs, leads to microdeletion of varying lengths of DNA, with varying proximal and distal endpoints, at varying frequencies, and with varying clinical consequences. The three most common that occur in the male with spermatogenic impairment are termed AZFc, AZFb, and AZFb/c (Fig. 15.1). These are not "nonoverlapping" as previously believed, but the acronyms still persist even though they could also be referred to by their molecular nomenclature: b2/b4, P5/proximal P1, and P5/distal P1, respectively [55].

Of the three, AZFc (b2/b4) is the most common, being present in 1 in 4000 men overall, 13% of NOA males, and 6% of severely oligospermic men [68,69]. Spanning 3.5 Mb, an AZFc microdeletion begins in the distal aspect of the P3 palindrome where the second of the 229 kb "blue" amplicons is located and extends to the P1 palindrome where the fourth of the "blue" amplicons resides [54]. It is these two amplicons, direct repeats of each other, which undergo ectopic homologous recombination with elimination of several genes that inhabit the intervening chromosomal material. There are four copies of the *DAZ* gene here (two *DAZ* genes form the P2 palindrome [reading in opposite directions from a central core] with a duplicate of this pair found upstream in P3) [70,71]. *DAZ* encodes an RNA-binding protein that may activate silent mRNAs during the early stages of meiosis, as its expression appears to be primarily in spermatogonia [72,73]. The genetically active material in the AZFc region may not be critical for meiotic recombination but "in the absence of the AZF region, the transient zygotene stage is extended, and chromosome condensation is reduced" [74].

Oates *et al.* clinically characterized men with AZFc microdeletions as follows [75]: **Men with an AZFc microdeletion have quantitatively impaired spermatogenesis, whereas the quality of any sperm produced appears normal in terms of fertilization, embryo development, and term pregnancy** [76]. Natural paternity is rare, and most men present with NOA or severe oligospermia and consequent sterility or infertility [77]. The spectrum of spermatogenic deficiency is a tight one, ranging from no spermatozoa found on TESE to markedly reduced numbers of sperm in the ejaculate (typically no higher than 5×10^6/mL). In the 42 men studied, 62% were azoospermic (2/3 had sperm found on subsequent TESE or testis biopsy), and 38% were severely oligospermic. Therefore, 81% had spermatozoa that could be employed in conjunction with

ICSI to try to achieve biological paternity (infertility) while 19% of the group overall had no sperm available from either the ejaculate or testis tissue (sterility). Genes in the AZFc region of the Y chromosome appear to be spermatogenesis-specific, in that their loss did not lead to any somatic health consequences or testicular abnormalities, such as cryptorchidism or germ cell neoplasia, in either the subject or his conceived offspring. Heretofore, nearly all AZFc microdeletions were de novo, although with the recent introduction of ICSI they can be passed from father to son. Whatever low level of spermatogenesis exists appears to be temporally fairly stable. For an individual harboring an AZFc microdeletion, history, physical examination, and hormonal parameters do not forecast the ultimate level of his sperm production. **The predicted reproductive spectrum of all male offspring should reflect that described above for AZFc microdeleted men, but their level of future spermatozoal production may not necessarily be the same as their fathers'** [75] (Fig. 15.2). **If the male partner of an infertile couple is found to have an AZFc microdeletion by Y-chromosomal microdeletion assay, the couple has several options to consider. They may choose to avoid use of his sperm. They may decide to use either his ejaculated or testis-derived sperm for ICSI and accept the random outcome vis-à-vis male or female offspring. Finally, they may decide to employ preimplantation genetic screening to discard male embryos and transfer only female embryos, thereby**

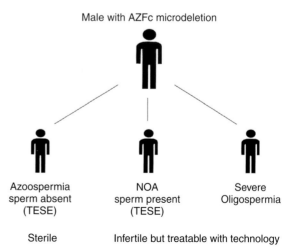

Male with AZFc microdeletion

Azoospermia
sperm absent
(TESE)

NOA
sperm present
(TESE)

Severe
Oligospermia

Sterile

Infertile but treatable with technology

Fig. 15.2. Predicted spectrum of spermatogenic deficiency in sons of male with AZFc microdeletion.

eliminating the propagation of an AZFc microdeletion and its resultant infertility/sterility [78].

As above, within the P5 and P1 palindromes are sequences that lend themselves to ectopic homologous recombination. Beginning in P5 and ending in either the proximal or distal aspect of P1, clinically significant microdeletions may occur, and are known as AZFb or AZFb/c, respectively (Fig. 15.1). The AZFb microdeletion is 6.2 Mb in length while the more extensive AZFb/c microdeletion is 7.7 Mb long [55]. **As can be seen, all three are overlapping – they do not involve spatially distant and distinct stretches of the Y chromosome. If either an AZFb or AZFb/c microdeletion is found in a man with NOA (1–3% of such men), there is little chance that sperm will be retrievable from testis tissue, and a Y-chromosomal microdeletion assay will, therefore, be prognostic and should be obtained prior to any surgical intervention [67].**

Other structural anomalies

Many other structural anomalies involving the Y chromosome may be found on karyotypic analysis, and they are important to identify in the infertile male [79]. A Y-chromosomal microdeletion assay is a necessary complementary test, because it will determine whether the MSY involving the AZFa region, as well as that stretch containing palindromes P5–P1 (the AZFb/AZFc area), is present. If not, then spermatogenesis will not be possible and no surgical intervention is necessary. For example, ring Y, designated r(Y), results from circularization of a Y whose terminal ends are lost, with consequent fusion of the arms [80]. Most cases present as mosaics 46,X,r(Y)/45,X, and the phenotype is variable, ranging from Turner syndrome to normal male external genitalia with azoospermia. The final phenotype depends not only on the percentage of cells that contain the r(Y) but also on the amount of chromosomal material lost [81]. The more material lost, the less likely it is that the r(Y) will be transmitted through mitotic stages to future cell lines, and the higher the percentage of 45,X cells. In addition, if the spermatogenic regions of MSY are missing, sperm production will not occur and azoospermia will result [82]. Other Y-chromosomal abnormalities may include isodicentric Y (two short arms, two centromeres, and a fused, truncated long arm), truncated Y, and various mosaic states with a 45,X cell line [1]. As for r(Y), a Y-chromosomal microdeletion assay must be obtained as a complementary test to determine if the replicative mishap eliminated the AZF regions. If

so, no TESE is needed. Occurring more often in the oligospermic population, reciprocal and Robertsonian translocations may be found on karyotypic analysis as well [83]. Preimplantation genetic analysis may improve chances for a live birth, and genetic counseling should be offered [84].

In summary, a karyotype and Y-chromosomal microdeletion assay should be obtained as complementary tests in all NOA and severely oligospermic men prior to ICSI and the use of ejaculated or testicular sperm. Prognosis and planning are optimized with any informative result.

Endocrine genetic defects causing male infertility

Androgen biosynthesis, metabolism, and androgen receptor signal transduction pathway abnormalities

The role of androgens

In the 1930s, testosterone (T) was recognized as the main circulating androgen secreted by the testis, the majority bound to sex hormone-binding globulin and albumin in dynamic equilibrium with unbound hormone. The free, bioavailable testosterone unbound to protein represents only 1–2% of total testosterone in the serum [85]. Testosterone and other steroids are lipophilic and enter both target and nontarget cells through passive diffusion [86]. It elicits activity within cells that express a functional androgen receptor. Depending upon the target tissue, T may be 5α-reduced to 5α-dihydrotestosterone (DHT) by the enzyme 5α-reductase. Testosterone and DHT are the major steroids that bind to the androgen receptor (AR) (described below). In some target organs, such as the prostate, the main androgen bound to the AR is DHT [87], while in other tissues, such as the Wolffian duct or testis, testosterone is the preferred ligand. Just one AR gene is known, notwithstanding the tissue-specific differential preference for one of these two ligands.

Androgen biosynthesis

Steroidogenic acute regulatory (StAR) protein (reviewed by [88,89]) is the rate-limiting step for androgen biosynthesis in particular and all steroids in general. StAR mediates the transfer of cholesterol from the outer to the inner mitochondrial membrane. Subsequently, cholesterol is converted by the cholesterol side-chain cleavage enzyme, cytochrome P450scc, to pregnenolone (the precursor for sex steroids, glucocorticoids, and mineralocorticoids) [90].

Mutations in the StAR gene result in congenital lipoid adrenal hyperplasia (CLAH) [91,92]. CLAH patients are unable to synthesize adrenal and gonadal steroids and, if untreated, die within a few weeks of birth. A similar phenotype is observed in StAR-deficient mouse tissues from StAR$^{-/-}$ mice [93]. As individuals with CLAH do not synthesize steroids, the phenotype is severe. Deficiencies of any of the enzymes required for the normal synthesis of testosterone can impact reproductive development and function. For example, males with 17β-hydroxysteroid dehydrogenase type 3 deficiency will be classified as females at birth, but when they reach puberty they will develop male secondary sex characteristics [94]. Male pseudohermaphroditism can occur with deficiency of testicular 17,20-desmolase [95–97]. Of note, steroid biosynthesis defects can be secondary to deficiencies of peptide hormones such as leptin [98].

Androgen action is required for male reproduction
Androgen action requires a functioning intracellular nuclear receptor that is a member of the steroid receptor superfamily. **As a member of the steroid receptor superfamily, the protein is characterized by a ligand-binding domain, a DNA-binding domain, and a transactivation domain** (reviewed in [99]). Indeed, the protein and its functional domains have been studied in detail over the past 40 years. The AR is a ligand-activated transcription factor present in all tissues responsive to testosterone or DHT. Located in the cytoplasm in the absence of androgen, it binds androgen with high affinity and specificity. Binding then initiates a series of events that include receptor activation, translocation to the nucleus, and interaction with the chromatin, where it ultimately modulates transcriptional regulation of specific gene expression (reviewed in [100]). Complicating our understanding of steroid receptor action, ligand-independent activation of receptor is observed under some conditions, for example as a result of activation by growth factors, such as interleukin 6 in prostate cancer [101]. In addition, it appears that the receptor needs to work in concert with a number of coactivators and corepressors, as well as transcription factors (reviewed in [102]). **Quite simply, from a clinical perspective, a functioning androgen receptor is necessary for optimal development of the embryonic and fetal male genital tract, as well as for the regulation of testicular, epididymal, prostate,** and seminal vesicle activity in the adult. Other targets of androgens include the muscle, skin, bone, and kidneys. **In the adult, spermatogenesis requires testosterone acting through the AR in the Sertoli cell, which in turn mediates reduction division during germ cell meiosis.** Androgens are also necessary for normal spermatid differentiation and play an important role in the epididymis, where spermatozoa acquire motility. Androgens maintain the differentiated function of the prostate and seminal vesicles and their secretions. Without androgens and a functional receptor, the male will not be reproductively viable. These processes and the consequences of deficiencies of AR action are described below.

Testosterone mediates normal male development
Leydig cells in the fetal primordial gonad secrete testosterone, which acts to maintain the Wolffian duct structures. The Wolffian duct differentiates into the adult seminal vesicles, vasa deferentia, and the distal two-thirds of the epididymides. Testosterone also acts in the fetal Sertoli cell to induce the production of anti-Müllerian hormone (AMH), also known as Müllerian-inhibiting substance (MIS). AMH/MIS is a peptide hormone that causes regression of Müllerian duct structures (the embryonic precursors of the fallopian tubes, uterus, and the upper two-thirds of the vagina in a female). First postulated by Jost in 1953 [103], it was years before a useful assay for this activity was developed, and it was not until the 1970s that AMH secretion was localized to the Sertoli cells [104–106] and later sequenced and cloned [107]. The combined actions of AMH and testosterone prevent differentiation of the primordial gonad into an ovary. Testosterone mediates the second phase of testicular descent during fetal development. In short, testosterone acts to drive development towards phenotypic maleness.

Testosterone is required for spermatogenesis
Testosterone alone qualitatively (but not quantitatively) maintains spermatogenesis in the absence of gonadotropins [101,108,109]. The action of testosterone on spermatogenesis is primarily mediated through the AR in the Sertoli cell, and to a lesser extent in the Leydig cell and the peritubular myoid cell (PM) [101,102,108–110]. Despite the absolute requirement for testosterone during spermatogenesis, the steroid does not act directly on the developing germ cells (although authors have debated whether androgen receptors are present in the germ cells [111,112]), suggesting that

spermatogenesis requires complex intercellular paracrine interactions. Using a technique called targeted gene deletion in a mouse model, AR was selectively knocked out in Sertoli [101,108,109,111], germ cell [108,111], or peritubular myoid cells [102] to define the contribution of androgen action to spermatogenesis in each testicular cell type. As one might predict, germ-cell-targeted deletion of the AR had no effect on spermatogenesis [108,111,112]. Germ cells from mice lacking functional androgen receptors could complete spermatogenesis after spermatogonial stem cell transplantation [111]. Mice lacking Sertoli-cell AR display incomplete germ cell development with a meiotic arrest at the second reduction division and lowered serum testosterone levels. These deficiencies result in azoospermia and infertility [101,108,109,113]. In contrast, mice lacking peritubular myoid-cell AR after cell-specific targeted deletion are oligospermic. Contractility of the peritubular myoid is deficient, impairing sperm release from the seminiferous tubules [102]. Mutations in the androgen receptor can cause androgen insensitivity.

Androgen insensitivity in the human directly affects male reproductive development and function

The three main clinical phenotypes resulting from androgen insensitivity are defined as complete, partial, and minimal androgen insensitivity (CAIS, PAIS, and MAIS). Kennedy syndrome, also known as X-linked spinal and bulbar muscular atrophy (SBMA), is a form of androgen insensitivity associated with aging, which results in reduced fertility. These diseases also include Reifenstein syndrome, testicular feminization (male pseudohermaphroditism), Lub syndrome, and Rosewater syndrome [114]. The androgen insensitivity syndromes are considered to represent disorders of sexual differentiation. Nevertheless, today physicians recognize that androgen resistance can be present in men who are undervirilized or infertile.

Complete androgen insensitivity (CAIS) or testicular feminization

Phenotypic female, genotypic 46,XY individuals who lack a functional AR display complete androgen insensitivity syndrome (CAIS) [115]. CAIS can result from AR gene deletion, but more commonly point mutations in the gene result in a loss of function of the protein. The Androgen Receptor Gene Mutations website (androgendb.mcgill.ca) provides a useful summary of the naturally occurring mutations identified to date in the androgen receptor [116]. Despite isolated case reports prior to 1953 [117], the first report of CAIS is

often attributed to Morris in that year [118]. The CAIS individuals are 46,XY pseudohermaphrodites (genotypic males) displaying an unambiguously female appearance. Female external genitalia develop because, despite high circulating testosterone levels, the tissues are resistant to androgen action. Thus DHT-dependent masculinization of the external genital primordia is absent. Patients with CAIS have underdeveloped labia, a blind-ending vagina, and paucity of axillary or pubic hair. Because the labial or abdominal testes continue to produce AMH, the uterus, ovaries, and fallopian tubes are absent. CAIS occurs in about 2–5/100 000 births [119], and these patients are sterile.

Partial androgen insensitivity (PAIS): a broad spectrum of phenotypic and functional abnormalities

The androgen receptor mutation in these patients impairs or changes the receptor function to varying degrees. Patients with PAIS exhibit a range of congenital genitourinary defects in combinations of varying severity including hypospadias, microphallus, cryptorchidism, gynecomastia, and infertility. At one extreme, the external genitalia resemble those associated with a nearly normal female phenotype, except for clitoromegaly and/or posterior labial fusion. At the other extreme, the genitalia may resemble those of a morphologically normal male but the scrotum or phallus may be small, or there may be simple coronal hypospadias or a prominent midline raphe of the scrotum. Reifenstein first reported this syndrome [120]. In some ways these patients can present significant clinical challenges because of their partial response to androgens. Infertility may result, due to the failure of normal male development. In the less severe cases early and continuous testosterone treatment can improve the chances of fertility.

Minimal androgen insensitivity syndrome (MAIS): mild phenotypic abnormalities

The phenotypic spectrum of deficiencies in MAIS, like those found in CAIS, varies markedly between patients. Infertility, azoospermia, micropenis, or gynecomastia may be present. Nearly 30 years ago Aiman proposed that azoospermia is linked to AIS [121]. At about the same time Larrea recognized a familial syndrome characterized by microphallus and gynecomastia and androgen insensitivity [122]. Quigley proposed a slightly more complex but similar classification of seven grades of AIS [114]. Simply put, some mutations vary AR function in a manner analogous to a rheostat causing mild functional deficiencies that in some cases can be overcome with increased levels of androgen [123].

X-linked spinal and bulbar muscular atrophy (SBMA): a triplet repeat disease associated with diminished male reproductive fitness

A gene polymorphism underlies Kennedy syndrome (SBMA). SBMA is a chronic, progressive neuromuscular disorder. It was discovered that AR from affected patients contains an expanded polyglutamine tract in exon 1 from 40 to 62 CAG triplets or longer [124]. SBMA, like other triplet repeat or CAG/polyglutamine disorders, is defined by neuronal intranuclear inclusion thought to represent misfolded AR. Weakness of the proximal limb muscles, with atrophy and fasciculations, is characteristic. Bulbar signs may include perioral fasciculations, a nasal quality of the voice, and recurrent aspiration. Partial androgen insensitivity is present, particularly with aging, with symptoms of gynecomastia, testicular atrophy, and decreased fertility. Typically, postmortem studies of SBMA males reveal abnormal testicular histology characterized by marked seminiferous tubule atrophy, and absence of germinal cells [125,126]. Because this is an adult-onset syndrome (except for instances of extremely long polyglutamine repeat lengths), the patient may have been fertile and virile as a young man, but in middle age develop progressive evidence of insensitivity. The use of assisted reproductive technologies to overcome the infertility of Kennedy syndrome patients must be undertaken with care. The disease is characterized by a phenomenon known as "anticipation." With each successive generation the repeat length tends to increase in length with an earlier age of onset and greater severity of symptoms. Preimplantation genetic diagnosis or other prenatal genetic diagnostic procedure is required to ensure that the offspring will not be affected.

The association of glutamine polymorphisms in the AR with male infertility is controversial

There is an inverse relationship between the length of the normally polymorphic polyglutamine repeat length and AR transcriptional activity [127,128]. This observation has led to the hypothesis that CAG length may correlate with male infertility. This hypothesis was confirmed by initial investigations [129–133], but it was not corroborated by Swedish [134], German [135], Dutch [136], and Danish [137] population studies. These discrepancies created confusion and led to the hypothesis that CAG repeat expansion leads to reduced fertility in Asian but not European populations,

possibly because of exposure to different environmental factors in the two populations. A recent meta-analysis of the combined data in the literature reveals that there is an association between increased androgen receptor CAG length and male infertility. An inverse relationship between the number of CAG and number of sperm is observed in some [129–133,138] but not all studies [134–137]. This controversy reflects the relative proportion of men with nonobstructive azoospermia in the infertile study population [133].

Additional evidence that AR defects are associated with male infertility

Abnormal AR function was described by Aiman *et al.* in three unrelated infertile patients who displayed a decrease of about 50% in high-affinity dihydrotestosterone binding capacity of cultured genital skin fibroblasts when they were compared with normal men [121]. To identify infertile men with AR abnormalities, an androgen sensitivity index (nmol/L serum testosterone times IU/L serum luteinizing hormone) was employed. Several of the infertile patients tested displayed an elevation in this value [139,140]. Others defined AR deficiencies in idiopathic azoospermic/oligospermic men using simple receptor binding assays with cultured genital skin fibroblasts. It was reported that 40% of these men had a decreased level of ^{3}H–DHT binding, similar to that found in patients with PAIS or CAIS [141]. Nevertheless, the relationship between abnormal AR activity and infertility remains controversial [142], and this type of functional analysis is never routinely performed on infertile men.

Molecular analysis of AR in idiopathic infertility [143–145] suggests that AR mutations are present in up to 10% of the patients, although the functional consequences of these mutations have not always been defined. Of the seven infertility-associated mutations [116,146], an analysis of the possible mechanism of action of the mutant receptor has been undertaken in one case (Met886Val) [85]. This study suggested that a functional element near M886 played a role, not in ligand-binding, but in interdomain and coactivator interactions. This mutation caused a 50% decrease in transcriptional activity and was associated with abnormal interactions between the COOH and NH_2-terminal regions of AR, and between AR and the transcriptional intermediary factor TIF-2 [143].

Disorders of steroid metabolism

5α-reductase deficiency is one of the best-known disorders of steroid metabolism leading to an intersex condition. In this case, testosterone cannot be metabo-lized to dihydrotestosterone. Thus the testis is normally developed but the Wolffian duct derivatives are female, as are the external genitalia. At puberty, the "female" undergoes a remarkable transformation to maleness with the high levels of androgen produced. Groups of patients with this genetic syndrome are more com-monly found in several distinct areas of the world, such as the Dominican Republic [147,148] .

Disorders of sexual development.

Individuals with ambiguous genitalia and/or sec-ondary sex characteristics (intersex and gonadal dys-genesis syndromes) may result from chromosomal and gonadal disorders, endocrine abnormalities, and genetic defects. Although not as common as crypt-orchidism and hypospadias, these disorders present significant challenges for physicians, parents, and, eventually, the afflicted individuals with respect to sur-gical correction, management, and, in some instances, gender assignment.

Approximately 1% of male infants are born with genital disorders, either cryptorchidism or hypo-spadias, placing them among the most common birth defects. Normal testicular descent and pen-ile development require appropriate function of the hypothalamic–pituitary–gonadal axis, with andro-gen action ultimately mediated through the androgen receptor. Recognized disorders along this pathway (anencephaly, Kallmann syndrome, testosterone bio-synthetic defects, androgen receptor abnormalities) exhibit cryptorchidism and/or hypospadias or incom-plete penile development (e.g., micropenis). Many of these syndromes, especially those involved in normal androgen action, have been shown to be the result of discrete genetic abnormalities. Nevertheless, while both hypospadias and cryptorchidism may be associated with disorders of gonadal differentiation and develop-ment, as well as endocrine abnormalities, they may also result from other genetic defects of development.

Genetic disorders of sex determination and development

The diagnosis, and in some cases the treatment, of many of the disorders of sex determination are the responsi-bility of the pediatric urologist. Understandably, these disorders are associated not only with infertility but also with considerable social, physiological, and psy-chological issues for the individuals and their families. An unresolved consequence of such genital anomalies

involves the impact of diagnosis on later male repro-ductive function and the effect of specific therapies altering that adult outcome. The molecular mecha-nisms responsible for normal genital tract develop-ment, as well as the genetic abnormalities associated with abnormal development, continue to be defined as the various molecular models developed in the laboratory provide ways to predictably alter urogenital morphogenesis.

Intersex

Currently, intersex is divided into four main categor-ies: female pseudohermaphroditism (FPH), mixed or pure gonadal dysgenesis (GD), true hermaph-roditism (TH), and male pseudohermaphroditism (MPH) [149]. True hermaphrodites have both ovarian and testicular gonadal tissue, and variable genitalia. There are many other syndromes that are manifested as incomplete masculinization, masculinized females, or patients with sex reversal in whom the genotypic sex is not the phenotypic sex. Intersex conditions can arise as a result of structural or numerical chromosomal defects (discussed above), genetic defects, or hormo-nal, gonadal or end-organ insensitivity or dysfunction. In some patients, the defect may result from a local response to a systemic endocrinopathy, while in oth-ers the defect may reflect a developmental abnormality acting locally (reviewed in [149]).

Gonadal development and intersex

The Wilms' tumor suppressor gene (*WT1*) initiates the development of the gonads, and its absence results in gonadal agenesis. The orphan receptor steroidogenic factor 1 is a key regulator of the development of the endocrine system as it is expressed in the embryonic gonads and adrenals. It regulates the expression of the cytochrome p450 hydroxylases, DAX-1 and AMH. The expression of the Y-chromosome gene, *SRY*, is one of the earliest signals in the genital ridge. It leads to the partial differentiation of the cells destined to be the Sertoli cells and thus to initiation of the differentiation of the testis [150]. Studies of human XX males who are *SRY*– suggest that the SRY protein plays a role in the repression of transcription (reviewed in [150]). Desert hedgehog (*DHH*) plays an early role in the differentia-tion of the pre-Sertoli cells and the fetal Leydig cells. *PTGDS*, which regulates the expression of prostag-landin D_2, acts to aid in the recruitment of cells to the Sertoli cell lineage. Other genes, such as *FGF9*, work downstream of *SRY* but upstream of *SOX9*. The next stage of differentiation results from the expression of

SOX9, which leads to continued development of the testis. During embryogenesis, the complex pathway of gene expression is highly regulated, ultimately leading to the development of a testis or ovary. Not surprisingly, given this complexity, the molecular basis for over 75% of human sex-reversal syndromes remains unknown, although a number of candidate genes have been identified on the basis of microarray analysis (reviewed in [150]). A greater understanding of sex determination in the mouse is expected to enhance rapidly our understanding of the human syndromes.

Mixed gonadal dysgenesis

Mixed gonadal dysgenesis is the most common intersex condition. It may result from a chromosome defect that can be identified by a karyotype analysis, although these are not always informative. The most common karyotype observed, the 45,X/46,XY mosaic, may result from the loss of a Y chromosome early in embryonic development. However, 33% of patients have a normal karyotype, suggesting that factors other than sex-chromosomal aneuploidy may be involved. The testes lack germ cells and, when intra-abdominal, have an increased risk of malignancy [151]. Dysgenetic gonads are surgically removed.

Hypospadias

Hypospadias is defined by abnormal anterior urethral development in which the urethral opening is located proximal to the tip of the glans penis. This defect occurs during urethral development (8–20 weeks of gestation in humans) and the opening may be on the ventrum of the glans proximal to the tip of the glans penis or as proximal as the scrotum or perineum. Hypospadias of some degree occurs in about 1/300 male births. Androgen receptor mutations may be associated with hypospadias, even distal hypospadias, although this is rare.

Genes potentially associated with hypospadias

Misregulated expression of genes in the genital tubercle during development is thought to be involved in human hypospadias. These include transforming growth factor beta (TGF-β) (β1, β receptor 3) and the associated genes in this signal transduction pathway. *ATF3* is one candidate shown to be estrogen-regulated. The SMAD proteins 3 and 4 are downstream signaling proteins and form a heterodimer with *ATF3*. A series of growth factors are also involved, such as fibroblast growth factor 1 (FGF1), FGF8, bone morphogenic protein 2 (BMP2), BMP4, BMP7, frizzled (FZD1),

WNT5A, sonic hedgehog (SHH) and homeobox type genes (muscle segment homolog homeobox [*MSX1*], *HOXA13*, *HOXD13*) and other genes such as thrombospondin 4 (*THBS4*) and wingless-type mouse mammary tumor virus integration site family member 5A (reviewed in [152]). On the basis of microarray studies, a number of other candidate genes are identified in the human, and these range from genes involved in cell signaling to those involved in transcriptional regulation, cell cycling, and even transport [152].

Steroid receptor pathway defects in hypospadias

A number of candidate genes associated with hypospadias have been identified recently. Both the estrogen and androgen receptor keys are involved in some types of hypospadias. One such candidate is activating transcription factor 3, an estradiol-regulated gene. Expression of this gene is increased in human foreskin from children with hypospadias, and in mouse models, the expression is up-regulated by estrogen-like compounds [153]. Polymorphisms in the estrogen receptor genes (1 and 2) are associated with varied risks of hypospadias [154]. Not surprisingly, maternal/fetal exposure to endocrine-disrupting chemicals has been implicated in some of these cases [155–157].

Cryptorchidism

Cryptorchidism, or failure of testicular descent, occurs in about 3% of full-term newborn boys. Its prevalence decreases to about 1% by six months of age. It may be either bilateral or unilateral, and testis location is defined at the time of surgery as intra-abdominal (9%), peeping testis (20%), tubercle (42%), upper scrotum (8%), superficial inguinal pouch/ectopic (12%), absent or atrophic (9%). Sometimes found in association with hypospadias, cryptorchidism is also associated with the presence of a patent processus vaginalis, abnormal epididymis, cerebral palsy, mental retardation, Wilms' tumor, and abdominal wall defects (e.g., gastroschisis, omphalocele, prune belly) (reviewed by Sumfest *et al.*, emedicine.medscape.com/article/438378-overview). Usually, it presents as an isolated defect. There are two main phases of testicular descent. The first phase occurs when the abdominal testis moves to the inguinal ring. The second phase is usually thought to be androgen-regulated. In the adult, it presents a risk of malignancy as well as infertility.

Insl3

The insulin-like 3 hormone (INSL3), also known as Ley I-L (Leydig insulin-like) and Rlf (relaxin-like factor), is the main testicular hormone that induces gubernacu-lar development [158,159]. Animal studies showed that deficiency of INSL3 resulted in the testis and genital tract being freely mobile within the abdomen because there were no cranial or caudal attachments of the testis to the inguinal region. The protein is similar to relaxin, a hormone produced by the ovaries and pros-tate. A number of groups have looked for mutations of *INSL3*, and results are controversial. However, several mutations have been identified and shown to impair the function of the protein [160–169].

Great gene (lgr8)

A mouse model of cryptorchidism was identified after a transgene insertional mutation caused high intra-abdominal cryptorchidism in homozygous males. A candidate gene, *Great* (G-protein-coupled recep-tor affecting testis descent), was identified within the transgene integration site. GREAT is a member of a group of receptors that show homology to the glyco-protein hormone receptors. The gene encodes a seven transmembrane receptor that is highly expressed in the gubernaculum, the ligament that controls testicular movement during development. With targeted dele-tion of this gene in a mouse model, gubernacula fail to differentiate. Mutation screening of the human *GREAT* gene in 60 cryptorchid patients revealed a unique mis-sense mutation (T222P) in the ectodomain of the GREAT receptor in one of the patients, implicating the gene in the etiology in some cases of cryptorchidism in humans [165–167].

Androgens and their cognate receptor

The second phase of testicular descent is andro-gen-regulated. In response to LH, testosterone regulates the involution of the suspensory ligament and is involved in the inguinoscrotal phase of des-cent. Not surprisingly, alterations in androgen sen-sitivity and the signaling pathway of the androgen receptor, as well as endocrine imbalance, can be asso-ciated with cryptorchidism. The section on androgen insensitivity reviews these pathways. Antiandrogen treatment during development, and, potentially, expo-sures to endocrine-disrupting chemicals or agents with estrogen-like properties, may be involved in cryptorchidism [170].

Steroid biosynthetic pathways and metabolism deficiencies

Deficiencies of 21α-hydroxylase or 11β-hydroxylase (elevated 17OHP), 3β-hydroxysteroid dehydrogenase

[3β-HSD] (increased DHEA : andro ratio), 17α-hydroxylase (increased P : 17OHP ratio), 17,20 lyase (increased 17OHP: andro ratio), 17β-HSD (increased andro : T ratio), and 5α-reductase (increased T : DHT ratio) may be associated with cryptorchidism or hypospadias. Congenital adrenal hyperplasia (CAH) accounts for about 80% of the masculinized females [149], and 90% of these result from a 21-hydroxylase deficiency. Less common causes of CAH include defects in 11β-hydroxylase, 3β-HSD, and P450 aromatase. As a result of the deficiency, the androgenic steroid pre-cursors accumulate, and masculinization of the female occurs. CAH is a particular concern because of the possibility of salt-wasting and low glucocorticoid and mineralocorticoid levels.

Androgen exposure during development

Maternal CAH or androgenic drug administration (e.g., danazol, anabolic steroids), or the presence of an androgen-producing tumor, can masculinize an other-wise normal female fetus [149].

Syndromes that adversely affect the extratesticular ductal system
Congenital bilateral absence of the vas deferens (CBAVD)

CBAVD is found in 1% of infertile males and in up to 6% of those with obstructive azoospermia [171,172]. **CBAVD has two genetic etiologies: one involves mutations in the same genes that underlie cystic fibrosis and the second involves unknown genetic mechanisms controlling mesonephric duct differ-entiation** [173,174]. Physical examination reveals normal testis size and consistency, as spermatogenesis is unaffected. The caput epididymidis, made up of the efferent ductules, is always present and will be full and firm, as it is distended with fluid from the testis. The corpus and cauda are occasionally found as well. The vasa are absent bilaterally to palpation. Since the semi-nal vesicles are typically absent or atrophic, although occasionally large and cystic, the ejaculate consists only of prostatic fluid and is thin, watery, of low volume (0.6 mL), and low pH (6.5). The seminal vesicle anoma-lies can be imaged by transrectal ultrasound [175]. For men with CBAVD, pulmonary and pancreatic func-tions are fine [176,177].

Cystic fibrosis (CF) is a common autosomal reces-sive disorder that afflicts 1 in 1600 people of Northern European descent [178]. CF occurs with less frequency in those with other geographic or ethnic backgrounds, and so CF mutation analysis should be population-specific [179,180]. The most life-threatening and morbid clinical component of CF is the obstructive pulmonary disease resulting from thickened, tenacious respiratory secretions that begin a cycle of repetitive infections in the small airways and alveoli [181]. Patients with CF may require lung transplantation.

For similar biochemical reasons, the pancreatic exocrine system may fail. This is a less morbid issue because of the availability of oral pancreatic enzyme replacement. Abnormalities of the reproductive ductal structures are similar to those described above [182]. Spermatogenesis is intrinsically normal.

CF and most cases of CBAVD result from mutations in both maternal and paternal copies of the CFTR genes that encode for the cystic fibrosis transmembrane conductance regulator protein. CFTR is crucial for the maintenance of viscosity and fluidity of epithelial secretions through regulation of proper sodium/chloride balance. If the total functional CFTR pool is reduced by 50%, as occurs in people with either the maternal or the paternal allele mutated, but not both, clinical disease is not apparent. This is the "carrier" state, found in approximately 1 in 20 people of Northern European descent. When both CFTR alleles are abnormal, clinical disease may be present, showing a wide phenotypic spectrum from the mildest expression (CBAVD) to the most pronounced (CF diagnosed in infancy) with intermediate forms as well (e.g., CBAVD and sinusitis) [183,184]. Common to all, however, is vasal absence [182,185]. Clinical disease is determined by the combination of the two mutations. Two "severe" mutations, each dramatically altering the function or quantity of CFTR, will lead to clinical CF. Two "mild" mutations may result in only CBAVD if the individual is male. What is most commonly found in CBAVD, however, is a combination of "severe" and "mild" mutations. A three-base-pair deletion, termed ΔF508, is the most common mutation found worldwide in both CF and CBAVD [186]. The resultant CFTR is functionally handicapped and ineffective. When the patient is ΔF508 homozygous, clinical CF will be manifest. An intron 8 anomaly, termed 5T, coupled with ΔF508 is the most common combination underlying CBAVD [187]. In intron 8, there is a string of five, seven, or nine thymidines. If the pre-mRNA contains either seven or nine thymidines, splicing efficiency is optimal and the exon 9 derivative is intact and present in the mature mRNA.

If only five thymidines are present, splicing efficiency is less than optimal and many mature mRNAs will be missing exon 9 derivatives, the final protein being significantly abnormal. Therefore, the presence of 5T leads to a quantitative reduction in the amount of normal CFTR.

In males with CBAVD, at least one mutation can be found in 80%. The second mutation is presumed to be present but not detectable in those who are not compound heterozygotes on initial testing [188]. Males with CFTR-mutation-based CBAVD have normal renal anatomy. Mesonephric duct differentiation is thought to be normal in the early stages of embryogenesis, and it may be only later in fetal life or early in infancy that the vasa deferentia and seminal vesicles become atretic. **The male of each couple should be tested to determine his mutational status. If a male with newly defined CBAVD is indeed on the cystic fibrosis spectrum, then any associated ailments, e.g., chronic sinusitis or occasional pneumonias, may be viewed in a different light and be treated subsequently in a different way. In addition, the male most likely has reproductive-age siblings and it is important to define for their family unit the CF mutations that each of them may have inherited.** Each brother may also have CBAVD. Since surgical or percutaneous sperm retrieval can be used to harvest sperm for use with ICSI, the female partner should be tested as well prior to any intervention [189]. If she is a carrier of a CF mutation, preimplantation genetic diagnosis can be employed to prevent the transfer of any embryos that will be predicted to have CF or CBAVD [190]. Sperm aspiration procedures coupled with ICSI should not be performed until the appropriate genetic evaluation and counseling have been carried out lest a child with clinical CF or a male with CBAVD be born [191,192] (Fig. 15.3).

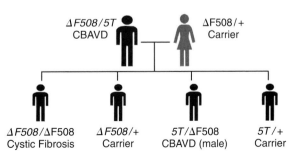

Fig. 15.3. Possible outcomes for offspring: paternal CBAVD (ΔF508/5T), maternal carrier (ΔF508 / +).

Failure of appropriate mesonephric duct differentiation may underlie a second genetic etiology, as posited by McCallum *et al.* [173]. At week 7 or so of gestation, the mesonephric duct splits into its two derivatives. The reproductive ductal portion will give rise to the distal two-thirds of the epididymis, the entire vas deferens (convoluted, straight, and ampullary segments), the seminal vesicle, and the ejaculatory duct. The caput epididymidis derives from the degenerating mesonephros and the prostate from the urogenital sinus. The urinary portion will give rise to the ureteral bud, which induces the metanephric blastema, the combination forming the kidney, the intrarenal collecting system, and the entirety of the ureter [193]. If an isolated insult occurs to one of the developing mesonephric ducts prior to week 7 of gestation, the kidney and reproductive ductal structures may be absent on that side, but the contralateral anatomy should be normal. If, however, there is a genetic anomaly that compromises mesonephric duct differentiation, both sides may be affected. At its most severe, this is perhaps the mechanism responsible for bilateral renal agenesis and Potter syndrome. In a slightly less severe form, perhaps this is the mechanism responsible for unilateral renal agenesis and bilateral vasal agenesis – one renal unit has developed and the patient is able to grow, mature, and present later in life with infertility. *CFTR* mutations will not be found in any higher frequency than in the general population because they are not the underlying genetic etiology. Genetic counseling should be offered and the couple informed that the genetic basis is unknown but that a possible outcome is bilateral renal agenesis for any offspring conceived [173].

Finally, a small number of azoospermic men with a low-volume, low-pH ejaculate and a palpable vas deferens on one side may have the same *CFTR* mutation spectrum as CBAVD men. and they should be tested [194]. They actually have bilateral vasal disease, as the palpable vas will be found to be non-patent somewhere along its course, scrotal, inguinal, or pelvic. Partner testing is mandatory.

Persistent Müllerian duct syndrome

AMH, also called Müllerian-inhibiting substance (MIS), is another TGF-β superfamily member essential during male fetal sex determination. AMH null males develop Müllerian duct derivatives, encompassing oviducts, a uterus, and a vagina, in addition to a complete male reproductive system [195,196]. Although these AMH null mice have testes that are fully descended and produce functional sperm, the null male is rendered infertile due to the presence of female reproductive organs that interfere with sperm transfer. The receptor type II mutant males develop as a phenocopy of the ligand-deficient male mice, developing internally as pseudohermaphrodites [197]. In contrast to the complexity of the other TGF-β gene family signaling pathways, AMH targeting provides evidence for only one ligand for the type II receptor. In humans, deficiency of either AMH or its receptor function results in a hernia inguinalis and cryptorchidism due to the presence of the Müllerian derivatives/remnants that effectively block testicular descent during development.

Prune belly syndrome

Prune belly syndrome consists of three types of congenital anomalies. Namely, the abdominal wall musculature is absent or deficient, the urinary tract is dilated, and cryptorchidism is present. It also can be associated with other more complex syndromes. In its complete form, it is a relatively rare occurrence (1/40,000 live births). Deletion of hepatocyte nuclear factor 1β (*HNF1β*), a gene involved in early embryogenesis and associated with a number of renal diseases, has been reported in one case of complete prune belly syndrome [198]. In other cases, it has been associated with complex structural chromosome defects [199–201].

Young syndrome

In 1970, the urologist Young identified a genetic linkage between bronchiectasis and absent vas deferens [202]. Also known as the Barry–Perkins–Young syndrome, it is characterized by chronic sinopulmonary infection and male infertility. Handelsman *et al.* suggested that this syndrome is as common as Klinefelter, although the overall incidence is not clear [203].

Defects of the hypothalamic–pituitary–gonadal axis

The hypothalamic–pituitary–gonadal (HPG) axis controls human sexual maturation and spermatogenesis. Disruption of any step of this highly regulated endocrine pathway can severely impair male sexual development and fertility. Albeit relatively rare in the population, mutations, small deletions, or polymorphic expansions within the regulatory genes involved in the biosynthesis of hormones, growth factors, the androgen receptors, and their associated signal transduction pathways can profoundly affect male reproductive development and function. Consequently, the genetic defects of the HPG axis must be considered in the evaluation and treatment of male infertility.

Hypogonadotropic hypogonadism

Hypogonadotropic hypogonadism (HH) is characterized by a decreased output of GnRH and low circulating levels of FSH and LH, resulting in deficient androgen secretion and spermatogenesis in the testis [204].

Kallmann syndrome

The hypothalamus secretes gonadotropin-releasing hormone (GnRH) which regulates the production of FSH and LH by the pituitary gonadotropes. Kallmann syndrome results from a failure of the GnRH-releasing neurons to migrate to the olfactory lobe during development. There are X-linked, autosomal dominant, and autosomal recessive forms of HH that occur in approximately 1 in 10 000–60 000 live births [205]. Kallmann syndrome represents the most common X-linked hypogonadotropic hypogonadism disorder in male infertility. A mutation in the X-linked *KAL1* gene encoding anosmin 1, which encodes a neural cell adhesion glycoprotein molecule found in some embryonic extracellular matrices, is the basis for the sex-linked form of the disease. Less commonly, structural chromosomal defects resulting in the loss of regions of the X chromosome may encompass the *KAL1* gene and result in a genomic form of familial X-linked Kallmann syndrome [206]. In contrast, one form of autosomal dominant HH results from mutations in the fibroblast growth factor receptor 1 gene (*FGFR1* or *KAL2*) [205]. The phenotypes observed can vary widely even within a given family with the identical mutation. In addition to the classical fibroblast growth factors, this receptor binds a number of adhesion molecules such as N-cadherin and LI [205]. Accordingly there are a number of other candidate genes that have been implicated but not shown to be causative. Loss-of-function mutations in the gene encoding a G-protein-coupled receptor, the prokineticin receptor 2 gene (*PROKR2* or *PROK2*), were reported in two sporadic cases of Kallmann syndrome, although this was a rare finding [207].

Not surprisingly, in patients with Kallmann syndrome puberty usually is delayed or does not occur. Because of the lack of GnRH, patients present with no serum gonadotropins, small, nonfunctioning testes, and a short penis. Although infertility may represent the only phenotypic abnormality, anosmia may be present due to the developmental failure of the olfactory bulb. In some cases congenital deafness, asymmetry of the cranium and face, cleft palate, cerebellar dysfunction, cryptorchidism, and renal abnormalities may be present. Hormone replacement is necessary, and spermatogenesis and subsequent fertility occur with coordinated gonadotropin stimulation [208]. Interestingly, in a recent study of a series of patients with idiopathic hypogonadotropic hypogonadism a subgroup showed sustained reversal of their hypogonadotropic hypogonadism following treatment cessation [209]. Despite oligospermia, with appropriate endocrine supplementation the majority of these patients can achieve fatherhood without the need for assisted reproduction.

Other gene defects causing hypogonadotropic hypogonadism

Dax1

DAX1, an X-chromosome-linked gene, encodes an orphan member of the steroid receptor superfamily required for the development of the hypothalamus, pituitary, adrenal glands, and gonads [210]. The protein also maintains the integrity of the testicular epithelium and spermatogenesis. *DAX1* mutations are associated with hypogonadotropic hypogonadism together with congenital adrenal hyperplasia, which may result in early infant death caused by an electrolyte imbalance.

Gonadotropic-releasing hormone receptor (GnRHR)

GNRHR, which encodes the gonadotropic-releasing hormone receptor located on pituitary gonadotropes, can be mutated in patients with hypogonadotropic hypogonadism. At least 21 different loss-of-function mutations have been identified in humans over the past 10 years [211].

Nasal embryonic LHRH factor (NELF)

NELF is a protein that guides the migration of the olfactory axon and the gonadotropin-releasing hormone neurons during development. Mutations in the gene encoding this protein are known but rare causes of hypogonadotropic hypogonadism [212].

GPR54 or kisspeptin

GPR54 is a G-protein-coupled member of the rhodopsin receptor family and kisspeptin 1 is a known agonist for this receptor [213]. Kisspeptin induces the secretion of the gonadotropins in a number of species and is thought to act on the GnRH neurons of the hypothalamus. Loss-of-function mutations of *GPR54* were identified in several patients with idiopathic hypogonadotropic hypogonadism, albeit rarely. Conversely, an activating mutation was identified in a Brazilian girl with precocious puberty [214]. This pathway plays an important role in the regulation of both puberty and the maintenance of reproductive function.

Convertase 1

Convertase 1, an endopeptidase encoded by the *PC1* gene, is involved in GnRH secretion and the release of the precursor of GnRH by the hypothalamus [215]. This gene is involved in the post-translational processing of prohormones and neuropeptides. Mutation in *PC1* is associated with hypogonadotropic hypogonadism with obesity and diabetes.

Prader–Willi syndrome

Prader–Willi syndrome is one of the leading genetic causes of obesity. Excessive appetite is characteristic. Prader–Willi, which can be associated with mild or moderate mental retardation and infantile hypotonia, can also present with hypogonadotropic hypogonadism. Sexual development is impaired or retarded, and testicular dysgenesis may be present, in part as a result of cryptorchidism. Rarely, precocious puberty is seen [216]. The most common cause is the deletion of the paternally derived chromosome 15q11–q13. Less commonly, it is found when maternal uniparental disomy (two maternal copies) of this locus occurs [217,218].

Defects in the gonadotropins and their receptors

FSH and LH are two key hormones produced by the testis that are necessary for male reproductive function. **These gonadotropins are dimeric molecules composed of an α subunit common to both human chorionic gonadotropin (hCG) and thyroid-stimulating hormone (TSH). The β subunits differ and provide specificity of action.**

Mutations in FSH and LH subunits

Mutations in the FSH and LH subunits can underlie male infertility. The phenotypes may vary from complete virilization failure to less severe forms of hypogonadism. Because LH acts on the Leydig cell to stimulate androgen production, androgen deficiency, with its associated developmental and functional features, occurs [219]. Less commonly, deficiencies in FSH occur in subfertile males. Although FSH β-subunit mutations have been suggested, they are rarely found in infertile men [220].

LH and FSH receptors

The LH and FSH receptors mediate the actions of these gonadotropins in the Leydig and Sertoli cells, respectively. Gene mutation causing LH receptor deficiency is rare in humans, but targeted deletion of LH receptor in the mouse results in male infertility, and the mice display the anatomical features of hypogonadism [221]. In contrast, constitutive activation of the LH receptor leads to male precocious pseudopuberty (but not infertility later in life), whereas pseudohermaphroditism and Leydig cell agenesis are the clinical phenotypes of LH resistance [222,223]. On the other hand, less is known about the FSH receptors; a mutation has been reported in a hypophysectomized man who is fertile, and in other men the incidence is rare [224,225].

Disorders that affect sperm function
Globozoospermia

Globozoospermia, or "round-headed sperm," is a severe form of teratozoospermia. The sperm heads appear round because there is no acrosome present. The presence of globozoospermia can be complete or incomplete, with varying percentages of round heads. Complete or total globozoospermia results in infertility. Partial globozoospermia occurs with varying degrees of normal sperm, and natural conception may result. Dam *et al.* reported on three of six brothers in an Ashkenazi Jewish family with a homozygous mutation in *SPATA16*, a spermatogenesis-specific gene [226]. Based upon SNP analysis, second- or third-degree consanguinity was present and a region of chromosome 3q26 of interest was identified with about 50 known genes. Within this region was the spermatogenesis-associated 16 (*SPATA16*) gene expressed only in human testis. A mutation was identified and expected to cause a splicing defect, but that could not be confirmed because testicular tissue was not available. Nevertheless, this defect was not observed in a small group of unrelated men with globozoospermia, and other candidate genes for globozoospermia are known from mouse models, including *Gopc*, which encodes a Golgi-associated protein, or the HIV-1 Rev binding protein gene (*Hrb*) [227–230]. Targeted gene deletion of casein kinase 2 alpha catalytic subunit, *Csnk2a2*, results in round-headed sperm in mice [231]. In a case report of two men with globozoospermia, polymorphisms in the *HRB*, *GOPC*, and *CSNK2A2* genes may have been associated with their globozoospermia, although the authors admit that complex trait-associated SNPs remain difficult to study [227].

Primary ciliary dyskinesia

Primary ciliary dyskinesia causes sperm abnormalities resulting from axonemal ultrastructural defects affecting the structure of the cilia/flagellum. The patients show bronchiectasis and a defect in sperm tails causing a motility defect. Kartagener syndrome, one type of ciliary dyskinesia, is among the syndromic forms of asthenospermia commonly found in combination with situs inversus. Absent or shortened dynein arms in the sperm tail are found in more than half of the men with primary ciliary dyskinesia or Kartagener syndrome. Kartagener is due to mutations in the dynein genes [232]. These include the *DNAI1*, *DNHH5*, *TXNDC3*, and *DNAH11* genes found on chromosomes 9, 5, 7, and 7, respectively. Another candidate identified by linkage analysis (genes not yet cloned) was found on chromosome 16 (type 5). In one patient with asthenospermia, a heterozygous mutation in the tektin-t gene was found [233]. Clearly the etiology is multifactorial.

Conclusion

In conclusion, fast-paced evolution of advanced reproductive therapies has allowed the achievement of biological paternity by men who, heretofore, would never have been permitted by nature to procreate. It is important to strive to identify the genetic mishaps that have rendered a particular male either severely oligospermic or azoospermic. Finding a genetic basis before applying any type of surgical or in-vitro technology allows counseling of the couple with regard to immediate, intermediate, and long-term issues that they should be aware of and consider before moving forward. Will a testis tissue extraction in an azoospermic male be worthwhile to even carry out in an attempt to find sperm for ICSI – an *immediate* concern? If an AZFa or AZFb/c microdeletion is found as the proximate cause of the azoospermia, the answer is no – sperm will not be found, and no operative intervention is necessary or appropriate. If a karyotype reveals a translocation in a severely oligospermic patient, preimplantation genetic diagnosis can be employed to maximize ICSI success by identifying and transferring only those embryos that may lead to a genetically healthy offspring – an *intermediate* time-frame issue. Equally important, though, are the many *long-term* consequences and outcomes that we must consider before blindly applying therapy that compensates for defects in the father but that may pass disease or abnormalities along to his offspring or even the following generation. An AZFc microdeletion will render a son infertile or sterile – a situation that is preventable with preimplantation screening and transfer of only female embryos. What are the ultimate health effects on the children of patients when we treat globozoospermia, primary ciliary dyskinesia, and idiopathic severe oligospermia? This is a legitimate question that we must continue to try to answer as we get better and better at bypassing nature's restrictions on conception.

Acknowledgments

Supported in part by Grants No. 2P01 HD 36289, AUAF, and the National Institutes of Health Cooperative Centers Program in Reproductive Research (U54 HD07495) from the National Institutes of Health.

References

[1] Van Assche E, Bonduelle M, Tournaye H, *et al.* Cytogenetics of infertile men. *Hum Reprod* 1996; **11**: 1–26.

[2] Barr ML. The natural history of Klinefelter's syndrome. *Fertil Steril* 1966; **17**: 429–41.

[3] Becker KL, Hoffman DL, Underdahl LO, Mason HL. Klinefelter's syndrome: clinical and laboratory findings in 50 patients. *Arch Intern Med* 1966; **118**: 314–21.

[4] Oates RD. Clinical and diagnostic features of patients with suspected Klinefelter syndrome. *J Androl* 2003; **24**: 49–50.

[5] Visootsak J, Graham JM. Klinefelter syndrome and other sex chromosomal aneuploidies. *Orphanet J Rare Dis* 2006; **1**: 42.

[6] Lowe X, Eskenazi B, Nelson DO, *et al.* Frequency of XY sperm increases with age in fathers of boys with Klinefelter syndrome. *Am J Hum Genet* 2001; **69**: 1046–54.

[7] Eskenazi B, Wyrobek AJ, Kidd SA, *et al.* Sperm aneuploidy in fathers of children with paternally and maternally inherited Klinefelter syndrome. *Hum Reprod* 2002; **17**: 576–83.

[8] Arnedo N, Templado C, Sanchez-Blanque Y, Rajmil O, Nogues C. Sperm aneuploidy in fathers of Klinefelter's syndrome offspring assessed by multicolour fluorescent in situ hybridization using probes for chromosomes 6, 13, 18, 21, 22, X and Y. *Hum Reprod* 2006; **21**: 524–8.

[9] Aksglaede L, Petersen JH, Main KM, Skakkebaek NE, Juul A. High normal testosterone levels in infants with non-mosaic Klinefelter's syndrome. *Eur J Endocrinol* 2007; **157**: 345–50.

[10] Yoshida A, Miura K, Nagao K, *et al.* Sexual function and clinical features of patients with Klinefelter's

syndrome with the chief complaint of male infertility. *Int J Androl* 1997; **20**: 80–5.

[11] Tomasi PA, Oates R, Brown L, Delitala G, Page DC. The pituitary–testicular axis in Klinefelter's syndrome and in oligo-azoospermic patients with and without deletions of the Y chromosome long arm. *Clin Endocrinol (Oxf)* 2003; **59**: 214–22.

[12] Aksglaede L, Andersson AM, Jorgensen N, *et al*. Primary testicular failure in Klinefelter's syndrome: the use of bivariate luteinizing hormone–testosterone reference charts. *Clin Endocrinol (Oxf)* 2007; **66**: 276–81.

[13] Swerdlow AJ, Schoemaker MJ, Higgins CD, Wright AF, Jacobs PA. Cancer incidence and mortality in men with Klinefelter syndrome: a cohort study. *J Natl Cancer Inst* 2005; **97**: 1204–10.

[14] Aguirre D, Nieto K, Lazos M, *et al*. Extragonadal germ cell tumors are often associated with Klinefelter syndrome. *Hum Pathol* 2006; **37**: 477–80.

[15] Juul A, Aksglaede L, Lund AM, *et al*. Preserved fertility in a non-mosaic Klinefelter patient with a mutation in the fibroblast growth factor receptor 3 gene: case report. *Hum Reprod* 2007; **22**: 1907–11.

[16] Denschlag D, Tempfer C, Kunze M, Wolff G, Keck C. Assisted reproductive techniques in patients with Klinefelter syndrome: A critical review. *Fertil Steril* 2004; **82**: 775–9.

[17] Gonsalves J, Turek PJ, Schlegel PN, *et al*. Recombination in men with Klinefelter syndrome. *Reproduction* 2005; **130**: 223–9.

[18] Schiff JD, Palermo GD, Veeck LL, *et al*. Success of testicular sperm extraction [corrected] and intracytoplasmic sperm injection in men with Klinefelter syndrome. *J Clin Endocrinol Metab* 2005; **90**: 6263–7.

[19] Bourne H, Stern K, Clarke G, *et al*. Delivery of normal twins following the intracytoplasmic injection of spermatozoa from a patient with 47,XXY Klinefelter's syndrome. *Hum Reprod* 1997; **12**: 2447–50.

[20] Hinney B, Guttenbach M, Schmid M, Engel W, Michelmann HW. Pregnancy after intracytoplasmic sperm injection with sperm from a man with a 47,XXY Klinefelter's karyotype. *Fertil Steril* 1997; **68**: 718–20.

[21] Komori S, Horiuchi I, Hamada Y, *et al*. Birth of healthy neonates after intracytoplasmic injection of ejaculated or testicular spermatozoa from men with nonmosaic Klinefelter's syndrome: a report of 2 cases. *J Reprod Med* 2004; **49**: 126–30.

[22] Kahraman S, Findikli N, Berkil H, *et al*. Results of preimplantation genetic diagnosis in patients with Klinefelter's syndrome. *Reprod Biomed Online* 2003; **7**: 346–52.

[23] Tachdjian G, Frydman N, Morichon-Delvallez N, *et al*. Reproductive genetic counselling in non-mosaic 47,XXY patients: implications for preimplantation or prenatal diagnosis: Case report and review. *Hum Reprod* 2003; **18**: 271–5.

[24] Morel F, Bernicot I, Herry A, *et al*. An increased incidence of autosomal aneuploidies in spermatozoa from a patient with Klinefelter's syndrome. *Fertil Steril* 2003; **79** (Suppl 3): 1644–6.

[25] Ron-El R, Strassburger D, Gelman-Kohan S, *et al*. A 47,XXY fetus conceived after ICSI of spermatozoa from a patient with non-mosaic Klinefelter's syndrome: case report. *Hum Reprod* 2000; **15**: 1804–6.

[26] Blanco J, Egozcue J, Vidal F. Meiotic behavior of the sex chromosomes in three patients with sex chromosome anomalies (47,XXY, mosaic 46,XY/47,XXY and 47,XYY) assessed by fluorescence in-situ hybridization. *Hum Reprod.* 2001; **16**: 887–92.

[27] Bergere M, Wainer R, Nataf V, *et al*. Biopsied testis cells of four 47,XXY patients: fluorescence in-situ hybridization and ICSI results. *Hum Reprod.* 2002; **17**: 32–7.

[28] Foresta C, Galeazzi C, Bettella A, *et al*. Analysis of meiosis in intratesticular germ cells from subjects affected by classic Klinefelter's syndrome. *J Clin Endocrinol Metab* 1999; **84**: 3807–10.

[29] Madgar I, Dor J, Weissenberg R, *et al*. Prognostic value of the clinical and laboratory evaluation in patients with nonmosaic Klinefelter syndrome who are receiving assisted reproductive therapy. *Fertil Steril* 2002; **77**: 1167–9.

[30] Lin YM, Huang WJ, Lin JS, Kuo PL. Progressive depletion of germ cells in a man with nonmosaic Klinefelter's syndrome: optimal time for sperm recovery. *Urology* 2004; **63**: 380–1.

[31] Okada H, Goda K, Yamamoto Y, *et al*. Age as a limiting factor for successful sperm retrieval in patients with nonmosaic Klinefelter's syndrome. *Fertil Steril* 2005; **84**: 1662–4.

[32] Okada H, Goda K, Muto S, *et al*. Four pregnancies in nonmosaic Klinefelter's syndrome using cryopreserved–thawed testicular spermatozoa. *Fertil Steril* 2005; **84**: 1508.

[33] Okada H, Shirakawa T, Ishikawa T, *et al*. Serum testosterone levels in patients with nonmosaic Klinefelter syndrome after testicular sperm extraction for intracytoplasmic sperm injection. *Fertil Steril* 2004; **82**: 237–8.

[34] Ramasamy R, Yagan N, Schlegel PN. Structural and functional changes to the testis after conventional versus microdissection testicular sperm extraction. *Urology* 2005; **65**: 1190–4.

[35] Damani MN, Mittal R, Oates RD. Testicular tissue extraction in a young male with 47,XXY Klinefelter's

syndrome: potential strategy for preservation of fertility. *Fertil Steril* 2001; **76**: 1054–6.

[36] Aksglaede L, Wikstrom AM, Rajpert-De Meyts E, *et al*. Natural history of seminiferous tubule degeneration in Klinefelter syndrome. *Hum Reprod Update* 2006; **12**: 39–48.

[37] Wikstrom AM, Dunkel L, Wickman S, Norjavaara E, Ankarberg-Lindgren C, Raivio T. Are adolescent boys with Klinefelter syndrome androgen deficient? A longitudinal study of Finnish 47,XXY boys. *Pediatr Res* 2006; **59**: 854–9.

[38] Bojesen A, Gravholt CH. Klinefelter syndrome in clinical practice. *Nat Clin Pract Urol* 2007; **4**: 192–204.

[39] de la Chapelle A. Nature and origin of males with XX sex chromosomes. *Am J Hum Genet* 1972; **24**: 71–105.

[40] Schiebel K, Winkelmann M, Mertz A, *et al*. Abnormal XY interchange between a novel isolated protein kinase gene, PRKY, and its homologue, PRKX, accounts for one third of all (Y+)XX males and (Y–)XY females. *Hum Mol Genet* 1997; **6**: 1985–9.

[41] Rajender S, Rajani V, Gupta NJ, *et al*. SRY-negative 46,XX male with normal genitals, complete masculinization and infertility. *Mol Hum Reprod* 2006; **12**: 341–6.

[42] Grigorescu-Sido A, Heinrich U, Grigorescu-Sido P, *et al*. Three new 46,XX male patients: a clinical, cytogenetic and molecular analysis. *J Pediatr Endocrinol Metab* 2005; **18**: 197–203.

[43] Vorona E, Zitzmann M, Gromoll J, Schuring AN, Nieschlag E. Clinical, endocrinologic and epigenetic features of the 46, XX male syndrome compared to 47,XXY Klinefelter patients. *J Clin Endocrinol Metab* 2007; **92**: 3458–65.

[44] Linden MG, Bender BG, Robinson A. Intrauterine diagnosis of sex chromosome aneuploidy. *Obstet Gynecol* 1996; **87**: 468–75.

[45] Wong EC, Ferguson KA, Chow V, Ma S. Sperm aneuploidy and meiotic sex chromosome configurations in an infertile XYY male. *Hum Reprod* 2008; **23**: 374–8.

[46] Milazzo JP, Rives N, Mousset-Simeon N, Mace B. Chromosome constitution and apoptosis of immature germ cells present in sperm of two 47,XYY infertile males. *Hum Reprod* 2006; **21**: 1749–58.

[47] Wang JY, Samura O, Zhen DK, *et al*. Fluorescence in-situ hybridization analysis of chromosomal constitution in spermatozoa from a mosaic 47,XYY/46,XY male. *Mol Hum Reprod*. Jul 2000; **6**: 665–8.

[48] Tilford CA, Kuroda-Kawaguchi T, Skaletsky H, *et al*. A physical map of the human Y chromosome. *Nature* 2001; **409**: 943–5.

[49] Graves JA, Wakefield MJ, Toder R. The origin and evolution of the pseudoautosomal regions of human sex chromosomes. *Hum Mol Genet* 1998; **7**: 1991–6.

[50] Ciccodicola A, D'Esposito M, Esposito T, *et al*. Differentially regulated and evolved genes in the fully sequenced Xq/Yq pseudoautosomal region. *Hum Mol Genet* 2000; **9**: 395–401.

[51] Wilhelm D, Palmer S, Koopman P. Sex determination and gonadal development in mammals. *Physiol Rev* 2007; **87**: 1–28.

[52] Skaletsky H, Kuroda-Kawaguchi T, Minx PJ, *et al*. The male-specific region of the human Y chromosome is a mosaic of discrete sequence classes. *Nature* 2003; **423**: 825–37.

[53] Jobling MA, Tyler-Smith C. The human Y chromosome: an evolutionary marker comes of age. *Nat Rev Genet* 2003; **4**: 598–612.

[54] Kuroda-Kawaguchi T, Skaletsky H, Brown LG, *et al*. The AZFc region of the Y chromosome features massive palindromes and uniform recurrent deletions in infertile men. *Nat Genet* 2001; **29**: 279–86.

[55] Repping S, Skaletsky H, Lange J, *et al*. Recombination between palindromes P5 and P1 on the human Y chromosome causes massive deletions and spermatogenic failure. *Am J Hum Genet* 2002; **71**: 906–22.

[56] Tiepolo L, Zuffardi O. Localization of factors controlling spermatogenesis in the nonfluorescent portion of the human Y chromosome long arm. *Hum Genet* 1976; **38**: 119–24.

[57] Lin YM, Teng YN, Lee PC, *et al*. AZFa candidate gene deletions in Taiwanese patients with spermatogenic failure. *J Formos Med Assoc* 2001; **100**: 592–7.

[58] Hurles ME, Willey D, Matthews L, Hussain SS. Origins of chromosomal rearrangement hotspots in the human genome: Evidence from the AZFa deletion hotspots. *Genome Biol* 2004; **5**: R55.

[59] Kamp C, Hirschmann P, Voss H, Huellen K, Vogt PH. Two long homologous retroviral sequence blocks in proximal Yq11 cause AZFa microdeletions as a result of intrachromosomal recombination events. *Hum Mol Genet* 2000; **9**: 2563–72.

[60] Sun C, Skaletsky H, Rozen S, *et al*. Deletion of azoospermia factor a (AZFa) region of human Y chromosome caused by recombination between HERV15 proviruses. *Hum Mol Genet* 2000; **9**: 2291–6.

[61] Wimmer R, Kirsch S, Weber A, Rappold GA, Schempp W. The Azoospermia region AZFa: an evolutionar y view. *Cytogenet Genome Res* 2002; **99**: 146–50.

[62] Session DR, Lee GS, Wolgemuth DJ. Characterization of D1Pas1, a mouse autosomal homologue of the human AZFa region DBY, as a nuclear protein in spermatogenic cells. *Fertil Steril* 2001; **76**: 804–11.

[63] Ditton HJ, Zimmer J, Kamp C, Rajpert-De Meyts E, Vogt PH. The AZFa gene DBY (DDX3Y) is widely transcribed but the protein is limited to the male germ cells by translation control. *Hum Mol Genet* 2004; **13**: 2333–41.

[64] Sun C, Skaletsky H, Birren B, *et al.* An azoospermic man with a de novo point mutation in the Y-chromosomal gene USP9Y. *Nat Genet* 1999; **23**: 429–32.

[65] Krausz C, Degl'Innocenti S, Nuti F, *et al.* Natural transmission of USP9Y gene mutations: A new perspective on the role of AZFa genes in male fertility. *Hum Mol Genet* 2006; **15**: 2673–81.

[66] Blagosklonova O, Fellmann F, Clavequin MC, Roux C, Bresson JL. AZFa deletions in Sertoli cell-only syndrome: A retrospective study. *Mol Hum Reprod* 2000; **6**: 795–9.

[67] Hopps CV, Mielnik A, Goldstein M, Palermo GD, Rosenwaks Z, Schlegel PN. Detection of sperm in men with Y chromosome microdeletions of the AZFa, AZFb and AZFc regions. *Hum Reprod* 2003; **18**: 1660–5.

[68] Reijo R, Lee TY, Salo P, *et al.* Diverse spermatogenic defects in humans caused by Y chromosome deletions encompassing a novel RNA-binding protein gene. *Nat Genet* 1995; **10**: 383–93.

[69] Reijo RJ, Alagappan R, Patrizio P, Page DC. Severe oligospermia resulting from deletions of the azoospermia factor gene on Y chromosome. *Lancet* 1996; **347**: 1290–3.

[70] Saxena R, de Vries JW, Repping S, *et al.* Four DAZ genes in two clusters found in the AZFc region of the human Y chromosome. *Genomics* 2000; **67**: 256–67.

[71] Lepretre AC, Patrat C, Mitchell M, Jouannet P, Bienvenu T. No partial DAZ deletions but frequent gene conversion events on the Y chromosome of fertile men. *J Assist Reprod Genet* 2005; **22**: 141–8.

[72] Menke DB, Mutter GL, Page DC. Expression of DAZ, an azoospermia factor candidate, in human spermatogonia. *Am J Hum Genet* 1997; **60**: 237–41.

[73] Collier B, Gorgoni B, Loveridge C, Cooke HJ, Gray NK. The DAZL family proteins are PABP-binding proteins that regulate translation in germ cells. *Embo J* 2005; **24**: 2656–66.

[74] Geoffroy-Siraudin C, Aknin-Seiffer I, Metzler-Guillemain C, *et al.* Meiotic abnormalities in patients bearing complete AZFc deletion of Y chromosome. *Hum Reprod* 2007; **22**: 1567–72.

[75] Oates RD, Silber S, Brown LG, Page DC. Clinical characterization of 42 oligospermic or azoospermic men with microdeletion of the AZFc region of the Y chromosome, and of 18 children conceived via ICSI. *Hum Reprod* 2002; **17**: 2813–24.

[76] Mulhall JP, Reijo R, Alagappan R, *et al.* Azoospermic men with deletion of the DAZ gene cluster are capable of completing spermatogenesis: Fertilization, normal embryonic development and pregnancy occur when retrieved testicular spermatozoa are used for intracytoplasmic sperm injection. *Hum Reprod* 1997; **12**: 503–8.

[77] Kuhnert B, Gromoll J, Kostova E, *et al.* Case report: natural transmission of an AZFc Y-chromosomal microdeletion from father to his sons. *Hum Reprod* 2004; **19**: 886–8.

[78] Stouffs K, Lissens W, Tournaye H, Van Steirteghem A, Liebaers I. The choice and outcome of the fertility treatment of 38 couples in whom the male partner has a Yq microdeletion. *Hum Reprod* 2005; **20**: 1887–96.

[79] Faure AK, Aknin-Seifer I, Satre V, *et al.* Fine mapping of re-arranged Y chromosome in three infertile patients with non-obstructive azoospermia/cryptozoospermia. *Hum Reprod* 2007; **22**: 1854–60.

[80] Arnedo N, Nogues C, Bosch M, Templado C. Mitotic and meiotic behaviour of a naturally transmitted ring Y chromosome: reproductive risk evaluation. *Hum Reprod* 2005; **20**: 462–8.

[81] Hsu LY. Phenotype/karyotype correlations of Y chromosome aneuploidy with emphasis on structural aberrations in postnatally diagnosed cases. *Am J Med Genet* 1994; **53**: 108–40.

[82] Carvalho FM, Wolfgramm EV, Degasperi I, *et al.* Molecular cytogenetic analysis of a ring-Y infertile male patient. *Genet Mol Res* 2007; **6**: 59–66.

[83] Mau-Holzmann UA. Somatic chromosomal abnormalities in infertile men and women. *Cytogenet Genome Res* 2005; **111**: 317–36.

[84] Otani T, Roche M, Mizuike M, Colls P, Escudero T, Munne S. Preimplantation genetic diagnosis significantly improves the pregnancy outcome of translocation carriers with a history of recurrent miscarriage and unsuccessful pregnancies. *Reprod Biomed Online* 2006; **13**: 869–74.

[85] Pardridge WM. Serum bioavailability of sex steroid hormones. *Clin Endocrinol Metab* 1986; **15**: 259–78.

[86] Lasnitzki I, Franklin HR, Wilson JD. The mechanism of androgen uptake and concentration by rat ventral prostate in organ culture. *J Endocrinol* 1974; **60**: 81–90.

[87] Bruchovsky N, Wilson JD. The conversion of testosterone to 5-alpha-androstan-17-beta-ol-3-one by rat prostate in vivo and in vitro. *J Biol Chem* 1968; **243**: 2012–21.

[88] Stocco DM, Clark BJ. Regulation of the acute production of steroids in steroidogenic cells. *Endocr Rev* 1996; **17**: 221–44.

[89] Stocco DM. StAR protein and the regulation of steroid hormone biosynthesis. *Annu Rev Physiol* 2001; **63**: 193–213.

[90] Clark BJ, Wells J, King SR, Stocco DM. The purification, cloning, and expression of a novel luteinizing hormone-induced mitochondrial protein in MA-10 mouse Leydig tumor cells: characterization of the steroidogenic acute regulatory protein (StAR). *J Biol Chem* 1994; **269**: 28314–22.

[91] Tee MK, Lin D, Sugawara T, *et al*. T→A transversion 11 bp from a splice acceptor site in the human gene for steroidogenic acute regulatory protein causes congenital lipoid adrenal hyperplasia. *Hum Mol Genet* 1995; **4**: 2299–305.

[92] Bose HS, Sugawara T, Strauss JF, Miller WL. The pathophysiology and genetics of congenital lipoid adrenal hyperplasia. International Congenital Lipoid Adrenal Hyperplasia Consortium. *N Engl J Med* 1996; **335**: 1870–8.

[93] Caron KM, Soo SC, Wetsel WC, Stocco DM, Clark BJ, Parker KL. Targeted disruption of the mouse gene encoding steroidogenic acute regulatory protein provides insights into congenital lipoid adrenal hyperplasia. *Proc Natl Acad Sci U S A* 1997; **94**: 11540–5.

[94] Faienza MF, Giordani L, Delvecchio M, Cavallo L. Clinical, endocrine, and molecular findings in 17β-hydroxysteroid dehydrogenase type 3 deficiency. *J Endocrinol Invest* 2008; **31**: 85–91.

[95] Zachmann M, Werder EA, Prader A. Two types of male pseudohermaphroditism due to 17,20-desmolase deficiency. *J Clin Endocrinol Metab* 1982; **55**: 487–90.

[96] Goebelsmann U, Zachmann M, Davajan V, *et al*. Male pseudohermaphroditism consistent with 17,20-desmolase deficiency. *Gynecol Invest* 1976; **7**: 138–56.

[97] Zachmann M, Vollmin JA, Hamilton W, Prader A. Steroid 17,20-desmolase deficiency: a new cause of male pseudohermaphroditism. *Clin Endocrinol (Oxf)* 1972; **1**: 369–85.

[98] Barash IA, Cheung CC, Weigle DS, *et al*. Leptin is a metabolic signal to the reproductive system. *Endocrinology* 1996; **137**: 3144–7.

[99] Vornberger W, Prins G, Musto NA, Suarez-Quian CA. Androgen receptor distribution in rat testis: new implications for androgen regulation of spermatogenesis. *Endocrinology* 1994 May; **134**: 2307–16.

[100] Maiti S, Meistrich ML, Wilson G, *et al*. Irradiation selectively inhibits expression from the androgen-dependent Pem homeobox gene promoter in sertoli cells. *Endocrinology* 2001; **142**: 1567–77.

[101] Chang C, Chen YT, Yeh SD, *et al*. Infertility with defective spermatogenesis and hypotestosteronemia in male mice lacking the androgen receptor in Sertoli cells. *Proc Natl Acad Sci U S A* 2004; **101**: 6876–81.

[102] Zhang C, Yeh S, Chen YT, *et al*. Oligozoospermia with normal fertility in male mice lacking the androgen receptor in testis peritubular myoid cells. *Proc Natl Acad Sci U S A* 2006; **103**: 17718–23.

[103] Jost A. Problems of fetal endocrinology: the gonadal and hypophyseal hormones. *Recent Prog Horm Res* 1953; **8**: 379–418.

[104] Picard JY, Josso N. Purification of testicular anti-Mullerian hormone allowing direct visualization of the pure glycoprotein and determination of yield and purification factor. *Mol Cell Endocrinol* 1984; **34**: 23–9.

[105] Vigier B, Picard JY, Tran D, Legeai L, Josso N. Production of anti-Mullerian hormone: another homology between Sertoli and granulosa cells. *Endocrinology* 1984; **114**: 1315–20.

[106] Donahoe PK, Ito Y, Price JM, Hendren WH III. Mullerian inhibiting substance activity in bovine fetal, newborn and prepubertal testes. *Biol Reprod* 1977; **16**: 238–43.

[107] Cate RL, Mattaliano RJ, Hession C, *et al*. Isolation of the bovine and human genes for Mullerian inhibiting substance and expression of the human gene in animal cells. *Cell* 1986; **45**: 685–98.

[108] Tsai MY, Yeh SD, Wang RS, *et al*. Differential effects of spermatogenesis and fertility in mice lacking androgen receptor in individual testis cells. *Proc Natl Acad Sci U S A* 2006; **103**: 18975–80.

[109] De GK, Swinnen JV, Saunders PT, *et al*. A Sertoli cell-selective knockout of the androgen receptor causes spermatogenic arrest in meiosis. *Proc Natl Acad Sci U S A* 2004; **101**: 1327–32.

[110] Xu Q, Lin HY, Yeh SD, *et al*. Infertility with defective spermatogenesis and steroidogenesis in male mice lacking androgen receptor in Leydig cells. *Endocrine* 2007; **32**: 96–106.

[111] Johnston DS, Russell LD, Friel PJ, Griswold MD. Murine germ cells do not require functional androgen receptors to complete spermatogenesis following spermatogonial stem cell transplantation. *Endocrinology* 2001; **142**: 2405–8.

[112] Zhou X, Kudo A, Kawakami H, Hirano H. Immunohistochemical localization of androgen receptor in mouse testicular germ cells during fetal and postnatal development. *Anat Rec* 1996; **245**: 509–18.

[113] Tan KA, De GK, Atanassova N, *et al*. The role of androgens in Sertoli cell proliferation and functional maturation: studies in mice with total or Sertoli cell-selective ablation of the androgen receptor. *Endocrinology* 2005; **146**: 2674–83.

[114] Quigley CA, De BA, Marschke KB, *et al*. Androgen receptor defects: historical, clinical, and molecular perspectives. *Endocr Rev* 1995; **16**: 271–321.

[115] Griffin JE, McPhaul MJ, Russell LD, Wilson JD. The androgen resistance syndromes: Steroid 5 alpha reductase-2 deficiency, testicular feminization and related disorders. In: Scriver CS, Beaudet AL, Sly WS, Valle D, eds. *The Metabolic and Molecular Bases of Inherited Diseases.* New York, NY: McGraw-Hill, 2001: 4117–46.

[116] Gottlieb B, Lehvaslaiho H, Beitel LK, *et al.* The Androgen Receptor Gene Mutations Database. *Nucleic Acids Res* 1998; **26**: 234–8.

[117] Petterson G, Bonnier G. Inherited sex mosaic in men. *Hereditas* 1937; **23**: 49–69.

[118] Morris JM. The syndrome of testicular feminization in male pseudohermaphrodites. *Am J Obstet Gynecol* 1953; **65**: 1192–211.

[119] Bangsboll S, Qvist I, Lebech PE, Lewinsky M. Testicular feminization syndrome and associated gonadal tumors in Denmark. *Acta Obstet Gynecol Scand* 1992; **71**: 63–6.

[120] Reifenstein EC. Herditary familial hypogonadism. *Proc Am Fed Clin Res* 1947; **3**: 86.

[121] Aiman J, Griffin JE, Gazak JM, Wilson JD, MacDonald PC. Androgen insensitivity as a cause of infertility in otherwise normal men. *N Engl J Med* 1979; **300**: 223–7.

[122] Larrea F, Benavides G, Scaglia H, *et al.* Gynecomastia as a familial incomplete male pseudohermaphroditism type 1: a limited androgen resistance syndrome. *J Clin Endocrinol Metab* 1978; **46**: 961–70.

[123] McPhaul MJ, Marcelli M, Tilley WD, *et al.* Molecular basis of androgen resistance in a family with a qualitative abnormality of the androgen receptor and responsive to high-dose androgen therapy. *J Clin Invest* 1991; **87**: 1413–21.

[124] La Spada AR, Wilson EM, Lubahn DB, Harding AE, Fischbeck KH. Androgen receptor gene mutations in X-linked spinal and bulbar muscular atrophy. *Nature* 1991; **352**: 77–9.

[125] MacLean HE, Gonzales M, Greenland KJ, Warne GL, Zajac JD. Age-dependent differences in androgen binding affinity in a family with spinal and bulbar muscular atrophy. *Neurol Res* 2005; **27**: 548–51.

[126] McManamny P, Chy HS, Finkelstein DI, *et al.* A mouse model of spinal and bulbar muscular atrophy. *Hum Mol Genet* 2002; **11**: 2103–11.

[127] Mhatre AN, Trifiro MA, Kaufman M, *et al.* Reduced transcriptional regulatory competence of the androgen receptor in X-linked spinal and bulbar muscular atrophy. *Nat Genet* 1993; **5**: 184–8.

[128] Choong CS, Kemppainen JA, Zhou ZX, Wilson EM. Reduced androgen receptor gene expression with first exon CAG repeat expansion. *Mol Endocrinol* 1996; **10**: 1527–35.

[129] von ES, Syska A, Gromoll J, *et al.* Inverse correlation between sperm concentration and number of androgen receptor CAG repeats in normal men. *J Clin Endocrinol Metab* 2001; **86**: 2585–90.

[130] Tut TG, Ghadessy FJ, Trifiro MA, Pinsky L, Yong EL. Long polyglutamine tracts in the androgen receptor are associated with reduced trans-activation, impaired sperm production, and male infertility. *J Clin Endocrinol Metab* 1997; **82**: 3777–82.

[131] Dowsing AT, Yong EL, Clark M, *et al.* Linkage between male infertility and trinucleotide repeat expansion in the androgen-receptor gene. *Lancet* 1999; **354**: 640–3.

[132] Yoshida KI, Yano M, Chiba K, Honda M, Kitahara S. CAG repeat length in the androgen receptor gene is enhanced in patients with idiopathic azoospermia. *Urology* 1999; **54**: 1078–81.

[133] Casella R, Maduro MR, Misfud A, *et al.* Androgen receptor gene polyglutamine length is associated with testicular histology in infertile patients. *J Urol* 2003; **169**: 224–7.

[134] Giwercman YL, Xu C, Arver S, Pousette A, Reneland R. No association between the androgen receptor gene CAG repeat and impaired sperm production in Swedish men. *Clin Genet* 1998; **54**: 435–6.

[135] Dadze S, Wieland C, Jakubiczka S, *et al.* The size of the CAG repeat in exon 1 of the androgen receptor gene shows no significant relationship to impaired spermatogenesis in an infertile Caucasoid sample of German origin. *Mol Hum Reprod* 2000; **6**: 207–14.

[136] Van GR, Van HK, Kiemeney L, *et al.* Is increased CAG repeat length in the androgen receptor gene a risk factor for male subfertility? *J Urol* 2002; **167**: 621–3.

[137] Rajpert-De ME, Leffers H, Petersen JH, *et al.* CAG repeat length in androgen-receptor gene and reproductive variables in fertile and infertile men. *Lancet* 2002; **359**: 44–6.

[138] Mifsud A, Sim CK, Boettger-Tong H, *et al.* Trinucleotide (CAG) repeat polymorphisms in the androgen receptor gene: molecular markers of risk for male infertility. *Fertil Steril* 2001; **75**: 275–81.

[139] Migeon CJ, Brown TR, Lanes R, *et al.* A clinical syndrome of mild androgen insensitivity. *J Clin Endocrinol Metab* 1984; **59**: 672–8.

[140] Warne GL, Gyorki S, Risbridger GP, Khalid BA, Funder JW. Correlations between fibroblast androgen receptor levels and clinical features in abnormal male sexual differentiation and infertility. *Aust N Z J Med* 1983; **13**: 335–41.

[141] Aiman J, Griffin JE. The frequency of androgen receptor deficiency in infertile men. *J Clin Endocrinol Metab* 1982; **54**: 725–32.

[142] Bouchard P, Wright F, Portois MC, Couzinet B, Schaison G, Mowszowicz I. Androgen insensitivity

in oligospermic men: a reappraisal. *J Clin Endocrinol Metab* 1986; **63**: 1242–6.

[143] Ghadessy FJ, Lim J, Abdullah AA, *et al*. Oligospermic infertility associated with an androgen receptor mutation that disrupts interdomain and coactivator (TIF2) interactions. *J Clin Invest* 1999; **103**: 1517–25.

[144] Giwercman YL, Nikoshkov A, Bystrom B, *et al*. A novel mutation (N233K) in the transactivating domain and the N756S mutation in the ligand binding domain of the androgen receptor gene are associated with male infertility. *Clin Endocrinol (Oxf)* 2001; **54**: 827–34.

[145] Ferlin A, Vinanzi C, Garolla A, *et al*. Male infertility and androgen receptor gene mutations: Clinical features and identification of seven novel mutations. *Clin Endocrinol (Oxf)* 2006; **65**: 606–10.

[146] Gottlieb B, Lombroso R, Beitel LK, Trifiro MA. Molecular pathology of the androgen receptor in male (in)fertility. *Reprod Biomed Online* 2005; **10**: 42–8.

[147] Imperato-McGinley J, Guerrero L, Gautier T, German JL, Peterson RE. Steroid 5alpha-reductase deficiency in man. An inherited form of male pseudohermaphroditism. *Birth Defects Orig Artic Ser* 1975; **11**: 91–103.

[148] Leshin M, Griffin JE, Wilson JD. Hereditary male pseudohermaphroditism associated with an unstable form of 5α-reductase. *J Clin Invest* 1978; **62**: 685–91.

[149] Nelson CP, Gearhart JP. Current views on evaluation, management, and gender assignment of the intersex infant. *Nat Clin Pract Urol* 2004; **1**: 38–43.

[150] Beverdam A, Koopman P. Expression profiling of purified mouse gonadal somatic cells during the critical time window of sex determination reveals novel candidate genes for human sexual dysgenesis syndromes. *Hum Mol Genet* 2006; **15**: 417–31.

[151] Wegner HE, Ferszt A, Wegner RD, Dieckmann KP. Mixed gonadal dysgenesis: a rare cause of primary infertility. Report of 2 cases and review of the literature. *Urologe A* 1994; **33**: 342–6.

[152] Willingham E, Baskin LS. Candidate genes and their response to environmental agents in the etiology of hypospadias. *Nat Clin Pract Urol* 2007; **4**: 270–9.

[153] Liu B, Lin G, Willingham E, *et al*. Estradiol upregulates activating transcription factor 3, a candidate gene in the etiology of hypospadias. *Pediatr Dev Pathol* 2007; **10**: 446–54.

[154] Ban S, Sata F, Kurahashi N, *et al*. Genetic polymorphisms of ESR1 and ESR2 that may influence estrogen activity and the risk of hypospadias. *Hum Reprod* 2008; **23**: 1466–71.

[155] Hsieh MH, Breyer BN, Eisenberg ML, Baskin LS. Associations among hypospadias, cryptorchidism, anogenital distance, and endocrine disruption. *Curr Urol Rep* 2008; **9**: 137–42.

[156] Hsieh MH, Grantham EC, Liu B, *et al*. In utero exposure to benzophenone-2 causes hypospadias through an estrogen receptor dependent mechanism. *J Urol* 2007; **178**: 1637–42.

[157] Agras K, Shiroyanagi Y, Baskin LS. Progesterone receptors in the developing genital tubercle: Implications for the endocrine disruptor hypothesis as the etiology of hypospadias. *J Urol* 2007; **178**: 722–7.

[158] Zimmermann S, Steding G, Emmen JM, *et al*. Targeted disruption of the Insl3 gene causes bilateral cryptorchidism. *Mol Endocrinol* 1999; **13**: 681–91.

[159] Nef S, Parada LF. Cryptorchidism in mice mutant for Insl3. *Nat Genet* 1999; **22**: 295–9.

[160] Nuti F, Marinari E, Erdei E, *et al*. The leucine-rich repeat-containing G protein-coupled receptor 8 gene T222P mutation does not cause cryptorchidism. *J Clin Endocrinol Metab* 2008; **93**: 1072–6.

[161] Tomboc M, Lee PA, Mitwally MF, Schneck FX, Bellinger M, Witchel SF. Insulin-like 3/relaxin-like factor gene mutations are associated with cryptorchidism. *J Clin Endocrinol Metab* 2000; **85**: 4013–18.

[162] Marin P, Ferlin A, Moro E, Garolla A, Foresta C. Different insulin-like 3 (INSL3) gene mutations not associated with human cryptorchidism. *J Endocrinol Invest* 2001; **24**: RC13–15.

[163] Marin P, Ferlin A, Moro E, *et al*. Novel insulin-like 3 (INSL3) gene mutation associated with human cryptorchidism. *Am J Med Genet* 2001; **103**: 348–9.

[164] Baker LA, Nef S, Nguyen MT, *et al*. The insulin-3 gene: Lack of a genetic basis for human cryptorchidism. *J Urol* 2002; **167**: 2534–7.

[165] Bogatcheva NV, Agoulnik AI. INSL3/LGR8 role in testicular descent and cryptorchidism. *Reprod Biomed Online* 2005; **10**: 49–54.

[166] Bogatcheva NV, Truong A, Feng S, *et al*. GREAT/LGR8 is the only receptor for insulin-like 3 peptide. *Mol Endocrinol* 2003; **17**: 2639–46.

[167] Gorlov IP, Kamat A, Bogatcheva NV, *et al*. Mutations of the GREAT gene cause cryptorchidism. *Hum Mol Genet* 2002; **11**: 2309–18.

[168] Ferlin A, Simonato M, Bartoloni L, *et al*. The INSL3-LGR8/GREAT ligand–receptor pair in human cryptorchidism. *J Clin Endocrinol Metab* 2003; **88**: 4273–9.

[169] Canto P, Escudero I, Soderlund D, *et al*. A novel mutation of the insulin-like 3 gene in patients with cryptorchidism. *J Hum Genet* 2003; **48**: 86–90.

[170] Toppari J, Virtanen H, Skakkebaek NE, Main KM. Environmental effects on hormonal regulation of testicular descent. *J Steroid Biochem Mol Biol* 2006; **102**: 184–6.

[171] Grangeia A, Niel F, Carvalho F, et al. Characterization of cystic fibrosis conductance transmembrane regulator gene mutations and IVS8 poly(T) variants in Portuguese patients with congenital absence of the vas deferens. Hum Reprod 2004; 19: 2502–8.

[172] Ferlin A, Raicu F, Gatta V, Zuccarello D, Palka G, Foresta C. Male infertility: role of genetic background. Reprod Biomed Online 2007; 14: 734–45.

[173] McCallum T, Milunsky J, Munarriz R, et al. Unilateral renal agenesis associated with congenital bilateral absence of the vas deferens: Phenotypic findings and genetic considerations. Hum Reprod 2001; 16: 282–8.

[174] Southern KW. Cystic fibrosis and formes frustes of CFTR-related disease. Respiration 2007; 74: 241–51.

[175] Kuligowska E, Baker CE, Oates RD. Male infertility: role of transrectal US in diagnosis and management. Radiology 1992; 185: 353–60.

[176] Oates RD, Amos JA. The genetic basis of congenital bilateral absence of the vas deferens and cystic fibrosis. J Androl 1994; 15: 1–8.

[177] Colin AA, Sawyer SM, Mickle JE, et al. Pulmonary function and clinical observations in men with congenital bilateral absence of the vas deferens. Chest 1996; 110: 440–5.

[178] Strausbaugh SD, Davis PB. Cystic fibrosis: a review of epidemiology and pathobiology. Clin Chest Med 2007; 28: 279–88.

[179] Dayangac D, Erdem H, Yilmaz E, et al. Mutations of the CFTR gene in Turkish patients with congenital bilateral absence of the vas deferens. Hum Reprod 2004; 19: 1094–100.

[180] Sakamoto H, Yajima T, Suzuki K, Ogawa Y. Cystic fibrosis transmembrane conductance regulator (CFTR) gene mutation associated with a congenital bilateral absence of vas deferens. Int J Urol 2008; 15: 270–1.

[181] Wilschanski M, Dupuis A, Ellis L, et al. Mutations in the cystic fibrosis transmembrane regulator gene and in vivo transepithelial potentials. Am J Respir Crit Care Med 2006; 174: 787–94.

[182] McCallum TJ, Milunsky JM, Cunningham DL, et al. Fertility in men with cystic fibrosis: An update on current surgical practices and outcomes. Chest 2000; 118: 1059–62.

[183] Samli H, Samli MM, Yilmaz E, Imirzalioglu N. Clinical, andrological and genetic characteristics of patients with congenital bilateral absence of vas deferens (CBAVD). Arch Androl 2006; 52: 471–7.

[184] Boyle MP. Adult cystic fibrosis. JAMA 2007; 298: 1787–93.

[185] Rutherford AJ. Male infertility and cystic fibrosis. J R Soc Med 2007; 100 (Suppl 47): 29–34.

[186] Uzun S, Gokce S, Wagner K. Cystic fibrosis transmembrane conductance regulator gene mutations in infertile males with congenital bilateral absence of the vas deferens. Tohoku J Exp Med 2005; 207: 279–85.

[187] Lebo RV, Grody WW. Variable penetrance and expressivity of the splice altering 5T sequence in the cystic fibrosis gene. Genet Test 2007; 11: 32–44.

[188] Claustres M. Molecular pathology of the CFTR locus in male infertility. Reprod Biomed Online 2005; 10: 14–41.

[189] Committee Abpp. Report on evaluation of the azoospermic male. Fertil Steril 2006; 86 (5 Suppl): S210–15.

[190] Keymolen K, Goossens V, De Rycke M, et al. Clinical outcome of preimplantation genetic diagnosis for cystic fibrosis: the Brussels' experience. Eur J Hum Genet 2007; 15: 752–8.

[191] Oates RD, Lobel SA, Harris DH, et al. Efficacy of intracytoplasmic sperm injection using intentionally cryopreserved epididymal spermatozoa. Hum Reprod 1996; 11: 133–8.

[192] Phillipson GT, Petrucco OM, Matthews CD. Congenital bilateral absence of the vas deferens, cystic fibrosis mutation analysis and intracytoplasmic sperm injection. Hum Reprod 2000; 15: 431–5.

[193] George FW, Wilson JD. Embryology of the genital tract. In: Walsh PC, Retik AB, Stamey TA, Vaughan ED, eds. Campbell's Urology, 6th edn. Philadelphia, PA: Saunders, 1992: Vol. 2, 1496–508.

[194] Mickle J, Milunsky A, Amos JA, Oates RD. Congenital unilateral absence of the vas deferens: a heterogeneous disorder with two distinct subpopulations based upon aetiology and mutational status of the cystic fibrosis gene. Hum Reprod 1995; 10: 1728–35.

[195] Behringer RR, Finegold MJ, Cate RL. Mullerian-inhibiting substance function during mammalian sexual development. Cell 1994; 79: 415–25.

[196] Behringer RR. The in vivo roles of mullerian-inhibiting substance. Curr Top Dev Biol 1994; 29: 171–87.

[197] Mishina Y, Rey R, Finegold MJ, et al. Genetic analysis of the Mullerian-inhibiting substance signal transduction pathway in mammalian sexual differentiation. Genes Dev 1996; 10: 2577–87.

[198] Murray PJ, Thomas K, Mulgrew CJ, et al. Whole gene deletion of the hepatocyte nuclear factor-1β gene in a patient with the prune-belly syndrome. Nephrol Dial Transplant 2008; 23: 2412–15.

[199] Guillen DR, Lowichik A, Schneider NR, et al. Prune-belly syndrome and other anomalies in a stillborn fetus with a ring X chromosome lacking XIST. Am J Med Genet 1997; 70: 32–6.

[200] Ramos FJ, Donald-McGinn DM, Emanuel BS, Zackai EH. Tricho-rhino-phalangeal syndrome type II (Langer-Giedion) with persistent cloaca and prune belly sequence in a girl with 8q interstitial deletion. *Am J Med Genet* 1992; **44**: 790–4.

[201] Donnenfeld AE, Conard KA, Roberts NS, Borns PF, Zackai EH. Melnick–Needles syndrome in males: a lethal multiple congenital anomalies syndrome. *Am J Med Genet* 1987; **27**: 159–73.

[202] Young D. Surgical treatment of male infertility. *J Reprod Fertil* 1970; **23**: 541–2.

[203] Handelsman DJ, Conway AJ, Boylan LM, Turtle JR. Young's syndrome: obstructive azoospermia and chronic sinopulmonary infections. *N Engl J Med* 1984; **310**: 3–9.

[204] Seminara SB, Oliveira LM, Beranova M, Hayes FJ, Crowley WF. Genetics of hypogonadotropic hypogonadism. *J Endocrinol Invest* 2000; **23**: 560–5.

[205] Tsai PS, Gill JC. Mechanisms of disease: insights into X-linked and autosomal-dominant Kallmann syndrome. *Nat Clin Pract Endocrinol Metab* 2006; **2**: 160–71.

[206] Hershkovitz E, Loewenthal N, Peretz A, Parvari R. Testicular expressed genes are missing in familial X-linked Kallmann syndrome due to two large different deletions in daughter's X chromosomes. *Horm Res* 2008; **69**: 276–83.

[207] Leroy C, Fouveaut C, Leclercq S, et al. Biallelic mutations in the prokineticin-2 gene in two sporadic cases of Kallmann syndrome. *Eur J Hum Genet* 2008; **16**: 865–8.

[208] Sigman M. Assisted reproductive technics for the treatment of male factor infertility. *R I Med J* 1991; **74**: 591–6.

[209] Raivio T, Falardeau J, Dwyer A, et al. Reversal of idiopathic hypogonadotropic hypogonadism. *N Engl J Med* 2007; **357**: 863–73.

[210] Burris TP, Guo W, McCabe ER. The gene responsible for adrenal hypoplasia congenita, DAX-1, encodes a nuclear hormone receptor that defines a new class within the superfamily. *Recent Prog Horm Res* 1996; **51** : 241–59.

[211] Bedecarrats GY, Kaiser UB. Mutations in the human gonadotropin-releasing hormone receptor: insights into receptor biology and function. *Semin Reprod Med* 2007; **25**: 368–78.

[212] Miura K, Acierno JS, Seminara SB. Characterization of the human nasal embryonic LHRH factor gene, NELF, and a mutation screening among 65 patients with idiopathic hypogonadotropic hypogonadism (IHH). *J Hum Genet* 2004; **49**: 265–8.

[213] Seminara SB. Kisspeptin in reproduction. *Semin Reprod Med* 2007; **25**: 337–43.

[214] Teles MG, Bianco SD, Brito VN, et al. A GPR54-activating mutation in a patient with central precocious puberty. *N Engl J Med* 2008; **358**: 709–15.

[215] Jackson RS, Creemers JW, Ohagi S, et al. Obesity and impaired prohormone processing associated with mutations in the human prohormone convertase 1 gene. *Nat Genet* 1997; **16**: 303–6.

[216] Crino A, Di Giorgio G, Schiaffini R, et al. Central precocious puberty and growth hormone deficiency in a boy with Prader–Willi syndrome. *Eur J Pediatr* 2008; **167**: 1455–8.

[217] Smeets DF, Hamel BC, Nelen MR, et al. Prader–Willi syndrome and Angelman syndrome in cousins from a family with a translocation between chromosomes 6 and 15. *N Engl J Med* 1992; **326**: 807–11.

[218] Burman P, Ritzen EM, Lindgren AC. Endocrine dysfunction in Prader–Willi syndrome: a review with special reference to GH. *Endocr Rev* 2001; **22**: 787–99.

[219] Huhtaniemi I. The Parkes lecture. Mutations of gonadotrophin and gonadotrophin receptor genes: what do they teach us about reproductive physiology? *J Reprod Fertil* 2000; **119**: 173–86.

[220] Layman LC, Porto AL, Xie J, et al. FSH beta gene mutations in a female with partial breast development and a male sibling with normal puberty and azoospermia. *J Clin Endocrinol Metab* 2002; **87**: 3702–7.

[221] Lei ZM, Mishra S, Zou W, et al. Targeted disruption of luteinizing hormone/human chorionic gonadotropin receptor gene. *Mol Endocrinol* 2001; **15**: 184–200.

[222] Wu SM, Hallermeier KM, Laue L, et al. Inactivation of the luteinizing hormone/chorionic gonadotropin receptor by an insertional mutation in Leydig cell hypoplasia. *Mol Endocrinol* 1998; **12**: 1651–60.

[223] Wu RH, Rosenfeld R, Fukushima D. Hypogonadism and Leydig cell hypoplasia unresponsive to human luteinizing hormone (hLH). *Am J Med Sci* 1984; **287**: 23–5.

[224] Gromoll J, Simoni M, Nordhoff V, et al. Functional and clinical consequences of mutations in the FSH receptor. *Mol Cell Endocrinol* 1996; **125**: 177–82.

[225] Song GJ, Park YS, Lee HS, et al. Mutation screening of the FSH receptor gene in infertile men. *Mol Cells* 2001; **12**: 292–7.

[226] Dam AH, Koscinski I, Kremer JA, et al. Homozygous mutation in SPATA16 is associated with male infertility in human globozoospermia. *Am J Hum Genet* 2007; **81**: 813–20.

[227] Christensen GL, Ivanov IP, Atkins JF, Campbell B, Carrell DT. Identification of polymorphisms in the Hrb, GOPC, and Csnk2a2 genes in two men with globozoospermia. *J Androl* 2006; **27**: 11–15.

[228] Suzuki-Toyota F, Ito C, Toyama Y, *et al*. The coiled tail of the round-headed spermatozoa appears during epididymal passage in GOPC-deficient mice. *Arch Histol Cytol* 2004; **67**: 361–71.

[229] Ito C, Suzuki-Toyota F, Maekawa M, *et al*. Failure to assemble the peri-nuclear structures in GOPC deficient spermatids as found in round-headed spermatozoa. *Arch Histol Cytol* 2004; **67**: 349–60.

[230] Yao R, Ito C, Natsume Y, *et al*. Lack of acrosome formation in mice lacking a Golgi protein, GOPC. *Proc Natl Acad Sci U S A* 2002; **99**: 11211–16.

[231] Xu X, Toselli PA, Russell LD, Seldin DC. Globozoospermia in mice lacking the casein kinase II α' catalytic subunit. *Nat Genet* 1999; **23**: 118–21.

[232] Zuccarello D, Ferlin A, Cazzadore C, *et al*. Mutations in dynein genes in patients affected by isolated non-syndromic asthenozoospermia. *Hum Reprod* 2008 **23**: 1957–62.

[233] Zuccarello D, Ferlin A, Garolla A, *et al*. A possible association of a human tektin-t gene mutation (A229V) with isolated non-syndromic asthenozoospermia: Case report. *Hum Reprod* 2008; **23**: 996–1001.

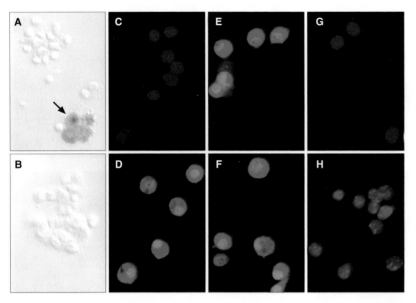

Fig. 3.3. Characteristics of stem Leydig cells (SLCs). Freshly isolated SLCs contaminated by fetal Leydig cells (FLCs) are shown in panel A with a cluster of FLCs stained strongly for 3β-HSD (arrow). After negative immunoselection to eliminate LHR-positive cells and positive selection of PDGFRα-expressing cells, none of the cells stained for 3β-HSD (Panel B). LHR[neg] PDGFRα[pos] SLCs did not stain for 3β-HSD (C) or LHR (G). They were, however, positively stained for PDGFRα (D), c-kit (E), LIFR (F), and GATA4 (H). DAPI staining (blue) was used to provide nuclear contrast. (From Ge RS, *et al*. In search of rat stem Leydig cells: identification, isolation, and lineage-specific development. *Proc Natl Acad Sci U S A* 2006; **103**: 2719–24, with permission of the publisher.)

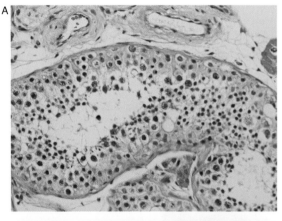

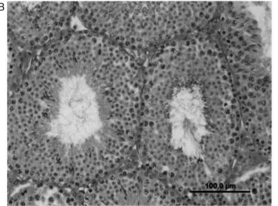

Fig. 4.2. Light microscope images of sections of the (A) human and (B) rodent testis. Hematoxylin and eosin staining (× 40).

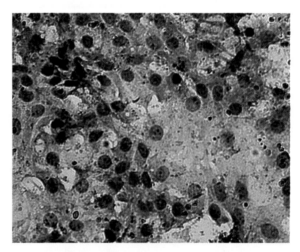

Fig. 4.3. Light microscope images of mouse Sertoli cells in culture 5 days post harvest. DAPI staining (× 40).

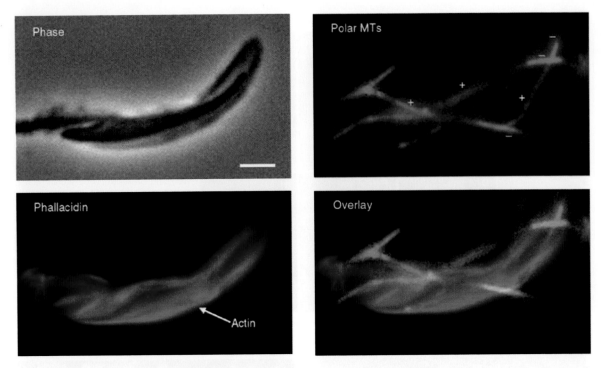

Fig. 4.10. Phase-contrast image of polarity-marked microtubules bound to ectoplasmic specializations. Overlay images of actin (to show the presence of the ectoplasmic specialization) and the polarity-marked microtubules attached to the junction plaque as well as an overlay of the polar microtubules on the ectoplasmic specialization. Actin = red, polar microtubules = green. Bar = 2.5 μm. (Reprinted with permission from Guttman JA *et al.* Dynein and plus-end microtubule-dependent motors are associated with specialized Sertoli cell junction plaques (ectoplasmic specializations). *J Cell Sci* 2000; **113**: 2167–76.)

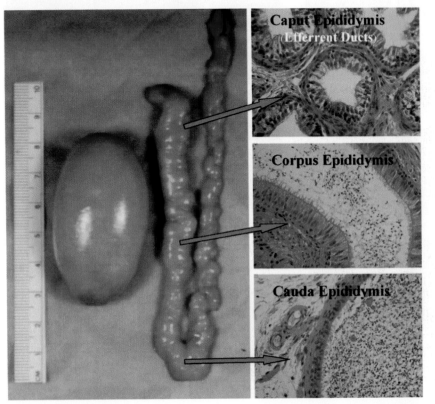

Fig. 6.3. The histology of the adult human epididymis. Much of the caput epididymidis is actually efferent duct tubule, of which there are several leading to the single true epididymal tubule. Based on histological appearance, there are six types of ciliated efferent duct tubule [13], of which only type 2 is illustrated. In the midcorpus region there is a single, highly coiled epididymal tubule with a tall, columnar, stereociliated epithelium. Sperm concentration is increasing in the epididymal lumen. In the cauda epididymidis, a short, stereociliated epithelium surrounds the large tubule lumen full of densely packed spermatozoa.

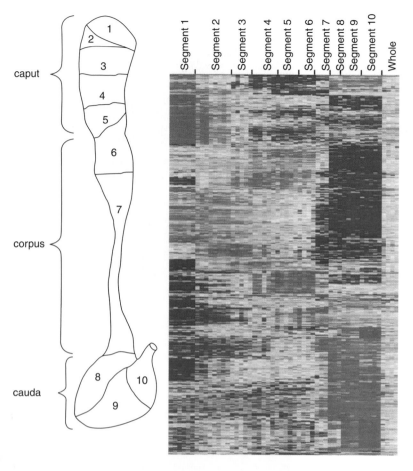

Segment 1 | Segment 2 | Segment 3 | Segment 4 | Segment 5 | Segment 6 | Segment 7 | Segment 8 | Segment 9 | Segment 10 | Whole

caput

corpus

cauda

1
2
3
4
5
6
7
8 9 10

Fig. 6.5. Illustration of the segments of the mouse epididymis and gene expression patterns in each segment. Left: schematic of segmentation; segments consist of lobules of coiled tubule separated by connective tissue septa. Right: heat map of the 1100 most highly regulated genes in the different epididymal segments as determined by microarray analysis of gene expression in each segment [34]. Colors indicate relative expression level: red, high; white, moderate; blue, low. Results from multiple microarray analyses (3–6) of each segment are displayed. These results indicate that individual segments or groups of contiguous segments can be unique in their gene expression profiles, which implies a functional difference between those segments.

Fig. 8.1 (below) The developmental stages of meiotic prophase I demonstrated by antibody immunofluorescence. Within these spermatocytes, antisera were directed against SCP3 (synaptonemal complex protein 3; SCs, red), MLH1 (Mut-L homolog 1; MLH1 foci, yellow), and CREST antigens (centromeres, blue). Cells are in the following stages of meiotic prophase: (A) leptotene; (B) early zygotene; (C) late zygotene; (D) early pachytene, with arrowhead indicating the sex chromosomes (X and Y); (E) late pachytene, with arrowhead indicating the desynapsed sex chromosomes; and (F) diplotene. Magnification × 1000. (From Gonsalves J *et al.* Defective recombination in infertile men. *Hum Mol Genet* 2004, **13**: 2875–83, by permission of Oxford University Press.)

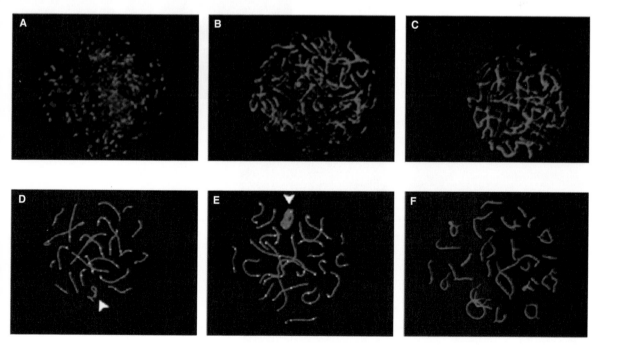

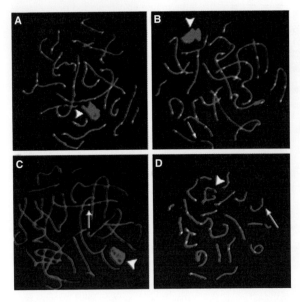

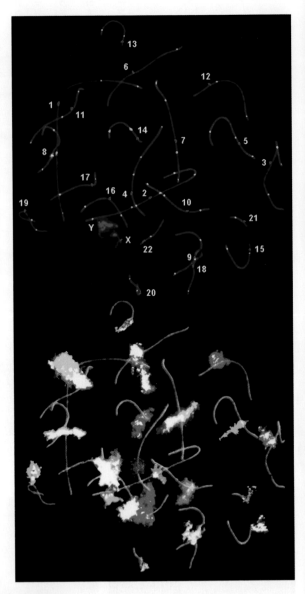

Fig. 8.2. Pachytene spermatocytes from men in (A) control, (B) obstructive and (C & D) nonobstructive azoospermia groups. (SCs, red; MLH1 foci, yellow; centromeres, blue). The sex chromosomes are indicated (arrowheads in A–D). There are several areas of faulty recombination noted: the arrow in (B) indicates a chromosomal bivalent with incomplete synapsis; the arrow in (C) indicates one of only a few SCs in this spermatocyte with any MLH1 foci; the arrow in (D) indicates a bivalent with no MLH1 foci in the SC. Magnification × 1000. (From Gonsalves J *et al.* Defective recombination in infertile men. *Hum Mol Genet* 2004, **13**: 2875–83, by permission of Oxford University Press.)

Fig. 8.3 (right) (Upper) Human pachytene spermatocyte with SCs shown in red, centromeres in blue, and MLH1 foci in yellow. (Lower) Subsequent cenM-FISH analysis allows identification of individual chromosomes so that recombination (MLH1) foci can be analyzed for each SC on each chromosome. (From Sun F *et al.* Variation in MLH1 distribution in recombination maps for individual chromosomes from human males. *Hum Mol Genet* 2006; **15**: 2376–91, by permission of Oxford University Press.)

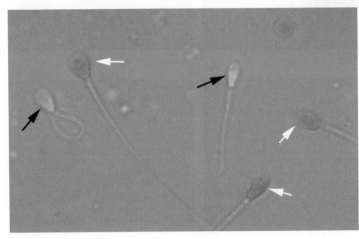

Fig. 11.1. Sperm viability stain with eosin Y. Live sperm do not take up the stain (dark arrows) while nonviable sperm stain orange-yellow (white arrows).

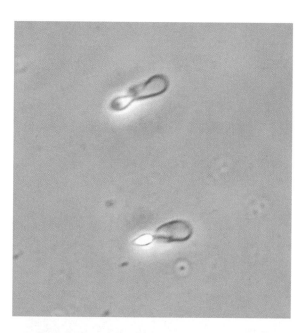

Fig. 11.2. Hypo-osmotic swelling test. Viable sperm demonstrate tail swelling, which appears as coiled tails.

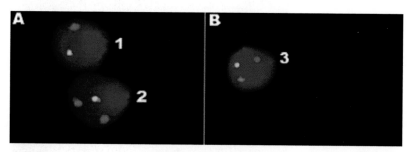

Fig. 11.3. Images of three human sperm nuclei hybridized with chromosome-specific probes (chromosome X labeled in yellow, Y in green, and 21 in red). Sperm #1 is a normal X-bearing sperm (with a single chromosome X and a single chromosome 21 signal), sperm #2 is an autosomal disomic sperm (i.e., X,21,21) and sperm #3 is a sex chromosome disomic sperm (X,Y,21).

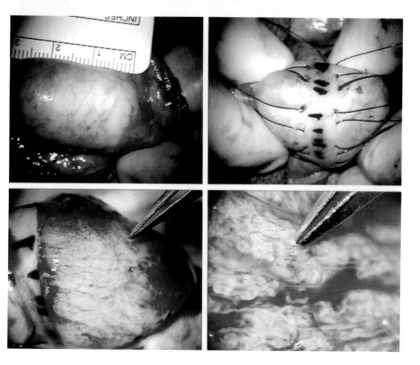

Fig. 13.1. Images from microdissection TESE (testicular sperm extraction). *Top left:* testis delivered into field, ruler for scale. *Top right:* preparation for incision in tunica albuginea; holding stitches of 5–0 chromic placed in tunica; horizontal incision marked. *Bottom left:* incision in tunica albuginea made, testis bivalved. *Bottom right:* image of same field through operative microscope ($\times$ 25), demonstrating tubules for extraction.

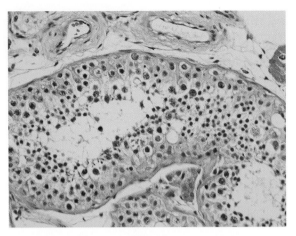

Fig. 13.2. Light-microscope image of a section of the human testis (× 200). Hematoxylin and eosin (H&E) staining.

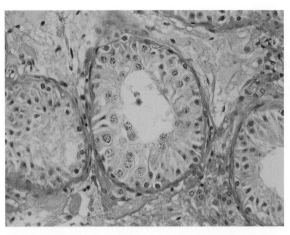

Fig. 13.5. Early maturation arrest at the level of the primary spermatocyte (× 500). Hematoxylin and eosin (H&E) staining.

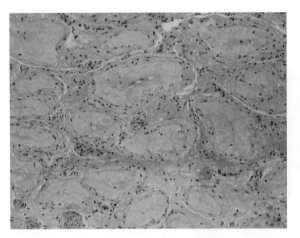

Fig. 13.3. Basement membrane hyalinization with associated peritubular fibrosis (× 200). Hematoxylin and eosin (H&E) staining.

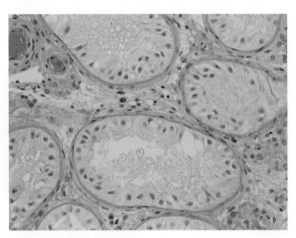

Fig. 13.6. Sertoli-cell-only or germinal cell aplasia. Empty tubules with the exception of Sertoli cells with characteristic round nucleus and tripartite nucleolus (× 500). Hematoxylin and eosin (H&E) staining.

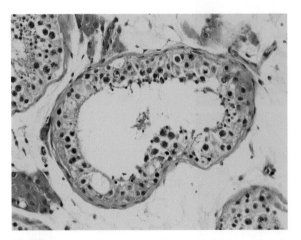

Fig. 13.4. Hypospermatogenesis. Decreased numbers of germ cells, with only some elongate spermatids noted (× 500). Hematoxylin and eosin (H&E) staining.

Centrosome Disposition vs. Meiotic Spindle Assembly

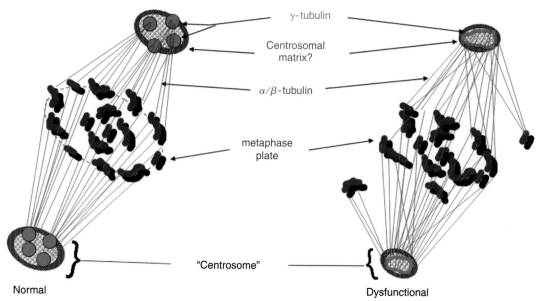

γ-tubulin

Centrosomal matrix?

α/β-tubulin

metaphase plate

"Centrosome"

Normal   Dysfunctional

Fig. 19.5 (above) Schematic representation of the meiotic spindle in normal younger (left) and older (right) preovulatory oocyte. In the normal spindle, the microtubule nucleating centers in each centrosome are distinct, and there are multiple sites per spindle pole. In the aneuploid conditions, the nucleating centers are indistinct, almost ring-like. It is speculated that the capture of chromosomes may be abnormal due to this condition, leading to an increased propensity to aneuploidy. (From Battaglia D *et al*. Changes in centrosomal domains during meiotic maturation in the human oocyte. *Mol Hum Reprod* 1997; **2**: 845–51.)

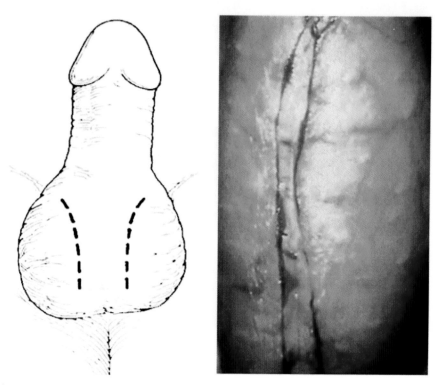

Fig. 22.1. Vertical hemiscrotal incision used for delivery of the testicle.

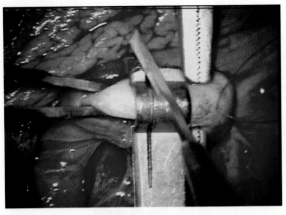

Fig. 22.2. Dividing the vas deferens, using a nerve holder for stabilization.

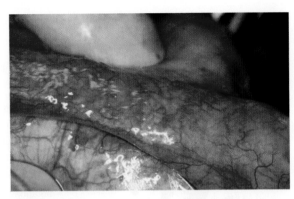

Fig. 22.5. Dilated epididymal tubules visualized under the operating microscope.

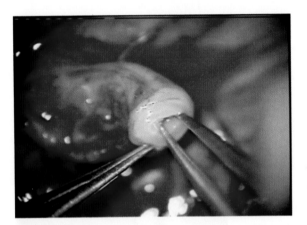

Fig. 22.3. Gentle dilation of the testicular end of the vas deferens.

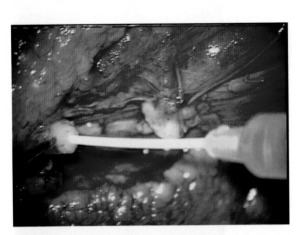

Fig. 22.4. Vasal sperm aspiration using an angiocatheter and syringe.

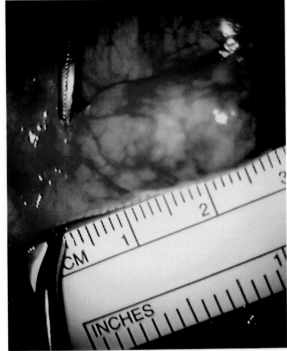

Fig. 22.6. Hypoplastic epididymis in patient with CBAVD.

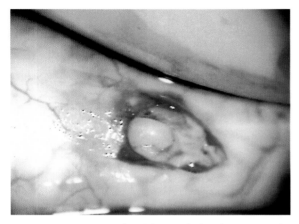

Fig. 22.7. Appearance of epididymal tubules after opening the tunica of the epididymis.

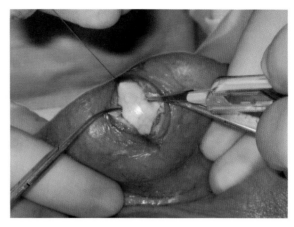

Fig. 22.10. Testicle is stabilized using a holding suture. An opening is made in the tunica albuginea. The holding suture may then be used to close the tunica albuginea.

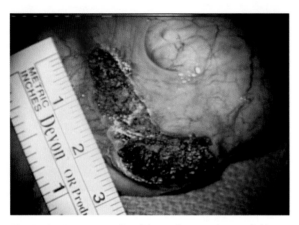

Fig. 22.8. Appearance of epididymis after completion of obliterative MESA.

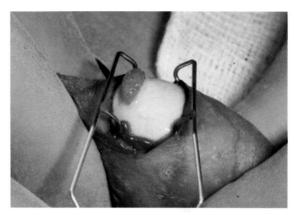

Fig. 22.11. Eyelid retractor can be used as a self-retaining retractor. Seminiferous tubules are easily extruded using light manual pressure.

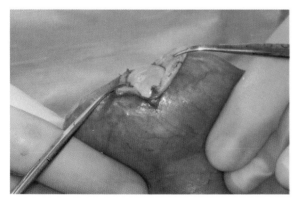

Fig. 22.9. Small transverse incision used to access the testis for testicular sperm retrieval.

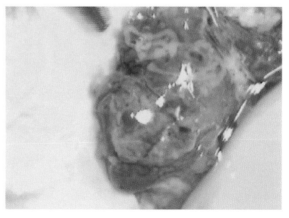

Fig. 22.13. Appearance of dissected testicular tissue during microdissection TESE with prominent seminiferous tubules containing sperm. (Courtesy of Peter N. Schlegel MD.)

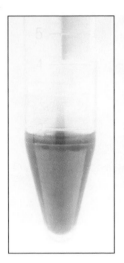

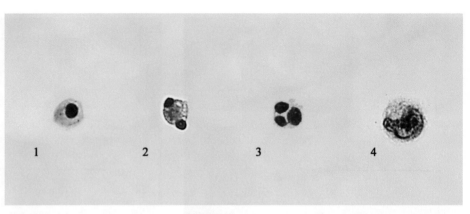

Fig. 33.1. Comparison of leukocytes and sperm precursors: (1) spermatocyte; (2) spermatid; (3) polymorphonuclear leukocyte (PMN) – note nuclear bridges; (4) monocyte – note large U-shaped nucleus, foamy cytoplasm.

Fig.26.9. Twenty-seven percent of men with SCI have brown-colored semen. The brown color is not related to semen stasis from infrequency of ejaculation.

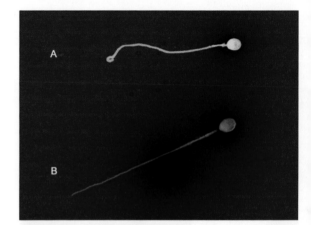

Fig. 33.5. Sperm viability using eosin–nigrosin staining: (A) live (white) cell – excludes the stain; (B) dead (pink) cell – takes up the stain.

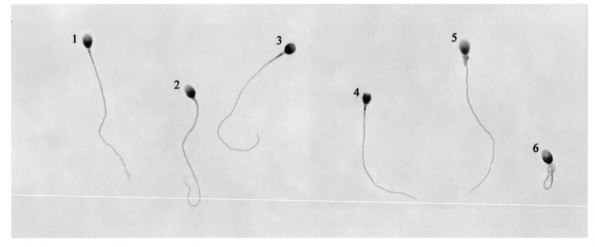

Fig. 33.7. Examples of normal and abnormal sperm: (1) normal sperm; (2) normal sperm; (3) borderline abnormal head (normal for WHO 3rd, abnormal for strict/WHO 4th); (4) abnormal head (small, small acrosome, irregular), normal midpiece and tail; (5) abnormal midpiece (thick), normal head and tail; (5) abnormal tail (coiled), normal head and midpiece.

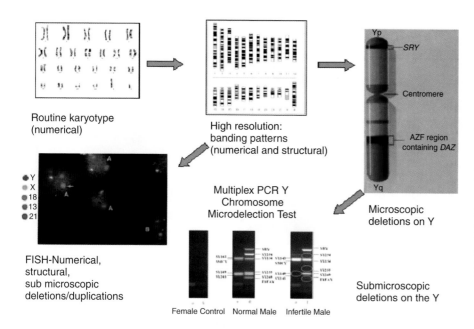

Fig. 41.1. Genetic advances and the diagnosis of male infertility. The routine karyotype first provided information concerning numerical defects of chromosomes, and later technological advances allowed large translocations, insertions, and deletions to be observed as well. The development of polymerase chain reaction (PCR), the sequencing of the human genome, and fluorescence in-situ hybridization (FISH) has permitted previously unrecognized genetic causes of male infertility to be realized. With each new technological advance our ability to diagnose genetic causes of male infertility has improved.

Routine karyotype
(numerical)

High resolution:
banding patterns
(numerical and structural)

Microscopic
deletions on Y

FISH-Numerical,
structural,
sub microscopic
deletions/duplications

Multiplex PCR Y
Chromosome
Microdelection Test

Female Control   Normal Male   Infertile Male

Submicroscopic
deletions on the Y

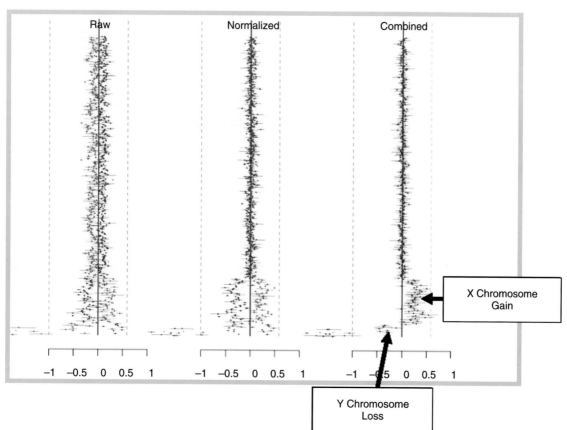

Fig. 41.2. Demonstration of the principles of chromosome microarray analysis. A region of chromosome gain is shown in blue and a loss in red, with the normal regions shown in green. Depicted is a schematic diagram of the data showing that female DNA stained red and male DNA stained green was competitively hybridized to a DNA assay of oligonucleotides spanning specific regions of each human chromosome, including the Y chromosome. The figure shows that the female DNA lacked the Y chromosome (as expected) but had a duplication of the X chromosome, as it should because the DNA is from a female.

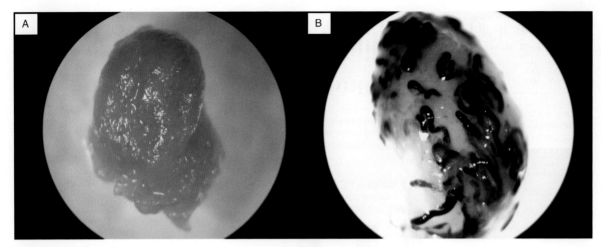

Fig. 41.3. Spermatogonial stem cell transplantation into Sertoli-cell-only histology mouse recipient testis. Spermatogonial stem cells from cryptorchid Rosa26 mouse testis expressing the *LacZ* transgene were enriched based upon exclusion of rhodamine dye and flow cytometry to select the cells that excluded the rhodamine dye. These cells were transplanted by microinjection via the efferent ducts and backwashing the testis of a TAF4b-deficient mouse with a Sertoli-cell-only histology. The cells engrafted, colonized the seminiferous tubules, and spermatogenesis was restored. (A) a noninjected control TAF4b-deficient testis; (B) a TAF4b testis four months after transplantation of the Rosa26 spermatogonial stem cells. The cell fate of the transplanted cells within the recipient seminiferous tubules is evident by the blue staining demonstrating the presence of the *LacZ* transgene [68].

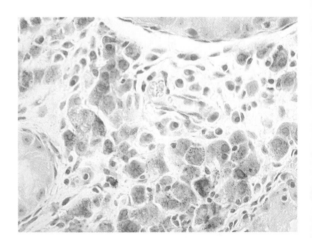

Fig. 41.4. Successful engraftment and colonization of transplanted Leydig cell progenitors into the interstitial space. Adult Leydig stem cell progenitors from the testis of Rosa26 male mice expressing the *LacZ* transgene were enriched by flow cytometry based upon exclusion of Hoechst 33342 dye and transplanted into a Wv mouse testis. The testicular section is stained to show the expression of the β-galactosidase transgene (blue) and counterstained with hematoxylin and eosin (pink) as described by Lo *et al.* [67].

Chapter 16

Immunologic infertility

Thomas J. Walsh and Paul J. Turek

Introduction

A basic understanding of immunity dates to ancient Greece, when King Mithridates VI, in an effort to avoid assassination, attempted to "vaccinate" himself against lethal poisons by consuming small amounts of the same [1]. Intellectual interest in the immune system was generated by Dr. Peter Medawar, who won the Nobel Prize in 1960 for his description of immune tolerance [2].The presence of autoantibodies to sperm was first described by Rumke in 1953, when it was hypothesized that antibodies could be a potential cause of infertility and abnormal semen parameters [3].

Today, although our understanding of the human immune system and its interplay with states of fertility has greatly improved, many questions remain unanswered. **Immunity to male sperm is unique among potential causes of infertility, as it may be generated by either partner, yet culminates in the same result: the impediment or destruction of sperm, or impaired oocyte fertilization.** This chapter summarizes normal immune function and its relationship to immunologic infertility. We begin with an overview of immune system components and include a description of the humoral and cellular arms of immunity as well as other mediators of immunity. We discuss the initiation of an immune response to sperm, and how this response is diagnosed and quantified. Finally, we review treatments available to immunologically infertile men.

Normal immune system function

The normal immune system identifies and destroys "foreign" material, or antigen, within the body. To accomplish this complex task, and to serve its important role as a barrier to infection or invasion, the immune system distinguishes "self" from "nonself," maintains a memory of this recognition, and diversifies its response to a changing environment of antigenic

challenges. This elaborate system responds to all antigens encountered during the life of an individual, yet requires only 1–2% of the human genome to function. **The immune response comprises two arms: the cell-mediated response and the antibody-mediated, or "humoral," response** [4]. A problem that has intrigued immunologists for decades is how we achieve immunological "tolerance" or acceptance of self antigens during development. The role of the thymus in controlling self-reactivity is well established. However, in interesting new work in humans and animal models, it has become apparent that **the thymus produces various, nonthymic, organ-specific proteins during development, called "self shadowing," which insures that the immune system does not react to individual body tissues** [5]. **Notably, it appears that a defect in the thymus of even one of those proteins is capable of inducing spontaneous, multiorgan, autoimmune syndromes** [6]. It is through such mechanisms that our immune system naturally learns to differentiate self from nonself. Similarly, failure of these mechanisms can lead to destructive autoimmune syndromes. A simplified overview of immune system structure is outlined in Figure 16.1.

Cell-mediated immunity

Many cells are involved in the generation of a cell-mediated immune response. These include cells that entrap, digest, and present foreign antigens, and those that generate antibodies to modulate the immune response (Table 16.1). Proliferation of immune cells occurs in response to an antigenic challenge. The process typically begins with the phagocytosis and engulfment of foreign material and the presentation of digested antigen by **antigen-presenting cells (APCs)** to the immune system in association with **type II major histocompatability (MHC) proteins** on the cell surface. Alternatively, the APC can be directly

Infertility in the Male, 4th edition, ed. Larry I. Lipshultz, Stuart S. Howards, and Craig S. Niederberger. Published by Cambridge University Press. © Cambridge University Press 2009.

Table 16.1. Cell types and mediators in cell-mediated immunity

Cell Type	Description	Associated factors
Monocyte, macrophage	Effect: phagocytosis, cell lysis, antigen presentation Location/derivation: tissue	Interleukin (IL)-1, tumor necrosis factor (TNF), lysozyme, prostaglandins (PG), complement, oxidative products
Neutrophil	Effect: migratory, phagocytosis, cell lysis, primary responder in acute inflammation Location/derivation: tissue	Oxidative products, prostaglandin E_2 (PGE$_2$), collagenase, elastase, proteases, histaminase
T lymphocyte	Effect: response to antigens in association with class I & II MHC Multiple subtypes: helper, suppressor, cytotoxic, memory Location/derivation: tissue	ILs 2–6, interferon (IFN)-γ, TNF, serine proteases
B lymphocyte	Effect: antibody production Location/derivation: reside in lymph organs and secretory surfaces/bone marrow	Immunoglobulins (Ig) – all classes
Natural killer (NK) cell	Effect: specific and nonspecific cytotoxicity, antigen presentation Location/derivation: tissue	IL-1, IL-2, colony stimulating factor, IFN-γ, TNF
Mast cell	Effect: fixed IgE binding Location/derivation: fixed in tissue (vasculature, lymph, stroma)	Histamine, serotonin, proteolytic enzymes, chemotactic factors
Basophil	Effect: mobile IgE binding Location/derivation: circulate throughout body	Histamine, serotonin, proteolytic enzymes, chemotactic factors
Eosinophil	Effect: secretory granule release, cytotoxicity, IgE & G binding, complement fixation Location/derivation: sites of increased parasite concentration	Leukotrienes, PGE$_2$, superoxide, phospholipidase, kinases

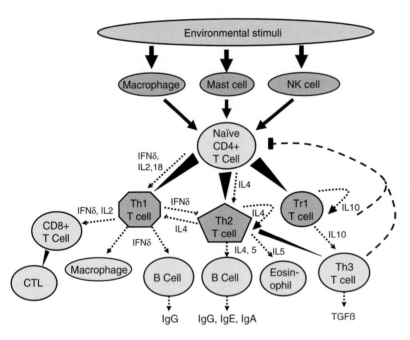

Fig. 16.1. Simplified view of the "bow-tie" architecture of the human immune system. Salient features include the central role of CD4+ T cells, the involvement of many cytokines, and the presence of negative feedback to prevent autoimmunity. In response to stimuli, CD4+ T cells become Th1, Th2, or Tr1 cells depending upon the cytokine profile induced by the stimulus. Th1 cells produce cytotoxic T cells (CTL, cell-mediated immunity) and some B cells, while Th2 cells produce mainly B cells (humoral immunity). Negative feedback is initiated by the Tr1 and Th3 cells. IFN, interferon; IL, interleukin; NK, natural killer.

infected by viruses and certain types of bacteria, which also permit antigen presentation to the immune system. Recognition of this antigen–MHC complex by specific lymphocytes triggers a cascade of events, leading ultimately to both cellular proliferation and release of immune mediators, including cytokines (Fig. 16.1, Table 16.2).

Once identified by the cellular immune system, antigen is eliminated through various pathways.

Direct contact of antigen with certain immune cells can result in immediate destruction; these cells include cytotoxic T cells ("killer T cells"), natural killer cells (NK cells), and macrophages. **Antigen can also be eliminated by antibodies in a process known as antibody-dependent cell-mediated cytotoxicity (ADCC). Lastly, antigen can be coated with antibody or "opsonized" and subsequently destroyed by the complement cascade. In the absence of complement**

Table 16.2. Cytokine type and function

Cytokine	Description	Function
Interferon (IFN)	Alpha, beta, and gamma subtypes; produced by macrophages, neutrophils, and T lymphocytes	Augments killing of virus infected cells, regulates cell surface MHC expression
Interleukins (IL)	IL-1 through IL-12 subtypes; glycoproteins produced by lymphocytes	Promotes immune cell activation and chemoattraction. Growth factors
Tumor necrosis factor (TNF)	Alpha and beta subtypes; produced by lymphocytes and macrophages	Induces tumor cell apoptosis, B lymphocyte activation, antigen induction
Low molecular weight immunomodulators (LMWI)	Thymosins, muramyldipeptides, pyrimidones	Augments lymphocyte killing, induces interferon production, antiviral killing, and tumor cell lysis

MHC, major histocompatiblity complex proteins.

proteins, opsonized antigen is destroyed by the cellular immune system [1,7].

Humoral immunity

Antibodies, also known as immunoglobulins, form the basis for vaccination theory. They are the soluble mediators of immunity. Antibodies are glycoproteins synthesized and secreted by B lymphocytes that have been activated to become plasma cells. Each antibody molecule is composed of two light chains and two heavy chains (Fig. 16.2). Together, these components define the function (Fab region) and type (Fc region) of each antibody. Most antibodies are monomers, with single Fab and Fc regions; IgM, a pentomer, is the exception to this rule. Five different antibody types exist, each with unique functionality and distribution in the body (Table 16.3). Unlike the cellular response, antibody recognition of antigen requires neither cellular digestion nor association of antigen with MHC proteins. As such, **the humoral immune system is suited to the destruction of whole, extracellular antigens, including most bacteria, larger parasites, and viruses.** Similar to the cellular response, antigens are eliminated via multiple pathways after recognition, including through complement, linkage to cellular immunity and phagocytosis, initiation of a mast cell response, local and systemic inflammation (allergic response), and lymphocyte binding and killing.

Although the cellular and humoral systems are described as distinct arms of immunity, these systems make up an intricately intertwined system, and one that is redundant, self-augmenting, and exquisitely specific [8].

Other mediators of immunity

Other secreted factors play key roles in integrating and augmenting the immune response. These **cytokines are non-immunoglobulin effector molecules that are synthesized and secreted by lymphocytes and other immune cells** [9]. Many cytokines exist, with distinct functions that serve to regulate both arms of the immune response to antigen (Fig. 16.1; Table 16.2). **As important mediators of inflammation, they play a distinct role in modulating interactions between the reproductive and immune systems** [7,10].

Regional or mucosal immunity

It is evident that various mucosal tissues within the body contain their own localized or regional immune systems. These local immune systems may function separately from systemic immunity, as demonstrated in Figure 16.3. They are characterized by the secretion of immunoglobulin A (IgA) at the mucosal surfaces of the gut, respiratory system, and genitourinary tracts. The concept of **common mucosal immunity stems from the fact that activated lymphocytes from the gut can disseminate immunity to other, distant, mucosal sites, and is the basis for research on orally administered vaccinations** [11]. Since it is not apparent that male immune infertility is associated with a measurable activation of generalized immunity, **the idea of a geographically restricted, mucosal immune system in the reproductive tract is conceptually attractive.** This is supported by the fact that antisperm antibodies are often present on sperm but not in serum of men with immune infertility. The sites of origin of mucosal immunity within the genitourinary tract are still undefined [12].

Testicular immunology

It is important to understand how the immune system functions in the male genital tract, as **the testes are unique and considered an immunologically**

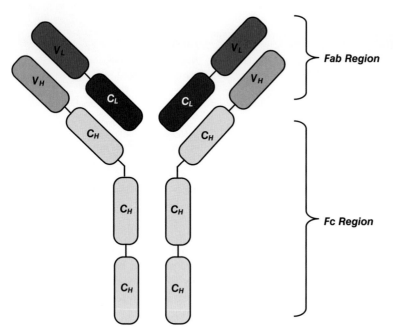

Fig. 16.2. Antibody anatomy. Each antibody molecule consists of variable light chain (V_L), constant light chain (C_L), variable heavy chain (V_H), and constant heavy chain (C_H) structures. These chains are further grouped into Fab and Fc regions. Antibody "type" is determined by the Fc region, and antibody binding "specificity" to antigen is determined by the Fab region.

Table 16.3. Antibody type, distribution, and function

Antibody type	Prevalence	Description	Function and location
IgG	75% of antibodies	Monomer form	Secondary humoral response
IgA	15% of antibodies	Monomer or dimer forms	Primary antibody in secretions
IgM	10% of antibodies	Pentomer forms	Primary humoral response, complement fixation
IgE	0.3% of antibodies	Monomer form	Induction of allergic response
IgD	0.003% of antibodies	Monomer form	Soluble humoral immunity, function unclear

"privileged" site in the body. Immune reactions easily induced in other organ systems appear to be qualitatively different (decreased) in the testis [13]. This is likely related to the unique way in which the immune system views sperm. **The immune system develops tolerance to self antigens during embryologic development**, well before the initiation of spermatogenesis [2]. At puberty, meiosis begins in the testis with synchronized waves of sperm production. **As germ cells take a haploid form, new cell-surface antigens are expressed that are novel to the immune system** [1]. As a result, mature spermatozoa appear "foreign" to the immune system. Despite the novelty of sperm proteins, it is surprising that autoimmunity to sperm does not occur more often than observed in the adult male [14].

How is this immunological "sanctuary" maintained? Electron microscopic and immunohistochemical studies have shown lymphocytes and macrophages in the spaces between seminiferous tubules, but not

within the tubules. This has led to the hypothesis that a **"blood–testis barrier" exists [15,16]. This barrier, more appropriately termed the "blood–seminiferous tubule barrier," has two components: an anatomic, or mechanical, barrier and a functional barrier.** The mechanical barrier is created by muscle-like myoid cells that surround seminiferous tubules and that have been shown in rodent models to exclude large molecules including immunoglobulins [17–20]. **The most important component of this barrier consists of synaptic tight junctions that form between Sertoli cells** [16]. These specialized attachments preclude the passage of large molecules and lymphocytes between cells. The occlusive nature of tight junctions has been confirmed by tracer studies, in which large molecules can access the basal, but not adluminal, compartment of the seminiferous tubule [17,21,22].

But even this mechanical barrier may be insufficient to guard developing spermatozoa [1]. Tight

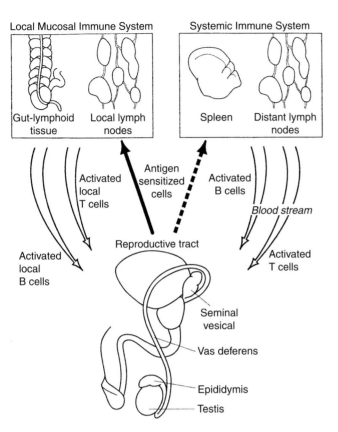

Local Mucosal Immune System

Gut-lymphoid tissue | Local lymph nodes

Systemic Immune System

Spleen | Distant lymph nodes

Activated local T cells

Antigen sensitized cells

Activated B cells

Blood stream

Activated local B cells

Reproductive tract

Activated T cells

Seminal vesical

Vas deferens

Epididymis

Testis

Fig. 16.3. Systemic and mucosal immunity in the reproductive tract. Both local (mucosal) and systemic immune systems may "see" sperm antigens through sensitized antigen-presenting cells. Each immune system then delivers activated T and B lymphocytes that manifest characteristic cellular and antibody responses. The local, mucosal immune response may play the larger role in reproductive tract immunity. (Used with permission from Turek PJ. Infections, immunity and male infertility. *Infert Reprod Clin North Am* 1999; **10**: 1.)

junctions vary in density throughout the reproductive tract. This is best exemplified in the ductuli efferentes, where tight junctions do not surround epithelial cells. The resultant gaps allow large molecules to traverse the germinal epithelium, and gain exposure to the adluminal compartment [23,24]. In guinea pigs, labeled antisperm IgG injected intravascularly has been found bound to sperm in both the rete testis and efferent tubules [19,25]. Thus, **while the mechanical barrier contributes to immune isolation of the testis, other "functional" components must also exist.**

The functional barrier appears to involve suppression of immunoreactivity and down-regulation of the cell-mediated immunity. Three mechanisms likely work in concert to protect sperm from destruction. First, lymphocytes are diverted by the vascular endothelium and are not allowed to accumulate in anatomically vulnerable regions in germinal epithelium [26]. Second, these vulnerable regions harbor mainly T suppressor cells [15,23]. Third, sperm antigens may be improperly presented to lymphocytes, impairing the immune response. This may be due to deficiencies in the association between antigens and the human leukocyte

antigen (HLA) system, or to defects in HLA proteins [23,27]. By these mechanisms immunoreactivity is impaired and the functional barrier is maintained.

Immunologic tolerance may also play a role in the functional testis barrier. Tung and colleagues have proposed that **within the anatomically weaker areas (rete testis, efferent tubule, epididymis) there is a small, continuous leak of sperm antigens** [14]. **This leak generates T suppressor cells and immune tolerance, similar to desensitization protocols for common environmental allergens.** However, with larger antigenic challenges, a true immune response results. In animal models of autoimmune orchitis, the orchitis begins in the rete testes [28,29], suggesting that this area is a site of antigen leak. Since experimental orchitis can also be induced by injecting activated T cells intravascularly, it is apparent that physical barriers need not be breached to allow lymphocyte access to sperm antigens. **Cytokines may also contribute to immune tolerance** [10], **specifically interferon γ, soluble Fc receptor, and transforming growth factor β** [1,30]. Hormones, and in particular androgens, also appear to regulate immunity [31]. Finally, the seminal plasma may provide an immunologically privileged environment for ejaculated sperm within the female genital tract [32–35]. Thus immune tolerance to sperm is complex and likely to involve many immune system components, with overall regulation driven by genetically conferred characteristics [36–40].

Mechanisms of immunologic infertility

Sperm antigenicity

Autoimmunity to the germline takes one of two forms: testis-specific or antispermatogenic [1]. **Testis-specific antigens are those that induce an organ-confined immune response, culminating in orchitis, and exemplified most stereotypically by mumps orchitis.** While not specific to the germinal epithelium or to sperm, this form of autoimmunity may cause severe, generalized inflammation of the testes, with destruction of both interstitial and epithelial components. **Antispermatogenic autoantigens induce autoimmunity to the germinal epithelium, resulting in a specific decline in sperm production due to germ cell destruction.** However, it is still unclear which surface antigens lead to autoimmunity. Interestingly, certain HLA antigens that play a key role in other autoimmune syndromes are demonstrably absent from germ cells.

Using monoclonal antibody technology, many sperm autoantigens have been identified in animal models [41,42]. These cell-surface molecules have important functions, including the regulation of spermatogenesis. Studies of human sperm have corroborated that some of these are autoantigens [32,43]. The **fertilization antigen 1 (FA-1)** is a large surface glycoprotein that may regulate sperm and zona pellucida interaction [44]. Antibodies directed against FA-1 prevent fertilization but do not impair sperm motility [45]. Other theories regarding sperm antigenicity have been proposed, including that men who develop antisperm antibodies may possess more highly immunogenic antigens than men without antisperm antibodies. Clearly, the antigens involved in generating autoimmune infertility are heterogeneous and, as such, have a variable impact on sperm production and function [1].

The study of sperm antigenicity is difficult, and the limitations in our understanding should be addressed. First, much of our current knowledge on this subject is derived from animal models. Caution should be exercised in translating these studies to humans, as not all antigens found in animals are present in humans. Second, it is important to recognize that

"cross-reactivity" may also play a role in autoimmunity, whereby an antibody to a particular molecule could also bind a completely different molecule with the same physical characteristics. Cross-reactivity may cause (a) the false identification of antigens that do not generate an autoimmune response, and (b) the production of antibodies to microorganisms or drugs that inadvertently cross-react with sperm antigens [46]. Another issue is that testis antigenicity is a highly dynamic characteristic. As sperm mature within the germinal epithelium, antigens are gained and lost. So antigens on primary spermatogonia may differ from those on spermatids, and carry different clinical implications [47,48]. Lastly, antisperm antibodies may also recognize internal antigens in addition to cell-surface antigens of sperm that are thought to have little clinical importance [49].

Antibody-mediated sperm autoimmunity

The ability of sperm to induce antibodies has been known for a century, yet only in the last 50 years have we come to realize the implications for infertility. **Up to 12% of men undergoing evaluation for infertility will have antisperm antibodies (ASA) [1,50]. ASAs have been found in serum, seminal plasma, and bound directly to sperm. The implication of serum antibodies is unclear,** given that they must first transudate to the seminal fluid before sperm binding can occur. Although it could be postulated that serum antibodies act as a marker of immune infertility, their clinical importance remains uncertain. **Antibodies within the seminal plasma are found both free and bound to sperm.** Bound antibodies may have a higher avidity for particular sperm antigens than those that are free. Ultimately, the binding of antibodies is related to the concentrations of both antibodies and antigens, as well as to the binding constants of the antibodies themselves [1].

Immune activation and antibody production

Recall that antibodies are produced by plasma cells activated by T-helper cells in response to recognition of antigen–MHC complex. **Antibody production is classified as primary or secondary, depending upon the event that led to immune activation [51]. "Primary" or "idiopathic" implies an unknown etiology of antibody production, whereas "secondary" implies a known traumatic, inflammatory, or obstructive** event that culminated in exposure of autoantigens to the immune system.

Although several theories have been proposed to explain pathologic ASA production, most involve a breach of the anatomic or functional blood–testis barrier. **Physical disruption of the barrier can occur in a variety of conditions, including testicular trauma, biopsy, vasectomy, or other testis, epididymal, or vasal surgery. Less obvious causes of ASA production include orchitis, testis cancer, torsion, cryptorchidism, and varicocele, all of which have been correlated with ASA production** [52]. For simplicity, each condition has been categorized once in Table 16.4, although several could easily find residence in multiple categories. Although the production of ASA in conjunction with many of these conditions has been studied in animal models, not all associations have been demonstrated in humans. Further, **the causal links between these exposures, ASA production, and infertility have not been demonstrated** [1].

Amongst the exposures in Table 16.4, several have been studied in greater depth and merit further discussion. Following vasectomy, 50–80% of men will have serum levels of ASA. These levels are observed as early as two months following the procedure, tend to peak at one year, and decline by year 2 [52,53]. Antibodies have been reported as late as 20 years after vasectomy [54]. Despite their presence, ASAs after vasectomy have very little clinical impact, since many men, despite elevated serum levels of antibody, are able to conceive normally following vasectomy reversal [55,56]. Individuals with unilateral or bilateral genital tract obstruction appear to be at increased risk for ASA production. Elevated ASA titers have been found in 81% of men with obstruction, compared to 10% of men with other causes of infertility [1,57,58]. Inflammatory conditions such as orchitis and prostatitis may also be associated with ASA production, but there is less evidence of that association [1,59–63]. **Assays for ASA in infertile men have found that men with varicoceles are two times more likely to have ASA titers than men without varicoceles** [64,65]. ASA production has also been demonstrated in men who have undergone testis biopsy [66]. Lastly, genetics may influence ASA production, including the possibility that a predisposition for autoimmunity occurs with defects in thymic development [5]. In addition, there is evidence that men with ASA are more likely to possess a particular HLA marker, namely HLA-B28 [67,68].

Table 16.4. Conditions linked with antisperm antibodies

| **Obstruction** |
| Vasectomy and reversal |
| Idiopathic epididymal obstruction |
| Ejaculatory duct obstruction |
| Congenital absence of the vas deferens |
| **Inflammation** |
| Orchitis |
| Venereal disease |
| Prostatitis |
| Cancer |
| **Thermal** |
| Varicocele |
| Cryptorchidism |
| Hot baths, tubs |
| **Trauma** |
| Coital |
| Torsion |
| Testis biopsy |
| Oral, rectal exposure |
| **Genetic** |
| Thymic maldevelopment |
| HLA-B28 haplotype |

In cases of post-testicular obstruction or reproductive tract surgery, the substantial release of sperm antigens may inoculate the immune system, with plasma cell differentiation and ASA production. Unlike in states of immune tolerance, this "bolus" exposure of sperm antigens overwhelms the steady-state immunosuppression in the functional blood–testis barrier. In addition to direct vascular exposure of antigen, peritoneal and gastrointestinal exposures resulting from trauma and lymphatic drainage may also foster antibody production [69–71].

Once an autoimmune response is initiated, many antibody types can be generated. However, only **IgG, IgM, and IgA** have been shown to be directed against sperm. Although IgM ASAs have been found in the seminal plasma, its large, pentomer structure likely prevents transudation to semen; therefore its role in immune infertility probably is limited [72]. IgG is produced locally in the genital tract as well as transudated from serum, where it is produced in large quantities [73]. Only 1% of serum IgG is observed in the seminal plasma, and most IgG production results from systemic antigen inoculation [74]. The presence of IgG in the seminal plasma despite absent serum levels suggests a mechanism for in-situ, local production as well [75]. IgA is found in the seminal plasma but virtually never in serum. Based upon this and our understanding of IgA behavior in other organ systems, it is likely generated by local antigen inoculation. The exact location of IgG and IgA antibody production in the reproductive tract is unknown [76,77].

Mechanisms of antibody-mediated infertility

Once antibodies are generated, infertility may be caused by mechanisms beyond simply a decrease in sperm concentration. **Antibodies may impair sperm motility, passage through the female reproductive tract, and the capacity for sperm to properly interact with the oocyte during fertilization** [78]. Antibody binding to sperm may prevent penetration of the cervical mucus, and forms the basis of the cervical mucus test. **When more than 50% of sperm are antibody-bound, the probability of adequate numbers of sperm penetrating cervical mucus is significantly reduced** [79]. Experimental studies suggest that the Fc region of IgA binds receptors within the mucus, impairing forward progression [80]. **Sperm bound by antibody can also cause agglutination, which decreases their efficient passage through the cervical mucus.** These interactions are caused predominantly by IgA as opposed to IgG antibody, suggesting that the local antibody response may have a greater role in autoimmunity than the systemic antibody response [51,81]. **Female antisperm antibodies may also cause poor sperm mucus penetration.** In this case, sperm are quickly immobilized in the mucus after targeting by resident antibodies [71].

In addition to inhibited passage through the mucus, **antibody-bound sperm may also be targets for destruction.** Sperm opsonization occurs throughout the female genital tract, including in the uterine cavity, fallopian tubes, and intraperitoneally. Once opsonization has occurred, sperm are phagocytosed or fixed by the complement, and then lysed [82].

Antisperm antibodies may also prevent normal gamete interaction by preventing normal binding to the zona pellucida. The interaction between sperm and egg is highly regulated by specific receptor–ligand binding. Opsonized sperm may be unable to bind appropriately to the oocyte because of **steric interference.** Clinically, this suggests that head-directed antibodies may be more deleterious than tail-directed antibodies for infertility [83]. An example of this is disruption of the normal sperm–zona interaction and subsequent fertilization with antibodies directed against the FA-1 receptor [44,45].

Oocyte penetration by sperm may also be affected by ASA. In-vitro experiments in which sperm have been incubated with the sera of ASA-positive men have demonstrated that ASA-coated sperm only poorly penetrate zona-free hamster eggs [84]. Interestingly, this effect only occurs with antisperm IgG and IgM, but not IgA, which has led to the thought that complement fixation is key in preventing oocyte penetration [85].

The capacity of ASA to induce spontaneous abortion in affected couples has been suggested but has not been definitively shown. In experimental models, following the fusion of human sperm with hamster, rabbit, and mouse oocytes, the formed zygotes promptly begin to express sperm-derived surface antigens [86–88]. Expression of these antigens could conceivably make the embryo susceptible to opsonization by antisperm antibodies [78]. The most likely result from this is failed implantation and perceived infertility rather than recurrent abortion [1].

Cell-mediated sperm autoimmunity

Cell-mediated autoimmune infertility is difficult to demonstrate. However, several lines of evidence suggest that it may be important for infertility. Although ASAs are present in many cases of immune infertility, they are conspicuously absent in others, suggesting that **ASAs may be only a small component of the autoimmune response.** Clinically, this may be what is observed with spermatic cord torsion. Despite an obviously ischemic and necrotic testis and the release of a germ cell inoculum from this damage, significant ASA titers are rarely demonstrated afterwards. This occurs despite an active immunologic assault on the contralateral testis, characterized by pro-inflammatory cell infiltration and release of inflammatory mediators [89,90].

Investigators have also attempted to quantify the cellular immune response in patients with a history of surgically repaired cryptorchidism. In this study, subject macrophages were purified and combined with homologous sperm to assess macrophage reactivity. Half of the patients with unilateral cryptorchidism and 80% of those with bilateral disease demonstrated immunoreactivity [91]. While this study suffered from small numbers and the lack of a true control group, it suggests an active cellular immune response in this at-risk patient population.

Could pyospermia or leukocytospermia also be a manifestation of cellular immunity to sperm? Immunohistochemical studies of the male reproductive tract clearly demonstrate immunologically active cells within the testicular interstitium and seminal fluid, but their impact on sperm function is poorly understood [92–94]. Pyospermia, the elevation of white blood cells in seminal fluid, is also present in many men with infertility, and in-vitro studies have demonstrated poor oocyte penetration in such cases [47,95]. **However, while there may be associations between certain seminal white blood cell types and abnormal semen parameters, there is insufficient evidence to link cellular autoimmunity with pyospermia** [92].

Experimental models also support the role of cell-mediated sperm autoimmunity. The experimental allergic orchitis model (EAO), developed in murines, rats, and rabbits by injecting homologous sperm antigen intraperitoneally into naive animals [1], demonstrates profound cellular infiltrates and destruction of the germinal epithelium in the naive testes [25]. That similar outcomes are possible with injection of activated T cells alone implies the critical role of the cellular immune system in this condition.

Cytokines, the soluble mediators of inflammation, are most likely linked to any autoimmune response to sperm. Impairments of sperm motility and hamster egg penetration have been observed in sperm exposed to cytokines such as **interferon γ, tumor necrosis factor**, and the supernatant of activated lymphocytes [92,96]. In addition, the leukocytes of vasectomy patients, when stimulated with sperm in vitro, have augmented cytokine production compared with those of men without vasectomy [97,98]. **Attempts to measure cytokines in seminal plasma have proven difficult, likely because of the abundance of proteolytic enzymes that degrade them** [23].

Diagnosing immunologic infertility
Tests of antibody-mediated immunity
The diagnosis of antibody-mediated infertility lacks a pathognomonic clinical picture. However, an ASA assay should be obtained when:
(1) the semen analysis shows sperm **agglutination or clumping** in the absence of clinical infection;
(2) low sperm motility exists, with history of **testis injury or surgery**;
(3) there is confirmation that increased round cells are **leukocytes**;

(4) **sperm "shaking"** is observed on sperm–cervical mucus contact testing;
(5) **poor penetration of mucus** is observed on a postcoital test;
(6) there is **unexplained infertility**.

Immunologically mediated infertility is subtle and usually presents as unexplained infertility. During the male evaluation, attempts should be made to elucidate potential exposures that could predispose to ASA production.

Despite attempts to correlate routine semen parameters with ASA, no specific set of parameters is truly predictive [92,99]. In particular, neither sperm concentration nor viability is associated with ASA presence [100]. Decreased sperm motility can be caused by antibody coating of sperm, but other causes such as varicocele should be excluded [101]. Additionally, sperm that are bound by antibody are more likely to clump and be observed as agglutination. Unfortunately, agglutination is nonspecific, and can also be due to infection [102].

Examination of sperm behavior in cervical mucus, although not commonly performed, may help to identify ASA. Postcoital and cervical mucus penetration testing assess the capacity of sperm to penetrate cervical mucus. The finding of sperm that are shaking back and forth, without forward progression, may indicate ASA production [103,104].

Several variables should be considered with ASA testing. As one might suspect, the greater the percentage of sperm coated by antibody, the greater the likelihood of infertility. Evidence to date indicates that a threshold is reached when over 50% of sperm are bound by antibody. Below this value, clinical studies demonstrate that postcoital tests approximate fertile controls [105]. The location of antibody binding to sperm, or antibody "binding geography," may also differentially affect sperm function. Whereas **tail-directed sperm antibodies are more likely to impair motility and cause agglutination, sperm head-directed antibodies may preferentially affect zona binding and fertilization**, as suggested by immobilization and penetration assays [1].

Antisperm antibody detection has evolved considerably since the first serum agglutination assays were used in the 1950s [106]. Contemporary assays employ various methodologies with differing sensitivities and clinical implications (Table 16.5) [106–115]. **In choosing an ASA assay, three important characteristics should be considered: (1) the body compartment in which ASAs are being measured, (2) which antibody classes are detected, and (3) how sperm are**

Table 16.5. Assays for the detection of antisperm antibodies

Technique	Compartment	Method	Reference
Gel agglutination test	Serum	Agglutination	Kibrick et al., 1952 [106]
Tray slide agglutination test	Serum/sperm	Microagglutination	Franklin and Dukes, 1964 [107]
Sperm immobilization test	Serum	Immobilization	Fjallbrant et al., 1968 [108]
Immunofluorescence	Processed sperm	Antibody fluorescence	Hjort and Hansen, 1971 [109]
Microtray agglutination test	Serum/sperm	Microagglutination	Friberg, 1974 [110]
Mixed agglutination reaction	Sperm	Agglutination of erythrocytes	Jager et al., 1978 [111]
Radiolabeled antiglobulin test	Sperm	Radioimmune assay	Haas et al., 1980 [112[
Immunobead test	Sperm	Agglutination of beads	Bronson et al., 1981 [113]
ELISA	Fixed sperm	Colorimetry	Zanchetta et al., 1982 [114]
Flow cytometry	Sperm	Antibody fluorescence	Garner et al., 1986 [115]

prepared for the assay. Although ASAs are detectable in both serum and seminal plasma, consensus is that **antibodies bound to sperm within the semen are the most important.** As a result, assays for sperm-bound antibodies are considered the most relevant. Moreover, since only **IgG and IgA** are found in significant quantities within the reproductive tract, incorporating these antibody classes into the ASA assay is important [51]. Lastly, although historically sperm were processed prior to ASA testing, contemporary assays use **fresh, motile sperm** to ensure that only surface antigens, and not confounding internal antigens, are identified [116].

Currently, the most popular tests to identify ASA are the **immunobead test (IBT)** and the **mixed agglutination reaction (MAR)** [71]. The IBT identifies immunoglobulins on the sperm surface by directing bead-bound antibody to the Fc portion of the ASA. Based upon the pattern of immunobead binding, this assay determines the proportion of sperm in the sample that are antibody-bound, the class of antibody bound, and the location on sperm where the antibody is bound [49,71,100]. The MAR test uses similar principles of monoclonal antibody technology but employs sheep erythrocytes instead of immunobeads to detect and localize antibody-bound sperm. Unfortunately, by any current methodology, **the lower limit of detection of sperm antibodies is not known,** and thus the clinical relevance of these assays is limited.

Tests of cell-mediated immunity

Despite the idea that cell-mediated immunity plays a pivotal role in the pathology of immune infertility, few assays exist to quantify its role [1]. This reflects not only the complexity of the cellular immune system, but also our lack of understanding of the exact cellular components that mediate infertility. A leukocyte migration assay has been described for the detection of delayed hypersensitivity to sperm [117,118]. Isolated peripheral blood leukocytes from either partner are mixed with sperm, and leukocyte migration through the gel is assessed by video analysis. In mixtures where there is sperm–leukocyte reaction, leukocyte movement is inhibited. Early work with this assay examined antisperm reactivity in women [119]. In a subsequent evaluation of fertile and infertile men with abnormal semen analyses, the same investigators found that all men with normal semen analyses had a normal assay result, whereas 53% of asthenospermic men ($n = 32$, < 50% motility) and 25% of men with oligoasthenospermia ($n = 24$, < 20 million sperm/mL and < 50% motility) had abnormal indices indicative of a cellular immune response to sperm [118]. More useful assays for the detection of cell-mediated immune infertility will undoubtedly arise as our understanding of autoimmunity improves.

Treatment of immunologic infertility

Condoms

Condom use represents a simple means by which continual inoculation of the female partner with sperm antigens is prevented. Although easy to use, with good supportive theory, no studies have demonstrated a decrease in ASA titers with condom use. More importantly, there is no correlation between a history of rigorous condom use and increased pregnancy rates [1,119].

Systemic immunosuppression

Similar to other autoimmune diseases, suppression of the immune system is a cornerstone of autoimmune infertility treatment. The most common pharmacologic agents employed for immune suppression are corticosteroids. **Corticosteroids prevent the chemotaxis of inflammatory cells, impede cytokine release, decrease antibody production, and even weaken antigen–antibody association** [120]. Although the exact molecular mechanisms by which corticosteroids act is not fully understood, it is clear that they have a suppressive effect upon both the humoral and cellular arms of immunity.

More than a dozen studies, performed over the last four decades, have investigated the effect of steroid treatment on in-vivo conception rates. The results of treatment appear encouraging, with natural pregnancy rates ranging from 9% to 50% during treatment [1]. Unfortunately, the vast majority of studies do not have an appropriate nontreatment or placebo control group, and therefore the results are difficult to interpret. **Importantly, two randomized controlled trials of steroid use as a treatment of immune infertility have been performed.** The first was completed in 1987 by Haas and Manganiello, who randomized 20 patients with presumed immune infertility to treatment with high-dose methylprednisolone for seven days, cyclically for three months, versus no treatment [121]. Although a 15% overall pregnancy rate was achieved, the authors failed to find a difference in semen parameters or pregnancy rates between groups, and concluded that high-dose steroids were not beneficial for this diagnosis. In 1990, Hendry and colleagues randomized 43 couples to treatment of twice-daily doses of prednisone 20 mg, on days 1–10 of the menstrual cycle for a total of nine months followed by a washout period and crossover [122]. The authors found that those men undergoing treatment were three times more likely to achieve conception than those receiving placebo (31% vs. 9%). While neither semen parameters nor serum antibody titers differed between treatment groups, titers of antibodies in the seminal fluid declined precipitously (often becoming undetectable) in the treatment group. The reasons for the disparity between these two studies are not entirely clear; one issue may be that the Haas and Manganiello study did not include sufficient follow-up (3 months) to adequately assess natural pregnancy rates. Overall, this suggests that long-term, moderate doses of steroids may be more beneficial in the reduction of ASA, and the achievement of pregnancy.

Important clinical considerations in the use of steroids to treat autoimmune infertility are potential side effects. **Mild side effects include acne, dyspepsia, skin rashes, fluid retention, and mood changes in approximately 60% of patients** [122]. Unfortunately, there

have been at least two reported cases of **aseptic necrosis of the hip** [123,124]. Both occurred in patients on high-dose methylprednisolone; however, aseptic necrosis is generally considered an idiosyncratic reaction that is not dose-related.

The last two decades have seen a significant rise in the use of novel immunosuppressive agents in organ transplant recipients and patients with autoimmune disease. However, very few of these agents have been investigated as treatments for immune infertility. Cyclosporin, a member of the calcineurin family of immunosuppressant agents, has been used for decades to prevent graft rejection in transplant recipients, through its inhibition of T-lymphocyte activity, humoral immunity, and cytokine production [125]. Bouloux *et al.* performed a pilot study of nine men with immune infertility by treating with cyclosporine for nine months, but failed to show a significant decline in ASA titers [126]. Although one-third of subjects achieved pregnancy, there was no control group, making the results difficult to interpret. There is still hope, however, that newer, less toxic immunosuppressive agents will find a place in the treatment of immune infertility.

Sperm washing

The goal of sperm washing is to remove bound antibody. Several techniques have been described to remove ASA from seminal fluid as well as from sperm. However, the dissociation of tightly bound antibodies can be difficult. **While rapid dilutional washing of the seminal fluid may remove unbound antibodies, it has little impact upon those that are already bound** [127,128]. Detergent-based washes may remove antibodies but can severely damage sperm [129]. Enzymatic cleaning has been described using a protease specific to the Fc region of IgA [101]. Cleaning by this method reduces immunobead binding and increases cervical mucus penetration. However, because the protease is not active against a second isoform of IgA, not all antibody is removed. Additionally, given the site of cleavage on the antibody, portions of the antibody remain on sperm, thus negating the effects of the digestion. To be effective, all sperm washing techniques should be combined with intrauterine insemination (IUI), or with higher levels of assisted reproduction.

Intrauterine insemination (IUI)

One cause of immune-mediated infertility is the inability of opsonized sperm to adequately penetrate the cervical mucus [80]. The rationale for IUI in this situation is to place more sperm beyond the cervix in the female reproductive tract, sperm that would have been caught in cervical mucus due to ASA [71,130]. Given that antibody-bound sperm may have a shorter survival time within the female genital tract, accurate estimation of ovulation could improve the success of this technique [131].

Unfortunately, **there are no controlled, prospective studies of IUI in treating immune infertility.** However, retrospective case reviews suggest that IUI, combined with ovulatory stimulation, may be successful. Margalloth and colleagues implemented IUI in a cohort of couples with poor postcoital tests, and found pregnancy rates of 5%, 9.7%, and 14.3% per cycle with unstimulated, clomiphene citrate, and gonadotropin-stimulated IUI, respectively [132]. Additionally, these authors found decreased pregnancy rates in cases in which antibodies were directed to the sperm head, when compared to those directed to the tail. Other investigators have reported pregnancy rates ranging from 14% to 25% per cycle using washed sperm with IUI [133–135]. While encouraging, two of these series included data on only eight patients, while the third included only seven. Further, these studies used serum and not sperm-bound ASA to make a diagnosis of immunologic infertility. Kremer and colleagues performed IUI in 15 patients with ASA, and achieved pregnancy in 20% per cycle [136]. However, Glazener and colleagues studied a cohort of 19 couples with ASA by immunobead testing and compared IUI pregnancy rates to a similar cohort without immune infertility and obtained no pregnancies in the ASA group, but a 26% pregnancy rate per cycle in the non-ASA group [137]. In a larger retrospective review, Agarwal performed IUI in 45 couples in which the male partner demonstrated ASA [138]. Thirty-three percent of these couples achieved pregnancy with IUI, compared to 19% of couples undergoing IUI for other reasons. In summary, **although case-series studies suggest a benefit of IUI for ASA, the lack of randomized controlled trials investigating this issue makes it difficult to draw hard conclusions about the role of IUI in immune infertility.** Given this, **IUI is best suited for treatment of infertility when there is evidence of a cervical mucus problem**, whether it is due to antibodies or not, as demonstrated by the inability of sperm to penetrate the cervical mucus.

In-vitro fertilization

In-vitro fertilization (IVF) refers to the co-incubation of harvested ova and processed sperm followed by fertilization within the laboratory and subsequent transfer of embryos to the uterus. Relatively low numbers of sperm (100 000/oocyte) are required for successful IVF in cases of female-factor infertility, thus making it useful for male-factor infertility as well. **When IVF is used to treat immune infertility, the fertilization and pregnancy rates are lower than those observed for other indications, with overall pregnancy rates ranging from 14% to 35% per cycle** [1]. The impact of ASA type and degree of sperm binding on IVF success has been investigated. Clarke and colleagues performed IVF in 17 cases of immune infertility, and divided them into two cohorts: (1) men with both IgA and IgG bound to >80% of sperm (immunobead assay), and (2) men with <80% of sperm bound by IgA only [139]. In the former group, fertilization and pregnancy were achieved in only 27% and 0% per cycle, respectively. In the latter group, with less antibody burden, fertilization and pregnancy rates were 72% and 67% per cycle, respectively. These results clearly suggest that **extensive binding by both isotypes of ASA impede IVF success.** Confirming these findings, Junk and colleagues, in a small series of patients, observed a mean normal fertilization rate of 30% in cases of IgA- and IgG-bound sperm (immunobead assay), compared to 79% in cases in which sperm were bound by either but not both antibody classes [140]. More recently, Lahteenmaki et al assessed the efficacy of treating men with immunologic infertility with low-dose prednisone prior to IVF [141]. Fifty-three men, assessed with the mixed agglutination reaction assay, were grouped into placebo or prednisone arms. They found no significant differences in either fertilization rates (35% vs. 39% in treatment and placebo groups, respectively) or pregnancy rates (29% vs. 35%). **In cases of female-derived ASA, IVF offers fertilization and pregnancy rates comparable to those associated with other diagnoses for which IVF is indicated** [142–145].

IVF–ICSI

In cases in which immune infertility is not overcome by IVF, intracytoplasmic sperm injection (ICSI) may be used. With this technique, individual sperm are aspirated into a microscopic pipette after mechanical immobilization by crushing the sperm tail. The sperm are injected directly through the zona pellucida covering the unfertilized oocyte, through the perivitelline space that separates the oocyte from the zona pellucida, and directly into the egg cytoplasm. With ICSI, the numerical sperm requirement for egg fertilization is as low as one viable sperm for each retrieved oocyte [140]. ICSI reliably allows viable sperm with limited intrinsic fertilizing capacity, including "immature" sperm obtained surgically, to fertilize eggs. While it has been used to overcome many forms of severe male-factor infertility, ICSI also has the potential to overcome antibody-mediated infertility by bypassing the interaction between sperm and the zona pellucida and oocyte membrane [146]. Lahteenmaki *et al.* retrospectively compared IVF and ICSI fertilization rates among several groups of patients: 22 couples who had ICSI for (MAR-positive) antisperm antibodies, 20 couples who used ICSI for other reasons (MAR-negative), and 37 MAR-positive couples who had IVF alone [141]. Normal fertilization rates were similar between MAR-positive and MAR-negative couples with ICSI (79% vs. 68%), but were significantly greater in ICSI than in IVF alone in MAR-positive couples (79% vs. 44%). Similarly high ICSI fertilization rates in ASA cases have been obtained by other investigators [147]. Interestingly, these **studies have also observed that embryo quality is poorer in ASA-positive than in ASA-negative ICSI cases, suggesting that ASA may affect post-fertilization events.** Despite this apparent relationship between ASA presence and fertilization, the positive predictive value for pre-procedure ASA tests to predict low fertilization rates (< 50%) is only 25% [148].

Summary

Immunologic infertility is caused by an abnormal immune response to sperm. Both the humoral and cellular arms of the immune system play a causal role in this form of autoimmunity. Despite three decades of impressive advances in our understanding of the immune system, the immunopathology leading to infertility is still poorly understood. Contributing to this problem are a lack of properly controlled experiments, the use of many, heterogeneous assays to diagnose immune infertility, and the need to oversimplify a complex immunologic network for clinical purposes. Although certain clinical conditions and semen analysis parameters are suggestive of autoimmune infertility, they are by no means pathognomic. For this reason, clinicians should keep in mind other potential causes of male infertility in addition to autoimmune infertility. Given the advances in our understanding of the immune system and in the treatment of organ transplant patients, the promise is great for new diagnostic tools and novel treatments for immune infertility in the future.

References

[1] Turek PJ, Lipshultz LI. Immunologic infertility. *Urol Clin North Am* 1994; **21**: 447–68.

[2] Billingham RE, Brent L, Medawar PB. Actively acquired tolerance of foreign cells. *Nature* 1953; **172**: 603–6.

[3] Rumke P. The presence of sperm antibodies in serum of two patients with oligozoospermia. *Vox Sang* 1954; **4**: 135–40.

[4] Yunis E. The cellular and humoral basis of the immune response. *Semin Arthritis Rheum* 1983; **13** (1 Suppl 1): 89–93.

[5] Anderson MS, Venanzi ES, Klein L, *et al*. Projection of an immunological self shadow within the thymus by the aire protein. *Science* 2002; **298**: 1395–401.

[6] DeVoss J, Hou Y, Johannes K, *et al*. Spontaneous autoimmunity prevented by thymic expression of a single self-antigen. *J Exp Med* 2006; **203**: 2727–35.

[7] Parkin J, Cohen B. An overview of the immune system. *Lancet* 2001; **357**: 1777–89.

[8] Kimber I, Dearman RJ. Immune responses: adverse versus non-adverse effects. *Toxicol Pathol* 2002; **30**: 54–8.

[9] Gery I, Gershon RK, Waksman BH. Potentiation of the T-lymphocyte response to mitogens. I. The responding cell. *J Exp Med* 1972; **136**: 128–42.

[10] Ben-Rafael Z, Orvieto R. Cytokines: involvement in reproduction. *Fertil Steril* 1992; **58**: 1093–9.

[11] Holmgren J, Czerkinsky C, Lycke N, Svennerholm AM. Mucosal immunity: implications for vaccine development. *Immunobiology* 1992; **184**: 157–79.

[12] Parr MB, Ren HP, Russell LD, Prins GS, Parr EL. Urethral glands of the male mouse contain secretory component and immunoglobulin A plasma cells and are targets of testosterone. *Biol Reprod* 1992; **47**: 1031–9.

[13] Whitmore WF, Karsh L, Gittes RF. The role of germinal epithelium and spermatogenesis in the privileged survival of intratesticular grafts. *J Urol* 1985; **134**: 782–6.

[14] Tung KSK. Autoimmunity of the testis. In: Dhindsa DS, Schumacher GFB, eds. *Immunological Aspects of Infertility and Fertility Regulation*. New York, NY: Elsevier-North Holland, 1980; 33–91.

[15] el-Demiry MI, Hargreave TB, Busuttil A, *et al*. Lymphocyte sub-populations in the male genital tract. *Br J Urol* 1985; **57**: 769–74.

[16] Gilula NB, Fawcett DW, Aoki A. The Sertoli cell occluding junctions and gap junctions in mature and developing mammalian testis. *Dev Biol* 1976; **50**: 142–68.

[17] Dym M, Fawcett DW. The blood–testis barrier in the rat and the physiological compartmentation of the seminiferous epithelium. *Biol Reprod* 1970; **3**: 308–26.

[18] Fawcett DW, Leak LV, Heidger PM. Electron microscopic observations on the structural components of the blood–testis barrier. *J Reprod Fertil Suppl* 1970; **10**: 105–22.

[19] Tung KS, Unanue ER, Dixon FJ. Pathogenesis of experimental allergic orchitis. II. The role of antibody. *J Immunol* 1971; **106**: 1463–72.

[20] Tung KS, Unanue ER, Dixon FJ. Pathogenesis of experimental allergic orchitis. I. Transfer with immune lymph node cells. *J Immunol* 1971; **106**: 1453–62.

[21] Connell CJ. A freeze-fracture and lanthanum tracer study of the complex junction between Sertoli cells of the canine testis. *J Cell Biol* 1978; **76**: 57–75.

[22] Neaves WB. Advances in physiology, biochemistry and function. In: Johnson AD, Gomes WR, Vandemark NL, eds. *The Testis*. New York, NY: Academic Press, 1977: 125.

[23] Anderson DJ, Hill JA. Cell-mediated immunity in infertility. *Am J Reprod Immunol Microbiol* 1988; **17**: 22–30.

[24] Suzuki F, Nagano T. Regional differentiation of cell junctions in the excurrent duct epithelium of the rat testis as revealed by freeze-fracture. *Anat Rec* 1978; **191**: 503–19.

[25] Brown PC, Dorling J, Glynn LE. Ultrastructural changes in experimental allergic orchitis in guinea-pigs. *J Pathol* 1972; **106**: 229–33.

[26] Mahi-Brown CA, Yule TD, Tung KS. Evidence for active immunological regulation in prevention of testicular autoimmune disease independent of the blood–testis barrier. *Am J Reprod Immunol Microbiol* 1988; **16**: 165–70.

[27] Jenkins MK, Pardoll DM, Mizuguchi J, Chused TM, Schwartz RH. Molecular events in the induction of a nonresponsive state in interleukin 2-producing helper T-lymphocyte clones. *Proc Natl Acad Sci U S A* 1987; **84**: 5409–13.

[28] Mahi-Brown CA, Yule TD, Tung KS. Adoptive transfer of murine autoimmune orchitis to naive recipients with immune lymphocytes. *Cell Immunol* 1987; **106**: 408–19.

[29] Tung KS, Yule TD, Mahi-Brown CA, Listrom MB. Distribution of histopathology and Ia positive cells in actively induced and passively transferred experimental autoimmune orchitis. *J Immunol* 1987; **138**: 752–9.

[30] Perussia B, Kobayashi M, Rossi ME, Anegon I, Trinchieri G. Immune interferon enhances functional properties of human granulocytes: Role of Fc receptors and effect of lymphotoxin, tumor necrosis factor, and granulocyte-macrophage colony-stimulating factor. *J Immunol* 1987; **138**: 765–74.

[31] Diemer T, Hales DB, Weidner W. Immune–endocrine interactions and Leydig cell function: The role of cytokines. *Andrologia* 2003; **35**: 55–63.

[32] Alexander NJ, Anderson DJ. Immunology of semen. *Fertil Steril* 1987; **47**: 192–205.

[33] Lord EM, Sensabaugh GF, Stites DP. Immunosuppressive activity of human seminal plasma. I. Inhibition of in vitro lymphocyte activation. *J Immunol* 1977; **118**: 1704–11.

[34] Petersen BH, Lammel CJ, Stites DP, Brooks GF. Human seminal plasma inhibition of complement. *J Lab Clin Med* 1980; **96**: 582–91.

[35] Sedor J, Callahan HJ, Perussia B, Lattime EC, Hirsch IH. Soluble Fc gamma RIII (CD16) and immunoglobulin G levels in seminal plasma of men with immunological infertility. *J Androl* 1993; **14**: 187–93.

[36] Fritz TE, Lombard SA, Tyler SA, Morris WP. Pathology and familial incidence of orchitis and its relation to thyroiditis in a closed beagle colony. *Exp Mol Pathol* 1976; **24**: 142–58.

[37] Teuscher C, Smith SM, Goldberg EH, Shearer GM, Tung KS. Experimental allergic orchitis in mice. I. Genetic control of susceptibility and resistance to induction of autoimmune orchitis. *Immunogenetics* 1985; **22**: 323–33.

[38] Tung KS, Ellis L, Teuscher C, *et al*. The black mink (Mustela vison): a natural model of immunologic male infertility. *J Exp Med* 1981; **154**: 1016–32.

[39] Madrigal JA, Yunis EJ, Anderson DJ. Qualitative differences in sperm antibody responses in mice of different inbred strains and sexes. *J Reprod Immunol* 1986; **9**: 175–86.

[40] Mathur S, Neff MR, Williamson HO, *et al*. Sperm antibodies and human leukocyte antigens in couples with early spontaneous abortions. *Int J Fertil* 1987; **32**: 59–65.

[41] Anderson DJ, Narayan P, DeWolf WC. Major histocompatibility antigens are not detectable on post-meiotic human testicular germ cells. *J Immunol* 1984; **133**: 1962–5.

[42] Haas GG, Nahhas F. Failure to identify HLA ABC and Dr antigens on human sperm. *Am J Reprod Immunol Microbiol* 1986; **10**: 39–46.

[43] Gilbert BR, Witkin SS, Goldstein M. Immunology of male fertility. *AUA Update Series* 1990; **9**: Lesson 8, 590

[44] Naz RK, Alexander NJ, Isahakia M, Hamilton MS. Monoclonal antibody to a human germ cell membrane glycoprotein that inhibits fertilization. *Science* 1984; **225**: 342–4.

[45] Naz RK, Brazil C, Overstreet JW. Effects of antibodies to sperm surface fertilization antigen-1 on human sperm-zona pellucida interaction. *Fertil Steril* 1992; **57**: 1304–10.

[46] Tung KS, Cooke WD, McCarty TA, Robitaille P. Human sperm antigens and antisperm antibodies. II. Age-related incidence of antisperm antibodies. *Clin Exp Immunol* 1976; **25**: 73–9.

[47] Berger RE, Karp LE, Williamson RA, *et al*. The relationship of pyospermia and seminal fluid bacteriology to sperm function as reflected in the sperm penetration assay. *Fertil Steril* 1982; **37**: 557–64.

[48] Kapur DK, Ahuja GK. Immunocytochemistry of male reproductive organs. *Arch Androl* 1989; **23**: 169–83.

[49] Bronson R, Cooper G, Rosenfeld D. Sperm antibodies: their role in infertility. *Fertil Steril* 1984; **42**: 171–83.

[50] Hendry WF, Morgan H, Stedronska J. The clinical significance of antisperm antibodies in male subfertility. *Br J Urol* 1977; **49**: 757–62.

[51] Hendry WF. The significance of antisperm antibodies: measurement and management. *Clin Endocrinol (Oxf)* 1992; **36**: 219–21.

[52] Haas GG. Antibody-mediated causes of male infertility. *Urol Clin North Am* 1987; **14**: 539–50.

[53] Ansbacher R. Humoral sperm antibodies: a 10-year follow-up of vas-ligated men. *Fertil Steril* 1981; **36**: 222–4.

[54] Kremer J, Jager S. The sperm–cervical mucus contact test: a preliminary report. *Fertil Steril* 1976; **27**: 335–40.

[55] Royle MG, Parslow JM, Kingscott MM, Wallace DM, Hendry WF. Reversal of vasectomy: The effects of sperm antibodies on subsequent fertility. *Br J Urol* 1981; **53**: 654–9.

[56] Sullivan MJ, Howe GE. Correlation of circulating antisperm antibodies to functional success in vasovasostomy. *J Urol* 1977; **117**: 189–91.

[57] Girgis SM, Ekladious EM, Iskander R, El-Dakhly R, Girgis FN. Sperm antibodies in serum and semen in men with bilateral congenital absence of the vas deferens. *Arch Androl* 1982; **8**: 301–5.

[58] Hendry WF, Parslow JM, Stedronska J, Wallace DM. The diagnosis of unilateral testicular obstruction in subfertile males. *Br J Urol* 1982; **54**: 774–9.

[59] Andrada JA, von der Walde F, Hoschoian JC, Comini E, Mancini E. Immunological studies in patients with mumps orchitis. *Andrologia* 1977; **9**: 207–15.

[60] Andrada JA, Von der Walde FE, Andrada EC. Immunologic studies of male infertility. *Immunol Ser* 1990; **52**: 345–78.

[61] Jarow JP, Kirkland JA, Assimos DG. Association of antisperm antibodies with chronic nonbacterial prostatitis. *Urology* 1990; **36**: 154–6.

[62] Mathur S, Baker ER, Williamson HO, *et al*. Clinical significance of sperm antibodies in infertility. *Fertil Steril* 1981; **36**: 486–95.

[63] Witkin SS, Zelikovsky G. Immunosuppression and sperm antibody formation in men with prostatitis. *J Clin Lab Immunol* 1986; **21**: 7–10.

[64] Gilbert BR, Witkin SS, Goldstein M. Correlation of sperm-bound immunoglobulins with impaired semen analysis in infertile men with varicoceles. *Fertil Steril* 1989; **52**: 469–73.

[65] Golomb J, Vardinon N, Homonnai ZT, Braf Z, Yust I. Demonstration of antispermatozoal antibodies in varicocele-related infertility with an enzyme-linked immunosorbent assay (ELISA). *Fertil Steril* 1986; **45**: 397–402.

[66] Hjort T, Husted S, Linnet-Jepsen P. The effect of testis biopsy on autosensitization against spermatozoal antigens. *Clin Exp Immunol* 1974; **18**: 201–12.

[67] Hancock RJ, Duncan D, Carey S, Cockett AT, May A. Anti-sperm antibodies, HLA antigens, and semen analysis. *Lancet* 1983; **2**: 847–8.

[68] Law HY, Bodmer WF, Mathews JD, Skegg DC. The immune response to vasectomy and its relation to the HLA system. *Tissue Antigens* 1979; **14**: 115–39.

[69] Bronson RA, Cooper GW, Rosenfeld DL, *et al*. Comparison of antisperm antibodies in homosexual and infertile men with autoimmunity to spermatozoa [abstract]. Society for Gynecologic Investigation, Washington, DC, 1983.

[70] Wolff H, Schill WB. Antisperm antibodies in infertile and homosexual men: relationship to serologic and clinical findings. *Fertil Steril* 1985; **44**: 673–7.

[71] Bronson RA. Antisperm antibodies: a critical evaluation and clinical guidelines. *J Reprod Immunol* 1999; **45**: 159–83.

[72] Rumke P. The origin of immunoglobulins in semen. *Clin Exp Immunol* 1974; **17**: 287–97.

[73] Haas GG. Male fertility and immunity. In: Lipshultz LI, Howards SS, eds. *Infertility in the Male*. St. Louis, MO:, Mosby Year Book, 1991: 277–96.

[74] Haas GG, Cunningham ME. Identification of antibody-laden sperm by cytofluorometry. *Fertil Steril* 1984; **42**: 606–13.

[75] Haas GG, Schreiber AD, Blasco L. The incidence of sperm-associated immunoglobulin and C3, the third component of complement, in infertile men. *Fertil Steril* 1983; **39**: 542–7.

[76] Uehling DT. Secretory IgA in seminal fluid. *Fertil Steril* 1971; **22**: 769–73.

[77] Witkin SS, Zelikovsky G, Good RA, Day NK. Demonstration of 11S IgA antibody to spermatozoa in human seminal fluid. *Clin Exp Immunol* 1981; **44**: 368–74.

[78] Cropp CS, Schlaff WD. Antisperm antibodies. *Arch Immunol Ther Exp (Warsz)* 1990; **38**: 31–46.

[79] Fjallbrant B. Cervical mucus penetration by human spermatozoa treated with anti-spermatozoal antibodies from rabbit and man. *Acta Obstet Gynecol Scand* 1969; **48**: 71–84.

[80] Jager S, Kremer J. Immunological aspects of male infertility. *Ann Biol Clin (Paris)* 1987; **45**: 340–5.

[81] Jager S, Kremer J, Kuiken J, van Slochteren-Draaisma T. Immunoglobulin class of antispermatozoal antibodies from infertile men and inhibition of in vitro

sperm penetration into cervical mucus. *Int J Androl* 1980; **3**: 1–14.

[82] Witkin SS, Bongiovanni AM, Berkeley A, Ledger WJ, Toth A. Detection and characterization of immune complexes in the circulation of infertile women. *Fertil Steril* 1984; **42**: 384–8.

[83] Bronson RA, Cooper GW, Rosenfeld DL. Sperm-specific isoantibodies and autoantibodies inhibit the binding of human sperm to the human zona pellucida. *Fertil Steril* 1982; **38**: 724–9.

[84] Abdel-Latif A, Mathur S, Rust PF, *et al.* Cytotoxic sperm antibodies inhibit sperm penetration of zona-free hamster eggs. *Fertil Steril* 1986; **45**: 542–9.

[85] Bronson RA, Cooper GW, Rosenfeld DL. Complement-mediated effects of sperm head-directed human antibodies on the ability of human spermatozoa to penetrate zona-free hamster eggs. *Fertil Steril* 1983; **40**: 91–5.

[86] Johnson LV, Calarco PG. Mammalian preimplantation development: the cell surface. *Anat Rec* 1980; **196**: 201–19.

[87] Menge AC, Fleming CH. Detection of sperm antigens on mouse ova and early embryos. *Dev Biol* 1978; **63**: 111–17.

[88] O'Rand MG. The presence of sperm-specific surface isoantigens on the egg following fertilization. *J Exp Zool* 1977; **202**: 267–73.

[89] Walsh TJ, Joyner BD. Evaluation of the pediatric patient with a non-traumatic acute scrotum. *AUA Update Series* 2005; **24**: Lesson 12, 97.

[90] Anderson MJ, Dunn JK, Lipshultz LI, Coburn M. Semen quality and endocrine parameters after acute testicular torsion. *J Urol* 1992; **147**: 1545–50.

[91] Singer R, Dickerman Z, Sagiv M, Laron Z, Livni E. Endocrinological parameters and cell-mediated immunity postoperation for cryptorchidism. *Arch Androl* 1988; **20**: 153–7.

[92] Anderson DJ. Cell-mediated immunity and inflammatory processes in male infertility. *Arch Immunol Ther Exp (Warsz)* 1990; **38**: 79–86.

[93] el-Demiry MI, Young H, Elton RA, *et al.* Leucocytes in the ejaculate from fertile and infertile men. *Br J Urol* 1986; **58**: 715–20.

[94] Wolff H, Anderson DJ. Immunohistologic characterization and quantitation of leukocyte subpopulations in human semen. *Fertil Steril* 1988; **49**: 497–504.

[95] Maruyama DK, Hale RW, Rogers BJ. Effects of white blood cells on the in vitro penetration of zona-free hamster eggs by human spermatozoa. *J Androl* 1985; **6**: 127–35.

[96] Hill JA, Haimovici F, Politch JA, Anderson DJ. Effects of soluble products of activated lymphocytes and macrophages (lymphokines and monokines) on human sperm motion parameters. *Fertil Steril* 1987; **47**: 460–5.

[97] Anderson DJ, Alexander NJ, Fulgham DL, Vandenbark AA, Burger DR. Immunity to tumor-associated antigens in vasectomized men. *J Natl Cancer Inst* 1982; **69**: 551–5.

[98] Nagarkatti PS, Rao SS. Cell-mediated immunity to homologous spermatozoa following vasectomy in the human male. *Clin Exp Immunol* 1976; **26**: 239–42.

[99] Cookson MS, Witt MA, Kimball KT, Grantmyre JE, Lipshultz LI. Can semen analysis predict the presence of antisperm antibodies in patients with primary infertility? *World J Urol* 1995; **13**: 318–22.

[100] Clarke GN, Elliott PJ, Smaila C. Detection of sperm antibodies in semen using the immunobead test: a survey of 813 consecutive patients. *Am J Reprod Immunol Microbiol* 1985; **7**: 118–23.

[101] Bronson RA, Cooper GW, Rosenfeld DL, Gilbert JV, Plaut AG. The effect of an IgA1 protease on immunoglobulins bound to the sperm surface and sperm cervical mucus penetrating ability. *Fertil Steril* 1987; **47**: 985–91.

[102] Hekman A, Rumke P. The antigens of human seminal plasma: with special reference to lactoferrin as a spermatozoa-coating antigen. *Fertil Steril* 1969; **20**: 312–23.

[103] Haas GG. The inhibitory effect of sperm-associated immunoglobulins on cervical mucus penetration. *Fertil Steril* 1986; **46**: 334–7.

[104] Kremer J, Jager S. Sperm–cervical mucus interaction, in particular in the presence of antispermatozoal antibodies. *Hum Reprod* 1988; **3**: 69–73.

[105] Bronson RA, Cooper GW, Rosenfeld DL. Autoimmunity to spermatozoa: effect on sperm penetration of cervical mucus as reflected by postcoital testing. *Fertil Steril* 1984; **41**: 609–14.

[106] Kibrick S, Belding DL, Merrill B. Methods for the detection of antibodies against mammalian spermatozoa. I. A modified macroscopic agglutination test. *Fertil Steril* 1952; **3**: 419–29.

[107] Franklin RR, Dukes CD. Antispermatozoal antibody and unexplained infertility. *Am J Obstet Gynecol* 1964; **89**: 6–9.

[108] Fjallbrant B. Studies on sera from men with sperm antibodies. *Acta Obstet Gynecol Scand* 1969; **48**: 131–46.

[109] Hjort T, Hansen KB. Immunofluorescent studies on human spermatozoa. I. The detection of different spermatozoal antibodies and their occurrence in normal and infertile women. *Clin Exp Immunol* 1971; **8**: 9–23.

[110] Friberg J. A simple and sensitive micro-method for demonstration of sperm-agglutinating activity in serum from infertile men and women. *Acta Obstet Gynecol Scand Suppl* 1974; (36): 21–9.

[111] Jager S, Kremer J, van Slochteren-Draaisma T. A simple method of screening for antisperm antibodies in the human male: detection of spermatozoal surface

IgG with the direct mixed antiglobulin reaction carried out on untreated fresh human semen. *Int J Fertil* 1978; **23**: 12–21.

[112] Haas GG, Cines DB, Schreiber AD. Immunologic infertility: identification of patients with antisperm antibody. *N Engl J Med* 1980; **303**: 722–7.

[113] Bronson RA, Cooper GW, Rosenfeld DL. Membrane-bound sperm specific antibodies: their role in infertility. In: Vogel H, Jagiello GJ, eds. *Bioregulators of Reproduction*. New York, NY: Academic Press, 1981: 521–7.

[114] Zanchetta R, Busolo F, Mastrogiacomo I. The enzyme-linked immunosorbent assay for detection of the antispermatozoal antibodies. *Fertil Steril* 1982; **38**: 730–4.

[115] Garner DL, Pinkel D, Johnson LA, Pace MM. Assessment of spermatozoal function using dual fluorescent staining and flow cytometric analyses. *Biol Reprod* 1986; **34**: 127–38.

[116] Haas GG, DeBault LE, D'Cruz O, Shuey R. The effect of fixatives and/or air-drying on the plasma and acrosomal membranes of human sperm. *Fertil Steril* 1988; **50**: 487–92.

[117] Dimitrov DG, Sedlak R, Nouza K, Kinsky R. A quantitative objective method for the evaluation of anti-sperm cell-mediated immunity in humans. *J Immunol Methods* 1992; **154**: 147–53.

[118] Dimitrov DG, Urbanek V, Zverina J, et al. Correlation of asthenozoospermia with increased antisperm cell-mediated immunity in men from infertile couples. *J Reprod Immunol* 1994; **27**: 3–12.

[119] Bujas M, Beric B, Kapamadzija A. Incidence of infertility of immune origin in a group of marriages with unexplained infertility. *Hum Reprod* 1988; **3**: 301–2.

[120] Rosse WF. Quantitative immunology of immune hemolytic anemia: II. The relationship of cell-bound antibody to hemolysis and the effect of treatment. *J Clin Invest* 1971; **50**: 734–43.

[121] Haas GG, Manganiello P. A double-blind, placebo-controlled study of the use of methylprednisolone in infertile men with sperm-associated immunoglobulins. *Fertil Steril* 1987; **47**: 295–301.

[122] Hendry WF, Hughes L, Scammell G, Pryor JP, Hargreave TB. Comparison of prednisolone and placebo in subfertile men with antibodies to spermatozoa. *Lancet* 1990; **335**: 85–8.

[123] Hendry WF. Bilateral aseptic necrosis of femoral heads following intermittent high-dose steroid therapy. *Fertil Steril* 1982; **38**: 120.

[124] Shulman JF, Shulman S. Methylprednisolone treatment of immunologic infertility in male. *Fertil Steril* 1982; **38**: 591–9.

[125] Morris PJ. Cyclosporine, FK-506 and other drugs in organ transplantation. *Curr Opin Immunol* 1991; **3**: 748–51.

[126] Bouloux PM, Wass JA, Parslow JM, Hendry WF, Besser GM. Effect of cyclosporin A in male autoimmune infertility. *Fertil Steril* 1986; **46**: 81–5.

[127] Adeghe AJ. Effect of washing on sperm surface autoantibodies. *Br J Urol* 1987; **60**: 360–3.

[128] Haas GG, D'Cruz OJ, Denum BM. Effect of repeated washing on sperm-bound immunoglobulin G. *J Androl* 1988; **9**: 190–6.

[129] Alexander NJ. Treatment for antisperm antibodies: voodoo or victory? *Fertil Steril* 1990; **53**: 602–3.

[130] Nachtigall RD, Faure N, Glass RH. Artificial insemination of husband's sperm. *Fertil Steril* 1979; **32**: 141–7.

[131] London SN, Haney AF, Weinberg JB. Macrophages and infertility: Enhancement of human macrophage-mediated sperm killing by antisperm antibodies. *Fertil Steril* 1985; **43**: 274–8.

[132] Margalloth EJ, Sauter E, Bronson RA, et al. Intrauterine insemination as treatment for antisperm antibodies in the female. *Fertil Steril* 1988; **50**: 441–6.

[133] Ulstein M. Fertility of husbands at homologous insemination. *Acta Obstet Gynecol Scand* 1973; **52**: 5–8.

[134] Shulman S, Harlin B, Davis P, Reyniak JV. Immune infertility and new approaches to treatment. *Fertil Steril* 1978; **29**: 309–13.

[135] Confino E, Friberg J, Dudkiewicz AB, Gleicher N. Intrauterine inseminations with washed human spermatozoa. *Fertil Steril* 1986; **46**: 55–60.

[136] Kremer J, Jager S, Kuiken J. Treatment of infertility caused by antisperm antibodies. *Int J Fertil* 1978; **23**: 270–6.

[137] Glazener CM, Coulson C, Lambert PA, et al. The value of artificial insemination with husband's semen in infertility due to failure of postcoital sperm-mucus penetration –controlled trial of treatment. *Br J Obstet Gynaecol* 1987; **94**: 774–8.

[138] Agarwal A. Treatment of immunological infertility by sperm washing and intrauterine insemination. *Arch Androl* 1992; **29**: 207–13.

[139] Clarke GN, Lopata A, McBain JC, Baker HW, Johnston WI. Effect of sperm antibodies in males on human in vitro fertilization (IVF). *Am J Reprod Immunol Microbiol* 1985; **8**: 62–6.

[140] Junk SM, Matson PL, Yovich JM, Bootsma B, Yovich JL. The fertilization of human oocytes by spermatozoa from men with antispermatozoal antibodies in semen. *J In Vitro Fert Embryo Transf* 1986; **3**: 350–2.

[141] Lahteenmaki A, Reima I, Hovatta O. Treatment of severe male immunological infertility by intracytoplasmic sperm injection. *Hum Reprod* 1995; **10**: 2824–8.

[142] Vazquez-Levin MH, Notrica JA, Polak de Fried E. Male immunologic infertility: sperm performance on in vitro fertilization. *Fertil Steril* 1997; **68**: 675–81.

[143] Hershlag A, Napolitano B, Cangemi C, Scholl G, Rosenfeld D. The value of routine screening of female serum for antisperm antibodies in assisted reproductive technology cycles. *Fertil Steril* 1994; **61**: 867–71.

[144] Vazquez-Levin M, Kaplan P, Guzman I, *et al.* The effect of female antisperm antibodies on in vitro fertilization, early embryonic development, and pregnancy outcome. *Fertil Steril* 1991; **56**: 84–8.

[145] Daitoh T, Kamada M, Yamano S, *et al.* High implantation rate and consequently high pregnancy rate by in vitro fertilization-embryo transfer treatment in infertile women with antisperm antibody. *Fertil Steril* 1995; **63**: 87–91.

[146] Kamada M, Yamano S, Senuma M, *et al.* Semen analysis and antisperm antibody. *Arch Androl* 1998; **40**: 117–28.

[147] Nagy ZP, Verheyen G, Liu J, *et al.* Results of 55 intracytoplasmic sperm injection cycles in the treatment of male-immunological infertility. *Hum Reprod* 1995; **10**: 1775–80.

[148] Culligan PJ, Crane MM, Boone WR, *et al.* Validity and cost-effectiveness of antisperm antibody testing before in vitro fertilization. *Fertil Steril* 1998; **69**: 894–8.

The effect of genital tract infection and inflammation on male infertility

Sanjay S. Kasturi, E. Charles Osterberg, Justin Tannir, and Robert E. Brannigan

Introduction

Infection and inflammation of the male reproductive tract are complex clinical conditions that can negatively affect reproductive potential. In this chapter, we discuss sites of genitourinary tract infections, infectious organisms, the numerous ways in which leukocytes may impair male reproduction, and the diagnosis and treatment of leukocytospermia and bacteriospermia. For the purpose of this chapter, leukocytospermia refers to the World Health Organization threshold of ≥ 1×10^6 white blood cells/mL in the semen.

Genital tract infections

The male genital tract proximal to the urethra is typically sterile, and several components of the male reproductive system are immunologically sequestered [1,2]. Without a fully competent immune response, the genital tract may be prone to infections. These infections may be either bacterial or viral, and manifest in acute, chronic, or subclinical processes. **Infections of the male genitourinary (GU) tract can adversely impact male fertility by impairing spermatogenesis, disrupting sperm function, causing obstruction of the genital ductal system, inhibiting accessory gland function, or causing inflammation secondary to leukocyte response** [1,3].

Acute infections of the genital tract are indicated by patient history and can present with irritative voiding symptoms, urethral discharge, orchialgia, or painful ejaculation. **Traditional diagnostic criteria consist of two or more of the following parameters: (1) history of GU infection and/or abnormal rectal examination, (2) abnormal expressed prostatic secretions and/or urinary sediment after prostatic massage, (3) ≥ 10^3 bacteria/mL ejaculate, or (4) ≥ 10^6 leukocytes/mL ejaculate** [4].

Subclinical infections are more difficult to recognize and diagnose than acute infections. This is true not only because patients are largely asymptomatic, but also because some of these infections may actually represent contamination from commensal, nonpathogenic organisms. Additionally, due to antibacterial effects of semen, there are limitations in culturing all potential pathogenic organisms [1,5]. Several investigators have demonstrated that bacterial isolates from semen of men in subfertile couples are often commensal, nonpathogenic organisms. Furthermore, these isolates often do not correlate with leukocytospermia (WHO) or pregnancy rates [6,7].

Sites of infection

Urethritis

Infections of the urethra are most commonly due to sexually transmitted pathogens, and they are separated into two broad categories: gonococcal urethritis (due to *Neisseria gonorrhoeae*) and nongonococcal urethritis (*Chlamydia trachomatis*, Mycoplasma species, *Trichomonas vaginalis*) (Fig. 17.1). Patients with urethritis typically present with urethral discharge and dysuria. However, asymptomatic carrier states may occur, especially in partners of those with known infections. The proper diagnostic workup of suspected urethritis includes: (1) Gram stains of a urethral smear, (2) leukocyte quantification of a first-void urine sample, and (3) specific isolation techniques such as endourethral culture, PCR, or ELISA [8]. Based on these modalities, a urethral Gram stain containing > 4 leukocytes per microscopic field (×1000) or a first-void urine sample smear containing > 15 leukocytes per microscopic field (×400) is regarded as a positive result [9,10]. Consideration should be given to empiric treatment for both gonococcal and nongonococcal

Infertility in the Male, 4th edition, ed. Larry I. Lipshultz, Stuart S. Howards, and Craig S. Niederberger. Published by Cambridge University Press. © Cambridge University Press 2009.

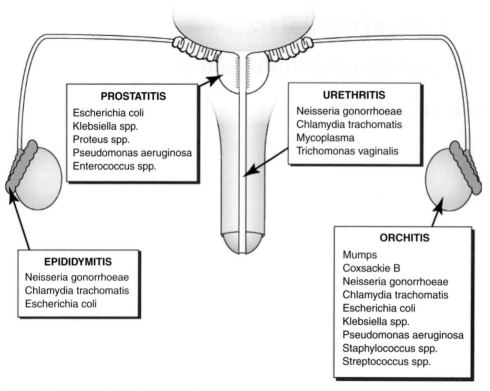

Fig. 17.1. Sites of infection and common pathogens in the male genitourinary tract.

organisms when a diagnosis of urethritis is suspected, as co-infection is common and the responsible pathogens are often unknown at the time of initial evaluation. Typically, a one-time dose of ceftriaxone and a week of doxycycline therapy are recommended [11] or one 2 g dose of azithromycin.

Prostatitis

Drach *et al.* described the first widely used classification system for prostatitis. Briefly, the authors presented four classes based on localization techniques and clinical correlates: acute bacterial prostatitis (ABP), chronic bacterial prostatitis (CBP), nonbacterial prostatitis (NBP), and prostatodynia (Pd) [12]. This classification is no longer commonly employed, and the National Institutes of Health (NIH) system is now preferred. **The NIH system categorizes prostatitis into four main divisions: type I – acute bacterial, type II – chronic bacterial, type III – chronic (abacterial) prostatitis/chronic pelvic pain syndrome (CP/CPPS), and type IV – asymptomatic inflammatory** [13]. Type I prostatitis is generally the result of ascending urinary tract infection (UTI) of typical uropathogenic organisms.

Patients usually present with constitutional symptoms, perineal or prostatic pain, and voiding complaints [14]. Complications include prostatic abscess, especially in immunocompromised patients and diabetics. A long-term course of antibiotics for 2–3 weeks is the mainstay of treatment for uncomplicated cases. Type II prostatitis is defined as prostatic inflammation and recurrent UTI with a bacterial pathogen localized to the prostate. Common pathogens include *E. coli* and other UTI-causing Gram-negative organisms (*Klebsiella* spp., *Proteus* spp., *P. aeruginosa*, *Enterococcus* spp.) [15] (Fig. 17.1). Unlike type I prostatitis, type II prostatitis is typically not associated with fever. However, both type I and type II prostatitis are often alleviated with antibiotics. Treatment requires extended therapy (as long as 6–12 weeks) with antibiotics that are lipophilic, thus able to penetrate the prostate. Trimethoprim-sulfamethoxazole and fluoroquinolones [15] are examples of antibiotics usually effective in this setting. Care must be taken in administering prolonged courses of fluoroquinolones, because of the increased risk of associated tendonitis and tendon rupture [16]. Type III prostatitis or CP/CPPS is a complex entity consisting of prostatic pain and voiding difficulties, with 90% of symptomatic prostatitis patients grouped into this category [13]. Type III prostatitis is further divided into type IIIA and type IIIB. Type IIIA, or inflammatory type, presents with leukocytosis on expressed prostatic secretions (EPS) or post-prostatic massage urinalysis. Type IIIB, or noninflammatory, is also known as Pd. Interestingly, Nickels et al. demonstrated that a 12-week course of antimicrobial therapy does alleviate symptoms in CP/CPPS [17], despite the absence of documented bacterial infection that defines this condition. Lastly, type IV prostatitis is an incidental finding on prostate biopsy or expressed prostatic secretions. The effect of prostatitis on male fertility will be discussed later in this chapter.

Epididymitis

Epididymitis is one of the most common causes of acute scrotum, presenting with ipsilateral scrotal swelling and pain. Systemic symptoms such as fever and leukocytosis are seen in 30–50% of patients [18]. The organism responsible for the infection typically is dependent on patient demographics. **Sexually active men under the age of 35 are often infected with C. trachomatis or N. gonorrhoeae, with accompanying symptoms of urethritis** (Fig. 17.1). In many patients, exposure to the organism may have occurred several months before presentation [10]. Chlamydia accounts for two-thirds of the total cases of urethritis in these men and is two to three times more common than gonorrhea [19]. Similar to urethritis, co-infection is not uncommon in epididymitis, occurring in approximately 30% of cases [19]. **For men over 35 years of age, men with recent urinary tract instrumentation or surgery, or men with anatomical abnormalities, E. coli is often the etiological organism causing epididymitis** [10]. Treatment of epididymitis should be pathogen-specific, with consideration given to patient demographics during initial evaluation.

In the case of acute epididymitis, several authors have observed that both sperm concentration and forward motility are transiently impaired [20,21]. However, with appropriate antibiotic treatment, decreased semen parameters and impaired sperm function often normalize [21].

Orchitis

Viruses represent a significant reproductive tract pathogen, capable of causing testicular inflammation and infection. These infections typically arise via hematogenous routes rather than by contiguous spread (Fig. 17.1). Paramyxovirus, which causes mumps, is one viral agent capable of inducing significant GU pathology. **Mumps infrequently involves the testicles in prepubertal boys, though orchitis occurs in approximately 20% of affected postpubertal males** [22]. Testicular pain and enlargement typically occur 4–6 days after the onset of parotitis, but testicular involvement is subclinical in 30–40% of cases. Orchitis is bilateral in approximately 30% of affected patients. Historical data reveal associated infertility rates of 25% in bilateral disease, but this problem is uncommon today due to the advent of the mumps vaccine [22,23]. Testicular atrophy is observed in 30–50% of patients with mumps orchitis, and infertility may be an associated long-term consequence [19]. Like paramyxovirus, coxsackie B virus may also result in viral orchitis similar to mumps [22].

Bacterial orchitis, unlike viral orchitis, often results from contiguous spread of infection from the epididymis. Common pathogens include N. gonorrhoeae/C. trachomatis, Gram-negative bacilli (E. coli, K. pneumoniae, P. aeruginosa), and Gram-positive cocci (staphylococci and streptococci) (Fig. 17.1). Patients may present with fever, testicular pain and swelling, and often an acute, reactive hydrocele [22]. Medical management is similar to that administered in the case of epididymitis, as treatment is pathogen-specific with consideration to the given patient demographic. Surgical intervention is indicated for testicular infarction or abscess [22].

Specific bacterial infections of the male genital tract

Neisseria gonorrhoeae

N. gonorrhoeae is a common cause of urethritis in America [24]. Although most affected males are symptomatic, as many as 10% of men with N. gonorrhoeae urethritis are asymptomatic [25]. Ascending infections in men involving genitourinary tract structures other than the urethra are rare (estimated at less than 1%), but when epididymitis or orchitis does occur, testicular damage or excurrent ductal obstruction can result. In a study of 184 men seen at an infertility clinic, patients with a prior remote history of N. gonorrhoeae had significantly more seminal leukocytes than those without such a history (2×10^6/mL vs. 0.5×10^6, $P < 0.0013$) [26].

Chlamydia trachomatis

C. trachomatis is the most common cause of nongonococcal urethritis and acute epididymitis in men

of reproductive age, and is also the most common sexually transmitted disease in industrial nations [27]. Ten to twenty-five percent of infected men may be asymptomatic with chronic, subclinical disease [28]. Infertility may arise because *C. trachomatis* is an obligate intracellular organism capable of causing a variety of pathological changes including epididymitis, orchitis, testicular atrophy, genital ductal obstruction, germinal epithelial cell damage, and blood–testis barrier breakdown leading to antisperm antibody production [1,29]. This bacterium exists in two forms – the reticulate body (RB) and the elementary body (EB). As an RB, *C. trachomatis* actively replicates in host cells, while the inactive EB serves as an extracellular agent of transmission. Immunologic laboratory techniques for diagnosis are targeted against EB antigens [1]. Hosseinzadeh *et al.* demonstrated that EBs cause increased tyrosine phosphorylation of sperm proteins, possibly impairing sperm capacitation and function [30]. Interestingly, subsequent data revealed that co-incubation of human spermatozoa and *C. trachomatis* EBs causes decreased motility and increased premature sperm death [31]. The spermicidal effects of EBs are mediated specifically by lipopolysaccharide (LPS), ultimately resulting in apoptosis [32,33]. In sum, EBs represent an important mediator of *C. trachomatis*-induced pathophysiology.

The relationship between *C. trachomatis* infection and semen quality is an actively debated topic (Table 17.1) [34–49]. Multiple studies have demonstrated a detrimental impact on semen parameters [34–36] and stimulation of antisperm antibody (ASA) production [37,38]. However, other investigators have found no relationship between chlamydial infections and semen parameters, ASA production, sperm penetration, or leukocytospermia [39,40–47]. Several authors suggest these discrepancies may be explained by the lack of uniformity and reliability in the diagnostic methods employed in these various studies, i.e., cultures (ejaculates and urethral swabs), enzyme-linked immunoassays to chlamydial antigens, and serum and semen antibodies [29,49]. Efforts to diagnose chlamydial infections are further hampered by the fact that seminal plasma inhibits cell culture techniques [50] and the host antibody response is not specific to *C. trachomatis* [51]. More recently, molecular amplification techniques consisting of polymerase chain reaction (PCR) and ligase chain reaction (LCR) have come to represent the tests of choice for diagnosing chlamydial infections [52]. Eggert-Kruse *et al.* demonstrated no effect on semen parameters in men from

infertile couples diagnosed with chlamydia using LCR compared to normal controls [48]. In a study of men undergoing an infertility evaluation, Hosseinzadeh *et al.* also noted that semen presenting as PCR-positive for chlamydia was not associated with impairment of sperm motility [49]. However, the authors did report a twofold increased incidence of leukocytospermia in PCR positive semen samples.

Mycoplasma

Four species of mycoplasma exist, two of which are pathogenic in human beings: *Mycoplasma hominis* and *Ureaplasma urealyticum*. *U. urealyticum* is a significant cause of urethritis, and is believed to be responsible for up to 25% of nongonococcal urethritis [1,5]. Similar to other bacterial causes of urethritis, mycoplasma infections may present acutely or remain subclinical, and the actual impact of *U. urealyticum* and *M. hominis* on male fertility is controversial (Tables 17.2, 17.3) [53–67].

Gnarpe and Friberg initially demonstrated that, although *U. urealyticum* is present in both fertile and infertile couples, it is more prevalent in the latter [53]. Furthermore, Swenson *et al.* found that infertile males with *U. urealyticum* infections had significantly improved sperm motility following treatment [66]. Additionally, Toth *et al.* demonstrated that couples in whom the male's *U. urealyticum* infection was cleared with doxycycline experienced significantly higher pregnancy rates than couples with persistent male infection [67]. However, sperm count and overall semen quality were not significantly different between the two groups.

Other authors have noted that men with *U. urealyticum* infections have reduced sperm count with reduced concentration, motility, and morphology [54–56]. Rose and Scott demonstrated that semen samples with mycoplasma (*U. urealyticum* and *M. hominis*) had decreased motility, morphology, hyperactivation, and acrosome reactivity when compared with controls [68]. A more recent in-vitro study also noted decreased motility and increased membrane alterations on the basis of the hypo-osmotic swelling test [69]. Lastly, Reichart *et al.* demonstrated that *U. urealyticum* is associated with increased sperm chromatin and DNA damage on the basis of both in-vitro studies (semen from normospermic men inoculated with *U. urealyticum*) and in-vivo studies (semen culture positive for *U. urealyticum*) [70]. The authors hypothesized that these changes may ultimately affect embryogenesis. In

Table 17.1. Studies investigating chlamydial infections in asymptomatic males attending infertility clinics

Reference	*n*	Detection method	Prevalence	Findings
Studies supporting a role for chlamydia				
Custo, 1989 [34]	1023	EIA	9%	Men with *C. trachomatis* infection had a significantly higher incidence of abnormal "semen scores" than healthy controls + symptomatic men infected with common pathogens + symptomatic men without infection
Wolff, 1991 [35]	209 prevalence analysis 331 semen Analysis	EIA for seminal antibodies	15.4%	Reduced ejaculate volume and progressive sperm motility in *C. trachomatis* antibody-positive patients with higher seminal inflammation (> 250 ng PMN elastase/mL) than those with lower inflammation (< 250 ng PMN elastase/mL)
Cengiz, 1997 [36]	284	EIA for seminal antibodies	12.6%	Significant differences in density, morphology, motility, and viability between antibody-positive and antibody-negative patients
Witkin, 1995 [37]	227	EIA for seminal and serum IgA and IgG antibodies	IgA 24.7% (semen), 14.5% (serum) IgG 10.9% (semen), 21.5% (serum)	Men with antichlamydial IgA in their semen had a lower median sperm count than those without ASA strongly correlated to antichlamydial IgA in semen
Munoz, 1995 [38]	48	EIA for seminal and serum IgA and IgG antibodies	IgA 29.2% (semen) IgG 8.3% (semen)	Men with seminal antichlyamdial IgA had elevated seminal concentrations of specific T-cell population than men without No differences in semen parameters in patients with antichlamydial antibodies (IgA and/or IgG) than men without
Studies refuting a role for chlamydia				
Close, 1987 [39]	270	Micro-IF of serum	5.9%	No difference in sperm count, motility, forward progress, % ovals, number of leukocytes, SPA, or serum ASA between patients seropostive and seronegative for *C. trachomatis*
Nagy, 1989 [40]	184	McCoy culture with Lugol stain	14.1%	No difference in cell count, motility, morphology, bovine mucus penetration, and HOS in infected and noninfected groups
Rujis, 1990 [41]	184	Direct IF of urethral smear, serum and seminal antibody titers	Smears 2.8%	No association between chlamydial antibody titers and sperm count, motility, morphology, leukocytes, MAR, SCMC results
Soffer, 1990 [42]	175	McCoy culture and Iodine stain	7%	No differences in mean motility index, total sperm count, normal form percentage between infected and noninfected groups Seminal ASA activity was elevated in cases of positive culture (both *C. trachomatis* and mycoplasma)
Bjercke, 1992 [43]	100	EIA for seminal and serum IgA and serum IgG	IgA 24% (semen) serum IgA/IgG not reported	No difference in sperm concentration, total sperm count, motility (several parameters), and morphology
Dieterle, 1995 [44]	50	*C. trachomatis* PCR and direct DNA probing	10%	No association between the detection of *C. trachomatis* (PCR or DNA probing) and chlamydial antibodies in serum or semen No association between chlamydial antibodies in serum or semen and mean sperm concentration, progressive motility, morphology, and serum ASA
Eggert-Kruse, 1996 [45]	197	EIA of semen (both IgA and IgG)	IgA 18.8% IgG 8.1%	No association between seminal chlamydial antibodies and sperm count, motility, morphology, viability, MAR, SCMPT, and PCT

Table 17.1. continued

Reference	n	Detection method	Prevalence	Findings
Eggert-Kruse, 1997 [46]	1317	Indirect immunofluorescence assay (IFA)	12.6%	No association between seminal chlamydial antibodies and sperm count, motility, morphology, MAR, SCMPT, and PCT
Habermann, 1999 [47]	207	EIA of semen	IgA 18.8% IgG 15.5%	No difference in sperm parameters, leukocytes, and MAR in patients with and without chlamydial antibodies
Eggert-Kruse, 2003 [48]	707	LCR of semen and urine samples	1.8%	No association between chlamydial infection by LCR and sperm count, motility, morphology, viability, MAR, and SCMPT
Hosseinzadeh, 2004 [49]	642	LCR/PCR of semen samples	4.9%	Men whose ejaculates were PCR-positive for chlamydial DNA had a higher mean concentration of leukocytes and twice the prevalence of leukocytospermia compared with those whose ejaculates were PCR-negative No difference in sperm concentration, % motile sperm, or % normal morphology in men PCR-positive and men PCR-negative for chlamydia

ASA, antisperm antibody; DNA, deoxyribonucleic acid; EIA, enzyme immunoassay; HOS, hypo-osmotic swelling; IF, immunofluorescence; Ig, immunoglobulin (IgG typically found in serum, IgA typically found in secretions); LCR, ligase chain reaction; MAR, mixed agglutination reaction; PCR, polymerized chain reaction; PCT, postcoital testing; PMN, polymorphonuclear leukocyte; SCMC, sperm–cervical mucus contact; SCMP, sperm cervical mucus penetration test.

Table 17.2. Studies investigating mycoplasma infections in males attending infertility clinics

Reference	n	Detection method	Prevalence	Findings
Studies supporting a role for mycoplasma				
Gnarpe, 1972 [53]	A: 36 infertile couples B: 19 infertile couples	Culture[a]	Patient groups A: 85% B: 95% Controls C: 23% D: 26%	UU was isolated in higher frequencies in the couples with infertility (A: primary infertility; B: ASA detected in female partners) than in the two control groups (C: pregnant women; D: men married to pregnant women)
Fowlkes, 1975 [54]	625 male partners of infertile couples with > 10⁶/mL semen	Culture	39%	Patients with UU infections had changes in their distribution curves toward lower total sperm counts and lower motility than infertile patients free of UU infections Patients with UU infections had a significant increase in the aberrant sperm forms compared with infertile patients free of UU infections
Upadhyaya, 1984 [55]	280 attending a fertility clinic	Culture	50%	Patient with UU infections had significantly lower sperm concentrations UU infection did not affect sperm motility, viability, or morphology
Naessens, 1986 [56]	120 men attending an infertility clinic	Culture	33%	Isolation of UU was significantly correlated with lower sperm counts and abnormal motility, but was not correlated with sperm morphology
Kalugdan, 1996 [57]	34 males	PCR–ELISA	29.4%	Mycoplasma-positive sperm[b] demonstrated decreased oocyte penetration capacity compared with mycoplasma-negative sperm
Studies refuting a role for mycoplasma				
De Louvois, 1974 [58]	120 infertile couples	Culture	*M. hominis* Fertile 13.2% Infertile 14.7% *U. urealyticum* Fertile 52.6% Infertile 57.2	Mycoplasma was not more prevalent in infertile versus fertile couples

Table 17.2. continued

Reference	n	Detection method	Prevalence	Findings
Harrison, 1975 [59]	120 infertile couples; 27 couples conceived during the 1 year of study	Culture	*M. hominis* Conception(+): 18% Conception(−): 18% *U. urealyticum* Conception(+): 63% Conception(−): 56%	Mycoplasma was not more prevalent in infertile couples who conceived versus those who did not conceive
Desai, 1980 [60]	150 infertile couples	Culture	Couples: 46% Men: 32.6%	No statistical difference in sperm count, motility, and morphology between infertile patients with and without UU infections
Cintron, 1981 [61]	96 male partners of infertile couples	Culture	45%	No statistical difference in sperm count, motility, and morphology between infertile patients with and without UU infections
Lewis, 1981 [62]	31 men attending an infertility clinic	Culture	58%	No statistical difference in the distribution of "normal" and "abnormal" semen analyses between infertile patients with and without UU infections
Shalhoub, 1986 [63]	76 male partners of infertile couples and 22 fertile controls	Culture	Fertile: 27% Infertile: 21%	No statistical difference in sperm count, motility, morphology, BCMP, and SPA between infertile patients with and without UU infections
de Jong, 1990 [64]	569 infertile men 75 fertile controls	Culture	Fertile: 5.3% Infertile: 7%	UU was not more prevalent in infertile versus fertile couples No statistical difference in sperm count, motility, and morphology between infertile men with and without UU
Ombelet, 1997 [65]	143 infertile couples 144 fertile couples	Culture	*M. hominis* Fertile: 1.4% Infertile 2.9% *U. urealyticum* Fertile: 7.6% Infertile: 12.5%	No further investigations of mycoplasma infection were performed

ASA, antisperm antibodies; BCMP, Bovine cervical mucous penetration; ELISA, enzyme-linked immunosorbent assay; PCR, polymerized chain reaction; SPA, hamster sperm penetration assay; UU, *U. urealyticum*.
[a] Various semen culture methods were employed by the different studies.
[b] Processed by the 48 hr TEST (TES and Tris) yolk buffer method.

Table 17.3. Studies investigating treatment of mycoplasma infections in males attending infertility clinics

Reference	n	Detection method	Treatment course	Findings
Swenson, 1979 [66]	73 men with infection attending an infertility clinic	Culture	Both partners: tetracycline 250mg QID or doxycycline 100mg BID for 30 days	The 64 patients successfully treated for UU had a significant improvement in sperm motility (speed of forward progression and % motility) In the 64 patients successfully treated for UU, the median percentage of motile cells increased from 35% to 50% following treatment
Toth, 1983 [67]	161 men with infection attending an infertility clinic	Culture	Both partners: doxycycline 100mg BID for 28 days	In couples treated for UU infection, eradication of UU in the male partner resulted in significantly more pregnancies than in couples whose male partner did not clear the infection (60% vs. 5%)
Harrison, 1975 [59]	88 couples with primary infertility	Culture	30 couples: doxycycline 100mg BID 28 couples: placebo 30 couples: no intervention (28 days for all)	In couples treated for mycoplasma infection, doxycycline therapy was shown to clear infection (96% eradication rate) but did not affect conception rates in those treated versus controls

UU, *U. urealyticum*.

sum, mycoplasma may lead to infertility by impairing sperm function and genetic integrity.

Several authors have examined the pathological interaction between mycoplasma and sperm. Gnarpe and Friberg observed that *U. urealyticum* attached directly to spermatozoa. This finding has been confirmed by others using electron micrography, noting specific attachment to the sperm head and midpiece regions [69,71,72]. As a result of this direct interaction, sperm motility may be impaired. Furthermore, Busolo and Zanchetta observed decreased hamster egg penetration in vitro (using viable sperm cultured with *U. urealyticum*) [73]. Kalugdan *et al.* corroborated these results by comparing penetration of zona-free hamster oocytes using "mycoplasma-positive sperm" and "mycoplasma-negative sperm." Mycoplasma positivity or negativity was determined by extracting sperm DNA from washed semen samples and assaying for mycoplasma DNA using PCR [57]. These last two studies suggest that direct attachment of mycoplasma to sperm may impair sperm penetration of eggs. Interestingly, Potts *et al.* demonstrated that semen samples from men presenting for a chronic prostatitis evaluation who were culture-positive for *U. urealyticum* had significantly elevated reactive oxygen species (ROS) compared with those who were culture-negative [74]. Therefore, ROS may also lead to damaged sperm membranes and DNA, providing additional mechanisms for fertility impairment.

In contrast to the above findings, de Louvois *et al.* did not observe an increased incidence of *U. urealyticum* or *M. hominis* in infertile versus fertile couples [58]. Harrison *et al.* noted that in 120 couples presenting for infertility evaluation, infection with *U. urealyticum* or *M. hominis* did not affect the rate of conception during 12 months of follow-up [59]. Additionally, in a subgroup of 88 patients with primary infertility, doxycycline therapy was shown to clear infection but did not affect conception rates. More recently, de Jong *et al.* and Ombelet *et al.* noted no difference between the frequency of *U. urealyticum* in the semen of infertile and fertile men [64,65]. Furthermore, several studies demonstrated no statistical difference in sperm count, motility, or morphology when infertile patients with and without *U. urealyticum* infections were compared [60–62]. These results were corroborated by Shalhoub *et al.*, who found no significant differences in semen parameters, mucus penetration, or oocyte penetration between semen samples with and without *U. urealyticum* [63]. **Although the impact of mycoplasma on male-factor fertility is controversial, several studies suggest that the adverse effects on sperm function arise from ROS production, DNA damage, and direct attachment of mycoplasma to spermatozoa. Therefore, treating patients with an appropriate course of antimicrobial therapy such as doxycycline should be considered, as doxycycline eradicates infection in the majority of cases** [58,59,64,67].

In regard to in-vitro fertilization (IVF), current data suggest that adverse outcomes (decreased pregnancy rates) associated with *U. urealyticum* infection in couples are secondary to endometritis associated with *U. urealyticum* infection [75,76]. As a result, treatment of male partners with *U. urealyticum* infection prior to IVF is still recommended [77].

The methods employed to detect *U. urealyticum* have evolved over time. Classically, genital tract samples were inoculated in broth with an indicator system utilizing the presence of urease in *U. urealyticum*. As urea is metabolized into ammonia and ultimately ammonium, the pH of the medium is increased, resulting in a color change of the indicator system. This color change corresponds to adequate bacterial replication. At this point, the broth is subcultured on selective solid media for final identification. In recent years, PCR techniques (targeted to the urease gene) have offered faster alternatives to culture for the diagnosis of mycoplasma. Blanchard *et al.* reported a 97.3% sensitivity and a 72% specificity of PCR compared to culture (considered the "gold standard") in 250 genital swabs from 181 male and female patients [78]. Furthermore, Teng *et al.* reported a higher sensitivity for *U. urealyticum* detection with PCR (semen, urine, urethral swabs, or prostatic secretions) than culture in males with urethritis or infertility [79]. However, Povlsen *et al.* reported only a 64% sensitivity and a 99% specificity for *U. urealyticum* detection with PCR compared to culture in male urogenital swabs [80]. Of note, Blanchard states that patient samples may contain substances that inhibit PCR, as suggested by increased PCR sensitivity with dilution of specimens. This finding may account for the decreased sensitivity of PCR versus culture. Further studies employing PCR for *U. urealyticum* detection in infertile males are needed to help clarify this issue.

Gram-negative infections

Gram-negative infections, in particular *E. coli*, are the most common cause of nongonococcal bacterial infections of the male genital tract. While these infections are often symptomatic, they may manifest as subclinical epididymitis or prostatitis [1,2,81]. In aggregate, the numerous clinical studies examining the effects of *E. coli* on male fertility do not support detrimental associations. Fowler and Mariano could not detect *E. coli* in any ejaculates of 62 male partners of infertile couples using IgA antibodies targeted against eight common O-antigens [82]. Hiller *et al.* isolated *E. coli* by culture in less than 10% of semen samples from 37 males attending an infertility clinic; however, no association with sperm dysfunction or leukocytospermia was observed [83]. Naessens *et al.* noted similar results in 120 male infertility patients [56]. Furthermore, Ombelet *et al.* observed no difference in the prevalence of *E. coli* when comparing 144 fertile males with 143 subfertile males [65]. More recently, Esfandiari *et al.* found no correlation between Gram-negative bacteria (Enterobacteriaceae family) and sperm characteristics in 80 infertile men with asymptomatic leukocytospermia [84]. These studies collectively suggest that the presence of *E. coli* in the semen of infertile males often represents benign colonization or sample contamination rather than an infectious cause of infertility.

Despite the lack of a definitive association between *E. coli* and male fertility impairment from the clinical literature, several basic science studies demonstrate that *E. coli* binds to sperm and causes ultrastructural damage and sperm agglutination. Collectively, these changes result in decreased sperm motility and penetration. Teague *et al.* first reported that *E. coli* obtained from urinary and cervical cultures, when added to semen from healthy volunteers, resulted in agglutination of spermatozoa and decreased motility [85]. These effects were found to be independent of endotoxin or lipopolysaccharide (LPS). Wolff *et al.* incubated sperm from healthy donors with *E. coli* isolated from the ejaculates of male infertility patients. They observed sperm agglutination due to direct adherence of *E. coli* to sperm mediated by mannose-binding proteins [86]. Interestingly, reversal of mannose-mediated agglutination yielded return of sperm motility. El-Mulla *et al.* demonstrated decreased inducibility of the acrosome reaction due to *E. coli* in an in-vitro experiment [87]. Studies by Diemer *et al.* suggest that at prolonged incubation times *E. coli* exerts irreversible damage to both acrosomal and tail architecture [88,89]. Though these results suggest a role for *E. coli* in male infertility, high concentrations of *E. coli* were used (1 : 1 ratio with sperm), and therefore they may not be clinically relevant [89].

Overall, the incidence of Gram-negative infections is low in young men [1,3]. While several in-vitro studies suggest mechanisms for male fertility impairment by Gram-negative organisms, a paucity of similar findings in the clinical literature suggests that these organisms may have limited male reproductive pathogenicity.

Trichomonas vaginalis

T. vaginalis is a sexually transmitted protozoan organism that accounts for a minority of nongonococcal urethritis cases [1]. Tuttle *et al.* demonstrated that, in an in-vitro environment, sperm incubated with *T. vaginalis* had diminished motility that significantly decreased over time [90]. In subsequent in-vitro studies, Jarecki-Black *et al.* isolated a spermicidal protein released by *T. vaginalis* [91]. Furthermore, Gopalkrishnan *et al.* reported that *T. vaginalis*-positive semen from asymptomatic men (4.4% of cases) demonstrated decreased sperm motility, decreased morphology, altered membrane integrity, and increased viscosity versus controls. Treatment with a single course of metronidazole resulted in significantly improved semen parameters in 50% of patients [92]. Interestingly, Lloyd *et al.* recently described the first case of *T. vaginalis* orchitis associated with oligoasthenoteratozoospermia and hypogonadism diagnosed during testicular sperm extraction [93]. These limited data suggest that *T. vaginalis* may impair sperm function, though the clinical utility of screening for *T. vaginalis* remains to be seen.

Viruses

Viruses may impact male fertility by stimulating direct cytotoxic immune mechanisms and indirect inflammatory processes (Table 17.4) [94–102]. They can infect the genitourinary system via the bloodstream or, less commonly, via the urethra. Viruses depend on host cells for replication, and these pathogens are capable of invading epithelial, neuronal, and immune cells present in the genitourinary tract [3]. Viruses are effectively detected in semen by sensitive and specific DNA amplification techniques including PCR and LCR.

The herpesvirus family consists of herpes simplex virus (HSV) types 1 and 2, cytomegalovirus (CMV), Epstein–Barr virus (EBV), varicella-zoster virus (VZV), and human herpes virus (HHV) types 6, 7, and 8. These viruses are collectively responsible for an array of disease processes ranging from simple rashes to malignancy. Krause *et al.* evaluated the presence of HSV, CMV, and EBV in the semen of infertile men with

Table 17.4. Studies investigating viral infections in asymptomatic males attending infertility clinics

Reference	Virus(es)	Detection method	Study population (*n*)	Prevalence	Findings
Krause, 2002 [94]	HSV, CMV, EBV	Serum IgG and IgM serology	Male infertility patients with (130) and without leukocytospermia (80)	(+) Leukocytospermia: HSV IgM: 10% (−) Leukocytospermia: HSV IgM: 1.25%	Of all the viruses and antibody isotypes, only IgM against HSV was more prevalent in patients with leukocytospermia than those without
Kapranos, 2003 [95]	HSV, CMV, EBV	DNA PCR	Men attending an infertility clinic (113)	HSV: 49.5% CMV: 7.1% EBV: 16.8%	HSV, but not CMV or EBV, was associated with decreased mean sperm count and mean sperm motility
Shen, 1994 [96]	CMV	DNA PCR	Male partners of infertile couples (217)	32.7%	Associations with semen parameters or sperm function were not studied
Yang, 1995 [97]	CMV	CMV IgG serum serology and DNA PCR of semen samples	Infertile couples (250)	IgG: 98.9% DNA PCR: 33.5%	In males, no effects on semen quality were observed
Levy, 1997 [98]	CMV	CMV IgG serum serology and DNA PCR of semen samples	Male partners of infertile couples (81) tested for serology and 70 separate semen samples from CMV IgG positive patients for PCR analysis	IgG: 58% DNA PCR: 2.85%	Authors recommend screening for CMV-seropositive patients followed by viral PCR detection in semen due to potential risk of congenital CMV infection
Bezold, 2002 [99]	Herpesvirus types: EBV, HSV, CMV, HHV 6–8, VZV	DNA PCR	Men seeking fertility evaluation (252)	All types: 17.1% EBV: 7.1% HSV: 3.2% CMV: 3.6% HHV 6: 4% HHV 7: 0.4% HHV 8: 0% VZV: 0%	Patients with EBV-positive PCR had higher seminal granulocytes than those without No associations between any virus and sperm count, motility, and morphology Authors also recommend screening for HSV and CMV due to potential risk of congenital infections
Green, 1991 [100]	HPV 11 & 16	DNA PCR	Men attending an STD clinic (27) and a fertility clinic (104)	STD clinic: 85% Fertility clinic: HPV total: 41% HPV 11: 22% HPV 16: 33% HPV 11&16: 14%	Associations with semen parameters or sperm function were not studied
Lai, 1997 [101]	HPV 16 & 18	DNA & RNA PCR	Men attending a fertility clinic (24)	HPV 16 DNA: 25% RNA: 8% HPV 18 DNA: 46% RNA: 8%	Higher rate of asthenospermia in patients infected with either HPV than in patients without infection Certain aspects of motility were significantly lower in the specimens with HPV than in those without
Martorell, 2005 [102]	HPV (multiple types)	DNA PCR from paraffin embedded sections	Patients with azoospermia undergoing testicular biopsy (185)	6.48%	Further studies indicate that Sertoli, Leydig, and possibly germinal cells harbored the HPV infections

CMV, cytomegalovirus; DNA, deoxyribonucleic acid; EBV, Epstein–Barr virus; HHV, human herpes virus; HPV, human papillomavirus; HSV, herpes simplex virus; Ig, immunoglobulin (IgG typically found in serum, IgA typically found in secretions); PCR, polymerized chain reaction; STD, sexually transmitted disease; VZV, varicella-zoster virus.

and without leukocytospermia [94]. Through the use of serum serologies, the authors noted significantly more patients with serum IgM antibodies against HSV when comparing infertile men with leukocytospermia with controls (10.8 vs. 1.25, $P < 0.05$). However, when they compared HSV DNA PCR on semen samples from infertile men with leukocytospermia to semen samples from infertile men without leukocytospermia, they found no such association. More recently, Kapranos et al. employed PCR detection of HSV virus in the semen of 113 men attending an infertility clinic [95]. The investigators detected HSV in 49.5% of samples and reported significantly decreased sperm concentration and motility in HSV-positive patients versus HSV-negative patients. CMV and EBV were also studied, but neither impacted semen parameters.

Yang et al. studied the presence of CMV in 250 infertile couples in Taiwan using blood serologies and DNA hybridization techniques. While the authors demonstrated 98.9% prevalence of anti-CMV IgG in the serum from males, they detected viral shedding in only 33.5% of semen samples using DNA hybridization techniques [97]. The authors reported that viral shedding of CMV in semen did not affect semen quality. In a similar study of 81 infertile couples in France, Levy et al. noted the presence of anti-CMV IgG serologies in 58% of men and 62% of women [98]. However, in 70 semen samples of those with anti-CMV IgG positive serologies, only two semen samples were positive for CMV DNA through amplification. The difference in these two studies is largely attributed to patient demographics (France vs. Taiwan), and the full effects of CMV on reproductive health remain to be determined.

In a study by Bezold et al., herpesviruses were detected in 17% of 252 semen samples from men undergoing an infertility evaluation [99]. EBV was the most common (7.1% of samples), and was associated with increased concentrations of granulocytes. However, no associations between EBV infection and impaired semen parameters or sexual gland dysfunction (e.g., fructose assay for seminal vesicles) were demonstrated.

The relationship of human papillomavirus (HPV) to male fertility is intriguing, considering the role of HPV in genital warts (types 6 and 11) and penile carcinoma (types 16 and 18). Through DNA PCR of semen, Green et al. reported a 41% prevalence of seminal HPV in a total of 104 men attending a fertility clinic [100]. **In another study of 24 men attending a fertility clinic, Lai et al. demonstrated that patients infected with HPV type 16 or 18 detected by PCR in semen had a significantly higher rate of asthenospermia than patients without HPV infection (75% vs. 8%, $P = 0.008$) [101].** No such differences were observed regarding sperm concentration or morphology when comparing patients with and without seminal HPV. More recently, Martorell et al. isolated HPV by PCR in 6.48% of 185 paraffin-embedded testicular biopsies of men with nonobstructive azoospermia versus 0% of healthy controls (autopsies) [102]. However, each of the 12 patients identified with HPV infection had other probable etiologies for azoospermia (e.g., chemotherapy effects, etc.). At this time, the relationship between HPV and male infertility is unclear, given the available data.

Infection with human immunodeficiency virus (HIV) is a significant cause of morbidity and mortality worldwide, with disease progression resulting in acquired immunodeficiency syndrome (AIDS). The isolation of HIV in human semen is well documented [3], and thus represents a potential pathogen to sperm development and function (Table 17.5) [103–110]. Krieger et al. demonstrated that semen specimens from 21 men seropositive for HIV did not significantly differ from those of seronegative semen donors [103]. However, the authors demonstrated that the three study patients with AIDS had leukocytospermia and microscopically abnormal sperm forms. **Several subsequent investigations corroborate these data, as early HIV infections are generally not associated with abnormalities in semen parameters. However, with disease progression to AIDS (i.e., CD4+ count < 200 cells/mm^3 or symptomatic disease), significant seminal abnormalities (impaired concentration, morphology, motility, viscosity) and leukocytospermia are often evident** [104–107,111]. Using regression analysis, Dondero et al. demonstrated correlations between peripheral blood CD4+ lymphocyte count, sperm motility ($r = 0.45$, $P < 0.05$), and abnormal sperm morphology ($r = -0.51$, $P < 0.05$) in 21 HIV seropositive males [107].

Treatment of HIV with the antiretroviral zidovudine (AZT) is not associated with detrimental changes in semen parameters [103,104], and in some reports AZT therapy has been shown to result in decreased seminal leukocytes [106] and titers of seminal HIV-1 [105]. Dulioust et al. studied 189 HIV-infected men without AIDS, a majority (94%) of whom were taking one or more antiretrovirals [108]. These otherwise

Table 17.5. Studies investigating the effects of HIV, AIDS, and antiretrovirals on male fertility

Reference	Study population (n)	Symptomatic HIV (n)	AIDS (n)	Patients receiving treatment (%)	Findings
Krieger, 1991 [103]	24 HIV-positive males	5	3	12 (50%)	No difference in sperm count, morphology, motility, or WBCs in HIV semen samples compared to controls Zidovudine treatment did not affect semen parameters Three patients with AIDS had grossly visible leukocytospermia, spermophagy, and abnormal sperm form by light and electron microscopy
Crittenden, 1992 [104]	39 HIV-positive males	9	8	9 (49%)	HIV-positive males had decreased motile sperm, more round cells Serum CD4 count and CD4 percentage of HIV patients was positively correlated to proportion of motile sperm
Anderson, 1992 [105]	95 HIV-positive males	47 with AIDS or symptoms	47 with AIDS or symptoms	31 (33%)	9% of HIV-positive males had positive HIV semen cultures Serum CD4 < 200/µL, symptomatic disease, and elevated seminal WBC (>1x10⁶/ml) were associated with HIV detection in semen Zidovudine treatment was associated with decreased detection of HIV in semen
Politch, 1992 [106]	166 HIV-positive males	NA	55	80 (48%)	HIV-positive males with CD4 counts > 200/µL and patients with zidovudine therapy (regardless of CD4 count) had normal semen parameters Untreated HIV-positive males with CD4 counts < 200/µL had decreased sperm count and concentration and increased % of abnormal sperm forms
Dondero, 1996 [107]	21 HIV-positive males	None	None	16 (76%)	No difference in sperm density, motility, and viscosity in HIV patients compared to controls HIV patients had a higher number of WBCs and spermophage cells than controls Serum CD4 count of HIV patients was positively correlated to sperm motility and inversely correlated to abnormal sperm
Dulioust, 2002 [108]	189 HIV-positive males requesting ART	None	None	177 (94%)	HIV-positive males had decreased total sperm count, decreased % of rapidly progressive sperm, decreased ejaculated volumes, and increased nonsperm cells compared with controls These results may be due to antiretroviral treatment
Nicopoullos, 2004 [109]	106 HIV-positive males requesting ART (IUI)	None	None	74 (55.6%)	HIV-positive males had decreased sperm concentration, total count, progressive motility, normal morphology, and ejaculate volume compared to controls A significant positive correlation was observed between CD4 count and sperm concentration, total count, motility, progressive motility, and post-preparation concentration⁹ A significant negative correlation was observed between CD4 count with normal sperm morphology of both raw and post-preparation samples VL < 1000 copies/mL and the use of antiretrovirals significantly improved IUI outcomes

Table 17.5. continued

Reference	Study population (n)	Symptomatic HIV (n)	AIDS (n)	Patients receiving treatment (%)	Findings
Bujan, 2007 [110]	190 HIV-positive males attending a fertility clinic	None	None	172 (91%)	HIV-positive males had decreased total sperm motile count, % progressive spermatozoa, polynuclear cell count, and ejaculate volume versus controls. HIV-positive males had increased seminal pH value and multiple anomaly index[b] versus controls. These results may be due to antiretroviral treatment

AIDS, acquired immunodeficiency syndrome; ART, assisted reproductive technology; CD, cluster of differentiation; HIV, human immunodeficiency virus; IUI, intrauterine insemination; VL, viral load; WBC, white blood cell.
[a] Sperm washing of HIV for IUI
[b] Mean number of anomalies per abnormal spermatozoon

healthy HIV patients had significant abnormalities in their semen parameters compared to age-matched seronegative controls, leading the authors to suggest a possible association between antiretrovirals and impaired semen quality [108]. A more recent study by Bujan et al. supports this conclusion; however, the authors did not find a correlation between duration of antiretroviral treatment and semen parameters [110].

The era of highly active antiretroviral therapy (HAART) has dramatically changed the lives of patients with HIV, resulting in increased life expectancy and improved quality of life. With the advent of HIV sperm washing techniques, parenthood has been achieved by male HIV patients using assisted reproductive technology (ART). Sperm washing is based on the principle that the HIV virus is found in seminal plasma and seminal leukocytes, but is not associated with sperm [112,113]. Semen samples are centrifuged multiple times using density gradient separation techniques, and this is followed by sperm swim-up procedures to isolate viable sperm [114]. The sperm isolate is then tested for HIV by nucleic acid amplification techniques, with Marina et al. noting HIV detection in 6% of samples and, more recently, Persico et al. reporting 0% detection rates [115,116]. **In a comprehensive review of the literature, Gilling-Smith et al. did not find any cases of seroconversion in female partners or children born in over 3000 cycles of sperm washing from HIV-infected males utilized in conjunction with ART** [117].

With respect to ART, Nicopoullos et al. demonstrated that the use of antiretrovirals and undetectable viral loads significantly improved the outcome of intrauterine insemination with sperm washing [109]. Antiretrovirals may indeed decrease HIV in semen, thereby inhibiting HIV-mediated sperm dysfunction. However, additional studies are needed to determine if, at higher concentrations or longer duration of use, antiretrovirals themselves may lead to inhibited sperm function.

Leukocytospermia and male-factor infertility
Mediators of inflammation

Immune cells present in human semen

The testes are immunologically sequestered organs, and as such represent an unusual deviation from the meticulous regulation imposed on the human body by the immune system. This sequestration is achieved through Sertoli cells intimately linked by tight junctions, forming the blood–testis barrier. Additionally, the molecular milieu of the testicle may also result in immunological tolerance. Therefore, the presence of abnormal concentrations of leukocytes within the male reproductive tract may represent a pathophysiological process contributing to male infertility (Table 17.6) [4,118–133].

Several groups have investigated WBC subpopulations in the semen of fertile and infertile men (Table 17.7) [121,125,126,134]. El-Demiry and colleagues used monoclonal antibodies (mAb) to characterize the lymphocyte subpopulations along

Table 17.6. Prevalence of leukocytospermia among infertile men

Reference	Detection method	Type of WBC	Threshold	Prevalence	n	Sperm parameters
Endtz, 1974 [118]	Peroxidase	PMN	0.5×10^6/mL	24%	300	Not investigated
Comhaire, 1980 [4]	Peroxidase	PMN	1×10^6/mL	13%	500	Not investigated
Jochum, 1986 [119]	PMN-elastase	PMN	1000 ng/mL	19%	163	No effects on sperm count and morphology
Wolff, 1988 [120]	PMN-elastase	PMN	1000 ng/mL	15%	118	Not investigated
Wolff, 1988 [121]	Immunohistology	All	1×10^6/mL	24%	118	Not investigated
Wolff, 1990 [122]	Immunohistology	All	1×10^6/mL	23%	179	↓Total sperm number, % motility, sperm velocity, motility index, total motile sperm
Gonzales, 1992 [123]	Giemsa/ Papanicoulau	All	1×10^6/mL	38%	280	↓Sperm count,[a] % motile sperm, % sperm vitality
Tomlinson, 1992 [124]	Immunohistology	All	1×10^6/mL	5%	351	Not associated with reduced semen quality or conception rates
Kung, 1993 [125]	Immunohistology	All	1×10^6/mL	2%	49	Inverse correlation to morph and motility
Tomlinson, 1993 [126]	Immunohistology	All	1×10^6/mL	3%	512	↑Ideal forms, ↓ head defects, ↓ oligospermia
Wang, 1994 [127]	Immunohistology	All	1×10^6/mL	8%	101	Not investigated
Yanushpolksy, 1995 [128]	Peroxidase	PMN	0.5×10^6/mL	11%	1710	↓Conc
			1×10^6/mL	7%		–
			2×10^6/mL	4%		↓Morph
Arata, 2000 [129]	Peroxidase	PMN	1×10^6/mL	32%	62	↓Conc, motility, HOS
Kaleli, 2000 [130]	Peroxidase	PMN	1×10^6/mL	72%	219	↑Conc, HOS, acrosome reaction
Sharma, 2001 [131]	Peroxidase	PMN	1×10^6/mL	9%	271	↑ROS
Saleh, 2002 [132]	Peroxidase	PMN	1×10^6/mL	33%	48	↑ROS, DNA damage, ↓motility
Aziz, 2004 [133]	Peroxidase	PMN	1×10^6/mL	36%	56	↓ Sperm structural integrity

Conc, concentration; DNA, deoxyribonucleic acid; HOS, hypo-osmotic swelling; Morph, morphology; PMN, polymorphonuclear leukocyte; ROS, reactive oxygen species; WBC, white blood cell.
[a] Only in the presence of hypofunctional seminal vesicles as assayed by fructose levels
(Adapted from Anderson DJ. The effect of genital tract infection and inflammation on male infertility. In: Lipshultz LI, Howards SS, eds. *Infertility in the Male*, 3rd edn. St. Louis, MO: Mosby Year Book, 1997: 326–35.)

the genital tract of normal men and men with infertility [135]. The authors demonstrated the presence of predominantly CD8+ suppressor/cytotoxic T cells in the epithelial lining of the prostate, seminal vesicle, vas deferens, and epididymis. While no lymphocytes were present in testis biopsies from normal men, all 10 testicular biopsies from infertile men demonstrated T lymphocytes between the fibrous tunica propria and the germinal epithelium of the seminiferous tubules.

Additionally, aggregates of leukocytes were seen in the interstitium of the testis. This suggests that in normal tissue, cellular mechanisms and an intact blood–testis barrier prevent immune responses to sperm antigens. Wolff and Anderson characterized leukocyte subpopulations (granulocytes, monocytes/macrophages, CD4+ T lymphocytes, CD8+ T lymphocytes, B lymphocytes) by mAb in the semen of 17 fertile and 51 infertile patients [121]. The study demonstrated that infertile

Table 17.7. WBC subpopulations in semen of fertile and infertile men

	Wolff, 1988 [121] Mean(±SEM)/ejaculate[a] n = 17 (fertile men)	Wolff, 1988 [121] Mean(±SEM)/ejaculate[a] n = 51 (infertile men)	Kung, 1993 [125] Mean(±SEM)/ejaculate[a] n = 16 (fertile men)	Kung, 1993 [125] Mean(±SEM)/ejaculate[a] n = 51 (infertile men)	Tomlinson, 1993 [126] Mean(±SEM)/mL n = 229 (infertile men)	Aitken, 1994 [134] Mean(±SEM)/mL n = 120[b] (infertile men)
Total WBC	1 636 365 (4 966 260)[c]	7 199 090 (19 612 917)	385 708 (343 191)[d]	385 513 (997 398)	132 800 (26 900)	391 900 (90 500)
Granulocyte	1 348 160 (4 799 149)[c]	5 407 075 (16 387 801)	261 562 (384 941)	343 159 (482 179)	67 000 (14 600)	396 900 (76 000)
Monocyte/macrophage	175 897 (288 476)	978 557 (1 788 724)	47 541 (146 258)	53 450 (137 152)	23 900 (3 200)	38 300 (20 100)
CD4+ T lymphocyte	9 205 (13 804)	155 505 (555 658)	52 066 (105 511)	52 020 (103 149)	940 (160)	60 600 (15 800)[e]
CD8+ T lymphocyte	6 250 (13 521)[c]	86 112 (211 047)	0 (0)	6 685 (26 637)	1170 (180)	
B lymphocyte	2 737 (6 869)	88 634 (415 199)	28 427 (57 44)	13 838 (46 811)	1620 (460)	37 700 (9 800)

WBC, white blood cells.

[a] WBC/ejaculate = ((WBC/field)/(sperm/field)) × (sperm/ejaculate).
[b] Further differentiation of WBC subtypes was performed in 91 patients.
[c] Wolff, 1988: significantly different between fertile and infertile groups by Kolmogorow–Smirnov test (P < 0.05).
[d] Kung, 1993: No difference in any WBC appreciated between fertile and infertile groups.
[e] Total T lymphocytes only, not CD4+ or CD8+ subpopulations.
(Adapted from Keck C et al. Seminal tract infections: impact on male fertility and treatment options. Hum Reprod Update. 1998; **4**: 891–903.)

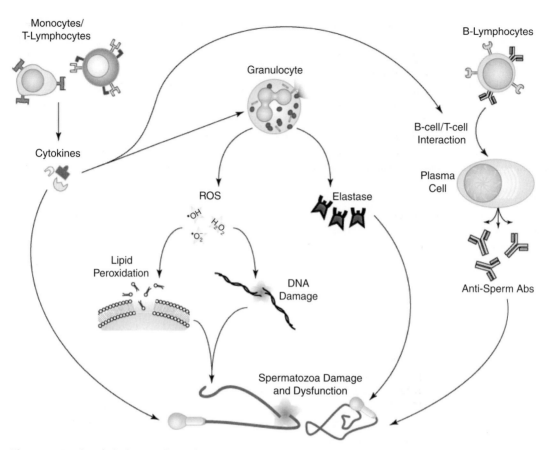

Fig. 17.2. Paradigm for leukocyte subpopulation interaction in infertile men with leukocytospermia.

men had significantly more seminal leukocytes than fertile men, with granulocytes representing the most prevalent subpopulation in both cases. Semen of infertile men also demonstrated significantly more granulocytes and CD8+ T lymphocytes. Finally, significantly more men in the infertile group than in the fertile group had leukocytospermia. **In total, these studies suggest that increased concentrations of leukocytes in the genital tract and semen are associated with infertility.** In Figure 17.2 we present a paradigm detailing the numerous mechanisms by which subpopulations of leukocytes can disrupt normal spermatogenesis and sperm function.

Several authors have noted a negative correlation between the presence of seminal leukocytes and other semen analysis parameters. Wolff and colleagues reported that infertile men with leukocytospermia (mAb) had significant reductions in total sperm number and parameters of motility (percent sperm motility, motility index, total motile sperm, and sperm

velocity) [122]. Furthermore, Arata et al. found that in semen of infertile men, leukocyte concentration (peroxidase) was negatively correlated with sperm morphology, motility, and hypo-osmotic swelling [129]. Other investigators have noted adverse effects of leukocytospermia on semen parameters only in the presence of seminal vesicle dysfunction (low fructose value corrected for sperm count) [123]. Aitken et al. noted that semen parameters were not negatively influenced by the presence of leukocytes; sperm function was only negatively impacted in washed sperm preparations contaminated by leukocytes. The authors postulated that these effects may be attributable to the antioxidative properties of seminal plasma, missing in the washed samples [134]. More recently, Aziz et al. demonstrated that infertile men with leukocytospermia (peroxidase) had worse sperm motility and morphology than both infertile men without leukocytospermia and fertile controls [133]. The authors also noted significant negative correlations between leukocyte concentration, percentage sperm motility, and various indices of morphology.

Several authors have reported adverse effects of leukocytes on the sperm penetration assay (SPA). Berger et al. first reported that the concentrations of leukocytes, granulocytes, and lymphocytes all correlated with abnormal SPA assay results (< 11% eggs penetrated) [136]. Maruyama et al. demonstrated that in fertile donors the human spermatozoa penetration of zona-free hamster oocytes decreased in the presence of the donors' own plasma-purified leukocytes [137]. Interestingly, in infertile patients with more than 3×10^6 leukocytes/mL, the penetration rates increased with the removal of seminal leukocytes. In contrast to these studies, Aitken et al. found no correlation between the concentration or total number of leukocytes and hamster oocyte penetration in men attending an infertility clinic [134]. However, as briefly mentioned above, leukocyte contamination of washed sperm preparations significantly decreased penetration, suggesting a protective role of seminal plasma.

Granulocyte concentration in semen has been specifically investigated, since granulocytes are the predominant leukocyte subset in fertile and infertile men with leukocytospermia [122,126,134,138,139]. Yanushpolsky and associates reported that in semen samples of 1710 male partners of infertile couples, granulocyte concentrations (peroxidase) greater than 5×10^5 cells/mL and 2×10^6 cells/mL were associated with significant differences in sperm concentration and morphology, respectively [140]. The authors also found a robust correlation between the number of granulocytes and the percent of samples with less than 10^7 motile sperm per ejaculate ($r = 0.94$, $P < 0.0001$). These results are corroborated by Thomas et al., who demonstrated that in 79 male patients attending a fertility clinic, seminal granulocyte concentrations (peroxidase) greater than 5×10^5 cells /mL and 1×10^6 cells/ mL were both associated with a significantly lower percentage normal sperm morphology than seminal granulocyte concentrations below these values [141]. The authors also noted a negative correlation between granulocyte concentration and normal morphology ($r = -0.27$, $P < 0.01$).

The clinical relevance of leukocytospermia in regard to male fertility is controversial, as other reports argue against detrimental effects of leukocytes on spermatozoa. In a study of 120 men attending an infertility clinic, Aitken et al. demonstrated that leukocytospermia (WHO) had no influence on sperm morphology, motility, oocyte penetration, or acrosome reaction [134]. In two separate studies, el-Demiry and colleagues demonstrated that semen of fertile men had higher concentrations of leukocytes and granulocytes than semen from sub/infertile men [138,139]. The authors suggest that leukocytes in the semen may represent both a nonspecific defense mechanism and a scavenging system for damaged, dead, and immature sperm. In a prospective study, Tomlinson et al. investigated the effects of leukocytes on seminal parameters and pregnancy outcomes in 229 patients with male-factor infertility [126]. The authors found that although granulocyte and macrophage concentration had modest negative correlations with the percentage of spermatozoa head defects ($r = -0.17$, $P < 0.001$, and $r = -0.15$, $P < 0.01$, respectively), these subpopulations and total leukocytes were not associated with motility or sperm density. In fact, leukocytes were positively correlated with percent "ideal forms" (morphology index). Furthermore, total granulocytes in semen were predictive of pregnancy (over a two-year period). These results are corroborated by Kaleli et al., who demonstrated a positive association between leukocyte concentration and sperm concentration and function [130]. In total, these findings suggest a potential protective role of leukocytes, especially granulocytes, in sperm quality.

Oxidative stress and reactive oxygen species

Oxidative stress is a fundamental pathophysiological process mediated by oxygen and oxygen derivatives known as reactive oxygen species (ROS). Prominent examples of ROS include hydroxyl peroxide, superoxide anion, hydroxyl radical, peroxyl radical, and the hypochlorite radical. ROS are classified as free radical molecules because they harbor an unpaired electron. They are inherently unstable and highly reactive. **ROS serve normal physiological roles in cellular messaging systems. However, in pathological states, the inherent reactivity of ROS overwhelms endogenous antioxidant systems and is the principal force mediating oxidative stress-induced cellular damage** [142]. This process is well documented in a variety of disease states, including cardiovascular, autoimmune, and infectious processes.

In the context of the testicular microenvironment, two cell populations are involved in the production of ROS: spermatozoa (especially damaged spermatozoa) and seminal leukocytes – most notably granulocytes [143–145]. Recently, immature spermatozoa within the ejaculates of male subjects were also shown to produce more ROS than mature spermatozoa. Some have suggested that this finding may adversely impact male fertility potential as the immature sperm migrate from the seminiferous tubules to the epididymis [146,147]. However, granulocytes are responsible for the majority of the ROS burden, contributing an estimated 10^3 greater magnitude than contributed by spermatozoa [148,149]. In regard to the pathogenesis of male-factor infertility, oxidative stress results in lipid peroxidation (LPO) of the sperm membrane with resultant membrane dysfunction and DNA damage.

Several studies have established that chemically induced oxidative stress results in LPO of the sperm membrane with abnormal changes in membrane composition, significant impairment in sperm motility, and disordered sperm–oocyte fusion [150–153]. ROS may decrease sperm motility through axonemal damage and depletion of ATP [154]. Furthermore, LPO appears to be significantly accelerated in damaged and defective spermatozoa [150,153]. Addition of seminal plasma, endogenous protective enzymes (superoxide dismutase, catalase), and antioxidants has been shown to inhibit subsequent damage by LPO and, in certain cases, to reverse LPO-induced dysfunction in vitro [150,153].

Similar results have been demonstrated using human spermatozoa incubated with ROS-producing activated human granulocytes [148,149,155]. Studies investigating semen samples from male patients undergoing infertility evaluations demonstrated significant associations between ROS production and impaired sperm function [143–145,150]. A prospective study by Aitken et al. revealed that ROS levels were negatively correlated to both sperm–oocyte fusion (zona-free hamster oocyte penetration test) and in-vivo fertility [156]. Zalata et al. demonstrated that in semen of infertile men, leukocytospermia (peroxidase) was positively correlated to oxidative stress ($r = 0.79$, $P < 0.001$) and negatively correlated to acrosin (enzyme involved in the acrosome reaction) activity ($r = -0.71$, $P < 0.001$) [157]. Overall, an inverse correlation between oxidative stress and acrosin activity was also reported ($r = -0.89$, $P < 0.001$). Most recently, in a retrospective study of 132 patients, Agarwal et al. demonstrated a significant association between ROS levels (10^4 cpm/20×10^6 sperm) and male-factor infertility (OR = 4.25, $P = 0.0034$) [158].

Several investigators have reported that leukocyte-induced oxidative stress is only associated with sperm dysfunction in washed spermatozoa preparations, which are devoid of seminal plasma [134,143]. This observation is supported by studies of infertile couples undergoing IVF in which leukocyte contamination of sperm preparations (i.e., lacking seminal plasma) resulted in elevated levels of ROS, decreased sperm motility, and decreased fertilization capacity [148,159]. Several lines of investigation demonstrate the protective role of seminal plasma against oxidative stress-induced sperm dysfunction [153,155]. The seminal plasma of infertile men also has lower levels of total antioxidant capacity, lower levels of individual antioxidants, and correspondingly higher levels of lipid peroxidation than seminal plasma from fertile controls [160–162].

As mentioned above, DNA damage results from oxidative stress and, in turn, decreases the genetic viability of spermatozoa. Kodama et al. demonstrated that spermatozoal DNA from infertile males demonstrated greater oxidative damage than controls [163]. This is corroborated by basic science data from an in-vitro study of NADPH-induced generation of ROS demonstrating increased sperm DNA fragmentation [164]. Both studies also revealed beneficial effects from in-vitro antioxidants on oxidative DNA damage, although each study had varying results depending on the antioxidant used and the source of the oxidative damage. As previously described, ROS production by immature spermatozoa may cause DNA damage in addition to increased LPO in mature spermatozoa during sperm migration [147,165]. Alvarez et al. examined male subjects with leukocytospermia and demonstrated a significant increase in sperm DNA damage versus healthy donors and patients without leukocytospermia [165]. Erenpreiss et al. also noted similar results, finding that semen from infertile men with leukocytospermia (peroxidase) and abnormal semen parameters was associated with increased DNA damage compared to semen from patients with leukocytospermia and normal semen parameters [166]. This growing body of literature suggests that leukocytospermia may increase DNA damage in infertile men via ROS.

Several studies have directly demonstrated the detrimental effects of leukocyte production of ROS on semen parameters and sperm function (Table 17.8) [131,132,134,143,165]. As mentioned previously, Aitken et al. demonstrated that leukocyte production of ROS inhibited oocyte fusion in sperm preparations devoid of seminal plasma in 120 male patients attending an infertility clinic [134]. Furthermore, in a

Table 17.8. Association of leukocyte concentration with reactive oxygen species production in semen of infertile men

Reference	n	Leukocyte detection method	ROS assay	Correlation between leukocytes and ROS	Relevant findings
Aitken, 1994 [134]	120	Immuno-histochemistry	Chemiluminescence	$r = 0.78$ ($P < 0.001$) in washed[a] sperm preparations contaminated by leukocytes	In patients attending an infertility clinic, leukocyte contamination of washed sperm preparations resulted in decreased oocyte penetration
Aitken, 1995 [143]	115	Immunohisto-chemistry	Chemiluminescence	$r = 0.729$ ($P < 0.001$) in intact semen samples $r = 0.840$ ($P < 0.001$) in washed sperm preparations	In infertile subjects, leukocyte-produced ROS were detected in *intact* human semen samples, but no significant correlations were noted between semen parameters (motility, morphology, sperm concentration and total count) or sperm function (penetration assays) and either ROS or leukocyte population. In infertile subjects, leukocytes in *washed* sperm preparations resulted in decreased sperm motility, increased ROS, and increased LPO versus controls
Sharma, 2001 [131]	271	Peroxidase test	ROS–TAC[b]	$r = -0.39$ ($P < 0.001$)	Oxidative stress increased with an increase in WBC count even when WBC was much less than 1×10^6/mL. Significant negative correlation between oxidative stress and sperm concentration, motility, and morphology
Saleh, 2002 [132]	48	Peroxidase test	ROS–TAC	$r = -0.56$ ($P < 0.001$)	Levels of spontaneous and induced ROS production in pure-sperm suspensions (free of leukocytes) from the infertile men with leukocytospermia were higher compared to infertile men without leukocytospermia and to control group
Alvarez, 2002 [165]	74	Peroxidase test	Chemiluminescence	$r^2 = 0.64$ ($P < 0.004$)[c]	In patients attending an infertility clinic, subjects with leukocytospermia demonstrated increased sperm DNA damage versus subjects without leukocytospermia or healthy donors

DNA, deoxyribonucleic acid; LPO, lipid peroxidation; ROS, reactive oxygen species; TAC, total antioxidant capacity; WBC, white blood cells.
[a] Free of seminal plasma.
[b] ROS–TAC inversely correlated to oxidative stress, accounts for a negative correlation to leukocytes compared to chemiluminescence.
[c] Spermatozoa at a certain stage of maturation isolated by density gradient centrifugation.

subsequent study by Aitken *et al.* of 66 infertile males and 49 healthy donors, the authors found that leukocyte production of ROS in unwashed semen samples was not correlated with seminal parameters or sperm function [143]. These results suggest that seminal plasma protects against leukocyte-produced ROS. It should be noted that these studies employed chemiluminescence to assay ROS. More recently, Sharma *et al.* introduced the reactive oxygen species–total antioxidant capacity (ROS–TAC) score, which measures sperm ROS and seminal TAC chemiluminescence as well [167]. The composite ROS–TAC values are inversely correlated with the level of oxidative stress. In a subsequent study employing ROS–TAC, Sharma et al. demonstrated a moderate correlation between the concentration of leukocytes (peroxidase) and ROS in 271 men attending an infertility clinic [131]. A similar study examining infertile men with and without leukocytospermia and healthy controls also noted a correlation between leukocyte concentration (peroxidase) and oxidative stress via ROS–TAC [132]. The authors noted that men with leukocytospermia had decreased sperm motility, presumably from LPO, and increased DNA damage – both supporting the concept of cellular injury arising from oxidative stress.

Leukocyte production of nitric oxide (NO) and other reactive nitrogen intermediates (RNI) constitutes another chemical mediator system studied in relation to sperm function. Spermatozoa are able to produce NO for physiological functions [168,169], but NO can also react with the superoxide anion forming the highly reactive peroxynitrite (ONOO) anion, resulting in cytotoxicity [170]. Toxicity from these molecules is believed to arise from inhibition of cellular aerobic respiration, and has been demonstrated in spermatozoa [171]. In-vitro studies revealed that incubating sperm with low concentrations (nM) of sodium nitroprusside (NO donor) enhanced sperm motility and viability and decreased LPO [172]. In contrast, high concentrations adversely affected sperm motility [124,171,173]. Sperm incubations with other NO donors support the deleterious effects of NO [171,173]. Nitrite is a stable end product of NO and has been used as an assay of NO production. Nobunaga et al. demonstrated that semen from infertile men with leukocytospermia (peroxidase) had significantly elevated levels of nitrite compared to semen from infertile men without leukocytospermia, and semen from fertile controls [174]. However, Revelli et al. reported that semen samples from men seen at a fertility clinic revealed no correlation between nitrite concentration and leukocyte concentration (anti-CD45 antibody) or sperm motility [175].

Elastase

As previously discussed, leukocytes in semen from infertile men may result in cellular spermatozoal damage through the release of ROS. Since granulocytes are the major constituent of seminal leukocytes, other mediators of granulocyte-induced cellular damage

may be present in the semen of infertile men with leukocytospermia.

Wolff et al. demonstrated that in 118 male patients with infertility, concentrations of granulocyte elastase were positively correlated to white blood cell (WBC) concentrations (measured by immunohistochemistry) ($r = 0.755$) [120]. These results were corroborated by studies finding elevated levels of granulocyte elastase in infertile men with leukocytospermia [176,177]. Furthermore, Rajasekaran et al. found that granulocyte elastase was not significantly elevated in infertile men without leukocytospermia compared to normal fertile controls, but was significantly elevated in infertile men with leukocytospermia compared to both of these other two groups. These results were verified in a subsequent study by the authors, with an even more rigid definition of leukocytospermia (2×10^6 leukocytes/mL) [178].

More recently, Zorn et al. found that granulocyte elastase in semen at a cutoff concentration of ≥ 290 ng/mL is an accurate predictor of leukocytospermia-associated genital tract inflammation (sensitivity 79.5%, specificity 74.4%) [179]. In findings similar to those of Wolff et al., the authors also noted a positive but less robust correlation between granulocyte-elastase concentration and leukocyte concentration in 312 infertile male patients ($r = 0.330$). Although Zorn et al. found no correlation between granulocyte elastase and ROS concentration, Henkel and Schill did find a positive correlation between these two parameters in a study of 176 men attending an infertility clinic ($r = 0.613$, $P < 0.0001$) [180]. Zorn et al. also demonstrated a negative correlation between granulocyte-elastase concentrations and sperm DNA damage ($r = -0.194$, $P = 0.024$) suggesting a possible unexpected protective role for granulocyte elastase [179]. No association was found between semen parameters and granulocyte-elastase concentrations. Interestingly, the authors also noted a higher concentration of granulocyte elastase in men whose female partners had tubal damage than in men whose female partners had no tubal damage.

Cytokines

Cytokines are the principle molecular signals of the immune system and are released by both lymphocytes and monocytes. Certain cytokines activate cellular proliferation and inflammatory mechanisms, ultimately resulting in oxidative stress, while others act in direct opposition to inflammation. If leukocytospermia results in increased oxidative stress, then a preponderance of increased pro-inflammatory and decreased anti-inflammatory cytokines with resulting impairment of sperm function should be appreciated. In fact, Hill *et al.* demonstrated that incubating spermatozoa with supernatant from activated peripheral blood leukocytes significantly decreased sperm motility [181].

Rajasekaran *et al.* noted that seminal plasma of infertile men with leukocytospermia (Papanicolaou stain and granulocyte-elastase assay) had significantly elevated levels of IL-2 and IL-8 compared to seminal plasma of infertile men without leukocytospermia and of fertile controls. IL-2 activates and induces proliferation of T-helper cell lymphocytes; this suggests a possible role for cell-mediated immunity. The authors also noted that IL-8 but not IL-2 was significantly related to ROS levels (chemiluminescence, $r = 0.704$). Since IL-8 is a granulocyte chemoattractant, these results strengthen the argument for leukocytospermia-induced ROS production. Other studies also demonstrated increased levels of IL-8 in infertile men with leukocytospermia (mostly granulocytes) [182,183]. Furthermore, Shimoya *et al.* demonstrated a significant correlation between and IL-8 and granulocyte-elastase levels ($r = 0.688, P < 0.001$).

Tumor necrosis factor α (TNF-α), IL-1, and IL-6 are all pro-inflammatory cytokines. TNF-α was found to be elevated in infertile men with leukocytospermia compared to infertile men without leukocytospermia [182,184] and fertile controls [184]. It should be noted that Maegawa *et al.* used granulocyte-elastase concentrations greater than 1000 ng/mL to define leukocytospermia, whereas Omu *et al.* used Papanicolaou staining and WHO criteria to measure and define leukocytospermia. Hill *et al.* reported that spermatozoa incubated with TNF-α and interferon γ demonstrated decreased motility [181]. Taken together, these studies suggest that TNF-α is elevated in infertile men with leukocytospermia, and that this elevation leads to impaired sperm function.

Several other investigators also noted increased concentrations of IL-6 in semen of men with leukocytospermia (fertility status unknown) [185] and infertile men [186] compared to those in fertile controls. Naz *et al.* showed that the elevation of IL-6 in infertile men was significantly correlated with detrimental effects on sperm number, motility, and penetration. Furthermore, IL-6 concentrations were demonstrated to be greater in infertile men with leukocytospermia than in fertile

controls and infertile men without leukocytospermia [187,188]. Comhaire *et al.* also noted that IL-1β concentrations were elevated in men with leukocytospermia when compared to those in controls [185]. Interestingly, TNF-α, IL-1α, and IL-1β were all shown to stimulate significant production of ROS by sperm from fertile donors in an in-vitro setting [189].

Not all pro-inflammatory cytokines contribute to fertility difficulties in males with leukocytospermia. Naz *et al.* reported higher levels of IL-12 in fertile men than in infertile men with leukocytospermia [190] and infertile men without leukocytospermia [190,191]. IL-12, which is released by activated macrophages, has no currently known role in leukocytospermia-associated infertility. However, other signaling molecules associated with monocyte activity, such as monocyte chemotactic and activating factor (MCAF) and tissue factor (TF), have been shown to be elevated in semen of infertile men with leukocytospermia when compared with semen of infertile men without leukocytospermia and with that of fertile controls [187,188].

Lastly, certain cytokines antagonize the inflammatory process and serve to regulate the immune response. Two such anti-inflammatory cytokines, IL-4 and IL-10, were demonstrated to be significantly lower in infertile men with and without leukocytospermia than in fertile controls [178,184].

The studies described suggest that pro-inflammatory cytokines are increased in infertile men with leukocytospermia and may impair sperm function, and they suggest an important role for both monocytes and lymphocytes in the pathophysiology of leukocytospermia. The release of cytokines from these cells activates the immune system, specifically triggering the proliferation and activation of T lymphocytes, B lymphocytes, granulocytes, and macrophages. Ultimately, a cascade of inflammatory changes leads to impaired sperm function.

Antisperm antibodies

Antisperm antibodies (ASA) are present in 3–12% of men seeking evaluation at infertility clinics. **ASA interfere with fertilization via several mechanisms: agglutination of sperm, prevention of cervical mucus penetration, and inhibition of sperm–oocyte interaction/fusion** [192]. Production of ASA is postulated to result from three basic changes in the affected patient: namely, the breakdown of the blood–testis barrier, inoculation of the host with sperm antigens, and failure of immunosuppression. Infections of the genital tract, such as acute and chronic prostatitis, are well-known risk factors for ASA generation [192]. However, the data regarding the risk associated with leukocytospermia are less well characterized.

Wolff *et al.* noted no association between leukocytospermia (mAb) and ASA in 179 infertile patients [122]. These results have been corroborated by subsequent studies [126,193,194]. Gonzalez *et al.* also demonstrated no overall association between leukocytospermia and ASA [195]. However, the authors did note that in the setting of seminal vesicle dysfunction, infertile patients with leukocytospermia had a significant increase in ASA compared with patients with leukocytospermia and normal seminal vesicle function and patients without leukocytospermia. This suggests a possible association between seminal vesicle function and immune regulation.

Paschke and colleagues demonstrated in a cohort of 1189 men evaluated for infertility that leukocytospermia (peroxidase) was significantly correlated to mixed agglutination reaction (MAR) IgG and IgA results [196]. Other studies have reported a high prevalence of ASA in infertile men with leukocytospermia [184,195]. Only Omu *et al.* distinguished between microbial and nonmicrobial (idiopathic) causes of leukocytospermia, and the authors noted a higher prevalence of ASA in men with microbial than in those with non-microbial leukocytospermia. Both groups had a higher prevalence of ASA than fertile controls.

More recently, Eggert-Kruse *et al.* demonstrated that IgA antibodies against human 60 kDa heat shock protein (HSP60) were significantly associated with leukocytospermia (mAb) [197]. Heat shock proteins are chaperone proteins that respond to environmental stress and represent a cellular injury response mechanism. Antibodies against HSP may result in sperm that are more susceptible to oxidative stress, thus potentially contributing to infertility. Although Eggert-Kruse *et al.* reported that the presence of anti-HSP60 antibodies was not associated with abnormal semen parameters or sperm function, HSPs may represent another target of leukocytospermia pathology. HSP impairment may not be detected on routine semen analysis or sperm function testing, but it may result in impaired intracellular responses to oxidative stress.

Humoral immunity mediated by T-helper and B lymphocytes (rather than granulocytes) drives the production of ASA, with B cells detected in 20–59% of semen samples of infertile patients [120,126]. In the testicular microenvironment, the release of cytokines such as IL-1, IL-2, and IL-6 (discussed above), together with T-helper cells, may activate and differentiate these localized B cells into plasma cells and induce production of ASA.

Detection of leukocytospermia

Currently, the WHO defines leukocytospermia as $\geq 1 \times 10^6$ WBCs/mL semen. This recommendation is derived from Comhaire's threshold of 1×10^6 peroxidase-positive leukocytes per mL semen for the diagnosis of male adnexitis (male accessory gland inflammation) [4]. Several tests available to identify and quantify seminal leukocytes are discussed below.

Histology/morphology

Round cell counts

The concept of "round cells" is important when considering leukocyte quantification. **Round cells refer to the similar morphology shared by both seminal WBCs and immature germ cells when viewed under phase microscopy.** In a study of 108 males of infertile couples, Eggert-Kruse *et al.* demonstrated that a majority of round cells were immature germ cells, while less than 5% were WBCs (range 0–58%, median 3%) [198]. Interestingly, Sigman and Lopes noted that in 627 men presenting for an infertility evaluation, leukocytospermia was present in 35% of semen samples with excessive round cells (> 10/hpf or 1×10^6/mL) [23]. The authors concluded that the majority of patients with excessive round cells do not have leukocytospermia. However, the two are not mutually exclusive. Quantification of round cells by phase microscopy alone is not an accurate method for the determination of leukocytospermia.

Bryan–Leishman

The Bryan–Leishman stain was developed by Couture *et al.* in 1976 [199]. Comparison of the Bryan–Leishman test with immunohistochemistry overestimates lymphocytes and underestimates granulocytes in semen smears [200].

Peroxidase/Endtz

The peroxidase test, or Endtz test, was first described by Endtz in 1974. This test stains for the peroxidase enzyme present in granulocytes and thus measures only this subpopulation of the WBCs [118]. Because granulocytes are typically the most prevalent WBC found in semen, the peroxidase test is clinically useful and recommended by the WHO for granulocyte detection [201].

In a study of 87 men undergoing an infertility evaluation and 25 controls, Potlich et al. demonstrated a robust correlation between peroxidase and immuno-histology for WBC enumeration ($r = 0.70$, $P < 0.0001$) [202]. However, the authors noted that WBC concentrations as measured by immunohistology were significantly higher than those measured by peroxidase testing. In fact, leukocytospermia was detected in 8.9% of samples assayed by peroxidase, whereas this number rose to 15.2% of samples when immunohistology was employed. Overall, the peroxidase test had a sensitivity of 58.8% and a specificity of close to 100% when compared to the "gold standard" of immunohistology.

Immunological techniques

Immunohistology

The "gold standard" for WBC detection and quantification is immunohistology. Immunohistology employs monoclonal antibodies (mAb) targeted against WBC surface markers [203]. For instance, antibodies directed against the common leukocyte antigen CD45 will detect granulocytes, macrophages, and lymphocytes. Additionally, mAb may be targeted against WBC sub-population-specific cell markers (e.g., CD15 detects granulocytes). Visualization methods of mAb-stained specimens often employ direct color contrasts between positive and negative cells (e.g., positive-red vs. negative-blue). Alternatively, immunofluorescence (mAb-stained cells emit a colored light) may be utilized [204]. Overall, immunohistology provides the most accurate means of leukocyte detection and quantification.

Flow cytometry

Flow cytometry, when used in conjunction with monoclonal antibodies, can provide rapid analysis of scant WBC subpopulations without purification procedures. Leukocytes, monocytes, and granulocytes are differentiated using the light-scatter properties of the WBCs and the density of the leukocyte marker antibody, CD45. CD45 has low affinity for granulocytes, higher affinity for monocytes, and the highest affinity for lymphocytes. Ricci et al. demonstrated a strong correlation between flow cytometry (using mAbs against CD45 and CD53) and the peroxidase test ($r = 0.619$, $P < 0.0001$) and the elastase test ($r = 0.542$, $P < 0.0001$). When compared with flow cytometry, the peroxidase test had 58.8% sensitivity and a 92.8% specificity in detecting leukocytospermia, while the elastase test had a 78.8% sensitivity and 75% specificity [205].

Products of leukocytes/inflammatory markers

Elastase

Granulocyte elastase is an enzyme specific to activated granulocytes, and it can be detected in fresh or frozen–thawed seminal plasma by immunoassay. Elastase levels are generally categorized into three groups: < 250 ng/mL = no inflammation; 250–1000 ng/mL = intermediate range; and > 1,000 ng/mL = genital tract inflammation [119]. Wolff et al. found that elastase detection using ELISA correlated strongly with immunohistochemical means of granulocyte detection [120]. Henkel et al. found a strong correlation between granulocyte elastase and ROS production ($r = 0.613$, $P = 0.0001$) [180]. Granulocyte-elastase assessment results in an objective measure of activated seminal granulocytes, but the large cost associated with using ELISA may deter its use. Furthermore, elastase indicates male adnexitis, and may therefore represent a better indicator of inflammation than seminal WBC counts.

Chemiluminescence

Chemiluminescence (CL) is an indirect method for leukocyte detection, as it quantifies leukocyte production of ROS. In its most basic form, CL involves a molecular probe (luminol), which emits light in the presence of ROS. A luminometer measures and quantifies this signal, which is proportional to the amount of ROS. Leino et al. demonstrated a high degree of correlation ($r = 0.932$, $P < 0.001$) between CL and peroxidase methods for WBC detection [206]. Limitations of this technique include the fact that CL is based on the metabolic products of viable cells only and the expense of a luminometer, which may preclude widespread use of this assay.

The above tests demonstrate the various methods of identifying leukocytospermia. The peroxidase test and granulocyte-elastase test appear to be useful screening methods for leukocytospermia detection. For more careful evaluation of leukocytospermia, immunohistochemistry is a highly accurate, but more timely and costly, method of leukocyte detection.

Treatment of leukocytospermia

Several treatment options exist to protect spermatozoa from the deleterious effects of leukocytes and therefore optimize semen quality. **The four major pharmacologic approaches are antimicrobial therapy to treat clinical or subclinical infection, anti-inflammatory medications (such as COX-2 inhibitors), antioxidant therapy to minimize associated oxidative stress, and antihistamines to stabilize mast cells.**

Antibiotics

A great deal of evidence supports the use of antibiotics to reduce leukocytospermia. In addition to treating infection, the goal of therapy is to restore sperm quality via an increase in sperm velocity, sperm number, percent motility, and total motile sperm. However, the use of antibiotics is not without risk. Many antibiotics have been implicated in negatively affecting fertility status. Nitrofurans, macrolides, aminoglycosides, tetracyclines, and sulfa drugs have all been linked to infertility. Schlegel *et al.* suggest that extrinsic factors, such as antibiotic use, may play a role in the 10–15% of couples demonstrating primary infertility [207].

Branigan *et al.* conducted a prospective cohort study of men experiencing unexplained infertility of at least one year's duration [208]. Using a Bryan–Leishman stain, the authors identified those patients with WHO-defined leukocytospermia. Subjects were then randomly assigned to either a nontreatment group or a treatment group receiving 100 mg doxycycline twice daily for seven days, followed by 100 mg once a day for 21 days. The female partner of each male was treated simultaneously with 100 mg doxycycline twice daily for five days, followed by 100 mg once a day for five more days. The males were advised to ejaculate frequently (at least every third day). The authors found a 53% pregnancy rate (over six months) in female partners of leukocytospermic men who were responsive to treatment. This pregnancy rate was significantly higher than that of leukocytospermic men who did not respond to treatment (6%), leukocytospermic men who did not receive treatment (6%), and even men without leukocytospermia (12%). No statistically significant differences in sperm concentration, sperm motility, or percent normal sperm morphology were seen between the men who responded to treatment and the other groups, either before or after therapy. The authors concluded that leukocytospermia that responds to antibiotic therapy is suggestive of a bacterial etiology [208], and this subgroup of leukocytospermic patients enjoys markedly improved pregnancy rates with antibiotic treatment.

Yamamoto *et al.* examined 263 males attending an infertility clinic. Of these patients, 48 co-expressed both > 10 WBCs/hpf on EPS and $> 1 \times 10^6$ WBCs/mL in semen [209]. These men then underwent randomization into either (1) no treatment, (2) trimethoprim 80 mg, sulfamethoxazole 400 mg orally twice per day, or (3) trimethoprim 80 mg, sulfamethoxazole 400 mg orally twice per day, plus instruction to ejaculate at least once every three days for a month. The baseline frequency of ejaculation for all patients before initiation of the study was 5 ± 1.3 times (range 2–10) per month. The authors found that after one month of treatment, 56% of men in group 2 and 76% of men in group 3 achieved resolution of their leukocytospermia, compared to only 6.7% in the group 1, the no-treatment group. Resolution was significantly higher for both treatment groups when compared to group 1 by chi-square analysis ($P < 0.05$ for group 2; $P < 0.01$ for group 3). While the authors reported an increase in frequency of ejaculation from 5 to 10 times per month for patients in group 3 during the treatment phase, they did not report any data on frequency of ejaculation for patients in either group 1 or group 2 during the treatment phase. Thus, frequency of ejaculation was not truly controlled for, which somewhat limits our ability to draw conclusions regarding this parameter.

Omu *et al.* examined the effects of antibiotics on semen parameters, seminal total antioxidant activity, vitamins A and E, T-helper cytokines, and ASA in infertile men with leukocytospermia (hematoxylin/eosin stain) and/or bacteriospermia [210]. Patients were identified as (1) leukocytospermic with seminal bacteria, (2) leukocytospermic without any seminal bacteria, and (3) fertile controls. Preceding treatment with antibiotics, sperm concentrations and sperm motility were significantly higher in fertile controls than in the two leukocytospermic groups. Also, total antioxidant activity was highest in the control group (3.2 ± 1.4 mmol/L), lower in the purely leukocytospermic group (1.7 ± 1.3), and lowest in the bacteriospermic and leukocytospermic group (1.1 ± 0.3). Likewise, inflammatory T-helper cytokines (IL-8 and IL-2) were significantly higher in men with bacteriospermia and leukocytospermia than in controls, while anti-inflammatory IL-4 was higher in controls. ASA were more prevalent in the group with bacteriospermia and leukocytospermia than in the group with leukocytospermia only. Patients in group 1 received antibiotic therapy, and following treatment the authors found significant improvement in sperm concentration and motility. Antibiotic therapy also improved total antioxidant activity ($P < 0.02$) and reduced IL-2 ($P < 0.03$) and IL-8 ($P < 0.05$) levels, but increased IL-4 ($P < 0.01$). No differences in ASA levels were found. The authors concluded that antibiotic therapy benefits affected patients by reducing pro-inflammatory cytokines and oxidative stress.

Though these trials do show beneficial effects of antibiotics on the resolution of leukocytospermia, improvement in semen parameters, and increased pregnancy rates, some important points should be noted. The trials used basic histology, not peroxidase or mAb staining methods, to identify leukocytes. Also, the etiology of leukocytospermia is of importance (i.e., infection, abacterial, autoimmunity). Branigan et al. did not distinguish between men with or without bacteriospermia, while Omu et al. treated only those with leukocytospermia and bacteriospermia and not those with leukocytospermia alone.

Yanushpolsky et al. conducted a prospective randomized controlled study of leukocytospermic males and their partners who together had experienced unexplained infertility and no evidence of genital infection [128]. Identification of leukocytospermia was conducted in accordance with WHO standards using peroxidase testing. Subjects were randomly assigned to groups in which: (1) patients and their partners received 100 mg oral dose of doxycycline twice per day for 14 days, (2) patients and their partners received trimethoprim 160 mg/sulfamethoxazole 800 mg orally twice per 14 days, or (3) patients received no therapy. The authors demonstrated no statistically significant differences in the WBC count between the two groups treated with antibiotics. Furthermore, Yanushpolsky et al. found that semen parameters did not statistically improve after antibiotic treatment; this led the authors to conclude that antibiotic treatment does not provide benefit to asymptomatic leukocytospermic males.

Erel et al. conducted a randomized controlled trial of 70 male partners of infertile couples [211]. After detection of leukocytospermia ($> 1 \times 10^6$ WBCs/mL) by peroxidase staining, subjects were randomly assigned to one of three groups: (1) a placebo group, (2) a group that received 100 mg of doxycycline twice a day for 10 days, and (3) a group that received 100 mg of doxycycline twice a day for 10 days plus two injections of 0.5 g ceftriaxone intramuscularly. The authors found no statistically significant differences between the three groups for age, duration of infertility, sperm concentration, sperm motility, or sperm morphology at baseline. Following treatment, groups 2 and 3 had statistically significant reduction of WBC counts compared to baseline. However, there was no statistical difference in the resolution of leukocytospermia cases between treatment groups and the control group over a four-week period. Furthermore, antibiotic treatment did not improve sperm concentration, motility, or

morphology. This suggests that while antibiotics may help improve seminal WBC concentrations, the treatments do not lead to improved semen parameters in asymptomatic leukocytospermic males.

The studies by Yanushpolsky et al. and Erel et al. both employed peroxidase staining of leukocytes and were structured as randomized controlled trials. Overall, these two studies demonstrate better methodology than the studies advocating the use of antibiotics. Furthermore, the choice of antibiotics is another important issue that must be considered when reviewing these studies. Most of the above trials employed a predetermined, empiric treatment regimen, whereas Omu et al. used culture sensitivities to guide therapy. **In summary, the efficacy of antibiotic treatment for isolated leukocytospermia remains in question.**

COX-2 inhibitors

Recently, Lackner et al. conducted a prospective non-randomized study examining the use of cyclooxygenase-2 (COX-2) inhibitors in 12 patients with abacterial leukocytospermia [212]. COX-2 inhibitors are anti-inflammatory medications that inhibit prostaglandin production. The patients were treated with valdecoxib 20 mg/day for two weeks. Following treatment, the authors found a reduction in leukocyte concentration from 5.5×10^6 WBCs/mL (interquartile range 3.3–6.8) to 1.0×10^6 WBCs/mL (interquartile range 0.3–2.0) ($P < 0.001$). Furthermore, sperm count was significantly increased, though motility and morphology did not improve. **Though the study was small, these results suggest a beneficial role for COX-2 inhibitors in patients with abacterial leukocytospermia.**

Antioxidants

Vicari et al. conducted a prospective study of men with chronic, abacterial prostatovesiculoepididymitis (PVE) [213]. Concurrently, subjects were also experiencing infertility of a median duration of seven years, as well as persistent leukocytospermia according to WHO standards. Subjects were randomly assigned to one of four groups: (1) carnitine therapy for four months, (2) nonsteroidal anti-inflammatory drugs (NSAIDs) for four months, (3) NSAIDS for two months followed by carnitine therapy for two months, and (4) NSAIDs simultaneously with carnitines for four months. Following treatment, the authors demonstrated improved sperm viability (%) and reduced seminal leukocyte concentration in all groups compared with pretreatment values. Interestingly, group 3 not only had the highest percentage of viable sperm but was also the only treatment group to demonstrate significantly increased forward motility (%). These effects observed in group 3 were complemented by the highest reduction of ROS production. Concomitant use of carnitines alongside NSAIDs in group 4 was less effective at reducing ROS. Lastly, and perhaps most importantly, group 3 had the highest pregnancy rate ($P < 0.01$). **While the literature regarding carnitine use in male infertility has been disappointing overall, this study suggests the use of carnitine following pretreatment with NSAIDs helps to optimize semen parameters, possibly by decreasing ROS. Additional studies need to be undertaken to corroborate the above findings.**

Antihistamines

Recently, Olivia and Multigner conducted an open, noncontrolled study of 55 men identified as having leukocytospermia ($> 1 \times 10^6$ WBCs/mL) by Giemsa staining [214]. After a 12-week course of ketotifen, these men were found to have reduced seminal WBC counts. Ketotifen is an antihistamine-like drug with mast cell stabilizing effects that inhibits WBC degranulation and the release of inflammatory mediators. After four weeks of ketotifen at 1 mg twice a day, the authors reported a reduction of WBCs from 5×10^6 WBCs/mL (interquartile range 2–6) to 0 WBCs/mL ($P < 0.0001$). Following therapy, sperm motility and sperm morphology significantly improved from pretreatment values. Olivia and Multigner did not find any differences between seminal volume, sperm concentration, and sperm count from ketotifen treatment after the 12-week therapy.

Spinal cord injury and leukocytospermia

Every year there are approximately 10 000 new cases of spinal cord injury (SCI) in the United States; the majority of victims are males in their reproductive years [215]. SCI results in impaired sexual function and fertility due to erectile dysfunction, ejaculatory dysfunction, and poor semen quality. **Regardless of the level and extent of SCI, semen analyses of male patients with SCI generally demonstrate normal sperm count with decreased motility and viability [216,217]. Though considerable debate exists as to the etiology of sperm impairment, the observed adverse changes are likely multifactorial and secondary to stasis of semen/sperm, scrotal hyperthermia, UTIs, ejaculatory reflux of urine, SCI-related testicular atrophy, SCI-related hypothalamic–pituitary–gonadal axis**

dysfunction, abnormal semen composition, and leukocytospermia [218].

Aird et al. compared the semen of nine men with chronic SCI (> 1 year) obtained via electroejaculation (both antegrade and retrograde) to semen from healthy donors [219]. Using monoclonal antibodies against leukocytes, the authors concluded that the increased percentage of leukocytes in semen of males with SCI was the result of concomitant UTIs, especially in retrograde samples. Furthermore, impairment of motility was not correlated with the number of leukocytes. Finally, granulocytes and macrophages were the predominant leukocyte subtypes, and the proportion of leukocytes in the semen of males with SCI was not related to level, extent, or duration of SCI. It should be appreciated that quality of retrograde semen samples is considered inferior to that of antegrade samples [220,221]. In a similar study, Trabulsi et al. compared antegrade semen samples (electroejaculation) of 17 males with SCI free of UTIs to age-matched controls [222]. The authors reported that the semen of men with SCI had significantly elevated total WBC-to-sperm ratios, granulocyte-to-sperm ratios, and macrophage-to-sperm ratios compared to semen of the control population. While this study demonstrated increased leukocytes in the semen of male SCI patients in the absence of UTI, the effects of increased leukocytes on semen parameters and sperm function were not assessed. Basu et al. also examined antegrade semen samples from 12 male patients with SCI free of UTIs compared with samples from eight healthy age-matched controls [223]. Unlike investigators in the previous studies, the authors used penile vibratory stimulation, not electroejaculation, for semen collection in men with SCI. Electroejaculation has been associated with decreased semen quality [217,220]. Flow cytometry was employed to detect seminal leukocytes. The authors found similar sperm concentrations in both groups, but impaired sperm motility and viability in the semen of men with SCI when compared with that of controls. Men with SCI also had significantly increased leukocytes, which were predominantly activated T-helper lymphocytes. Mature granulocytes were also significantly elevated in the semen of men with SCI.

As mentioned previously in this chapter, leukocyte-induced damage of sperm may be mediated by ROS. Interestingly, de Lamirande et al. demonstrated that men with SCI have higher levels of seminal ROS than infertile men without SCI and healthy controls [154].

Furthermore, there was an inverse correlation between percentage motility and ROS in men with SCI. These data are corroborated by Padron et al., who demonstrated that men with SCI had decreased sperm motility, impaired sperm morphology, increased seminal leukocytes (peroxidase test), and elevated ROS (chemiluminescence) when compared with healthy controls [224]. The levels of seminal ROS in men with SCI were also negatively correlated with sperm motility ($r = -0.46$ to -0.49, $P = 0.02$). Together, these studies suggest an important role for ROS in leukocyte-mediated sperm damage in men with SCI.

Collectively, the studies suggest that abnormal concentrations of leukocytes are a common finding in the semen of men with SCI. While the etiology of leukocytospermia is unclear in these men, the elevated concentration of WBCs may have a detrimental effect on sperm motility and viability through the production of ROS. Recently, Randall et al. reported that the prostates of men with both SCI and leukocytospermia do not harbor increased inflammatory changes, suggesting that the prostate is not the source of seminal leukocytes [225]. Indeed, other genital tract changes related to SCI may be driving the leukocyte response.

Prostatitis, male infertility, and leukocytospermia

The effect of prostatitis on male fertility is controversial. Much of this confusion is due to different classification systems and methods of diagnosis employed in various studies. Prior to the NIH classification system, several studies demonstrated decreased semen parameters in men with CP/CPPS. Christiansen et al. reported decreased sperm concentration, motility, morphology, and viability, and increased incidence of leukocytospermia, in men with chronic abacterial prostatovesiculitis versus controls ($P < 0.001$) [226]. However, leukocytospermia was not predictive of abnormal semen quality. These data are corroborated by Lieb et al., who also noted decreased sperm motility and morphology, and increased WBC concentration (Giemsa stain), in patients with CP/CPPS (NBP and Pd) versus controls ($P < 0.05$) [227]. In comparison to Leib, Krieger et al. examined differences in semen parameters between patients with NBP and Pd. The authors only noted decreased sperm motility in patients with NBP versus those with Pd [228]. Conversely, Weidner et al. did not report a difference in semen parameters among patients with CBP, NBP, Pd, or controls.

However, patients with CBP and NBP had significantly increased leukocytes (peroxidase) [229] ($P < 0.001$).

Since the introduction of the NIH classification, several authors have revisited this topic. Much of this research has focused on type III prostatitis or CP/CPPS. Pasqualotto et al. demonstrated that men with type III prostatitis had elevated seminal oxidative stress (ROS–TAC) versus controls [230]. Furthermore, sperm motility was impaired only in type III patients with leukocytospermia (peroxidase). Menkveld et al. demonstrated no difference in sperm concentration, motility, viability, and WHO morphology criteria between patients with type III prostatitis and controls [231]. However, further morphological investigation demonstrated that men with type IIIA had significantly elevated, elongated spermatozoal forms compared to those of controls. Taken together, elevated oxidative stress secondary to prostatic inflammation may be one mechanism for prostatitis-associated infertility. This is especially relevant for type IIIA prostatitis. However, Ludwig et al. found no association between leukocytospermia (peroxidase) and impaired semen parameters in men with type III prostatitis [176]. A more recent study by Motrich et al. suggests that an autoimmune response to prostatic antigens may result in infertility in men with type III prostatitis [232]. Further research is needed to delineate the relationship between CP/CPPS and male infertility.

Conclusion

In this chapter, we set out to provide a state-of-the-art overview of the impact of inflammation and infection on male reproductive function. The complex relationship between infection, inflammation, and male fertility has been incompletely elucidated to date. The literature clearly demonstrates that many organisms are pathogenic to male reproduction, sometimes rendering men severely and permanently debilitated in terms of fertility potential. Numerous studies have also shown that monocyte and T-lymphocyte release of cytokines stimulates B-cell production of ASA and granulocyte production of ROS and elastase, with detrimental effects on semen quality and sperm function. Patients with infection and inflammation of the genital tract are quite heterogeneous in terms of underlying etiologies and responses to therapy. While many excellent studies describing treatment outcomes with various therapies have been reported in this chapter, additional prospective, randomized clinical trials with clearly defined patient populations are needed to help clarify which treatments are truly beneficial and cost-effective.

References

[1] Bar-Chama N, Goluboff E, Fisch H. Infection and pyospermia in male infertility: is it really a problem? *Urol Clin North Am* 1994; **21**: 469–75.

[2] Anderson DJ. The effect of genital tract infection and inflammation on male infertility. In: Lipshultz LI, Howards SS, eds. *Infertility in the Male*, 3rd edn. St. Louis, MO: Mosby Year Book, 1997: 326–35.

[3] Keck C, Gerber-Schafer C, Clad A, Wilhelm C, Breckwoldt M. Seminal tract infections: impact on male fertility and treatment options. *Hum Reprod Update* 1998; **4**: 891–903.

[4] Comhaire F, Verschraegen G, Vermeulen L. Diagnosis of accessory gland infection and its possible role in male infertility. *Int J Androl* 1980; **3**: 32–45.

[5] Moskowitz MO, Mellinger BC. Sexually transmitted diseases and their relation to male infertility. *Urol Clin North Am* 1992; **19**: 35–45.

[6] Cottell E, Harrison RF, McCaffrey M, *et al.* Are seminal fluid microorganisms of significance or merely contaminants? *Fertil Steril* 2000; **74**: 465–70.

[7] Jennings MG, McGowan MP, Baker HW. Is conventional bacteriology useful in the management of male infertility? *Clin Reprod Fertil* 1986; **4**: 359–66.

[8] Krieger JN. Prostatitis, epididymitis, and orchitis. In: Mandell G, Bennett J, Dolin R, eds. *Mandell, Douglas, and Bennett's Principles of Infectious Disease*, 6th edn. Philadelphia, PA: Churchill-Livingstone, 2005: Section L, Chapter 105.

[9] Schiefer HG. Microbiology of male urethroadnexitis: diagnostic procedures and criteria for aetiologic classification. *Andrologia* 1998; 30 (Suppl) **1**: 7–13.

[10] Weidner W, Krause W, Ludwig M. Relevance of male accessory gland infection for subsequent fertility with special focus on prostatitis. *Hum Reprod Update* 1999; **5**: 421–32.

[11] Berger R, Lee JC. Sexually transmitted diseases: the classic diseases. In: Walsh PC, Retik AB, Vaughan ED, Wein AJ, eds. *Campbell's Urology*, 8th edn. Philadelphia, PA: Saunders, 2002: 1, 671–87.

[12] Drach GW, Fair WR, Meares EM, Stamey TA. Classification of benign diseases associated with prostatic pain: prostatitis or prostatodynia? *J Urol* 1978; **120**: 266.

[13] Krieger JN, Nyberg L, Nickel JC. NIH consensus definition and classification of prostatitis. *JAMA* 1999; **282**: 236–7.

[14] Hua VN, Schaeffer AJ. Acute and chronic prostatitis. *Med Clin North Am* 2004; **88**: 483–94.

[15] Nickel JC, Moon T. Chronic bacterial prostatitis: an evolving clinical enigma. *Urology* 2005; **66**: 2–8.

[16] Corrao G, Zambon A, Bertu L, *et al.* Evidence of tendinitis provoked by fluoroquinolone treatment: A case-control study. *Drug Saf* 2006; **29**: 889–96.

[17] Nickel JC, Downey J, Johnston B, Clark J. Predictors of patient response to antibiotic therapy for the chronic prostatitis/chronic pelvic pain syndrome: a prospective multicenter clinical trial. *J Urol* 2001; **165**: 1539–44.

[18] Rosenstein D, McAninch JW. Urologic emergencies. *Med Clin North Am* 2004; **88**: 495–518.

[19] Burgher SW. Acute scrotal pain. *Emerg Med Clin North Am* 1998; **16**: 781–809.

[20] Berger RE, Alexander ER, Harnisch JP, *et al.* Etiology, manifestations and therapy of acute epididymitis: prospective study of 50 cases. *J Urol* 1979; **121**: 750–4.

[21] Weidner W, Garbe C, Weissbach L, *et al.* Initial therapy of acute unilateral epididymitis using ofloxacin. II. Andrological findings. *Urologe A* 1990; **29**: 277–80.

[22] McCormick WM, Rein MF. Prostatitis, epididymitis, and orchitis. In: Mandell G, Bennett J, Dolin R, eds. *Mandell, Douglas, and Bennett's Principles of Infectious Disease*, 6th edn. Philadelphia, PA: Churchill-Livingstone, 2005.

[23] Sigman M, Lopes L. The correlation between round cells and white blood cells in the semen. *J Urol* 1993; **149**: 1338–40.

[24] Harnisch JP, Berger RE, Alexander ER, Monda G, Holmes KK. Aetiology of acute epididymitis. *Lancet* 1977; **1**: 819–21.

[25] Handsfield HH, Lipman TO, Harnisch JP, Tronca E, Holmes KK. Asymptomatic gonorrhea in men: diagnosis, natural course, prevalence and significance. *N Engl J Med* 1974; **290**: 117–23.

[26] Trum JW, Mol BW, Pannekoek Y, *et al.* Value of detecting leukocytospermia in the diagnosis of genital tract infection in subfertile men. *Fertil Steril* 1998; **70**: 315–19.

[27] Litvin YS, Nagler H. Infertility and genitourinary infections. *Infect Urol* 1992; **5**: 104–7.

[28] Karam GH, Martin DH, Flotte TR, *et al.* Asymptomatic Chlamydia trachomatis infections among sexually active men. *J Infect Dis* 1986; **154**: 900–3.

[29] Paavonen J, Eggert-Kruse W. Chlamydia trachomatis: impact on human reproduction. *Hum Reprod Update* 1999; **5**: 433–47.

[30] Hosseinzadeh S, Brewis IA, Pacey AA, Moore HD, Eley A. Coincubation of human spermatozoa with Chlamydia trachomatis in vitro causes increased tyrosine phosphorylation of sperm proteins. *Infect Immun* 2000; **68**: 4872–6.

[31] Hosseinzadeh S, Brewis IA, Eley A, Pacey AA. Co-incubation of human spermatozoa with Chlamydia trachomatis serovar E causes premature sperm death. *Hum Reprod* 2001; **16**: 293–9.

[32] Eley A, Hosseinzadeh S, Hakimi H, Geary I, Pacey AA. Apoptosis of ejaculated human sperm

is induced by co-incubation with Chlamydia trachomatis lipopolysaccharide. *Hum Reprod* 2005; **20**: 2601–7.

[33] Hosseinzadeh S, Pacey AA, Eley A. Chlamydia trachomatis-induced death of human spermatozoa is caused primarily by lipopolysaccharide. *J Med Microbiol* 2003; **52**: 193–200.

[34] Custo GM, Lauro V, Saitto C, Frongillo RF. Chlamydial infection and male infertility: an epidemiological study. *Arch Androl* 1989; **23**: 243–8.

[35] Wolff H, Neubert U, Zebhauser M, *et al.* Chlamydia trachomatis induces an inflammatory response in the male genital tract and is associated with altered semen quality. *Fertil Steril* 1991; **55**: 1017–19.

[36] Cengiz T, Aydoganli L, Baykam M, *et al.* Chlamydial infections and male infertility. *Int Urol Nephrol* 1997; **29**: 687–93.

[37] Witkin SS, Kligman I, Bongiovanni AM. Relationship between an asymptomatic male genital tract exposure to Chlamydia trachomatis and an autoimmune response to spermatozoa. *Hum Reprod* 1995; **10**: 2952–5.

[38] Munoz MG, Witkin SS. Autoimmunity to spermatozoa, asymptomatic Chlamydia trachomatis genital tract infection and gamma delta T lymphocytes in seminal fluid from the male partners of couples with unexplained infertility. *Hum Reprod* 1995; **10**: 1070–4.

[39] Close CE, Wang SP, Roberts PL, Berger RE. The relationship of infection with Chlamydia trachomatis to the parameters of male fertility and sperm autoimmunity. *Fertil Steril* 1987; **48**: 880–3.

[40] Nagy B, Corradi G, Vajda Z, Gimes R, Csomor S. The occurrence of Chlamydia trachomatis in the semen of men participating in an IVF programme. *Hum Reprod* 1989; **4**: 54–6.

[41] Ruijs GJ, Kauer FM, Jager S, *et al.* Is serology of any use when searching for correlations between Chlamydia trachomatis infection and male infertility? *Fertil Steril* 1990; **53**: 131–6.

[42] Soffer Y, Ron-El R, Golan A, *et al.* Male genital mycoplasmas and Chlamydia trachomatis culture: its relationship with accessory gland function, sperm quality, and autoimmunity. *Fertil Steril* 1990; **53**: 331–6.

[43] Bjercke S, Purvis K. Chlamydial serology in the investigation of infertility. *Hum Reprod* 1992; **7**: 621–4.

[44] Dieterle S, Mahony JB, Luinstra KE, Stibbe W. Chlamydial immunoglobulin IgG and IgA antibodies in serum and semen are not associated with the presence of Chlamydia trachomatis DNA or rRNA in semen from male partners of infertile couples. *Hum Reprod* 1995; **10**: 315–19.

[45] Eggert-Kruse W, Buhlinger-Gopfarth N, Rohr G, *et al.* Antibodies to chlamydia trachomatis in semen and

relationship with parameters of male fertility. *Hum Reprod* 1996; **11**: 1408–17.

[46] Eggert-Kruse W, Rohr G, Demirakca T, *et al.* Chlamydial serology in 1303 asymptomatic subfertile couples. *Hum Reprod* 1997; **12**: 1464–75.

[47] Habermann B, Krause W. Altered sperm function or sperm antibodies are not associated with chlamydial antibodies in infertile men with leucocytospermia. *J Eur Acad Dermatol Venereol* 1999; **12**: 25–9.

[48] Eggert-Kruse W, Rohr G, Kunt B, *et al.* Prevalence of Chlamydia trachomatis in subfertile couples. *Fertil Steril* 2003; **80**: 660–3.

[49] Hosseinzadeh S, Eley A, Pacey AA. Semen quality of men with asymptomatic chlamydial infection. *J Androl* 2004; **25**: 104–9.

[50] Mardh PA, Colleen S, Sylwan J. Inhibitory effect on the formation of chlamydial inclusions in McCoy cells by seminal fluid and some of its components. *Invest Urol* 1980; **17**: 510–13.

[51] Moss TR, Darougar S, Woodland RM, *et al.* Antibodies to Chlamydia species in patients attending a genitourinary clinic and the impact of antibodies to C. pneumoniae and C. psittaci on the sensitivity and the specificity of C. trachomatis serology tests. *Sex Transm Dis* 1993; **20**: 61–5.

[52] Black CM. Current methods of laboratory diagnosis of Chlamydia trachomatis infections. *Clin Microbiol Rev* 1997; **10**: 160–84.

[53] Gnarpe H, Friberg J. Mycoplasma and human reproductive failure. I. The occurrence of different Mycoplasmas in couples with reproductive failure. *Am J Obstet Gynecol* 1972; **114**: 727–31.

[54] Fowlkes DM, MacLeod J, O'Leary WM. T-mycoplasmas and human infertility: correlation of infection with alterations in seminal parameters. *Fertil Steril* 1975; **26**: 1212–18.

[55] Upadhyaya M, Hibbard BM, Walker SM. The effect of Ureaplasma urealyticum on semen characteristics. *Fertil Steril* 1984; **41**: 304–8.

[56] Naessens A, Foulon W, Debrucker P, Devroey P, Lauwers S. Recovery of microorganisms in semen and relationship to semen evaluation. *Fertil Steril* 1986; **45**: 101–5.

[57] Kalugdan T, Chan PJ, Seraj IM, King A. Polymerase chain reaction enzyme-linked immunosorbent assay detection of mycoplasma consensus gene in sperm with low oocyte penetration capacity. *Fertil Steril* 1996; **66**: 793–7.

[58] de Louvois J, Blades M, Harrison RF, Hurley R, Stanley VC. Frequency of mycoplasma in fertile and infertile couples. *Lancet* 1974; **1**: 1073–5.

[59] Harrison RF, de Louvois J, Blades M, Hurley R. Doxycycline treatment and human infertility. *Lancet* 1975; **1**: 605–7.

[60] Desai S, Cohen S, Khatamee M, Leiter E. Ureaplasma urealyticum (T-mycoplasma) infection: does it have a role in male infertility? *J Urol* 1980; **124**: 469–71.

[61] Cintron RD, Wortham JW, Acosta A. The association of semen factors with the recovery of Ureaplasma urealyticum. *Fertil Steril* 1981; **36**: 648–52.

[62] Lewis RW, Harrison RM, Domingue GJ. Culture of seminal fluid in a fertility clinic. *Fertil Steril* 1981; **35**: 194–8.

[63] Shalhoub D, Abdel-Latif A, Fredericks CM, Mathur S, Rust PF. Physiological integrity of human sperm in the presence of Ureaplasma urealyticum. *Arch Androl* 1986; **16**: 75–80.

[64] de Jong Z, Pontonnier F, Plante P, Perie N, Talazac N, Mansat A, Chabanon G. Comparison of the incidence of Ureaplasma urealyticum in infertile men and in donors of semen. *Eur Urol* 1990; **18**: 127–31.

[65] Ombelet W, Bosmans E, Janssen M, *et al.* Semen parameters in a fertile versus subfertile population: a need for change in the interpretation of semen testing. *Hum Reprod* 1997; **12**: 987–93.

[66] Swenson CE, Toth A, O'Leary WM. Ureaplasma urealyticum and human infertility: the effect of antibiotic therapy on semen quality. *Fertil Steril* 1979; **31**: 660–5.

[67] Toth A, Lesser ML, Brooks C, Labriola D. Subsequent pregnancies among 161 couples treated for T-mycoplasma genital-tract infection. *N Engl J Med* 1983; **308**: 505–7.

[68] Rose BI, Scott B. Sperm motility, morphology, hyperactivation, and ionophore-induced acrosome reactions after overnight incubation with mycoplasmas. *Fertil Steril* 1994; **61**: 341–8.

[69] Nunez-Calonge R, Caballero P, Redondo C, *et al.* Ureaplasma urealyticum reduces motility and induces membrane alterations in human spermatozoa. *Hum Reprod* 1998; **13**: 2756–61.

[70] Reichart M, Kahane I, Bartoov B. In vivo and in vitro impairment of human and ram sperm nuclear chromatin integrity by sexually transmitted Ureaplasma urealyticum infection. *Biol Reprod* 2000; **63**: 1041–8.

[71] Busolo F, Zanchetta R, Bertoloni G. Mycoplasmic localization patterns on spermatozoa from infertile men. *Fertil Steril* 1984; **42**: 412–17.

[72] Fowlkes DM, Dooher GB, O'Leary WM. Evidence by scanning electron microscopy for an association between spermatozoa and T-mycoplasmas in men of infertile marriage. *Fertil Steril* 1975; **26**: 1203–11.

[73] Busolo F, Zanchetta R. The effect of Mycoplasma hominis and Ureaplasma urealyticum on hamster egg in vitro penetration by human spermatozoa. *Fertil Steril* 1985; **43**: 110–14.

[74] Potts JM, Sharma R, Pasqualotto F, *et al.* Association of Ureaplasma urealyticum with abnormal reactive oxygen species levels and absence of leukocytospermia. *J Urol* 2000; **163**: 1775–8.

[75] Kanakas N, Mantzavinos T, Boufidou F, Koumentakou I, Creatsas G. Ureaplasma urealyticum in semen: is there any effect on in vitro fertilization outcome? *Fertil Steril* 1999; **71**: 523–7.

[77] Montagut JM, Lepretre S, Degoy J, Rousseau M. Ureaplasma in semen and IVF. *Hum Reprod* 1991; **6**: 727–9.

[77] Shalika S, Dugan K, Smith RD, Padilla SL. The effect of positive semen bacterial and Ureaplasma cultures on in-vitro fertilization success. *Hum Reprod* 1996; **11**: 2789–92.

[78] Blanchard A, Hentschel J, Duffy L, Baldus K, Cassell GH. Detection of Ureaplasma urealyticum by polymerase chain reaction in the urogenital tract of adults, in amniotic fluid, and in the respiratory tract of newborns. *Clin Infect Dis* 1993; 17 (Suppl) **1**: S148–53.

[79] Teng K, Li M, Yu W, Li H, Shen D, Liu D. Comparison of PCR with culture for detection of Ureaplasma urealyticum in clinical samples from patients with urogenital infections. *J Clin Microbiol* 1994; **32**: 2232–4.

[80] Povlsen K, Jensen JS, Lind I. Detection of Ureaplasma urealyticum by PCR and biovar determination by liquid hybridization. *J Clin Microbiol* 1998; **36**: 3211–16.

[81] Holmes KK, Handsfield HH, Wang SP, *et al.* Etiology of nongonococcal urethritis. *N Engl J Med* 1975; **292**: 1199–205.

[82] Fowler JE, Mariano M. Bacterial infection and male infertility: absence of immunoglobulin A with specificity for common Escherichia coli 0-serotypes in seminal fluid of infertile men. *J Urol* 1983; **130**: 171–4.

[83] Hillier SL, Rabe LK, Muller CH, *et al.* Relationship of bacteriologic characteristics to semen indices in men attending an infertility clinic. *Obstet Gynecol* 1990; **75**: 800–4.

[84] Esfandiari N, Saleh RA, Abdoos M, Rouzrokh A, Nazemian Z. Positive bacterial culture of semen from infertile men with asymptomatic leukocytospermia. *Int J Fertil Womens Med* 2002; **47**: 265–70.

[85] Teague NS, Boyarsky S, Glenn JF. Interference of human spermatozoa motility by Escherichia coli. *Fertil Steril* 1971; **22**: 281–5.

[86] Wolff H, Panhans A, Stolz W, Meurer M. Adherence of Escherichia coli to sperm: a mannose mediated phenomenon leading to agglutination of sperm and E. coli. *Fertil Steril* 1993; **60**: 154–8.

[87] el-Mulla KF, Kohn FM, Dandal M, *et al.* In vitro effect of Escherichia coli on human sperm acrosome reaction. *Arch Androl* 1996; **37**: 73–8.

[88] Diemer T, Huwe P, Michelmann HW, *et al.* Escherichia coli-induced alterations of human spermatozoa: an electron microscopy analysis. *Int J Androl* 2000; **23**: 178–86.

[89] Diemer T, Weidner W, Michelmann HW, *et al.* Influence of Escherichia coli on motility parameters of human spermatozoa in vitro. *Int J Androl* 1996; **19**: 271–7.

[90] Tuttle JP, Holbrook TW, Derrick FC. Interference of human spermatozoal motility by Trichomonas vaginalis. *J Urol* 1977; **118**: 1024–8.

[91] Jarecki-Black JC, Lushbaugh WB, Golosov L, Glassman AB. Trichomonas vaginalis: preliminary characterization of a sperm motility inhibiting factor. *Ann Clin Lab Sci* 1988; **18**: 484–9.

[92] Gopalkrishnan K, Hinduja IN, Kumar TC. Semen characteristics of asymptomatic males affected by Trichomonas vaginalis. *J In Vitro Fert Embryo Transf* 1990; **7**: 165–7.

[93] Lloyd GL, Case JR, De Frias D, Brannigan RE. Trichomonas vaginalis orchitis with associated severe oligoasthenoteratospermia and hypogonadism. *J Urol* 2003; **170**: 924.

[94] Krause W, Herbstreit F, Slenzka W. Are viral infections the cause of leukocytospermia? *Andrologia* 2002; **34**: 87–90.

[95] Kapranos N, Petrakou E, Anastasiadou C, Kotronias D. Detection of herpes simplex virus, cytomegalovirus, and Epstein–Barr virus in the semen of men attending an infertility clinic. *Fertil Steril* 2003; **79** (Suppl 3): 1566–70.

[96] Shen L, Zhang L, Zhang X. [An analysis of CMV infection in 115 cases with viral hepatitis.] *Zhonghua Yu Fang Yi Xue Za Zhi* 1996; **30**: 157–9.

[97] Yang YS, Ho HN, Chen HF, *et al.* Cytomegalovirus infection and viral shedding in the genital tract of infertile couples. *J Med Virol* 1995; **45**: 179–82.

[98] Levy R, Najioullah F, Keppi B, *et al.* Detection of cytomegalovirus in semen from a population of men seeking infertility evaluation. *Fertil Steril* 1997; **68**: 820–5.

[99] Bezold G, Schuster-Grusser A, Lange M, *et al.* Prevalence of human herpesvirus types 1–8 in the semen of infertility patients and correlation with semen parameters. *Fertil Steril* 2001; **76**: 416–18.

[100] Green J, Monteiro E, Bolton VN, Sanders P, Gibson PE. Detection of human papillomavirus DNA by PCR in semen from patients with and without penile warts. *Genitourin Med* 1991; **67**: 207–10.

[101] Lai YM, Lee JF, Huang HY, *et al.* The effect of human papillomavirus infection on sperm cell motility. *Fertil Steril* 1997; **67**: 1152–5.

[102] Martorell M, Gil-Salom M, Perez-Valles A, *et al.* Presence of human papillomavirus DNA in testicular biopsies from nonobstructive azoospermic men. *Arch Pathol Lab Med* 2005; **129**: 1132–6.

[103] Krieger JN, Coombs RW, Collier AC, *et al.* Fertility parameters in men infected with human immunodeficiency virus. *J Infect Dis* 1991; **164**: 464–9.

[104] Crittenden JA, Handelsman DJ, Stewart GJ. Semen analysis in human immunodeficiency virus infection. *Fertil Steril* 1992; **57**: 1294–9.

[105] Anderson DJ, O'Brien TR, Politch JA, *et al.* Effects of disease stage and zidovudine therapy on the detection of human immunodeficiency virus type 1 in semen. *JAMA* 1992; **267**: 2769–74.

[106] Politch JA, Mayer KH, Abbott AF, Anderson DJ. The effects of disease progression and zidovudine therapy on semen quality in human immunodeficiency virus type 1 seropositive men. *Fertil Steril* 1994; **61**: 922–8.

[107] Dondero F, Rossi T, D'Offizi G, *et al.* Semen analysis in HIV seropositive men and in subjects at high risk for HIV infection. *Hum Reprod* 1996; **11**: 765–8.

[108] Dulioust E, Du AL, Costagliola D, *et al.* Semen alterations in HIV-1 infected men. *Hum Reprod* 2002; **17**: 2112–18.

[109] Nicopoullos JD, Almeida PA, Ramsay JW, Gilling-Smith C. The effect of human immunodeficiency virus on sperm parameters and the outcome of intrauterine insemination following sperm washing. *Hum Reprod* 2004; **19**: 2289–97.

[110] Bujan L, Sergerie M, Moinard N, *et al.* Decreased semen volume and spermatozoa motility in HIV-1 infected patients under antiretroviral treatment. *J Androl* 2007; **28**: 444–52.

[111] Muller CH, Coombs RW, Krieger JN. Effects of clinical stage and immunological status on semen analysis results in human immunodeficiency virus type 1-seropositive men. *Andrologia* 1998; **30** (Suppl 1): 15–22.

[112] Kim LU, Johnson MR, Barton S, *et al.* Evaluation of sperm washing as a potential method of reducing HIV transmission in HIV-discordant couples wishing to have children. *AIDS* 1999; **13**: 645–51.

[113] Quayle AJ, Xu C, Mayer KH, Anderson DJ. T lymphocytes and macrophages, but not motile spermatozoa, are a significant source of human immunodeficiency virus in semen. *J Infect Dis* 1997; **176**: 960–8.

[114] Semprini AE, Levi-Setti P, Bozzo M, *et al.* Insemination of HIV-negative women with processed semen of HIV-positive partners. *Lancet* 1992; **340**: 1317–19.

[115] Marina S, Marina F, Alcolea R, *et al.* Human immunodeficiency virus type 1: serodiscordant couples can bear healthy children after undergoing intrauterine insemination. *Fertil Steril* 1998; **70**: 35–9.

[116] Persico T, Savasi V, Ferrazzi E, *et al.* Detection of human immunodeficiency virus-1 RNA and DNA by extractive and in situ PCR in unprocessed semen and seminal fractions isolated by semen-washing procedure. *Hum Reprod* 2006; **21**: 1525–30.

[117] Gilling-Smith C, Nicopoullos JD, Semprini AE, Frodsham LC. HIV and reproductive care: a review of current practice. *BJOG* 2006; **113**: 869–78.

[118] Endtz AW. A rapid staining method for differentiating granulocytes from "germinal cells" in Papanicolaou-stained semen. *Acta Cytol* 1974; **18**: 2–7.

[119] Jochum M, Pabst W, Schill WB. Granulocyte elastase as a sensitive diagnostic parameter of silent male genital tract inflammation. *Andrologia* 1986; **18**: 413–19.

[120] Wolff H, Anderson DJ. Evaluation of granulocyte elastase as a seminal plasma marker for leukocytospermia. *Fertil Steril* 1988; **50**: 129–32.

[121] Wolff H, Anderson DJ. Immunohistologic characterization and quantitation of leukocyte subpopulations in human semen. *Fertil Steril* 1988; **49**: 497–504.

[122] Wolff H, Politch JA, Martinez A, *et al.* Leukocytospermia is associated with poor semen quality. *Fertil Steril* 1990; **53**: 528–36.

[123] Gonzales GF, Kortebani G, Mazzolli AB. Leukocytospermia and function of the seminal vesicles on seminal quality. *Fertil Steril* 1992; **57**: 1058–65.

[124] Tomlinson MJ, White A, Barratt CL, Bolton AE, Cooke ID. The removal of morphologically abnormal sperm forms by phagocytes: a positive role for seminal leukocytes? *Hum Reprod* 1992; **7**: 517–22.

[125] Kung AW, Ho PC, Wang C. Seminal leucocyte subpopulations and sperm function in fertile and infertile Chinese men. *Int J Androl* 1993; **16**: 189–94.

[126] Tomlinson MJ, Barratt CL, Cooke ID. Prospective study of leukocytes and leukocyte subpopulations in semen suggests they are not a cause of male infertility. *Fertil Steril* 1993; **60**: 1069–75.

[127] Wang AW, Politch J, Anderson D. Leukocytospermia in male infertility patients in China. *Andrologia* 1994; **26**: 167–72.

[128] Yanushpolsky EH, Politch JA, Hill JA, Anderson DJ. Antibiotic therapy and leukocytospermia: a prospective, randomized, controlled study. *Fertil Steril* 1995; **63**: 142–7.

[129] Arata de Bellabarba G, Tortolero I, Villarroel V, *et al.* Nonsperm cells in human semen and their relationship with semen parameters. *Arch Androl* 2000; **45**: 131–6.

[130] Kaleli S, Ocer F, Irez T, Budak E, Aksu MF. Does leukocytospermia associate with poor semen parameters and sperm functions in male infertility? The role of different seminal leukocyte concentrations. *Eur J Obstet Gynecol Reprod Biol* 2000; **89**: 185–91.

[131] Sharma RK, Pasqualotto AE, Nelson DR, Thomas AJ, Agarwal A. Relationship between seminal white blood cell counts and oxidative stress in men treated at an infertility clinic. *J Androl* 2001; **22**: 575–83.

[132] Saleh RA, Agarwal A, Kandirali E, *et al.* Leukocytospermia is associated with increased reactive oxygen species production by human spermatozoa. *Fertil Steril* 2002; **78**: 1215–24.

[133] Aziz N, Agarwal A, Lewis-Jones I, Sharma RK, Thomas AJ. Novel associations between specific sperm morphological defects and leukocytospermia. *Fertil Steril* 2004; **82**: 621–7.

[134] Aitken RJ, West K, Buckingham D. Leukocytic infiltration into the human ejaculate and its association with semen quality, oxidative stress, and sperm function. *J Androl* 1994; **15**: 343–52.

[135] el-Demiry MI, Hargreave TB, Busuttil A, *et al.* Lymphocyte sub-populations in the male genital tract. *Br J Urol* 1985; **57**: 769–74.

[136] Berger RE, Karp LE, Williamson RA, *et al.* The relationship of pyospermia and seminal fluid bacteriology to sperm function as reflected in the sperm penetration assay. *Fertil Steril* 1982; **37**: 557–64.

[137] Maruyama DK, Hale RW, Rogers BJ. Effects of white blood cells on the in vitro penetration of zona-free hamster eggs by human spermatozoa. *J Androl* 1985; **6**: 127–35.

[138] el-Demiry MI, Hargreave TB, Busuttil A, James K, Chisholm GD. Identifying leucocytes and leucocyte subpopulations in semen using monoclonal antibody probes. *Urology* 1986; **28**: 492–6.

[139] el-Demiry MI, Young H, Elton RA, Hargreave TB, James K, Chisholm GD. Leucocytes in the ejaculate from fertile and infertile men. *Br J Urol* 1986; **58**: 715–20.

[140] Yanushpolsky EH, Politch JA, Hill JA, Anderson DJ. Is leukocytospermia clinically relevant? *Fertil Steril* 1996; **66**: 822–5.

[141] Thomas J, Fishel SB, Hall JA, *et al.* Increased polymorphonuclear granulocytes in seminal plasma in relation to sperm morphology. *Hum Reprod* 1997; **12**: 2418–21.

[142] Sharma RK, Agarwal A. Role of reactive oxygen species in male infertility. *Urology* 1996; **48**: 835–50.

[143] Aitken RJ, Buckingham DW, Brindle J, *et al.* Analysis of sperm movement in relation to the oxidative stress created by leukocytes in washed sperm preparations and seminal plasma. *Hum Reprod* 1995; **10**: 2061–71.

[144] Aitken RJ, West KM. Analysis of the relationship between reactive oxygen species production and leucocyte infiltration in fractions of human semen separated on Percoll gradients. *Int J Androl* 1990; **13**: 433–51.

[145] Iwasaki A, Gagnon C. Formation of reactive oxygen species in spermatozoa of infertile patients. *Fertil Steril* 1992; **57**: 409–16.

[146] Gil-Guzman E, Ollero M, Lopez MC, *et al.* Differential production of reactive oxygen species by

subsets of human spermatozoa at different stages of maturation. *Hum Reprod* 2001; **16**: 1922–30.

[147] Ollero M, Gil-Guzman E, Lopez MC, *et al.* Characterization of subsets of human spermatozoa at different stages of maturation: implications in the diagnosis and treatment of male infertility. *Hum Reprod* 2001; **16**: 1912–21.

[148] Krausz C, Mills C, Rogers S, Tan SL, Aitken RJ. Stimulation of oxidant generation by human sperm suspensions using phorbol esters and formyl peptides: relationships with motility and fertilization in vitro. *Fertil Steril* 1994; **62**: 599–605.

[149] Plante M, de Lamirande E, Gagnon C. Reactive oxygen species released by activated neutrophils, but not by deficient spermatozoa, are sufficient to affect normal sperm motility. *Fertil Steril* 1994; **62**: 387–93.

[150] Aitken RJ, Clarkson JS, Fishel S. Generation of reactive oxygen species, lipid peroxidation, and human sperm function. *Biol Reprod* 1989; **41**: 183–97.

[151] Aitken RJ, Buckingham D, Harkiss D. Use of a xanthine oxidase free radical generating system to investigate the cytotoxic effects of reactive oxygen species on human spermatozoa. *J Reprod Fertil* 1993; **97**: 441–50.

[152] Alvarez JG, Touchstone JC, Blasco L, Storey BT. Spontaneous lipid peroxidation and production of hydrogen peroxide and superoxide in human spermatozoa: superoxide dismutase as major enzyme protectant against oxygen toxicity. *J Androl* 1987; **8**: 338–48.

[153] Jones R, Mann T, Sherins R. Peroxidative breakdown of phospholipids in human spermatozoa, spermicidal properties of fatty acid peroxides, and protective action of seminal plasma. *Fertil Steril* 1979; **31**: 531–7.

[154] de Lamirande E, Leduc BE, Iwasaki A, Hassouna M, Gagnon C. Increased reactive oxygen species formation in semen of patients with spinal cord injury. *Fertil Steril* 1995; **63**: 637–42.

[155] Kovalski NN, de Lamirande E, Gagnon C. Reactive oxygen species generated by human neutrophils inhibit sperm motility: Protective effect of seminal plasma and scavengers. *Fertil Steril* 1992; **58**: 809–16.

[156] Aitken RJ, Irvine DS, Wu FC. Prospective analysis of sperm–oocyte fusion and reactive oxygen species generation as criteria for the diagnosis of infertility. *Am J Obstet Gynecol* 1991; **164**: 542–51.

[157] Zalata AA, Ahmed AH, Allamaneni SS, Comhaire FH, Agarwal A. Relationship between acrosin activity of human spermatozoa and oxidative stress. *Asian J Androl* 2004; **6**: 313–18.

[158] Agarwal A, Sharma RK, Nallella KP, *et al.* Reactive oxygen species as an independent marker of male factor infertility. *Fertil Steril* 2006; **86**: 878–85.

[159] Sukcharoen N, Keith J, Irvine DS, Aitken RJ. Predicting the fertilizing potential of human sperm suspensions in vitro: importance of sperm morphology and leukocyte contamination. *Fertil Steril* 1995; **63**: 1293–300.

[160] Lewis SE, Sterling ES, Young IS, Thompson W. Comparison of individual antioxidants of sperm and seminal plasma in fertile and infertile men. *Fertil Steril* 1997; **67**: 142–7.

[161] Lewis SE, Boyle PM, McKinney KA, Young IS, Thompson W. Total antioxidant capacity of seminal plasma is different in fertile and infertile men. *Fertil Steril* 1995; **64**: 868–70.

[162] Smith R, Vantman D, Ponce J, Escobar J, Lissi E. Total antioxidant capacity of human seminal plasma. *Hum Reprod* 1996; **11**: 1655–60.

[163] Kodama H, Yamaguchi R, Fukuda J, Kasai H, Tanaka T. Increased oxidative deoxyribonucleic acid damage in the spermatozoa of infertile male patients. *Fertil Steril* 1997; **68**: 519–24.

[164] Twigg J, Fulton N, Gomez E, Irvine DS, Aitken RJ. Analysis of the impact of intracellular reactive oxygen species generation on the structural and functional integrity of human spermatozoa: Lipid peroxidation, DNA fragmentation and effectiveness of antioxidants. *Hum Reprod* 1998; **13**: 1429–36.

[165] Alvarez JG, Sharma RK, Ollero M, *et al.* Increased DNA damage in sperm from leukocytospermic semen samples as determined by the sperm chromatin structure assay. *Fertil Steril* 2002; **78**: 319–29.

[166] Erenpreiss J, Hlevicka S, Zalkalns J, Erenpreisa J. Effect of leukocytospermia on sperm DNA integrity: a negative effect in abnormal semen samples. *J Androl* 2002; **23**: 717–23.

[167] Sharma RK, Pasqualotto FF, Nelson DR, Thomas AJ, Agarwal A. The reactive oxygen species–total antioxidant capacity score is a new measure of oxidative stress to predict male infertility. *Hum Reprod* 1999; **14**: 2801–7.

[168] Lewis SE, Donnelly ET, Sterling ES, *et al.* Nitric oxide synthase and nitrite production in human spermatozoa: Evidence that endogenous nitric oxide is beneficial to sperm motility. *Mol Hum Reprod* 1996; **2**: 873–8.

[169] O'Bryan MK, Zini A, Cheng CY, Schlegel PN. Human sperm endothelial nitric oxide synthase expression: correlation with sperm motility. *Fertil Steril* 1998; **70**: 1143–7.

[170] Beckman JS, Beckman TW, Chen J, Marshall PA, Freeman BA. Apparent hydroxyl radical production by peroxynitrite: implications for endothelial injury from nitric oxide and superoxide. *Proc Natl Acad Sci U S A* 1990; **87**: 1620–4.

[171] Weinberg JB, Doty E, Bonaventura J, Haney AF. Nitric oxide inhibition of human sperm motility. *Fertil Steril* 1995; **64**: 408–13.

327

[172] Hellstrom WJ, Bell M, Wang R, Sikka SC. Effect of sodium nitroprusside on sperm motility, viability, and lipid peroxidation. *Fertil Steril* 1994; **61**: 1117–22.

[173] Rosselli M, Dubey RK, Imthurn B, Macas E, Keller PJ. Effects of nitric oxide on human spermatozoa: evidence that nitric oxide decreases sperm motility and induces sperm toxicity. *Hum Reprod* 1995; **10**: 1786–90.

[174] Nobunaga T, Tokugawa Y, Hashimoto K, *et al.* Elevated nitric oxide concentration in the seminal plasma of infertile males: Nitric oxide inhibits sperm motility. *Am J Reprod Immunol* 1996; **36**: 193–7.

[175] Revelli A, Bergandi L, Massobrio M, *et al.* The concentration of nitrite in seminal plasma does not correlate with sperm concentration, sperm motility, leukocytospermia, or sperm culture. *Fertil Steril* 2001; **76**: 496–500.

[176] Ludwig M, Kummel C, Schroeder-Printzen I, Ringert RH, Weidner W. Evaluation of seminal plasma parameters in patients with chronic prostatitis or leukocytospermia. *Andrologia* 1998; **30** (Suppl 1): 41–7.

[177] Rajasekaran M, Hellstrom WJ, Naz RK, Sikka SC. Oxidative stress and interleukins in seminal plasma during leukocytospermia. *Fertil Steril* 1995; **64**: 166–71.

[178] Rajasekaran M, Hellstrom W, Sikka S. Quantitative assessment of cytokines (GRO alpha and IL-10) in human seminal plasma during genitourinary inflammation. *Am J Reprod Immunol* 1996; **36**: 90–5.

[179] Zorn B, Virant-Klun I, Meden-Vrtovec H. Semen granulocyte elastase: its relevance for the diagnosis and prognosis of silent genital tract inflammation. *Hum Reprod* 2000; **15**: 1978–84.

[180] Henkel R, Schill WB. Sperm separation in patients with urogenital infections. *Andrologia* 1998; **30** (Suppl 1): 91–7.

[181] Hill JA, Haimovici F, Politch JA, Anderson DJ. Effects of soluble products of activated lymphocytes and macrophages (lymphokines and monokines) on human sperm motion parameters. *Fertil Steril* 1987; **47**: 460–5.

[182] Maegawa M, Kamada M, Irahara M, *et al.* A repertoire of cytokines in human seminal plasma. *J Reprod Immunol* 2002; **54**: 33–42.

[183] Shimoya K, Matsuzaki N, Tsutsui T, *et al.* Detection of interleukin-8 (IL-8) in seminal plasma and elevated IL-8 in seminal plasma of infertile patients with leukospermia. *Fertil Steril* 1993; **59**: 885–8.

[184] Omu AE, Al-Qattan F, Al-Abdul-Hadi FM, Fatinikun MT, Fernandes S. Seminal immune response in infertile men with leukocytospermia: Effect on antioxidant activity. *Eur J Obstet Gynecol Reprod Biol* 1999; **86**: 195–202.

[185] Comhaire F, Bosmans E, Ombelet W, Punjabi U, Schoonjans F. Cytokines in semen of normal men and of patients with andrological diseases. *Am J Reprod Immunol* 1994; **31**: 99–103.

[186] Naz RK, Kaplan P. Increased levels of interleukin-6 in seminal plasma of infertile men. *J Androl* 1994; **15**: 220–7.

[187] Shimoya K, Matsuzaki N, Ida N, *et al.* Detection of monocyte chemotactic and activating factor (MCAF) and interleukin (IL)-6 in human seminal plasma and effect of leukospermia on these cytokine levels. *Am J Reprod Immunol* 1995; **34**: 311–16.

[188] Ohta S, Wada H, Gabazza EC, Nobori T, Fuse H. Evaluation of tissue factor antigen level in human seminal plasma. *Urol Res* 2002; **30**: 317–20.

[189] Buch JP, Kolon TF, Maulik N, Kreutzer DL, Das DK. Cytokines stimulate lipid membrane peroxidation of human sperm. *Fertil Steril* 1994; **62**: 186–8.

[190] Naz RK, Evans L, Armstrong JS, Sikka SC. Decreased levels of interleukin-12 are not correlated with leukocyte concentration and superoxide dismutase activity in semen of infertile men. *Arch Androl* 1998; **41**: 91–6.

[191] Naz RK, Evans L. Presence and modulation of interleukin-12 in seminal plasma of fertile and infertile men. *J Androl* 1998; **19**: 302–7.

[192] Turek PJ. Immunopathology and infertility. In: Lipshultz LI, Howards SS, eds. *Infertility in the Male*, 3rd edn. St. Louis, MO: Mosby Year Book, 1997: 305–25.

[193] Fedder J, Askjaer SA, Hjort T. Nonspermatozoal cells in semen: relationship to other semen parameters and fertility status of the couple. *Arch Androl* 1993; **31**: 95–103.

[194] Kortebani G, Gonzales GF, Barrera C, Mazzolli AB. Leucocyte populations in semen and male accessory gland function: relationship with antisperm antibodies and seminal quality. *Andrologia* 1992; **24**: 197–204.

[195] Gonzales GF, Kortebani G, Mazzolli AB. Effect of isotypes of antisperm antibodies on semen quality. *Int J Androl* 1992; **15**: 220–8.

[196] Paschke R, Schulze Bertelsbeck D, Bahrs S, Heinecke A, Behre HM. Seminal sperm antibodies exhibit an unstable spontaneous course and an increased incidence of leucocytospermia. *Int J Androl* 1994; **17**: 135–9.

[197] Eggert-Kruse W, Neuer A, Clussmann C, *et al.* Seminal antibodies to human 60kd heat shock protein (HSP 60) in male partners of subfertile couples. *Hum Reprod* 2002; **17**: 726–35.

[198] Eggert-Kruse W, Bellmann A, Rohr G, Tilgen W, Runnebaum B. Differentiation of round cells in semen by means of monoclonal antibodies and relationship with male fertility. *Fertil Steril* 1992; **58**: 1046–55.

[199] Couture M, Ulstein M, Leonard J, Paulsen CA. Improved staining method for differentiating

immature germ cells from white blood cells in human seminal fluid. *Andrologia* 1976; **8**: 61–6.

[200] Wolff H. The biologic significance of white blood cells in semen. *Fertil Steril* 1995; **63**: 1143–57.

[201] World Health Organization. *WHO Laboratory Manual for the Examination of Human Semen and Sperm–Cervical Mucus Interaction*, 4th edn. Cambridge: Cambridge University Press, 1999: 128.

[202] Politch JA, Wolff H, Hill JA, Anderson DJ. Comparison of methods to enumerate white blood cells in semen. *Fertil Steril* 1993; **60**: 372–5.

[203] Wolff H. Methods for the detection of male genital tract inflammation. *Andrologia* 1998; **30** (Suppl 1): 35–9.

[204] Villegas J, Schulz M, Vallejos V, *et al.* Indirect immunofluorescence using monoclonal antibodies for the detection of leukocytospermia: comparison with peroxidase staining. *Andrologia* 2002; **34**: 69–73.

[205] Ricci G, Presani G, Guaschino S, Simeone R, Perticarari S. Leukocyte detection in human semen using flow cytometry. *Hum Reprod* 2000; **15**: 1329–37.

[206] Leino L, Virkkunen P. An automated chemiluminescence test for diagnosis of leukocytospermia. *Int J Androl* 1991; **14**: 271–7.

[207] Schlegel PN, Chang TS, Marshall FF. Antibiotics: potential hazards to male fertility. *Fertil Steril* 1991; **55**: 235–42.

[208] Branigan EF, Spadoni LR, Muller CH. Identification and treatment of leukocytospermia in couples with unexplained infertility. *J Reprod Med* 1995; **40**: 625–9.

[209] Yamamoto M, Hibi H, Katsuno S, Miyake K. Antibiotic and ejaculation treatments improve resolution rate of leukocytospermia in infertile men with prostatitis. *Nagoya J Med Sci* 1995; **58**: 41–5.

[210] Omu AE, al-Othman S, Mohamad AS, al-Kaluwby NM, Fernandes S. Antibiotic therapy for seminal infection: effect on antioxidant activity and T-helper cytokines. *J Reprod Med* 1998; **43**: 857–64.

[211] Erel CT, Senturk LM, Demir F, Irez T, Ertungealp E. Antibiotic therapy in men with leukocytospermia. *Int J Fertil Womens Med* 1997; **42**: 206–10.

[212] Lackner JE, Herwig R, Schmidbauer J, *et al.* Correlation of leukocytospermia with clinical infection and the positive effect of antiinflammatory treatment on semen quality. *Fertil Steril* 2006; **86**: 601–5.

[213] Vicari E, La Vignera S, Calogero AE. Antioxidant treatment with carnitines is effective in infertile patients with prostatovesiculoepididymitis and elevated seminal leukocyte concentrations after treatment with nonsteroidal anti-inflammatory compounds. *Fertil Steril* 2002; **78**: 1203–8.

[214] Oliva A, Multigner L. Ketotifen improves sperm motility and sperm morphology in male patients with leukocytospermia and unexplained infertility. *Fertil Steril* 2006; **85**: 240–3.

[215] Devivo M. Epidemiology of spinal cord injury. In: Lin V, ed. *Spinal Cord Medicine: Principles and Practice*. New York, NY: Demos Medical Publishing, 2003: 79–85.

[216] Brackett NL, Nash MS, Lynne CM. Male fertility following spinal cord injury: facts and fiction. *Phys Ther* 1996; **76**: 1221–31.

[217] Brackett NL, Santa-Cruz C, Lynne CM. Sperm from spinal cord injured men lose motility faster than sperm from normal men: the effect is exacerbated at body compared to room temperature. *J Urol* 1997; **157**: 2150–3.

[218] Linsenmeyer TA, Perkash, I. Infertility in men with spinal cord injury. *Arch Phys Med Rehabil* 1991; **72**: 747–54.

[219] Aird IA, Vince GS, Bates MD, Johnson PM, Lewis-Jones ID. Leukocytes in semen from men with spinal cord injuries. *Fertil Steril* 1999; **72**: 97–103.

[220] Brackett NL, Lynne CM. The method of assisted ejaculation affects the outcome of semen quality studies in men with spinal cord injury: a review. *NeuroRehabilitation* 2000; **15**: 89–100.

[221] Brackett NL, Bloch WE, Lynne CM. Predictors of necrospermia in men with spinal cord injury. *J Urol* 1998; **159**: 844–7.

[222] Trabulsi EJ, Shupp-Byrne D, Sedor J, Hirsch IH. Leukocyte subtypes in electroejaculates of spinal cord injured men. *Arch Phys Med Rehabil* 2002; **83**: 31–4.

[223] Basu S, Lynne CM, Ruiz P, *et al.* Cytofluorographic identification of activated T-cell subpopulations in the semen of men with spinal cord injuries. *J Androl* 2002; **23**: 551–6.

[224] Padron OF, Brackett NL, Sharma RK, *et al.* Seminal reactive oxygen species and sperm motility and morphology in men with spinal cord injury. *Fertil Steril* 1997; **67**: 1115–20.

[225] Randall JM, Evans DH, Bird VG, *et al.* Leukocytospermia in spinal cord injured patients is not related to histological inflammatory changes in the prostate. *J Urol* 2003; **170**: 897–900.

[226] Christiansen E, Tollefsrud A, Purvis K. Sperm quality in men with chronic abacterial prostatovesiculitis verified by rectal ultrasonography. *Urology* 1991; **38**: 545–9.

[227]. Leib Z, Bartoov B, Eltes F, Servadio C. Reduced semen quality caused by chronic abacterial prostatitis: an enigma or reality? *Fertil Steril* 1994; **61**: 1109–16.

[228] Krieger JN, Berger RE, Ross SO, Rothman I, Muller CH. Seminal fluid findings in men with nonbacterial prostatitis and prostatodynia. *J Androl* 1996; **17**: 310–18.

[229] Weidner W, Jantos C, Schiefer HG, Haidl G, Friedrich HJ. Semen parameters in men with and without proven chronic prostatitis. *Arch Androl* 1991; **26**: 173–83.

[230] Pasqualotto FF, Sharma RK, Potts JM, *et al.* Seminal oxidative stress in patients with chronic prostatitis. *Urology* 2000; **55**: 881–5.

[231] Menkveld R, Huwe P, Ludwig M, Weidner W. Morphological sperm alternations in different types of prostatitis. *Andrologia* 2003; **35**: 288–93.

[232] Motrich RD, Maccioni M, Molina R, *et al.* Reduced semen quality in chronic prostatitis patients that have cellular autoimmune response to prostate antigens. *Hum Reprod* 2005; **20**: 2567–72.

Chapter 18

Varicocele

Harris M. Nagler and Aaron B. Grotas

Introduction

A varicocele is a dilation of the pampiniform plexus. Although the varicocele is generally regarded as the most common treatable cause of male infertility, it continues to be the focus of controversy. When does the varicocele cause male infertility? How should one diagnose a varicocele? If a varicocele does in fact cause infertility, how does it adversely affect spermatogenesis? When should varicoceles be corrected? And lastly, what is the best means of correcting a varicocele?

The incidence of varicoceles in the general population has been reported to be approximately 20% [1], but as many as 40% of men being evaluated for infertility have varicoceles [2]. The higher incidence of varicoceles in subfertile men has led to the belief that varicoceles cause infertility [3], and this belief has been supported by the documented beneficial effects of varicocelectomy [4–7]. Improvement in semen analyses [4–7], testicular size [8], and testicular histology have each been observed after varicocelectomy [9,10]. Analysis of reports reviewing thousands of infertile patients treated with varicocelectomy indicates that 50–80% of patients experience an improvement in semen variables, with 30–40% of patients initiating a pregnancy after the procedure. Nevertheless, skepticism has persisted, because the deleterious effects of the varicocele on spermatogenesis, as well as the beneficial effects after varicocelectomy, are unpredictable. The variable effect of the clinical varicocele has engendered further debate regarding the significance and treatment of the varicocele in the adolescent population. Those minimizing the importance of the varicocele have become emboldened by the improved success rates that are achieved by assisted reproductive techniques. **The debate between those treating male infertility and reproductive endocrinologists has been codified by the phrase, "to treat or to cure."**

This chapter reviews the current concepts and ongoing controversies regarding the pathophysiology, diagnosis, significance, and treatment of the varicocele.

Historical perspective

The varicocele and its association with infertility have been recognized for centuries. Celsius, in the first century AD, first described dilation of the scrotal veins and noted an association between the presence of a varicocele and testicular atrophy. The first notion that varicoceles were related to infertility appeared in 1856 when Curling reported that the testicle exhibited a decrease in the "secreting powers of the gland" when a varicocele was present [11]. In 1885, Barwell observed that the ipsilateral testis in patients with left-sided varicoceles was small and soft, and noted that the placement of a wire loop around the dilated scrotal veins was followed by the return of a normal-feeling testis [12]. However, the beneficial effects of varicocele ligation on male reproduction were not truly appreciated until 1889, when Bennet performed bilateral varicocelectomy in a patient who subsequently experienced improvement in semen quality [13]. In 1929, Macomber and Sanders reported in the *New England Journal of Medicine* the case of an oligospermic subfertile patient who underwent varicocele repair and became normospermic and fertile [14]. It was not until 1955, when Tulloch reported the results of a series of infertile men treated by varicocelectomy, that the procedure became the mainstay of treatment for male infertility [15,16]. **Since then, a causal relationship between the varicocele and impaired fertility has been assumed. Numerous uncontrolled studies have confirmed improved semen quality and pregnancy following varicocelectomy** [5,17,18]. The literature supporting the efficacy of varicocelectomy has been criticized, and will be fully reviewed below (see section on outcomes).

Infertility in the Male, 4th edition, ed. Larry I. Lipshultz, Stuart S. Howards, and Craig S. Niederberger. Published by Cambridge University Press. © Cambridge University Press 2009.

Recently, the World Health Organization assessed the influence of varicoceles on variables of fertility. This study identified varicoceles in 25.4% of men with abnormal semen compared with 11.7% of men with normal semen. The varicocele was associated with decreased testicular volume, impaired semen quality, and abnormal Leydig cell function [3]. **Although efficacy of varicocelectomy was not addressed by this report, the varicocele continues to be recognized as the major surgically correctable cause of male infertility.**

In spite of the ongoing controversy, varicoceles continue to be considered an important cause of male infertility. Varicocelectomy is widely accepted as an effective treatment, which results in significant improvement in semen parameters in a large percentage of men and improved spontaneous pregnancy rates.

Etiology and anatomy

As previously noted, varicoceles are dilations of the pampiniform plexus. Clinically, varicoceles occur most commonly as isolated left-sided lesions (75–95%). Although the incidence of bilateral varicoceles has historically been reported to be approximately 10%, recent data have indicated bilaterality in 30–80% of cases [7,16,19]. The isolated right-sided varicocele is uncommon, and causes concern regarding the possibility of an underlying retroperitoneal abnormality.

The apparent predisposition for the development of varicoceles on the left has been explained by the anatomy of the internal spermatic system. The left internal spermatic vein drains perpendicularly into the left renal vein, taking a course that is approximately 8–10 cm longer than the course of the right internal spermatic vein, which enters the vena cava. The greater length of the left internal spermatic vein results in increased hydrostatic pressure when the patient is in the upright position, thereby overcoming valvular mechanisms and resulting in backflow, venous dilation, and varicocele formation. Additionally, the right-angle insertion of the left spermatic vein into the renal vein allows for the direct transmission of left renal vein pressure to the spermatic vein. On the other hand, the right spermatic vein enters the vena cava at an oblique angle, protecting the vessel from pressure elevations within the inferior vena cava [20]. Shafik and Bedeir measured bilateral venous pressures in 30 control and 32 varicocele patients standing and performing a Valsalva maneuver [21]. The mean internal spermatic venous pressure in the varicocele group was 19.7 mmHg

greater in the standing position and 22 mmHg greater during the Valsalva maneuver than the pressures measured in the control group [22]. This finding supports the hypothesis that the varicocele is associated with increased hydrostatic pressures. **The assumption of a standing position results in overcoming the valvular system of the internal spermatic vein and can result in the formation of a varicocele.**

Increased hydrostatic pressure within the left internal spermatic vein may also result from compression of the left renal vein between the superior mesenteric artery and aorta, the so-called "nutcracker" phenomenon. Buschi and colleagues studied the anatomy of the left renal vein with computerized axial tomography scans and reported marked narrowing of the left renal vein as it crossed the aorta [23]. Proximal venous dilation was noted in 70% of all subjects, regardless of the presence or absence of a varicocele. Coolsaet supported this finding venographically, demonstrating compression of the left renal vein in 37 (55%) of 67 patients with a varicocele [24]. Whether renal vein compression is of clinical significance has not yet been demonstrated. It is likely that there may be several mechanisms by which varicoceles occur.

In an autopsy series reported in 1966, Ahlberg *et al.* demonstrated the potential significance of valvular abnormalities in the etiology of the varicocele [25]. They reported the absence of valves within the left internal spermatic vein in all cadavers with varicoceles, and the presence of numerous valves within the internal spermatic vein in all cadavers without varicoceles. They also found that the absence of valves was less common in the right internal spermatic vein. However, radiographic studies have demonstrated the right spermatic vein to reflux in 40–80% of patients with clinical left-sided varicoceles [18,26–28]. **Thus the absence or incompetence of valves appears to play a role in the etiology of the varicocele.** Since humans evolved to assume an upright position, these mechanisms may explain the development of the varicocele.

Although most varicoceles are thought to be related to abnormalities of the internal spermatic venous system, dilation of the external cremasteric system may also be clinically significant. Coolsaet demonstrated that partial obstruction of the left common iliac vein results in dilation of the external spermatic (cremasteric) venous system and pampiniform system [24] and, as a result, this pathway must be taken into consideration during varicocele repair. Chehval and Purcell carefully examined the external cremasteric vessels in 96 successive varicocele repairs performed via the inguinal approach [29]. The external cremasteric vein is normally 2–3 mm in diameter in the adult without a varicocele. Therefore, any vein greater than 4 mm in diameter was thought to be abnormally dilated and was ligated. Intraoperative examination revealed external cremasteric vein dilation greater than 4 mm in 49.5% of the varicoceles. If overlooked, persistence of the varicocele might have resulted. Therefore, they recommended routine inspection and ligation of the external cremasteric vein in all cases. Although the physiologic significance of these vessels has not been established, this concept has been widely embraced and has been invoked as a reason that the inguinal or subinguinal approach to varicocelectomy is preferable.

Pathophysiology

Many hypotheses have been proposed to explain the mechanism by which a varicocele may exert a deleterious effect on spermatogenesis and fertility. This quandary is further complicated by the fact that unilateral lesions appear to affect spermatogenesis bilaterally. However, recent data demonstrate that although unilateral varicoceles affect spermatogenesis, as evidenced by improved semen parameters after varicocelectomy, bilateral varicoceles and varicocelectomies are associated with even greater improvement [30]. This would appear to suggest a size-dependent effect of the varicocele on spermatogenesis. **The presence of bilateral varicoceles may be one manifestation of a clinically severe varicocele.** In this study, patients with bilateral varicoceles had a higher number of grade 3 varicoceles (21% vs. 9.6%). Importantly, patients undergoing bilateral varicocelectomy experience a greater improvement in sperm density and motility [30]. Though it did not significantly impact the results of the study, this information suggests that patients with larger varicoceles are predisposed to formation of varicoceles on the contralateral side. **Collateral pathways to the contralateral side can be found by way of the pudendal and cremasteric veins.**

Many of the theories of the pathophysiology of the varicocele are based upon the fact that in the presence of a varicocele venography demonstrates reflux of blood from the renal vein to the spermatic vein [26]. It has been hypothesized that the reflux of metabolic by-products of the adrenal glands and kidneys has a toxic effect on testicular function. A number of studies have examined potential differences between serum concentrations of various substances in the internal spermatic vein and the peripheral venous circulation. Ozbek *et al.* reported elevated levels of adrenomedullin in the internal spermatic vein of normal men compared with brachial vein levels in men with varicocele [31]. Adrenomedullin is a vasodilatory peptide secreted by the adrenal gland. Cohen *et al.* [32] and Comhaire and Vermeulen [33,34] reported increased catecholamine levels in the internal spermatic vein of patients with varicoceles. Other investigators were unable to confirm this finding [35–37]. Cortisol levels from the internal spermatic vein and peripheral venous blood of subfertile males have been found to be similar [36,38]. Ito *et al.* noted an elevation of prostaglandin E and prostaglandin F in the internal spermatic vein in patients with varicoceles [39]. Cockett *et al.* demonstrated higher levels of prostaglandin $F_{2\alpha}$ and serotonin in the spermatic veins of patients with varicoceles [4]. Although prostaglandins have been shown to have an antispermatogenic effect in animal models [40], their role in the pathophysiology of the varicocele remains to be defined. Harrison and colleagues investigated the role of adrenal reflux by creating experimental varicoceles in rhesus monkeys [41]. They reported that left adrenalectomy at the time of experimental varicocele induction did not alter the development of varicocele-related testicular changes. Turner and Lopez showed similar results in rats with experimentally induced varicoceles with or without left adrenalectomy [42]. Thus the adrenal gland metabolites and products do not appear to play a part in the effects of the varicocele on spermatogenesis. **The role of renal metabolites, however, has not been systematically investigated.**

Hormonal dysfunction

Altered testicular steroidogenesis has also been proposed as a mechanism by which the varicocele exerts its deleterious effects on spermatogenesis. Early reports by Comhaire and others have reported decreased plasma testosterone levels in patients with varicoceles [27,28]. Other investigators have shown that testosterone levels in peripheral venous or internal spermatic vein blood of patients with varicocele do not differ from those of normal men [25,36,43]. Swerdloff and Walsh evaluated the hypothalamic–pituitary–gonadal axis in patients with varicoceles [43]. There were significant differences in the unstimulated serum estradiol, follicle-stimulating hormone (FSH), luteinizing hormone (LH), and testosterone levels between infertile patients with varicoceles and controls. Pasqualotto *et al.* observed that FSH levels were significantly higher in infertile men with varicoceles (7.8 ± 7.6 IU/L) than in fertile men with varicoceles (3.5 ± 2.1 IU/L) or in fertile men without varicoceles (3.5 ± 1.9 IU/L) [44]. In their study, the testosterone levels did not differ. Most studies have not demonstrated a significant clinical correlation between varicoceles and decreased FSH levels. Gat and colleagues noted that both testosterone and free testosterone levels increased significantly after treatment of varicocele by embolization of the internal spermatic vein [45]. Although Su et al. have reported that testosterone levels are decreased in men with varicoceles, they did not suggest that this decrease results in abnormal spermatogenesis [46].

Hypothesizing that the adverse effects of varicoceles are related to disturbed hypothalamic–pituitary–gonadal axis function, numerous investigators have looked at gonadotropin-releasing hormone (GnRH) stimulation tests to predict response to varicocelectomy. O'Brien et al. were unable to demonstrate a correlation between a positive GnRH stimulation test and response to varicocelectomy, defined as semen parameter improvement or increased pregnancy rates [47]. Guarino, Tadini, and Bianchi reported that elevated basal and GnRH-stimulated FSH levels were associated with impaired preoperative semen parameters when compared to those in adolescents with varicoceles and normal semen parameters [48]. The authors advocate using FSH and GnRH stimulation to identify adolescents for varicocele repair. However, Fisch et al. concluded that elevated FSH levels in conjunction with an increased response to the GnRH stimulation test may represent a normal physiological response during adolescent development [49].

Although the varicocele may be associated with a subtle alteration in the hypothalamic–pituitary–gonadal axis, whether this is the mechanism of the effect of the varicocele or the result of the primary pathophysiologic effect of the varicocele is unclear.

Hypoxia and reactive oxygen species

Recently hypoxia and reactive oxidative species have been a focus of pathophysiology research. Human and experimental data suggest that apoptosis, hypoxia, and reactive oxygen species play a role in the pathophysiology of varicocele. In a rat varicocele model, Barqawi et al. demonstrated increased apoptosis in germ cells of varicocele animals compared to controls [50]. **The findings of this small study were not statistically significant but questioned the role of apoptosis in the pathophysiology of the varicocele.**

An earlier study by Nagler et al. showed increased microvascular hemodynamics in the varicocele in an experimental animal model [51]. Kilinç et al. examined hypoxia-inducible factor 1α (HIF-1α) [52]. This study evaluated microvessel density (MVD) increases as a measure of angiogenesis in response to hypoxia. Animals with experimentally induced varicoceles had a higher MVD, HIF-1α, and positive stained vascular endothelial growth factor (VEGF) when compared to animals subjected to sham surgery and control animals. This study demonstrates that experimental varicoceles induce hypoxia and angiogenesis. Lee et al. showed a sevenfold increase in internal spermatic vein levels of HIF-1α expression in patients undergoing varicocelectomy as compared to hernia (control) patients [53].

Varicoceles may also affect reactive oxygen species generation, rendering the testicle and/or the sperm unable to handle oxidative stress, and resulting in reactive oxygen species buildup. Hydrogen peroxide, free radicals, and superoxide anions have been reported in both semen and testicular biopsy specimens [54]. Hendin et al. analyzed spermatozoal reactive oxygen species and seminal plasma antioxidant capacity in men with varicocele and in controls [55]. Their data suggest that elevated reactive oxygen species and diminished total antioxidant capacity are associated with varicoceles. Since fertile and infertile men with varicoceles had the same changes, it is not clear whether these changes are related to the pathophysiology of the varicocele or its impact on fertility. Nitrotyrosine is another marker of oxidative stress. Romeo et al. found that adolescents with grade 2 and 3 varicoceles had similar peripheral plasma nitrotyrosine concentrations when compared to controls, even though nitrotyrosine levels in the spermatic veins were significantly elevated [56]. Shiraishi and Naito investigated the evidence of oxidative stress in men with varicoceles versus controls undergoing testes biopsy [57]. They found that patients with a varicocele had increased expression of 4-hydroxy-2-nonenal (4-HNE)-modified proteins, indicating the presence of oxidative stress and increased heme oxygenase 1, which is thought to fight oxidative stress in Leydig cells.

Oxidative stress has also been investigated as a mechanism by which DNA fragmentation is increased in association with varicoceles. Smith et al. found higher DNA fragmentation indices and positive TUNEL (terminal dUTP nick end-labeling) assays in patients with varicoceles than in controls. In addition, reactive oxygen species levels were also higher in the varicocele group [58].

Apoptosis

Since toxic agents and heavy metals accumulate in tissues undergoing apoptosis, several investigators have examined testicular tissue heavy-metal content in men with varicoceles [59]. In particular, cadmium has been implicated as a mediator of the toxic effects of cigarette smoking [60]. This heavy metal has also been detected both in animals with experimental varicoceles and, subsequently, in the seminal plasma of men with varicoceles. Benoff *et al.* demonstrated that higher levels of cadmium and apoptosis were present in the seminiferous tubules of men with varicoceles than in men with obstructive azoospermia. These abnormalities were also found in the contralateral testes even in men with isolated left varicoceles [61]. The authors suggested that cadmium levels are an indicator of a tissue's inability to handle oxidative stress, and that the buildup of the toxic metal exacerbates the deleterious effects of the varicocele. In addition, these authors suggested that cadmium levels and apoptosis rates may identify those patients with varicocele who have experienced irreversible testicular damage. This assertion remains controversial.

Hyperthermia

The detrimental effect of elevated temperature on sperm production was first noted by MacLeod and Hotchkiss in 1941 [62]. Further investigation was undertaken in 1973 by Zorgniotti and MacLeod [63], who compared scrotal temperatures in 50 oligospermic infertile varicocele patients with those of 35 control subjects. The control subjects had intrascrotal temperatures that were 0.6–0.8 °C lower than the intrascrotal temperatures of patients with varicoceles. Agger and Johnsen expanded on this study by measuring scrotal temperatures before and after varicocelectomy [9]. They found no difference in the scrotal temperatures in patients with preoperative sperm concentrations greater than 50 million/mL. However, the subpopulation of patients who had preoperative sperm concentrations less than 50 million/mL and postoperative counts greater than 50 million/mL experienced a decrease in scrotal temperatures of 0.5 °C after varicocelectomy.

Lewis and Harrison, using scrotal thermographic techniques, demonstrated higher scrotal temperatures in patients with varicoceles and abnormal spermatogenesis than in patients with varicoceles and normal semen analyses [10]. Comhaire and colleagues confirmed this observation, reporting increased scrotal temperatures in 37 of 39 patients with varicoceles and abnormal spermatogenesis [28]. However, an interesting study by Mieusset *et al.* showed that all infertile men with abnormal spermatogenesis, with or without a varicocele, had elevated testicular scrotal temperatures [64]. Goldstein and Eid measured intratesticular and scrotal temperatures in men with varicoceles [65]. **They found that, on average, temperatures in the testicle and both sides of the scrotum were elevated in men with unilateral varicoceles, confirming the findings of multiple animal studies.** Jung *et al.* showed a positive effect on motility, morphology, and concentration of sperm by using an external scrotal cooling device [66]. While men with elevated scrotal temperatures with or without varicoceles may suffer similar effects, the pathophysiology of the varicocele remains closely related to alterations in temperature.

Although research continues in the quest to understand the pathophysiology of the varicocele, definitive evidence remains elusive.

Testicular pathology associated with the varicocele

Although the etiology and pathophysiology of the varicocele remain enigmatic, gross testicular alterations associated with the varicocele are well documented. The earliest descriptions of the varicocele note its association with decreased testicular size [12,13]. The testes of subfertile males with varicoceles generally exhibit some degree of atrophy [67]. Marks and colleagues reported that 77% of subfertile patients with a varicocele had either unilateral or bilateral testicular atrophy [68]. Lipshultz and Corriere, using caliper measurements, showed that both the right and left testes of patients with varicoceles were significantly smaller than testes of patients with idiopathic oligospermia or those of normal patients [67]. It has been well documented that varicoceles are associated with macroscopic and microscopic testicular alterations. These changes are observed bilaterally even in the presence of unilateral clinical varicoceles [69].

Microscopic examination of both the right and left testes in patients with unilateral varicoceles and oligospermia shows thinning and sloughing of the germinal epithelium [70]. Spermatogenic arrest in the late spermatid stage may also be observed. Electron microscopic evaluation has demonstrated maturation arrest at the primary spermatocyte level, maloriented spermatids, and structurally abnormal Sertoli cell–germ cell junctional complexes [71–74]. These structural changes have been seen only in the adluminal compartment, with the Sertoli–Sertoli cell junctions remaining unchanged. Hadziselimovic et al. studied testicular biopsies of infertility patients with idiopathic left varicoceles and found endothelial proliferative lesions of the capillaries at the ultrastructural level [75]. These endothelial changes preceded the testicular tubular damage. **The reversibility of these changes postoperatively emphasized the deleterious effects of the varicocele as well as the potential benefit of varicocelectomy in the treatment of the infertile male.**

The effect of varicocelectomy on testicular histology was documented in a classic study by Johnsen and Agger [76]. These authors compared preoperative and postoperative testes biopsies in patients with varicoceles who were infertile and in patients with varicoceles who were fertile. This "masked" study showed that the infertile group had a significant increase in the number of seminiferous tubules containing "numerous" spermatozoa after varicocelectomy. Subsequent investigators have also demonstrated that gross and microscopic alterations occur in conjunction with the clinical varicocele [4,77,78]. Evidence of hypoxia, reactive oxygen species, and apoptosis in testicular histopathology specimens was discussed in the preceding section on pathophysiology.

Diagnosis
Physical examination
Inspection and palpation remains the cornerstone for the diagnosis of the scrotal varicocele. Most physicians will have little difficulty in recognizing large or moderate-sized varicoceles. The distended veins may appear as a vermiform bluish discoloration beneath the scrotal skin. On palpation, they have been described as a "bag of worms" by Dubin and Amelar [79]. The size of a varicocele is assessed by a simple grading system as proposed by Dubin and Amelar [80]. **"Large" (grade 3) varicoceles are visible through the scrotal skin; "moderate" (grade 2) varicoceles are easily palpable without a Valsalva maneuver; the "small" (grade 1) varicocele is palpable only with a concurrent Valsalva maneuver.** The small varicocele can be missed unless a thorough examination of the scrotum is performed, with the patient in both supine and upright positions. Since it has been reported by Dubin and Amelar that

the small varicocele may impair spermatogenesis as often as the large varicocele, it is important to carefully examine the scrotum of every man being evaluated for infertility. However, more recently, Steckel et al. reported that the size of a varicocele may be a factor in the degree of improvement in semen variables after varicocelectomy [81]. They observed that infertile men with larger varicoceles had poorer semen variables preoperatively, and that repair of large varicoceles resulted in greater improvement than repair of small or medium-sized varicoceles. Although several authors have supported this correlation, it is still important to identify all clinical varicoceles.

Examining the patient in a warm and comfortable environment facilitates the scrotal examination. A cool examining room may result in shrinkage and "tightening" of the scrotum, obscuring a varicocele. **A varicocele is most easily detected when the patient is upright and performing a Valsalva maneuver.** During this maneuver, the dilated scrotal varicosities become engorged and more prominent. Asymmetrical filling of the cord and/or a discrete pulse may be palpated when the cord is grasped above the testicle. The Valsalva maneuver may be associated with contraction of the cremasteric muscle, and with resultant thickening and shortening of the spermatic cord. This may be confused with retrograde filling of the pampiniform plexus observed with a varicocele. Gentle traction on the testicle during the Valsalva maneuver will prevent this phenomenon and minimize the likelihood of an incorrect diagnosis. Prolonged standing may also help to accentuate a varicocele. Recently Nagler and Zahalsky reported on a new maneuver, "the Nagler maneuver," which was reported to increase the detection of varicoceles. In this maneuver the abdomen is extended outward [82]. Venous reflux velocities were found to be greater with this maneuver than with the standard provocative maneuvers.

After the upright examination, the patient is re-examined in a supine position. Decompression of the varicocele may be appreciated. Persistence of cord fullness while the patient is in a supine position may be indicative of a cord lipoma, hernia, or other pathologic conditions rather than venous distension of a varicocele. A varicocele that results from renal vein obstruction secondary to a tumor may also persist when the patient is supine. The patient is again examined in the upright position. It is sometimes helpful to grasp the cord structures between the thumb and forefinger as the patient moves from the supine to the upright position. Release of this compression while the patient is standing may allow the examiner to appreciate an increase in cord thickness indicative of retrograde filling of a varicocele. Careful physical examination is mandatory for the accurate diagnosis of the varicocele.

Adjunctive diagnostic tests

Since the varicocele remains the most treatable cause of male-factor infertility, clinicians have used many techniques to aid in its diagnosis. The routine application of adjunctive tests has been questioned in the absence of proof of the efficacy of treating subclinical varicoceles. In general, these techniques should be used to supplement and confirm the diagnosis of a clinical varicocele rather than as primary methods of diagnosis.

Doppler examination

A pencil-probe Doppler stethoscope has been advocated as an adjunctive tool in the examination of the varicocele. Reflux, which is demonstrated with Valsalva, is believed to be indicative of a clinical varicocele. The presence of reflux is indicated by an auditory signal and can be visualized with a graphic representation. The patient is examined in the upright position. Ultrasonographic conducting gel is applied to the upper aspect of the scrotum. There should be complete acoustical silence prior to having the patient perform the Valsalva maneuver. If arterial pulsations are heard, changes in blood flow with Valsalva can be interpreted erroneously as being indicative of a varicocele. A varicocele may be diagnosed by a persistent and reproducible venous rush. The Doppler may also be utilized to assess for the presence of a small or subclinical right varicocele in the presence of a clinically apparent left varicocele. Doppler probes may also be used with a visual display, as described by Greenberg et al. [83,84]. This approach provides for documentation of the findings of the evaluation. Greenberg et al. were able to demonstrate Valsalva maneuver-induced reflux by Doppler examination in all patients studied ($n = 28$) with clinically apparent varicoceles [83]. Most modern series include real-time ultrasound examination rather than Doppler examination, since real-time ultrasound allows for more accurate assessment and measurement of the varicocele.

The significance of a positive test result in subfertile, oligospermic patients with a subclinical varicocele screened by Doppler is uncertain. Hirsh et al. demonstrated Valsalva maneuver-induced varicocele, Doppler-positive reflux in 83% of the left spermatic

veins and 59% of the right spermatic veins of 118 patients without clinical varicoceles [85]. There was no difference between the infertile and fertile men. Because of the high incidence of reflux induced by the Valsalva maneuver, many authors advocate assessing reflux during quiet respiration. Using this method, Hirsh et al. found reflux in 88% of patients with a clinical varicocele, whereas only 18% patients without a varicocele showed the same pattern [86]. In conclusion, the Doppler examination is an adjunct to the physical examination and may be used cautiously to confirm the findings of a physical examination, not to replace them.

If cord structures are normal by physical examination, a Doppler examination is not recommended. However, in our practice, when a clinical varicocele is found on one side, we examine the contralateral cord by Doppler to determine if a subclinical varicocele exists. Ultrasonography may be employed to confirm these findings. This is the only circumstance in which Doppler examination is used to determine the presence of "subclinical reflux." If a subclinical varicocele is appreciated, it is treated at the same time as the coexistent clinical varicocele. This approach is based on the observation that altered blood flow after varicocelectomy may unmask an underlying contralateral venous anomaly, resulting in clinical varicocele formation [72,87]. There is controversy regarding the incidence and clinical significance of bilateral varicoceles, especially if one is considered to be "subclinical." The importance of treating bilateral varicoceles when they exist has recently been highlighted by Libman et al. [30]. In this report, patients with bilateral varicoceles experienced greater improvement than those with unilateral varicoceles. Therefore it is incumbent upon the physician to be certain that bilateral varicoceles are not present prior to subjecting an individual to a surgical intervention.

Ultrasonography

Ultrasonography has become an increasingly useful modality in the diagnosis of varicoceles. As in the case of Doppler examination, the role that sonography will ultimately play in the evaluation of the subfertile male remains to be determined. Kondoh et al. advocate the routine use of sonography in the evaluation of varicoceles [88]. In the subset of patients with a clinical left-sided varicocele, the literature supports the use of sonography in the evaluation of the right side [86,89]. Studies suggest that subclinical right-sided varicoceles play a role in the pathogenesis of male infertility, and that bilateral surgical correction is warranted in these patients. This approach has been extrapolated to color-flow Doppler evaluation. Preliminary reports suggested that the repair of subclinical varicoceles diagnosed using color-flow Doppler sonography is associated with improved semen variables [62]. Although McClure and Hricak demonstrated improvement in sperm motility after repair of bilateral subclinical varicoceles [90], subclinical varicoceles are not thought to be of clinical significance [91]. Several papers have indicated that larger clinical varicoceles (grade 3) were associated with greater semen abnormalities [80,92]. Color-flow Doppler (CFD) sonography has been reported to be nearly as reliable as venography in diagnosing a varicocele, with a 90% accuracy rate. Chiou et al. describe a sensitivity of 93% and specificity of 85% for this technique when compared to physical examination; ultrasound detected all grade 2 and 3 varicoceles on physical examination as well [93]. **Therefore, color-flow Doppler appears to be a useful diagnostic modality in the diagnosis of the hard-to-palpate varicocele.** Zahalsky et al. discussed the role of CFD in diagnosis of varicoceles, and indicated that it is the most common diagnostic modality performed, with accuracy similar to that of invasive venography [94]. Further studies are needed to evaluate the role of CFD ultrasonography in the diagnosis of the subclinical varicocele. Mihmanli et al. detected 94 subclinical varicoceles when examining 208 testes in men with infertility and no clinical varicoceles [95]. The significance of the subclinical varicocele will be reviewed in the outcomes section below. **However, the widespread use of this ultrasound modality for screening of varicoceles cannot be advocated.**

Venography

Venography is usually performed only in conjunction with therapeutic occlusion or in research studies. It is performed using the Seldinger technique via the right femoral vein or right internal jugular vein [96]. Retrograde spermatic venography (Fig. 18.1) is generally regarded as the most sensitive technique for diagnosis of the scrotal varicocele; however, as with the Doppler, its specificity is controversial. When venography is performed in subfertile patients with palpable varicoceles, reflux is seen in nearly 100% of patients [26]. However, in subfertile patients without a palpable varicocele, left testicular reflux has been reported in 60–70% of patients [97]. Furthermore, this

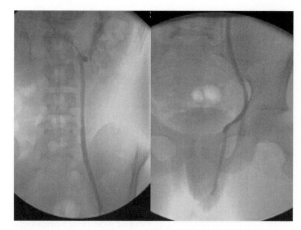

Fig. 18.1. Venogram demonstrating reflux into internal spermatic vein.

same study also reported a 70% incidence of right testicular vein reflux. Equally disturbing is the report by Netto et al. that demonstrated venographic reflux in 58% of men with varicoceles and abnormal semen, in 58% of men with varicoceles and normal semen, and in 33% of normal controls [98]. Although venography may be highly sensitive for reflux, its specificity and significance in reference to the clinical varicocele are unclear. Technical factors may be responsible for many false-positive venographic studies. If the catheter tip is placed in the proximal portion of the left testicular vein, thus bypassing a critical valve at the junction of the left testicular vein and left renal vein, a higher percentage of patients will demonstrate reflux [99]. Given the invasive nature of venography and the controversy regarding the significance of venographically demonstrated reflux, venography should not be used routinely to diagnose varicoceles in the oligospermic patient. The most appropriate indication for venography is the persistent varicocele in the postsurgical patient. In this instance, venography can be both diagnostic and therapeutic when veno-occlusion is performed with use of sclerosing agents [100], Gianturco coils [101], or detachable balloons [102] (as discussed in the following section). **Intraoperative venography has been used to identify persistent vessels after ligation of the internal spermatic veins, and has been reported to decrease the surgical failure rate** [103].

Additional diagnostic techniques

Scrotal thermography has been used to detect elevated temperatures associated with varicoceles. Contact thermography involves the application of a flexible film containing heat-sensitive liquid crystals. This is applied to the scrotum once the patient has been undressed and upright for five minutes in a room at normal temperature. The phallus is taped to the abdominal wall to prevent interference. The thermostrips of different colors correlate with different temperatures, allowing for easy interpretation by the operator [104]. Hirsh et al. reported the accuracy of scrotal thermography in detecting varicoceles to be similar to that of Doppler flow studies [86]. Comhaire et al. [28], Lewis and Harrison [105], Kormano et al. [106], and Pochaczevsky et al. [107] have also advocated the use of scrotal thermography in evaluating patients with suspected varicoceles. However, Mieusset et al. reported that increased scrotal temperatures were observed in infertile men with abnormal spermatogenesis without varicoceles [64]. Although scrotal thermography may also be used as an adjunctive test to confirm the clinical impression, it has not been widely employed.

Radionucleotide imaging

Radionucleotide imaging is familiar to urologists in the evaluation of renal function, and has also been employed in the diagnosis of varicoceles. Nuclear venography involves the injection of the radioisotope into a peripheral vein and subsequent acquisition of images with a gamma-ray scintillation camera focused on the retroperitoneum and scrotum. Although this technique involves intravenous injection of radioisotope, the procedure exposes the patient to minimal exposure to radiation compared to traditional venography [108]. Radionucleotide technetium-99m pertechnetate scintigraphy demonstrates varicoceles by "pooling" of radionucleotide within the dilated pampiniform plexus [109]. Paz and Melloul showed 93.5% correlation between physical examination and radionuclide demonstration of varicocele [110]. They were also able to demonstrate subclinical varicoceles and recurrent varicoceles. **Although effective, this technique is not widely employed.**

Therapeutic indications of varicocele repair
Infertility

The most common indication for varicocelectomy is infertility. However, the mere presence of a varicocele in a subfertile male is not a sole indication for varicocelectomy. One must be certain that the patient has no other causes for infertility and be assured by appropriate

gynecologic examination and evaluation that the partner has a normal fertility potential. Evaluation of the varicocele has been discussed in previous sections of this chapter.

Semen analysis

The detrimental effect of the varicocele on spermatogenesis in the subfertile male is most often reflected in abnormal seminal parameters. Infertile men with varicoceles may have abnormal semen quality, demonstrating reduced sperm counts (less than 20 million/mL), decreased motility, and/or abnormal morphology [18,111,112]. The varicocele appears to affect spermatogenesis, regardless of fertility status. Nagao et al. reported that although fertile men with varicoceles had higher sperm counts than infertile men with varicoceles, counts in both groups of men were significantly lower than in normal controls [113].

MacLeod in 1965 introduced the term "stress pattern" to reflect the altered morphology (increased numbers of immature cells and "tapered" forms) observed in association with a varicocele [111]. The stress pattern was defined as a semen analysis with greater than 15% tapered forms. MacLeod found this pattern in 90% of his infertile patients with a varicocele. Although the "stress pattern" came to be associated with the diagnosis of a varicocele, it is not pathognomonic of the varicocele but rather represents a nonspecific finding associated with abnormal spermatogenesis [112,114]. Ayodeji and Baker found no difference in morphology patterns between infertile patients with varicoceles and infertile patients without varicoceles [73]. Saypol demonstrated that subfertile men with varicoceles had the same percentage (5%) of tapered forms as infertile patients with idiopathic oligoasthenospermia [112]. Similarly, Rodriguez-Rigau et al. compared infertile patients, with and without varicoceles, and showed that the sperm counts, motility, and morphology were significantly associated with one another rather than with the presence or absence of a varicocele [114]. The percentage of "tapered" or amorphous forms observed was inversely associated with sperm counts, and was independent of the presence of a varicocele. In his original report in 1965, MacLeod recognized that there were other causes, such as certain viral illnesses or exposure to antispermatogenic medications, that may produce a stress pattern [111]. The "stress pattern," which was often interpreted as being pathognomonic for a varicocele, is indicative of abnormal testicular function, regardless of cause. Therefore, the term has been largely abandoned. An abnormal semen analysis in a man with a clinical varicocele and a normal partner is the most common indication for varicocelectomy.

The 1992 WHO study showed that 25.4% of men with abnormal semen parameters had a palpable varicocele, compared with only 11.7% of men with normal semen parameters [3]. This study suggested that the presence of a varicocele plays an integral role in the infertile male.

Symptomatic varicocele

Scrotal pain as a result of a varicocele is uncommon, but if it exists and is persistent, varicocelectomy may be of benefit. Symptomatic varicoceles are usually very large. Since varicocelectomy does not necessarily provide the desired relief, it is of paramount importance that other causes of scrotal and inguinal pain be considered before varicocelectomy is offered for relief of scrotal pain. Before scrotal pain is attributed to a varicocele, conservative measures such as scrotal support and the use of anti-inflammatory and analgesic agents should be taken. Patients may benefit from consultation with pain specialists. If persistent pain exists and there is no other indication, the varicocele may, with caution, be implicated. Karademir *et al.* demonstrated that 101 of 121 patients (83%) reported improvement in their scrotal pain in questionnaires answered after undergoing inguinal or subinguinal orchiectomy for scrotal pain [115]. Of these patients, 75% had complete resolution of pain while the remaining 25% had partial resolution. In another large study, high inguinal ligation was used in all patients presenting only with pain: 72 (82.8%) patients reported complete resolution; eight (9.2%) reported partial response; and seven (8%) had persistent pain [116]. Chawla *et al.* comment on reoperation on recurrent varicoceles for pain [117]. Relief of pain was noted in 10 of 11 patients who underwent subinguinal varicocelectomy for orchialgia. **The authors recommend reoperation for pain in patients who have a varicocele recurrence that fails conservative management.**

Pediatric/adolescent varicocele

Historically, the pediatric/adolescent varicocele has been left untreated unless it caused pain or gross testicular damage. However, in recent years, various authors have proposed that ligation of a varicocele during childhood or adolescence may improve the potential for future fertility [8,118,119]. The cornerstone of this approach to the adolescent varicocele is the acceptance of the basic tenet that the varicocele in the adult is associated with male-factor infertility. If one accepts this association, one would logically question the significance of the same process in the prepubertal or adolescent male. Does early ligation prevent subsequent testicular dysfunction?

There are several reports in the literature indicating that the childhood varicocele becomes apparent peripubertally. While the incidence of the prepubertal varicocele is 0–1%, the incidence of varicocele in adolescents is reported to be between 2% and 16% [8,100,119,120]. In males 15 years of age, the incidence has been reported to be as high as 20% [121]. This increased incidence is thought to be related to the physiologic changes that occur during puberty. With the onset of puberty, testicular mass increases significantly, accompanied by an increase in blood flow. This increased perfusion may unmask the venous abnormality responsible for varicocele formation [122].

Although previously unappreciated, it is clear that a varicocele in an adolescent is not a rare entity. Therefore it becomes imperative to establish its physiologic significance. Testicular biopsy results in peripubertal children with varicoceles have demonstrated damage similar to that seen in adults. Heinz *et al.* indicated that testicular histology was already abnormal in 12-year-old boys; more severe histologic abnormalities were seen in older adolescents [77]. Pozza *et al.* examined adolescents with varicoceles, and reported a 74% incidence of testicular atrophy and a 90% incidence of abnormal histology [123]. Therefore, histologic damage appears early in pubertal development and apparently progresses with time.

Lipshultz and Corriere indicated that the presence of the varicocele was associated with a loss of testicular mass that appeared to be progressive with age [67]. Their report was the first to raise the question of whether early ligation would arrest this process. Most authors have discussed testicular atrophy secondary to varicoceles. However, the pubescent testicle harboring a varicocele may suffer from growth retardation rather than atrophy [8,124]. This concept was suggested by Kass and Belman, who demonstrated a significant increase in testicular volume after varicocelectomy in adolescents (ages 11–19 years) [124]. They referred to this phenomenon as "catch-up" growth. Although these authors did not assess the effect of the varicocele or varicocelectomy on spermatogenesis, the reversal in growth retardation (testicular hypotrophy) was assumed to be a surrogate of testicular health and indicative of the removal of noxious stimulus effects of the varicocele.

In a recent survey of pediatricians, Kubal and colleagues noted that 85% of respondents referred patients with clinical varicoceles to a urologist [125]. However, the authors reported that 16.9% of pediatricians do not routinely examine genitalia of adolescent males; 10% of those who do perform testicular examinations fail to check for varicoceles. In addition, those that check for varicoceles do so either by visual inspection alone, with the patient in the supine position, or without Valsalva maneuvers. **Although the pediatricians are aware of varicoceles and their potential significance, they are ill-prepared to diagnose them.**

Two main parameters that have been utilized to dictate varicocele repair in the pediatric population are (1) size discrepancy between the affected testicle and the contralateral testicle and (2) the association of varicocele grade with testicular disparity. The significance of the size of the varicocele and its impact on testicular size has been confirmed by some and refuted by others. Thomas and Elder reported testicular growth arrest at the time of initial presentation to the pediatric urologist in approximately 30% of grade 2 varicoceles and 45% of grade 3 varicoceles [126]. These measurements were performed using calipers, as compared to other studies that use orchidometers or sonography. However, Alukal et al. found that the grade of varicocele did not correlate with the presence or degree of testicular disparity in adolescent males with varicoceles [127]. The authors acknowledged that eight urologists and several ultrasound technicians participated in the study, potentially creating variability in the classification of both varicocele grade and testicle size. **A recent report by Sakamoto et al. showed that in patients undergoing orchiectomy, ultrasound was superior to orchidometer in comparing testicular volume** [128].

Since Kass and Belman popularized the concept of "catch-up growth" following repair of pediatric varicoceles [124], there has been greater emphasis on varicocele repair in the adolescent. In a recent study by Greenfield et al., catch-up growth was demonstrated by caliper measurements in 30 of 36 patients (83%) who were evaluated after subinguinal varicocelectomy [129]. These authors also noted that 15% of younger patients without atrophy at the time of presentation subsequently developed disparity. This suggests that over time the deleterious effect of a varicocele may cause a disparity even if it is not present at the time of diagnosis.

Since a semen sample cannot easily be obtained from the majority of adolescents with a varicocele, it has been difficult to determine the frequency of testicular dysfunction in this group. Kass et al. reported that an abnormal response to GnRH stimulation can be demonstrated in almost one-third of adolescents with a varicocele, and they concluded that this finding indicates a functional disturbance of the testicle [130]. These authors postulated that an excessive release of LH after GnRH stimulation is an indirect indication of Leydig cell dysfunction, and an exaggerated FSH response indicates an abnormality of the seminiferous tubules. GnRH stimulation studies are not widely used.

In a controlled prospective study, Laven et al. repaired varicoceles in 34 boys and observed an increase in left testicular volume, whereas the 33 boys who were controls with varicoceles did not show this increase [131]. In addition, sperm concentrations significantly improved in the treatment group. It is important to note that all serum hormone levels were within the normal range in both groups. Cayan et al. measured semen parameters before and after subinguinal varicocelectomy in adolescents [132]. They reported improvement of semen parameters including concentration and motility.

The ultimate goal of the treatment of the pediatric varicocele is preservation of fertility. When assessing the implications of the pediatric varicocele, it is important to recognize that most men with varicoceles have normal fertility; only 13% of men with varicoceles will be infertile [112]. Studies of the pediatric varicocele have not enabled us to predict the group of adolescents with a varicocele who will have a fertility problem [133]. Because of the uncertainty about benefits in terms of future fertility and the risk of recurrence or surgical complications, most surgeons have adopted the position that the pediatric varicocele should be left untreated unless there is significant testicular asymmetry or retarded testicular growth (> 20% volume disparity) documented on serial examinations [124]. Testicular growth retardation, indicating a potentially significant pathologic lesion, has become a prime indication for varicocelectomy.

The controversy surrounding the adolescent varicocele must be carefully presented to any family seeking consultation. The decision to operate must be a joint decision based on the information available and the family's response to that information.

Secondary infertility

The role of varicoceles in infertility has been strongly implicated in males with secondary infertility. In a review of 2989 patients over a five-year period, Witt and Lipshultz determined that the varicocele is a progressive lesion which results in the loss of previously established fertility [134]. A series published by Gorelick and Goldstein supported this observation [135]. The approach to the individual with secondary infertility and a varicocele should not differ from that taken to the male with primary infertility and a varicocele. Varicocelectomy should be recommended when other factors contributing to infertility have been eliminated.

Non-infertility indications

Although the most common indication for varicocelectomy is infertility, there are other indications worthy of mention.

Cosmesis

Occasionally, a varicocele will cause a patient distress because of a disfigured appearance of the scrotum. This concern is generally more significant to young men with grade 3 varicoceles. Kubal *et al.* in their survey of pediatricians noted a 4% referral rate for varicocelectomy due to cosmetic concerns [125]. Raj and Wiener in a review of adolescent varicoceles addressed this concern but said that decisions to operate for cosmetic reasons are driven by patients rather than by recommendations of the surgeon [136].

Concern regarding future fertility

The work of Kubal and colleagues demonstrated the need to educate pediatricians about the significance of varicoceles in adolescents [125]. **As pediatricians become more aware of the significance of varicoceles, and are more inclined to refer patients with varicoceles to urologists, it is likely that more young adolescents and families will become concerned about yet untested future fertility.** As discussed above, there are several parameters that have been advocated to aid the patient and physician in the decision-making process. However, ultimately there continues to be uncertainty about the impact of a varicocele on an individual's subsequent fertility. Therefore, some families choose to undergo pre-emptive varicocelectomy whereas others choose observation.

Surgical treatment

Surgical varicocelectomy is the cornerstone of varicocele therapy. The goal of intervention is the complete

disruption of the internal spermatic venous drainage of the testicle while preserving the internal spermatic artery, vas deferens with its blood supply, and spermatic cord lymphatics. Several surgical approaches are available to accomplish a varicocelectomy. The approaches discussed below are in anatomic order in a cephalad direction rather than a reflection of the authors' preference. These include the scrotal approach, the subinguinal approach, the inguinal approach (modified Ivanissevich), the retroperitoneal approach (modified Palomo), and the laparoscopic approach (Fig. 18.2).

Scrotal approach

Mentioned only for completeness and historical accuracy, this approach has been abandoned because the complexity of the scrotal pampiniform plexus and its rich anastomotic network makes successful interruption less likely. Additionally, damage to the end testicular artery and resulting testicular ischemia are more likely because of the multiple sites of division and ligation. One would suspect that injury to the vas and/or artery would be similar to or less than rates in hydrocelectomy, which can range from 5% to 17% according to Zahalsky *et al.* [137]. **This technique is best avoided, because of its higher failure and complication rates.**

Subinguinal approach

The subinguinal approach is simply a modification of the inguinal approach. An oblique or transverse incision is made at the level of the external inguinal ring (Fig. 18.2). The external oblique fascia is not incised. This minimizes postoperative discomfort and reduces risk of ilioinguinal nerve injury. The spermatic cord is mobilized below the level of the external inguinal ring as it crosses over the pubic tubercle entering the scrotum. A smaller incision is usually made, leading to potentially greater difficulty in mobilizing the cord. Some advocate gently grasping the cord with a Babcock clamp and elevating it with gentle traction. We choose not to grasp the cord with an instrument, to minimize any possibility of a crush injury to the vas. Sheynkin *et al.* have demonstrated that minor compression of the vas can result in cicatrix and subsequent obstruction [138]. The cord can be easily mobilized through a 3 cm incision using blunt dissection with surgical peanuts. A Penrose drain is passed behind the spermatic cord for support, and the procedure performed in the same fashion as the inguinal approach. Marmar and Kim reported that morbidity with this procedure is less than that of inguinal

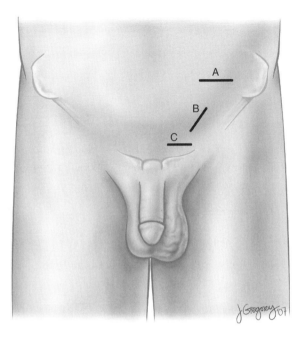

Fig. 18.2. Surgical varicocelectomy. (A) Retroperitoneal approach: a short transverse incision is made just medial to the anterior superior iliac spine at the level of the internal ring. (B) Inguinal approach: an oblique incision is made along the axis connecting the anterior superior spine and the pubic tubercle. (C) Subinguinal approach: an oblique or transverse incision is made at the level of the external inguinal ring.

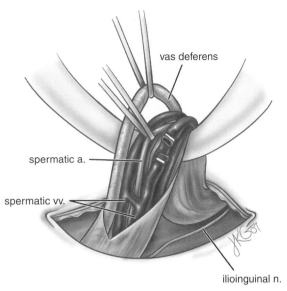

Fig. 18.3. Subinguinal approach. A Penrose drain is used to elevate the cord. The vas deferens and spermatic artery are placed under vessiloops to isolate and preserve them.

and retroperitoneal surgery, because the muscle layers and inguinal canal are not violated [139]. The external cremasteric vessels are easy to identify and, if abnormal, ligate at this level (Fig. 18.3). Because the internal spermatic venous system is more branched at this level, this approach is more tedious than the inguinal approach. **Due to the complexity at the cord at this level, microscopic technique is generally employed when a subinguinal varicocelectomy is performed.**

Inguinal approach: modified Ivanissevich

The inguinal approach exposes the internal spermatic vessels within the inguinal canal. As noted by Ivanissevich, this approach has several advantages over the retroperitoneal approach [140]. First, the urologic surgeon is quite comfortable with the anatomy within the inguinal canal. As the spermatic vein moves cephalad and approaches the internal inguinal ring, it will coalesce to form several larger vessels. This approach will also allow for identification of large external cremasteric vessels that may contribute to the varicocele.

Optical loupe magnification may be used for opening and closing the wound. An oblique incision is made parallel to the inguinal canal connecting the anterior superior iliac spine and the pubic tubercle. The medial aspect of the incision should be approximately two finger breadths above the symphysis pubis at the lateral edge of the scrotum (Fig. 18.2). Before the incision is made, the exact location of the external ring may be noted by invaginating the scrotal skin. The external oblique aponeurosis is exposed and incised in the direction of its fibers. Care is taken to avoid injury to the underlying ilioinguinal nerve. This procedure can be safely carried out by making a small stab through the fascia. The Metzenbaum scissors are then slid down to the external ring with the tips of the scissors elevated against the undersurface of the fascia. The scissors are then rotated 90° to expose a groove between the two blades; this is used as a guide for the knife in incising the fascia. The spermatic cord is then mobilized at the level of the pubic tubercle. A Penrose drain is passed beneath the cord, elevating it from the canal. The Penrose drain is also used to exclude the ilioinguinal nerve from the operative field (Fig. 18.4).

When the cremasteric fascia is incised, one should attempt to identify the artery using visual inspection and intraoperative Doppler ultrasound. The operating microscope is used to aid in the identification and preservation of the internal spermatic artery [141].

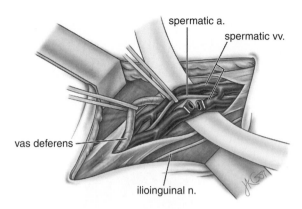

Fig. 18.4. Inguinal approach. The external oblique aponeurosis is incised and exposed. A Penrose drain is used to elevate the spermatic cord into the wound. The ilioinguinal nerve, vas deferens, and spermatic artery are placed under vessiloops to isolate and preserve them. Spermatic veins are then tied or clipped as depicted.

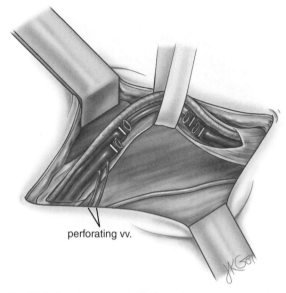

Fig. 18.5. Inguinal approach. The floor of the canal is exposed to identify perforating external cremasteric veins.

When the artery is identified, a vessiloop is utilized to isolate the artery from the area in which further dissection proceeds. With the artery protected, all venous channels are isolated and ligated with a nonabsorbable suture or clipped (Fig. 18.4). A representative segment may be excised.

Great care is taken to identify even small venous channels. These may be cauterized with bipolar forceps. The vas deferens is identified and its vasculature preserved. At this point, attention is redirected to the artery and surrounding veins, which have been encircled by the vessiloop. Meticulous dissection allows the surgeon to remove the rich anastomotic network of veins that is closely adherent to the spermatic artery. The artery is identified throughout the dissection both visually and via Doppler examination. Topical application of papaverine or bupivacaine will cause arterial dilation and may aid in the identification of the artery. When the artery has been cleared of the surrounding veins, its pulsations are immediately apparent. Lymphatic channels are generally clearly visualized. These should be preserved to minimize the incidence of hydrocele formation. After the spermatic cord has been fully explored, the cord is lifted out of the inguinal canal by gentle elevation of the Penrose drain (Fig. 18.5). The floor of the canal at the level of the external ring is inspected for any external cremasteric veins. These vessels perforate the canal to drain into the pudendal vein and, ultimately, the saphenous vein. These veins should be identified, since they may contribute to recurrent varices in a small proportion of patients. The external oblique fascia is closed with a continuous 3–0 chromic suture; the subcutaneous layer is approximated with interrupted 3–0 plain catgut. A subcuticular absorbable closure is used.

Goldstein and associates suggest that recurrent varicoceles are due to venous collaterals that bypass the inguinal portion of the spermatic cord, and therefore deliver the testicle through the inguinal incision to provide direct access to all avenues of testicular venous drainage [141]. The gubernaculum can be inspected for the presence of veins exiting the tunica vaginalis, which can then be cauterized, ligated, or clipped. This approach has not been widely accepted. Ramasamy and Schlegel have refuted this practice in a recent comparison of subinguinal varicocelectomy with or without testicular delivery [142]. **This study showed no benefit and a possible detriment of testicular delivery, based on better improvement of semen parameters without the addition of this extra step.**

Retroperitoneal approach: modified Palomo

The retroperitoneal approach or modified Palomo technique exposes the internal spermatic vein within the retroperitoneum after it exits the inguinal canal. A transverse abdominal incision is made just medial to the anterior superior iliac spine at the level of the internal ring (Fig. 18.2). The external oblique fascia is incised in the direction of the fibers, and the internal oblique muscle is incised and retracted cephalad. This

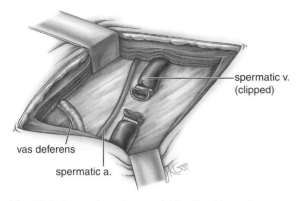

spermatic v.
(clipped)

vas deferens

spermatic a.

Fig. 18.6. Retroperitoneal approach. The dilated internal spermatic vein is identified and ligated just superior to the internal ring.

exposes the dilated internal spermatic vein, which is ligated and divided (Fig. 18.6). The dissection may proceed cephalad toward the renal vein to identify the collateral vessels. The vas deferens and spermatic vessels meet as they enter the internal ring, aiding in the identification of the internal spermatic vessels (Fig. 18.2). Although Palomo described ligating both the internal spermatic artery and veins [22], most authors believe that the artery should be preserved [143]. The theoretical advantage of this technique is that retroperitoneal ligation of the internal spermatic vein reduces the number of veins contributing to the varicocele and therefore minimizes the potential for recurrence of the varicocele. Cockett *et al.* [4] advocate this approach, on the premise that venous communications may occur between the left and right varicoceles at a level above the internal ring as described by Etriby *et al.* [144]. A major disadvantage of this technique is that it does not allow identification and ligation of the external cremasteric vessels. These vessels have been implicated as a cause of recurrent and persistent varicoceles after varicocelectomy [24,145]. Additionally, the approach is not familiar to most urologic surgeons. **This technique may be advantageous in patients with previous inguinal surgery, because it minimizes incidental injury to the testicular artery and ilioinguinal nerve.**

The Palomo technique has gained some popularity among pediatric urologists. In a comparison of several techniques, Pintus *et al.* advocated the original Palomo approach for pediatric varicocelectomy due to its low recurrence rate of less than 2% [146]. Kass and Reitelman wrote, "When surgery is necessary, the Palomo approach significantly decreases the risk of operative failure and has facilitated 'catch-up' growth of the left testis that is comparable to that after

artery-sparing procedures" [147]. Mass ligation of the internal spermatic vessels results in fewer persistent varicoceles than artery-sparing techniques [148].

Laparoscopic approach

The urologist's experience with pediatric and adult laparoscopy has progressed in recent years. It is now feasible for many urologists to execute this approach for the high ligation of the internal spermatic vein [149].

A Foley catheter is placed in all patients to avoid injury to the bladder. After routine preparation of the abdomen, a Veress needle is used to establish a pneumoperitoneum. Alternatively, a small peritoneotomy can be performed subumbilically, and a 10 mm trocar passed under direct vision. This allows for greater safety and faster insufflation. The laparoscopic camera is then passed through the subumbilical port. Under direct vision, one additional trocar (5 mm) is placed to the left of the midline and one trocar (5 mm) is placed to the right. The internal ring, vas deferens, and medial umbilical ligament can be readily identified. After identification of the iliac and epigastric vessels, the parietal peritoneum is opened lateral to the spermatic vessels. The internal spermatic artery can be identified by its appearance and pulsations. In addition, papaverine solution causing dilation can be used to enhance visualization of the artery [150]. The use of the Doppler probe introduced through one of the ports may aid in the localization of the spermatic artery [151]. The vessels are dissected free, and the vein is clipped with titanium clips both proximally and distally and cut between. Bilateral ligations can be performed by simply switching to the contralateral side. After careful inspection for hemostasis, the instruments are withdrawn and the carbon dioxide released. The fascia is closed with #1 polyglycolic acid suture, and the skin is reapproximated with an absorbable subcuticular suture. Patients may be discharged the same day [150].

Mehan and colleagues reported on 38 patients who underwent laparoscopic internal spermatic vein ligation [150]. Pregnancy was achieved in 16 (42%) of 38 patients. Of the 22 cases not achieving a pregnancy, nine (41%) had a 50% rise in sperm density, and eight of these (36%) had an increase in sperm viability and motility. Thirteen cases had no significant change. The only major complication reported was a hydrocele. The results of this study indicate that the procedure is physiologically equivalent to the retroperitoneal/ modified Palomo approach. Proponents of laparoscopic surgery assert that the technique affords a lower postoperative morbidity and faster return to normal activities. Donovan and Winfield performed 19 laparoscopic varicocelectomies in 14 patients (five bilateral) without any complications [151]. However, since the potential for significant morbidity from laparoscopy exceeds that of the extraperitoneal approach, this technique has not been widely embraced.

Ligation of the testicular artery during varicocelectomy does not always result in testicular atrophy because vascular communication between the testicular, cremasteric, and vasal arteries is present. Kass and Marcol reported that mass ligation of the internal spermatic vessels resulted in a lower rate of varicocele persistence than artery-sparing techniques [148]. Matsuda *et al.* reported that there was no significant difference between artery-preserving varicocelectomy and artery-ligating surgery when improvements in semen quality and postoperative pregnancy data were evaluated [152]. Similarly, Parrott and Hewatt showed that in the adolescent total ligation of the testicular vascular pedicle above the entrance of the vas deferens into the spermatic cord allowed for the "catch-up growth" of the smaller ipsilateral testes with low risk for recurrence of the varicocele [153]. Because the major complication of varicocelectomy is persistence of the varicocele, an argument can be made for not preserving the artery. Wright and Goldstein reported a diminished response (i.e., improvement in semen variables) after varicocelectomy when the testicular artery was divided [143]. However, since arterial injury may result in testicular atrophy in a small number of patients, and this complication is unpredictable, we recommend testicular artery preservation in all cases.

Nonsurgical treatment of varicoceles
Percutaneous venous occlusion

From 1952 until 1978, infertile men with varicoceles underwent surgical varicocelectomy only. In 1978, Lima and colleagues reported the use of transvenous sclerotherapy for ablation of varicoceles [154]. Techniques used to achieve transvenous occlusion of the internal spermatic veins have included the deployment of detachable balloons, Gianturco coils, and sclerotherapy, or a combination of these modalities (Fig. 18.7). Each of these techniques has its proponents. However, all these techniques share common advantages and disadvantages [101,155]. Each procedure can be performed on an outpatient basis with

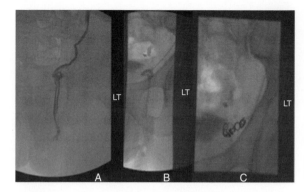

Fig. 18.7. Venogram demonstrates reflux into the internal spermatic veins (A and B). Coils are placed to embolize the varicocele.

intravenous sedation. They each afford a nonoperative approach to what historically has been treated surgically. Theoretically, recuperative time is minimized. The disadvantages of these techniques focus on patient discomfort with a nonsurgical approach to ablation of the internal spermatic veins. However, infertile patients are often reluctant to have any unnecessary exposure to radiation. They are also concerned with balloon or coil migration. Most importantly, they want to minimize the chances of recurrence and the possible need for an additional procedure, since the success rates for percutaneous venous occlusion are less than reported for surgical repair [1,7].

With the use of detachable balloons, either a femoral or a jugular approach is employed. The jugular approach allows easier access to the right internal spermatic vein, and is therefore employed with bilateral and right unilateral varicocele. The inguinal approach is generally preferred when treating isolated left-sided varicoceles. The use of detachable balloons affords the radiologist the ability to test the adequacy of the occlusion before releasing the balloon. However, since different-sized balloons may be required to achieve satisfactory occlusion, it is necessary to maintain an inventory of expensive balloons. Furthermore, there are isolated reports of balloon deflation and migration with time [156,157]. Although Gianturco coils are inexpensive, multiple coils may be required to achieve occlusion, and the adequacy of occlusion cannot be tested before the release of the coil [101]. Most invasive radiologists are comfortable with the utilization of coils. Sclerotherapy allows occlusion of smaller collateral venous channels, but this modality is cumbersome [158]. Sclerotherapy may also be used in conjunction with the coil occlusion technique.

Although embolization is a nonoperative approach to the varicocele, it is often difficult and more time-consuming than varicocelectomy. Pryor and Howards summarized the success of veno-occlusion, and reported that embolization is recognized to be technically unsuccessful at the time of the procedure in 27% of cases [1]. Additionally, when the procedure is considered technically successful, the recurrence rate after embolization is approximately 5%. Therefore the success rate for this procedure, taking into account both the occlusion rate (73%) and the nonrecurrence rate (95%), is only 69% [156]. Kaufman et al. reported recurrences in eight of 70 patients (11%) who had balloon occlusion of varicocele [157].

Currently, we use embolization for the treatment of surgical failures, in patients with previous inguinal surgery, or because of patient preference. Murray and associates reviewed the mechanism of recurrence after surgically treated and embolized varicoceles [145]. The surgical failures were easily treated with embolization, whereas 39% of the embolization failures were not amenable to repeat venographic occlusion. With the increased safety of local and regional ambulatory anesthesia, in addition to the greater "reliability" and efficiency of the operative procedure, varicocele ligation remains the procedure of choice for the primary treatment of the varicocele.

Antegrade sclerotheraphy

Antegrade sclerotherapy for the treatment of varicocele was originally described by Tauber in 1988 [159]. It is performed using local anesthesia. An incision is made high in the scrotum and the spermatic cord is isolated with a Penrose drain. The largest spermatic vein is cannulated using a catheter, and antegrade venography is performed using 5 mL of contrast medium. Sclerosing agent is mixed with air in 3 : 1 ratio (air block technique) and injected while the patient performs a Valsalva maneuver. In a randomized trial of Tauber sclerotherapy versus inguinal varicocelectomy, patients showed slightly better results for improvement of motility, although the two techniques were comparable in terms of other semen parameters. Each technique was associated with minimal perioperative and postoperative complications [160].

Testicular hypothermia device

Although the pathophysiology of the varicocele is unclear, the varicocele may exert its deleterious effects by increasing testicular temperature. This assumption

led to the development of the testicular hypothermia device (THD) [161]. The THD was an externally applied device that cooled the scrotum by evaporation of water, which was continuously applied to a cotton scrotal support. This technique was reported to lower scrotal temperatures by 2.3 °C. The THD was prescribed to 140 infertile patients with subfertile semen, elevated scrotal temperatures, and more than two years of unprotected intercourse with a presumed fertile partner [161]. The compliance rate was only 46%. Of the 64 remaining patients who wore the THD for at least 16 weeks, 66% exhibited improvements in semen parameters. A 27% pregnancy rate was reported in this study. Poor patient compliance, resulting from water leaks and general discomfort, limited the acceptance of and the usefulness of this noninvasive modality. Many patients prefer to undergo a procedure that theoretically will rectify the pathology in one "sitting" rather than wearing an uncomfortable device as a daily reminder of an already frustrating problem. Further study would be necessary to demonstrate the effectiveness of this approach. However, there have been no publications on this technique since 1987 [162].

Outcome analysis
Prognosis

This section presents the evaluable data for assessing the efficacy of varicocelectomy. Two large review studies and additional primary studies were available for analysis. Review of the literature was performed using MEDLINE, Ovid, and the Cochrane databases. Pryor and Howards assembled 15 papers evaluating the success of varicocele surgery [1]. Their review encompassed 2466 varicocelectomies. The overall rate of improvement in semen quality was 66% (range 51–78%), and the overall reported pregnancy rate was 43% (range 24–53%). An extensive review of the literature published by Schlesinger and Nagler concluded that varicocelectomy does have a beneficial effect on sperm density [163]. It was noted that motility and morphology may improve significantly after varicocelectomy when an associated rise in density was observed. Their review has been refined and expanded here, and the tables and discussion below reflect a comprehensive update of the Schlesinger and Nagler reviews (Tables 18.1–18.7) [164–173].

In spite of a considerable quantity of data demonstrating improved semen quality and pregnancy

Table 18.1. Randomized varicocelectomy trials: pregnancy rates

Study	Treated	Controls	Odds ratio	Semen parameters	Varicocele definition	Control group
Krause, 2002 [170]	16% (n = 31)	18% (n = 33)	0.875	Azoospermia excluded	Clinical only	
Unal, 2001 [168]	10% (n = 21)	5% (n = 21)	2.00		Subclinical only	Clomiphene citrate
Grasso, 2000 [171]	3% (n = 34)	6% (n = 34)	0.485		Subclinical only	
Nieschlag, 1998 [169]	29% (n = 62)	25% (n = 63)	1.20			More grade 1 varicoceles in control group 56% vs. 40%
Yamamoto, 1996 [172]	7% (n = 45)	10% (n = 40)	0.643		Subclinical only	
Madgar, 1995 [167]	60% (n = 20)	40% (n = 25)	13.5	Excluded azoospermia		
Breznik, 1993 [173]	34% (n = 43)	53% (n = 46)	0.449	Included patients with normal semen parameters		
Vermeulen, 1986 [165]	41% (n = 105)	53% (n = 30)	0.3029		Subclinical varicoceles grade included	44% of control group SC vs. 31% treated
Baker, 1985 [166]	47% (n = 283)	21% (n = 611)	3.21	Excluded azoospermia		
Nilsson, 1979 [164]	8% (n = 51)	18% (n = 45)	0.394	Included patients with normal semen parameters		

Table 18.2. Randomized varicocelectomy trials: sperm density

Study	Patients (n)	Comment	Intake sperm density	Follow-up sperm density	Significance
Krause, 2002 [170]	14	Sclerotherapy	11.7 ± 21.0	10.8 ± 22.5	NS
Unal, 2001 [168]	18	Controls	6.6 ± 33.1	8.8 ± 32.7	NS
	21	Varicocelectomy	47.9 ± 35.7	59.8 ± 50.1	NS
		Clomiphine citrate	51.6 ± 39.4	59.1 ± 46.0	NS
Grasso, 2000 [171]	34	Varicocelectomy	16.39	16	NS
	34	Controls	16.17	15.83	NS
Yamamoto, 1996 [172]	45	High ligation	15 ± 18.1	20.9 ± 18.9	NS
	40	Controls	15.1 ± 20.1	13.4 ± 16.8	
Madgar, 1995 [167]	25	Varicocelectomy	15[a]	32[a]	P < 0.05
	20	Controls	15[a]	15[a]	NS
Nilsson, 1979 [164]	51	Palomo	47 ± 41	49 ± 40	NS
	45	Controls	59 ± 43		

[a] Estimated from graphical representation of data in Madgar *et al.* [166]

rates following varicocelectomy, most of the studies are uncontrolled [164,165]. There have been many uncontrolled studies of the effect of varicocelectomy on infertility, but there have been only 10 randomized controlled studies. Four of these studies demonstrated improved sperm parameters and pregnancy rates [166–169]. However, six studies did not demonstrate

Table 18.3. Randomized varicocelectomy trials: motility

Study	Patients (n)	Comment	Intake motility	Postoperative motility	Significance
Krause, 2002 [170]	14	Treated with sclerotherapy	NA	-5.4 ± 22.1^{a}	NS
	18	Controls	NA	-2.1 ± 25.3^{a}	NS
Unal, 2001 [168]	21	Varicocelectomy	39.0 ± 14.0	$48.0 \pm 14.0‡$	NS
	21	Clomiphine citrate	43.8 ± 20.5	58.9 ± 13.6	NS
Grasso, 2000 [171]	34	Varicocelectomy	22.06 ± 2.83	22.99 ± 2.7	NS
	34	Controls	19.53 ± 5.12	20.49 ± 4.31	
Nieschlag, 1998 [169]	14	Sclerotherapy	NA	NA	
Yamamoto, 1996 [172]	45	High ligation	21.7 ± 15.1	23.2 ± 16.69	NS
	40	Controls	21.7 ± 13.2	21.5 ± 13	NS
Madgar, 1995 [167]	25	Varicocelectomy	30%	55%	$P < 0.001$
	20	Controls	30%	33%	NS
Nilsson, 1979 [164]	51	Palomo	32 ± 8	32 ± 7	NS
	45	Controls	31 ± 7		

^{a} data reported as change in motility

Table 18.4. Randomized varicocelectomy trials: morphology

Study	Patients (n)	Comment	Intake morphology % normal	Postoperative % normal	Significance
Krause, 2002 [170]	14	Treated with sclerotherapy	NA	NA	
	18	Untreated	NA	NA	
Unal, 2001 [168]	21	Varicocelectomy	$69.1 \pm 16.$	70.4 ± 12.4	NS
	21	Clomiphine citrate	64.3 ± 23.6	73.4 ± 9.8	NS
Grasso, 2000 [171]	34	Varicocelectomy	30.06 ± 3.01	29.99	NS
	34	Untreated	31.82 ± 3.25	31.94 ± 3.73	NS
Nieschlag, 1998 [169]			NA	NA	
Yamamoto, 1996 [172]	45	High ligation	31.5 ± 15.0	30 ± 8.5	NS
	40	No treatment	30.3 ± 8.5	30.5 ± 9.4	NS
Madgar, 1995 [167]	25	Varicocelectomy	27	40	$P < 0.005$
	20	Controls	25	27.5	NS
Nilsson, 1979 [164]	51	Palomo	42	42	N
	45	Controls	41		

benefit, or reported a deleterious effect on fertility [164,165,170–173].

One of the best randomized prospective studies of patients with varicoceles, comparing those treated surgically with those treated by observation alone, was performed by Madgar *et al.* [167]. This study clearly demonstrated that varicocelectomy improves sperm parameters and fertility rates. Several randomized

Table. 18.5. Uncontrolled varicocelectomy trials: sperm density

Study	Patients (n)	Comment	Intake sperm density	Postoperative density	Pregnancy rate	Significance
Hsieh, 2006	254	Ivanisevich	24.2 ± 18	41 ± 28	37%	P < 0.05
Marmar, 2005	60	Marmar	11.92 ± 8.80	19.93 ± 12.00		P < 0.01
Orhan, 2005	82	Ivanisevich	30 ± 8.3	33 ± 8.9	41%	
	65	Marmar	29 ± 8.5	32 ± 10.0	33%	
Pasqualotto, 2005	28	Germ cell aplasia	9.82 ± 5.9	12.05 ± 4.8	25%	P = 0.04
	32	Maturation arrest	19.97 ± 22.34	24.76 ± 16.9	53.8%	P = 0.08
Pasqualotto, 2005	28	≤ 5 veins ligated	38.87 ± 13.2	22.09 ±	No info	P = 0.03
	21	5–9	13.4 ± 4.6	12.9 ± 5.9	No info	P = 0.09
	12	≥ 10	13.28 ± 7.2	37.45 ± 13.2	No info	P = 0.04
Zini, 2005	37	Marmar	34.6 ± 6.0	38.4 ± 7.6	No info	P = 0.54
Gat, 2005	101	Embolization	0.22 ± 0.30	9.28 ± 1.2	No info	P < 0.001
	32	Azoospermia	0	3.81 ± 1.69	No info	P < 0.03
	31	Virtual azoospermia	0.054 ± 0.007	10.31 ± 1.87	No info	P < 0.001
	38	Severe oligoazoospermia	0.54 ± 0.04	12.11 ± 1.85		P < 0.001
Watanabe, 2005	50	High ligation	15.9 ± 19.8	28.8 ± 32.5	55.1% @ 5 years	P < 0.01
	33	Laparoscopic	21.9 ± 22.2	52.3 ± 55.4	48.9% @ 5 years	P < 0.01
	61	Marmar	23.5 ± 29.7	59.4 ± 50.2	56.4% @ 5 years	P < 0.01
Kibar, 2002	90	Subinguinal	22.1 ± 4.2	38.3 ± 6.1	No info	P < 0.00002
Onozawa, 2002	18	Observed	36.6 ± 31.9	41.9 ± 45.7	80%	P > 0.05
	26	Palomo	26.0 ± 28.8	34.6 ± 29.2	30%	P = 0.09
Jungwirth, 2000	272	Subinguinal micro	51.7 ± 4.2	64.3 ± 5.6		P < 0.0001 vs. control
	91	Grade 1	42.7 ± 6.1	41.7 ± 6.6		P < 0.01 vs. control
	71	Grade 2	44.4 ± 7.8	52.0 ± 7.7		P < 0.01 vs. control
	107	Grade 3	55.2 ± 16.9	89.2 ± 34.7		P < 0.01 vs. control
Vazquez-Levin, 1997	33	Microsurgical	35.2 ± 6.2	45.8 ± 8.0		
Nieschlag, 1995	47	Treated	16.5 ± 2.5	25.1 ± 4.1	25.5% (not sig from control group)	P = 0.008
Hirokawa, 1993	18		55.85 ± 6.9	67.47 ± 9.2		P < 0.05
	32		9.06 ± 1.09	19.57 ± 2.9		P < 0.01
Yavetz, 1992	43	Ivanissevich	13 ± 18	24		P < 0.01
	43	Bernardi	12 ± 13	15		NS
		Embolization	9 ± 10	18		P < 0.05

Table. 18.5. continued

Study	Patients (n)	Comment	Intake sperm density	Postoperative density	Pregnancy rate	Significance
Sayfran, 1992	28	Inguinal	54 ± 62	118 ± 121		P < 0.05
	36	Embolization	56 ± 65	68 ± 91		NS
	55	High ligation	47 ± 47	93.0 ± 12.9		P < 0.05
Rageth, 1992	33		9.92	15.11		P < 0.05
Mehan, 1992	33		20.96 ± 21.06	38.96 ± 26.05		Not calculated
Laven, 1992	27		47.4 ± 43.9	68.9 ± 46.2		P < 0.05
Goldstein, 1992	271		36.97	46.85		P < 0.001
Yarborough, 1989	13		14.1 ± 3.9	20.2 ± 5.8		P < 0.05
Parsch, 1989	72	Sclerosis	48.6 ± 61.8	65.6 ± 84.8		P < 0.05
	31	High ligation	40.9 ± 46.6	55.7 ± 64.9		P < 0.05
Okuyama, 1988	10	Treated		25.9 ± 11.8		–
	13			5 ± 20.7		P < 0.01
Nilsson, 1979	51		47 ± 41	49 ± 40		NS
Rodrigues-Rigau, 1978	24		17.02 ± 3.26	27.32 ± 6.8		P < 0.01
Johnsonen & Agger, 1978	21		44	100		P < 0.01

trials have been performed more recently, but they suffer from assorted weaknesses (Table 18.1) [164–173]. It is important to critically evaluate studies assessing the effectiveness of varicocelectomy in the treatment of infertility. Inclusion or exclusion criteria may have a significant impact on the reported results. For instance, Krause et al. [169], Madgar et al. [167], and Baker et al. [166] excluded men with azoospermia, while Breznik et al. [173] and Nilsson et al. [164] included men with normal semen parameters. Unal et al. [168], Grasso et al. [171], and Yamamoto et al. [172] included or focused exclusively on patients with subclinical varicoceles. Therefore, since different populations were included, a meta-analysis of the randomized data would be inherently flawed. In Tables 18.2–18.4 [164,167–172], we have analyzed the results of the randomized studies which presented evaluable data on specific semen parameters. Only two of six studies [167,168] showed improvement in sperm density (Table 18.2). The study by Madgar et al. [167] was the only one that demonstrated improvement in motility and morphology (Tables 18.3–18.4).

Prognostic variables

Despite the lack of good randomized data supporting varicocelectomy, numerous nonrandomized studies support its efficacy. Perhaps the most frequently quoted study is the early study by Dubin and Amelar [79]. They found a higher pregnancy rate postoperatively in patients with preoperative sperm densities greater than 10 million/mL. Brown reported similar findings [174]. However, Cockett et al. reported an increased pregnancy rate in patients with sperm concentrations less than 10 million/mL [4]. Each of these studies attempted to utilize sperm concentrations as prognostic indicators of efficacy. **In an attempt to identify prognostic factors predicting postoperative pregnancies, Marks and colleagues showed four preoperative variables to be of value** [68]. The absence of testicular atrophy was found to indicate a good prognosis: 56% of patients with normal testicular size established pregnancies, compared with a 33% pregnancy rate in patients with testicular atrophy. Patients with initial sperm counts of 50 million or more per ejaculate

Table 18.6. Uncontrolled varicocelectomy trials: motility

Study	Patients (n)	Comment	Intake motility	Postoperative motility	Significance
Hsieh, 2006	254	Ivanisevich	30 ± 18	47 ± 16	$P < 0.05$
Marmar, 2005	60		30.00 ± 12.10	44.02 ± 9.51	$P < 0.001$
Pasqualotto, 2005	28	Germ cell aplasia	44.3 ± 25.6	41.3 ± 19.6	$P = 0.09$
Pasqualotto, 2005	32	Maturation arrest	38.5 ± 23.1	42.4 ± 22.6	$P = 0.08$
Orhan, 2005	82	Ivanisevich	29 ± 8.4	35 ± 13.1	$P = 0.01$
	65	Marmar	29 ± 8	34 ± 13.1	$P = 0.01$
Pasqualotto, 2005	28	≤ 5 Veins ligated	45.9 ± 42.8	42.8 ± 21.3	$P = 0.09$
	21	5–9	35.4 ± 14.6	43.7 ± 18.3	$P = 0.09$
	12	≥ 10	39.7 ± 14.3	41.55 ± 15.7	$P = 0.09$
Zini, 2005	37	Marmar	20.9 ± 1.9	22.1 ± 2.6	NS
Gat, 2005	101	Embolization	8.78 ± 1.59	29.56 ± 2.0	$P < 0.01$
	32	Azoospermia	0	1.20 ± 3.62	$P < 0.01$
	31	Virtual azoospermia	6.07 ± 2.69	35.8 ± 2.76	$P < 0.01$
	38	Severe oligoazoospermia	13.96 ± 3.06	33.24 ± 3.13	< 0.01
Watanabe, 2005	50	High ligation	38.0 ± 22.1	39.1 ± 25.2	NS
	33	Laparoscopic	40.4 ± 18.8	42.5 ± 22.6	NS
	61	Marmar	32.4 ± 26.0	38.8 ± 26.2	NS
Kibar, 2002	90	Subinguinal	23.2 ± 2.2	45.1 ± 1.9	$P < 0.01$
Jungwirth, 2000	272	Subinguinal micro	17.4 ± 0.7^a	28.3 ± 1.3^a	$P < 0.001$
	91	Grade 1	19.9 ± 1.6^a	30.9 ± 1.8^a	$P < 0.01$
	71	Grade 2	16.5 ± 1.5^a	26.1 ± 1.7^a	$P < 0.001$
	107	Grade 3	17.2 ± 5.8^a	21.6 ± 60^a	NS^a
Vazquez-Levin, 1997	33	Microsurgical	26.4 ± 2.6	31.0 ± 2.1	NS
Sayfran, 1992	28	Inguinal	73 ± 48^b	97 ± 58^b	NS
	36	Embolization	62 ± 45^b	82 ± 57^b	NS
	55	High ligation	71 ± 51^b	88 ± 54^b	NS
Rageth, 1992	33		35.6	37.57	NS
Laven, 1992	27		54.3 ± 14	59.3 ± 9.9	NS
Goldstein, 1992	271		39.62	45.66	$P < 0.001$
Yarborough, 1989	13		36.7 ± 3.6	39.2 ± 4.4	NS
Parsch, 1989	72	Sclerosis	36 ± 14.6	40.3 ± 12.1	$P < 0.05$
	31	High ligation	39.2 ± 14.5	45.3 ± 10.8	$P < 0.05$
Okuyama, 1988	10	Treated		62.2 ± 15.3	$P < 0.01$
	13			30.7 ± 18.1	
Rodrigues-Rigau, 1978	24		41.2 ± 3.9	42.3 ± 5.1	NS

[a] forward progressive motility
[b] motility index

Table 18.7. Uncontrolled varicocelectomy trials: morphology

Study	Patients (*n*)	Comment	Intake morphology normal values	Postoperative morphology normal values	Significance
Hsieh, 2006	254	Ivanisevich	Not specified	Not specified	No significant improvement
Marmar, 2005	60	Marmar	14.65%	25.28%	$P < 0.001$
Orhan, 2005	82	Ivanisevich	$9.8 \pm 0.7\%$	$18 \pm 0.8\%$	$P < 0.001$
	65	Marmar	$9.0 \pm 0.5\%$	$17 \pm 0.6\%$	$P < 0.001$
Zini, 2005	37	Marmar	$21.2 \pm 1.8\%$	$23.4 \pm 1.6\%$	$P = 0.08$
Gat, 2005	101	Embolization	$3.79 \pm 0.74\%$	$13.72 \pm 1.37\%$	$P < 0.005$
Grober, 2004	334	Marmar	$35.8 \pm 1.4\%$	$37.7 \pm 1.5\%$	
Kibar, 2002	90	Subinguinal	$2.6 \pm 0.5\%$	$10.2 \pm 0.9\%$	$P < 0.0001$
Goldstein, 1992	271		48.42	52.1	$P < 0.001$
Yarborough, 1989	13		52.8 ± 2.4	55.9 ± 4.7	NS
Parsch, 1989	72	Sclerosis	32.6 ± 22	37.4 ± 20.7	$P < 0.05$
	31	High ligation	34.2 ± 23	42.2 ± 17.7	$P < 0.05$
Okuyama, 1988	10	Treated		71.9 ± 13.6	$P < 0.01$
	13			42.5 ± 17.7	–
Nilsson, 1979	51		44 ± 19	44 ± 13	NS
Johnsonen & Agger, 1978	21		46	53	$P < 0.025$

were significantly more likely to establish pregnancies after varicocelectomy. Thirty percent of patients with preoperative sperm motility of less than 60% initiated pregnancies postoperatively, whereas 60% of those with normal preoperative motility produced pregnancies. As expected, elevation of FSH was a poor prognostic indicator. In this study, only 25% of patients whose FSH was above 300 ng/mL achieved pregnancies, whereas 46% of patients with normal FSH levels (< 300 ng/mL) initiated pregnancies. The studies of Steckel *et al.* [81] and Dubin and Amelar [80] similarly found no relationship between the clinical grade of the varicocele and postoperative pregnancy rates despite improvements in semen variables. Tinga *et al.* studied the relationship between varicocele size and prognosis, and reported a significant relationship between the grade of the varicocele and semen quality improvement [175]. **However, they found no relationship between varicocele size and postoperative pregnancy rates.**

Standard semen analysis is limited in its ability to differentiate fertile from infertile males. In fact,

pregnancies attributed to alterations in semen variables may be unrelated. Other parameters have been used for the evaluation of varicocele efficacy. Rogers *et al.* attempted to demonstrate functional improvement after varicocelectomy using the sperm penetration assay [176]. In their study, 70% of those who achieved a pregnancy demonstrated improvement in the sperm penetration assay.

Reactive oxygen species have been implicated as mediators of the abnormal spermatogenesis observed in the presence of the varicocele [177]. In the pathophysiology section above, the relationship between apoptosis and cadmium levels was discussed. Preliminary data showed that the amount of cadmium in the testis biopsy was indicative of the extent of damage caused by varicoceles. The patients with low intratesticular cadmium levels prior to varicocelectomy were noted to have a greater improvement in sperm counts than those patients with higher cadmium levels [178]. Unfortunately, pregnancy data were not included in this study. Acrosome reaction via the acrobeads test has been used to assess sperm quality in a small study of infertility patients who underwent varicocelectomy [179]. The couples who achieved pregnancy ($n = 10$) had a statistically significant improvement in sperm acrosome status (using the acrobeads test) when compared to those who did not achieve pregnancy. The authors suggest that this test may provide a better method of testing for sperm function than standard semen parameters. More recently, attention has been directed to assessing sperm DNA integrity in male-factor infertility. Human sperm DNA damage or fragmentation may adversely affect fertility outcomes [180]. Zini et al. showed that the percentage of spermatozoa with DNA denaturation decreased following varicocelectomy to 24.6%, from 27.7% preoperatively ($P < 0.05$) [181]. While new tests of varicocele repair efficacy are being used, there is no adjunctive testing established that predicts the response to varicocelectomy.

Adjuvant hormonal therapy

The value of hormonal therapy after varicocelectomy is unclear. Dubin and Amelar reported that adjuvant human chorionic gonadotropin (hCG) resulted in better semen parameters and pregnancy rates in patients with counts less than 10 million/mL than in those treated with varicocelectomy alone [80]. These authors treated patients with sperm counts of less than 10 million/mL with injections of hCG, 4000 units intramuscularly twice weekly for 10 weeks. A 55% improvement in semen quality and a 45% pregnancy rate was observed. Cockett et al. used clomiphene citrate, 25 mg/day for 25 days with a five-day rest period, and reported a 53% pregnancy rate [4]. However, other authors using adjuvant clomiphene citrate reported no advantage [182,183]. Except in patients with a demonstrated gonadotropin deficiency, it is unclear whether exogenous hormones have an effect in the varicocele patient. Rodrigues-Netto recommends repeating the patient's endocrine studies two months after adjuvant endocrine therapy, and suggests that if an increase in FSH is noted without improvement in the semen analysis, therapy be discontinued [184]. Raman and Schlegel discussed the use of an aromatase inhibitor, testolactone, in infertile patients [185]. A subgroup of these patients ($n = 18$) had previously undergone a varicocelectomy. These patients showed an increase in testosterone-to-estradiol ratios (5.5 ± 0.5 vs. 11.8 ± 2.1, $P < 0.005$). While the authors did not discuss improvements in semen parameters or fertility for this group specifically, they demonstrated an increase in sperm concentration and motility index in men treated with the aromatase inhibitor. Results were recorded only for the 25 of 140 subfertile patients for whom semen analysis data were available. A prospective trial would be necessary to evaluate specifically the use of aromatase inhibitors to enhance the efficacy of varicocelectomy. Adjuvant therapy is empiric therapy and has not been definitively demonstrated to be effective.

Varicocelectomy and azoospermia

Although Tulloch's classic article reported the initiation of spermatogenesis in a man with azoospermia, azoospermia has generally been regarded as a contraindication to varicocelectomy [16]. Recently, there has been renewed interest in varicocelectomy in the azoospermic patient. Tables 18.8 through 18.10 present data for sperm density, motility, and morphology for azoospermic patients. Esteves and Glina biopsied all azoospermic men who underwent microsurgical varicocelectomy [186]. Improvement was observed after varicocelectomy in men with hypospermatogenesis (5 of 6), and maturation arrest (3 of 5), but not in the six men with Sertoli-cell-only syndrome. Testicular histology may predict technical success of varicocelectomy in the azoospermic patient. Even with the appearance of sperm in the ejaculate, it is likely that the infertile couple will require assisted reproductive technology.

Complications of varicocele therapy: surgical and venographic

Recurrence or persistence of varicocele after therapy is the most common complication of varicocele therapy. After surgical therapy, the recurrence rate has been reported to be between 0% and 20%. The recurrence after venographic techniques is reported to be between 2% and 12% [1]. In a recent series, 206 of 223 (92%) of attempted embolizations were technically feasible, and 172/206 patients (83.5%) showed complete resolution of the varicocele; however, 34/206 (16.5%) had evidence of recurrence [187]. Thus the reported technical "success rate" for embolization may be as low as 77% after six months of follow-up. This result does not compare favorably with the recurrence rates of any of the large historical or contemporary surgical series. In 1977, Dubin and Amelar reported on 986 patients who underwent varicocelectomy [79]. Recurrence was noted in one patient. Obviously, there is wide variation in surgical and venographic skills, and success rates will depend on the experience of the radiologist or surgeon. However, most urologic surgeons have extensive experience in operating within the inguinal canal. Most interventional

Table 18.8. Effect of varicocelectomy on sperm density in patients with azoospermia

Study	Patients (n)	Comment	Follow-up sperm density	Pregnancy rate	Significance
Gat, 2005	32	Azoospermia	3.81 ± 1.69	–	P < 0.03
	31	Virtual azoospermia	10.31 ± 1.87	–	P < 0.001
Esteves, 2005	17	Hypospermatogenesis	1.5	–	
Pasqualotto, 2003	15	Microsurgical repair	2.54	7%	
Kim, 1999	28	Microsurgical repair	1.2 ± 3.6	One via IUI One via TESE	
Matthews, 1998	22	Azoospermia	2.2 ± 1.1	14%	

Table 18.9. Effect of varicocelectomy on motilty in patients with azoospermia

Study	Patients (n)	Comment	Postoperative motility	Significance
Gat, 2005	32	Azoospermia	1.20 ± 3.62	P < 0.01
	31	Virtual azoospermia	35.8 ± 2.76	P < 0.01
Esteves, 2005	17	Hypospermatogenesis	0.8	
Pasqualotto, 2003	15	Microsurgical repair	18	
Kim, 1999	28	Microsurgical repair	19 ± 24	P < 0.001
Goldstein, 1998	22	Azoospermia	2.2 ± 1.1	P < 0.05

Table 18.10. Effect of varicocelectomy on morphology in patients with azoospermia

Study	Patients (n)	Comment	Follow-up sperm morphology	Signifcance
Gat, 2005	101	Embolization	13.72 ± 1.37%	P < 0.005
Esteves, 2005	17	Hypospermatogenesis	5.7%	
Pasqualotto, 2003	15	Microsurgical repair	2%	

radiologists are now adept at embolization techniques. There are complications that are specific to the various techniques. Surgical repair may be accompanied by hydrocele formations (3%), epididymitis (less than 1%), and, rarely, wound infections [79]. No recurrence was reported for contemporary microsurgical varicocelectomy, and hydrocele formation was 1.3% (5/304). With the retroperitoneal approach, the recurrence rates reported were 7% (8/109), and hydrocele formation was 6.4% (7/109) [188]. **In a retrospective review by Richardson and Nagler, of 368 varicocelectomies in patients not receiving perioperative antibiotics, the incidence of culture-documented wound infection was 0.5% [189].**

The major complication associated with balloon occlusion of varicoceles is balloon migration. This has been reported, but no clinical sequelae were noted [156,157]. Additionally, there are complications common to all invasive radiologic techniques. Contrast extravasation is the most common, but reactions are rare. Spermatic vein phlebitis and pain occur infrequently; inadvertent femoral artery puncture may also occur. The overall complication rate, as compiled by Pryor and Howards, is 11% [1].

Potential complications of the antegrade sclerotherapy technique include inability to cannulate the vein, testicular necrosis due to injection into the spermatic artery, and recurrence. In a randomized prospective study by Mazzoni et al., the recurrence rate after antegrade sclerotherapy was 4.5%, which was similar to the recurrence rate of 4.4% with their Palomo technique [190].

Conclusion

A review of the evolution of our understanding of the varicocele, as well as theories of its pathophysiology, makes us aware of our limited understanding of the mechanism by which the varicocele adversely affects spermatogenesis. While research in hypoxia and reactive oxygen species may provide new insights into the pathophysiology of the varicocele, our ability to assess the impact of an individual's varicocele on that individual's semen analysis and our ability to predict the response to varicocelectomy remain limited. Varicocelectomy remains a mainstay in the treatment of the infertile male. However, in the absence of controlled studies, clear predictive parameters remain problematic, both for the physician and for the patient.

References

[1] Pryor JL, Howards SS. Varicocele. *Urol Clin North Am* 1987; **14**: 499–513.

[2] Fretz PC, Sandlow JI. Varicocele: current concepts in pathophysiology, diagnosis, and treatment. *Urol Clin North Am* 2002; **29**: 921–37.

[3] World Health Organization. The influence of varicocele on parameters in a large group of men presenting to infertility clinics. *Fertil Steril* 1992; **57**: 1289–93.

[4] Cockett ATK, Takihara H, Consentino MJ. The varicocele. *Fertil Steril* 1984; **41**: 5–11.

[5] Newton R, Schinfeld JS, Schiff I. The effect of varicocelectomy on sperm count, motility, and conception rate. *Fertil Steril* 1980; **34**: 250–4.

[6] Rodrigues-Netto N, Fakiani EP, Lemos GC. Varicocele: clinical or surgical treatment? *Int J Fertil* 1984; **29**: 164–7.

[7] Saypol DC, Lipshultz LI, Howards SS. Varicocele. In: Lipshultz LI, Howards SS, eds. *Infertility in the Male*, 1st edn. New York, NY: Churchill Livingstone, 1983.

[8] Lyon RP, Marshall S, Scott MP. Varicocele in childhood and adolescence: implication in adulthood infertility. *Urology* 1982; **6**: 641–4.

[9] Agger P, Johnsen SG. Quantitative evaluation of testicular biopsies in varicocele. *Fertil Steril* 1978; **19**: 52–7.

[10] Lewis RW, Harrison RM. Contact scrotal thermography: application to problems of fertility. *J Urol* 1979; **122**: 40–2.

[11] Curling TB. *A Practical Treatise on the Disease of the Testis and of the Spermatic Cord and Scrotum*. Philadelphia, PA: Blanchard & Lea, 1856.

[12] Barwell R. 100 cases of varicocele treated by the subcutaneous wire loop. *Lancet* 1885; **1**: 978.

[13] Bennet WH. Varicocele, particularly with reference to its radical cure. *Lancet* 1889; **1**: 261–3.

[14] Macomber D, Sanders MB. The spermatozoa count: its value in the diagnosis, prognosis and treatment of sterility. *N Engl J Med* 1929; **200**: 981–4.

[15] Tulloch WS. A consideration of sterility factors in the light of subsequent pregnancies: subfertility in the male. *Trans Edinb Obstet Soc* 1952; **59**: 29–34.

[16] Tulloch WS. Varicocele in subfertility, results of treatment. *Br Med J* 1955; **2**: 356–8.

[17] Dubin L, Amelar RD. Varicocelectomy: 986 cases in a 12 year study. *Urology* 1977; **10**: 446–9.

[18] Greenberg SH, Lipshultz LI, Wein AJ. Experience with 425 subfertile male patients. *J Urol* 1978; **119**: 507–10.

[19] Gat Y, Bachar GN, Zukerman Z, Belenky A, Gornish M. Varicocele: a bilateral disease. *Fertil Steril* 2004; **81**(2): 424–9.

[20] Siegel Y, Gat Y, Bacher GN, Gornish M. A proposed anatomic typing of the right internal spermatic vein: Importance for percutaneous sclerotherapy of varicocele. *Cardiovasc Intervent Radiol* 2006; **29**(2): 192–7.

[21] Shafik A, Bedeir G. Venous tension patterns in cord veins in normal and varicocele individuals. *J Urol* 1980; **23**: 383–5.

[22] Palomo A. Radical cure of varicocele by a new technique: preliminary report. *J Urol* 1969; **61**: 604–7.

[23] Buschi N, Harrison RB, Norman A. Distended left renal vein: CT/sonographic normal variant. *AJR Am J Roentgenol* 1980; **135**: 339–42.

[24] Coolsaet BL. The varicocele syndrome: venography determining the optimal level for surgical management. *J Urol* 1980; **124**: 833–9.

[25] Ahlberg NE, Bartley O, Chidekel N. Right and left gonadal veins: an anatomic and statistical study. *Acta Radiol Diagn (Stockh)* 1966; **4**: 593–601.

[26] Ahlberg NE, Bartley O, Chidekel N, Fritjofsson A. Phlebography in varicocele scroti. *Acta Radiol Diagn (Stockh)* 1966; **4**: 517–28.

[27] Comhaire FH, Kunnen M, Nahoum C. Radiologic anatomy of the internal spermatic vein(s) in 200 retrograde venograms. *Int J Androl* 1981; **4**: 379–87.

[28] Comhaire F, Monteyne R, Kunnen M. The value of scrotal thermography as compared with selective retrograde venography in the internal spermatic vein for the diagnosis of "subclinical" varicocele. *Fertil Steril* 1976; **27**: 694–8.

[29] Chehval MJ, Purcell MH. Varicocelectomy: incidence of external spermatic vein involvement in the clinical varicocele. *Fertil Steril* 1992; **39**: 573–5.

[30] Libman J, Jarvi K, Lo K, Zini A. Beneficial effect of microsurgical varicocelectomy is superior for men with bilateral versus unilateral repair. *J Urol* 2006; **176**: 2602–5.

[31] Ozbek E, Yurekli M, Soylu A, Davarci M, Balbay MD. The role of adrenomedullin in varicocele and impotence. *BJU Int* 2000; **86**: 694–8.

[32] Cohen MS, Plaine L, Brown JS. The role of internal spermatic vein plasma catecholamine determinations in subfertile men with varicoceles. *Fertil Steril* 1975; **26**: 1243–9.

[33] Comhaire F, Vermeulen A. Varicoceles: cortisol and catecholamines. *Fertil Steril* 1974; **25**: 88–95.

[34] Comhaire F, Vermeulen A. Plasma testosterone in patients with varicocele and sexual inadequacy. *J Clin Endocrinol Metab* 1982; **40**: 824–9.

[35] Hudson RW, Hayes KA, Crawford VA>, McKay DE. Seminal plasma testosterone and dihydrotestosterone levels in males with varicoceles. *Int J Androl* 1983; **6**: 135–42.

[36] Hudson RW, Perez-Marrero RA,Crawford VA, McKay DE. Hormonal parameters of men with varicocele before and after varicocelectomy. *Fertil Steril* 1985; **43**: 905–10.

[37] Steeno O, Koumans J, De Moor P. Adrenal cortical hormones in the spermatic vein of 95 patients with left varicocele. *Andrologia* 1976; **8**: 101–4.

[38] Lindholmer C, Thulin L, Eliasson R. Concentrations of cortisol and renin in the internal spermatic vein of men with varicocele. *Andrologie* 1973; **5**: 21–2.

[39] Ito H, Fuse H,Minagawa H, Kawamura K,Murakami M, Shimazaki J. Internal spermatic vein prostaglandins in varicocele patients. *Fertil Steril* 1982; **37**: 218–22.

[40] Free ML, Jaffe RA. Dynamics of circulation in the testis of the conscious rat. *Am J Physiol* 1972; **223**: 241–8.

[41] Harrison RM, Lewis RW, Roberts JA. Pathophysiology of varicocele in nonhuman primates: long-term seminal and testicular changes. *Fertil Steril* 1986; **46**: 500–10.

[42] Turner T, Lopez TJ. Effects of experimental varicocele require neither adrenal contribution nor venous reflux. *J Urol* 1989; **142**: 1372–5.

[43] Swerdloff RS, Walsh PC. Pituitary and gonadal hormones in patients with varicocele. *Fertil Steril* 1975; **26**: 1006–12.

[44] Pasqualotto FF, Lucon AM, de Góes PM, *et al.* Relationship between the number of veins ligated in a varicocelectomy with testicular volume, hormonal levels and semen parameters outcome. *J Assist Reprod Genet* 2005; **22**: 245–9.

[45] Gat Y, Gornish M,Belenky A, Bachar GN. Elevation of serum testosterone and free testosterone after embolization of the internal spermatic vein for the treatment of varicocele in infertile men. *Hum Reprod* 2004; **19**: 2303–6.

[46] Su LM, Goldstein M, Schlegel PN. The effect of varicocelectomy on serum testosterone levels in infertile men with varicoceles. *J Urol* 1995; **154**: 1752–5.

[47] O'Brien J, Bowles B,Kamal KM, Jarvi K, Zini A. Does the gonadotropin-releasing hormone stimulation test predict clinical outcomes after microsurgical varicocelectomy? *Urology* 2004; **63**: 1143–7.

[48] Guarino N, Tadini B, Bianchi M. The adolescent varicocele: the crucial role of hormonal tests in selecting patients with testicular dysfunction. *J Pediatr Surg* 2003; **38**: 120–3.

[49] Fisch H, Hyun G, Hensle TW. Testicular growth and gonadotrophin response associated with varicocele repair in adolescent males. *BJU Int* 2003; **91**: 75–8.

[50] Barqawi A, Caruso A, Meacham RB. Experimental varicocele induces testicular germ cell apoptosis in the rat. *J Urol* 2004; **171**: 501–3.

[51] Nagler HM, Tomashefsky P, Zippe CD. Microvascular hemodynamic observations in the experimental varicocele. Paper presented at the American Urologic Association Meeting, Boston, MA, 1998.

[52] Kilinç F, Kayaselcuk F, Aygun C, *et al.* Experimental varicocele induces hypoxia inducible factor-1α, vascular endothelial growth factor expression and angiogenesis in the rat testis. *J Urol* 2004; **172**: 1188–91.

[53] Lee JD, Jeng SY, Lee TH. Increased expression of hypoxia-inducible factor-1α in the internal spermatic vein of patients with varicocele. *J Urol* 2006; **175**: 1045–8.

[54] Santoro G, Romero C. Normal and varicocele testis in adolescents. *Asian J Androl* 2001; **3**: 259–62.

[55] Hendin BN, Kolettis PN, Sharma RK, Thomas AJ, Agarwal A. Varicocele is associated with elevated spermatozoal reactive oxygen species production and diminished seminal plasma antioxidant capacity. *J Urol* 1999; **161**: 1831–4.

[56] Romeo C, Ientile R, Impellizzeri P, *et al.* Preliminary report on nitric oxide-mediated oxidative damage in adolescent varicocele. *Hum Reprod* 2003; **18**: 26–9.

[57] Shiraishi K, Naito K. Increased expression of Leydig cell haem oxygenase-1 preserves spermatogenesis in varicocele. *Hum Reprod* 2005; **20**: 2608–13.

[58] Smith R, Kaune H, Parodi D, *et al.* Increased sperm DNA damage in patients with varicocele: relationship with seminal oxidative stress. *Hum Reprod* 2006; **21**: 986–93.

[59] Ku JH, Shim HB, Kim SW, Paick JS. The role of apoptosis in the pathogenesis of varicocele. *BJU Int* 2005; **96**: 1092–6.

[60] Nawrot T, Plusquin M, Hogervorst J, *et al.* Environmental exposure to cadmium and risk of cancer: a prospective population-based study. *Lancet Oncol* 2006; 7: 119–26.

[61] Benoff S, Goodwin LO, Millan C, *et al.* Deletions in L-type calcium channel alpha1 subunit testicular

transcripts correlate with testicular cadmium and apoptosis in infertile men with varicoceles. *Fertil Steril* 2005; **83**: 622–34.

[62] MacLeod J, Hotchkiss RS. The effect of hyperpyrexia on spermatozoa counts in men. *Endocrinology* 1941; **28**: 780–4.

[63] Zorgniotti AW, MacLeod J. Studies in temperature, human semen quality, and varicocele. *Fertil Steril* 1973; **24**: 854–63.

[64] Mieusset R, Bujan L, Mondinat C, *et al*. Association of scrotal hyperthermia with impaired spermatogenesis in infertile men. *Fertil Steril* 1987; **48**: 1006–11.

[65] Goldstein M, Eid F. Elevation of intratesticular and scrotal skin surface temperature in men with varicocele. *J Urol* 1989; **142**: 743–5.

[66] Jung A, Eberl M, Schill W. Improvement of semen quality by nocturnal scrotal cooling and moderate behavioural change to reduce genital heat stress in men with oligoasthenoteratozoospermia. *Reproduction* 2001; **121**: 595–603.

[67] Lipshultz LI, Corriere JN. Progressive testicular atrophy in the varicocele patient. *J Urol* 1977; **117**: 175–6.

[68] Marks JL, McMahon R, Lipshultz LI. Predictive parameters of successful varicocele repair. *J Urol* 1986; **136**: 609–12.

[69] Dubin L, Hotchkiss RS. Testis biopsy in subfertile men with varicocele. *Fertil Steril* 1969; **20**: 51–7.

[70] Jones MA, Sharp GH, Trainer TD. The adolescent varicocele: a histopathologic study of 13 testicular biopsies. *Am J Clin Pathol* 1988; **89**: 321–8.

[71] Kim ED, Leibman BB, Grinblat DM, Lipshultz LI. Varicocele repair improves semen parameters in azoospermic men with spermatogenic failure. *J Urol* 1999; **162**: 737–40.

[72] Amelar RD, Dubin L. Right varicocelectomy in selected infertile patients who have failed to improve after previous left varicocelectomy. *Fertil Steril* 1987; **47**: 833–7.

[73] Ayodeji O, Baker HWG. Is there a specific abnormality of sperm morphology in men with varicoceles? *Fertil Steril* 1986; **45**: 839–42.

[74] Cameron DF, Snydle FE. Ultrastructural surface characteristics of seminiferous tubules from men with varicocele. *Andrologia* 1982; **14**: 425–33.

[75] Hadziselimovic F, Herzog B, Liebundgut B, Jenny P, Buser M. Testicular and vascular changes in children and adults with varicocele. *J Urol* 1989; **142**: 583–5.

[76] Johnsen SG, Agger P. Quantitative evaluation of testicular biopsies before and after operation for varicocele. *Fertil Steril* 1978; **29**: 58–63.

[77] Hienz HA, Voggenthaler J, Weissbach L. Histological findings in testes with varicocele during childhood

and their therapeutic consequences. *Eur J Pediatr* 1980; **133**: 139–46.

[78] Kass EJ, Chandra RS, Belman AB. Testicular histology in the adolescent with a varicocele. *Pediatrics* 1987; **79**: 996–8.

[79] Dubin L, Amelar RD. The varicocele and infertility. In: Amelar RD, Dubin L, Walsh PC, eds. *Male Infertility*. Philadelphia, PA: Saunders, 1977: 57–68.

[80] Dubin L, Amelar RD. Varicocele size and results of varicocelectomy in selected subfertile men with varicocele. *Fertil Steril* 1970; **21**: 606–9.

[81] Steckel J, Dicker AP, Goldstein M. Relationship between varicocele size and response to varicocelectomy. *J Urol* 1993; **149**: 769–71.

[82] Nagler HM, Zahalksy MP. The Nagler maneuver: a reliable physical examination technique to distinguish varicoceles. Presented at the American Urologic Association Meeting, 2003.

[83] Greenberg SH, Lipshultz LI, Morganroth J, Wein AJ. The use of the Doppler stethoscope in the evaluation of varicoceles. *J Urol* 1977; **117**: 296–8.

[84] Greenberg SH, Lipshultz LI, Wein AI. A preliminary report on "subclinical varicocele": diagnosis by Doppler ultrasonic stethoscope. Examination and initial results of surgical therapy. *J Reprod Med* 1979; **22**: 77–81.

[85] Hirsh AV, Cameron KM, Tyler JP, Simpson J, Pryor JP. The Doppler assessment of varicoceles and internal spermatic vein reflux in infertile men. *Br J Urol* 1980; **52**: 50–6.

[86] Hirsh AV, Kellett MJ, Robertson G, Pryor JP. Doppler flow studies, venography and thermography in the evaluation of varicoceles of fertile and subfertile men. *Br J Urol* 1980; **52**: 560–5.

[87] Amelar RD, Dubin L. Therapeutic implications of left, right, and bilateral varicocelectomy. *Urology* 1987; **30**: 53–9.

[88] Kondoh N, Meguro N, Matsumiya K, *et al*. Significance of subclinical varicocele detected by scrotal sonography in male infertility: a preliminary report. *J Urol* 1993; **150**: 1158–60.

[89] Eskew LA, Watson NE, Wolfman N, *et al*. Ultrasonographic diagnosis of varicoceles. *Fertil Steril* 1993; **60**: 693–7.

[90] McClure RD, Hricak H. Scrotal ultrasound in the infertile man: detection of subclinical unilateral and bilateral varicoceles. *J Urol* 1986; **135**: 711–15.

[91] Jarow JP, Ogle SR, Eskew LA. Seminal improvement following repair of ultrasound detected subclinical varicoceles. *J Urol* 1996; **155**: 1287–90.

[92] Scherr D, Goldstein M. Related articles, comparison of bilateral versus unilateral varicocelectomy in men with palpable bilateral varicoceles. *J Urol* 1999; **162**: 85–8.

[93] Chiou RK, Anderson JC, Wobig RK, *et al.* Color Doppler ultrasound criteria to diagnose varicoceles: correlation of a new scoring system with physical examination. *Urology* 1997; **50**: 953–6.

[94] Zahalsky M, Berman A, Nagler HM. Current US techniques for evaluating male infertility. *Contemp Urol* 2005; **17** (4): 52–8.

[95] Mihmanli I, Kurugoglu S, Cantasdemir M, *et al.* Color Doppler ultrasound in subclinical varicocele: an attempt to determine new criteria. *Eur J Ultrasound* 2000; **12**: 43–8.

[96] Sigman M, Jarow JP. Male infertily. In: Walsh PC, Retik AB, Vaughan ED, Wein AJ, eds. *Campbell's Urology*, 8th edn. Philadelphia, PA: Saunders, 2002; 2: 1475–515.

[97] Narayan P, Gonzalez R, Amplatz K. Varicocele and male subfertility. Paper presented at the American Fertility Society, Houston, March 1980.

[98] Netto Júnior NR, Lerner JS, Paolini RM, de Góes GM. Varicocele: the value of reflux in the spermatic vein. *Int J Fertil* 1980; **25**: 71–4.

[99] Nadel SN, Hutchins GM, Albertsen PC, White RI. Valves of the internal spermatic vein: potential for misdiagnosis of varicoceles by venography. *Fertil Steril* 1984; **41**: 479–81.

[100] Seyferth W, Jecht E, Zeitler E. Percutaneous sclerotherapy of varicoceles. *Radiology* 1981; **139**: 335–40.

[101] Morag B, Rubinstein ZJ, Goldwasser B, Yerushalmi A, Lunnenfeld B. Percutaneous venography and occlusion in the management of spermatic varicoceles. *AJR Am J Roentgenol* 1984; **143**: 635–40.

[102] Walsh PC, White RI. Balloon occlusion of the internal spermatic vein for the treatment of varicoceles. *JAMA* 1981; **246**: 1701–2.

[103] Hart RR, Rushton HG, Belman AB. Intraoperative spermatic venography during varicocele surgery in adolescents. *J Urol* 1992; **148**: l514–16.

[104] Gat Y, Bachar GN, Zukerman Z, Belenky A, Gorenish M. Physical examination may miss the diagnosis of bilateral varicocele: a comparative study of 4 diagnostic modalities. *J Urol* 2004; **172**: 1414–17.

[105] Lewis RW, Harrison RM. Contact scrotal thermography. II. Use in the infertile male. *Fertil Steril* 1980; **34**: 259–63.

[106] Kormano M, Kahanpää K, Svinhufvud U, Tähti E.. Thermography of varicocele. *Fertil Steril* 1970; **21**: 558–64.

[107] Pochaczevsky R, Lee WJ, Mallett E. Management of male infertility: roles of contact thermography, spermatic venography, and embolization. *AJR Am J Roentgenol* 1986; **147**: 97–102.

[108] Harris JD, McConnell BJ, Lipshultz LI, McConnell RW, Conoley PH.. Radioisotope angiography in diagnosis of varicocele. *Urology* 1980; **16**(1): 69–72.

[109] Wheatley JK, Fajman WA, Witten FR. Clinical experience with the radioisotope varicocele scan as a screening method for the detection of subclinical varicoceles. *J Urol* 1982; **128**: 57–9.

[110] Paz A, Melloul M. Comparison of radionuclide scrotal blood-pool index versus gonadal venography in the diagnosis of varicocele. *J Nucl Med* 1998; **39**: 1069–74.

[111] MacLeod J. Seminal cytology in the presence of varicocele. *Fertil Steril* 1965; **16**: 735–57.

[112] Saypol DC. Varicocele. *J Androl* 1981; **2**: 61–71.

[113] Nagao RR, Plymate SR, Berger RE, Perin EB, Paulsen CA.. Comparison of gonadal function between fertile and infertile men with varicoceles. *Fertil Steril* 1986; **46**: 930–3.

[114] Rodriguez-Rigau LJ, Smith KD, Steinberger E. Varicocele and the morphology of spermatozoa. *Fertil Steril* 1981; **35**: 54–7.

[115] Karademir K, Senkul T, Baykal K, *et al.* Evaluation of the role of varicocelectomy including external spermatic vein ligation in patients with scrotal pain. *Int J Urol* 2005; **12**: 484–8.

[116] Yeniyol CO, Tuna A, Yener H, Zeyrek N, Tilki A. High ligation to treat pain in varicocele. *Int Urol Nephrol* 2003; **35**(1): 65–8.

[117] Chawla A, Kulkarni G, Kamal K, Zini A. Microsurgical varicocelectomy for recurrent or persistent varicoceles associated with orchalgia. *Urology* 2005; **66**: 1072–4.

[118] Hudson RW, Perez-Marrero RA, Crawford VA, McKay DE. Hormonal parameters in incidental varicoceles and those causing infertility. *Fertil Steril* 1976; **45**: 692–700.

[119] Buch JP, Cromie WJ. Evaluation and treatment of the preadolescent varicocele. *Urol Clin North Am* 1985; **12**: 3–12.

[120] Oster J. Varicocele in children and adolescents: an investigation of the incidence among Danish school children.. *Scand J Urol Nephrol* 1971; **5**: 27–32.

[121] Homer JS. The varicocele: a survey amongst secondary school boys. *Med Officer* 1960; **104**: 377.

[122] Reitelman C, Burbige KA, Sawczuk IS, Hensle TW. Diagnosis and surgical correction of the pediatric varicocele. *J Urol* 1987; **138**: 1038–40.

[123] Pozza D, D'Ottavio G, Masci P, Coia L, Zappavigna D. Left varicocele at puberty. *Urology* 1983; **3**: 271–4.

[124] Kass EJ, Belman AB. Reversal of testicular growth by varicocele ligation. *J Urol* 1987; **137**: 475–6.

[125] Kubal A, Nagler HM, Zahalsky M, Budak M. The adolescent varicocele: diagnostic and treatment patterns of pediatricians. A public health concern? *J Urol* 2004; **171**: 411–13.

[126] Thomas JC, Elder JS. Testicular growth arrest and adolescent varicocele: does varicocele size make a difference? *J Urol* 2002; **168**: 1689–91.

[127] Alukal JP, Zurakowski D, Atala A, *et al.* Testicular hypotrophy does not correlate with grade of adolescent varicocele. *J Urol* 2005; **174**: 2367–70.

[128] Sakamoto H, Saito K, Ogawa Y, Yoshida H. Testicular volume measurements using Prader orchidometer versus ultrasonography in patients with infertility. *Urology* 2007; **69**: 158–62.

[129] Greenfield SP, Seville P, Wan J. Experience with varicoceles in children and young adults. *J Urol* 2002; **168**: 1684–8.

[130] Kass EJ, Freitas JE, Salisz JA, Steinert BW. Pituitary gonadal dysfunction in adolescents with varicocele. *Urology* 1993; **42**: 179–81.

[131] Laven JS, Haans LC, Mali WP, *et al.* Effects of varicocele treatment in adolescents: a randomized study. *Fertil Steril* 1992; **58**: 756–62.

[132] Cayan S, Acar D, Ulger S, Akbay E. Adolescent varicocele repair: long-term results and comparison of surgical techniques according to optical magnification use in 100 cases at a single university hospital. *J Urol* 2005; **174**: 2003–6.

[133] Sawczuk IS, Hensle TW, Burbige KA, Nagler HM. Varicoceles: effect on testicular volume in prepubertal and pubertal males. *Urology* 1993; **41**: 466–8.

[134] Witt MA, Lipshultz LI. Varicocele: a progressive or static lesion? *J Urol* 1993; **42**: 541–3.

[135] Gorelick N, Goldstein M. Loss of fertility in men with varicocele. *Fertil Steril* 1993; **59**: 613–16.

[136] Raj GV, Wiener JS. Facing the dilemma of adolescent varicoceles. *Contemp Urol* 2004; **16** (7): 23–33.

[137] Zahalsky MP, Berman AJ, Nagler HM. Evaluating the risk of epididymal injury during hydrocelectomy and spermatocelectomy. *J Urol* 2004; **171**: 2291–2.

[138] Sheynkin YR, Hendin BN, Schlegel PN, Goldstein M. Microsurgical repair of iatrogenic injury to the vas deferens. *J Urol* 1998; **159**: 139–41.

[139] Marmar JL, Kim Y. Subinguinal microsurgical varicocelectomy: a technical critique and statistical analysis of semen and pregnancy data. *J Urol* 1994; **152**: 1127–32.

[140] Ivanissevich O. Left varicocele due to reflux: experience with 4,470 cases in forty-two years. *J Int Coll Surg* 1960; **34**: 742–55.

[141] Goldstein M, Gilbert BR, Dicker AP, Dwosh J, Gnecco C. Microsurgical inguinal varicocelectomy with delivery of the testis: an artery and lymphatic sparing technique. *J Urol* 1992; **148**: 1808–11.

[142] Ramasamy R, Schlegel PN. Microsurgical inguinal varicocelectomy with and without testicular delivery. *Urology* 2006; **68**: 1323–6.

[143] Wright EJ, Goldstein M. Ligation of the testicular artery during microsurgical varicocelectomy: Incidence and implications. Abstract presented at the 89th Annual Meeting of the American Urological Association, May 1994.

[144] Etriby AA, Ibrahim AA, Mahmoud KZ, Elhaggar S. Subfertility and varicocele. I. Venogram demonstration of anastomosis sites in subfertile men. *Fertil Steril* 1975; **26**: 1013–17.

[145] Murray RR, Mitchell SE, Kadir S, *et al.* Comparison of recurrent varicocele anatomy following surgery and percutaneous balloon occlusion. *J Urol* 1986; **135**: 286–9.

[146] Pintus C, Rodriguez Matas MJ, Manzoni C, Nanni L, Perrelli L. Varicocele in pediatric patients: comparative assessment of different therapeutic approaches. *Urology* 2001; **57**: 157–8.

[147] Kass EJ, Reitelman C. Adolescent varicocele. *Urol Clin North Am* 1995; **22**: 151–9.

[148] Kass EJ, Marcol B. Results of varicocele surgery in adolescents: a comparison of techniques. *J Urol* 1992; **148**: 694–6.

[149] Gerber GS, Rukstalis DB, Levine LA, Chodak GW. Current and future roles of laparoscopic surgery in urology. *Urology* 1993; **41** (1 Suppl): 5–9.

[150] Mehan DJ, Andrus CH, Parra RO. Laparoscopic internal spermatic vein ligation: report of a new technique. *Fertil Steril* 1992; **58**: 1263–6.

[151] Donovan JF, Winfield HN. Laparoscopic varix ligation. *J Urol* 1992; **147**: 77–81.

[152] Matsuda T, Horii Y, Yoshida O. Should the testicular artery be preserved at varicocelectomy? *J Urol* 1993; **149**: 1357–60.

[153] Parrott TS, Hewatt L. Ligation of the testicular artery and vein in adolescent varicocele. *J Urol* 1994; **152**: 791–3.

[154] Lima SS, Castro MP, Costa OF. A new method for the treatment of varicocele. *Andrologia* 1978; **10**: 103–6.

[155] Halden W, White RI. Outpatient embolotherapy of varicocele. *Urol Clin North Am* 1987; **13**: 137–44.

[156] Formanek A, Rusnak B, Zollikofer C, *et al.* Embolization of the spermatic vein for treatment of infertility: A new approach. *Radiology* 1981; **139**: 315–21.

[157] Kaufman SL, Kadir S, Barth KH, *et al.* Mechanisms of recurrent varicocele after balloon occlusion or surgical ligation of the internal spermatic vein. *Radiology* 1983; **147**: 435–40.

[158] Comhaire FH, Kunnen M. Factors affecting the probability of conception after treatment of subfertile men with varicocele by transcatheter embolization with Bucrylate. *Fertil Steril* 1985; **43**: 781–6.

[159] Tauber R, Johnsen N. Antegrade scrotal sclerotherapy for the treatment of varicocele: technique and late results. *J Urol* 1994; **151**: 386–90.

[160] Zucchi A, *et al.* Treatment of varicocele: randomized prospective study on open surgery versus Tauber antegrade sclerotherapy. *J Androl* 2005; **26**: 328–32.

[161] Zorgniotti AW, Sealton AI. Chronic scrotal hypothermia: treatment outcome in 90 couples

with poor semen. Abstract presented at the Annual Meeting of the American Fertility Society, Toronto, ON, Canada, September 1986.

[162] Kaufman DG, Nagler HM. Specific nonsurgical therapy in male infertility. *Urol Clin North Am* 1987; **14**: 489–98.

[163] Schlesinger MH, Wilets IF, Nagler HM. Treatment outcome after varicocelectomy: a critical analysis. *Urol Clin North Am* 1994; **21**: 517–29.

[164] Nilsson S, Edvinsson A, Nilsson B. Improvement of semen and pregnancy rate after ligation and division of the internal spermatic vein: fact or fiction? *Br J Urol* 1979; **51**: 591–6.

[165] Vermeulen A, Vandeweghe MN, Deslypere JP. Prognosis of subfertility in men with corrected or uncorrected varicocele. *J Androl* 1986; **7**: 147–55.

[166] Baker HW, Burger HG, de Kretser DM, *et al.* Testicular vein ligation and fertility in men with varicoceles. *Br Med J* 1985; **291**: 1678–80.

[167] Madgar I, Weissenberg R, Lunenfeld B, Karasik A, Goldwasser B. Controlled trial of high spermatic vein ligation for varicocele in infertile men. *Fertil Steril* 1995; **63**: 120–4.

[168] Unal D, Yeni E, Verit A, Karatas OF. Clomiphene citrate versus varicocelectomy in treatment of subclinical varicocele: a prospective randomized study. *Int J Urol* 2001; **8**: 227–30.

[169] Nieschlag E, Hertle L, Fischedick A, Abshagen K, Behre HM. Update on treatment of varicocele: Counseling as effective as occlusion of the vena spermatica. *Hum Reprod* 1998; **13**: 2147–50.

[170] Krause W, Mulle, H, Schafer H, Weidner W. Does treatment of varicocele improve male fertility? Results of the "Deutsche Varikozelenstudie" a multicenter study of 14 collaborating centers. *Andrologia* 2002; **34**: 4–171.

[171] Grasso M, Lania M, Castelli M, *et al.* Low-grade left varicocele in patients over 30 years old: the effect of spermatic vein ligation on fertility. *BJU Int* 2000; **85**: 305–7.

[172] Yamamoto M, Hibi H, Hirata Y, Miyake K, Ishigaki T. Effect of varicocelectomy on sperm parameters and pregnancy rate in patients with subclinical varicocele: a randomized prospective controlled study. *J Urol* 1996; **155**: 1636–8.

[173] Breznik R, Vlaisavljevic V, Borko E. Treatment of varicocele and male fertility. *Arch Androl* 1993; **30**: 157–60.

[174] Brown JS. Varicocelectomy in the subfertile male: a ten year experience with 295 cases. *Fertil Steril* 1976; **27**: 1046–53.

[175] Tinga DJ, Jager S, Bruijnen CL, Kremer J, Mensink HJ. Factors related to semen improvement and fertility after varicocele operation. *Fertil Steril* 1984; **41**: 404–10.

[176] Rogers BJ, Mygatt GG, Soderdahl DW, Hale RW. Monitoring of suspected infertile men with varicocele by the sperm penetration assay. *Fertil Steril* 1985; **44**: 800–5.

[177] Allamaneni SS, Naughton CK, Sharma RK, Thomas AJ, Agarwal A. Increased seminal reactive oxygen species levels in patients with varicoceles correlate with varicocele grade but not with testis size. *Fertil Steril* 2004; **82**: 1684–6.

[178] Bennoff S, Millan C, Hurley I, Napolitano B, Marmar JL. Bilateral increased apoptosis and bilateral accumulation of cadmium in infertile men with left varicocele. *Hum Reprod* 2004; **19**: 616–27.

[179] Fuse H, Iwasaki M, Mizuno I, Ikehara-Kawauchi Y. Evaluation of acrosome reactivity using the Acrobeads test in varicocele patients: findings before and after treatment. *Arch Androl* 2003; **49**: 1–6.

[180] O'Brien J, Zini A. Sperm DNA integrity and male infertility. *Urology* 2005; **65**: 16–22.

[181] Zini A, Blumenfeld A, Libman J, Willis J. Beneficial effect of microsurgical varicocelectomy on human sperm DNA integrity. *Hum Reprod* 2005; **20**: 1018–21.

[182] Lewis RW, Harrison RM. Diagnosis and treatment of varicocele. *Clin Obstet Gynecol* 1982; **25**: 501–23.

[183] Newton R, Schinfeld JS, Schiff I. Clomiphene treatment of infertile men: failure of response with idiopathic oligospermia. *Fertil Steril* 1980; **34**: 399–400.

[184] Rodrigues-Netto N. Varicocele: fact or fiction? In: Paulson JD, Negro-Vilar A, Lucena E, Martini L, eds. *Andrology: Male Fertility and Sterility*. Orlando, FL: Academic Press, 1986.

[185] Raman JD, Schlegel PN. Aromatase inhibitors for male infertility. *J Urol* 2002; **167**: 624–9.

[186] Esteves SC, Glina S. Recovery of spermatogenesis after microsurgical subinguinal varicocele repair in azoospermic men based on testicular histology. *Int Braz J Urol* 2005; **31**: 541–8.

[187] Gazzera C, *et al.* Radiological treatment of male varicocele: technical, clinical, seminal and dosimetric aspects. *Radiol Med* 2006; **111**: 449–58.

[188] Ghanem H, Anis T, El-Nashar A, Shamloul R. Subinguinal microvaricocelectomy versus retroperitoneal varicocelectomy: comparative study of complications and surgical outcome. *Urology* 2004; **64**: 1005–9.

[189] Richardson I, Nagler HM. Prophylactic antibiotics are not necessary for microsurgical varicocelectomy. Presented at New York Academy of Medicine Valentine Essay Contest, New York, 2007.

[190] Mazzoni G, Spagnoli A, Lucchetti MC, *et al.* Adolescent varicocele: Tauber antegrade sclerotherapy versus Palomo repair. *J Urol* 2001; **166**: 1462–4.

Chapter 19

Evaluation of female infertility for the non-gynecologist

R. Dale McClure and Nancy A. Klein

Introduction

Reproductive difficulties encountered by couples are receiving increasing attention both in the news media and in public discussion. Several factors are responsible for this. Discoveries in biology have led to major advances in the availability and efficacy of infertility treatments, such as in-vitro fertilization (IVF) and assisted reproductive technologies (ART), providing new avenues of hope for the infertile couple. **Socioeconomic and demographic trends over the past few decades have resulted in increasing numbers of women attempting pregnancy at a more advanced age, when they are biologically less fertile.** These trends include greater focus on education and careers among women, tendency to delay marriage, increased numbers of second marriages, and readily available and acceptable contraceptive methods. Advances in information technology have greatly improved access to information for couples seeking pregnancy, and improved access to treatment has also contributed to a higher number of couples seeking infertility care. Because infertility problems are more visible and socially acceptable, couples tend to be evaluated and treated earlier, when success rates are higher. Although little has changed in our knowledge about the diagnosis and underlying pathophysiology of infertility, significant advances in treatment have led to a focus on early screening and diagnosis, leading to treatment that is more proactive, specific, and effective.

Couples should be considered as a unit and be evaluated in a parallel manner until a significant problem is uncovered. Although partners are often being cared for by different physicians, they should be interviewed together whenever possible, especially during the initial visit. This allows the physician to gain information regarding their dynamics as a couple as well as their individual motivation, and it helps to identify and alleviate the stress the infertility investigation

tends to elicit. At all times during the infertility evaluation, the couple should feel free to question the indication, rationale, and outcomes of various diagnostic and therapeutic maneuvers. An explanation of the fundamental aspects of both male and female reproductive biology helps to achieve this goal.

The diagnostic evaluation of the female should proceed in a logical, timely, and cost-effective sequence to elucidate possible causes of the infertility. Communication between the physicians treating the female and the male allows a workup that is both efficient and appropriate and avoids unnecessary tests and procedures. Our role as physicians is to provide accurate information, dispel myths regarding fertility, and provide emotional support and counseling, while remaining conscious of the couple's medical and financial limitations. Whether the infertility evaluation is carried out by the urologist, andrologist, or primary care provider, an understanding of the basic components of female infertility evaluation and prognostic factors is essential to providing appropriate counseling and/or referral.

Causes of infertility

Eighty-five percent of couples with regular, unprotected intercourse conceive within one year [1]. Those failing to achieve pregnancy within this time frame usually should commence investigation. Earlier investigation is indicated in women over age 35, those with a history of pelvic infections or surgery, infertility with a previous partner, known abnormalities of the uterus or fallopian tubes, prior treatment with gonadotoxic agents, history of endometriosis, and menstrual cycle abnormalities suggestive of ovulatory dysfunction. Partners of men with obviously poor semen quality or men who are candidates for surgical correction of obstructive azoospermia (e.g., vasectomy reversal) should receive a basic evaluation to assess whether there are factors

Infertility in the Male, 4th edition, ed. Larry I. Lipshultz, Stuart S. Howards, and Craig S. Niederberger. Published by Cambridge University Press. © Cambridge University Press 2009.

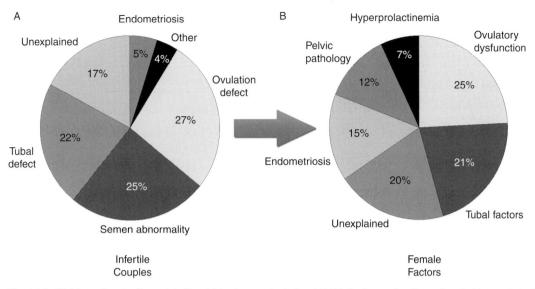

Fig. 19.1. (A) Primary female diagnosis in 21 published reports including 14 141 infertile couples. (Reproduced with permission from Collins HA. Unexplained infertility. In: Key WR *et al.*, eds. *Infertility: Evaluation and Treatment.* Philadelphia, PA: Saunders 1995: 249–62.) (B) Primary female infertility diagnoses in 8500 infertile couples using a standardized diagnostic protocol. (With permission from *Recent Advances in Medically Assisted Conception.* WHO Technical Report Series 820, 1992.)

that may warrant consideration of early ART (e.g., tubal disease, endometriosis, greater female age, or decreased ovarian reserve). In these cases, primary treatment with IVF and surgical sperm retrieval may be warranted.

Human reproduction is a complex process that can be broken down into several components, any one of which could affect fertility. A comprehensive assessment of each of these components is paramount, as many couples are found to have a combination of factors contributing to their infertility. Sperm of optimal quality must be deposited near the cervix at the time of ovulation, ascend into the fallopian tube and have the capability to fertilize the oocyte (male factor). The cervix must be able to capture, filter, and release sperm into the uterus and fallopian tubes (cervical factor). Ovulation of a mature oocyte must occur on a regular, predictable basis (ovulatory factor). The peritoneal cavity must allow normal sperm/oocyte interaction and normal anatomical relationships between the distal tube and the ovarian surface (peritoneal factor). The fallopian tubes must be able to capture the ovulated ova and allow for normal transport of sperm and embryos (tubal factor). Finally, the uterus must provide a hospitable environment with normal configuration, blood supply, and hormonal preparation to allow implantation and early embryo development (uterine factor).

An accurate estimate of the prevalence of various infertility diagnoses is difficult to ascertain, because of variability in the extent of evaluation and the coexistence of multiple infertility factors. In an excellent quantitative analysis of the causes of female infertility, Collins reviewed 21 published results of 14 141 infertile couples (Fig. 19.1A) [2]. The primary diagnoses of these individuals were ovulatory disorders (27%), abnormal semen parameters (25%), tubal defects (22%), endometriosis (5%), others (4%), and unexplained (17%). The World Health Organization, using a standardized diagnostic protocol, conducted a study of 8500 couples, looking at diseases in the male and female (Fig. 19.1B) [3]. **The diseases most often identified in the female were ovulatory disorders (25%), pelvic adhesions (12%), tubal occlusion or abnormality (21%), hyperprolactinemia (7%), and endometriosis (15%).**

History and physical

The cornerstone of the workup of the infertile female is a careful history and physical examination. An infertility questionnaire that addresses most of the important historical points is extremely useful (Table 19.1) [4,5]. Age, duration of infertility, and past reproductive history (infertility, gravidity, pregnancy outcome) are useful in determining prognosis. The history should include detailed information about menstrual regularity, flow, cycle interval (normal generally 21–35 days), and the incidence and frequency of unscheduled

Table 19.1. History

Gravity, parity and pregnancy outcomes or complications
Cycle length and characteristics, onset and severity of dysmenorrhea
Coital frequency, and any sexual dysfunction
Duration of infertility and results of any previous evaluation and treatment
Past surgery and past or current medical illnesses
Previous abnormal Pap smears and subsequent treatment
Current medications and allergies
Occupation and use of tobacco, alcohol, and recreational drugs
Family history of birth defects, mental retardation, early menopause, or reproductive failure
Symptoms of thyroid disease, pelvic or abdominal pain, galactorrhea, hirsutism, and dyspareunia

Table 19.2. Physical examination

Weight and body mass index
Thyroid abnormalities
Breast secretions
Androgen excess, e.g., hirsutism
Pelvic or abdominal tenderness or organ enlargement
Vaginal or cervical abnormality, secretions, or discharge
Size, shape, and mobility of uterus
Adnexal mass or tenderness
Cul de sac mass, tenderness, or nodularity

bleeding. Previous gynecologic procedures, such as cervical conization, treatment of septic abortion, and pelvic surgery may implicate an anatomical cause of infertility. Symptoms of possible endocrinopathy, such as hyper- or hypothyroidism, galactorrhea, hirsutism, acne, or insulin-resistance should be elicited. History of eating disorders, excessive exercise, unusual weight gain or loss, and past or current exposures to gonadotoxic agents such as smoking, chemotherapy, or radiation should also be identified. Severe or progressive dysmenorrhea and dyspareunia may suggest endometriosis. A history of previous pelvic surgery, septic abortion, ruptured appendix, or sexually transmitted diseases may raise the suspicion for tubal or peritoneal disease. A history of alcohol or recreational drug abuse, excessive caffeine intake, or tobacco smoking may also adversely affect reproductive potential. Finally, inquiry into the frequency and timing of intercourse and erectile or ejaculatory dysfunction may uncover other correctable causes of infertility.

Although a non-gynecologist (e.g., urologist or andrologist) would not be carrying out the physical examination, many findings may be obtained from the female during the initial interview. Abnormal body mass index, galactorrhea, thyromegaly, signs of androgen excess (e.g., hirsutism, acne, clitoromegaly), Cushingoid features, and acanthosis nigricans may support suspicion of endocrinopathy associated with ovulatory dysfunction. On pelvic examination, the size and position of the uterus and ovaries, appearance of the cervical os and mucus, and presence of tenderness or nodularity may suggest the presence of fibroids, cysts, or endometriosis. **In the majority of cases, however, physical examination will be completely normal;** therefore, **associated imaging of pelvic anatomy and/or hormonal assessment will be indicated to detect or confirm abnormalities** (Table 19.2) [4].

Measuring clinical success

Most reproductive endocrinologists use the concept of fecundability in addition to discussing pregnancy rates. Fecundability is the probability of achieving pregnancy in one menstrual cycle (approximately 0.20–0.25 in healthy young couples) [6]. A similar concept, fecundity, is the ability to achieve a pregnancy that results in a live birth in one menstrual cycle [7]. **Fecundability is a valuable clinical and scientific concept, as it creates the framework for the quantitative analysis of fertility potential.** It also provides a convenient quantitative estimate of the efficacy of various fertility options. For instance, an infertile couple with an estimated fecundability of 0.04 may choose a low-cost treatment (e.g., clomiphene citrate plus intrauterine insemination) that increases the fecundability to approximately 0.08, or a more expensive treatment (e.g., IVF) that may increase the fecundability to 0.35 [5,8].

It must also be remembered that not all pregnancies produce a live birth. "Occult" pregnancy is defined as a pregnancy that terminates so quickly after implantation that there is no clinical suspicion of its existence [9]. A "chemical" pregnancy, on the other hand, occurs in the presence of a clinical suspicion of a pregnancy with a confirmation of an elevated human chorionic gonadotropin (hCG) when there is no evidence of the pregnancy detected by early first-trimester ultrasound. In a prospective study of couples attempting to conceive, 31% of all pregnancies were lost, and 41% of these were categorized as occult [9]. **The proportion of clinically recognized pregnancies that result in spontaneous abortion is approximately 15%, increasing significantly according to the age of the female partner** [10].

Factors affecting prognosis

Factors affecting prognosis in couples with infertility include prior fertility history, duration of infertility, diagnosis, and age. **The most important factor affecting prognosis is the age of the female partner.** As women near the end of the fourth decade, there is a steady and pronounced decline in the incidence of conception and live birth, whereas the incidence of early spontaneous abortion rises. This decline occurs in spite of the fact that most women maintain regular ovulatory function until within 1–2 years of menopause (average age 51). Ovulatory frequency remains high (95%) in menstruating women aged 40–55 until the onset of oligomenorrhea, when the percentage of ovulatory cycles drops significantly [11]. Women experience their highest reproductive potential in their early 20s, with a gradual decline thereafter until the late 30s, when the rate of decline becomes more pronounced (Fig. 19.2). Evidence for the effect of female age on natural fecundity rates was provided by Menken and Larsen, who reported birth and spontaneous abortion rates for married couples in seven populations meeting the following criteria: (1) marriage later in life is relatively common, (2) contraception is not practiced, (3) premarital conceptions rarely occur, and (4) accurate birth records are available [12]. These data

demonstrated that the fecundity of the couple is much more dependent upon the age of the female than that of the male, with the percentage of married women remaining childless rising steadily with age: 6% at age 20–24, 9% at age 25–29, 15% at age 30–34, 30% at age 35–39, and 64% at age 40–44. In these populations, the average age of women at the birth of the last child ranges between 39 and 42 [13]. Pregnancy rates reported for donor insemination cycles (eliminating the variables of coital frequency and fertility of the male) also illustrate this phenomenon. Data from a French registry of donor sperm insemination cycles in 2193 women married to azoospermic men demonstrated that cumulative conception rates declined significantly after the age of 30 [14].

The impact of female age on fertility is also evident in pregnancy and live birth rates after ART. In addition to producing fewer eggs and embryos, older women produce embryos that are less likely to implant than those derived from the oocytes of younger women. According to the 2004 CDC report of ART success rates in the United States, a striking age-associated decline in pregnancy rates per embryo transfer and a corresponding increase in miscarriage rates are observed (Fig. 19.3) [8]. The low delivery rates per embryo transfer observed in older women are particularly striking, in that only women who had adequate response

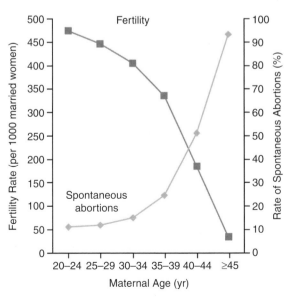

Fig. 19.2. Live birth and spontaneous abortion rates according to female age. (From Heffner L. Advanced maternal age: how old is too old? *N Engl J Med* 2004; **351**: 1927–9, with permission. Copyright © 2004 Massachusetts Medical Society. All rights reserved.)

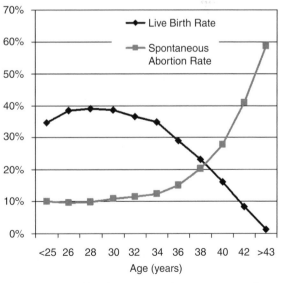

Fig. 19.3. Live birth and spontaneous abortion rates per embryo transfer in fresh, nondonor in-vitro fertilization cycles according to female age reported to the Centers for Disease Control, 2004. (From *2004 Assisted Reproductive Technology Success Rates: National Summary and Fertility Clinic Reports*. US Department of Health and Human Services, Centers for Disease Control and Prevention, 2006.)

to stimulation and embryos available for transfer were included. There was no age-related decrease in pregnancy rates for recipients of donor oocytes (Fig. 19.4) [8], and donor-egg IVF pregnancy and delivery rates have been shown to correspond to the age of the donor, rather than the recipient [15]. **The absence of an age-related decline in live birth rates in oocyte-donation IVF cycles provides compelling evidence that infertility related to advancing maternal age is almost entirely related to changes in oocyte quality.**

Oocytes from normal women in their early 40s exhibit abnormalities in microtubule and chromosome placement at the metaphase stage of meiosis II (Fig. 19.5) [16,17], and higher rates of single chromatid abnormalities are reported in oocytes derived from older infertility patients following ovarian hyperstimulation [18]. Fluorescence in-situ hybridization of blastomeres obtained from cleavage-stage embryos derived in IVF cycles reveals a high proportion of aneuploidy, with a striking increase in prevalence after age 35 [19]. The incidence of spontaneous abortions, largely due to chromosomal abnormalities, also increases significantly with advancing maternal age. Oocyte abnormalities account for the rise in the incidence of chromosome abnormalities observed in liveborn infants, from about 1/500 for women under 30 to 1/270 at age 30, 1/80 at age 35, 1/60 at age 40, and 1/20 at age 45 [20].

Although much more subtle, there is also a slight decline in fecundity according to the age of the male partner. The decreased rates of conception observed in natural populations are generally thought to be due to changes in coital frequency and/or increased incidence of erectile or ejaculatory dysfunction [12]. However, a recent report of the influence of paternal age on pregnancy rates in IVF cycles confirmed a statistically significant decrease in pregnancy rates in older men when controlling for female age [21]. Interestingly, investigators also observed a combined effect, wherein the lowest pregnancy rates were observed when both the male and female partners were older. In spite of these observations, counseling and treatment of the infertile couple is seldom influenced by the age of the male partner, except in consideration of nonmedical issues such as the health and longevity of the prospective father.

The profound impact of maternal age is an important consideration in the evaluation of the infertile couple, in counseling, and in determining the time line for evaluation and treatment. The initial approach to evaluation, as well as the long-term plan for treatment,

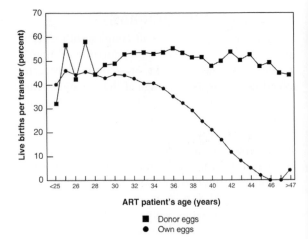

Fig. 19.4. Live birth rates per embryo transfer in fresh, nondonor (circles) and donor (squares) in-vitro fertilization cycles according to age of the woman undergoing transfer, CDC 2004. (From *2004 Assisted Reproductive Technology Success Rates: National Summary and Fertility Clinic Reports.* US Department of Health and Human Services, Centers for Disease Control and Prevention, 2006.)

should be modified appropriately when an older couple is being treated.

Ovulatory factor

In order to understand hormonal assessment of the female as well as assessment of ovarian function, it is important to have a basic understanding of menstrual cycle physiology. Normal ovulation is the result of coordinated stimuli and feedback between the hypothalamus, pituitary, and ovary. Gonadotropin-releasing hormone (GnRH) is released in a pulsatile fashion by the hypothalamus, stimulating release of follicle-stimulating hormone (FSH) and luteinizing hormone (LH). The frequency of pulsation determines the ratio of LH and FSH secreted, with higher-frequency, lower-amplitude pulses occurring in the follicular phase [22]. Pituitary gonadotropin secretion is influenced by the serum level of ovarian hormones, which exert both positive and negative feedback on both the hypothalamus and pituitary. **Because of the dynamic nature of ovarian hormone and gonadotropin secretion across the menstrual cycle, it is critical to measure these hormones at specified times relative to the menstrual period (early follicular phase – FSH, LH, and estradiol; luteal phase – progesterone).** Figure 19.6 depicts serum levels of gonadotropins and ovarian steroids determined daily over 1.5 menstrual cycles, normalized to the LH surge in normal, ovulatory women in

Centrosome Disposition vs. Meiotic Spindle Assembly

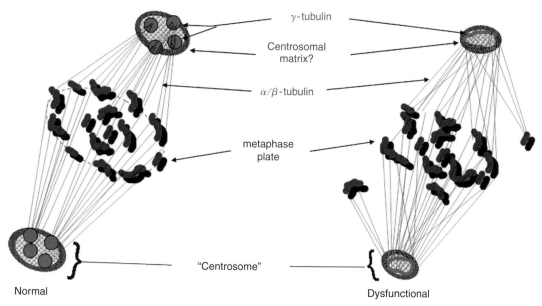

γ-tubulin

Centrosomal matrix?

α/β-tubulin

metaphase plate

"Centrosome"

Normal

Dysfunctional

Fig. 19.5. Schematic representation of the meiotic spindle in normal younger (left) and older (right) preovulatory oocyte. In the normal spindle, the microtubule nucleating centers in each centrosome are distinct, and there are multiple sites per spindle pole. In the aneuploid conditions, the nucleating centers are indistinct, almost ring-like. It is speculated that the capture of chromosomes may be abnormal due to this condition, leading to an increased propensity to aneuploidy. (From Battaglia D *et al.* Changes in centrosomal domains during meiotic maturation in the human oocyte. *Mol Hum Reprod* 1997; **2**: 845–51.) *See color plate section.*

two age groups (20–25 and 40–45). The only significant age-related difference between the two age groups is elevation of FSH throughout the menstrual cycle in the older age group, most pronounced in the early follicular phase [23].

Most ovulatory disturbances can be ascertained by simple history alone. Ovulatory women report regular menses, generally 21–35 days in length. Longer cycles may be ovulatory; however, the incidence of anovulation is high in cycles longer than 35 days, especially when the interval and/or flow are irregular. Other subjective signs of ovulation include ovulatory pain (mittelschmertz), cervical mucus changes (increased quantity, clarity, and "egg white" consistency), luteal-phase mastalgia, and other premenstrual symptoms. Dysmenorrhea is more common and pronounced in ovulatory than in anovulatory cycles.

Ovulatory cycles are associated with a shift in the basal body temperature (BBT) coinciding with the LH surge (Fig. 19.7). This thermal shift is associated with progesterone secretion, falling just prior to onset of menses, except during conception cycles, when the elevated temperature is maintained. While easy and inexpensive, BBTs are inherently inaccurate, difficult to read, and tedious, and ovulation can be determined only retrospectively. Because of these limitations, the BBT has been largely replaced by urinary assays available for home detection of the LH surge, providing reliable and prospective evidence of ovulation. A serum progesterone level of > 3 ng/mL is considered confirmatory of ovulation. **The follicular phase length (time to ovulation) varies significantly among women with variable menstrual cycle length, whereas the luteal phase length is relatively stable, generally about 14 days.** Therefore, the proper timing of the progesterone assessment is approximately one week prior to expected menses (e.g., day 21 of a 28-day cycle, day 28 of a 35-day cycle, etc.). Ultrasound monitoring may also be used to document dominant follicle development and collapse, although this is an expensive and usually unnecessary approach. Finally, endometrial biopsy in the luteal phase showing secretory histological changes is another means by which to verify ovulation, though it is not used clinically for this purpose.

For patients with obvious ovulatory dysfunction (oligomenorrhea or amenorrhea), medical evaluation

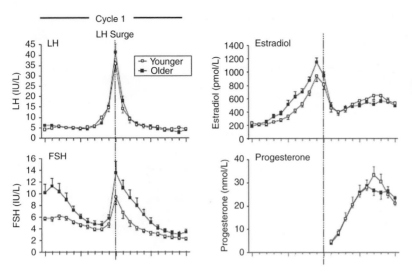

Fig. 19.6. Serum levels of follicle-stimulating hormone (FSH), luteinizing hormone (LH), estradiol, and progesterone determined in normal, ovulatory women in two age groups (20–25, open squares; 40–45, closed squares). Data are normalized to the day of peak LH (LH surge). FSH levels are significantly elevated throughout the menstrual cycle in the older age group (*P* < 0.05). There are no significant differences in levels of the other hormones between the two age groups. (From Klein NA *et al*. Age-related analysis of inhibin A, inhibin B, and activin A relative to the intercycle monotropic follicle-stimulating hormone rise in normal ovulatory women. *J Clin Endocrinol Metab* 2004; **89**: 2977–81, with permission. Copyright 2004, The Endocrine Society.)

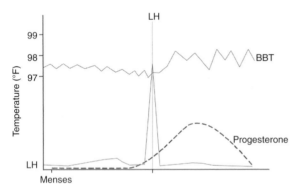

Fig. 19.7. Schematic representation of the biphasic thermal shift in basal body temperature (BBT) corresponding to the peak in luteinizing hormone (LH). Vertical line, LH surge.

of potential underlying causes should include screening for thyroid disease (TSH) and hyperprolactinemia. Women with clinical signs of androgen excess should also be screened for elevated testosterone and dehydroepiandrosterone sulfate (DHEA-S) and 21-hydroxylase deficiency (17-hydroxyprogesterone). Ultrasound may provide supportive, but not diagnostic, evidence of polycystic ovarian syndrome (PCOS). This common condition is characterized by clinical or laboratory evidence of androgen excess associated with chronic anovulation, and bilateral ovarian enlargement with multiple small antral follicles (< 10 mm) apparent on ultrasound. Women with stigmata of Cushing syndrome should be evaluated with a 24-hour free urinary cortisol or dexamethasone suppression test.

A progestin challenge test (administration of 5–10 days of medroxyprogesterone acetate, micronized progesterone, or a single injection of 100 mg progesterone-in-oil) serves as a clinical measure of estrogen status – a positive withdrawal bleed indicates prior endometrial estrogen exposure. **Failure to withdraw indicates hypoestrogenemia, due either to ovarian failure or to hypogonadotropic states.** Ovarian as opposed to hypothalamic–pituitary etiologies of amenorrhea can be distinguished by obtaining a serum FSH level, with FSH elevation being indicative of ovarian failure. Women with secondary amenorrhea who have a negative progestin challenge, normal FSH, and history of previous uterine instrumentation should be further assessed with another progestin challenge after exogenous estrogen administration to exclude Asherman syndrome (partial or complete obliteration of the endometrial cavity by intrauterine synechia).

Qualitative abnormalities in ovarian stimulation and hormone secretion can also occur in ovulatory women. This endocrinopathy most frequently presents as a shortening of the luteal phase associated with decreased integrated luteal phase progesterone secretion. This condition, referred to as "luteal phase deficiency" (LPD) may contribute to infertility or early pregnancy failure due to inadequate endometrial preparation for implantation. This deficiency is the subject of some debate, and does not appear to constitute a major cause of infertility. However, patients with obvious deficiency in progesterone production may benefit from either luteal progesterone supplementation or augmentation through ovulation induction. Methods used to diagnose LPD include observation of a luteal phase less than 11 days according to BBT or urinary LH detection, endometrial biopsy, and evaluation of serial progesterone levels. For many years, the "gold standard" was considered to be a late luteal phase endometrial biopsy; the histological appearance of the endometrial glands and stroma change daily throughout the luteal phase, correlating with the number of days of progesterone exposure. However, biopsy is uncomfortable, expensive, and subjective; therefore, it is not a commonly used diagnostic tool. Jordan *et al.* reported that three serum progesterone levels obtained over a five-day period from the fifth to the ninth day of the LH surge correlate better with daily progesterone levels than endometrial biopsy [24]. A combined level of 30 ng/mL (or average level $\geq$ 10 ng/mL) is considered the normal limit.

Cervical factor

In order for fertilization to occur, the cervix must serve as a conduit and reservoir for sperm. Prior to ovulation, elevated estradiol acts on the endocervical epithelium to increase the saline content of the cervical mucus in addition to changing the population of leukocytes present. Patients with anatomical (e.g., prior conization), inflammatory (e.g., cervicitis), and hormonal (e.g., patients on clomiphene citrate, with its antiestrogenic properties) disorders of cervical mucus production may have inadequate quantity and quality of cervical mucus for normal sperm transport. **Although very uncommon, cervical-factor infertility as an isolated factor is an easily treated cause of infertility through intrauterine insemination, which effectively bypasses the cervix.** Evaluation of the cervix is best done by visual inspection of the os and of the character of cervical mucus – clarity, quantity, spinnbarkeit, and cellularity – just prior to and during ovulation. Mucopurulent discharge, a sign of cervicitis, should be further evaluated with cultures for chlamydia and gonorrhea. The postcoital test is another means by which to assess the sperm–mucus interaction, serving as a measure of the quality of mucus and/or a screen for evidence of antisperm antibodies. A sample of cervical mucus is obtained between 2 and 18 hours after intercourse in the immediate preovulatory phase and examined microscopically for the presence of progressively motile sperm. However, due to low predictive value and poor specificity, this test remains controversial and is infrequently performed.

Tubal factor

An important part of the basic infertility evaluation is assessment of fallopian tube patency. A hysterosalpingogram, or HSG, is the most frequently utilized modality for tubal assessment (Fig. 19.8). Performed in the early to mid-follicular phase, an HSG consists of injection of iodinated contrast through a cannula or catheter placed into the endocervical canal or lower uterine segment while observation takes place through continuous or intermittent fluoroscopy. A tenaculum is often placed on the cervix to allow manipulation of uterine position so that the best images can be obtained. Information gained includes the shape and size of the uterine cavity, proximal and distal tubal patency, and caliber and mucosal pattern of the ampullary portion. Other findings may include filling defects within the uterus representing polyps, fibroids, or synechiae, congenital anomalies, salpingitis isthmica nodosa, and loculation of contrast outside the tubes suggesting the presence of pelvic adhesions. Intravasation into the myometrium may be associated with the presence of myomas, adenomyosis, or retained products of conception. Proximal tubal occlusion usually cannot be distinguished from spasm of the myometrium surrounding the interstitial portion of the tube. Repeat HSG, selective tubal cannulation, or laparoscopy is necessary to distinguish between a true and functional proximal tubal occlusion.

Contrast used in HSGs can be either water- or oil-based. Oil-based contrast has been discouraged by some because of concern about embolization after intravasation or granuloma formation in cases of distal tubal occlusion. However, low molecular weight oil-based contrast can be used without any evidence of serious or long-term side effects. **A meta-analysis of studies using either oil- or water-based contrast confirmed the phenomenon of a therapeutic effect when oil-based contrast was used** [25]. Furthermore, a randomized trial of tubal flushing with oil-based contrast in patients with laparoscopically confirmed endometriosis demonstrated a significant increase in pregnancy and live birth rates [26]. The mechanism for this improved fecundity rate is unclear. Another advantage of oil-based contrast is the potential to utilize a delayed film to document retained contrast in an occluded tube or to confirm normal intraperitoneal distribution and/or spill when the initial study is equivocal. Advantages of water-based contrast include better delineation of mucosal patterns within the fallopian tube and no concern about intravasation.

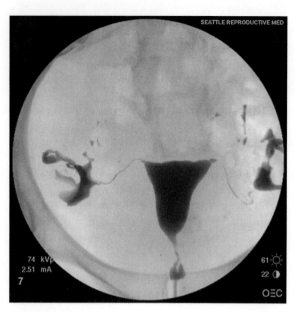

Fig. 19.8. Normal hysterosalpingogram using an oil-based contrast (ethiodol).

When HSG findings are abnormal or equivocal, laparoscopy is indicated for definitive assessment of fallopian tube status and for delineating the etiology of tubal occlusion. In some cases, a serum chlamydia titer is helpful in determining the likelihood of tubal pathology or intraperitoneal adhesions. In the case of hydrosalpinx, laparoscopy may also serve as a therapeutic measure. **Patients who are prepared to enter into IVF treatment are encouraged to undergo salpingectomy because of the very low pregnancy rates after neosalpingostomy, high rate of recurrent occlusion, risk of ectopic pregnancy, and, finally, decreased success rates after IVF when a hydrosalpinx is present** [27,28]. Neosalpingostomy in experienced hands is associated with a cumulative pregnancy rate as high as 25% [29]. However, because of superior pregnancy rates achieved with IVF (up to 40% live births per initiated cycle [CDC]), surgical repair of distal tubal occlusion generally is reserved for patients with relatively mild tubal disease or those who are opposed to IVF because of philosophical, financial, or religious concerns. Several studies have confirmed lower pregnancy rates and higher rates of spontaneous abortion after IVF when hyprosalpinx is present [27,28]. Other studies have shown that these differences are eliminated when salpingectomy or proximal tubal occlusion is performed [30].

Uterine factor

Both congenital and acquired abnormalities of the uterine cavity may affect the likelihood of pregnancy and/or pregnancy outcome. In-utero DES exposure, which may result in a classic T-shaped uterus, as well as abnormalities of formation or fusion of the uterine horns and uterine septae constitute abnormalities that have implications primarily in pregnancy outcome. Acquired defects include leiomyomata, endometrial polyps, and intrauterine synechiae. The size of the defect, location, and extent of distortion of the uterine cavity determine their likelihood to impair reproductive function. **A careful assessment of the uterine cavity should therefore be included in the female evaluation.**

There are three modalities commonly used to evaluate the uterine cavity: HSG, saline infusion sonohysterography (SIS), and hysteroscopy. HSG is usually the first-line test, as the assessment of the uterine cavity and fallopian tube status may be ascertained simultaneously. When the tubal status is not in question (e.g., after prior tubal ligation or salpingectomy), SIS is a simple and cost-effective way to assess the uterus. Saline is infused into the uterine cavity during real-time ultrasound assessment through a small catheter that has been placed into the cervical canal or uterus. Distension of the cavity provides an outline of the uterine contour and highlights filling defects such as polyps. Hysteroscopy is a direct inspection of the uterine cavity, and may allow for simultaneous resection of intrauterine pathology. Flexible, 3 mm hysteroscopes allow for efficient and usually painless inspection of the uterine cavity in the office setting. In most cases, uterine pathology can be easily identified by any one or a combination of these procedures. In some cases, however, MRI may be a useful adjunct, particularly when evaluating uterine anomalies that have a noncommunicating component, evaluating the size and location of larger myomas, and helping to distinguish between uterine fibroids and adenomyosis. Patients with congenital abnormalities such as bicornuate or septate uteri should also have MRI, US, or CT/IVP to assess renal anatomy because of the high incidence of urinary tract anomalies in these patients [31].

Peritoneal factor

A small subgroup of infertile women may be found to have normal HSG, pelvic exam, and ultrasound in spite of the presence of peritoneal factors such as tubal or ovarian adhesions or endometriosis. Therefore, patients with unexplained infertility or failure to conceive with conventional infertility treatment may benefit from laparoscopy to determine the presence and extent of endometriosis or adhesions. **Because of the increased utility of ART in these patients, and the relatively disappointing improvement in outcome after surgical treatment, laparoscopy is included less frequently in the routine evaluation of the infertile couple, with many couples choosing to go directly to ART.**

Assessment of ovarian reserve

Ovarian reserve is defined as the capacity of the ovaries to respond to gonadotropin stimulation. Women at birth are endowed with a finite number of follicles, the majority of which expire due to atresia. There is a progressive decline in the number of follicles with age, with an apparently accelerated rate of disappearance after the age of 37 [32,33]. **Whereas the correlation between egg quality and chronological age is very strong, there is significant variability in ovarian reserve among women at any given age.**

As women age, shortening of the follicular phase length (time to ovulation) is observed, constituting a clinical sign of decreasing ovarian reserve [23,34]. However, even when these clinical signs are present, studies in normal women indicate normal and often supraphysiologic ovarian secretion of both estradiol and progesterone until significant menstrual irregularity associated with the perimenopause occurs [35]. For this reason, many patients and practitioners may be falsely reassured by the continued presence of normal menstrual cycles and peripheral steroid concentrations. Therefore, a formal assessment of ovarian reserve is indicated to detect a woman's "relative reproductive age" as well as her potential to benefit from therapies involving controlled ovarian hyperstimulation.

Indirect measures of ovarian reserve include early follicular phase FSH, estradiol, inhibin B, and anti-Müllerian hormone levels. Recently, the antral follicle count (the number of follicles between 2 and 10 mm that can be measured on transvaginal ultrasound) has emerged as a predictor of stimulation quality in ART cycles [36,37]. The mainstay of ovarian reserve testing is determination of early follicular phase serum FSH and estradiol, traditionally on day 3 of the menstrual cycle. **Because estradiol inhibits FSH secretion, it is essential to obtain both hormones in order to interpret the FSH result with accuracy.** FSH levels below 10 IU/L are usually indicative of normal ovarian reserve, whereas levels of 10–15 suggest compromised ovarian reserve. Levels above 15 IU/L usually indicate a severe diminution of ovarian reserve, with most patients in this range failing to respond sufficiently to exogenous gonadotropins. Estradiol levels above 80 pg/mL are abnormal and provide an independent predictor of decreased ovarian reserve, probably due to early selection and maturation of a dominant follicle [23]. Variability cycle to cycle and between assay standards limits somewhat the predictive value of this test [38, 39]. Furthermore, many women with compromised ovarian reserve have normal day-3 FSH and estradiol levels. These patients may be detected by employing the clomiphene citrate challenge test, in which clomiphene is administered days 5 through 9 with a second FSH determination on day 10 [40]. Elevation of the day-10, stimulated FSH also predicts poor response to gonadotropin stimulation.

Newer measures of ovarian reserve include measurement of inhibin B [41] and anti-Müllerian hormone [42]. Both are secreted by the pool of small growing follicles and correlate very well with response to ovarian stimulation with gonadotropins. Although these hormones may prove to have higher specificity and sensitivity as markers of ovarian reserve, the assays are not as readily available and the normal ranges are less well established. In general, they add little to the clinical assessment of ovarian reserve. Ultrasound assessment of antral follicle count correlates with chronological age, is noninvasive, and may be assessed at any phase of the menstrual cycle. Antral follicle count determined in normal women at various ages demonstrates the same age-related decline as that seen in reports of nongrowing follicles, with an apparent increase in the rate of disappearance by age 40 [43] (Figs. 19.9, 19.10). **Antral follicle count demonstrates minimal inter-cycle variability [44], and has been found to be superior to FSH testing in predicting IVF outcome [45,46].**

Although ovarian reserve has traditionally been defined as the capacity of the ovaries to respond to gonadotropins, it is debated that abnormal ovarian reserve testing may also reflect a compromise in oocyte quality as well as oocyte quantity. El-Toukhy demonstrated that young patients with elevated FSH levels had poor ART outcome, arguing that youth and supposed good oocyte quality were not protective [47]. However, young patients with elevated FSH levels

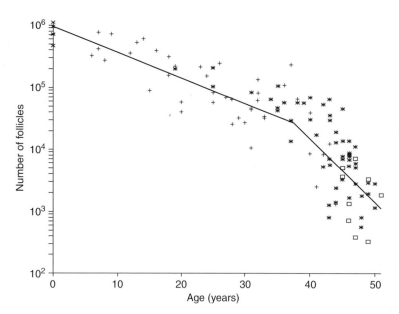

Fig. 19.9. Depiction of the declining follicle numbers determined in normal ovarian pairs from birth to age 51. (From Faddy MJ *et al.* Accelerated disappearance of ovarian follicles in mid-life: implications for forecasting menopause. *Hum Reprod* 1992; **7**: 1342–46, with permission.)

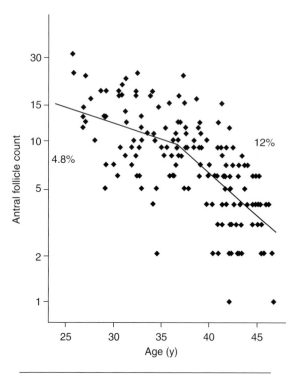

Scheffer. Antral follicle counts. Fertil Steril 1999.

Fig. 19.10. The number of antral follicles 2–10 mm determined by transvaginal ultrasound according to age. (From Scheffer GJ *et al.* Antral follicle counts by transvaginal ultrasonography are related to age in women with proven natural fertility. *Fertil Steril* 1999; **72**: 845–51, with permission. Copyright © 1999 American Society for Reproductive Medicine.)

had significantly higher implantation rates than older patients with normal FSH levels. FSH and antral follicle counts have more predictive value for quantitative outcome measures, such as gonadotropin requirement, number of oocytes, number of embryos, and cancellation rates, than for qualitative outcome such as implantation and pregnancy rates. A recent meta-analysis has suggested that the antral follicle count predicts ovarian response, but not pregnancy [48].

Ovarian reserve testing should be offered routinely to women over 35, as well as to those with unexplained infertility or failure to respond to conventional infertility treatment, and to those contemplating ART therapy. Risk factors for premature loss of ovarian reserve include prior ovarian infection, surgery, exposure to chemotherapy or radiation, family history of early menopause, family history of fragile X syndrome, and smoking. These patients, as well as those with clinical indicators of reduced ovarian reserve (recent onset of cycle irregularity or early ovulation), should have early assessment of ovarian reserve. Women with reduced ovarian reserve may have less benefit from ART; however, younger women may wish to be more aggressive and utilize ART sooner when decreased ovarian reserve is identified.

Summary

The guiding principle of evaluating infertility is to focus on the couple while practicing simultaneous evaluations. For that reason, the goal of this chapter has been to provide the non-gynecologist with a better understanding of female reproductive physiology and the appropriate workup of the female. This knowledge should facilitate productive communication between the treating professionals and lead to a more logical, cost-effective, and timely evaluation and treatment plan. The profound impact of maternal age on fertility potential must be an important consideration when treating the older couple.

References

[1] Guttmacher AF. Factors affecting normal expectancy of conception. *JAMA* 1956; **161**: 855–60.

[2] Collins HA. Unexplained infertility. In: Key WR, Chang RJ, Rebar RW, Soules MR, eds. *Infertility: Evaluation and Treatment.* Philadelphia, PA: Saunders, 1995: 249–62.

[3] World Health Organization. Recent advances in medically assisted conception. *World Health Organ Tech Rep Ser* 1992; **820**: 1–111.

[4] American Society for Reproductive Medicine. Optimal evaluation of the infertile female: a Practice Committee report. Birmingham, AL: ASRM, 2000.

[5] Barbieri RL. Female infertility. In: Strauss JF, Barbieri RL, eds. *Yen & Jaffe's Reproductive Medicine Endocrinology.* St. Louis, MO: Saunders, 2004: 633–88.

[6] Leridon H, Spira A. Problems in measuring the effectiveness of infertility therapy. *Fertil Steril* 1984; **41**: 580–6.

[7] Evers J. Female subfertility. *Lancet* 2002; **360**: 151–9.

[8] Centers for Disease Control, and Prevention. *2004 Assisted Reproductive Technology Success Rates: National Summary and Fertility Clinic Reports.* Atlanta, GA: CDC, US Department of Health and Human Services, 2006.

[9] Zinaman MJ, Clegg ED, Brown CC, O'Connor J, Selevan SG. Estimates of human fertility and pregnancy loss. *Fertil Steril* 1996; **65**: 503–9.

[10] Stein Z. A woman's age, childbearing and child rearing. *Am J Epidemiol* 1985; **121**: 327–42.

[11] Metcalf M. Incidence of ovulatory cycles in women approaching the menopause. *J Biosoc Sci* 1979; **11**: 39–48.

[12] Menken J, Trussell J, Larsen U. Age and infertility. *Science* 1986; **233**: 1389–94.

[13] Tietze C. Reproductive span and rate of reproduction among Hutterite women. *Fertil Steril* 1957; **8**: 89–97.

[14] Schwartz D, Mayaux MJ. Female fecundity as a function of age: results of artificial insemination in 2193 nulliparous women with azoospermic husbands. Federation CECOS. *N Engl J Med* 1982; **306**: 404–6.

[15] Balmaceda J, Bernardini L, Ciuffardi I, *et al.* Oocyte donation in humans: a model to study the effect of age on embryo implantation rate. *Hum Reprod* 1994; **9**: 2160–3.

[16] Battaglia D, Klein NA Soules MR. Changes in centrosomal domains during meiotic maturation in the human oocyte. *Mol Hum Reprod* 1997; **2**: 845–51.

[17] Battaglia D, Goodwin P, Klein N, Soules M. Influence of maternal age on meiotic spindle assembly in oocytes from naturally cycling women. *Human Reprod* 1996; **11**: 2217–22.

[18] Pellestor F, Andreo B, Arnal F, Humeau C, Demaille J. Maternal aging and chromosomal abnormalities: New data drawn from in vitro unfertilized human oocytes. *Hum Genet* 2003; **112**: 195–203.

[19] Platteau P, Staessen C, Michiels A, *et al.* Preimplantation genetive diagnosis for aneuploidy screening in women older than 37 years. *Fertil Steril* 2005; **84**: 319–24.

[20] Hook E. Rates of chromosomal abnormalities at different maternal ages. *Obstet Gynecol* 1981; **58**: 282–5.

[21] de La Rochebrochard E, de Mouzon J, Thepot F, Thonneau P, French National Ivf Registry (FIVNAT) Association. Fathers over 40 and increased failure to conceive: the lessons of *in vitro* fertilization in France. *Fertil Steril* 2006; **85**: 1420–4.

[22] Yen SSC, Tsai CC, Naftolin F, VandenBerg G, Ajabor L. Pulsatile patterns of gonadotropin release in subjects with and without ovarian function. *J Clin Endocrinol Metab* 1972; **34**: 671.

[23] Klein N, Battaglia D, Fujimoto V, *et al.* Reproductive aging: accelerated follicular development associated a monotropic follicle stimulating hormone rise in normal older women. *J Clin Endocrinol Metab* 1996; **81**: 1038–45.

[24] Jordan J, Craig K, Clifton DK, Soules MR. Luteal phase defect: the sensitivity and specificity of diagnostic methods in common clinical use. *Fertil Steril* 1994; **62**: 54–62.

[25] Johnson N, Vandekerckhove P, Watson A, *et al.* Tubal flushing for subfertility. *Cochrane Database Syst Rev* 2005; (2): CD003718.

[26] Johnson NP, Farquhar CM, Hadden WE, *et al.* The FLUSH trial: flushing with lipiodol for unexplained (and endometriosis-related) subfertility by hysterosalpingography. A randomized trial. *Hum Reprod* 2004; **19**: 2043–51.

[27] Strandell A, Waldenstrom U, Nilsson L, Hamberger L. Hydrosalpinx reduces *in-vitro* fertilization/embryo transfer pregnancy rates. *Hum Reprod* 1994; **9**: 861–3.

[28] Camus E, Poncelet C, Goffinet F, *et al.* Pregnancy rates after in-vitro fertilization in cases of tubal infertility with and without hydrosalpinx: a meta-analysis of published comparative studies. *Hum Reprod* 1999; **14**: 1243–9.

[29] Gomel V, McComb PF. Microsurgery for tubal infertility. *J Reprod Med* 2006; **51**: 177–84.

[30] Johnson NP, Mak W, Sowter MC. Surgical treatment for tubal disease in women due to undergo *in vitro* fertilisation. *Cochrane Database Syst Rev* 2001; (3): CD002125.

[31] Braun-Quentin C, Billes C, Bowing B, Kozot D. MURCS association: case report and review. *J Med Genet* 1996; **33**: 618–20.

[32] Gougeon A, Ecochard R, Thalabard J. Age-related changes of the population of human ovarian follicles: increase in the disappearance rate of non-growing and early-growing follicles in aging women. *Biol Reprod* 1994; **50**: 653–63.

[33] Richardson S, Senikas V, Nelson J. Follicular depletion during the menopausal transition: Evidence for accelerated loss and ultimate exhaustion. *J Clin Endocrinol Metab* 1987; **65**: 1231–7.

[34] Lenton E, Landgren B, Sexton L, Harper R. Normal variation in the length of follicular phase of the menstrual cycle: effect of chronological age. *Br J Obstet Gynaecol* 1984; **91**: 681–4.

[35] Lee S, Lenton E, Sexton L, Cooke I. The effect of age on the cyclical patterns of plasma LH, FSH, oestradiol and progesterone in women with regular menstrual cycles. *Hum Reprod* 1988; **3**: 851–5.

[36] Chang MY, Chiang CH, Hseih TT, Soong YK, Hsu KH. Use of the antral follicle count to predict the outcome of assisted reproductive technologies. *Fertil Steril* 1998; **69**: 505–10.

[37] Frattarelli JL, Lauria-Costa DF, Miller BT, Bergh PA, Scott RT. Basal antral follicle number and mean ovarian diameter predict cycle cancellation and ovarian responsiveness in assisted reproductive technology cycles. *Fertil Steril* 2000; **74**: 512–17.

[38] Schipper I, de Jong FH, Fauser BC. Lack of correlation between maximum early follicular phase serum follicle stimulating hormone concentrations and menstrual cycle characteristics in women under the age of 35 years. *Hum Reprod* 1998; **13**: 1442–8.

[39] van Rooij IA, Bancsi LH, Broekmans FJ, *et al.* Women older than 40 years of age and those

with elevated follicle-stimulating hormone levels differ in poor response rate and embryo quality in *in vitro* fertilization. *Fertil Steril* 2003; **79**: 482–8.

[40] Tanbo T, Dale PO, Lunde O, Norman N, Abyholm T. Prediction of response to controlled ovarian hyperstimulation: a comparison of basal and clomiphene citrate-stimulated follicle-stimulating hormone levels. *Fertil Steril* 1992; **57**: 819–24.

[41] Lockwood G. The diagnostic value of inhibin in infertility evaluation. *Semin Reprod Med* 2004; **22**: 195–208.

[42] Visser JA, de Jong FH, Laven JS, Themmen AP. Anti-Mullerian hormone: a new marker for ovarian function. *Reproduction* 2006; **131**: 1–9.

[43] Scheffer, GJ, Broeksmans, FJ, Dorland M, *et al.* Antral follicle counts by transvaginal ultrasonography are related to age in women with proven natural fertility. *Fertil Steril* 1999; **72**: 845–51.

[44] Kwee J, Schats R, McDonnell J, Lambalk CB, Schoemaker J. Intercycle variability of ovarian reserve tests: Results of a prospective randomized study. *Hum Reprod* 2004; **19**: 590–5.

[45] Nahum R, Shifren JL, Chang Y, *et al.* Antral follicle assessment as a tool for predicting outcome in IVF: is it a better predictor than age and FSH? *J Assist Reprod Genet* 2001; **18**: 151–5.

[46] Bancsi LF, Broekmans FJ, Eijkemans MJ, *et al.* Predictors of poor ovarian response in in vitro fertilization: A prospective study comparing basal markers of ovarian reserve. *Fertil Steril* 2002; **77**: 328–36.

[47] El-Toukhy T, Khalaf Y, Hart R, Taylor A, Braude P. Young age does not protect against the adverse effects of reduced ovarian reserve: an eight year study. *Hum Reprod* 2002; **17**: 1519–24.

[48] Hendriks DJ, Mol BW, Bancsi LF, te Velde ER, Broekmans FJ. Antral follicle count in the prediction of poor ovarian response and pregnancy rate after in vitro fertilization: a meta-analysis and comparison with basal follicle-stimulating hormone level. *Fertil Steril* 2005; **83**: 291–301.

Chapter 20

The use of ultrasound and radiologic imaging in the diagnosis of male infertility

Saleh Binsaleh, Myles Margolis, Keith Jarvi, and Kirk C. Lo

Introduction

Almost 50% of all causes of infertility can be attributed to a male factor. Hypofertile men are being investigated increasingly in an effort to find a treatable cause or to rule out more serious underlying conditions such as cancer.

Common causes of male infertility include varicocele, obstruction due to epididymal blockage, vasal or seminal vesicle agenesis, and ejaculatory duct obstruction. Other conditions such as cryptorchidism, testicular tumors, testicular microlithiasis, pituitary adenoma, and renal disorders may be identified during the infertility workup.

Imaging studies such as ultrasound scan (US), computed tomography (CT), magnetic resonance imaging (MRI), angiography, nuclear scans, and thermographs are used in the workup of infertile men. With the refinement and the introduction of newer imaging modalities, reliable adjuncts to clinical examination can be obtained to facilitate or to confirm a suspected cause in male infertility. In this chapter, various imaging modalities in the workup of male infertility will be summarized, with emphasis on indications and outcome interpretation.

Imaging for commonly identified causes in male infertility

The conditions outlined below are commonly identified causes for oligospermia and azoospermia, and are the usual targets for imaging investigations.

Varicocele

Varicoceles are dilated testicular veins caused by reflux of blood. A "significant" varicocele is a *clinical* diagnosis, and a clinically palpable varicocele is graded 1, 2, or 3 according to severity [1]. Physical examination

sometimes can be limited, thus hindering varicocele detection. This is obvious in patients with a thick scrotum, a history of previous surgery, or altered anatomy such as concomitant hydrocele. These limitations have been demonstrated in a multicenter study sponsored by the World Health Organization [2]. In this study of 141 men with subfertility, the sensitivity of clinical examination for the detection of a varicocele was approximately 50%, with a false-positive rate of 23%, when compared with venography.

Various diagnostic studies have been used in an effort to maximize our ability to diagnose and/or to confirm a suspicious diagnosis of varicocele that is not clear by physical examination. **These include color Doppler ultrasound (CDUS), which has now become the most reliable noninvasive test to detect nonpalpable reflux. Other modalities not in common use nowadays due to their decreased sensitivity and/or specificity to diagnose varicocele are Doppler stethoscope, scrotal contact thermography, and radionuclide angiography. Spermatic venography is considered by many as the gold standard for varicocele diagnosis.** This belief is based on the assumption that venography is not subject to technical variation and perturbation of technique. However, this is not necessarily the case. Pryor and Howards noted that the absence of technical standardization in venography could result in the appearance of reflux in any patient [3]. Moreover, the test is expensive, invasive, time-consuming, and occasionally incomplete because it may not be possible to catheterize the right internal spermatic vein in up to 5% of cases [4]. For interpretation, a normal venogram is one in which a single testicular vein is seen up to the inguinal ligament and into the spermatic cord; there may be a few divisions as part of the pampiniform plexus. If a varicocele is present, the internal spermatic vein will be enlarged and there will

Infertility in the Male, 4th edition, ed. Larry I. Lipshultz, Stuart S. Howards, and Craig S. Niederberger. Published by Cambridge University Press. © Cambridge University Press 2009.

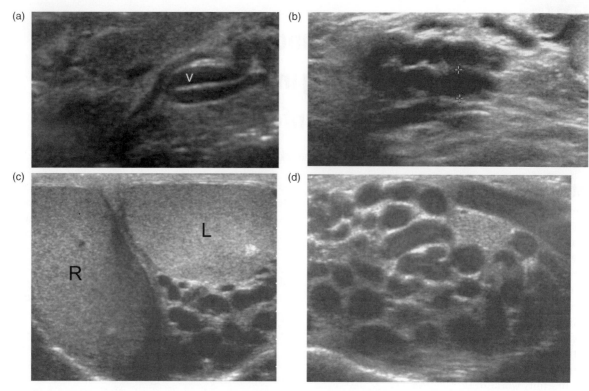

Fig. 20.1. Ultrasound images of varicocele. (a) Sagittal image of the left scrotum, showing mildly dilated veins (V), largest 3 mm. (b) Sagittal image of a moderate varicocele, 4 mm in maximal diameter (between cursors). (c) Transverse image of normal testis (R, right; L, left), and a large left varicocele deep to the left. (d) Sagittal image of the large left varicocele [same patient as in (C)], consisting of numerous tortuous and dilated veins.

be reflux into the abdominal, inguinal, scrotal, or pelvic portions of the spermatic vein. There will also be venous collateralization and anastomotic channels [5]. At present, spermatic venography is performed either in the assessment of difficult or uncertain cases or, more commonly, before definitive treatment by venous embolization (discussed later).

As mentioned above, CDUS has become the most frequently used imaging modality for varicocele detection. Ultrasound studies of spermatic veins have suggested that the presence of multiple large veins (> 3 mm) and reversal of blood flow with Valsalva maneuver indicate the presence of a varicocele [6–8]. Jarow et al found that men who underwent varicocelectomy with the largest vein measuring over 3 mm had significant improvement in sperm counts and motility compared with those with varicoceles less than 3 mm [9]. Preoperative ultrasound-measured reversal of flow during Valsalva (reflux) also predicted success of varicocelectomy (Fig. 20.1).

Chiou et al. compared spermatic vein diameter with physical examination and found that this commonly accepted ultrasound criterion for varicocele (maximal vein diameter ≥ 3 mm) had a sensitivity of 53% and a specificity of 91% compared with physical examination [10]. However, studies comparing ultrasound with spermatic venography obtained conflicting results in assessing the reliability of ultrasound in diagnosing varicoceles. The sensitivity and specificity are high (92% and 100%, respectively) when venography is carried out selectively [11], and lower (70% and 55%) when contrast medium is injected into the left renal vein or the inferior vena cava [12].

CDUS has superseded grayscale imaging alone. It is more sensitive than clinical examination and can detect up to 93% of the reflux subsequently confirmed by spermatic venography [13]. However, the significance of nonpalpable "color reflux" has been questioned. Meacham et al. studied 34 young volunteers with normal sperm counts and found that CDUS was positive in half of those with no palpable varicoceles [14]. Furthermore, Cvitanic et al. reported reflux in 64% of surgically treated patients (in whom varicoceles were no longer palpable in 91%) and in 42% of volunteers with no palpable varicocele and with normal sperm counts [15]. Both authors concluded that the significance of reflux on CDUS, in the absence of palpable varicocele (subclinical), remains to be determined. Jarow in a meta-analysis found no benefit in treating subclinical varicoceles [16]. On the other hand, Pasqualotto et al. found that the repair of right-sided subclinical varicocele resulted in significant improvement in seminal parameters in patients with clinical left varicocele compared to those in patients with left-sided varicocelectomy only [17].

Some investigators postulate that in order to identify a significant nonpalpable varicocele, reflux detected by CDUS must be quantified; the CDUS does not accurately quantify reflux, because it is difficult to calculate the duration of reflux or to assess its amplitude during straining [18]. To measure the duration of reflux accurately, pulsed-mode Doppler ultrasound is preferable [4]. **Ultrasound-detected reflux can be classified into three categories. Brief reflux lasts less than a second and is physiological. Permanent reflux lasts more than two seconds and has a plateau aspect throughout the abdominal strain.** This reflux type is nonpalpable in only 20% of cases and does not correlate with the diameter of the spermatic vein [4]. **The third type, intermediate reflux, is not palpable, lasts 1–2 seconds, in most cases keeps decreasing during the Valsalva maneuver, and stops before the end of the maneuver. It has been suggested that, in the absence of palpable varicocele, only permanent reflux should be termed a subclinical varicocele, because the Doppler findings and change after treatment are identical to those of palpable varicoceles** [4].

Finally, the detection of an isolated right-sided varicocele is rare and, if seen, warrants imaging of the abdomen and pelvis to rule out retroperitoneal mass.

In summary, accurate diagnosis of varicocele is important because correct treatment may lead to resolution of symptoms and improvement in semen parameters in subfertile patients. **At present a significant varicocele that warrants treatment is one that is clinically palpable, and until further evidence indicates otherwise, routine imaging to detect subclinical varicocele is not recommended unless the physical examination is inconclusive.**

Epididymal obstruction

This condition may account for 7–14% of cases of azoospermia or severe oligospermia [19]. It can be congenital or acquired. Jarvi et al. reported that at least 47% of otherwise healthy men with idiopathic epididymal obstruction had a cystic fibrosis transmembrane conductance regulator (CFTR) gene mutation [20]. The diagnosis is suspected in severely oligospermic or azoospermic patients with a normal testicular volume, normal FSH level, and normal ejaculate volume with alkaline pH. Epididymal enlargement can sometimes be clinically palpated [19].

Scrotal and transrectal ultrasound (TRUS) have been used to investigate epididymal obstruction. On scrotal ultrasound, the epididymis can have a hypoechoic or hyperechoic appearance corresponding to the sequelae of epididymitis. The epididymal tube can be dilated, with or without spermatocele (Fig. 20.2). Dilation less commonly involves the efferent ducts or the rete testis. Therefore, imaging is of limited value when the epididymides are enlarged on palpation. Marked post-infectious sclerosis can mask this dilation [18]. Similarly, in nonazoospermic patients, only ultrasound with high-frequency probes (10–14 MHz) can detect partial epididymal obstruction that can be the cause of hypofertility [21]. On TRUS, the caudal junction of the vas deferens and seminal vesicles can be normal or show signs of chronic prostatitis [18].

In clinical practice, epididymal obstruction is a diagnosis of exclusion, and imaging studies are not generally indicated. However, in certain circumstances ultrasound may aid in confirmation of a diagnosis.

Congenital absence of the vas deferens

Men with vasal or epididymal abnormalities, typically in combination with low-volume azoospermia, are at risk for cystic fibrosis (CF) gene mutations. If the vas deferens is not palpable, CF gene mutation testing is recommended. The most commonly encountered condition in this category is cystic fibrosis transmembrane conductance regulator (CFTR) gene mutation. Between 50% and 82% of men with congenital bilateral absence of the vas deferens (CBAVD), and approximately 43% of those with congenital unilateral absence (CUAVD), will have at least one detectable CFTR gene mutation [22,23]. Furthermore, 98% of men with CF present with CBAVD [24].

CUAVD should not adversely affect fertility except when there is contralateral testicular pathology such as torsion, varicocele, or cryptorchidism. However, a partial contralateral Wolffian abnormality can be observed, with low-volume azoospermia. The vas can still be palpated in the scrotum but terminates either in the anterior wall of the pelvis or by crossing the midline to merge with the contralateral seminal vesicle if present [25,26].

In CBAVD the diagnosis is established clinically by the absence of the two vasa deferentia on palpation. The semen volume is usually below 1 mL, with an acidic pH. **Scrotal ultrasound may show dilation of the efferent ducts, with the head of the epididymis stopping abruptly at the junction of the body and tail. TRUS may show the absence of ampullae of vas deferens** [27]. **Seminal vesicle (SV) abnormalities are observed in 90% of cases** (Fig. 20.3) [28]. They can be absent bilaterally in approximately 40% of cases, while in the remaining 60% one or both vesicles

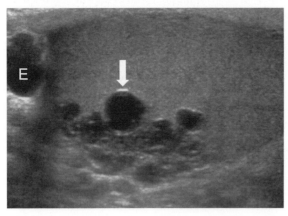

Fig. 20.2. Sagittal ultrasound scan of an epididymal head cyst (E), and cystic dilation of the rete testis (arrow).

are visible with variable ultrasonographic abnormalities (hypoplasia, vesicular cyst, calcifications, and hyperechoic appearance) (Figs. 20.4, 20.5). In 10% of cases the seminal vesicles are normal. MRI is helpful in tracing the vas in the pelvic region (Fig. 20.6). Another constant finding in patients with CBAVD is a diffuse hyposignal activity of the entire prostatic peripheral zone seen only by MRI, the cause of which is still unknown [27].

Incomplete forms, with preservation of the body and tail of the epididymis or one seminal vesicle and its corresponding ejaculatory duct, can be seen [27]. These incomplete forms explain how the volume of semen can be only moderately reduced (1.5–2 mL), the pH can be alkaline, and even one vas deferens can be palpated in rare cases of CBAVD [18].

Renal ultrasound is routinely performed in the workup of congenital vasal agenesis. Schlegel et al. observed that renal agenesis is evident in about 11% of men with bilateral and 26% of infertile men with unilateral congenital absence of the vas deferens [23]. **Ipsilateral renal ectopia, crossed-fused renal ectopia, and horseshoe kidneys have also been observed.** When the renal anomalies coexist with congenital vasal agenesis, genetic mutation is rarely found [29].

Ejaculatory duct obstruction (EDO)

Patients with ductal obstruction have azoospermia when obstruction is complete, or severe oligospermia if the obstruction is partial. Clinically, bilateral vasa deferentia are palpable in the scrotum, and, similar to CBAVD, are associated with small ejaculate volume with acidic pH, and little or no seminal fructose. The cause can be congenital or acquired [30]. The most

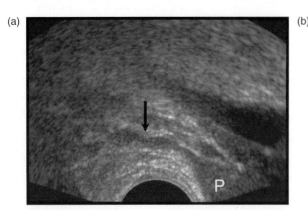
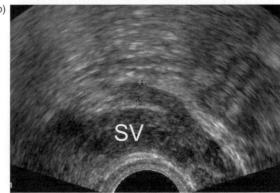

Fig. 20.3. (a) Transverse TRUS image just cranial to the prostate (P) of a markedly atrophic right seminal vesicle and absent vas deferens in a patient with CBAVD. (b) TRUS image of a normal right seminal vesicle (SV) and vas deferens joining its medial aspect.

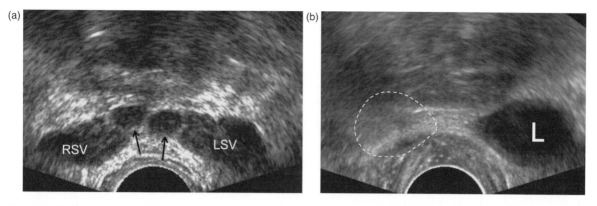

Fig. 20.4. (a) Transverse midline TRUS image of normal seminal vesicles (RSV, right; LSV, left) and vas deference (arrows). (b) TRUS image of a dilated left seminal vesicle (L) and absence of the right (dotted line outlining its expected position). No vas was seen on either side.

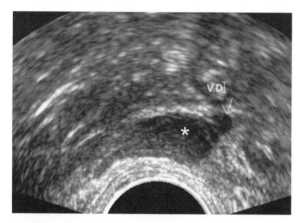

Fig. 20 5. Transverse TRUS image of a solitary and atrophic left seminal vesicle (asterisk), and a single blind-ended vas entering aberrantly into its lateral aspect (VD and arrow).

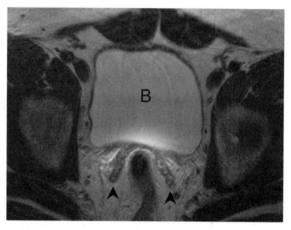

Fig. 20.6. Transverse MR image of bilaterally atrophic seminal vesicles (arrowheads) and absent vas (B, bladder).

frequent congenital cause is compression by median cysts, followed by mega seminal vesicles in patients with adult polycystic kidney disease. Acquired causes include distal inflammatory stenoses of the ejaculatory ducts (Fig. 20.7).

Previously, vasography was commonly used to demonstrate seminal tract obstruction and to define the level of a block within or outside the vas, but the procedure is an invasive technique, is technically difficult, and in itself may result in damage to the vas deferens. The role of imaging is to identify and occasionally treat the cause of the obstruction [18].

Median cysts

These cysts are classified into two categories: those that contain semen and those that do not [31]. These types sometimes can be difficult to distinguish from each other. **The cysts containing semen are of Wolffian origin, and those that do not are of Müllerian or utricular origin and are the most frequent.** While both can originate in the verumontanum or slightly proximal to it, Müllerian cysts often extend above the base of the prostate. **Cysts of the utricle generally measure no more than 15 mm on the long axis. They are strictly median, while extraprostatic Müllerian cysts can be more laterally located in their extraprostatic portion.** Cysts containing semen originate in the ejaculatory ducts and have the same sonographic appearance as non-Wolffian cysts. They are congenital but can be secondary to distal stenosis of the ducts [32]. A Wolffian cyst may not contain semen if there is also an epididymal obstruction occurring secondarily when the distal stenosis has been long-standing [33].

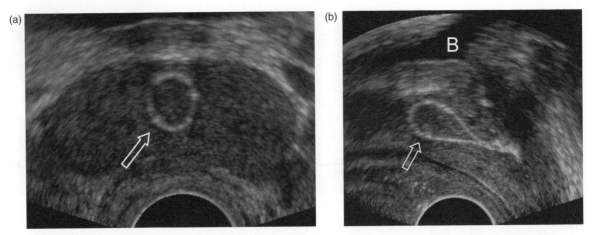

Fig. 20.7. (a) Transverse TRUS image of the prostate shows a peripherally calcified ejaculatory duct cyst, with internal low-level echogenic debris (arrow). (b) Sagittal TRUS image of the same cyst (arrow) showing the typical teardrop shape, pointing towards the urethra (B, bladder).

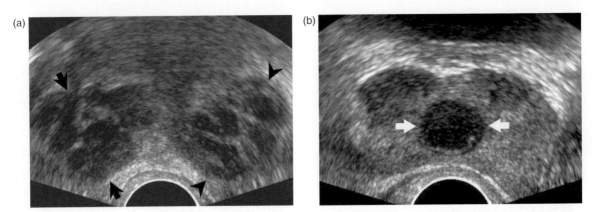

Fig. 20.8. (a) Transverse TRUS of symmetrically distended seminal vesicles (between arrowheads). (b) Transverse TRUS, more inferiorly through the prostate, of a 1.2 cm midline cyst (arrows).

Median cysts are obstructive when they compress the ejaculatory ducts (Fig. 20.8). This is often difficult to show by imaging, because dilation of the vesicles or vas ampullae is not the rule. **Diagnosis of a compressive cyst is** therefore **based on clinical findings, i.e., azoospermia or severe oligospermia with reduced ejaculate volume.** In selected cases, when TRUS fails to detect distension proximal to the cyst, dilation can be confirmed by MRI.

Distal inflammatory stenosis of the ejaculatory ducts

The diagnosis is suggested by TRUS if there is marked dilation proximal to the obstruction. Stones can be present in one or both ejaculatory ducts (Fig. 20.9). A more proximal obstruction is likely to be associated with the distal obstruction if scrotal sonography or palpation shows dilated epididymides; this

can be confirmed by vasogram, as shown by Pryor and Hendry, who reported multifocal stenoses on the vas deferens in 20% of patients with ejaculatory duct obstruction [30]. An alternative, developed by Jarow [34], is to puncture the seminal vesicles under TRUS guidance and check for the presence of motile sperm, which indicates absence of a more proximal obstruction. Absence of motile sperm would indicate that azoospermia is not due to the distal obstruction alone. It has been also shown that transrectal vesiculography and retrograde opacification could be performed to assess the normal patency of the vas deferens [35,36], but this can only be done immediately prior to endoscopic resection. Endorectal MRI can be used to assess the length of stenosis.

Selection of patients with an isolated EDO, without combined proximal obstruction, probably improves

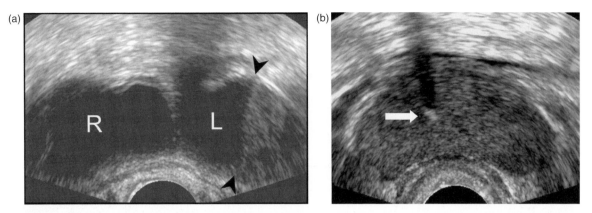

Fig. 20.9. (a) Midline transverse TRUS of cystic dilation of both seminal vesicles (R, right; L, left). Note the debris-fluid level in the left SV, layering laterally due to the patient's left lateral decubitus position (along line between arrowheads). (b) Transverse TRUS of prostate in the same patient with a tiny echogenic right ejaculatory duct calcification (arrow), demonstrating acoustic shadowing deep to it.

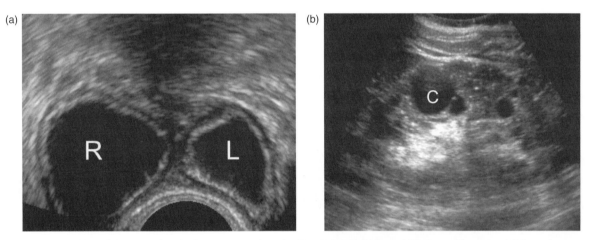

Fig. 20.10 (a) TRUS midline image of markedly cystic seminal vesicles (R, right; L, left). (b) Sagittal US of one of this patient's kidneys shows innumerable anechoic cysts, the largest labeled (C), and allows for a diagnosis of bilateral polycystic kidney disease.

results of transurethral resection of the ejaculatory duct (TURED), which restores a normal sperm count in only 20–60% of azoospermic patients [37,38].

Mega seminal vesicles and functional causes of ejaculatory duct obstruction

The obstruction in this rare condition is due to a disorder of seminal vesicle contractions. The atonic seminal vesicles can be seen in men with diabetic neuropathy. Patients with polycystic kidney disease can have mega vesicles (Fig. 20.10). **Diagnosis is established by vasography showing mega vesicles with no visible obstruction.**

Partial ejaculatory duct obstruction

This condition can be difficult to diagnose. Clinically, patients present with oligospermia. Although there is

no definite preoperative diagnosis test to prove partial EDO, the combination of a volume of ejaculate less than 1.5 mL and seminal vesicle enlargement (anterior–posterior diameter > 15 mm), along with roundish anechoic areas of seminal vesicles, has been suggested to be a reliable sign of partial EDO [39]. Endorectal MRI can be helpful in selected cases, as it can detect moderate dilation of the seminal vesicles when TRUS fails to find distension [27], but this sign has not been validated. TRUS-guided puncture of the seminal vesicles to confirm sperm retention has been used in these patients, but validity of the test has not been verified. Endoscopic treatment by TURED remains the only confirmatory test, and it can be therapeutic. Improvement of ejaculate volume and percentage of sperm count and motility can be

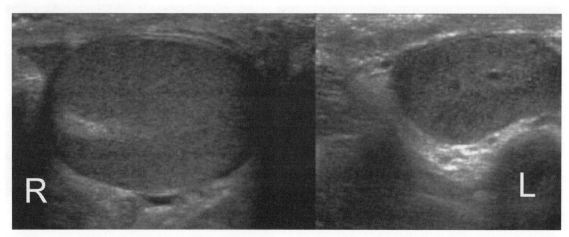

Fig. 20.11. Split-screen US image of both testicles, taken with identical magnification. The right (R) is normal in size and location; the left (L) is undescended, in the inguinal canal, small and heterogeneous.

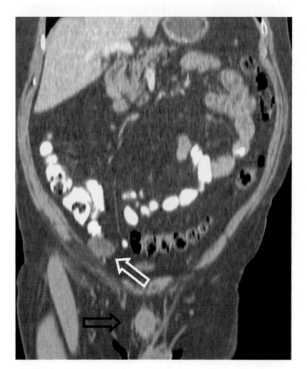

Fig. 20.12. Coronal MR image of an undescended right testicle, just above the inguinal canal (white arrow). Note the absence of normal cord structures in the right hemiscrotum (black arrow).

seen in approximately 60% of cases [38,40]. However, a complete EDO can occur in 4% of cases following ED resection [40].

Cryptorchidism

History of cryptorchidism (undescended testis or UDT) is a definite cause of hypofertility. This condition

(UDT) is also associated with a 14-times increased risk of subsequently developing a testis tumor; 7–10% of patients with a testicular tumor have a history of undescended testis. Patients with bilateral undescended testis and unilateral testicular carcinoma have an increased risk of testicular tumor in the remaining testis [41]. Early detection of testicular tumor is the goal of scrotal ultrasound in these patients.

Ultrasound is particularly useful in localizing the inguinal undescended testis (Fig. 20.11), **but is more limited in detecting intra-abdominal testis** [42]. Intra-abdominal testis is frequently atrophic and obscured by overlying structures during ultrasound. **Among other imaging modalities, MRI is considered advantageous for detecting intra-abdominal testis** [43], **and it avoids the ionizing radiation associated with CT scans** (Figs. 20.12, 20.13, 20.14).

Other conditions

These conditions can be seen during imaging workups of infertile males or during workups of other conditions not related directly to infertility.

Scrotal masses

It has been suggested that infertility, testis cancer, undescended testis, and hypospadias are part of the testicular dysgenesis syndrome that result from disturbed prenatal testicular development [44]. In one series testicular tumor was detected in 7.5% of azoospermic males [45], and others found a 20-fold greater incidence of testicular cancer in infertile men with abnormal semen analysis than in the general population [46].

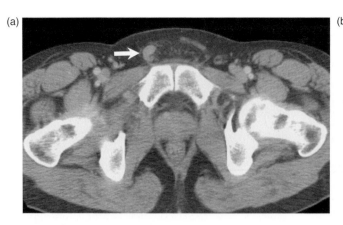

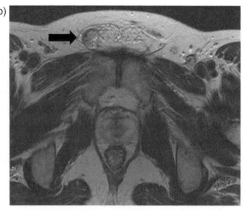

Fig. 20.13. (a & b) Axial CT and MR images of an undescended, atrophic right testicle in the lower inguinal canal (arrows).

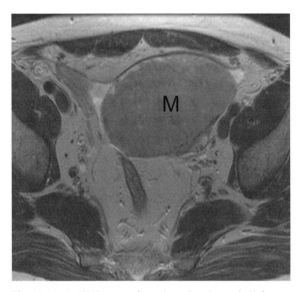

Fig. 20.14. Axial MR image of an enlarged, undescended left pelvic testicle replaced by a tumor mass (M).

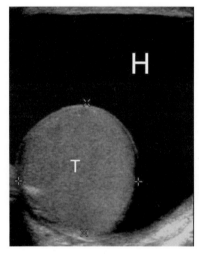

Fig. 20.15. Transverse scrotal US of a normal testicle (T) and a large, anechoic hydrocele (H).

The initial determination of a scrotal mass as intratesticular or extratesticular is important. Malignant extratesticular masses are rare, whereas intratesticular solid masses must be considered malignant until proved otherwise [43]. Ultrasound is extremely sensitive in detecting scrotal masses. The most common extratesticular scrotal masses include inguinal hernias, hydrocele, epididymal masses, and varicoceles. Hydrocele is a fluid collection between the testis and the tunica vaginalis, and generally not related to male subfertility (Fig. 20.15). Cystic masses of the epididymis include the simple epididymal cyst and the often larger, multilocular spermatocele. Most epididymal cysts involve the head of the epididymis, but

they can also involve the epididymal tail or body [43]. Spermatoceles contain spermatozoa, whereas epididymal cysts contain clear fluid (Fig. 20.16). Ultrasound cannot dependably differentiate between these two entities [47]. Epididymal solid masses are usually adenomatoid – a benign tumor that is considered the most common paratesticular tumor [48]. These tumors are believed to arise from the mesothelium [49]. Surgical intervention for epididymal masses is not recommended unless they are growing, symptomatic, or causing infertility, which is seen rarely when the mass causes tubular obstruction [50]. If palpated, scrotal ultrasound is indicated to rule out an associated testicular mass.

Malignant germ cell tumors constitute 90–95% of intratesticular primary tumors. Their appearance

383

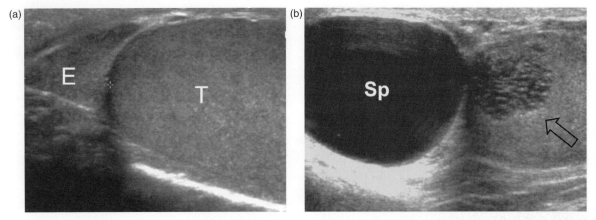

Fig. 20.16. (a) Sagittal scrotal US of a normal epididymal head (E) and normal upper testicle (T). (b) US image of a large supratesticular cyst representing a spermatocele (Sp), and dilated rete testis (arrow).

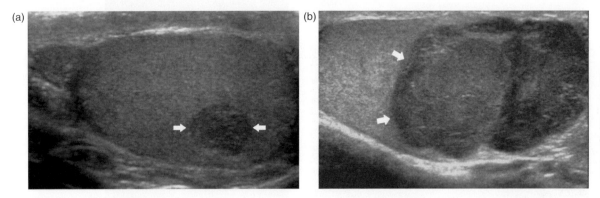

Fig. 20.17. (a) Scrotal US of a small testicular malignancy, contained within the testicular capsule (arrows). (b) A larger testicular tumor replacing the inferior two-thirds (arrows depicting its upper margin), with extracapsular spread inferiorly.

on ultrasound is variable, usually as a hypoechoic hypervascular lesion (Fig. 20.17).

Seminoma is the most common cancer of the testis in adults and the most common tumor associated with cryptorchidism [51]. On ultrasound they may appear as hypoechoic round masses with areas of necrosis. Embryonal cell carcinoma is also hypoechoic but it is more non-homogeneous, less defined on ultrasonography because of cyst formation and hemorrhage, and may contain areas of calcification. On ultrasonography, teratomas appear as hypoechoic masses and commonly have foci of increased echogenicity due to calcifications. Cystic components are also common. Choriocarcinomas are rare small tumors that usually are associated with calcifications and bleeding, which gives them a heterogeneous appearance on ultrasonography.

Lymphoma is one of the most frequently seen testicular tumors in older men. It is the most frequent bilateral testicular neoplasm, accounting for up to 7% of testicular neoplasms. The second most frequent testicular metastatic cancer is leukemia. **The ultrasonographic appearance of lymphoma and leukemia is generally that of a hypoechoic mass with or without testicular enlargement, and the testicular contour is generally preserved [52]. Leydig and Sertoli cell tumors are gonadal stromal tumors. They are hypoechoic on ultrasonography and typically benign (Fig. 20.18). They commonly have cystic areas and cannot be differentiated from malignant lesions on ultrasonography [53].**

Intratesticular cysts include cysts of the tunica albuginea, tubular ectasia of the rete testis, and testicular cysts. They have the typical appearance of other cysts: well-defined anechoic structures with increased through-transmission. Evaluation of the wall for solid components to exclude a cystic

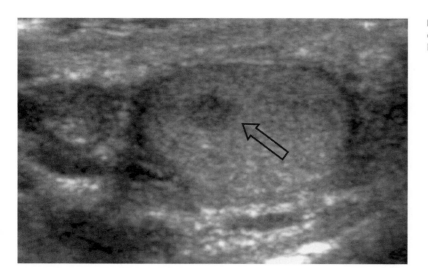

Fig. 20.18. Sagittal US of a small testicle containing a 5mm pathologically proven Leydig cell tumor (arrow).

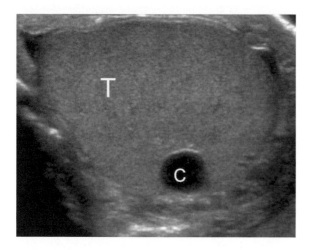

Fig. 20.19. Transverse US of a benign testicular cyst (C). Note its thin, smooth wall, and anechoic contents (T, testicle).

neoplasm must be performed carefully (Fig. 20.19). Tubular ectasia of the rete testis is a benign entity that is important to identify on ultrasonography, because it can be confused with a tumor, leading to unnecessary intervention. Ultrasonographic findings are those of hypoechoic branching cystic configurations in the mediastinum testis (Fig. 20.20). These findings may be associated with a spermatocele visualized in the same testes. Tubular ectasia tends to occur in an older group than does malignancy and is frequently bilateral. The etiology is thought to involve infection or trauma [43].

Diagnostic ultrasound and MRI are highly sensitive for detecting intratesticular masses, but

their specificity is low [54]. **Consequently, imaging modalities are unable to differentiate benign from malignant lesions using appearance or size criteria, and exploratory surgery is still the only way to exclude malignancy by a histopathological analysis.** Muller *et al.* reviewed the histology of 20 incidental intratesticular masses of ≤ 5 mm in diameter and found them benign in 80% of cases [55], although some nodules as small as 3 mm were found to be malignant.

Whether men with infertility should have screening ultrasound for small testicular masses is controversial. Since testicular cancer is a curable disease if detected early, some believe in the advantage of routine use of scrotal ultrasound in the workup of infertile men [56,57]. For others this is not the standard of care as there is no evidence that detection of nonpalpable small tumors provides better cancer control or prognosis than early detection of palpable lesions.

Testicular microlithiasis (TM)

TM is characterized by the presence of numerous punctate calcifications within the testis. The calcifications arise from degeneration of the cells lining the seminiferous tubules [42]. This condition can be observed in 1/2100 cases in autopsy series [58], and in 1/125–1/168 of testicular biopsies [58,59]. Up to 23% of patients with TM consult for hypofertility. TM is 10 times more common in patients with history of undescended testis.

Scrotal ultrasound is diagnostic. **Typically, there are small echogenic foci (1–2 mm large), uniformly**

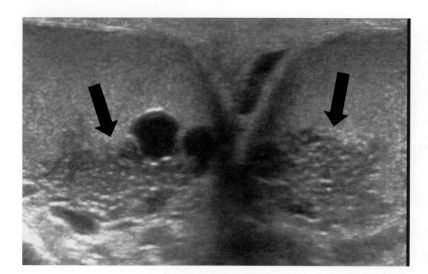

Fig. 20.20. Transverse midline scrotal US of bilaterally dilated rete testis (arrows), not to be confused with neoplasia.

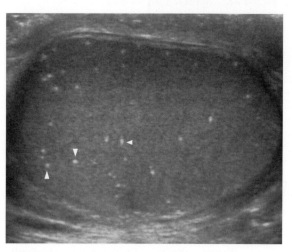

Fig. 20.21. Sagittal scrotal US of multiple tiny echogenic testicular foci (arrowheads point out a few) representing microlithiasis.

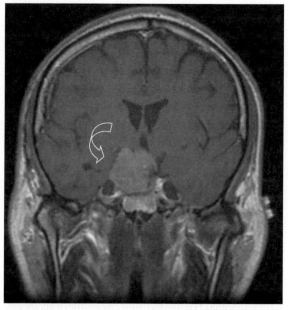

Fig. 20.22. Coronal MRI of the sella turcica shows a large pituitary adenoma (curved arrow).

distributed in the testis, and bilaterally, in most cases [60]. **Most of them show no acoustic shadowing, likely due to their tiny size (Fig. 20.21). In 29% of cases, microliths can be predominantly clustered peripherally in the testis. According to the number of microliths per testis (5–10, 10–20, >20), TM has been classified as grade 1, 2, and 3, respectively.**

The frequency of germ cell tumors in patients with TM has been estimated in several series between 21% and 45% [60–63]. However, detection bias was suspected as many of these patients had presented with a scrotal mass, which artificially increases the rate of TM-associated malignancy. Recently, Rashid *et al.* reviewed all published data and found no higher risk

of developing testis cancer in patients with TM [64]. A direct relationship between TM and subsequent development of a testicular tumor during follow-up has been reported in only two cases [65,66]. Tumor risk is thus not yet entirely known, and it has been suggested that limited microlithiasis with fewer than five microliths is probably not a factor predisposing to malignancy, making follow-up unnecessary in these patients [67]. Similarly, there is no definite proof that TM by itself can cause hypofertility.

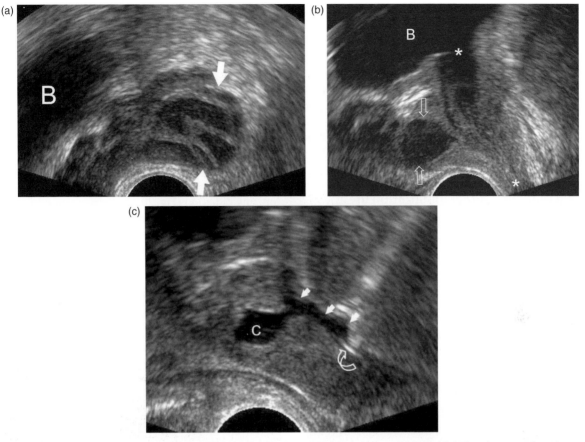

Fig. 20.23. (a) Transverse TRUS image of a dilated left seminal vesicle 2 cm thick (between arrows) (B, bladder). The other seminal vesicle (not shown) had a similar appearance. (b) Sagittal TRUS image of the prostate shows the obstructing midline cyst (between arrows) (B, bladder; urethral course is along a line between asterisks). (c) Sagittal midline TRUS image immediately following transurethral resection of the ejaculatory dust cyst (C, cyst; arrows outline fluid-filled prostatic urethra communicating with the unroofed cyst; curved arrow shows the echogenic tip of the cystoscope just inferior to the cyst).

Pituitary adenoma

It is estimated that 10% of all intracranial tumors are pituitary adenomas but are too small or endocrinologically inactive to be detected clinically. Prolactin-producing adenomas, a cause for male and female infertility, account for 70% of all pituitary adenomas [68]. **Imaging technology, in particular cranial MRI, enables accurate diagnosis and localization** (Fig. 20.22).

Renal disorders

Unilateral renal agenesis can be suspected in cases of CBAVD or CUAVD. Similarly, polycystic kidneys can be associated with epididymal (18%) and seminal vesicle cysts (39%) [69]. Renal ultrasound should be performed routinely at the time of TRUS when such cystic findings are identified.

Use of imaging for treatment guidance

Imaging techniques can be used to treat or to guide therapy in some cases of male infertility.

Image-guided treatment of obstructive conditions

In obstructive azoospermia, TRUS can be used to guide median cyst puncture and seminal vesicle aspiration in cases of suspected ejaculatory duct obstruction (EDO) (Fig. 20.23). **TRUS-guided echo-enhanced seminal vesiculography in combination with TURED is considered the best imaging method when treating EDO [70]. With this technique the ejaculatory ducts and level of obstruction can be located successfully,** and the operator is able to direct the incisional line with real-time TRUS and hence maximize accuracy and minimize possible complications. Direct vesiculography and image-guided balloon placement and ejaculatory duct dilation have also been described. Such balloon dilation is particularly suited to those with partial obstruction or extraprostatic obstruction [71,72]. TRUS or endorectal MRI can be used to assess the distance between the posterior wall of the prostatic urethra and the wall of the ducts before undertaking TURED.

Percutaneous angioembolization of varicocele

Angiographically guided embolization of the testicular veins frequently is used to treat varicoceles. The procedure typically is performed with the patient under local anesthesia with or without conscious sedation. Venous access is obtained by puncturing the right common femoral vein under ultrasound guidance; the jugular vein offers an alternative route of access. With a coaxial system, a 5 F sheath is placed into the common

femoral vein. A 5 F catheter and hydrophilic guide-wires are then advanced into the inferior vena cava (IVC) and the renal vein on the left or, occasionally, directly into the testicular vein on the right as it enters the IVC. Access to the right renal vein may be difficult in some cases, necessitating the use of an angled catheter or eventually access via the internal jugular vein. Occasionally the basilic vein may be used as an access point [5]. The catheter is advanced into the testicular vein over the guide-wire. Contrast medium is then injected and images obtained. Limited images should be obtained over the testes due to their sensitivity to ionizing radiation (Fig. 20.24). Subsequent occlusion is accomplished with sclerosing agents or via embolization using coils (Fig. 20.25) or detachable balloons [4]. Coils are usually deployed starting distally at the

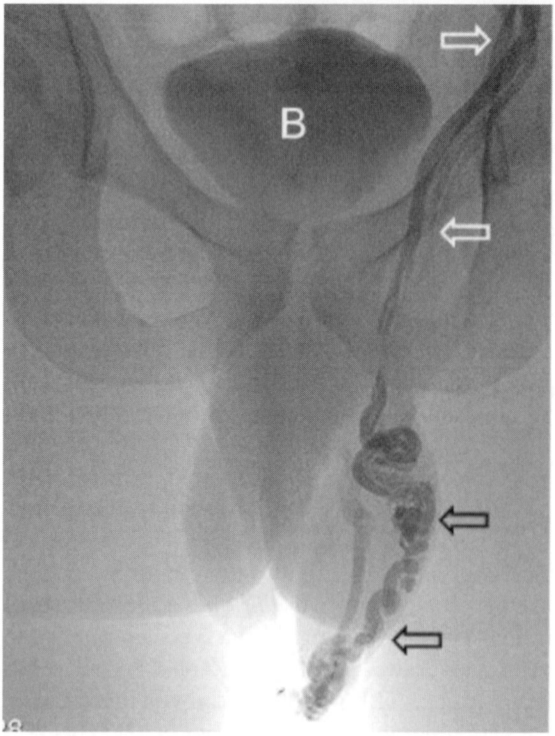

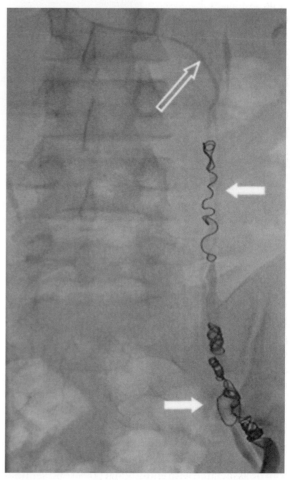

Fig. 20.24. Antero-posterior radiograph obtained during left testicular venogram. Multiple dilated and refluxing veins, at the level of the scrotum (black arrows) and at the lower pelvic–inguinal level (white arrows) (B, contrast-filled bladder).

Fig. 20.25. Antero-posterior radiograph obtained during left testicular angio-embolization for varicocele. Multiple embolization coils have been deployed within the venous lumen (solid arrows), via a transjugular angiographic catheter (open arrow).

level of the inguinal ligament and progressing proximally [73]. Coil migration is rare and usually is related to coil release too near to the renal vein [4]. Sclerosing agents such as sodium tetradecyl sulfate, hypertonic glucose solution, or biological glue may also be used for embolization. If used, it is imperative that reflux into the pampiniform plexus be prevented by external pressure at the inguinal crease before the sclerosant is injected. Thrombosis of the pampiniform plexus by the sclerosing agent is possible, and although it occurs in less than 5% of patients it is troublesome and requires treatment with anti-inflammatory agents and antibiotics [74].

Image-guided sperm retrieval

Scrotal ultrasound can also be helpful to guide testicular sperm aspiration in azoospermic patients. Belenky *et al.* evaluated 39 azoospermic men who underwent testicular sperm aspiration, 16 under sonographic guidance and 23 with no imaging guidance [75]. The ultrasound group had fewer complications and more successful retrievals, although no difference was found between the two groups in pregnancy rate. Similarly, the testicular vascularity index distribution obtained by scrotal power Doppler ultrasound can be used to predict sites with the greatest potential for spermatogenesis for sperm retrieval during microscopic testicular sperm extraction (micro-TESE). This technique is based on the hypothesis that spermatogenesis is more likely to occur in regions that are well perfused with oxygenated blood [76].

Infertility with no established indications for imaging

Some conditions associated with male infertility may not benefit from investigative imaging . These include idiopathic infertility, hypogonadotropic hypogonadism, diagnosed testicular failure, genetic causes of male infertility, or immunological causes, unless an underlying scrotal or upper urinary tract infection, urinary tract anomaly, stones, or tumors are suspected.

References

[1] Dubin L, Amelar RD. Varicocele size and results of varicocelectomy in selected subfertile men with varicocele. *Fertil Steril* 1970; **21**: 606–9.

[2] World Health Organization. Comparison among different methods for the diagnosis of varicocele. *Fertil Steril* 1985; **43**: 575–82.

[3] Pryor JL, Howards SS. Varicocele. *Urol Clin North Am* 1987; **14**: 499–513.

[4] Cornud F, Belin X, Amar E, et al. Varicocele: strategies in diagnosis and treatment. *Eur Radiol* 1999; **9**: 536–45.

[5] Beddy P, Geoghegan T, Browne RF, Torreggiani WC. Testicular varicoceles. *Clin Radiol* 2005; **60**: 1248–55.

[6] Rifkin MD, Foy PM, Kurtz AB, Pasto ME, Goldberg BB. The role of diagnostic ultrasonography in varicocele evaluation. *J Ultrasound Med* 1983; **2**: 271–5.

[7] McClure RD, Hricak H. Scrotal ultrasound in the infertile man: detection of subclinical unilateral and bilateral varicoceles. *J Urol* 1986; **135**: 711–15.

[8] Wolverson MK, Houttuin E, Heiberg E, Sundaram M, Gregory J. High-resolution real-time sonography of scrotal varicocele. *AJR Am J Roentgenol* 1983; **141**: 775–9.

[9] Jarow JP, Ogle SR, Eskew LA. Seminal improvement following repair of ultrasound detected subclinical varicoceles. *J Urol* 1996; **155**: 1287–90.

[10] Chiou RK, Anderson JC, Wobig RK, et al. Color Doppler ultrasound criteria to diagnose varicoceles: correlation of a new scoring system with physical examination. *Urology* 1997; **50**: 953–6.

[11] Hamm B, Fobbe F, Sorensen R, Felsenberg D. Varicoceles: combined sonography and thermography in diagnosis and posttherapeutic evaluation. *Radiology* 1986; **160**: 419–24.

[12] Eskew LA, Watson NE, Wolfman N, et al. Ultrasonographic diagnosis of varicoceles. *Fertil Steril* 1993; **60**: 693–7.

[13] Petros J, Andriole G, Middleton W. Correlation of testicular color doppler ultrasonography, physical examination and venography in the detection of left varicoceles in men with infertility. *J Urol* 1991; **145**: 785–8.

[14] Meacham RB, Townsend RR, Rademacher D, Drose JA. The incidence of varicoceles in the general population when evaluated by physical examination, grey-scale sonography, and colour doppler sonography. *J Urol* 1994; **151**: 1535–8.

[15] Cvitanic OA, Cronan JJ, Sigman M, Landau ST. Varicoceles: Postoperative prevalence: a prospective study with color Doppler US. *Radiology* 1993; **187**: 711–14.

[16] Jarow JP. Effects of varicocele on male fertility. *Hum Reprod Update* 2001; 7: 59–64.

[17] Pasqualotto FF, Lucon AM, de Goes PM, et al. Is it worthwhile to operate on subclinical right varicocele in patients with grade II–III varicocele in the left testicle? *J Assist Reprod Genet* 2005; **22**: 227–31.

[18] Cornud F, Amar E, Hamida K, Helenon O, Moreau JF. Ultrasound findings in male hypofertility and impotence. *Eur Radiol* 2001; **11**: 2126–36.

[19] Bellaish J. Medical aspects of male sterilities. In: Papiernik E, Rozenbaum H, Belaish-Allart J, eds. *Gynecology*. Paris: Flammarion Medicine-Sciences, 1990: 381–94.

[20] Jarvi K, Zielenski J, Wilschanski M, *et al.* Cystic fibrosis transmembrane conductance regulator and obstructive azoospermia. *Lancet* 1995; **345**: 1578.

[21] Schoysman R. Epididymal oligospermia. *Reprod Nutr Dev* 1988; **28**: 1339–45.

[22] Anguiano A, Oates RD, Amos JA, *et al.* Congenital bilateral absence of the vas deferens: a primarily genital form of cystic fibrosis. *JAMA* 1992; **267**: 1794–7.

[23] Schlegel P, Shin D, Goldstein M. Urogenital anomalies in men with congenital absence of the vas deferens. *J Urol* 1996; **155**: 1644–8.

[24] Bienvenu T, Claustres M. Molecular basis of cystic fibrosis and congenital bilateral agenesis of vas deferens. *Contracep Fertil Sex* 1996; **24**: 495–500.

[25] Hall S, Oates R. Unilateral absence of the scrotal vas deferens associated with contralateral mesonephric duct anomalies resulting in infertility: laboratory, physical and radiographic findings, and therapeutic alternatives. *Urology* 1993; **150**: 1161–4.

[26] Kuligowska E, Baker CE, Oates RD. Male infertility: role of transrectal US in diagnosis and management. *Radiology* 1992; **185**: 353–60.

[27] Cornud F, Belin X, Delafontaine D, *et al.* Imaging of obstructive azoospermia. *Eur Radiol* 1997; **7**: 1079–85.

[28] Carter SS, Shinohara K, Lipshultz LI. Transrectal ultrasonography in disorders of the seminal vesicles and ejaculatory ducts. *Urol Clin North Am* 1989; **16**: 773–90.

[29] Augarten A, Yahav Y, Kerem BS, *et al.* Congenital bilateral absence of vas deferens in the absence of cystic fibrosis. *Lancet* 1994; **344**: 1473–4.

[30] Pryor JP, Hendry WF. Ejaculatory duct obstruction in subfertile males: analysis of 87 patients. *Fertil Steril* 1991; **56**: 725–30.

[31] Nghiem HT, Kellman GM, Sandberg SA, Craig BM. Cystic lesions of the prostate. *Radiographics* 1990; **10**: 635–50.

[32] Goluboff ET, Stifelman MD, Fisch H. Ejaculatory duct obstruction in the infertile male. *Urology* 1995; **45**: 925–31.

[33] Silber SJ. Ejaculatory duct obstruction. *J Urol* 1980; **124**: 294–7.

[34] Jarow JP. Seminal vesicle aspiration in the management of patients with ejaculatory duct obstruction. *J Urol* 1994; **152**: 899–901.

[35] Jones TR, Zagoria RJ, Jarow JP. Transrectal US-guided seminal vesiculography. *Radiology* 1997; **205**: 276–8.

[36] Riedenklau E, Buch JP, Jarow JP. Diagnosis of vasal obstruction with seminal vesiculography: An alternative to vasography in select patients. *Fertil Steril* 1995; **64**: 1224–7.

[37] Aggour A, Mostafa H, Maged W. Endoscopic management of ejaculatory duct obstruction. *Int Urol Nephrol* 1998; **30**: 481–5.

[38] Meacham RB, Hellerstein DK, Lipshultz LI. Evaluation and treatment of ejaculatory duct obstruction in the infertile male. *Fertil Steril* 1993; **59**: 393–7.

[39] Colpi GM, Negri L, Nappi RE, Chinea B. Is transrectal ultrasonography a reliable diagnostic approach in ejaculatory duct sub-obstruction? *Hum Reprod* 1997; **12**: 2186–91.

[40] Turek PJ, Magana JO, Lipshultz LI. Semen parameters before and after transurethral surgery for ejaculatory duct obstruction. *J Urol* 1996; **155**: 1291–3.

[41] Narayan P. Cancer and infertility. In: Tanagho EA, Lue TF, McClure RD, eds. *Contemporary Management of Impotence and Infertility*. Baltimore, MD: Williams and Wilkins, 1998: 348–56.

[42] Ragheb D, Higgins JL. Ultrasonography of the scrotum: technique, anatomy, and pathologic entities. *J Ultrasound Med* 2002; **21**: 171–85.

[43] Sarihan H, Sari A, Abes M, Dinc H. Nonpalpable undescending testis: value of magnetic resonance imaging. *Minerva Urol Nefrol* 1998; **50**: 233–6.

[44] Bay K, Asklund C, Skakkebaek NE, Andersson AM. Testicular dysgenesis syndrome: Possible role of endocrine disrupters. *Best Pract Res Clin Endocrinol Metab* 2006; **20**: 77–90.

[45] Mancini M, Carmignani L, Gazzano G, *et al.* High prevalence of testicular cancer in azoospermic men without spermatogenesis. *Hum Reprod* 2007; **22**: 1042–6.

[46] Raman JD, Nobert CF, Goldstein M. Increased incidence of testicular cancer in men presenting with infertility and abnormal semen analysis. *J Urol* 2005; **174**: 1819–22.

[47] Tessler FN, Tublin ME, Rifkin MD. Ultrasound assessment of testicular and paratesticular masses. *J Clin Ultrasound* 1996; **24**: 423–36.

[48] Mostofi FK, Price EB Jr. Tumors of the male genital system. In: Firminger HI, ed. *Atlas of Tumor Pathology.* Washington, DC: Armed Forces Institute of Pathology, 1973: 144–51.

[49] Delahunt B, Eble JN, King D, *et al.* Immunohistochemical evidence for mesothelial origin of paratesticular adenomatoid tumor. *Histopathology* 2000; **36**: 109–15.

[50] Horstman WG, Sands JP, Hooper DG. Adenomatoid tumor of testicle. *Urology* 1992; **40**: 359–61.

[51] Howlett DC, Marchbank ND, Sallomi DF. Ultrasound of the testis. *Clin Radiol* 2000; **55**: 595–601.

[52] Bree RL, Hoang DT. Scrotal ultrasound. *Radiol Clin North Am* 1996; **34**: 1183–205.

[53] Krone KD, Carroll BA. Scrotal ultrasound. *Radiol Clin North Am* 1985; **23**: 121–39.

[54] Coret A, Leibovitch I, Heyman Z, Goldwasser B, Itzchak Y. Ultrasonographic evaluation and clinical correlation of intratesticular lesions: a series of 39 cases. *Br J Urol* 1995; **76**: 216–19.

[55] Muller T, Gozzi C, Akkad T, *et al.* Management of incidental impalpable intratesticular masses of ≤5 mm in diameter. *BJU Int* 2006; **98**: 1001–4.

[56] Pierik FH, Dohle GR, van Muiswinkel JM, Vreeburg JT, Weber RF. Is routine scrotal ultrasound advantageous in infertile men? *J Urol* 1999; **162**: 1618–20.

[57] Sakamoto H, Saito K, Shichizyo T, *et al.* Color Doppler ultrasonography as a routine clinical examination in male infertility. *Int J Urol* 2006; **13**: 1073–8.

[58] Nistal M, Paniagua R, Diez-Pardo JA. Testicular microlithiasis in 2 children with bilateral cryptorchidism. *J Urol* 1979; **121**: 535–7.

[59] Sasagawa I, Nakada T, Kazama T, *et al.* Testicular microlithiasis in male infertility. *Urol Int* 1988; **43**: 368–9.

[60] Backus ML, Mack LA, Middleton WD, *et al.* Testicular microlithiasis: Imaging appearances and pathologic correlation. *Radiology* 1994; **192**: 781–5.

[61] Cast JE, Nelson WM, Early AS, *et al.* Testicular microlithiasis: Prevalence and tumor risk in a population referred for scrotal sonography. *AJR Am J Roentgenol* 2000; **175**: 1703–6.

[62] Hobarth K, Susani M, Szabo N, Kratzik C. Incidence of testicular microlithiasis. *Urology* 1992; **40**: 464–7.

[63] Ganem JP, Workman KR, Shaban SF. Testicular microlithiasis is associated with testicular pathology. *Urology* 1999; **53**: 209–13.

[64] Rashid HH, Cos LR, Weinberg E, Messing EM. Testicular microlithiasis: a review and its association with testicular cancer. *Urol Oncol* 2004; **22**: 285–9.

[65] Winter TC, Zunkel DE, Mack LA. Testicular carcinoma in a patient with previously demonstrated testicular microlithiasis. *J Urol* 1996; **155**: 648.

[66] Gooding GA. Detection of testicular microlithiasis by sonography. *AJR Am J Roentgenol* 1997; **168**: 281–2.

[67] Bennett HF, Middleton WD, Bullock AD, Teefey SA. Testicular microlithiasis: US follow-up. *Radiology* 2001; **218**: 359–63.

[68] Franks S, Jacobs HS, Nabarro JD. Studies of prolactin in pituitary disease. *J Endocrinol* 1975; **67**: 55P.

[69] Belet U, Danaci M, Sarikaya S, *et al.* Prevalence of epididymal, seminal vesicle, prostate, and testicular cysts in autosomal dominant polycystic kidney disease. *Urology* 2002; **60**: 138–41.

[70] Apaydin E, Killi RM, Turna B, Semerci B, Nazli O. Transrectal ultrasonography-guided echo-enhanced seminal vesiculography in combination with transurethral resection of the ejaculatory ducts. *BJU Int* 2004; **93**: 1110–12.

[71] Jarow JP, Zagoria RJ. Antegrade ejaculatory duct recanalization and dilation. *Urology* 1995; **46**: 743–6.

[72] Lawler LP, Cosin O, Jarow JP, Kim HS. Transrectal US-guided seminal vesiculography and ejaculatory duct recanalization and balloon dilation for treatment of chronic pelvic pain. *J Vasc Interv Radiol* 2006; **17**: 169–73.

[73] Iaccarino V. Nonsurgical treatment of varicocele: trans-catheter sclerotherapy of gonadal veins. *Ann Radiol (Paris)* 1980; **23**: 369–70.

[74] Thomas AJ Jr, Geisinger MA. Current management of varicoceles. *Urol Clin North Am* 1990; **17**: 893–907.

[75] Belenky A, Avrech OM, Bachar GN, *et al.* Ultrasound-guided testicular sperm aspiration in azoospermic patients: a new sperm retrieval method for intracytoplasmic sperm injection. *J Clin Ultrasound* 2001; **29**: 339–43.

[76] Eytan O, Har-Toov J, Fait G, *et al.* Vascularity index distribution within the testis: a technique for guiding testicular sperm extraction. *Ultrasound Med Biol* 2001; **27**: 1171–6.

Microsurgical treatment of male infertility

Edmund S. Sabanegh Jr. and Anthony J. Thomas Jr.

Introduction

Microsurgical reconstruction of the male genital tract has dramatically improved over the past 100 years, and today it is one of the most successful and gratifying therapies for the management of male infertility. Over 7% of patients with primary infertility will have ductal obstruction, which is potentially correctible with surgical reconstruction. The safety and efficacy of vasectomy as a means of birth control has been a double-edged sword. As many as 5% of men will eventually request a restoration of fertility because of changing life circumstances such as remarriage, change in goals, or death of a child.

Recognition of ductal obstruction has long fueled an interest in innovative approaches to restore genital tract patency. Martin *et al.*, in 1903, first reported a technique to treat epididymal obstruction by anastomosing the vas to the epididymis in a side-to-side fashion with fine silver wire in a patient with a history of gonococcal epididymitis [1]. More than 30 years later, Hagner described his surgical outcomes using Martin's technique and reported patency in over 60% of patients [2]. This fistula technique remained the standard for nearly 75 years, until advances in technique and instrumentation made direct, single-tubule anastomosis feasible. In a similar fashion, Quinby performed the first reportedly successful vasectomy reversal in 1919 using a strand of silkworm gut as a stent.

These pioneers and many others provided the rich soil from which the innovations of today have grown. There has been a reassuring pattern of incremental improvements in surgical decision making and technique followed by careful critical analysis of results to support these refinements.

This chapter focuses on the salient features of ductal obstruction of the male genital tract to allow the identification of the appropriate candidates for microsurgical treatment. Surgical preparation and techniques are described in detail, along with a critical review of outcomes. Finally, the chapter examines the role of microsurgical reconstruction in the era of assisted reproductive technology.

Anatomy, physiology, and pathology of the excurrent ductal system

To secure an understanding of the surgical procedures utilized to restore patency of the excurrent ducts, it is critical to understand the anatomy and physiology of the male reproductive system. Spermatozoa are produced within the seminiferous tubules and released into the lumen. The terminal ends of these tubules drain into the rete testis, an area within the posterior mediastinum of the testis where a network of anastomosing ducts consolidates into the efferent ducts. These 6–8 efferent ducts derive from the degeneration of the mesonephric duct and become the caput, or head, of the epididymis. This marks the beginning of the epididymal tubule, a highly convoluted thinwalled structure measuring approximately 3 m in length, tightly coiled to a 4–5 cm long structure that is positioned posterior and lateral on each testis. The epididymis is divided into the head or caput, the midbody or corpus, and the tail or cauda. At the termination of the cauda epididymidis, the tubule is invested with a thick muscular wall marking the beginning of the vas deferens. During ejaculation, the sympathetic nervous system mediates contractions of the muscular wall of the vas, propelling sperm toward the ampulla of the vas. The vas deferens traverses the inguinal canal and enters the retroperitoneum, where it crosses in front of the ureter and behind the medial umbilical ligament. Within the retrovesical space it becomes more dilated to form the ampulla of the vas. The terminal narrow segment, the ejaculatory duct, enters the prostate and ends in the prostatic urethra in the verumontanum.

Infertility in the Male, 4th edition, ed. Larry I. Lipshultz, Stuart S. Howards, and Craig S. Niederberger. Published by Cambridge University Press. © Cambridge University Press 2009.

The epididymis provides four vital functions: sperm maturation, transport, concentration, and storage. It is in the area of sperm maturation that the epididymis has the largest potential implication for microsurgical outcomes. While the exact mechanism of epididymal-derived maturation remains unknown, it is well recognized that transit through the proximal portion of the epididymis is critical to sperm function (i.e., fertilization potential). Animal studies have shown that the increase in progressive sperm motility and fertilizing capability is dramatically greater in sperm taken from the cauda than from the caput epididymidis [3,4]. Similar work in humans has shown that the **chances for fertility after vasoepididymostomy increase with the length of the epididymis that the sperm were able to transit** [5,6]. The cauda epididymidis does not appear to have a significant role in sperm development but does function as an area of sperm storage before ejaculation.

Obstruction may occur anywhere along the course of the excurrent ducts. The etiologies of obstruction are often divided by their causative nature into *congenital, inflammatory, traumatic, iatrogenic,* and *idiopathic.*

In the setting of congenital obstruction, there often may be hypoplasia of the seminal vesicles or absence of the vas deferens and a major portion of the distal epididymis. This condition, called vasal agenesis, can be unilateral or bilateral. Approximately two-thirds of men with bilateral vasal agenesis will be found to have at least one genetic mutation that is observed in the cystic fibrosis population (*CFTR* or cystic fibrosis transmembrane regulator gene). Most of these patients have no phenotypic manifestations of cystic fibrosis. Because of the associated absence of the seminal vesicles in conjunction with bilateral vasal agenesis, they will have low-ejaculate-volume azoospermia with semen that does not coagulate, as well as low or absent fructose in the seminal plasma. Most of these patients are candidates for surgical or percutaneous sperm harvesting and intracytoplasmic sperm injection.

In contrast, obstruction of the excretory ducts secondary to infection may be surgically correctable. Tuberculous epididymitis is rare and can result in epididymal occlusion and azoospermia. Prompt antituberculin therapy potentially can maintain a man's fertility and obviate the need for microsurgical repair. Gonorrheal epididymitis was a frequent cause of obstructive epididymitis in the past, although this has become relatively rare in the antibiotic era. Today, it is more common to have epididymal scarring as a result of bacterial epididymitis from organisms such as *Chlamydia.*

Trauma to the epididymis is a relatively uncommon cause of an epididymal obstruction, but it may occur as a result of blunt or penetrating injury. Iatrogenic injuries are more common, occurring after procedures such as spermatocelectomy, hydrocelectomy, or even testis biopsy [7].

Elective vasectomy is the leading cause of obstructive azoospermia and subsequent infertility. While usually a single, focal obstructive site, the development of high intraluminal pressures after a vasectomy can result in rupture of the delicate epididymal tubule, with secondary obstruction in the epididymis. This phenomenon is more frequent in patients who underwent their vasectomy more than 10 years earlier, and in those who have had a prior unsuccessful vasectomy reversal procedure [8]. In a similar fashion, long-term obstruction associated with iatrogenic vasal injuries from prior surgery such as pediatric inguinal herniorrhaphies can also result in secondary epididymal obstructions.

Men with obstruction of the excretory ducts proximal to the ejaculatory ducts will have normal-volume azoospermia and normal testicular size. Leydig cell function, serum follicle-stimulating hormone (FSH), and luteinizing hormone (LH) levels usually will be normal. Despite these findings, restoration of genital tract patency does not always restore fertility. Growing evidence supports the belief that adverse testicular histology develops after vasectomy in most species studied. Guinea pigs can show extensive alterations, attributed to autoimmune orchitis [9,10]. Rabbits manifest severe testicular alterations with immune complex deposition around the seminiferous tubules [11], and long-term vasectomized monkeys show orchitis, germ cell aplasia, and immune deposits [12–14]. Some strains of rats have bilateral reduction of seminiferous tubular diameter even after a unilateral vasectomy [15]. The p53-Bax-dependent apoptosis of germ cells has been implicated as a possible mechanism for disrupted spermatogenesis after vasectomy in the rat [16]. A variety of histologic findings in the testes of vasectomized men have been reported to include degeneration of spermatids [17], thickened basement membranes [18,19] and increased phagocytosis by Sertoli cells [20]. Quantitative morphometric analysis of testicular histology in men after vasectomy has revealed dilation of the seminiferous tubules, interstitial fibrosis, and reductions in the seminiferous cell population [21]. A more recent study confirmed these findings, and demonstrated that the severity of the interstitial fibrosis inversely correlated with vasovasostomy outcomes [22]. **Regardless of the mechanism, it is becoming clear that vasectomy induces permanent changes in the testes that may inhibit the restoration of fertility in some patients.**

Reconstructive procedures
Preoperative assessment

Prior to considering a surgical procedure, all patients should have a complete medical history and physical examination. The history should include an assessment of any prior conceptions with current or prior partners. Prior history of childhood inguinal or scrotal surgery can provide important information regarding possible site and cause of genital tract obstruction. A history of epididymitis or sexually transmitted infection can suggest an occult epididymal obstruction. Physical examination should include a careful assessment of the scrotal contents with documentation of testicular size and consistency. The vas deferens should be easily palpable and assessed for thickness and induration. The epididymides should be palpated for induration. In the patient who has not previously had a vasectomy, at least two semen analyses should be obtained to document normal-volume azoospermia. In addition, serum FSH and testosterone levels should be evaluated to document a normal hypothalamic–pituitary–gonadal axis. Patients who have atretic or nonpalpable vas deferens should be tested for gene mutations in the cystic fibrosis transmembrane regulator gene [23]. Partners of surgical candidates should have a gynecological evaluation to ensure that there are no concurrent female-factor fertility problems or general health issues that need to be corrected, or that contraindicate the establishment of a pregnancy.

Men requesting a vasectomy reversal require no further workup or additional procedures as long as their scrotal examination reveals at least one normal-sized testicle and they have not developed any fertility-impacting medical conditions since their vasectomy. If there is any question regarding the presence of normal sperm production, a testis biopsy may be performed in advance of the reconstruction.

For men who have not previously had a vasectomy, proof of adequate sperm production can be provided from a testis biopsy at the same time as the planned reconstruction. A vasogram can also be performed to confirm patency or obstruction of the vas deferens and/

or ejaculatory duct. A vasogram can easily be obtained by isolating the straight portion of the vas deferens and passing a 30-gauge lymphangiogram needle (No. 6657, Becton-Dickinson Co., Franklin Lakes, NJ) directly into the lumen. Alternatively, the vas can be carefully hemitransected and a 24-gauge angiocatheter inserted into the vas lumen. A one-to-one mixture of 5 mL of contrast (Renografin 60®) and saline is injected in the vas in an antegrade fashion. A common practice is for the surgeon to cannulate the abdominal vas deferens and perfuse with saline, for example with a 24-gauge Angiocath catheter attached to a syringe. If the fluid flows easily, abdominal vasal patency is confirmed and radiography is not required. Likewise, the surgeon may pass a monofilament nonabsorbable suture, such as 4–0 Prolene, through the abdominal vas to confirm patency without radiography, and if obstruction is encountered, its precise position may be determined by the length of suture passed. A radiograph is obtained to confirm patency of the vasa deferentia, seminal vesicles, and ejaculatory ducts. The vasogram should not be performed before the time of definitive reconstruction, since this may cause scarring of the vas and render subsequent reparative surgery more difficult.

Intraoperative sperm cryopreservation can be offered to patients as part of their preoperative counseling. It is easily performed in conjunction with a reconstruction, and offers the potential for assisted reproduction if the anastomosis should fail and they remain azoospermic.

Type of reconstruction: vasovasostomy versus vasoepididymostomy

While most men with primary excurrent ductal obstruction will be obstructed at the level of the epididymis and can only be corrected with a vasoepididymostomy, patients who have had a vasectomy can be obstructed at the level of the prior vasectomy site as well as within the epididymis. **The choice of reconstruction in vasectomized men depends on a number of factors including the obstructive interval, the quality of the fluid from the proximal vas at the time of surgery, and the surgeon's microsurgical experience.** Epididymal obstruction rarely occurs within four years of a vasectomy, but is present in more than 60% of patients on one or both sides after 15 years of vasal obstruction [24]. The absence of fluid, or thick, viscous, paste-like fluid, is indicative of an epididymal obstruction, and such patients require a vasoepididymostomy for their reconstruction.

Using the data from the authors' institution, Parekattil *et al.* developed a linear regression algorithm based on time since vasectomy and patient age to predict if a vasoepididymostomy would be required in vasectomy reversal [25]. The equation for the vasoepididymostomy prediction score was (age × 0.31) + (obstructive interval × 0.94). If the score was greater than 20, then a vasoepididymostomy was predicted on one or both sides, based on a retrospective analysis of 483 patients. The score was intentionally set for a 100% sensitivity to allow urologists who were not comfortable performing a vasoepididymostomy to identify this population preoperatively and refer to someone who had the appropriate experience with this procedure. This model was subsequently validated in a multicenter retrospective and prospective review of 345 vasectomy reversal patients [26].

Operative planning

Microsurgical reconstructions are typically performed as an ambulatory outpatient procedure. For vasectomy reversal when the obstructive interval is shorter (less than 10 years), it is reasonable to perform the surgery under local anesthesia with sedation, since it is unlikely to require a vasoepididymal anastomosis. The skin is injected with 1% lidocaine. Once the vas is isolated, 0.25% bupivacaine is injected into the vasal sheath to allow an extended duration of anesthesia. In the setting where a vasoepididymostomy is contemplated, or in patients whose level of anxiety might make a local anesthetic procedure problematic, a general anesthetic or continuous epidural anesthesia is preferred. Minimal intravenous hydration is provided during the procedure to avoid bladder distension, since a Foley catheter is not usually utilized during these operations.

When the patient is anesthetized, careful positioning is beneficial, because these are prolonged procedures. The surgeon pads pressure points, and overextension may be minimized by abducting the patient's arms at 45° angles from the body. The anesthesiologist can consider a soft doughnut pad beneath the patient's head and occasional shifting of the head position to prevent pressure-related alopecia. While the literature is not definitive on deep venous thrombosis prophylaxis, sequential compression hose may be considered. As postoperative infections from scrotal surgery are uncommon, the surgeon may or may not recommend a broad-spectrum antibiotic, such as a cephalosporin, 30 minutes before the start of surgery.

At the start of the procedure, the vas is isolated over the vasectomy defect using a towel clip through the scrotal skin. A vertical surgical incision is centered over each hemiscrotum to allow for extension into the groin if more extensive mobilization of the vas is required. In the case where a vasovasostomy is anticipated, these incisions are 1–2 cm in length to allow only the vas ends to be delivered through the skin incision. If a vasoepididymostomy will be required, or if a long vasal defect is appreciated, a longer skin incision is made to allow delivery of the testis.

Vasovasostomy reconstructive techniques

After completion of a vertical scrotal incision as described above, blunt and sharp dissection is used in the region of the prior vasectomy to dissect the vas with its vascular pedicle from the surrounding tissue (Fig. 21.1A). Microsurgical bipolar or battery-operated disposable thermal cautery units can be used to obtain meticulous hemostasis while minimizing collateral cautery injury. After the vas deferens has been sufficiently mobilized, but before the vas is cut, the vasal vascular pedicle is ligated with 6–0 nylon at a point

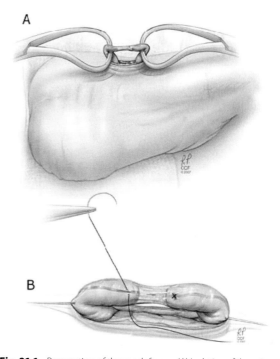

Fig. 21.1. Preparation of the vas deferens. (A) Isolation of the prior vasectomy site with delivery through the skin incision. (B) Vasal holding sutures with ligation of the vascular pedicle adjacent to intended anastomosis sites.

about 1 mm from the site of planned transection. A 6–0 nylon suture is placed in the periadventitial tissue at the base of each vas about 3 cm from the vasal end to act as a holding suture (Fig. 21.1B) to lift and maintain the vas ends above skin level. The vas is cut across in a perpendicular fashion proximal to the vasectomy site. The vas ends must be resected back to normal healthy tissue to minimize the chance of early postoperative stenosis. Fluid from the proximal vas is expressed and examined under high-power light microscopy. **While the presence of complete spermatozoa is associated with the best prognosis for future fertility, copious clear fluid without spermatozoa also portends a good outcome** [27].

Vasovasostomy may be performed using optical loupes or an operative microscope. Macrosurgical techniques which do not use any optical magnification have been described in the past. These procedures suffer from higher rates of failure and are now of a historic nature. Two of the most widely accepted techniques, the modified one-layer and the multilayer vasal anastomosis, will be described below. These methods have proved to be equally effective with regard to patency and pregnancy when performed by an experienced surgeon [27]. The one-layer anastomosis is useful when the vasovasostomy is to be performed in the straight portion of the vas deferens and there is minimal discrepancy in luminal size between the proximal and distal ends. The multilayer technique offers great precision in approximating the lumen of each end of the vas, particularly when there are widely discrepant luminal diameters.

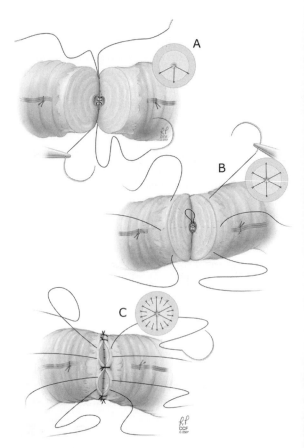

Fig. 21.2. Modified one-layer vasovasostomy. (A) Placement of three full-thickness 9–0 nylon sutures in the posterior aspect of the ends of the vas deferens. (B) Additional three full-thickness 9–0 nylon sutures in the anterior aspect. (C) Completion of the anastomosis with interrupted 9–0 nylon seromuscular sutures between the full-thickness stitches.

Modified one-layer vasovasostomy

First popularized by Schmidt [28], and later modified [27], this anastomosis can be performed under either loupe or microscopic magnification. The healthy vasal ends are prepared as described above and approximated in preparation for anastomosis. The distal lumen can be gently dilated with the tip of the jeweler's forceps to allow a more symmetric luminal diameter. Some surgeons place the ends of the vas in an approximating clamp to facilitate the anastomosis. It has been our practice to secure the 6–0 nylon vasal holding sutures to the operative drape in a fashion to allow performance of a tension-free anastomosis. Starting posteriorly, a 9–0 nylon suture is passed through the entire thickness of the vas deferens, puncturing in sequence the serosa of the proximal segment, though the muscularis and into the edge of the mucosa; then to the mucosa of the distal

end, muscularis, and out through the distal serosa. This suture is tied. Two additional full-thickness 9–0 nylon sutures are placed on each side of the 9–0 nylon suture (Fig. 21.2A). Three full-thickness 9–0 sutures are then placed in the anterior aspect and tied (Fig. 21.2B). The anastomosis is completed by placing 9–0 nylon seromuscular sutures between the previously placed full-thickness sutures (Fig. 21.2C).

Multilayer vasovasostomy

This technique is modified from the formal two-layer anastomosis, popularized and refined by Silber [29]. With this anastomosis, three separate layers are approximated: luminal, seromuscular, and periadventitial. The precision of this procedure necessitates the use of a microscope, and it should be performed by surgeons with the appropriate skill set. The vasal ends

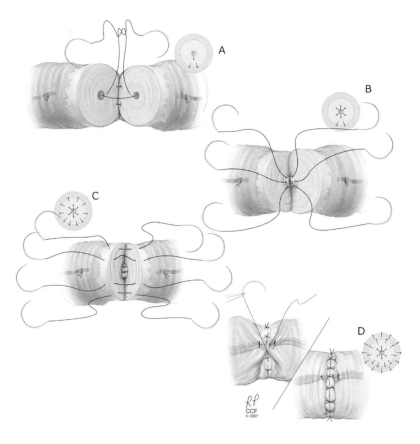

Fig. 21.3. Multilayer vasovasostomy (inset diagrams show inner and outer suture locations). (A) Two 9–0 nylon seromuscular sutures have been placed in 5 and 7 o'clock positions of vasal ends and tied. The first 10–0 nylon mucosal suture has been placed posteriorly. Note double-armed suture, which facilitates precise in-to-out placement of mucosal sutures. (B) Additional 10–0 nylon mucosal sutures placed in anterior aspect. (C) Anastomosis is completed with outer 9–0 nylon seromuscular sutures, with tied mucosal sutures visible deep to suture placement. (D) Third layer of 9–0 nylon suture is used to approximate the loose periadventitial layer adjacent to the vas ends.

are prepared in a similar fashion as described for the modified one-layer anastomosis. With two 9–0 nylon sutures, the posterior vasal ends are brought together at the 5 and 7 o'clock positions, incorporating only adventitia and muscularis (Fig. 21.3A). These sutures serve to stabilize the anastomosis in advance of placing the delicate luminal stitches. A double-armed 10–0 nylon suture is then passed inside to out through the mucosal edges of each vas end at the 6 o'clock position (Fig. 21.3A). This suture is tied, and six or seven additional 10–0 nylon luminal stitches are placed circumferentially (Fig. 21.3B). Because of the difference in luminal diameter between the dilated proximal vas lumen and the smaller distal vas lumen, sutures should be spaced to allow careful alignment of the lumen, avoiding bunching of the luminal edges. Suture ends should be cut closely to the knot to avoid protrusion of the suture tails into the seromuscular region. Once the luminal layer is completed, a 9–0 nylon is passed through the seromuscular tissue at the 12 o'clock position. Four additional equally spaced sutures of 9–0 nylon are placed on both sides of the 12 o'clock suture to complete the seromuscular layer (Fig. 21.3C). A

third layer of 9–0 nylon suture is used to approximate the loose periadventitial layer adjacent to the vas ends (Fig. 21.3D).

Other vasovasostomy anastomotic techniques

While the microsurgical anastomosis remains the gold standard, a variety of other anastomotic techniques have been utilized with varying degrees of success. These approaches seek to shorten operative time and reduce experience requirements for the surgeon while maintaining or improving upon surgical outcomes. In many respects, they reflect the prevailing trends in general urology today.

With the growing interest in robotic-assisted surgical procedures, it is not surprising that this technology has been applied to microsurgery. Motion downscaling software allows the surgeon to use both dominant and nondominant hands without discernible tremors. The da Vinci Surgical System (Intuitive Surgical, Mountain View, CA) was used in our laboratory for ex-vivo vasovasostomies with human vas deferens [30]. While the mean operative times were higher for the robotic-assisted anastomosis than for the microsurgical procedure in this small series, the time was decreasing with each successive procedure. Patency rates were comparable to those of the microsurgical anastomosis. Excellent patency rates were also noted in robotic-assisted vasovasostomies and vasoepididymostomies in the rat model [31]. Similar findings have been described with robotic-assisted ovarian tubal reanastomoses [32,33].

Research efforts have also focused on the development of methods to produce vasal anastomosis while minimizing suture placement. Fibrin glue has shown promise as a tissue adhesive in a variety of surgical applications, including reproductive microsurgery. Animal studies using fibrin glue sealant for vasovasostomies have consistently shown patency rates comparable to those of microsurgical anastomosis with reduced operative times [34–39]. Shekarriz *et al.* reported fibrin glue-assisted vasoepididymostomy in the rat model [40]. This technique allowed similar patency rates to standard end-to-side microsurgical anastomoses but with marked reduction in surgical times as compared to those with conventional reconstruction. Ho *et al.* reported the first series of patients receiving fibrin glue vasovasostomy [41]. In their small series, fibrin glue was applied as a sealant after placement of three transmural microsurgical anastomotic sutures. Patency and pregnancy rates were 86% and 52%, respectively, with mean operative times of 79 minutes. Similarly, small studies have utilized the carbon dioxide laser to successfully spot-weld the vasal anastomosis [42,43]. These techniques may offer some intraoperative time savings without compromising success rates. Only larger series and longer study duration can establish whether fibrin glue and laser welding will be enduring methods for vasal reconstruction.

Complex vasal reconstructions

Special approaches for reconstruction are indicated when the vasal obstruction is outside of the scrotum, or when a solitary functioning testis has an irreparable ductal system or no ductal system in conjunction with a poorly functioning contralateral testis that has normal ductal anatomy. Extrascrotal vasal obstruction is most commonly associated with vasal injury from hernia repairs occurring in infancy or early childhood. Recently, there have also been reports noting vasal obstruction from laparoscopic and open mesh herniorrhaphies in adults [44]. Pediatric surgical injuries are not usually noticed at the time of injury but diagnosed

decades later when the patient reaches reproductive age. **As many as 27% of subfertile male patients with a history of childhood inguinal hernia repair have unilateral vas deferens obstruction from injury** [45]. If only one vas is obstructed and the contralateral testis and vas are functioning normally, the patient's fertility may be unimpaired and the obstruction never diagnosed. If there are bilateral injuries to the vas or a hypofunctioning contralateral testis, repair of the vas deferens in the inguinal canal or retroperitoneum is indicated. If this repair cannot be performed, because of absence of or severe damage to the vas, consideration should be given to performing a crossover procedure to utilize a contralateral normal ductal system to drain the obstructed testis.

Occult vasal injury is suggested by a history of pediatric inguinal or retroperitoneal surgery in conjunction with a normal-sized testis and a distended or indurated epididymis. The scrotal vas deferens may feel normal or thickened. At the time of surgical correction, a testis biopsy is indicated to confirm active spermatogenesis in the normal-size testis. A vasogram will demonstrate a dilated vas lumen ending blindly at the level of the internal ring or in the retroperitoneum (Fig. 21.4). To locate the proximal end of the vas deferens, an incision should be made parallel to the inguinal canal and over the area of the internal ring. On occasion, if the vasal obstruction is over the lower area of the inguinal canal, such as at the level of the external ring, the scrotal incision used for the biopsy can be extended up over the external ring to allow repair. The proximal end of the vas can be isolated and a 6–0 nylon holding suture placed in the seromuscular layer to allow easy identification of the lower portion of the vas. Usually, a fibrous band extends from the end of the vas, and, if followed carefully, this will lead to the abdominal end of the vas deferens. Care must be taken to avoid disrupting this band, since it can be very difficult to find the proximal end of the vas if the "trail" is interrupted. Once the distal and proximal vasal ends have been mobilized with their vascular pedicles, the ends are brought to the skin level for a single or multilayer vasovasostomy. Prior to this procedure, fluid from the testicular end of the vas deferens is examined for sperm. As with vasectomy reversal patients, there may be secondary epididymal obstructions. If no sperm are seen, the inguinal vasovasostomy can still be performed, with the understanding that the patient may require a subsequent vasoepididymostomy in 3–6 months if he has persistent azoospermia. Inguinal vasovasostomies are

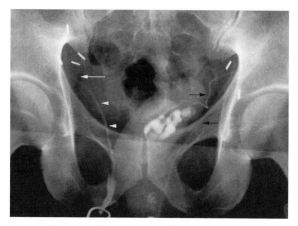

Fig. 21.4. Right vasogram with internal ring obstruction from prior herniorraphy. Note normal contralateral vasogram.

challenging surgical procedures, largely because of the dense fibrotic reaction that may encase the vasal ends, making it difficult to mobilize an adequate vasal length. One group utilizes laparoscopic mobilization of the vas deferens to facilitate the inguinal anastomosis [46]. **Inguinal reconstructions can have patency and pregnancy rates that are comparable to those with scrotal vasovasostomies** [47].

Alternatively, the patient can be evaluated for a crossover procedure if the contralateral vas deferens is normal but the contralateral testis is atrophic. Although this combination of circumstances is not common, one review noted these findings at scrotal exploration in 6% of azoospermic patients [48]. The normal vas deferens can be mobilized with its vascular pedicle and tunneled through the scrotal septum to anastomose either with the vas deferens, if present, or directly to the epididymis. Contemporary series of crossover vasovasostomies have reported moderate success for the management of complex obstructions [49,50]. The authors reported their early series of crossover vasoepididymostomies, and noted mean sperm concentrations over 15 million/mL in 89% of patients [51].

Patients who previously have had an unsuccessful vasectomy reversal present a special challenge for surgical reconstruction. These patients often have a marked vasal desmoplastic reaction as well as a shorter length of usable vas deferens. The vas may need to be mobilized by extending the scrotal incision onto the lower inguinal region to facilitate dissection of the vas up to the inguinal canal. This can create 3–4 cm of additional vasal length and avoid the creation of a high-riding testicle due to the short vasal length. In addition,

these patients have a very high likelihood of a secondary epididymal obstruction. In our series of repeat vasectomy reversals, 73% of the patients required a vasoepididymostomy on at least one side [8], versus only 4% in initial reconstructions [27].

Vasovasostomy results

While there is a plethora of series reviewing vasovasostomy success rates, it is difficult to compare the surgical outcomes because of a lack of standardized obstructive intervals, coexisting female-factor infertility, and differences in surgical algorithms in the choice of vasovasostomy and vasoepididymostomy. **Microsurgical vasovasostomy with either a single-layer or multilayer technique produces superior results with regard to both patency and pregnancy when compared with surgery done without magnification** (Table 21.1) [27,29,52–56].

A variety of preoperative and intraoperative factors have been identified that can affect the success rates for vasovasostomy [57]. In a large multicenter review of vasectomy reversal procedures, Belker *et al.* related the time of obstruction to the success of the surgery (Table 21.2) [27]. These results were confirmed by a Cox regression analysis of 1902 vasovasostomies, which demonstrated that when more than nine years had elapsed since a vasectomy the chance of a successful reversal decreased to less than 60% of the success rates achieved when reconstruction took place within three years after vasectomy [58]. A history of a prior unsuccessful vasectomy reversal was not a negative predictor for repeat procedure success. Pregnancy and patency rates were comparable to those with initial reconstruction series when examined at equivalent intervals of obstruction [59].

The partner's age is an additional factor that affects the eventual success of vasectomy reversal. Fuchs and Burt reported that the pregnancy rate was 64% in partners who were less than 30 years of age and dropped progressively to 28% in women aged 40 or older [24]. The overall pregnancy rates seemed to favor vasectomy reversal over intracytoplasmic sperm injection until spouses were over age 35, when both techniques were associated with dropping success rates. Kolettis *et al.* reported similar pregnancy rates for vasectomy reversal in a study of couples with spouses age 35 or older [60]. Others have found good pregnancy rates until spousal age reaches 40 years old [61].

Intraoperatively, vasal fluid quality is a predictor of eventual outcome. **When clear fluid with motile sperm**

Table 21.1. Vasovasostomy series

Author	Year	Microsurgery	Patients (n)	Patency (%)	Pregnancy (%)
Derrick [52] [a]	1973	No	1600	38	19
Silber [29]	1977	Yes	126	90	76
Lee [53]	1980	No	41	90	46
		Yes	26	96	54
Soonawala [54]	1984	No	194	81	44
		Yes	339	89	63
Belker [27]	1991	Yes	1247	86	52
Kabalin [55]	1991	No	111	79	36
Fox [56]	1994	Yes	103	84	48

[a] Survey of practicing urologists

Table 21.2. Obstructive interval vs. outcomes [27]

Obstructive interval (years)	Patency (%)	Pregnancy (%)
< 3	97	76
3–8	88	53
9–14	79	44
≥ 15	71	30

was noted at the time of surgery, 94% of patients had a return of sperm to their ejaculate, as opposed to only 60% when no sperm were noted in the vasal fluid [27]. When sperm were absent from the intraoperative vasal fluid, patency and pregnancy results correlated with characteristics of vasal fluid with copious clear fluid portending the best outcomes. The absence of fluid or a thick, inspissated fluid suggests an epididymal obstruction, and a vasoepididymostomy should be considered.

Vasoepididymostomy reconstructive techniques

Once the vasa are proved patent and the testis shown to be actively producing sperm by biopsy, the blockage must lie somewhere in between these structures. Obstruction at the rete testis or the efferent ducts ("empty epididymis syndrome") is uncommon. In most, the obstruction will be found within the epididymis and therefore is potentially correctable. After delivery of the testis and epididymis through a vertical scrotal incision, the epididymis is examined, and often the site of obstruction is readily apparent because of a sudden change in caliber of the tubule from distended to flat. Sometimes, the area of obstruction is demarcated by a blue-brown discoloration just beneath the epididymal tunic. This lipofuchsin stain represents sperm extravasation and breakdown near the site of obstruction. Ultimately, the area of obstruction must be confirmed by examination of the fluid within the epididymal tubule. Beginning in the tail of the epididymis, exploration is carried out systematically, moving proximal until normal-appearing motile or nonmotile sperm are found. To do this, a 1 cm incision is made in the epididymal tunic using curved microscissors. This window allows exposure of multiple epididymal tubule loops (Fig. 21.6A). A single loop is identified and carefully isolated from the surrounding tubules. The method of opening the tubule is determined by the choice of anastomotic technique, as will be described below.

A variety of methods for anastomosing the vas deferens to the epididymis have been described [62]. The original technique involved the creation of a fistulous communication between multiple incised epididymal loops and the opened lumen of the vas deferens. Patency and pregnancy rates were low by contemporary standards [48, 63,64], and this procedure has largely been abandoned. Lespinasse modified this technique and attempted to create a precise epididymal tubule-to-vas anastomosis [65]. Without the aid of magnification, he exposed loops of epididymal tubule and passed a fine suture through a single loop which he brought through the mucosal surface of the vas. The suture was brought out through the skin, and removed at a later time when it had eroded the epididymal tubule into the vas.

The next major advance was described by Silber in 1978 [66]. He reported his technique of end-to-end single tubule anastomosis, representing the first true microsurgical approach to vasoepididymal reconstruction. With this method, the end of the epididymis was serially cut off until reaching a point just above the obstruction identified by free flow of sperm-containing

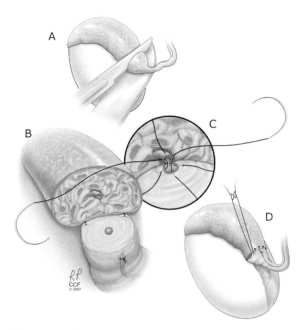

Fig. 21.5. End-to-end vasoepididymostomy. (A) Epididymis is serially transected starting distally until a sperm-laden tubule is identified. (B) Two 9–0 nylon sutures are placed in the 5 and 7 o'clock positions to approximate the seromuscular wall of the end of the vas with the cut edge of the epididymal tunic. (C) Four 10–0 nylon double-armed sutures are placed in quadrant fashion between the epididymal and vasal mucosa. (D) Anastomosis is completed with additional 9–0 nylon sutures between the epididymal tunic and the seromuscular wall of the vas deferens.

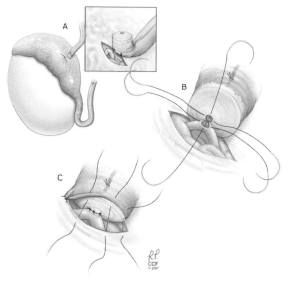

Fig. 21.6. End-to-side vasoepididymostomy. (A) Epididymal tunic is incised, exposing a loop of epididymal tubule. Inset: Epididymal tubule is opened along dotted line in figure. Seromuscular wall of the vas deferens is secured to the cut edge of the epididymal tunic with two 9–0 nylon sutures placed in the 5 and 7 o'clock positions. (B) Quadrant double-armed 10–0 nylon sutures are placed in an in-to-out fashion in the epididymal and vasal mucosa. (C) After the inner 10–0 sutures are tied, 9–0 nylon interrupted sutures are used to approximate the epididymal tunic to the seromuscular layer of the vas.

fluid from a single cut tubule (Fig. 21.5A). The cut end of the distal vas was then brought into opposition with the portion of the cut tubule exuding sperm, and two 9–0 nylon sutures were placed at the 5 and 7 o'clock positions of the seromuscular surface of the vas, to secure the cut end of the distal vas to the epididymal tunica (Fig. 21.5B). Next, four double-armed 10–0 nylon sutures were placed in a quadrant fashion between the mucosa of the vas and the epididymal tubule (Fig. 21.5C). These sutures were not tied until all had been positioned. Finally, the seromuscular vasal layer was approximated to the epididymal tunic layer with several interrupted 9–0 nylon sutures (Fig. 21.5D).

Others described a modification to this technique using an end-to-side anastomosis [67,68]. This circumvented some of the problems with the end-to-end technique since it did not require resection of the epididymis while facilitating identification of the patent epididymal tubule and minimizing bleeding. Instead of completely transecting the epididymis, a microknife is used to make a 0.5–1 mm incision in the side of a single epididymal tubule. With the tubule opened and sperm

presence confirmed, a single 10–0 nylon suture is placed outside-in at the lateral border of the cut mucosal edge. This acts as an identification suture for use later with the anastomosis. The vas is secured to the epididymal tunic with two 9–0 nylon sutures at the 5 and 7 o'clock positions (Fig. 21.6A). Next, three or four double-armed 10–0 nylon sutures are placed in a quadrant fashion through the edge of the epididymal tubule (Fig. 21.6B). The sutures are placed in the corresponding quadrant of the vasal mucosa and tied. The anastomosis is completed with additional 9–0 nylon sutures between the epididymal tunic and the seromuscular layer of the vas deferens (Fig. 21.6C). Finally, several 9–0 nylon sutures are used to anchor the vas deferens to the parietal layer of the tunica vaginalis. These final sutures serve to prevent direct tension on the anastomosis, and are placed well away from the vasoepididymostomy site.

Most recently, intussusception vasoepididymostomy, first described by Berger [69], with several subsequent modifications by others [70,71], has been gaining popularity. The intent of this technique is to allow the precision of the standard end-to-side anastomosis

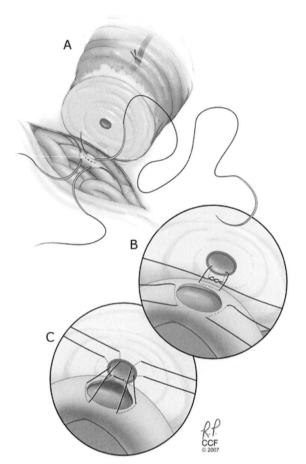

Fig. 21.7. Intussusception end-to-side vasoepidymostomy. (A) Three double-armed 10–0 nylon sutures are placed in a triangulated fashion in the epididymal loop. The needles are left in place until all have been placed to avoid decompressing the tubule, which could make suture placement more difficult. Tubule is incised along dotted line after suture placement. (B) Ends of the sutures are placed in-to-out in the vasal mucosa. (C) Sutures are tied to allow intussusception of the epididymal tubule into the vas lumen.

while simplifying and minimizing the microsuture placement. It differs from the end-to-side technique in that the lumen is opened after the sutures are positioned in the epididymal tubule and, once opened, the loop is drawn into the vasal lumen with the sutures rather than approximated to it. As with the end-to-side anastomosis, a small window is created in the epididymal tunic to allow extrusion of dilated epididymal loops. An appropriate loop is chosen and freed with sharp dissection from surrounding loops so that it can easily be pulled into the vasal lumen without tension. The end of the vas deferens is secured to the opened tunic with two 9–0 nylon sutures, as was performed with the

end-to-side anastomosis. Three double-armed 10–0 nylon sutures are placed in a triangular configuration in the desired epididymal loop (Fig. 21.7A). The epididymal tubule is carefully opened between the positioned sutures. Once sperm is confirmed in the epididymal fluid, the needles are passed through the corresponding areas of the lumen of the vas in an inside-out fashion. The sutures are then tied, creating an invagination of the epididymal loop into the vasal lumen (Fig. 21.7B,C). Finally, additional 9–0 nylon sutures are placed to approximate the seromuscular layer of the vas to the epididymal tunic.

Vasoepididymostomy results

Vasoepididymostomy results vary significantly, depending on the experience level of the surgeon, the level of the epididymal obstruction, and the reproductive capacity of the partner. Table 21.3 summarizes the contemporary patency and pregnancy rates for vasoepididymal anastomoses [63,69,70,72–75]. **Unlike vasovasostomies, which may demonstrate patency within weeks of surgery, vasoepididymostomy patients may only begin to have sperm in their ejaculate 3–6 months after surgery, and even longer in some cases.** For this reason, vasoepididymal anastomoses are not judged to be technical failures until at least 12 months have elapsed [62,76].

Tricks of the trade

Several additional techniques are worthy of special emphasis. One of the biggest challenges facing the surgeon who undertakes vasoepididymostomies or redo reconstructions is to obtain adequate vasal length to ensure a tension-free anastomosis. To obtain this length, the vas is placed on mild traction using the 6–0 Prolene seromuscular holding suture. This allows the loose tissue to be separated from the vas and small vessels cauterized with a bipolar or thermal cautery unit while preserving the vascular pedicle associated with the vas. The incision can be extended cephalad to the level of the pubic tubercle, allowing further exposure of the vas. Additional mobility can be obtained by pushing away the adherent tissue using a small blunt periosteal elevator or Kitner retractor. If necessary, the incision can be extended to the internal inguinal ring and the external oblique fascia incised to allow additional mobility. On the other end, the tail and proximal epididymis can also be freed to gain additional length. This maneuver requires great care to avoid devascularization of the epididymis but can provide an additional centimeter or so of length for the difficult vasoepididymal anastomosis.

Table 21.3. Vasoepididymostomy outcomes

Author	Year	Patients (n)	Anastomosis	Patency (%)	Pregnancy (%)
Dubin [63]	1985	46	End-to-end	39	13
Silber [72]	1989	139	End-to-end	78	56
Dewire [73]	1995	137	End-to-side	79	50
Berger [69]	1998	12	Intussusception	92	Not reported
Marmar [70]	2000	9	Intussusception	78	22
Chan [74]	2005	68	Intussusception	84	40
Schiff [75] [a]	2005	153	End-to-end	73	20
			End-to-side	74	40
			3-suture intuss	84	46
			2-suture intuss	80	44

[a] $P < 0.05$ comparing patency rates between intussusception techniques and end-to-end or end-to-side vasoepididymostomies. No statistically significant differences in pregnancy rates between techniques.

Extensive scrotal reconstructions, especially repeat procedures, potentially can injure the testicular blood supply and possibly result in testicular atrophy. Fortunately, this is a rare complication, but it is more likely if there has been a compromise of the vasculature from previous scrotal surgery, varicocele ligation, or hernia repair. In this setting, we use a Doppler ultrasonic probe (VTI Surgical Doppler ref. #108100 and a disposable neurosurgical Doppler probe, manufactured by Vascular Technology, Inc, Lowell, MA) to identify the arterial supply and facilitate extensive dissections.

Microsurgery in the era of assisted reproduction

An analysis of microsurgical reconstruction would not be complete unless placed in the context of developments in assisted reproductive technologies. Palermo *et al.* reported the first pregnancies from intracytoplasmic sperm injection in 1992 [77], and its use has revolutionized the management of some causes of male infertility. The success of the technique has driven some to suggest it for treatment of all causes of infertility, regardless of etiology. However, to do so would overlook a variety of safety issues related to ovulation induction, including ovarian hyperstimulation, which, while fortunately rare, can be a life-threatening complication [78,79]. A safety issue of more significance relates to the high incidence of multiple births, with the associated costs and complications of these pregnancies, as up to 40% of these pregnancies are twins, triplets, or even higher order [82]. While there does not appear to be a significant increase in the major chromosomal malformation

rate, there remain troubling reports concerning a higher incidence of minor malformations in the children resulting from intracytoplasmic sperm injection [81–87]. It remains to be seen if this elevated risk is related to the treatment itself, or to underlying genetic issues in the patients choosing assisted reproduction. Additionally, economic analyses strongly favor the use of microsurgical reconstructions over intracytoplasmic sperm injection for the treatment of the majority of patients with obstructive azoospermia [88,89].

Summary

Exciting advances in microsurgical technique, optical magnification, and surgical equipment have allowed the restoration of genital tract patency in patients with excurrent ductal obstruction. Ultimately, outcomes remain dependent on the surgeons' experience with their chosen techniques. Regardless of the surgical anastomosis method used, the surgeon who undertakes vasectomy reversal must be prepared for and facile with vasoepididymostomy techniques, since there is a significant likelihood this will be routinely called for in these patients.

References

[1] Martin E, Benton Carnett J, Valentine Levi J, *et al.* The surgical treatment of sterility due to obstruction at the epididymis together with a study of the morphology of human sperm. *Univ Penn Med Bull* 1902; **15**: 1.

[2] Hagner F. The operative treatment of sterility in the male. *JAMA* 1936; **107**: 1851–5.

[3] Hinrichsen MJ, Blaquier JA. Evidence supporting the existence of sperm maturation in the human epididymis. *J Reprod Fertil* 1980; **60**: 291–4.

[4] Lacham O, Trounson A. Fertilizing capacity of epididymal and testicular spermatozoa microinjected under the zona pellucida of the mouse oocyte. *Mol Reprod Dev* 1991; **29**: 85–93.

[5] Silber SJ. Apparent fertility of human spermatozoa from the caput epididymidis. *J Androl* 1989; **10**: 263–9.

[6] Schlegel PN, Goldstein M. Microsurgical vasoepididymostomy: refinements and results. *J Urol* 1993; **150**: 1165–8.

[7] Hopps CV, Goldstein M. Microsurgical reconstruction of iatrogenic injuries to the epididymis from hydrocelectomy. *J Urol* 2006; **176**: 2077–9.

[8] Hernandez J, Sabanegh ES. Repeat vasectomy reversal after initial failure: overall results and predictors for success. *J Urol* 1999; **161**: 1153–6.

[9] Tung KS. Allergic orchitis lesions are adoptively transferred from vasoligated guinea pigs to syngeneic recipients. *Science* 1978; **201**: 833–5.

[10] Tung KS, Alexander NJ. Immunopathologic studies on vasectomized guinea pigs. *Biol Reprod* 1977; **17**: 241–54.

[11] Bigazzi PE, Kosuda LL, Hsu KC, Andres GA. Immune complex orchitis in vasectomized rabbits. *J Exp Med* 1976; **143**: 382–404.

[12] Tung KS, Alexander NJ. Monocytic orchitis and aspermatogenesis in normal and vasectomized rhesus macaques (Macaca mulatta). *Am J Pathol* 1980; **101**: 17–29.

[13] Hadley MA, Dym M. Spermatogenesis in the vasectomized monkey: quantitative analysis. *Anat Rec* 1983; **205**: 381–6.

[14] Heidger PM, Roberts JA, Chapman ES, *et al*. Vasectomy in rhesus monkeys. III. Light microscopic studies of testicular morphology. *Urology* 1978; **11**: 148–52.

[15] West DA, Chehval MJ, Winkelmann T, Martin SA. Effect of vasovasostomy on contralateral testicular damage associated with unilateral vasectomy in mature and immature Lewis rats. *Fertil Steril* 2000; **73**: 238–41.

[16] Shiraishi K, Naito K, Yoshida K. Vasectomy impairs spermatogenesis through germ cell apoptosis mediated by p53-Bax pathway in rat. *J Urol* 2001; **166**: 1565–71.

[17] Kubota R. Electron microscopic studies on the testis after vasectomy in rats and men. *Jpn J Urol* 1969; **60**: 373–97.

[18] Bigazzi PE, Alexander NJ, Silber SJ. Studies on testicular biopsies from vasectomized men. In: Lepow IH, Crozier R, eds. *Vasectomy: Immunologic and Pathologic Effects in Animals and Man*. New York, NY: Academic Press, 1979.

[19] McVicar CM, O'Neill DA, McClure N, *et al*. Effects of vasectomy on spermatogenesis and fertility outcome after testicular sperm extraction combined with ICSI. *Hum Reprod* 2005; **20**: 2795–800.

[20] Hagedoorn JP, Davis JE. Fine structure of seminiferous tubules after vasectomy in man. *Pathologist* 1974; **17**: 236–42.

[21] Jarow JP, Budin RE, Dym M, *et al*. Quantitative pathologic changes in the human testis after vasectomy: a controlled study. *N Engl J Med* 1985; **313**: 1252–6.

[22] Shiraishi K, Takihara H, Naito K. Influence of interstitial fibrosis on spermatogenesis after vasectomy and vasovasostomy. *Contraception* 2002; **65**: 245–9.

[23] Samli H, Samli MM, Yilmaz E, Imirzalioglu N. Clinical, andrological and genetic characteristics of patients with congenital bilateral absence of vas deferens (CBAVD). *Arch Androl* 2006; **52**: 471–7.

[24] Fuchs EF, Burt RA. Vasectomy reversal performed 15 years or more after vasectomy: correlation of pregnancy outcome with partner age and with pregnancy results of in vitro fertilization with intracytoplasmic sperm injection. *Fertil Steril* 2002; **77**: 516–19.

[25] Parekattil SJ, Kuang W, Agarwal A, Thomas AJ. Model to predict if a vasoepididymostomy will be required for vasectomy reversal. *J Urol* 2005; **173**: 1681–4.

[26] Parekattil SJ, Kuang W, Kolettis PN, *et al*. Multi-institutional validation of vasectomy reversal predictor. *J Urol* 2006; **175**: 247–9.

[27] Belker AM, Thomas AJ, Fuchs EF, Konnak JW, Sharlip ID. Results of 1,469 microsurgical vasectomy reversals by the Vasovasostomy Study Group. *J Urol* 1991; **145**: 505–11.

[28] Schmidt SS. Vasovasostomy. *Urol Clin North Am* 1978; **5**: 585–92.

[29] Silber SJ. Microscopic vasectomy reversal. *Fertil Steril* 1977; **28**: 1191–202.

[30] Kuang W, Shin PR, Matin S, Thomas AJ. Initial evaluation of robotic technology for microsurgical vasovasostomy. *J Urol* 2004; **171**: 300–3.

[31] Schiff J, Li PS, Goldstein M. Robotic microsurgical vasovasostomy and vasoepididymostomy: a prospective randomized study in a rat model. *J Urol* 2004; **171**: 1720–5.

[32] Degueldre M, Vandromme J, Huong PT, Cadière GB. Robotically assisted laparoscopic microsurgical tubal reanastomosis: a feasibility study. *Fertil Steril* 2000; **74**: 1020–3.

[33] Falcone T, Goldberg JM, Margossian H, Stevens L. Robotic-assisted laparoscopic microsurgical tubal anastomosis: a human pilot study. *Fertil Steril* 2000; **73**: 1040–2.

[34] Bach D, Distelmaier W, Weissbach L. Animal experiments on reanastomosis of the vas deferens using fibrin glue. *Urol Res* 1980; **8**: 29–36.

[35] Silverstein JI, Mellinger BC. Fibrin glue vasal anastomosis compared to conventional sutured vasovasostomy in the rat. *J Urol* 1991; **145**: 1288–91.

[36] Weiss JN, Mellinger BC. Fertility rates with delayed fibrin glue: vasovasostomy in rats. *Fertil Steril* 1992; **57**: 908–11.

[37] Ball RA, Steinberg J, Wilson LA, Loughlin KR. Comparison of vasovasostomy techniques in rats utilizing conventional microsurgical suture, carbon dioxide laser, and fibrin tissue adhesives. *Urology* 1993; **41**: 479–83.

[38] Niederberger C, Ross LS, Mackenzie B, Schacht MJ, Cho Y. Vasovasostomy in rabbits using fibrin adhesive prepared from a single human source. *J Urol* 1993; **149**: 183–5.

[39] Shekarriz M, Pomer S, Staehler G. Fibrin-glue vasovasostomy as an alternative to the conventional two-layer suture technique? *Investig Urol (Berl)* 1994; **5**: 253–5.

[40] Shekarriz BM, Thomas AJ, Sabanegh E, Kononov A, Levin HS. Fibrin-glue assisted vasoepididymostomy: a comparison to standard end-to-side microsurgical vasoepididymostomy in the rat model. *J Urol* 1997; **158**: 1602–5.

[41] Ho KL, Witte MN, Bird ET, Hakim S. Fibrin glue assisted 3-suture vasovasostomy. *J Urol* 2005; **174**: 1360–3.

[42] Alefelder J, Philipp J, Engelmann UH, Senge T. Stented laser-welded vasovasostomy in the rat: Comparison of Nd: YAG and CO2 lasers. *J Reconstr Microsurg* 1991; **7**: 317–20.

[43] Rosemberg SK. Further clinical experience with CO2 laser in microsurgical vasovasostomy. *Urology* 1988; **32**: 225–7.

[44] Shin D, Lipshultz LI, Goldstein M, *et al.* Herniorrhaphy with polypropylene mesh causing inguinal vasal obstruction: a preventable cause of obstructive azoospermia. *Ann Surg* 2005; **241**: 553–8.

[45] Matsuda T, Horii Y, Yoshida O. Unilateral obstruction of the vas deferens caused by childhood inguinal herniorrhaphy in male infertility patients. *Fertil Steril* 1992; **58**: 609–13.

[46] Kim A, Shin D, Martin TV, Honig SC. Laparoscopic mobilization of the retroperitoneal vas deferens for microscopic inguinal vasovasostomy. *J Urol* 2004; **172**: 1948–9.

[47] Matsuda T, Muguruma K, Hiura Y, *et al.* Seminal tract obstruction caused by childhood inguinal herniorrhaphy: results of microsurgical reanastomosis. *J Urol* 1998; **159**: 837–40.

[48] Hendry WF, Parslow JM, Stedronska J. Exploratory scrototomy in 168 azoospermic males. *Br J Urol* 1983; **55**: 785–91.

[49] Lizza EF, Marmar JL, Schmidt SS, *et al.* Transseptal crossed vasovasostomy. *J Urol* 1985; **134**: 1131–2.

[50] Hamidinia A. Transvasovasostomy: an alternative operation for obstructive azoospermia. *J Urol* 1988; **140**: 1545–8.

[51] Sabanegh E, Thomas AJ. Effectiveness of crossover transseptal vasoepididymostomy in treating complex obstructive azoospermia. *Fertil Steril* 1995; **63**: 392–5.

[52] Derrick FC, Yarbrough W, D'Agostino J. Vasovasostomy: results of questionnaire of members of the American Urological Association. *J Urol* 1973; **110**: 556–7.

[53] Lee L, McLoughlin MG. Vasovasostomy: a comparison of macroscopic and microscopic techniques at one institution. *Fertil Steril* 1980; **33**: 54–5.

[54] Soonawala F, Lal S. Microsurgery in vasovasostomy. *Indian J Urol* 1984; **1**: 104–9.

[55] Kabalin JN, Kessler R. Macroscopic vasovasostomy re-examined. *Urology* 1991; **38**: 135–8.

[56] Fox M. Vasectomy reversal: microsurgery for best results. *Br J Urol* 1994; **73**: 449–53.

[57] Nagler HM, Rotman M. Predictive parameters for microsurgical reconstruction. *Urol Clin North Am* 2002; **29**: 913–19.

[58] Holman CD, Wisniewski ZS, Semmens JB, Rouse IL, Bass AJ. Population-based outcomes after 28,246 in-hospital vasectomies and 1,902 vasovasostomies in Western Australia. *BJU Int* 2000; **86**: 1043–9.

[59] Hernandez J, Sabanegh ES. Repeat vasectomy reversal after initial failure: Overall results and predictors for success. *J Urol* 1999; **161**: 1153–6.

[60] Kolettis PN, Sabanegh ES, Nalesnik JG, *et al.* Pregnancy outcomes after vasectomy reversal for female partners 35 years old or older. *J Urol* 2003; **169**: 2250–2.

[61] Gerrard ER, Sandlow JI, Oster RA, *et al.* Effect of female partner age on pregnancy rates after vasectomy reversal. *Fertil Steril* 2007; **87**: 1340–4.

[62] Schoysman R. Vaso-epididymostomy: a survey of techniques and results with considerations of delay of appearance of spermatozoa after surgery. *Acta Eur Fertil* 1990; **21**: 239–45.

[63] Dubin L, Amelar RD. Magnified surgery for epididymovasostomy. *Urology* 1984; **23**: 525–8.

[64] Schoysman RJ, Bedford JM. The role of the human epididymis in sperm maturation and sperm storage as reflected in the consequences of epididymovasostomy. *Fertil Steril* 1986; **46**: 293–9.

[65] Lespinasse V. Obstructive sterility in the male: treatment by direct vaso-epididymostomy. *JAMA* 1918; **70**: 448–50.

[66] Silber SJ. Microscopic vasoepididymostomy: specific microanastomosis to the epididymal tubule. *Fertil Steril* 1978; **30**: 565–71.

[67] Fogdestam I, Fall M, Nilsson S. Microsurgical epididymovasostomy in the treatment of occlusive azoospermia. *Fertil Steril* 1986; **46**: 925–9.

[68] Thomas AJ. Vasoepididymostomy. *Urol Clin North Am* 1987; **14**: 527–38.

[69] Berger RE. Triangulation end-to-side vasoepididymostomy. *J Urol* 1998; **159**: 1951–3.

[70] Marmar JL. Modified vasoepididymostomy with simultaneous double needle placement, tubulotomy and tubular invagination. *J Urol* 2000; **163**: 483–6.

[71] Chan PT, Li PS, Goldstein M. Microsurgical vasoepididymostomy: a prospective randomized study of 3 intussusception techniques in rats. *J Urol* 2003; **169**: 1924–9.

[72] Silber SJ. Results of microsurgical vasoepididymostomy: role of epididymis in sperm maturation. *Hum Reprod* 1989; **4**: 298–303.

[73] Dewire D, Thomas A. Microsurgical end-to-side vasoepididymostomy. In: Goldstein M, ed. *Surgery of Male Fertility*. Philadelphia, PA: Saunders, 1995: 128–34.

[74] Chan PT, Brandell RA, Goldstein M. Prospective analysis of outcomes after microsurgical intussusception vasoepididymostomy. *BJU Int* 2005; **96**: 598–601.

[75] Schiff J, Chan P, Li PS, Finkelberg S, Goldstein M. Outcome and late failures compared in 4 techniques of microsurgical vasoepididymostomy in 153 consecutive men. *J Urol* 2005; **174**: 651–5.

[76] Jarow JP, Sigman M, Buch JP, Oates RD. Delayed appearance of sperm after end-to-side vasoepididymostomy. *J Urol* 1995; **153**: 1156–8.

[77] Palermo G, Joris H, Devroey P, Van Steirteghem AC. Pregnancies after intracytoplasmic injection of single spermatozoon into an oocyte. *Lancet* 1992; **340**: 17–18.

[78] Schenker JG, Ezra Y. Complications of assisted reproductive techniques. *Fertil Steril* 1994; **61**: 411–22.

[79] Lenton E, Soltan A, Hewitt J, *et al.* Induction of ovulation in women undergoing assisted reproductive techniques: recombinant human FSH (follitropin alpha) versus highly purified urinary FSH (urofollitropin HP). *Hum Reprod* 2000; **15**: 1021–7.

[80] Goldfarb JM, Austin C, Lisbona H, Peskin B, Clapp M. Cost-effectiveness of in vitro fertilization. *Obstet Gynecol* 1996; **87**: 18–21.

[81] Van Steirteghem A, Tournaye H, Van der Elst J, *et al.* Intracytoplasmic sperm injection three years after the birth of the first ICSI child. *Hum Reprod* 1995; **10**: 2527–8.

[82] De Jonge CJ, Pierce J. Intracytoplasmic sperm injection: what kind of reproduction is being assisted? *Hum Reprod* 1995; **10**: 2518–20.

[83] Patrizio P. Intracytoplasmic sperm injection (ICSI): potential genetic concerns. *Hum Reprod* 1995; **10**: 2520–3.

[84] Hansen M, Kurinczuk JJ, Bower C, Webb S. The risk of major birth defects after intracytoplasmic sperm injection and in vitro fertilization. *N Engl J Med* 2002; **346**: 725–30.

[85] Olson CK, Keppler-Noreuil KM, Romitti PA, *et al.* In vitro fertilization is associated with an increase in major birth defects. *Fertil Steril* 2005; **84**: 1308–15.

[86] Sanchez-Albisua I, Borell-Kost S, Mau-Holzmann UA, Licht P, Krägeloh-Mann I. Increased frequency of severe major anomalies in children conceived by intracytoplasmic sperm injection. *Dev Med Child Neurol* 2007; **49**: 129–34.

[87] Schieve LA, Rasmussen SA, Buck GM, *et al.* Are children born after assisted reproductive technology at increased risk for adverse health outcomes? *Obstet Gynecol* 2004; **103**: 1154–63.

[88] Kolettis PN, Thomas AJ. Vasoepididymostomy for vasectomy reversal: a critical assessment in the era of intracytoplasmic sperm injection. *J Urol* 1997; **158**: 467–70.

[89] Meng MV, Greene KL, Turek PJ. Surgery or assisted reproduction? A decision analysis of treatment costs in male infertility. *J Urol* 2005; **174**: 1926–31.

Chapter 22

Techniques of sperm retrieval

Edward Karpman and Daniel H. Williams IV

Introduction

The development of in-vitro fertilization using intracy-toplasmic sperm injection (IVF/ICSI) in 1992 revolutionized the management of male infertility. After the successful use of this combination, testicular biopsy became not only a diagnostic procedure to measure the degree of spermatogenesis, but also a therapeutic technique to retrieve sperm for IVF/ICSI. Earlier attempts to utilize testicular or epididymal sperm with conventional IVF had met with disappointing results, and couples were left with limited options of using donor sperm and artificial insemination or adoption.

Along with this new technology of IVF/ICSI came a need for simplified but more sophisticated sperm retrieval techniques. The demand for less invasive ways to retrieve sperm in patients with abundant sperm production (e.g., congenital absence of the vas deferens, reproductive tract obstruction) encouraged the development of minimally invasive surgical approaches such as percutaneous epididymal sperm aspiration and testis sperm aspiration or extraction. The ability of IVF/ICSI to overcome even the most difficult cases of male-factor infertility, such as nonobstructive azoospermia, led to the development of more sophisticated sperm retrieval techniques such as microdissection testicular sperm extraction in those patients with severely impaired spermatogenesis. The literature is replete with variations on these techniques for surgical sperm retrieval, and they allow reproductive urologists to choose for their patients the approach that will yield the greatest number of high-quality sperm while minimizing damage to the reproductive tract.

After establishing IVF/ICSI as a powerful tool for the treatment of male-factor infertility, many IVF centers began focusing on refining their technique in order to optimize outcomes for their patients. Additional pressure to produce high-quality results came about after the establishment in 1985 of mandatory reporting

of IVF success rates by individual centers in the USA to the Society for Assisted Reproductive Technology. This mandatory reporting is available for public scrutiny, and concern for market pressures has driven IVF centers to critically evaluate their own success rates. Optimizing IVF/ICSI success rates meant evaluating the sources of sperm retrieval (testicular or epididymal) and the success achieved with fresh versus frozen–thawed sperm, amongst other variables.

The goal of this chapter is to provide a comprehensive review of the available techniques for sperm retrieval, along with a brief description of the subtleties of each surgery. Following the description is a critical assessment of the outcomes associated with the various techniques, based on the published literature and the experience of the authors.

Pre-retrieval preparation

Patients are asked to discontinue any medications or supplements that may have an antiplatelet effect for at least one week prior to the procedure. **Appropriate infectious disease laboratory tests (HIV, HTLV, hepatitis, syphilis, etc.) are evaluated prior to the retrieval date to ensure that a specimen can be cryopreserved in the general population tanks, or to determine whether a quarantine tank will be required.** A responsible adult is requested to accompany the patient to and from the planned sperm retrieval procedure. Barring unforeseen circumstances, sperm procurement procedures are done on an outpatient basis. The physicians and technologists providing IVF/ICSI are made aware that a sperm retrieval is taking place and are involved with tissue examination and transportation of the specimens from the site of retrieval to the reproductive laboratory. Often, an embryologist or technician from the reproductive medicine center is present to examine specimens intraoperatively and to provide the appropriate transport media and supplies.

Infertility in the Male, 4th edition, ed. Larry I. Lipshultz, Stuart S. Howards, and Craig S. Niederberger. Published by Cambridge University Press. © Cambridge University Press 2009.

A bench microscope is available to examine specimens intraoperatively prior to transport.

Regardless of the method employed, sperm retrieval requires anesthesia. Conscious sedation, local, regional, or general anesthesia may be used. The specific type of anesthesia used depends on how sperm are procured as well as on both the surgeon's and the patient's preferences. For local anesthesia, the testicle and scrotal skin are anesthetized by infiltrating the spermatic cord and skin with a mixture of short- and long-acting local anesthetics. Conscious sedation in an office setting requires that the surgeon and the office staff be trained and certified in such techniques. The office is equipped to provide monitoring such as continuous pulse oximetry, serial blood pressures, and recording levels of patient consciousness. A "crash cart" is immediately available, and office staff is trained and certified to perform basic life support and advanced cardiac life support. If sperm retrieval is performed in a surgery center or hospital setting, the anesthesia of choice is administered by an anesthesiologist.

Patients are instructed to abstain from sexual activity for 2–3 days prior to sperm retrieval, and are asked not to shave prior to their procedure. However, a recent meta-analysis reported no difference in surgical site infections when patients are clipped or shaved one day before surgery or on the day of surgery [1]. A pre-procedure antibiotic with appropriate Gram-positive coverage is administered thirty minutes prior to incision [2–4]. If intravenous access is available, IV antibiotics are given. If a local anesthetic only is used, then an oral antibiotic is given. Patients are placed in the supine position. After the induction of anesthesia, the scrotal skin is shaved, prepped, and draped in the standard sterile fashion.

Vasal sperm
Indications
In the setting of normal spermatogenesis and vasal obstruction – either iatrogenic or congenital – sperm may be aspirated from the lumen of the testicular end of the vas deferens. Vasal sperm have completed their transit through the epididymis, presumably reaching full maturation and reproductive potential. **When indicated or desired by an infertile couple, vasal sperm may be procured at the time of vasectomy reversal for backup in case of short-term or long-term technical failure. Other potential indications to harvest vasal sperm include vasal occlusion after vasectomy, inguinal hernia repair with mesh, radical prostatectomy, or finding of vasal abnormalities in the setting of cystic fibrosis transmembrane regulator gene mutations.**

Technique
The authors prefer a vertical hemiscrotal incision carried through the dartos fibers to the level of the tunica vaginalis (Fig. 22.1), but any incision proximal to the vas deferens may be used. The dartos fibers are swept away bluntly, and the testicle is delivered from the hemiscrotum. Hemostasis is obtained with electrocautery. The operating microscope is used for optimal visualization of vital structures. The vas deferens is identified below the site of obstruction. Curved iris scissors and a needle-tipped bovie are used to isolate the vas deferens. A fine hemostat is placed under the testicular end of the vas deferens and the obstructed end of the vas is held with a fine-toothed pickup. A 5–0 holding stitch is placed on the testicular end of the vas deferens. A #3 nerve holder stabilizes the vas deferens, which is then transected with a straight blade (Fig. 22.2). The obstructed end of the vas is then tied with a 3–0 free tie for hemostasis. Bipolar electrocautery is used for hemostasis. The testicular end of the vas deferens is held with 0.12 pickups, while the lumen of the vas deferens is gently dilated with dilating jeweler's forceps (Fig. 22.3). The epididymis and vas deferens are gently manipulated while the vasal fluid is aspirated with a 1 mL tuberculin syringe with an angiocatheter (Fig. 22.4).

Each syringe is primed with a small amount of sperm wash media or human tubal fluid. Each syringe is transferred to the surgical scrub nurse, who replaces the used syringe with an empty syringe primed with media. The scrub nurse collects all vasal aspirates in a separate vial, which ultimately will be passed off the surgical field to the embryologist. Once adequate fluid has been expressed, a small drop is examined under light microscopy for the presence of motile sperm. At this anatomic level, only motile sperm are viable and adequate for IVF/ICSI or cryopreservation. Once the surgeon and embryologist determine that adequate numbers of viable sperm have been obtained, then the testicular end of the vas deferens is tied with a 3–0 free tie. Meticulous hemostasis is obtained with bipolar electrocautery. The testicle is replaced in the hemiscrotum. The dartos layer is closed with a running 3–0 suture. The skin edges are reapproximated with interrupted 3–0 sutures in a horizontal mattress fashion.

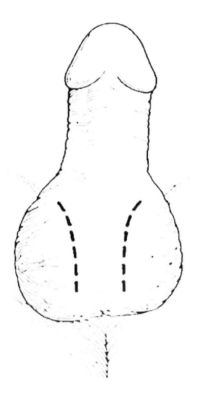

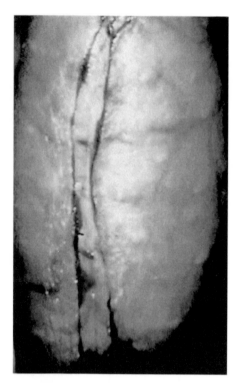

Fig. 22.1. Vertical hemiscrotal incision used for delivery of the testicle. *See color plate section.*

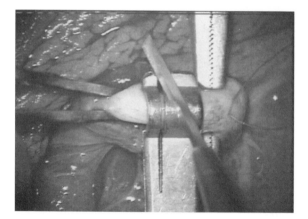

Fig. 22.2. Dividing the vas deferens, using a nerve holder for stabilization. *See color plate section.*

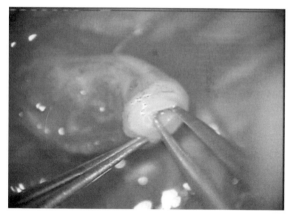

Fig. 22.3. Gentle dilation of the testicular end of the vas deferens. *See color plate section.*

Sterile dressings, fluffs, and a scrotal supporter are applied.

Vasal sperm are preferred in all patients who have vasal occlusion secondary to a vasectomy or prostatectomy, since this represents the most mature sperm and does not risk damaging the epididymis for future sperm retrieval. **Vasal sperm are used only when motile sperm can be identified in the specimen.**

Epididymal sperm
Indications

Indications for epididymal sperm procurement are similar to those for vasal sperm. Epididymal sperm aspiration may be pursued when it is known or deduced that testicular function is normal in the presence of obstructive azoospermia. **Common indications to**

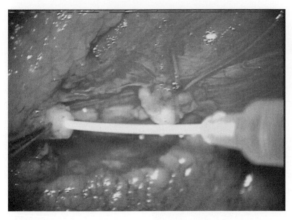

Fig. 22.4. Vasal sperm aspiration using an angiocatheter and syringe. *See color plate section.*

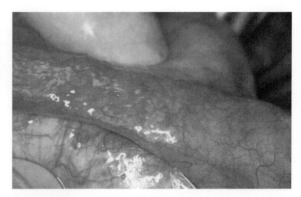

Fig. 22.5. Dilated epididymal tubules visualized under the operating microscope. *See color plate section.*

harvest epididymal sperm include congenital bilateral absence of the vas deferens and vasal occlusion after vasectomy in patients who either are not candidates for or do not desire microsurgical reconstruction. It should be noted that because outcomes in ICSI are similar when sperm are derived from the testis, these are also indications for testicular sperm extraction.

Techniques

Microsurgical epididymal sperm aspiration (MESA)

Various techniques of epididymal sperm aspiration have been described [5,6]. The authors prefer an obliterative approach in order to maximize sperm extraction. Obliterative MESA involves removing motile sperm from all possible sites of the epididymis to be used for immediate assisted reproductive techniques and for cryopreservation for subsequent IVF cycles. **Patients are counseled that in the event that no motile epididymal sperm are found, testicular sperm extraction is indicated.** A general anesthetic is preferred for MESA.

The testicle is delivered from the scrotum. The tunica vaginalis is opened to expose the tunica albuginea and epididymis. Hemostats are placed on the edges of the tunica vaginalis for easier identification at the end of the procedure. The operating microscope at 20–25× is used for optimal visualization and localization of epididymal tubules (Fig. 22.5). The epididymis is carefully inspected for dilated tubules and for a potential secondary epididymal "blowout," which might be seen after vasectomy. For patients

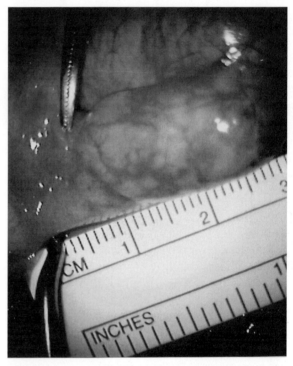

Fig. 22.6. Hypoplastic epididymis in patient with CBAVD. *See color plate section.*

with congenital bilateral absence of the vas deferens (CBAVD), the epididymis is examined and measured because the size of usable epididymis in these patients is variable (Fig. 22.6). Curved vasoepididymostomy scissors are used to open the tunica of the epididymis and isolate the dilated epididymal tubules. Indigo carmine irrigation can facilitate visualization of the tubules. Dissection begins at the tail of the epididymis and proceeds towards the caput. Once a

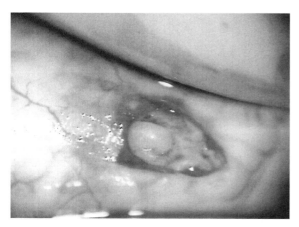

Fig. 22.7. Appearance of epididymal tubules after opening the tunica of the epididymis. *See color plate section.*

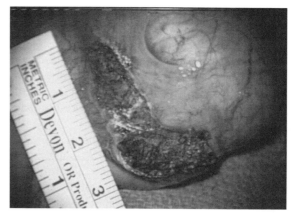

Fig. 22.8. Appearance of epididymis after completion of obliterative MESA. *See color plate section.*

tubule is isolated (Fig. 22.7), it is opened with a fine ophthalmologic blade or the vasoepididymostomy scissors. The epididymal fluid is aspirated and examined under light microscopy. If motile sperm are seen, the fluid may be collected for cryopreservation. **If no motile sperm are present, a more proximal tubule is isolated and opened.** The fluid at the new site is again aspirated and examined. This process is repeated until motile sperm are found. If no motile sperm are seen up to the level of the rete testis, then testicular sperm extraction is performed.

Obliterative MESA is performed by opening all dilated tubules containing motile sperm with the ophthalmologic blade. The surgeon squeezes the epididymis so as to minimize bleeding while the epididymal fluid is flushed with a 1 mL tuberculin syringe primed with human tubal fluid or sperm wash media. This technique continues from the point of finding motile sperm towards the head of the epididymis. Once all of the epididymal tubules have been opened and fluid has been aspirated to the satisfaction of the surgeon and the embryologist, the entire epididymis is obliterated with electrocautery until hemostasis is obtained. The tunica vaginalis may be closed with a running 3–0 suture, or a hydrocelectomy may be performed, at the surgeon's discretion. The testicle is delivered back into the hemiscrotum, which is closed.

Obliterative MESA (Fig. 22.8) typically is performed bilaterally in a single session so as to maximize sperm procurement while anesthetizing the patient only once. The decision to perform a unilateral obliterative MESA only is based on preoperative patient counseling as well as intraoperative findings.

Mini-MESA

As for obliterative MESA, general anesthesia is preferred for mini-MESA. However, conscious sedation with a spermatic cord block may be used. A 1 cm incision is made on the upper scrotal skin, and the tunica vaginalis is opened [7]. A self-retaining retractor, such as a pediatric eyelid retractor, is placed. The testicle is maintained within the hemiscrotum, and the epididymis is rotated into the field. A 7–0 Prolene stay suture is placed in the tunica of the epididymis. With the operating microscope at 20–25 optical magnification, a single epididymal tubule is isolated and opened with a fine ophthalmologic blade or the vasoepididymostomy scissors. Epididymal fluid is then aspirated with a fine-tipped angiocatheter. **As in the obliterative MESA technique, inspection of epididymal tubules begins at the cauda and progresses proximally toward the head of the epididymis.** The fluid is examined under light microscopy. Individual epididymal tubules are closed with interrupted 10–0 nylon sutures, and the epididymal tunic is closed with interrupted 9–0 nylon sutures. Meticulous hemostasis is obtained with bipolar electrocautery and the scrotum is closed in layers. If adequate amounts of motile sperm are not obtained, the procedure is repeated on the contralateral side.

Percutaneous epididymal sperm aspiration (PESA)

PESA may be performed to obtain sperm for IVF/ICSI [8,9]. It can be done with a local anesthetic in an office setting. Conscious sedation or premedication with an analgesic and/or anxiolytic agent may be administered. **The advantages of this technique over**

MESA may include lower costs, less post-procedure pain, and no need for a general anesthetic. The disadvantages include procurement of fewer sperm for IVF/ICSI, the potential for increased bleeding, since the aspiration needle is passed blindly, multiple times, into vascular structures, and the inability to examine for sites of bleeding or to administer electrocautery.

After a spermatic cord block and local anesthetic are administered, the epididymis is isolated and held by the surgeon's nondominant hand. **If the epididymis does not feel full, or if it is difficult to palpate, testicular extraction should be considered in lieu of PESA, as these findings suggest either that the epididymis is not obstructed or that a secondary epididymal "blowout" has occurred.** A 23-gauge butterfly needle connected to a 10 mL syringe is used. A vacuum is created in the needle tubing by placing a hemostat close to the butterfly needle, withdrawing the syringe plunger to create the vacuum, and placing a second hemostat on the tubing closer to the syringe. The plunger is released and attention is turned to the PESA.

A butterfly needle is inserted into the epididymis to stabilize it, and the hemostat closest to the needle is released. A small amount of epididymal tissue and fluid should be visible in the needle tubing. With the needle in place, the steps to create the vacuum in the needle tubing are repeated so that multiple aspirations may be performed. If necessary, the needle is withdrawn and replaced in a separate site until adequate tissue and fluid are obtained. The sample is examined under light microscopy by the embryologist, and if it is deemed adequate the procedure is ended. After the butterfly needle is withdrawn, direct pressure is applied to the puncture site(s) to ensure adequate hemostasis.

Testicular sperm

Indications

For cases of severe male-factor infertility such as nonobstructive azoospermia, or for obstructive azoospermia, testicular sperm may be used for IVF/ICSI. Nonobstructive azoospermia can be the consequence of a number of genetic or environmental conditions including Klinefelter syndrome, Y-chromosome microdeletions, cryptorchidism, hypogonadism, varicocele, or mumps orchitis. Additionally, testicular sperm may offer superior outcomes over epididymal or ejaculated sperm in properly selected cases [10]. Evidence suggests

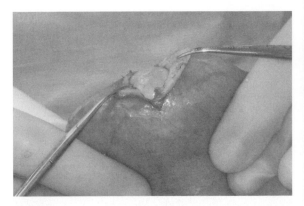

Fig. 22.9. Small transverse incision used to access the testis for testicular sperm retrieval. *See color plate section.*

that the outcomes of IVF/ICSI are improved in patients using testicular versus ejaculated sperm when multiple IVF attempts have failed and abnormal sperm DNA integrity is demonstrated [10].

Techniques

Testicular sperm extraction (TESE)/testicular mapping

General anesthesia is preferred for this procedure, although conscious sedation with a spermatic cord block may be used. **Magnification is recommended.** The preferred technique of the authors is similar to the open "window" technique [11]. The scrotum is shaved, prepped, and draped. If a testicular size discrepancy exists, the larger testicle is biopsied first. If the testes are of similar size and consistency, and if a varicocele is present, the side without the varicocele is biopsied first.

A 1–2 cm incision is made on the scrotal skin and carried through the dartos layer to the tunica vaginalis. The tunica vaginalis is grasped with fine-toothed pickups and opened sharply with curved iris scissors. Hemostats are placed on the edges of the tunica vaginalis. The opening in the tunica vaginalis is extended with electrocautery to expose the surface of the tunica albuginea (Fig. 22.9). **The testicle remains in the hemiscrotum.** A pediatric eyelid speculum may be placed underneath the tunica vaginalis as a retractor. The surface of the testicle is inspected for any abnormalities and for prominent vasculature. **Care is taken to avoid sub-tunical blood vessels.** A 5–0 holding stitch is placed in the tunica albuginea, and a #11 blade is used to open the tunica albuginea (Fig. 22.10). Seminiferous tubules are extruded and removed (Fig. 22.11). A piece of tissue is sent to the pathologist,

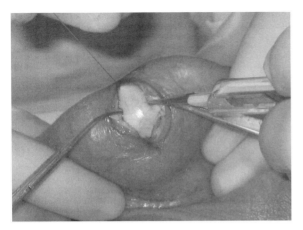

Fig. 22.10. Testicle is stabilized using a holding suture. An opening is made in the tunica albuginea. The holding suture may then be used to close the tunica albuginea. *See color plate section.*

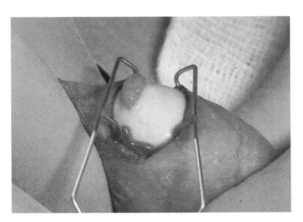

Fig. 22.11. Eyelid retractor can be used as a self-retaining retractor. Seminiferous tubules are easily extruded using light manual pressure. *See color plate section.*

and another piece is teased on a sterile slide with a drop of human tubal fluid or sperm wash media and examined under light microscopy. If sperm are seen, more tissue is taken from this area and given to the embryologist for use for IVF/ICSI. If no sperm are seen, then bipolar electrocautery is used for hemostasis, and the opening in the tunica albuginea is closed with the previously placed 5–0 suture in a running fashion. After this suture is tied, the ends are left long and a hemostat is placed on them to be used for retraction. The above procedure is repeated until sperm are found or until the upper, middle, and lower poles of the testicle have been adequately sampled. If no sperm are seen, the identical procedure is performed on the contralateral testicle. The wound is closed with a running 3–0 suture on the tunica vaginalis and a running

3–0 suture on the dartos layer; and the skin edges are reapproximated with interrupted 3–0 sutures in a horizontal mattress fashion. Sterile dressings, fluffs, and a scrotal supporter are placed.

Another testicular biopsy technique for nonobstructive azoospermia involves sampling multiple areas of the testis by fine-needle aspiration [12]. **With this technique, a "map" of the testicle may be constructed, which can be useful in directing future open sperm extractions.** For this mapping procedure, the scrotum is not opened. Rather, a spermatic cord block and wheals of local anesthetic are made on the scrotal skin. A 23-gauge needle attached to a 10 mL control syringe is passed into the testicle. While suction is applied, the needle is passed in and out of the testicle, and tissue is systematically obtained. In general, 4–12 samples are taken. The tissue is then examined for the presence or absence of sperm.

Microdissection testicular sperm extraction

In an effort to minimize the amount of testicular tissue removed during testicular sperm extraction (TESE) and to maximize the number of sperm harvested from the testicle, the technique of microdissection TESE was developed [13]. **Microdissection TESE (also referred to as "micro-TESE") has been shown to result in finding of sperm in a greater proportion of men with nonobstructive azoospermia than have random biopsies alone. Despite a single larger incision, this technique may result in less intratesticular reaction than a multiple biopsy approach [13–16]. Microdissection TESE also is effective in retrieving sperm when previous conventional biopsies showed no sperm [17].**

General anesthesia is preferred for this technique, given the extensive dissection and the need for high-powered 15–25 optical magnification with the operating microscope to optimally visualize vital structures. The testicle is delivered out of its respective hemiscrotum and the tunica vaginalis is opened. At the level of the midpole of the testis, the tunica albuginea is opened widely with the #11 blade, while the integrity of the testicular blood supply is maintained. The surgeon's nondominant hand holds the everted testicle while the dominant hand carefully and systematically dissects the seminiferous tubules under high-power magnification (Fig. 22.12). The bipolar electrocautery is used for dissection and meticulous hemostasis, and saline is used to irrigate the field for optimal visualization of bleeding vessels. **Seminiferous tubules that appear prominent**

413

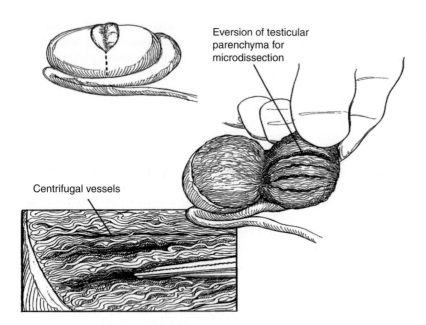

Eversion of testicular
parenchyma for
microdissection

Centrifugal vessels

Fig. 22.12. Schematic representation
of the microdissection TESE procedure.
(Courtesy of Peter N. Schlegel MD.)

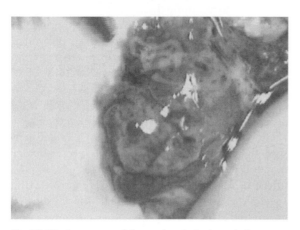

Fig. 22.13. Appearance of dissected testicular tissue during
microdissection TESE with prominent seminiferous tubules
containing sperm. (Courtesy of Peter N. Schlegel MD.) *See color plate
section.*

and full compared to the surrounding tubules
are harvested (Fig. 22.13). These small volumes of
higher-yield testicular tissue are excised, placed in
human tubal fluid, and passed off the operative field
to the experienced embryologist, who examines the
tissue under light microscopy, or sent to the tissue
processing laboratory. After sperm are found, or
when the dissection is complete, the tunica albuginea
is carefully closed with a running suture. The tunica
vaginalis is closed or a hydrocelectomy is performed.
The testicle is delivered back into the hemiscrotum

and the wound is closed. The procedure is performed
on the contralateral side if no sperm are found on
the first side, or if the surgeon prefers to maximize
sperm yield.

Testicular sperm aspiration (TESA)
Unlike TESE or micro-TESE, TESA is not recommended for patients with nonobstructive azoospermia except when used in conjunction with testicular mapping [18]. TESA is typically indicated in cases of obstructive azoospermia. Similar to PESA, TESA may be performed under a local anesthetic in an office setting. Conscious sedation or premedication with an analgesic and/or anxiolytic agent may be given. Two disadvantages of this minimally invasive technique are that fewer sperm are procured for IVF/ICSI and the sperm obtained are less mature than epididymal sperm. Since the aspiration or biopsy needle is passed blindly multiple times into the testicle, there is a potential for bleeding coupled with the inability to examine for bleeding sites or administer electrocautery.

After a spermatic cord block and local anesthetic are administered, the testis is held by the surgeon's nondominant hand. TESA is performed with a technique similar to that of PESA in that a 23-gauge butterfly needle connected to a 10 mL syringe is used. Some studies suggest improved yield with larger needles [19]. A vacuum is created in the needle, as described for PESA. A butterfly needle is inserted into the testis to stabilize it. The hemostat closest to the needle is then released.

A small number of seminiferous tubules are seen in the needle tubing. With the needle in place, the steps to create the vacuum in the needle tubing are repeated so that multiple aspirations may be performed. If necessary, the needle is withdrawn and replaced into a separate site until adequate tissue and fluid are obtained. The sample is examined under light microscopy by the embryologist, and if the sample is deemed adequate the procedure is ended. After the butterfly needle is withdrawn, direct pressure is applied to the puncture site(s) to ensure adequate hemostasis.

Post-retrieval care

Pain medication is provided as needed. Patients are instructed to apply ice packs to the scrotum for 24–48 hours, to abstain from sexual activity for at least three days, to keep their incision(s) dry for 24 hours, and to wear a scrotal supporter for at least 1–2 weeks until they are fully healed. Generally, oral antibiotics are continued empirically for 3–5 days, given the clean-contaminated environment of the surgical site, although some studies suggest that a single preoperative dose alone is adequate [2–4]. Patients are encouraged to return in 2–3 weeks for a postoperative wound check.

Outcomes
Surgical sperm retrieval success

The success of sperm retrieval depends on several factors, including the etiology of male-factor infertility, the technique used for sperm retrieval, the skill and experience of the individual surgeon, and the processing of the specimen after it has been retrieved. The actual outcome of IVF/ICSI in men with successful sperm retrieval is beyond the scope of this chapter.

The etiologic factors that require surgical sperm retrieval are very important in predicting the success of each type of procedure. Patients with obstructive azoospermia, by definition, have abundant sperm in both the testis and the epididymis that are available for surgical sperm retrieval by a wide range of techniques [20–23]. **Because of this, the Practice Committee of the American Society for Reproductive Medicine has stated in its recent guidelines that virtually all of the reported surgical sperm retrieval techniques are acceptable for patients with obstructive azoospermia** [24]. The success of surgical sperm retrieval is independent of the cause of obstructive azoospermia (i.e., congenital bilateral absence of the vas deferens,

elective sterilization, infection, iatrogenic injury). Consequently, male infertility specialists have tried to minimize the invasiveness of the procedures required to procure an adequate sample for multiple cycles of IVF/ICSI. Techniques to retrieve sperm from the epididymis (PESA) or testis (TESA, percutaneous biopsy or "PercBiopsy," and testicular fine-needle aspiration) via a percutaneous approach have been described.

Despite the universal prevalence of sperm in obstructive azoospermia, some of the minimally invasive surgical sperm retrieval techniques are not as effective as the standard open procedures in identifying sperm in patients with obstructive azoospermia. For example, the success rate of identifying sperm in obstructive azoospermia patients using PESA has been reported to be 41–91% of patients [20,22,25,26]. Additionally, in patients who have undergone a vasectomy, the success of surgical sperm retrieval using PESA was even lower (20%) when an epididymal cyst was found [22]. Epididymal cysts are found in 30% of patients after a vasectomy [27]. In all of these studies, men were found to have sperm on subsequent surgical sperm retrieval using standard open techniques or TESA.

Another instance of obstructive azoospermia in which PESA might yield lower success rates than open techniques is in patients with congenital bilateral absence of the vas deferens (CBAVD), especially when the absence is due to mutations of the cystic fibrosis transmembrane regulator gene. These patients often have poorly developed epididymal units in conjunction with the absence of vas deferens. The epididymal remnants can be limited to only a small epididymal head. In one study, success of PESA in cases of obstructive azoospermia due to CBAVD was observed to be 89%, and 95% in cases of vasectomy [28]. Additionally, recent evidence suggests that not all patients with cystic fibrosis transmembrane regulator gene mutations and reproductive tract anomalies have preserved spermatogenesis, further reducing the success of PESA in this subgroup of patients [29–31].

In contrast to results in patients with obstructive azoospermia, the success of surgical sperm retrieval is variable and significantly lower in patients with nonobstructive azoospermia, which can be caused by a broad spectrum of diseases. The incidence of finding mature sperm in the testicle in cases of nonobstructive azoospermia correlates highly with the underlying histopathologic diagnosis. For example, sperm are identified in 89.2% of patients with hypo-spermatogenesis, in 62.5% of those with maturation arrest, and in 16.3% of Sertoli-cell-only patients using a standard open testicular mapping technique, not exceeding four biopsies per testicle [32]. Using the testicular fine-needle aspiration technique, others have reported finding mature sperm in 95% of men with hypospermatogenesis, 46.4% of men with matu-ration arrest, and 48.3% of Sertoli-cell-only patients after undergoing a mean of 15 punctures per testicle [33]. Microdissection TESE is the latest and probably most promising technique for surgical sperm retrieval in nonobstructive azoospermia patients [13]. The reported sperm retrieval rate associated with micro-TESE is 81% in patients with hypospermatogen-esis, 44% in men with maturation arrest, and 41% in Sertoli-cell-only patients [15]. Knowledge of which surgical sperm retrieval is used in each individual eti-ology of nonobstructive azoospermia offers important prognostic information for both the couple undergo-ing IVF/ICSI and the reproductive endocrinologist. In even the most severe cases of testicular failure, as evi-denced by an FSH level greater than three times nor-mal, mature sperm are identified in 30% of the cases on a routine testicular biopsy [34].

Patients with several special conditions deserve particular attention as to their outcomes and type of sperm retrieval. These include patients with Klinefelter syndrome, Y-chromosome microdeletions, or undes-cended testes, and patients who have undergone chemotherapy or radiation for malignancy.

Klinefelter syndrome

Klinefelter syndrome represents the most common karyotypic abnormality associated with nonobstruct-ive azoospermia. These patients have sperm found at surgical sperm retrieval, with various success rates reported in the literature. **The largest series have shown a 48–66.6% success rate using TESE or TESA** [33,35]. Clinical parameters that can predict successful sperm retrieval include mosaic Klinefelter (47,XXY/ XY), normal facial hair pattern, and absent gyneco-mastia, according to one study [35]. Unfortunately, testicular size, FSH level, and testosterone level have shown inconsistent correlation with sperm recovery [35–37]. A unique approach of preoperative admin-istration of aromatase inhibitors or human chorionic gonadotropin followed by microdissection TESE was shown to be successful in 72% of Klinefelter patients undergoing surgical sperm retrieval [38].

Y-chromosome microdeletions

Y-chromosome microdeletions were found in up to 10.8% of men with infertility in several reported international studies [39–42]. Both complete and partial deletions of the azoospermia factor (AZF) locus have been described and subclassified into several regions (AZFa, AZFb, AZFc), and these are associated with various histologic patterns on testicu-lar biopsy. The impact on spermatogenesis is vari-able, and dependent on the specific region of deletion identified on the Y chromosome. Some men with Y-chromosome microdeletions will have sperm in the ejaculate whereas others will have azoospermia even on the most thorough inspection of testicular tissue. **One study investigating patients with vari-ous Y-chromosome microdeletions found an over-all success of 56% with surgical sperm retrieval** [43]. **The stratified results showed that only patients with pure AZFc deletions had successful sperm recovery.** Furthermore, the authors demonstrated that micro-dissection TESE was more successful than diagnostic biopsy in identifying sperm (75% vs. 45%). In patients with AZFa and AZFb deletions, no sperm for retrieval were found with either technique. However, caution should be used when recommending against surgical sperm retrieval in patients with AZFa or AZFb dele-tions, as the study group consisted of only 12 patients, limiting any generalized conclusion about these patients.

Cancer and chemotherapy or radiation therapy

Cancer and subsequent chemotherapy or radiation can cause azoospermia in young men still interested in fertility. Various types of cancer occur in men of reproductive age, but studies looking at the impact of these cancers on spermatogenesis have shown no sig-nificant impairment in pretreatment semen param-eters as compared to those of controls. One exception to this observation is seen in patients with testicular cancer. Various chemotherapeutics are used to treat cancer, and they have a variable impact on sperm-atogenesis and recovery of spermatogenesis after treatment. In men who remain azoospermic after chemotherapy, surgical sperm retrieval coupled with IVF/ICSI represents the only possibility for fathering a child genetically similar to both parents. **The suc-cess of surgical sperm retrieval in post-chemother-apy azoospermia is highly dependent on the type**

and duration of chemotherapy used. Consequently, there are no predictive models for sperm recovery rates in these patients. The histological patterns seen on testicular biopsy most often show Sertoli-cell-only syndrome, hypospermatogenesis, and maturation arrest, respectively [44,45]. **The success of surgical sperm retrieval in post-chemotherapy patients has been reported at 45% using either TESE or micro-dissection TESE in patients with an average age of 37.4 years, FSH 21.8 mIU/mL, and a mean testosterone level of 327 ng/dL. The histologic pattern was Sertoli-cell-only in 76% of the biopsies in this group of patients** [44]. Another study performed testicular mapping with fine-needle aspiration prior to TESE and reported a surgical retrieval rate of 65.2%. The patient characteristics were very similar to those in the previously described study, except for a much lower rate of Sertoli-cell-only (47.8%) found on testicular biopsy [45].

Cryptorchidism

Cryptorchidism is implicated in approximately 10% of cases of male infertility [46]. It accounts for 27% of all cases of azoospermia and 60% of cases of unexplained nonobstructive azoospermia [47]. Although there is a high incidence of azoospermia in patients who have undergone orchidopexy, many patients are still able to produce sperm of relatively normal quantity and quality. This group of patients represents another highly heterogeneous cohort when it comes to predicting the level of preserved spermatogenesis. Variables to be considered include the degree of cryptorchidism (abdominal, inguinal, high scrotal, ectopic), laterality (unilateral or bilateral), age at orchidopexy, and age of the patient when he seeks evaluation for a male-factor infertility. These patients represent the entire spectrum of histologic subtypes at the time of testicular biopsy [48–50]. **The success of surgical sperm retrieval has been reported to be between 51.9% and 74% in these series.** Looking at variables to predict success, Negri *et al.* reported patient age and FSH level as positive predictive variables in men who underwent TESE [48]. Raman *et al.* reported patient age at the time of orchidopexy and testicular volume as positive predictors in patients undergoing either TESE or micro-TESE [49]. In contrast, Vernaeve *et al.* reported that there were no clinical parameters that predicted successful sperm retrieval at the time of TESE in this subset of patients with azoospermia and history of orchidopexy [50].

Surgical volume and testicular tissue processing

The effect of individual surgeon experience on the outcomes of surgical procedures has been evaluated in many different fields of surgery. It is intuitive that surgeons who perform large numbers of a particular procedure will have better outcomes than their counterparts who perform the same procedure less frequently. This aspect of surgical outcomes has not been evaluated when it comes to surgical sperm retrieval, and likely represents one of the reasons for the disparities seen in reported sperm retrieval rates when similar procedures are compared.

Another often overlooked but important aspect of successful sperm retrieval is the impact of the processing of the tissue after it has been removed and identification of sperm within the specimen. A good example supporting this point is seen when evaluating samples in patients with known hypospermatogenesis. By definition, all of these patients should have sperm found during testicular sperm retrieval. However, even in the best of hands and with the most sophisticated techniques, the literature reports that efforts fall short of the universal identification of sperm. **The diligence and experience of the person or persons evaluating the tissue is critical to success in finding sperm.**

Special circumstances

One unique situation using testicular sperm for IVF/ICSI deserves mention. DNA damage to sperm may occur after the sperm separates from Sertoli cells [51]. Sperm with DNA damage may be associated with poorer outcomes in IVF/ICSI [52]. A novel solution to this problem of abnormal sperm DNA fragmentation employs sperm retrieved directly from the testicle, even when sperm are readily available in the ejaculate. In a small series of patients who had repeated IVF/ICSI failures and elevated DNA fragmentation indices, Greco *et al.* reported improved outcomes with IVF/ICSI when sperm were retrieved directly from the testicle [10]. Significant improvements in pregnancy (44.4% vs. 5.6%) and implantation rate (20.7% vs. 1.8%) were seen when the oocytes were fertilized with testicular sperm rather than ejaculated sperm. This initial report on the use of testicular sperm for patients with elevated sperm DNA damage is promising, and opens the door for further research and testing in this area. However, the results must be treated with caution, as the method to detect DNA fragmentation is under investigation, and the number of patients in the study is small.

Conclusion

Techniques for sperm retrieval have become an integral part of the surgical armamentarium of every reproductive urologist in the era of IVF/ICSI. Knowledge of and experience with the various procedures, along with an understanding of the relative success of each approach in individual situations, is important for any urologist counseling patients entering into an IVF/ICSI program. Not all techniques are equally suitable for all patients. The patient's underlying etiology of azoospermia or testicular failure, coupled with the urologist's and embryologist's expertise, are the critical determinants of successful sperm retrieval. PESA, TESA, and TESE have simplified the approach in patients with obstructive azoospermia, while more advanced techniques like testicular mapping and microdissection TESE have given new hope for patients with even the most severe cases of nonobstructive azoospermia.

References

[1] Tanner J, Woodings D, Moncaster K. Preoperative hair removal to reduce surgical site infection. *Cochrane Database Syst Rev* 2006; (3): CD004122.

[2] Woods RK, Dellinger EP. Current guidelines for antibiotic prophylaxis of surgical wounds. *Am Fam Physician* 1998; **57**: 2731–40.

[3] Amin M. Antibacterial prophylaxis in urology: a review. *Am J Med* 1992; **92**: 114–17S.

[4] Akalin HE. Surgical prophylaxis: the evolution of guidelines in an era of cost containment. *J Hosp Infect* 2002; **50** (Suppl A): S3–7.

[5] Schlegel PN, Berkeley AS, Goldstein M, *et al.* Epididymal micropuncture with *in vitro* fertilization and oocyte micromanipulation for the treatment of unreconstructable obstructive azoospermia. *Fertil Steril* 1994; **61**: 895–901.

[6] Temple-Smith PD, Southwick GJ, Yates CA, Trounson AO, de Kretser DM. Human pregnancy by *in vitro* fertilization (IVF) using sperm aspirated from the epididymis. *J In Vitro Fert Embryo Transf* 1985; **2**: 119–22.

[7] Nudell DM, Conaghan J, Pedersen RA, *et al.* The mini-micro-epididymal sperm aspiration for sperm retrieval: a study of urological outcomes. *Hum Reprod* 1998; **13**: 1260–5.

[8] Shrivastav P, Nadkarni P, Wensvoort S, Craft I. Percutaneous epididymal sperm aspiration for obstructive azoospermia. *Hum Reprod* 1994; **9**: 2058–61.

[9] Tsirigotis M, Pelekanos M, Yazdani N, *et al.* Simplified sperm retrieval and intracytoplasmic sperm injection in patients with azoospermia. *Br J Urol* 1995; **76**: 765–8.

[10] Greco E, Scarselli F, Iacobelli M, *et al.* Efficient treatment of infertility due to sperm DNA damage by ICSI with testicular spermatozoa. *Hum Reprod* 2005; **20**: 226–30.

[11] Coburn M, Wheeler T, Lipshultz LI. Testicular biopsy: its use and limitations. *Urol Clin North Am* 1987; **14**: 551–61.

[12] Turek PJ, Cha I, Ljung BM. Systematic fine-needle aspiration of the testis: correlation to biopsy and results of organ "mapping" for mature sperm in azoospermic men. *Urology* 1997; **49**: 743–8.

[13] Schlegel PN. Testicular sperm extraction: microdissection improves sperm yield with minimal tissue excision. *Hum Reprod* 1999; **14**: 131–5.

[14] Okada H, Dobashi M, Yamazaki T, *et al.* Conventional versus microdissection testicular sperm extraction for nonobstructive azoospermia. *J Urol* 2002; **168**: 1063–7.

[15] Ramasamy R, Yagan N, Schlegel PN. Structural and functional changes to the testis after conventional versus microdissection testicular sperm extraction. *Urology* 2005; **65**: 1190–4.

[16] Amer M, Ateyah A, Hany R, Zohdy W. Prospective comparative study between microsurgical and conventional testicular sperm extraction in non-obstructive azoospermia: follow-up by serial ultrasound examinations. *Hum Reprod* 2000; **15**: 653–6.

[17] Ramasamy R, Schlegel PN. Microdissection testicular sperm extraction: effect of prior biopsy on success of sperm retrieval. *J Urol* 2007; **177**: 1447–9.

[18] Turek PJ, Ljung BM, Cha I, Conaghan J. Diagnostic findings from testis fine needle aspiration mapping in obstructed and nonobstructed azoospermic men. *J Urol* 2000; **163**: 1709–16.

[19] Carpi A, Fabris FG, Todeschini G, Nardini V. Large-needle percutaneous aspiration biopsy of the testicle in men with nonobstructive azoospermia. *Fertil Steril* 2006; **86**: 464–5.

[20] Dohle GR, Ramos L, Pieters MH, Braat DD, Weber RF. Surgical sperm retrieval and intracytoplasmic sperm injection as treatment of obstructive azoospermia. *Hum Reprod* 1998; **13**: 620–3.

[21] Sheynkin YR, Ye Z, Menendez S, *et al.* Controlled comparison of percutaneous and microsurgical sperm retrieval in men with obstructive azoospermia. *Hum Reprod* 1998; **13**: 3086–9.

[22] Wood S, Vang E, Troup S, Kingsland CR, Lewis-Jones DI. Surgical sperm retrieval after previous vasectomy and failed reversal: clinical implications for *in vitro* fertilization. *BJU Int* 2002; **90**: 277–81.

[23] Friedler S, Raziel A, Strassburger D, *et al.* Factors influencing the outcome of ICSI in patients with obstructive and non-obstructive azoospermia: a comparative study. *Hum Reprod* 2002; **17**: 3114–21.

[24] Practice Committee of the American Society for Reproductive Medicine. Sperm retrieval for obstructive azoospermia. *Fertil Steril* 2006; **86**: S115–20.

[25] Rosenlund B, Westlander G, Wood M, *et al.* Sperm retrieval and fertilization in repeated percutaneous epididymal sperm aspiration. *Hum Reprod* 1998; **13**: 2805–7.

[26] Glina S, Fragoso JB, Martins FG, *et al.* Percutaneous epididymal sperm aspiration (PESA) in men with obstructive azoospermia. *Int Braz J Urol* 2003; **29**: 141–5.

[27] Reddy NM, Gerscovich EO, Jain KA, Le-Petross HT, Brock JM. Vasectomy-related changes on sonographic examination of the scrotum. *J Clin Ultrasound* 2004; **32**: 394–8.

[28] Meniru GI, Gorgy A, Podsiadly BT, Craft IL. Results of percutaneous epididymal sperm aspiration and intracytoplasmic sperm injection in two major groups of patients with obstructive azoospermia. *Hum Reprod* 1997; **12**: 2443–6.

[29] Meng MV, Black LD, Cha I, *et al.* Impaired spermatogenesis in men with congenital absence of the vas deferens. *Hum Reprod* 2001; **16**: 529–33.

[30] Black LD, Nudell DM, Cha I, Cherry AM, Turek PJ. Compound genetic factors as a cause of male infertility: Case report. *Hum Reprod* 2000; **15**: 449–51.

[31] Karpman E, Williams DH, Wilberforce S, Lipshultz LI. Compound genetic abnormalities in patients with cystic fibrosis transmembrane regulator gene mutation. *Fertil Steril* 2007; **87**: 1468.e5–8.

[32] Seo JT, Ko WJ. Predictive factors of successful testicular sperm recovery in non-obstructive azoospermia patients. *Int J Androl* 2001; **24**: 306–10.

[33] Lewin A, Reubinoff B, Porat-Katz A, *et al.* Testicular fine needle aspiration: the alternative method for sperm retrieval in non-obstructive azoospermia. *Hum Reprod* 1999; **14**: 1785–90.

[34] Kim ED, Gilbaugh JH, Patel VR, Turek PJ, Lipshultz LI. Testis biopsies frequently demonstrate sperm in men with azoospermia and significantly elevated follicle-stimulating hormone levels. *J Urol* 1997; **157**: 144–6.

[35] Vernaeve V, Staessen C, Verheyen G, *et al.* Can biological or clinical parameters predict testicular sperm recovery in 47,XXY Klinefelter's syndrome patients? *Hum Reprod* 2004; **19**: 1135–9.

[36] Madgar I, Dor J, Weissenberg R, *et al.* Prognostic value of the clinical and laboratory evaluation in patients with nonmosaic Klinefelter syndrome who

are receiving assisted reproductive therapy. *Fertil Steril* 2002; **77**: 1167–9.

[37] Westlander G, Ekerhovd E, Granberg S, *et al.* Testicular ultrasonography and extended chromosome analysis in men with nonmosaic Klinefelter syndrome: A prospective study of possible predictive factors for successful sperm recovery. *Fertil Steril* 2001; **75**: 1102–5.

[38] Schiff JD, Palermo GD, Veeck LL, *et al.* Success of testicular sperm extraction [corrected] and intracytoplasmic sperm injection in men with Klinefelter syndrome. *J Clin Endocrinol Metab* 2005; **90**: 6263–7.

[39] Pryor JL, Kent-First M, Muallem A, *et al.* Microdeletions in the Y chromosome of infertile men. *N Engl J Med* 1997; **336**: 534–9.

[40] Rucker GB, Mielnik A, King P, Goldstein M, Schlegel PN. Preoperative screening for genetic abnormalities in men with nonobstructive azoospermia before testicular sperm extraction. *J Urol* 1998; **160**: 2068–71.

[41] Foresta C, Garolla A, Bartoloni L, Bettella A, Ferlin A. Genetic abnormalities among severely oligospermic men who are candidates for intracytoplasmic sperm injection. *J Clin Endocrinol Metab* 2005; **90**: 152–6.

[42] Krausz C, Forti G, McElreavey K. The Y chromosome and male fertility and infertility. *Int J Androl* 2003; **26**: 70–5.

[43] Hopps CV, Mielnik A, Goldstein M, *et al.* Detection of sperm in men with Y chromosome microdeletions of the AZFa, AZFb and AZFc regions. *Hum Reprod* 2003; **18**: 1660–5.

[44] Chan PT, Palermo GD, Veeck LL, Rosenwaks Z, Schlegel PN. Testicular sperm extraction combined with intracytoplasmic sperm injection in the treatment of men with persistent azoospermia postchemotherapy. *Cancer* 2001; **92**: 1632–7.

[45] Damani MN, Master V, Meng MV, *et al.* Postchemotherapy ejaculatory azoospermia: Fatherhood with sperm from testis tissue with intracytoplasmic sperm injection. *J Clin Oncol* 2002; **20**: 930–6.

[46] Mieusset R, Bujan L, Massat G, Mansat A, Pontonnier F. Clinical and biological characteristics of infertile men with a history of cryptorchidism. *Hum Reprod* 1995; **10**: 613–19.

[47] Fedder J, Crüger D, Oestergaard B, Petersen GB. Etiology of azoospermia in 100 consecutive nonvasectomized men. *Fertil Steril* 2004; **82**: 1463–5.

[48] Negri L, Albani E, DiRocco M, *et al.* Testicular sperm extraction in azoospermic men submitted to bilateral orchidopexy. *Hum Reprod* 2003; **18**: 2534–9.

[49] Raman JD, Schlegel PN. Testicular sperm extraction with intracytoplasmic sperm injection is successful for the treatment of nonobstructive azoospermia

associated with cryptorchidism. *J Urol* 2003; **170**: 1287–90.

[50] Vernaeve V, Krikilion A, Verheyen G, *et al.* Outcome of testicular sperm recovery and ICSI in patients with non-obstructive azoospermia with a history of orchidopexy. *Hum Reprod* 2004; **19**: 2307–12.

[51] Tesarik J, Ubaldi F, Rienzi L, *et al.* Caspase-dependent and -independent DNA fragmentation in Sertoli and germ cells from men with primary testicular failure: relationship with histological diagnosis. *Hum Reprod* 2004; **19**: 254–61.

[52] Lopes S, Sun JG, Jurisicova A, Meriano J, Casper RF. Sperm deoxyribonucleic acid fragmentation is increased in poor-quality semen samples and correlates with failed fertilization in intracytoplasmic sperm injection. *Fertil Steril* 1998; **69**: 528–32.

Introduction

Ejaculatory duct obstruction has been identified as a possible cause for male-factor infertility since the late 1960s [1]. Interestingly in the authors' experience today, only a few of the men who are referred for further evaluation at a tertiary care center with the clinical picture of ejaculatory duct obstruction have been evaluated, nor has the diagnosis of obstruction even been considered. Making the diagnosis of partial ejaculatory duct obstruction can be clinically challenging, given the wide variation in its manifestations. Men with ejaculatory duct obstruction will have palpable vasa and normal testes on examination and normal hormonal evaluation. Semen analyses will vary, but will typically reveal low volume and azoospermia, or low concentration and/or motility, and sometimes necrospermia. In the past, the existence of partial ejaculatory duct obstruction has been challenged. However, with studies illustrating improvement of semen parameters in these cases after treatment, partial ejaculatory duct obstruction has been accepted as a clinical entity.

Ejaculatory duct obstruction frequently is incompletely evaluated, and a missed diagnosis is likely because it is an uncommon cause of male-factor infertility and not considered. The ejaculatory ducts may be obstructed by either congenital or acquired causes in 1–5% of infertile males [2–4]. Once the clinical picture of ejaculatory duct obstruction has been recognized, specialized testing will strengthen the diagnosis or rule out obstruction. Historically, obstruction has been evaluated by confirming normal spermatogenesis with testicular biopsy and then identifying the site of obstruction with vasography. Today, transrectal ultrasound (TRUS) is used to detect obstructing lesions and provide evidence of obstruction of the ejaculatory ducts in a noninvasive manner. In fact, screening studies using transrectal ultrasound of the prostate have found that 5% of the male population has ejaculatory cysts, though not all of them cause infertility [5]. Like many other men with infertility caused by obstruction, men with ejaculatory duct obstruction have multiple treatment options. Of these, transurethral resection of the ejaculatory ducts (TURED) offers men possible cure for their infertility. If left untreated, some lesions causing partial obstruction may progress to complete obstruction and azoospermia [6].

This chapter offers a discussion of basic normal ejaculatory duct embryology, anatomy, and physiology to lay a foundation for an understanding of the clinical findings and treatment of obstruction. Evaluation and treatment options for the patient with suspected ejaculatory duct obstruction will be discussed, as well as alternatives and potential complications of treatment.

Embryology, anatomy, and physiology

A comprehensive review of prostatic embryology and ejaculation physiology can be found in Chapters 1 and 9. However, a brief review may assist in the understanding of ejaculatory duct obstruction. The genital ductal system in males and females develops from the Wolffian (mesonephric) ducts and Müllerian (paramesonephric) ducts. These two ductal systems lie in close proximity to one another and adjacent to the undifferentiated gonads. The Wolffian duct develops and joins the urogenital sinus. From the Wolffian duct the ureteral bud forms. The caudal-most portion of the Wolffian duct is absorbed into the urogenital sinus, allowing the ureter and mesonephric duct to open separately into the urogenital sinus. **In the male the mesonephric duct continues to develop into the epididymis, vas deferens, seminal vesicle, and ejaculatory duct.** From along the posterior urogenital sinus, lateral to the verumontanum, five paired epithelial buds develop. These buds form above and below the mesonephric duct, forming the prostate as they grow into the mesenchyme. The Müllerian ducts develop

Infertility in the Male, 4th edition, ed. Larry I. Lipshultz, Stuart S. Howards, and Craig S. Niederberger. Published by Cambridge University Press. © Cambridge University Press 2009.

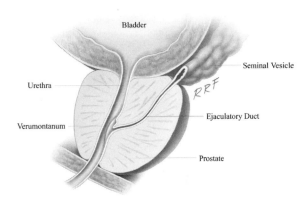

Fig. 23.1. Ejaculatory duct anatomy.

towards the urogenital sinus and in the female are destined to become the fallopian tubes, uterus, and the major portion of the vagina. Under the influence of anti-Müllerian hormone, secreted from the Sertoli cells in the primitive testis, the Müllerian structures involute. **The remnant Müllerian structures in the male are the prostatic utricle and appendix testis, and in some men remnant Müllerian duct structures can be found in the midline of the prostate as Müllerian duct cysts** [7].

In the adult male the prostatic utricle is normally found in the center of the verumontanum, and the ejaculatory ducts enter into the prostatic urethra as beveled orifices laterally on the verumontanum adjacent to the prostatic utricle (Fig. 23.1). Through the verumontanum the ducts are directed obliquely and downstream into the urethra, thereby minimizing the potential for reflux [8]. The major portion of the course of the ducts is lined with collagen, and the ducts function simply as a conduit for semen to exit the vasa and seminal vesicles during ejaculation. The diameter of the ejaculatory duct varies along its course, with the proximal portion measuring approximately 1.7 mm and the distal portion about 0.3 mm. In normal males, at the mid-portion of the duct, the average diameter is 0.6 ± 0.1 mm as measured by ultrasound and by microscopic anatomic studies of cadaveric and surgical specimens [8,9]. The ducts are typically between 1 and 2 cm long and enter the prostate at its base, coursing anteriorly and medially to reach the verumontanum. The ejaculatory ducts are contiguous with the seminal vesicles, which are joined at the origin of the ducts by the ampulla of the vas deferens [10,11].

During emission the sympathetic nervous system mediates contraction of the vas deferens and

seminal vesicles, with resultant emission of seminal fluid through the ejaculatory ducts and into the prostatic urethra. In normal ejaculation, the simultaneous closing of the bladder neck prevents retrograde ejaculation. Bladder neck closure is also controlled by sympathetic outflow. Ejaculation is the forceful expulsion of seminal fluid that occurs in response to rhythmic contractions of the bulbocavernosus and ischiocavernosus muscles of the pelvic floor. These striated muscle groups are under the control of the somatic nervous system.

Etiology

Causes of ejaculatory duct obstruction may be either congenital or acquired. Acquired causes include infections (sexually transmitted diseases, prostatic abscess, prostatitis, tuberculosis), tumors, ejaculatory duct calculi, and urethral catheterization, as well as iatrogenic trauma secondary to pediatric rectal surgery and transurethral procedures [12–14]. Congenital ejaculatory duct obstruction results from anomalies such as utricular, Müllerian, and Wolffian duct cysts, as well as congenital atresia or stenosis of the ejaculatory ducts [15]. Some unexplained cases of congenital ejaculatory duct obstruction might have genetic causes, because *CFTR* gene mutations found in some of these patients may represent a minor variant of cystic fibrosis [16].

Evaluation and diagnosis

The diagnosis of ejaculatory duct obstruction is established by documenting normal spermatogenesis and patent proximal excurrent ducts, including vas deferens, and establishing the point of distal obstruction. Evaluation of patients suspected of having ejaculatory duct obstruction starts with detailed history and physical examination. **The most common complaint in men presenting with ejaculatory duct obstruction is infertility, as most of these men are otherwise asymptomatic.** Other than infertility, men with ejaculatory duct obstruction may present with a variety of symptoms. In one study, patients with ultrasound findings of dilated seminal vesicles, prostatic cysts, or seminal vesicle or ejaculatory duct calculi were found to have hematospermia, perineal pain, and painful ejaculation [17]. Other symptoms occasionally associated with ejaculatory duct obstruction are pain radiating into testis, difficulties with bowel habits and tenesmus, change in the volume of ejaculate, and lower urinary symptoms consistent with bladder outlet obstruction. Patients presenting for evaluation of azoospermia may have a history of urinary tract infection, penile discharge, urethral trauma or manipulation, or decreasing ejaculate force or volume. Generally, a high degree of clinical suspicion is necessary to diagnose ejaculatory duct obstruction, because of the lack of specific symptoms associated with this condition.

Physical examination of men with ejaculatory duct obstruction in most cases is unremarkable. Occasionally, patients will have abnormal prostatic findings, such as a midline cystic mass or dilated seminal vesicles, suggesting possible anatomical abnormality and prompting further evaluation. Rarely, on scrotal examination men will have dilated vasa or epididymides. A routine hormonal profile is obtained to evaluate azoospermia or oligospermia, which in the case of ejaculatory duct obstruction usually reveals normal follicle-stimulating hormone (FSH), luteinizing hormone (LH), and testosterone, thus suggesting normal spermatogenesis [18].

Ejaculatory duct obstruction may be complete or partial, and men with partial obstruction will have varied presentations. The largest portion of the ejaculate is produced by the seminal vesicles, and when the ejaculatory ducts are obstructed the semen lacks those secretions. **Therefore, semen analyses in cases of complete ejaculatory duct obstruction will reveal low-volume (< 1 mL) azoospermia, and the ejaculate frequently will be watery and acidic (pH < 7) [19].** Absence of fructose in the semen is consistent with obstruction and lack of contribution of fluid from the seminal vesicles but is not always found in cases of ejaculatory obstruction. The differential diagnosis of complete ejaculatory duct obstruction should include congenital bilateral absence of the vas deference, failure of emission, and retrograde ejaculation [18]. Congenital bilateral absence of the vas deferens can be diagnosed with physical examination; postejaculatory urinalysis can rule out retrograde ejaculation, and failure of emission frequently may represent neurological causes. In cases of partial ejaculatory duct obstruction, semen parameters may vary, with the most frequent findings being low semen volume, oligospermia, or azoospermia, poor or absent sperm motility, and finally poor survival in vitro and failure to fertilize an egg [20,21].

The next step in the evaluation should include imaging modalities. The optimal diagnostic method has not been defined. Historically, vasography through a partial-thickness vasotomy was performed in the scrotal portion of the vas deferens [22]. This happens to be the most invasive diagnostic technique, as it involves scrotal incision and dissection of vas deferens. Partial vasotomy is then performed using intraoperative microscope and microsurgical technique. Vasal fluid obtained from vasotomy at the time of the procedure is examined microscopically. Presence of a significant amount of sperm confirms that spermatogenesis is present and proximal excurrent ducts are patent. Contrast medium injected using a 22- or 24-gauge angiocatheter into the abdominal portion of the vas deferens will either efflux into the bladder (indicating no obstruction) or fill dilated obstructed seminal vesicles. Methylene blue may be injected for a non-contrast vasography.

Contemporary evaluation and management of ejaculatory duct obstruction has been greatly simplified and streamlined by the use of high resolution transrectal ultrasound [19,23]. This has the advantage of being less invasive and less expensive than vasography. **The ultrasonographic diagnosis of ejaculatory duct obstruction is based upon the finding of dilation of the seminal vesicles** (Fig. 23.2) **and abnormalities in the region of the ejaculatory ducts.** Some additional findings include ejaculatory duct cysts, Müllerian duct remnants, and seminal vesicle or ejaculatory duct calculi (Fig. 23.3) [17]. Chronic obstruction of the ejaculatory ducts should, over time, produce dilation of the seminal vesicles and vasa. The size of the seminal vesicle on the ultrasound is determined by measuring its anteroposterior diameter. The normal size is thought to be up to 1.5 cm. Thus, ejaculatory duct obstruction should be suspected in men with seminal vesicle anteroposterior dimension greater than 1.5 cm [19]. Ejaculatory duct dilation (> 1.2 mm) may also be visualized by transrectal ultrasound in some cases of ejaculatory duct obstruction [24]. If the seminal vesicles are not dilated but the index of suspicion remains high for ejaculatory duct obstruction, seminal vesicle aspiration might bring additional diagnostic value. The finding of numerous sperm within the seminal vesicles of an azoospermic patient is suggestive of ejaculatory duct obstruction [25]. At the same time seminal vesiculography can be performed by injecting contrast medium into the seminal vesicles and obtaining dynamic images. In cases of ejaculatory duct obstruction, contrast fills the vasa retrograde and a vasogram is obtained. When there is no ejaculatory duct obstruction, contrast effluxes into the urethra through the ejaculatory ducts. Using the same transrectal access and ultrasound guiding technology, chromotubation may be done. Chromotubation

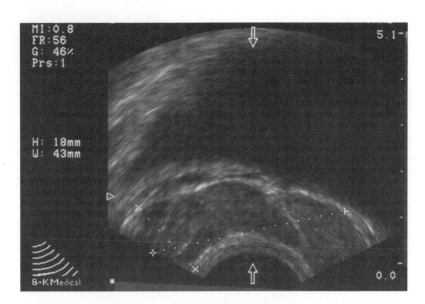

Fig. 23.2. High-resolution transrectal ultrasound of the prostate, demonstrating a dilated seminal vesicle with an anteroposterior size of 18 mm (in cross hatches).

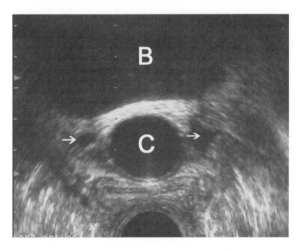

Fig. 23.3. High-resolution transrectal ultrasound of the prostate, demonstrating a Müllerian duct cyst (C), dilated ejaculatory ducts splayed laterally (arrows), and bladder (B).

is performed by injecting indigo carmine or diluted methylene blue into one seminal vesicle at a time in an antegrade fashion. Direct cystoscopic examination of the verumontanum and ejaculatory duct orifices follows the injection. Failure to visualize efflux of blue dye is usually thought to be suspicious for ejaculatory duct obstruction [26].

Purohit *et al.* studied different techniques to strengthen the diagnosis of ejaculatory duct obstruction and predict outcomes of transurethral resection of the ejaculatory ducts in men with findings consistent

with obstruction on semen analysis and initial transrectal ultrasound [26]. This study found that transrectal ultrasound alone has poor specificity for the evaluation of ejaculatory duct obstruction. **However, addition of such dynamic tests as seminal vesiculography or chromotubation more reliably predicted successful outcomes with transurethral resection of the ejaculatory ducts than did transrectal ultrasound or seminal vesicle aspiration for sperm alone.**

Engin *et al.* compared transrectal ultrasound to endorectal MR imaging for ejaculatory duct obstruction [27]. Prostatic cysts, ejaculatory duct dilation (>2 mm in width), ejaculatory duct calculi or calcifications, seminal vesicle dilation (anteroposterior diameter >15 mm), seminal vesicle hypo/agenesis (aneroposterior diameter <7 mm), seminal vesicle cysts (>5 mm), vasal agenesis, and chronic prostatitis (coarse calcifications, heterogeneity in prostate) were considered significant findings for obstruction of the seminal duct system. The authors concluded that ultrasound is a good method for initial evaluation of men suspected of having ejaculatory duct obstruction, and endorectal MRI should be reserved for selected patients in whom results of transrectal ultrasound are not conclusive. MRI allows better assessment of anatomical relationships between the structures of interest. High soft tissue contrast, multiplanar capability, the accuracy of determination of the localization of lesions, and characterization of the cystic lesions in T2-weighted images make endorectal MRI an ideal imaging method in the evaluation of some of these lesions that cannot be detected otherwise (Fig. 23.4) [27].

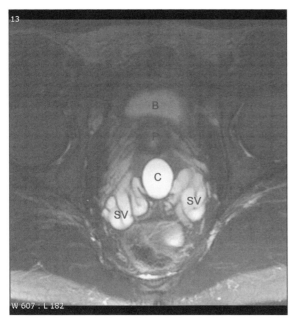

Fig. 23.4. Müllerian duct cyst (C), dilated seminal vesicles (SV), prostate (P), and bladder (B), as demonstrated on a T2-weighted MRI of the pelvis.

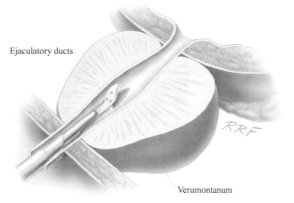

Fig. 23.5. Transurethral resection of ejaculatory ducts.

Management of ejaculatory duct obstruction

As with many other causes of male-factor infertility, there are multiple treatment options for infertile couples in whom the male partner has ejaculatory duct obstruction. To obtain improved chances at natural conception, men with ejaculatory duct obstruction may undergo transurethral resection of the ejaculatory ducts. For men with partial ejaculatory duct obstruction and motile sperm in the ejaculate, intrauterine insemination (IUI) or in-vitro fertilization (IVF) with or without intracytoplasmic sperm injection (ICSI) are treatment options, depending on individual semen parameters. For men who are azoospermic and suffer from ejaculatory duct obstruction, epididymal or testicular sperm extraction in conjunction with IVF/ICSI is an option to attain a pregnancy. **Before surgical therapy for correction of ejaculatory duct obstruction is undertaken a complete evaluation of the female partner should be performed, to exclude any female factors that may prevent natural conception.**

Transurethral resection of the ejaculatory ducts

Transurethral resection of the ejaculatory ducts (TURED) was first described by Farley and Barnes in

1973 [28]. In 1978, Porch reported the first pregnancy after a male with ejaculatory duct obstruction was treated with resection of the ejaculatory ducts [29]. Since these first reports, multiple different adjuncts to this procedure have been described to increase success rates, decrease morbidity, and avoid unnecessary resections. Transurethral resection of the ejaculatory ducts is carried out with the patient in the lithotomy position, usually under general or spinal anesthesia. Typically, opacification of the seminal vesicles and ejaculatory ducts is performed by either vasography or transrectal ultrasound-guided seminal vesiculography using contrast mixed with dilute methylene blue. The addition of one of these procedures lends multiple advantages. First, with each of these options fluid from either the vasa or the seminal vesicles can be sampled to confirm the presence of sperm, therefore confirming spermatogenesis in azoospermic males. Also, if sperm are present in the seminal vesicles at the time of seminal vesiculography the diagnosis of obstruction is supported. Vasography and seminal vesiculography may also confirm obstruction radiographically. Finally, inclusion of dilute methylene blue in the contrast media aids in guidance during resection. In patients with Müllerian or Wolffian cysts, simultaneous imaging with transrectal ultrasonography may also be helpful in guiding resection. **Resection of the ducts may be carried out with a standard 24 French resectoscope, resecting the proximal portion of the verumontanum (cephalad) to include the ejaculatory ducts** (Fig. 23.5). If a Müllerian or Wolffian duct cyst is present the cyst only needs to be unroofed to decompress the cyst and open the ejaculatory ducts (an optical urethrotome, Turner-Warwick, Collins hook, or Nd:YAG laser can also be used to unroof cystic lesions

425

Table 23.1. Success rates of transurethral resection of the ejaculatory ducts. Where possible, success rates of complete versus partial obstruction are differentiated [12,13,33–40]

Reference	Number of patients	Successful improvement of semen parameters	Successful pregnancy
Overall cases of ejaculatory duct obstruction			
Kadioglu, 2001 [33]	38	74%	13%
Turek, 1996 [34]	46	65%	20%
Meacham, 1993 [13]	24	50%	29%
Weintraub, 1993 [35]	5	80%	40%
Pryor, 1991 [12] [a]	12	83%	42%
Carson, 1984 [36]	4	75%	25%
Vicente, 1983 [37]	9	33%	11%
Amelar and Dubin, 1982 [38]	6	33%	17%
Complete obstruction			
Kadioglu, 2001 [33]	22	59%	9%
Turek, 1996 [34]	22	60%	18%
Partial obstruction			
Kadioglu, 2001 [33]	16	94%	19%
Netto, 1998 [39]	14	57%	43%
Turek, 1996 [34]	24	71%	40%
Goldwasser, 1985 [40]	4	75%	25%

[a] Only patients undergoing transurethral resection of the ejaculatory ducts were included in this table

[12,30–32]). If stenosis of the ducts or a calculus is the cause of obstruction, then resection must be carried out along the course of the ducts until the site of obstruction has been cleared. In both situations, relief of obstruction may be confirmed cystoscopically by direct visualization of efflux of methylene blue from the ducts either spontaneously or with gentle pressure on the seminal vesicles during a digital rectal examination. The use of cautery is minimized so as to avoid devascularization and stricturing of the ejaculatory ducts. A transurethral catheter is left for 24 hours and semen analysis is performed six weeks to three months post-resection.

Success rates of transurethral resection of the ejaculatory ducts

Overall, with TURED, approximately 50–90% of patients will experience improvement of semen parameters, and 9–43% of men will attain a natural pregnancy (Table 23.1) [12,13,33–40]. Several studies have tried to identify characteristics of men likely to have successful outcomes. Men with congenital causes for their obstruction do better with TURED than those with acquired causes for obstruction [39,40]. Better

outcomes have also occurred in men with partial ejaculatory duct obstruction than in those with complete ejaculatory duct obstruction [33]. **Also men with midline ejaculatory duct cysts and dilated seminal vesicles have been reported to have the greatest improvement in semen parameters** [33]. Interestingly, some patients (13%) may have improvement in semen volume with continued azoospermia [34], and a second site of obstruction may be a possibility in these men.

Potential complications of transurethral resection of the ejaculatory ducts

TURED has an overall complication rate of 20% [34]. Table 23.2 presents a complete list of potential complications [34,39,41–43]. **Stricturing of the resected ejaculatory ducts may represent the most significant complication in regard to fertility, and may occur immediately or in a delayed fashion.** A small fraction of men with partial ejaculatory duct obstruction and sperm in the ejaculate preoperatively may be rendered azoospermic with TURED [34,39]. Delayed stricture rates for this procedure may be significant, as demonstrated by Turek et al., who reported that 43%

Table 23.2. Potential complications of transurethral resection of ejaculatory ducts [34,39,41–43]

Potential complications of transurethral resection of the ejaculatory ducts
Retrograde ejaculation
Bladder neck contracture
Urine reflux into the ejaculatory ducts
Chronic or recurrent epididymitis
Delayed stricture of resected ejaculatory ducts
Postvoid dribbling
Urinary tract infection
Hematuria
Rectal injury
External sphincter injury and incontinence
Transient urinary retention

of patients with long-term follow-up ($n = 7$) and initial improvement in semen analysis exhibited declining semen parameters six months or more after surgery [34]. Orhan *et al.* describe a case of successful correction of secondary ejaculatory duct obstruction after transurethral resection of the ejaculatory ducts with a repeat TURED [44]. Reflux of urine into the seminal vesicles, likely secondary to resection of the normal antireflux mechanism of the ejaculatory ducts, may cause postvoid leakage of urine [34,41]. Also, contamination of semen with urine may impair sperm function and may explain lower than expected pregnancy rates in men with improvement of semen parameters [42]. Finally, reflux of urine into the ejaculatory ducts may lead to recurrent or chronic epididymitis.

Alternatives to transurethral resection of the ejaculatory ducts

Several alternatives to TURED exist for treatment of ejaculatory duct obstruction. Ejaculatory duct stones, which can be identified within an ejaculatory duct orifice at the time of cystoscopy, may be extracted, with resultant resolution of obstruction [45,46]. For patients with stenotic ejaculatory ducts, balloon dilation has also been described via a retrograde and antegrade approach. In retrograde approaches, partial resection of the verumontanum is sometimes necessary to allow access to the ducts [4]. In antegrade balloon dilation of the ejaculatory ducts, access to the ducts is achieved via transrectal ultrasound-guided seminal vesicle puncture to place the initial wire. This wire can then be

retrieved through the urethra with a rigid cystoscope to allow transurethral placement of the balloon dilator [47,48]. Currently, only case reports of balloon dilation of the ejaculatory ducts have been reported, and overall success rates for this procedure are not available. Couples who do not desire surgical correction of ejaculatory duct obstruction, or who have contributing female factors but still desire paternity, may consider epididymal or testicular sperm retrieval for use with an IVF/ICSI cycle (see Chapters 22 and 29). Couples should be reminded that adoption and donor insemination are options for all infertile couples to attain parenthood.

Summary

Ejaculatory duct obstruction is an uncommon but potentially correctable cause of male-factor infertility. Identification of patients with ejaculatory duct obstruction requires a high index of suspicion followed by a diagnosis supported by appropriate findings on physical examination, hormone studies, semen analysis, and transrectal ultrasound. There are multiple findings on transrectal ultrasound that support the diagnosis of obstruction, including dilated ejaculatory ducts, dilated seminal vesicles, ejaculatory duct stones, or prostatic cysts. Identification of sperm in aspirated seminal vesicle fluid or obstruction on seminal vesiculography or vasography can be used to confirm the diagnosis at the time of transurethral resection of ejaculatory ducts. Treatment of ejaculatory duct obstruction with TURED yields improvement of semen parameters in approximately 50–80% of patients and pregnancies in approximately 10–40% of couples. Complications of TURED include bleeding, infection, recurrent epididymitis, postvoid dribbling, retrograde ejaculation, and bladder neck contracture. Successful treatment may allow men who are azoospermic to conceive naturally, and in other cases may allow patients to graduate from one assisted reproductive technique, such as in-vitro fertilization, to less complex and expensive forms of assisted reproduction, such as intrauterine insemination [33].

References

[1] Girgis SM, Etriby A, El-Hefnawy H, Kahil S. Aspermia: a survey of 49 cases. *Fertil Steril* 1968; **19**: 580–8.

[2] Hendry WF, Pryor JP. Müllerian duct (prostatic utricle) cyst: diagnosis and treatment in subfertile males. *Br J Urol* 1992; **69**: 79–82.

[3] Jarow JP, Espeland MA, Lipshultz LI. Evaluation of the azoospermic patient. *J Urol* 1989; **142**: 62–5.

[4] Schlegel PN. Management of ejaculatory duct obstruction. In: Lipshultz LI, Howards SS, eds. *Infertility in the Male*, 3rd edn. St. Louis, MO: Mosby Year Book, 1997.

[5] Kim ED, Onel E, Honig SC, Lipshultz LI. The prevalence of cystic abnormalities of the prostate involving the ejaculatory ducts as detected by transrectal ultrasound. *Int Urol Nephrol* 1997; **29**: 647–52.

[6] Nagler HM, Rotman M, Zoltan E, Fisch H. The natural history of partial ejaculatory duct obstruction. *J Urol* 2002; **167**: 253–4.

[7] Sadler TW. Urogenital system. In: *Langman's Medical Embryology*. Baltimore, MD: Lippincott Williams and Wilkins, 2006: 229–56.

[8] Nguyen HT, Etzell J, Turek PJ. Normal human ejaculatory duct anatomy: a study of cadaveric and surgical specimens. *J Urol* 1996; **155**: 1639–42.

[9] Jarow JP. Transrectal ultrasonography of infertile men. *Fertil Steril* 1993; **60**: 1035–9.

[10] McCarthy JF, Fitter S, Klemperer P. Anatomical and histological study of the verumontanum with especial reference to the ejaculatory ducts. *J Urol* 1924; **17**: 1–16.

[11] McMahon S. An anatomic study by injection technique of the ejaculatory ducts and their relations. *J Urol* 1938; **39**: 422–43.

[12] Pryor JP, Hendry WF. Ejaculatory duct obstruction in subfertile males: analysis of 87 patients. *Fertil Steril* 1991; **56**: 725–30.

[13] Meacham RB, Hellerstein DK, Lipshultz LI. Evaluation and treatment of ejaculatory duct obstruction in the infertile male. *Fertil Steril* 1993; **59**: 393–7.

[14] Hellerstein DK, Meacham RB, Lipshultz LI. Transrectal ultrasound and partial ejaculatory duct obstruction in male infertility. *Urology* 1992; **39**: 449–52.

[15] Mayersak JS. Urogenital sinus-ejaculatory duct cyst: a case report with a proposed clinical classification and review of the literature. *J Urol* 1989; **142**: 1330–2.

[16] Meschede D, Dworniczak B, Behre HM, *et al.* CFTR gene mutations in men with bilateral ejaculatory-duct obstruction and anomalies of the seminal vesicles. *Am J Hum Genet* 1997 **61**: 1200–2.

[17] Littrup PJ, Lee F, McLeary RD, *et al.* Transrectal US of the seminal vesicles and ejaculatory ducts: clinical correlation. *Radiology*. 1988 **168**: 625–8.

[18] Jarow JP, Espeland MA, Lipshultz LI. Evaluation of the azoospermic patient. *J Urol* 1989; **142**: 62–5.

[19] Jarow JP. Transrectal ultrasonography in the diagnosis and management of ejaculatory duct obstruction. *J Androl* 1996; **17**: 467–72.

[20] Beiswanger JC, Deaton JL, Jarow JP. Partial ejaculatory duct obstruction causing early demise of sperm. *Urology* 1998; **51**: 125–7.

[21] Fisch H, Lambert SM, Goluboff ET. Management of ejaculatory duct obstruction: etiology, diagnosis, and treatment. *World J Urol* 2006; **24**: 604–10.

[22] Nagler HM, Thomas AJ Jr. Testicular biopsy and vasography in the evaluation of male infertility. *Urol Clin North Am* 1987; **14**: 167–76.

[23] Belker AM, Steinbock GS. Transrectal prostate ultrasonography as a diagnostic and therapeutic aid for ejaculatory duct obstruction. *J Urol* 1990; **144**: 356–8.

[24] Jarow JP. Transrectal ultrasonography of infertile men. *Fertil Steril* 1993; **60**: 1035–9.

[25] Jarow JP. Seminal vesicle aspiration in the management of patients with ejaculatory duct obstruction. *J Urol* 1994; **152**: 899–901.

[26] Purohit RS, Wu DS, Shinohara K, Turek PJ. A prospective comparison of 3 diagnostic methods to evaluate ejaculatory duct obstruction. *J Urol* 2004; **171**: 232–5.

[27] Engin G, Kadioglu A, Orhan I, Akdol S, Rozanes I. Transrectal US and endorectal MR imaging in partial and complete obstruction of the seminal duct system: a comparative study. *Acta Radiol* 2000; **41**: 288–95.

[28] Farley S, Barnes R. Stenosis of ejaculatory ducts treated by endoscopic resection. *J Urol* 1973; **109**: 664–6.

[29] Porch PP. Aspermia owing to obstruction of distal ejaculatory duct and treatment by transurethral resection. *J Urol* 1978; **119**: 141–2.

[30] Dik P, Lock TM, Schrier BP, ZeijlemakerBY, Boon TA. Transurethral marsupalization of a medial prostatic cyst in patients with prostatitis-like symptoms. *J Urol* 1996; **155**: 1301–4.

[31] Cornel EB, Dohle GR, Meuleman EJ. Transurethral deroofing of midline cyst for subfertile men. *Hum Reprod* 1999; **14**: 2297–300.

[32] Halpern EJ, Hirsch IH. Sonographically guided transurethral laser incision of a Müllerian duct cyst for treatment of ejaculatory duct obstruction . *AJR Am J Roentgenol* 2000; **175**: 77–8.

[33] Kadioglu A, Cayan S, Tefekli A, *et al.* Does response to treatment of ejaculatory duct obstruction in infertile men vary with pathology? *Fertil Steril* 2001; **76**: 138–42.

[34] Turek PJ, Magana JO, Lipshultz LI. Semen parameters before and after transurethral surgery for ejaculatory duct obstruction. *J Urol* 1996; **155**: 1291–3.

[35] Weintraub MP, De Mouy E, Hellstrom WJ. Newer modalities in the diagnosis and treatment of ejaculatory duct obstruction. *J Urol* 1993; **150**: 1150–4.

[36] Carson CC. Transurethral resection for ejaculatory duct stenosis and oligospermia. *Fertil Steril* 1984; **41**: 482–4.

[37] Vicente J, del Portillo L, Pomerol MM. Endoscopic surgery in distal obstruction of the ejaculatory ducts. *Eur Urol* 1983; **9**: 338.

[38] Amelar RD, Dubin L. Ejaculatory duct obstruction. In: Garcia CR, Mastroiani L, Amelar RD, Dubin L, eds. *Current Therapy of Infertility*. Trenton, NJ: BC Decker, 1982: 80–2.

[39] Netto NR, Esteves SC, Neves PA. Transurethral resection of partially obstructed ejaculatory ducts: seminal parameters and pregnancy outcomes according to the etiology of obstruction. *J Urol* 1998; **159**: 2048–53.

[40] Goldwasser BZ, Weinerth JL, Carson CC. Ejaculatory duct obstruction: the case for aggressive diagnosis and treatment. *J Urol* 1985; **134**: 964–6.

[41] Goluboff ET, Kaplan SA, Fisch H. Seminal vesicle urinary reflux as a complication of transurethral resection of ejaculatory ducts. *J Urol* 1995; **153**: 1234–5.

[42] Vazquez-Levin MH, Dressler KP, Nagler HM. Urine contamination of seminal fluid after transurethral resection of the ejaculatory ducts. *J Urol* 1994; **152**: 2049–52.

[43] Popken G, Wetterauer U, Schultze-Seemann W, Deckart A, Sommerkamp H. Transurethral resection of cystic and non-cystic ejaculatory duct obstructions. *Int J Androl* 1998; **21**: 196–200.

[44] Orhan I, Onur R, Ardicoglu A, Semercioz A, Koksal IT. Secondary ejaculatory duct obstruction: management by secondary transurethral resection of ejaculatory duct. *Arch Androl* 2005; **51**: 221–3.

[45] Conn IG, Peeling WB, Clements R. Complete resolution of a large seminal vesicle cyst: evidence for an obstructive aetiology. *Br J Urol* 1992; **69**: 636–9.

[46] Gordon Z, Monga M. Endoscopic extraction of an ejaculatory duct calculus to treat obstructive azoospermia. *J Endourol* 2001; **15**: 949–50.

[47] Jarow JP, Zagoria RJ. Antegrade ejaculatory duct recanalization and dilation. *Urology* 1995; **46**: 743–6.

[48] Lawler LP, Cosin O, Jarow JP, Kim HS. Transrectal US-guided seminal vesiculography and ejaculatory duct recanalization and balloon dilation for treatment of chronic pelvic pain. *J Vasc Interv Radiol* 2006; **17**: 169–73.

Nonsurgical treatment of male infertility: specific therapy

Jesse N. Mills and Randall B. Meacham

Introduction

Male-factor infertility is a multi-faceted problem. **Its treatment can be divided into surgical and nonsurgical modalities.** This chapter will focus on nonsurgical management. Once the etiology has been identified and surgical treatment has been ruled out, it is helpful to categorize nonsurgical therapy on the basis of the various factors potentially responsible for infertility. When the broad categories of male infertility are divided into pretesticular, intratesticular, and post-testicular, nonsurgical problems usually fall into either pretesticular or intratesticular causes, with a minority of post-testicular issues. Table 24.1 lists the various pretesticular, intratesticular, and post-testicular causes of infertility that are potentially amenable to a nonsurgical treatment option. The next part of this chapter will discuss targeted nonsurgical therapy for male-factor infertility. Many agents, prescription and over the counter, have been tried to improve semen parameters. One major development in the field of male infertility is the explosion of information and sales of fertility enhancement agents over the internet. To that end, we will briefly discuss some of the therapies patients may be exploring through this new medium.

Medications responsible for male-factor infertility

Many medications have been implicated as potential inhibitors of male fertility. **A careful history should include discussion of prescription drugs, over-the-counter medicines, and herbal supplements the man is taking. Additionally, a social history is important to rule out lifestyle factors such as tobacco, alcohol, and recreational drug use.** Many medications cause alterations in all categories of male infertility. Cimetidine, now an over-the-counter heartburn medication, suppresses the hypothalamic–pituitary–gonadal (HPG) axis in a reversible manner [1]. Cimetidine has also been linked to a reversible hyperprolactinemia [2]. Antihypertensives, as a class, can have myriad deleterious effects on male fertility. Calcium channel blockers interfere with the acrosome reaction [3]. Discontinuing calcium channel blockers can restore fertility in men using this type of medication. In the peripubertal mouse, calcium channel blockers at high doses cause spermatogenic arrest at the elongated spermatid stage [4]. Angiotensin-converting enzyme inhibitors do not appear to adversely affect fertility or sexual function, and therefore offer a good alternative for hypertensive subfertile men [5]. Spironolactone, a potassium-sparing diuretic, inhibits the HPG axis and blocks binding of dihydrotestosterone to its receptor. This inhibits spermatogenesis and reduces libido [5]. **A general rule of thumb for any male trying to conceive is to limit all medications, prescription or over the counter, when attempting conception.** When it is impossible to discontinue certain medications, such patients should seek out alternatives that are not as detrimental to fertility.

Illicit drugs, alcohol, and tobacco

Avoiding illicit drugs, drinking alcohol in moderation, and abstaining from tobacco products are good recommendations for any physician to make to a patient. In the subfertile male, this advice especially holds true. Consumption of marijuana has long been known to alter the HPG axis, decrease serum testosterone, and cause gynecomastia [6]. A direct spermatotoxic effect of marijuana has also been reported. Recent evidence demonstrates that human sperm express cannabinoid receptors. Stimulating these receptors with marijuana derivatives inhibits sperm motility, the acrosome reaction, and mitochondrial activity [7]. Its in-vivo effects are less well documented, but one could surmise that marijuana use should be avoided while attempting conception.

Infertility in the Male, 4th edition, ed. Larry I. Lipshultz, Stuart S. Howards, and Craig S. Niederberger. Published by Cambridge University Press. © Cambridge University Press 2009.

Table 24.1. Pretesticular, intratesticular, and post-testicular causes of infertility that are potentially amenable to a nonsurgical treatment option.

Pretesticular	Intratesticular	Post-testicular
Medications	Medications	Medications
Systemic infection	Genital tract infection	Genital tract infection
Hypogonadism	Hyperthermia	Ejaculatory dysfunction
Occupational exposures	Occupational exposures	Erectile dysfunction
Illicit drug use	Radiation therapy	

Alcohol use in the infertile male is a subject of some controversy. It is indisputable that alcoholism, with its hepatotoxic-induced estrogenic effects including gynecomastia, depressed libido, and erectile dysfunction, inhibits male fertility. Semen quality of social drinkers does not appear to be impaired, however [8]. Interestingly, animal studies show increased testicular apoptosis in rat germ cells treated with acute ingestion of ethanol [9]. It is not known what effect acute alcohol ingestion has on the human testis. **However, it may be prudent for men with marginal semen quality to abstain from alcohol during periods of attempted conception if no other causes of subfertility can be determined.**

Tobacco use poses a dramatic health risk that spans many organ systems. Its effects on infertility are less clear, but certainly any effort a physician exerts to encourage a man to quit smoking is worthwhile from a public health standpoint. One recent study demonstrated a dramatic decrease in seminal ascorbic acid levels in men who smoked over 20 cigarettes a day. Ascorbic acid is a potent antioxidant which is thought to protect sperm from oxidative damage. Additionally, in this study, high levels of ascorbic acid correlated positively with increased sperm concentration and percent motile sperm, and negatively with abnormal morphology [10]. Earlier studies have also shown that cigarette smoking perturbs sperm concentration, morphology, and motility [11].

Infections

Genitourinary infections in the male are an uncommon but potentially treatable source of infertility. *Chlamydia trachomatis* **has long been studied as a putative disrupter of male fertility**. Its exact role in male fertility, however, remains controversial. **It is by far the most prevalent sexually transmitted bacterial pathogen worldwide.** Up to 50% of men and 70% of women are asymptomatically infected with chlamydia. Couple this fact with the high prevalence of the disease

in men of reproductive age and one can see the motivation to investigate chlamydia as a source of unexplained infertility. It has been demonstrated that the elementary body form of chlamydia can enter the human sperm head. Once in the sperm, the elementary body transforms into the reticulate body and invades the nucleus. Once in the nucleus, the reticulate body "hijacks" the nuclear machinery to replicate. This is where our knowledge stops. We still do not understand how or if chlamydia impairs sperm function. One theory is that chlamydia causes urethritis, which leads to epididymo-orchitis. Epididymo-orchitis in turn is linked to obstructive infertility. Many studies have seen a correlation between high levels of antichlamydial antibodies and lower median sperm counts [12]. Chlamydia infection has also been shown to cause asthenospermia. Treatment with azithromycin or minocycline in infected men may improve sperm motility [13,14]. Does any of this translate to higher pregnancy rates? A recent prospective study of subfertile couples in an in-vitro fertilization program found no decreased success in the cohort of couples with either past or active chlamydial infection [15]. Men with azoospermia and cryptozoospermia were excluded without further workup from the study. This study also found no difference in sperm motility between infected and uninfected men. Prior to in-vitro fertilization (IVF) cycles, infected couples were treated with a 14-day course of doxycycline. This may explain how the researchers found no significant difference between infected and uninfected couples. It does not explain why no differences in motility were seen, however, as sperm samples were obtained from actively infected men. **The best evidence and common sense suggest that men with pyospermia, active urethral symptoms, or otherwise unexplained asthenospermia should be evaluated and, if necessary, treated for a chlamydial infection.**

The human immunodeficiency virus (HIV) and male infertility is becoming an area of increased interest as the advent of effective antiretroviral agents has dramatically improved life span and quality of life among infected individuals. Men with HIV may wish to become fathers. Sperm washing has increased the safety of conception with an infected male [16]. Infected men may have abnormal semen parameters, however, that can make conception more difficult. Leukocytospermia is almost always seen in men with HIV. HIV-positive men also have impaired sperm motility [17]. There are no data to confirm that spermatozoa are directly infected with HIV. The effect on male infertility of antiretroviral medications, the mainstay of HIV therapy, is not clear. One study noted minimal change in semen parameters in men before and after institution of HIV therapy. The effect of antiretroviral therapy on mitochondria may explain the impaired sperm motility seen in many studies. However, as previously noted, untreated men also have impaired semen motility [18]. Once sperm are harvested and washed, both intrauterine insemination (IUI) and intracytoplasmic sperm injection (ICSI) have been employed successfully, and there are strong proponents of each method.

Debate has smoldered for decades as to whether *Ureaplasma urealyticum* is pathogenic in urologic conditions ranging from infection to infertility. As a urethral pathogen, ureaplasma may be nothing more than an innocent colonizer. It is difficult to culture only ureaplasma without growing many other bacteria. One recent study from China found that men infected with ureaplasma had lower seminal pH and higher seminal viscosity [19]. This study did not look for the presence of commensurate bacteria, however. Further, no study has looked at fertility rates after treating the infection, so the clinical significance of infection remains uncertain.

Targeted therapy

Where much has been tried in the treatment of male infertility, much has failed. This section will review the many medical treatments that have been employed, and critically analyze what works and what does not. Clomiphene citrate has been used since the early 1990s to stimulate spermatogenesis in the man with nonobstructive azoospermia [20]. Clomiphene stimulates secretion of gonadotropin-releasing hormone (GnRH) from the hypothalamus, which, in turn, stimulates the release of gonadotropins from the anterior pituitary. The end result of this hormone cascade is increasing levels of intratesticular testosterone. A recent multicenter study looked at the effects of clomiphene on 42 men with nonobstructive azoospermia [21]. The men underwent pretreatment biopsy, and 42.9% had maturation arrest with 57.1% demonstrating hypospermatogenesis. Every-other-day dosing of 25–75 mg of clomiphene was given to titrate to a morning serum testosterone concentration between 600 and 800 ng/dL. Treatment continued for 3–9 months, and 64.3% of men demonstrated sperm in their ejaculate with a mean density of 3.8 million/mL. One couple went on to spontaneous pregnancy, while the remainder employed IVF or ICSI. The 35.7% of men who remained azoospermic underwent testicular biopsy and sperm extraction and were successful with ICSI. Clomiphene citrate may also be an effective therapy for men with hypogonadotropic hypogonadism (HH). A recent multicenter study evaluated 10 men with various etiologies of hypogonadotropic hypogonadism, eight of whom were azoospermic and two oligospermic [22]. Four of the 10 men were treated with clomiphene and six with either human chorionic gonadotropin (hCG) or a combination of hCG and follicle-stimulating hormone (FSH) for 3–6 months. Two of the clomiphene-treated men and two treated with hCG/FSH initiated pregnancies. Although this is a small study, it is encouraging that the rare infertile male with HH may benefit from clomiphene, a well-tolerated, relatively inexpensive oral medication.

Kallmann syndrome is a rare subset of HH associated with other midline defects including anosmia. The syndrome is inherited most commonly in an X-linked fashion but can also be transmitted in an autosomal dominant or autosomal recessive pattern. The X-linked form of Kallmann syndrome is tied to a defect in the *KAL1* gene, which codes for a neuronal adhesion molecule that guides migration of luteinizing hormone (LH)-secreting neurons to the basal hypothalamus. Spermatogenesis in men with Kallmann syndrome has traditionally and effectively been instituted with combination human chorionic gonadotropin/human menopausal gonadotropin (hCG and hMG). Therapy intended to initiate spermatogenesis begins with 2000 international units of hCG administered subcutaneously three times per week. If sperm are not present in the semen after six months of treatment, FSH therapy is started in the form of hMG, at 75 units subcutaneously three times weekly [23]. In a recent 30-year retrospective study in Japan, most patients achieved peak serum testosterone levels within 24 months using a dosing regimen of 3000 international units of hCG and 75 international units of hMG intramuscularly twice weekly for 12–48 months [24]. In this same study, which included both men with Kallmann's and men with other HH etiologies, sperm production was directly correlated with post-treatment testicular volume. Since men with Kallmann syndrome typically have small testicles secondary to the complete lack of endogenous pulsatile GnRH release, less than 36% of these men responded to therapy. GnRH infusion pumps have been employed in men with Kallmann syndrome with some degree of success. Pulsatile infusion-pump therapy consists of a portable pump with a reservoir filled with GnRH. A subcutaneous needle is inserted into the abdominal wall and GnRH is secreted in doses of 5–20 µg every two hours. The needle is changed every two days [25]. This therapy continues for four months or longer before sperm are seen in the ejaculate. Because of the cumbersome nature of this therapy, it generally is reserved for men who do not respond to gonadotropin therapy.

Another endocrine disorder, hyperprolactinemia, is also responsible for male infertility. Prolactin inhibits LH action on Leydig cells. Prolactin receptors are also present in the first layer of the seminiferous epithelium. This suggests prolactin also has a more direct effect on spermatogenesis, but it is not clear what that effect may be [26]. The first responsibility to a man presenting with hyperprolactinemia is to rule out more ominous causes of elevated hormone levels. **Although the incidence of a prolactin-secreting pituitary adenoma is low, it is the most common functional pituitary tumor.** In people between 20 and 50 years of age, prolactinoma is 10 times more common in women, but men more frequently present with mass effect symptoms such as headaches or ocular field defects suggestive of macroprolactinoma [27]. The initial workup of a man with an elevated serum prolactin level should include a careful history and review of systems, including questions about headaches, visual disturbances, galactorrhea, loss of libido, and erectile dysfunction. A baseline serum testosterone should also be drawn to monitor response to future therapy. Hyperprolactinemia usually causes hypogonadism, and treatment of the prolactinoma usually reverses the hypogonadism. Roughly one-third of men with hyperprolactinemia have a macroprolactinoma as evinced by mass effect symptoms [27]. Magnetic resonance imaging (MRI) of the brain, therefore, is warranted to determine the presence and size of the tumor. **Usually, a macroadenoma is greater than 1 cm in greatest dimension and has a concomitant serum prolactin level greater than 200 µg/L.** A microprolactinoma is less than 1 cm in greatest dimension on

MRI, and is typically associated with a serum prolactin level of 50 µg/L [28]. Treatment of prolactinomas usually depends on size. Patients with hyperprolactinemia and normal imaging studies, and those with microadenomas, can be treated with dopaminergic agonists such as bromocriptine or cabergoline. Cabergoline has stood up in multiple randomized prospective and retrospective trials as superior to bromocriptine with a more benign side-effect profile [27]. For microprolactinomas, cabergoline is dosed at 0.5 mg orally once weekly and titrated up to 0.5 mg orally twice weekly after the first week. Every six months, serum prolactin and testosterone levels should be drawn, and escalation of dosage up to 1 mg twice weekly can be made to keep serum prolactin levels under 15 µg/L [28]. Repeat MRI is sometimes performed. However, one can infer from symptom improvement and normalization of serum prolactin and testosterone that the tumor has shrunk.

Macroadenomas have warranted a referral to a neurosurgeon for transphenoidal or, more recently, endoscopic removal. However, recent studies suggest that even macroadenomas often can be successfully treated with dopaminergic agonists. A small study of 12 men with macroadenomas over 4 cm in size showed normalization of prolactin levels in 10 men after long-term (up to 84 months) cabergoline therapy [29]. Nine of the 12 men had visual field defects prior to treatment. After treatment, eight of the nine had either normal visual fields or improved visual fields. Eight of the 12 men had normalization of their serum testosterone after concluding treatment.

In addition to normalizing serum testosterone levels and improving erectile function and libido, medical therapy for prolactinomas can also improve semen analysis profiles. In one study, statistically significant improvements in sperm count were seen in hyperprolactinemic men treated with a six-month course of cabergoline [30].

L-carnitine has long been studied as a potential profertility agent. Several unproven mechanisms have been proposed for the efficacy of L-carnitine and its derivative, L-acetylcarnitine. First, it shuttles long-chain fatty acids into the mitochondria for intracellular energy production. It also binds acetyl groups for future energy production. There are also some data to support its role as an antioxidant. Men with idiopathic infertility have been shown to have low levels of seminal carnitine [31]. This observation led to the hypothesis that supplementing L-carnitine could result in improved fertility. A number of uncontrolled studies have demonstrated reasonable results and, with few to no side effects, L-carnitine has become a popular supplement during the past 10 years [32]. Increased scrutiny has fallen upon the early promising results, however. Two randomized controlled trials have been published over the past two years. An Italian study showed a modest improvement in sperm kinetics in men with idiopathic asthenospermia treated with L-carnitine and L-acetylcarnitine [33]. The study enrolled 60 men aged 20–40 who had sperm concentrations greater than 20 million/mL with motility less than 50% and normal morphology, 45 of them randomized to the treatment arm and 15 to the placebo. After six months of daily therapy, men in the combined L-carnitine and L-acetylcarnitine group had a 34.46% improvement of sperm total motility with standard deviations of 26.2%. The placebo group saw a 0.52% improvement with standard deviation of 17.43%. There were 12 spontaneous pregnancies during the nine-month observation period. Three of these pregnancies were achieved by men in the placebo arm. An American study did not demonstrate similarly positive results, however [34]. In a randomized, double-blind, placebo-controlled trial enrolling 21 men, 12 in the treatment arm, 9 in the control arm, L-carnitine was given for 24 weeks to infertile men between the ages of 18 to 65. The sperm count inclusion criterion was lower in this study, at greater than 5 million/mL. At 24 weeks, there was no statistically significant improvement in motility between study arms. There was one spontaneous pregnancy in the placebo arm and one assisted pregnancy in the treatment arm. Neither study described any significant side effects. With conflicting data, it is difficult to draw any meaningful conclusions. Commercially available preparations of L-carnitine and L-acetylcarnitine cost approximately $100 United States dollars per month. At treatment times of up to six months, this may pose a financial burden on infertile couples.

In addition to L-carnitine, many other supplements have been investigated as fertility aids. Zinc and folic acid supplementation appears to improve sperm concentrations in a subgroup of infertile men. A Dutch study randomized subfertile men (sperm concentration 5–20 million/mL) to a placebo arm, a daily zinc supplement arm (66 mg/day), a daily folic acid supplement arm (5 mg/day), and a combination arm of zinc and folic acid [35]. Median sperm concentrations in the pretreatment arm were 7.0 million/mL, and posttreatment they rose to 8.0 million/mL. Fertile men in this study also saw an increase in sperm concentrations

from 65.5 million/mL to 77.5 million/mL with a P-value < 0.01. The study did not follow the subfertile men to assess pregnancy rates, so these data remain intriguing but not necessarily clinically useful.

Environmental factors

Men are products of their environment. What men eat, where they live and work, and how they spend their leisure time can all influence the quality of their sperm. A careful patient history and counseling a patient to avoid harmful environmental exposures may be important to improve fertility outcomes.

Xenobiotics, compounds that are not naturally found in a biologic system, adversely affect semen in multitudinous ways. The chemical industry has introduced hundreds of xenobiotics to humans over the last half-century. Pesticides such as 1,2-dibromo-3-chloropropane (DBCP) interfere with sperm production and maturation in humans [36]. Men working in the agricultural industry, therefore, may be at risk for problems related to spermatogenesis. Additional organochlorine pesticides such as 1,1,1-trichloro-2,2-bis(p-chlorophenyl) ethane (DDT) all inhibit spermatogenesis. **Although DDT has been banned in the United States for nearly 40 years, it is still used in developing nations and will be entrenched in the soil for decades due to its long half-life.** The degradation product of DDT, dichlorodiphenyldichloroethylene (p,p'-DDE), binds to the estrogen receptor and also blocks androgen receptors. Few studies have looked at risks of human exposure to DDE. One Belgian study found decreased sperm concentration, motility, and morphology in subfertile men whose mothers had synchronously high serum concentrations of DDE [37]. This group was controlled for serum DDE concentrations in the affected males, smoking status, and alcohol consumption. It is unclear whether high maternal concentrations of DDE 25 years after conception correlates to maternal DDE levels at time of conception, but it raises more questions regarding the fragility of spermatogenesis and male reproductive development to xenobiotics. Methoxychlor, the pesticide that has replaced DDT in the United States, also exhibits antiandrogen effects and increases spermatogenic cell apoptosis in exposed mice. Vinclozolin, a fungicide used heavily in the wine industry, is another endocrine disruptor that affects both estrogenic and androgenic pathways. It is also known to impose transgenerational damage through the germline. In one particularly interesting study, male mice exposed to vinclozolin were bred to nonexposed females and the male offspring were examined for testicular development and semen analyses [38]. The offspring in the subsequent two unexposed generations had decreases in sperm motility and concentration similar to those in the father.

What is the clinical relevance of these xenobiotics? Many studies have looked at the global decrease in sperm concentration, and increasing incidence of testicular cancer and hypospadias, but no smoking gun has been discovered. A study by Swan investigated semen quality at four prenatal clinics in cities across the United States [39]. Men from the urban centers, Los Angeles, Minneapolis, and New York City, all showed higher sperm concentrations than men from the agricultural area of Columbia, Missouri. Multivariate analyses controlled for abstinence time, age, race, and history of smoking, fever, and sexually transmitted disease. A panel of pesticides was investigated in participants' serum, and all showed higher concentrations in the men from Missouri. Again, **no firm conclusion can be reached that pesticides cause alterations in sperm concentration and function, but it seems prudent to advise subfertile patients to avoid these exposures.**

Electromagnetic fields such as those created by cellular telephones have also been studied as causative factors in male infertility. Although it is difficult to control for all exposures, one can find some correlations between semen parameters and electromagnetic fields. Agarwal *et al.*, from the Cleveland Clinic, recently reported at a national reproductive medicine meeting that men who use a cellular telephone had a linear decline in sperm count, motility, viability, and morphology with increasing usage [40].

What's on the internet?

The internet has become an important part of life for most Americans. Many infertile couples seek information and support from thousands of different websites including academic, commercial, and personal sites. It is therefore important for the clinician to be familiar with what couples may be reading online. There are multiple nonprescription therapies for enhancing male fertility being advertised on the internet. Most of the formulations contain proprietary amounts of L-carnitine, zinc, selenium, and various vitamins. As discussed in a previous section, the efficacy of these supplements is not proven. To that end, the biggest concern about web-based infertility information and therapies is the inability of the consumer to judge veracity. A recent study by Zahalsky *et al.* highlights this situation [41]. The researchers typed "male infertility" into five popular internet search engines and categorized the first 20 resultant websites. **Nearly 70% of the websites were owned by either healthcare professionals or industry. Advertisement was the primary objective of over 70% of these sites. Close to 95% of the sites were targeted to people with no healthcare background.** The researchers then applied credibility criteria established by both the American Medical Association and a nonprofit organization, Health On the Net Foundation. A score of 6 is the highest achievable, and a score of less than 3 indicates a poorly credible site. Only 41.1% of all sites surveyed achieved a score of 4 or higher [41]. Patients will continue to access the internet; whether the information they glean is accurate or useful is quite variable. There currently are no regulations governing content on healthcare websites. It is therefore incumbent upon physicians to be aware of the resources available to their patients, so they can serve as advocates in this process.

References

[1] Van Thiel DH, Gavaler JS, Smith WI, Paul G. Hypothalamic–pituitary–gonadal dysfunction in men using cimetidine. *N Engl J Med* 1979; **300**: 1012–15.

[2] Okada H, Iwamoto T, Fujioka H, *et al.* Hyperprolactinaemia among infertile patients and its effect on sperm functions. *Andrologia* 1994; **28**: 197–202.

[3] Benoff S, Cooper GW, Hurley I, *et al.* The effect of calcium ion channel blockers on sperm fertilization potential, *Fertil Steril* 1994; **62**: 606–17.

[4] Lee JH, Kim H, Kim DH, Gye MC. Effects of calcium channel blockers on the spermatogenesis and gene expression in peripubertal mouse testis. *Arch Androl* 2006; **52**: 311–18.

[5] Monoski M, Nudell D, Lipshultz L. Effects of medical therapy, alcohol and smoking on male fertility. *Contemp Urol* 2002; **14** (6): 57–63.

[6] Kolodny RC, Masters WH, Kolodner RM, Toro G. Depression of plasma testosterone levels after chronic intensive marihuana use. *N Engl J Med* 1974; **290**: 872–4.

[7] Rossato M, Ion Popa F, Ferigo M, Clari G, Foresta C. Human sperm express cannabinoid receptor Cb1, the activation of which inhibits motility, acrosome reaction, and mitochondrial function. *J Clin Endocrinol Metab* 2005; **90**: 984–91.

[8] Nudell DM, Monoski MM, Lipshultz LI. Common medications and drugs: how they affect male fertility. *Urol Clin North Am* 2002; **29**: 965–73.

[9] Zhu Q, Meisinger J, Emanuele NV, *et al.* Ethanol exposure enhances apoptosis within the testes. *Alcohol Clin Exp Res* 2000; **24**: 1550–6.

[10] Mostafa T, Tawadrous G, Roaia MM, *et al*. Effect of smoking on seminal plasma ascorbic acid in infertile and fertile males. *Andrologia* 2006; **38**: 221–4.

[11] Dunphy BC, Barratt CL, von Tongelen BP, Cooke ID. Male cigarette smoking and fecundity in couples attending an infertility clinic. *Andrologia* 1991; **23**: 223–5.

[12] Gonzales GF, Muñoz G, Sánchez R, *et al*. Update on the impact of *Chlamydia trachomatis* infection on male fertility. *Andrologia* 2004; **36**: 1–23.

[13] Rezácová J, Masata J, Pribylová M, Drazd'áková M. *Chlamydia trachomatis* in men with impaired fertility. *Ceska Gynecol* 1999; **64**: 371–5.

[14] Malallah YA, Zissis NP. Effect in minocycline on the sperm count and activity in fertile men with high pus cell count in their seminal fluid. *J Chemother* 1992; **4**: 286–9.

[15] de Barbeyrac B, Papaxanthos-Roche A, Mathieu C, *et al*. *Chlamydia trachomatis* in subfertile couples undergoing an *in vitro* fertilization program: a prospective study. *Eur J Obstet Gynecol Reprod Biol* 2006; **129**: 46–53.

[16] Semprini AE, Levi-Setti P, Bozzo M, *et al*. Insemination of HIV-negative women with processed semen of HIV-positive partners. *Lancet* 1992; **340**: 1317–19.

[17] Umapathy E. STD/HIV association: effects on semen characteristics. *Arch Androl* 2005; **51**: 361–5.

[18] van Leeuwen E, Prins JM, Jurriaans S, *et al*. Reproduction and fertility in human immunodeficiency virus type-1 infection. *Hum Reprod Update* 2007; **13**: 197–206.

[19] Wang Y, Liang CL, Wu JQ, *et al*. Do *Ureaplasma urealyticum* infections in the genital tract affect semen quality? *Asian J Androl* 2006; **8**: 562–8.

[20] Akin JW. The use of clomiphene citrate in the treatment of azoospermia secondary to incomplete androgen resistance. *Fertil Steril* 1993; **59**: 223–7.

[21] Hussein A, Ozgok Y, Ross L, Niederberger C. Clomiphene administration for cases of nonobstructive azoospermia: a multicenter study. *J Androl* 2005; **26**: 787–91.

[22] Whitten SJ, Nangia AK, Kolettis PN. Select patients with hypogonadotropic hypogonadism may respond to treatment with clomiphene citrate. *Fertil Steril* 2006; **86**: 1664–8.

[23] Sigman M, Jarow JP. Male infertility. In: Walsh PC, Retik AB, Vaughan ED, Wein AJ, eds. *Campbell's Urology*, 8th edn. St. Louis, MO: Saunders, 2002: Vol 2, 1475–531.

[24] Miyagawa Y, Tsujimura A, Matsumiya K, *et al*. Outcome of gonadotropin therapy for male hypogonadotropic hypogonadism at university affiliated male infertility centers: a 30-year retrospective study. *J Urol* 2005; **173**: 2072–5.

[25] Zitzmann M, Nieschlag E. Hormone substitution in male hypogonadism. *Mol Cell Endocrinol* 2000; **161**: 73–88.

[26] Nishimura K, Matsumiya K, Tsuboniwa N, *et al*. Bromocriptine for infertile males with mild hyperprolactinemia: hormonal and spermatogenic effects. *Arch Androl* 1999; **43**: 207–13.

[27] Gillam MP, Molitch ME, Lombardi G, Colao A. Advances in the treatment of prolactinomas. *Endocr Rev* 2006; **27**: 485–534.

[28] Colao A, Vitale G, Cappabianca P, *et al*. Outcome of cabergoline treatment in men with prolactinoma: effects of a 24 month treatment on prolactin levels, tumor mass, recovery of pituitary function and semen analysis. *J Clin Endocrinol Metab* 2004; **89**: 1704–11.

[29] Shimon I, Benbassat C, Hadani M. Effectiveness of long-term cabergoline treatment for giant prolactinoma: study of 12 men. *Eur J Endocrinol* 2007; **156**: 225–31.

[30] De Rosa M, Ciccarelli A, Zarrilli S, *et al*. The treatment with cabergoline for 24 months normalizes the quality of seminal fluid in hyperprolactinaemic males. *Clin Endocrinol (Oxf)* 2006 ; **64**: 307–13.

[31] Zöpfgen A, Priem F, Sudhoff F, *et al*. Relationship between semen quality and the seminal plasma components carnitine, alpha-glucosidase, fructose, citrate and granulocyte elastase in infertile men compared with a normal population. *Hum Reprod* 2000; **15**: 840–5.

[32] Vitali G, Parente R, Melotti C. Carnitine supplementation in human idiopathic asthenospermia: clinical results. *Drugs Exp Clin Res* 1995; **21**: 157–9.

[33] Balercia G. Placebo-controlled double-blind randomized trial of the use of l-carnitine, l-acetylcarnitine, or combined l-carnitine and l-acetylcarnitine in men with idiopathic asthenozoospermia. *Fertil Steril* 2005; **84**: 662–71.

[34] Sigman M, Glass S, Campagnone J, Pryor JL. Carnitine for the treatment of idiopathic asthenospermia: a randomized, double-blind, placebo-controlled trial. *Fertil Steril* 2006; **85**: 1409–14.

[35] Ebisch IM, Pierik FH, DE Jong FH, Thomas CM, Steegers-Theunissen RP. Does folic acid and zinc sulphate intervention affect endocrine parameters and sperm characteristics in men? *Int J Androl* 2006; **29**: 339–45.

[36] Aitken RJ, Koopman P, Lewis SE. Seeds of concern. *Nature* 2004; **432**: 48–52.

[37] Charlier CJ, Foidart JM. Comparative study of dichlordiphenyldichlorethylene in blood and semen of two young male populations: lack of relationship to infertility, but evidence of high exposure of the mothers. *Reprod Toxicol* 2005; **20**: 215–20.

[38] Skinner M, Anway D. Seminiferous cord formation and germ-cell programming: epigenetic transgenerational actions of endocrine disruptors. *Ann N Y Acad Sci* 2005; **1061**: 18–32.

[39] Swan S. Semen quality in fertile US men in relation to geographical area and pesticide exposure. *Int J Androl* 2006; **29**: 62–8.

[40] Agarwal A, *et al.* Podium presentation. American Society for Reproductive Medicine (ASRM), New Orleans, LA, 2006.

[41] Zahalsky M, Wilson SR, Di Blasio CJ, Lam S, Nagler H. Male infertility on the internet: an analysis of web-based resources. *BJU Int* 2005; **95**: 481–4.

Chapter

25

Nonsurgical treatment of male infertility: empiric therapy

Karen E. Boyle

Introduction

In medicine, "empiric therapy" is a treatment initiated prior to the determination of a firm diagnosis. Empiric therapy is typically viewed as nonspecific intervention and is often based upon clinical concept and theory without proven efficacy. The term "empiric" is derived from the Greek word *empeirikos*, which means relying on experience only. **Such empiric medical therapy is commonly used not only in the treatment of patients with idiopathic male infertility but also inappropriately in patients who have an uncorrectable cause of their infertility, because the clinician is not aware that the infertility is not reversible, or is at a loss as to what to do in patients who have failed other treatments**.

When a diagnostic evaluation reveals no specific abnormalities to explain a man's infertility, he is said to have idiopathic infertility. Patients with idiopathic infertility not only are frustrated by having no explanation for their problem, but also are surprised by the scarcity of effective medical treatments to improve upon the production and quality of their sperm. The incidence of idiopathic infertility reported in the published retrospective reviews from male infertility clinics has ranged from 5% to 66%, with an average of 25% [1,2]. Idiopathic infertility, therefore, is often the "diagnosis" given to a large number of men seeking evaluation and treatment. Empiric therapy is the only available form of therapy for these patients.

Patients who have a known but untreatable cause of infertility, or patients who fail to respond adequately to specific treatments, are also candidates for such non-specific intervention. Many of the identifiable causes of infertility, including cryptorchidism, testicular torsion, and testicular failure, are not correctable with specific treatments now available. In addition, not all men improve after the application of specific treatments. All of these men are candidates for empiric forms of therapy. Therefore, empiric therapy might be offered

to any infertile man for whom a specific treatment is unavailable or in whom a specific treatment has failed. **Empiric medical therapy is not a specific medical therapy to treat endocrinopathies such as hypogonadotropic hypogonadism, congenital adrenal hyperplasia, hyperprolactinemia, or thyroid dysfunctions.**

A number of different medications have been proposed as empiric therapies for men with infertility. It is difficult, however, to assess the efficacy of these treatments, for a variety of reasons. Sperm quality and count can naturally, but dramatically, vary in the infertile male population. This group of patients is very heterogeneous in terms of etiology and baseline fertility status. Therefore, response to treatment may vary widely, depending on a variety of factors including patient selection, cause of infertility, and fertility status of the spouse.

Many male patients who are labeled as "subfertile" may actually be fertile if they are allowed more time to conceive or if problems in the spouse are resolved. In addition, spontaneous pregnancy rates, independent of any treatment, have been reported to be as high as 60% in couples with suspected male-factor infertility [3]. The inability to predict the spontaneous fertility potential of a patient population with any degree of accuracy makes it extremely important that treatments for infertility be evaluated by prospective, randomized, placebo-controlled clinical trials.

A lack of standardization in patient selection criteria, the extent of partner evaluation and treatment, the dosing regimen, treatment period, and the length of follow-up are just some of the other difficulties that exist in assessing the efficacy of empiric medical therapies. In addition, semen analysis results may vary significantly in an individual patient over time, and the definition of "therapeutic success" has varied from mere improvements in seminal parameters to pregnancy rates [4]. Since it is extremely difficult to satisfy

Infertility in the Male, 4th edition, ed. Larry I. Lipshultz, Stuart S. Howards, and Craig S. Niederberger. Published by Cambridge University Press. © Cambridge University Press 2009.

all of these criteria in the performance of a prospective, double-blinded, crossover, placebo-controlled, randomized study, most of the published studies represent a less than ideal assessment of empiric therapies.

This chapter will review the empiric therapies available today and discuss their mode of action, review published literature on outcomes available, and discuss the evidence for use and dosing recommendations. Tables throughout this chapter are limited to the results of controlled studies reported in the English-language literature.

With the exception of low-dose vitamin supplementation and aromatase inhibitors, empiric therapy is seldom recommended in the treatment of the infertile male. Instead, specific assisted reproductive techniques that have a measurable benefit are typically suggested to the couple with idiopathic male infertility.

Antiestrogen therapy

The hypothalamus is the site of production for the peptide hormone gonadotropin-releasing hormone (GnRH), which is secreted in a carefully timed pulsatile release. GnRH stimulates the synthesis and release of the gonadotropic hormones, luteinizing hormone (LH) and follicle-stimulating hormone (FSH), in the anterior pituitary. LH then stimulates the Leydig cells of the testes to produce testosterone. The current understanding of this hypothalamic–pituitary–gonadal (HPG) axis reveals an absolute dependence of spermatogenesis on normal serum testosterone levels. FSH is required for both the initiation of spermatogenesis and the maintenance of normal sperm production [5]. **Most empiric hormonal therapies are based upon the theory that increasing the amount of circulating testosterone and/or FSH will improve testicular function, specifically spermatogenesis.**

The intact HPG axis also depends on normal levels of circulating steroids (androgens and estrogens) for feedback inhibition of both hypothalamic and pituitary stimulation of the testis [6]. This negative feedback effect of androgens mostly occurs after their conversion to estrogens by aromatization either peripherally or at the target organ (hypothalamus or pituitary). **Therefore, antiestrogens and aromatase enzyme-inhibiting compounds can be used to block this negative feedback effect of steroids on the HPG axis without decreasing the effect of circulating androgens.**

With prevention of the important negative feedback of estrogens to the pituitary and hypothalamus,

LH and FSH release and GnRH stimulation are augmented. Since FSH is extremely important for the initiation and maintenance of spermatogenesis, an increase in FSH release may also further improve sperm production. This results in the stimulation of the testis by both LH and FSH, released by the pituitary gland in response to an increase in hypothalamic secretion of GnRH.

Clomiphene citrate and tamoxifen citrate are estrogen receptor blockers that have been used as empiric treatments for the idiopathic oligospermic male. Acting as competitive inhibitors of estrogen by reversibly binding to estrogen receptors, both can exert a mild estrogenic effect. **The effects of the antiandrogens on the fertility of men with idiopathic subfertility are not impressive. It is important to note, as discussed later, that although an improvement in sperm concentration may sometimes occur, there is little or no demonstrated effect on sperm motility or pregnancy rates.** Also important is that a large number of patients may have an impressive decline in sperm production while being treated by antiandrogens. Patients should be counseled about these potential risks and benefits prior to the initiation of treatment.

Clomiphene citrate

Clomiphene citrate is an analog of the nonsteroidal estrogen chlorotrianisene (TACE), and contains both a *cis* and a *trans* isomer [7]. The *trans* isomer has a predominant antiestrogenic effect, but a mild intrinsic estrogenic effect as well; the *cis* isomer is thought to have less estrogenic activity. Initially tested as a contraceptive agent, clomiphene citrate demonstrated a gonadotropin-inhibiting effect in early animal studies. However, when subsequent human studies showed that clomiphene citrate increased serum gonadotropins, it was tested as and continues to be used as a fertility drug in women.

Mellinger and Thompson first reported the study of clomiphene citrate in subfertile men in a 1966 study that yielded disappointing results [8]. Heller *et al.* then reported the effects of various dosages of clomiphene citrate on "normal" male volunteers [9]. All dosages tested increased both serum gonadotropins and testosterone. A dose of 400 mg/day had a deleterious effect and reduced the sperm count, whereas 50 mg/day resulted in an increased sperm count. Subsequent studies had conflicting results, however, and it was not until the 1977 report by Paulson *et al.* of a 40% pregnancy rate in a group of 32 subfertile men treated with

25 mg/day that clomiphene citrate became a popular drug for male infertility therapy [10].

More than 30 studies on the effect of clomiphene citrate on male reproductive function have been published in the English-language literature since 1964, although recent data are scarce. There have not been any prospective randomized controlled studies since 1992. Approximately two-thirds of these studies demonstrate a favorable response in seminal variables and/or fertility. However, of the nine studies that were controlled, only three demonstrated a favorable response (Table 25.1) [11–19]. Unfortunately, these eight studies used a variety of doses, dosing regimens, and treatment durations. In addition, there was great variation in the definition of oligospermia used by the investigators (20 million sperm/mL to 40 million sperm/mL), baseline gonadotropin levels in the patients studied, and the extent of evaluation of the spouse.

The only consistent finding in a study of clomiphene citrate was an increase in serum FSH, LH, and testosterone in all men treated with this drug [27]. Although improvement in sperm count was observed in up to 70% of men treated, and pregnancy rates ranged from 0% to 40%, these results have not been proven durable, and there is great variation in both study design and outcomes. Patients with normal baseline gonadotropin levels, without azoospermia, and no evidence of scarring on testicular biopsy, appear to be the most likely to respond positively to clomiphene citrate [28]. **Because an occasional patient will demonstrate worsening of sperm counts while receiving treatment, it is important to follow the semen parameters and serum hormonal values on a monthly basis.** A reasonable starting dose is 25 mg/day. Some men appear to be exquisitely sensitive to clomiphene citrate, whereas others may require higher doses before an appropriate hormonal response is obtained. Follow-up evaluation of patients receiving clomiphene citrate should include endocrine studies (testosterone and FSH), blood pressure monitoring, and semen analysis. The dosage should be adjusted in an effort to maximize serum FSH levels without increasing serum testosterone levels significantly above normal.

Paulson compared clomiphene citrate with cortisone acetate in 40 men and found a significant difference in response rates [12]. However, it is not clear whether this finding means that clomiphene citrate was beneficial or that cortisone had a deleterious effect. A study by Wang et al. showed a clear benefit of clomiphene citrate over placebo at a dose of 25 mg/day [15]. Check et al.

assessed the effects of clomiphene citrate in a group of male partners of couples with unexplained infertility [18]. In a controlled study of 100 men with normal semen parameters, they observed a significantly higher pregnancy rate in the group receiving clomiphene citrate 25 mg/day than in those receiving vitamin C, 58% versus 16%, respectively. However, the same group observed a significant deterioration in sperm morphology using strict criteria in a group of men with idiopathic oligospermia receiving clomiphene citrate 25 mg/day in a subsequent nonrandomized controlled study [29]. The remaining six studies demonstrated no significant difference between clomiphene citrate and placebo or vitamin C [11,13,14,16,17,19]. It is interesting to note the extreme variation of 0% to 44% in pregnancy rate among the different placebo groups. This may reflect differences in patient selection, fertility of the spouse, or duration of follow-up.

Hussein et al. conducted a multi-institutional study of 42 patients with nonobstructive azoospermia [30]. Initial testicular biopsy demonstrated maturation arrest in 42.9% and hypospermatogenesis in 57.1% of patients. Clomiphene citrate was administered, with the dose titrated to achieve serum testosterone levels between 600 and 800 ng/dL, and semen analyses were performed at periodic intervals. In patients remaining azoospermic on semen analysis, surgical testicular biopsy and sperm extraction were performed. After clomiphene citrate therapy, 64.3% of the patients demonstrated sperm in their semen analyses ranging from 1 to 16 million sperm/mL, with a mean sperm density of 3.8 million/mL. Sufficient sperm for intracytoplasmic sperm injection (ICSI) were retrieved by testicular sperm extraction in all patients, even though 35.7% remained azoospermic. **This study suggested considering a course of clomiphene citrate prior to surgical sperm retrieval in patients with nonobstructive azoospermia.**

The standard preparation of clomiphene citrate has intrinsic estrogenic effects despite a predominant antiestrogenic effect. Cisclomiphene, a relatively pure antiestrogen, has been tested with varying results. The only controlled study of cisclomiphene, by Wieland et al., did not demonstrate an effect significantly greater than that of placebo in 22 men with idiopathic oligospermia (Table 25.1) [20].

The side effects of clomiphene citrate are usually self-limited and may include visual disturbances, weight gain, and increased blood pressure. Gynecomastia after drug withdrawal has also been reported but is rare [31].

Table 25.1. Results of controlled studies of empiric medical therapy using cisclomiphene citrate, clomiphene citrate, tamoxifen citrate, and testolactone

Reference	Dosage	Duration of treatment (months)	No. of patients	Rate of seminal improvement (%)	Pregnancy rate (%)	Results[a]
Clomiphene citrate						
Foss et al., 1973 [11]	100 mg × 10 d/mo	3	114	NR	NR	Negative
	Placebo	3	114			
Paulson, 1979 [12]	25 mg × 25 d/mo	6	20	70	35	Positive
	Cortisone 10 mg/d	6	20	40	10	
Rönnberg, 1980 [13]	50 mg/d	3	27	78	10	Negative
	Placebo	3	29	21	3	
Abel et al., 1982 [14]	50 mg × 25 d/mo	9	98	0 0	17	Negative
	Vitamin C 200 mg/d	9	89		13	
Wang et al., 1983 [15]	25 mg/d	6–9	11	NR	36	Positive
	50 mg/d	6–9	18	NR	22	
	Placebo	6–9	7	NR	0	
Micic & Dotlic, 1985 [16]	50 mg/d	6–9	56	32 7	13	Negative
	No Rx	6–9	45		0	
Sokol et al., 1988 [17]	25 mg/d	12	23	NR	9	Negative
	Placebo	12	23	NR	44	
Check et al., 1989 [18]	25 mg/d	8	50	NR	58	Positive
	Vitamin C	8	50	NR	16	
WHO, 1992 [19]	25 mg/d	8	70	NR	10	Negative
	Placebo	8	71	NR	8	
Cisclomiphene citrate						
Wieland et al., 1972 [20]	5 mg/d 10 mg/d	3	6	17	17	Negative
	Placebo	3	5	40	0	Negative
		3	11	27	18	
Tamoxifen citrate						
Willis et al., 1977 [21]	10 mg/d	6	9	11	11	Negative
	Placebo	2	9	0	0	
Török, 1985 [22]	20 mg/d	3	27	NR	33	Negative
	Placebo	3	27	NR	25	
AinMelk et al., 1987 [23]	20 mg/d	6	16	NR	13	Negative
	Placebo	6	16	NR	0	
Krause et al., [24]	30 mg/d	3	39	NR	13	Negative
	Placebo	3	37	NR	8	
Testolactone						
Clark & Sherins, 1983 [25]	2 g/d	8	20	NR	0	Negative
	Placebo	8	20	NR	0	
Clark & Sherins, 1989 [26]	2 g/d	8	20	NR	0	Negative
	Placebo	8	20	NR		
Anastrozole						
Schlegel & Raman, 2002 [53]	1 mg/d testolactone 100–200 mg/day		140			Positive

NR, not reported; Rx, treatment; WHO, World Health Organization.
[a] Conclusion of authors as to whether drug therapy was more effective than placebo.

One study has suggested an association between clomiphene citrate therapy and testicular germ cell tumors [32], and another case report described a pulmonary embolism in a patient during clomiphene citrate therapy for infertility [33].

The overwhelming evidence suggests that clomiphene citrate is not an effective treatment for idiopathic infertility. Recent studies suggest that men with either partial androgen insensitivity or mild hypogonadotropic hypogonadism may be the best candidates for this treatment [34]. Patients should be counseled about the possible negative effects of treatment and be monitored with frequent testosterone and estradiol levels. Since a significant number of patients may in fact have a dramatic decline in sperm production on empiric therapy, patients should be counseled prior to the initiation of therapy. However, because some patients have responded favorably, there may be a subgroup of men in whom its use is appropriate, as recently documented by Hussein et al. [30]. Doses should be only 12.5–25 mg/day initially to avoid an excessive increase in serum testosterone.

Tamoxifen citrate

Another antiestrogen agent is tamoxifen citrate, which is commonly used in the treatment of women with metastatic carcinoma of the breast to prevent recurrence after surgery or radiation treatment, and as prophylaxis for patients at very high risk to develop breast cancer. It is thought to have less estrogenic activity than clomiphene citrate. Comhaire, in 1976, was the first to study this drug as a treatment for male infertility [35]. He reported a 20% pregnancy rate after treating men with idiopathic oligospermia for 6–11 months with 20 mg/day.

Between 1976 and 1993, 12 additional uncontrolled studies [36–47] and four controlled studies [21–24] on the effect of tamoxifen citrate were reported in the English-language literature. The majority of the uncontrolled studies showed an increase in sperm count, but very few demonstrated a change in motility or morphology. Pregnancy rates ranged from 17% to 40%. Dony et al. found equivalent hormonal and seminal variable effects when using either low-dose (5 to 10 mg/day) or high-dose (20 mg/day) tamoxifen therapy [40]. As with clomiphene citrate, patients with normal baseline gonadotropins are more likely to have a positive response, and patients with azoospermia rarely respond. In a study by Schieferstein et al. half of 210 men treated with tamoxifen demonstrated an objective increase in testicular volume based on ultrasonographic measurement [43].

None of the controlled studies investigating tamoxifen therapy has shown it to have any significant effect on pregnancy rate (Table 25.1) [21–24]. Interestingly, Török simultaneously conducted an open-label study on 20 patients in conjunction with his placebo-controlled study [22]. The open-label study demonstrated what appeared to be significant increases in total sperm counts and pregnancy rates. However, the double-blinded, placebo-controlled study did not confirm this finding.

Schill and Schillinger identified a subgroup of men who were thought to be the most likely candidates to have a positive response to tamoxifen citrate based on a one-week stimulation test [45]. Those who had no rise in FSH after receiving 40 mg/day of tamoxifen for one week tended to have a greater than 50% increase in sperm count.

Other recent work examining the combination of tamoxifen and testosterone undecanoate suggested improvement in semen and pregnancy rates when used to treat idiopathic oligospermia [48].

As is the case with clomiphene citrate, however, controlled studies of tamoxifen citrate do not demonstrate any efficacy, although further study may indeed reveal a subgroup of patients responsive to treatment.

Aromatase inhibitors

Aromatase inhibitors block the conversion of testosterone to estrogen. Leydig cells within the testis co-secrete testosterone and estradiol in response to gonadotropin secretion [49], but the major source of circulating estradiol in men is from peripheral conversion of androgens to estrogens by the aromatase enzyme in adipose tissue [50]. Despite the multiple sources of estradiol production, testosterone concentrations in the serum of an adult man are normally more than 100-fold higher than estradiol. As stated earlier, aromatization of androgens to estrogens within the hypothalamus appears to be necessary for steroidal inhibition of hypothalamic GnRH secretion. Testolactone lowers serum estradiol levels in men through the inhibition of the aromatase enzyme and does not have any intrinsic androgenic or estrogenic activity. Like tamoxifen, testolactone was originally used in the treatment of women with metastatic breast carcinoma. Testolactone has been found to be a safe and well-tolerated medication, and subsequently has been tested in men with idiopathic oligospermia. Testolactone theoretically can improve testicular function in two ways. Estradiol concentrations within peripheral serum and in the testis may be reduced by inhibition of estradiol production in adipose tissue and of the Leydig cells (potentially the Sertoli cells as well), respectively. In addition, testolactone, analogous to clomiphene citrate, stimulates gonadotropin secretion by the pituitary gland by blocking feedback inhibition.

In an uncontrolled study, Vigersky and Glass studied the effects of testolactone (1 g/day) in 10 oligospermic men [51]. They observed an increase in serum testosterone, a decrease in serum estradiol, and a dramatic rise in the androgen-to-estrogen ratio; gonadotropin secretion, whether basal or GnRH-stimulated, was unaffected. Eighty percent of men treated had an increase in sperm count, and 30% initiated a pregnancy. There was no change in sperm motility.

Clark and Sherins performed two randomized, double-blinded, crossover studies of testolactone (2 g/day) and did not observe a significant effect on fertility of testolactone over placebo (Table 25.1) [25,26]. However, the patients used in their study had very severe oligospermia, and the patients did not have any change in their hormone levels, suggesting there may have been a problem with the preparation used. As with the other drugs mentioned thus far, further studies are needed before the value of testolactone in the treatment of infertile men is determined. However, this drug may be considered in the management of obese patients with idiopathic infertility and high normal or elevated estradiol levels [52].

Schlegel and Raman examined the effect of anastrozole, a more selective aromatase inhibitor on the hormonal and semen parameters of infertile men with abnormal baseline testosterone-to-estradiol ratios [53]. One hundred forty subfertile men with abnormal testosterone-to-estradiol ratios were treated with 100–200 mg testolactone daily or 1 mg anastrozole daily. Men treated with testolactone had an increase in testosterone-to-estradiol ratios during therapy. This change was confirmed in subgroups of men with Klinefelter syndrome, a history of varicocele repair, and those with varicocele. A total of 12 oligospermic men had semen analysis before and during testolactone treatment, with an increase in sperm concentration (5.5 vs. 11.2 million sperm/mL, $P < 0.01$), motility (14.7% vs. 21.0%, $P < 0.05$), morphology (6.5% vs. 12.8%, $P = 0.05$), and motility index (606.3 vs. 1685.2 million motile sperm/ejaculate, respectively, $P < 0.05$). During anastrozole treatment, similar changes in the testosterone-to-estradiol ratios were seen (7.2 ± 0.3 vs. 18.1 ± 1.0, respectively, $P < 0.001$). This improvement of hormonal parameters was noted for all subgroups except

those patients with Klinefelter syndrome. A total of 25 oligospermic men with semen analysis before and during anastrozole treatment had an increase in semen volume (2.9 vs. 3.5 mL, $P < 0.05$), sperm concentration (5.5 vs. 15.6 million sperm/mL, $P < 0.001$) and motility index (832.8 vs. 2930.8 million motile sperm/ejaculate, respectively, $P < 0.005$). These changes were similar to those observed in men treated with testolactone. No significant difference in serum testosterone levels during treatment with testolactone and anastrozole was observed. However, the anastrozole treatment group did have a statistically better improvement of serum estradiol concentration and testosterone-to-estradiol ratios ($P < 0.001$). **Schlegel and Raman concluded that men who are infertile with a low serum testosterone-to-estradiol ratio can be treated with an aromatase inhibitor. With treatment, an increase in testosterone-to-estradiol ratio occurred in association with increased semen parameters.** Anastrozole and testolactone have similar effects on hormonal profiles and semen analysis. Anastrozole appears to be at least as effective as testolactone for treating men with abnormal testosterone-to-estradiol ratios, except for the subset with Klinefelter syndrome, who appeared to be more effectively treated with testolactone.

Gonadotropins

Exogenous gonadotropins, most commonly given as human chorionic gonadotropin (hCG) or human menopausal gonadotropin (hMG), and the newer recombinant human FSH now available, have been used in the treatment of men with idiopathic infertility. The initiation and maintenance of spermatogenesis, as well as the normal function of the male sex accessory glands, depend on the proper stimulation of the testis by gonadotropins secreted by the anterior pituitary gland. **Treatment of hypogonadotropic hypogonadism with exogenous gonadotropins or GnRH has produced remarkably good results compared with treatment of other male infertility problems** [54]. The results have led to the use of these hormones in subfertile men with either normal or elevated basal gonadotropin levels. The only rational argument for this therapy is that it is theoretically possible that infertile men might have either defective or inefficient production of bioactive LH or FSH, and would therefore benefit from exogenous hCG or hMG. However, defects in FSH production in infertile men have not been described [55].

Many agents have been available to raise the serum level of gonadotropins. The most common preparations used today are hCG and hMG; preparations used in the past were of questionable reliability. Both GnRH and synthetic GnRH analogs are now available, and they are also being studied in oligospermic men.

Human chorionic gonadotropin is comparable to LH in that it stimulates Leydig cell secretion of both testosterone and estradiol and subsequently suppresses FSH. Human menopausal gonadotropin has both LH and FSH activity and is the more expensive of the two drugs. Both hCG and hMG must be administered parenterally, and they have been used separately and together in various dosing regimens. One of the first reported studies using hCG alone, that of Glass and Holland, yielded surprisingly good results [56]. Among 20 men receiving 5000 IU hCG 2–3 times weekly for 1–3 months, 60% had improvement in seminal parameters, which resulted in a 35% pregnancy rate. In contrast, an early study by Lytton and Mroueh on the use of hMG alone had disappointing results: only 19% of the oligospermic men so treated had improvement in seminal parameters, and the subsequent pregnancy rate was only 13% [57].

Later studies using hMG alone have yielded improvement in seminal variables in 40–67% of patients [58–60]. However, pregnancy rates have remained poor, ranging from 0% to 17%. Similarly, the use of hCG alone has produced a wide range of results. Mehan and Chehval reported improvement in semen parameters in 53% of men with idiopathic oligospermia treated with 5000 IU hCG weekly; the pregnancy rate in this group was 30% [61]. Uncontrolled studies by Sherins [62] and Homonnai et al. [63] resulted in pregnancy rates of only 0% and 9%, respectively, after treatment with gonadotropins.

Dubin and Amelar used hCG (4000 IU twice weekly) as an adjuvant therapy in men with a baseline sperm count of less than 10 million/mL who underwent varicocelectomy [64]. Without adjuvant hCG therapy the pregnancy rate was only 23%, but it increased to 44% when hCG was administered in conjunction with varicocelectomy. Using a dose of hCG of 5000 IU per week, Mehan and Chehval confirmed this observation in a study of 40 men not responding to a varicocele repair and six men with an unrepaired varicocele [61]. The failed varicocelectomy group who received hCG had a 43% pregnancy rate, whereas the group with unrepaired varicocele who received hCG had a 0% pregnancy rate. Although promising, these results have not yet been substantiated by a randomized controlled study.

Exogenous FSH has been administered to men with idiopathic infertility who failed to achieve normal fertilization rates during an in-vitro fertilization (IVF) cycle. Acosta et al. administered 150 IU of pure human FSH three times weekly for a minimum of three months before the next attempt [65]. The fertilization rate increased from 2% before treatment to 54% after receipt of pure human FSH. They did not observe any significant changes in endocrine or semen analysis after therapy, and baseline FSH levels did not influence outcome. Some patients had significantly elevated baseline serum FSH levels. These results suggest that FSH may be improving the quality of sperm being produced without significantly affecting the conventionally measured semen variables. However, other investigators have demonstrated fertilization rates of 48–66% during the second cycle without any intervention in couples with idiopathic male-factor infertility who have failed to fertilize on the first IVF attempt [66,67]. As with studies of other medications, the absence of appropriate controls in this study of pure human FSH limits our ability to assess the true efficacy of this treatment.

The treatment of idiopathic oligospermia with a combination of both hCG and hMG has not been very successful. A controlled study by Knuth et al. demonstrated no significant benefit over placebo (Table 25.2) [68]. A review by Schill summarized the multiple studies evaluating the effects of hMG and hCG: patients with moderate oligospermia have a much better response rate than those with sperm densities below 10 million/L; improvement in seminal variables and pregnancy rate were 36% and 16%, respectively, in the moderately oligospermic group, and 20% and 8%, respectively, in the severely oligospermic group [75]. Namiki et al. identified a subgroup of patients with idiopathic infertility who were responders to combined gonadotropin therapy by measuring testicular FSH receptors [76]. FSH receptor-positive patients experienced a significant improvement in total motile count but were also found to have better baseline testicular histologic findings. The results of these two studies may reflect either the ability of these patients to respond to therapy or their underlying fertility potential independent of therapy. At this point, without demonstration of significantly better results, it is hard to justify the expense and effort involved in using these agents instead of the oral antiestrogens that achieve a similar result by stimulation of endogenous production of gonadotropins. However, antiestrogens

Table 25.2. Results of controlled studies of empiric medical therapy using gonadotropins, gonadotropin-releasing hormones (GnRH), and androgens

Reference	Dosage	Duration of treatment (months)	No. of patients	Rate of seminal improvement (%)	Pregnancy rate (%)	Results [a]
Gonadotropins						
Knuth et al., 1987 [68]	150 IU/d HMG 3 × wk plus 2500 IU HCG	3	17	NS	10	Negative
	Placebo	3	20		0	
GnRH						
Badenoch et al., 1988 [69]	1 µg Buserelin SC 2 × wk	3	7	NS	NR	Negative
	10 µg Buserelin SC 2 × wk	3	8	NS	NR	Negative
	Placebo	3	4		NR	
Crottaz et al., 1992 [70]	0.2 mg IN every 2 hrs	3	14	NS	36	Negative
	Placebo	3	14		21	
Androgens						
Aafges et al., 1993 [71]	Mesterolone 25 mg/d	6	59	NS	12	Negative
	Placebo	6	59		12	
Wang et al., 1983 [15]	Mesterolone 100 mg/d	6	12	NS	0	Negative
	Testosterone rebound	6	15	NS	0	Negative
	Placebo	6	7		0	
WHO., 1989 [72]	Mesterolone 150 mg/d	12	50	NS	19	Negative
	Mesterolone 75 mg/d	12	54	NS	12	Negative
	Placebo	12	53		11	
Comhaire, 1990 [73]	Testosterone 240 mg/d	3	10	NS	10	Negative
	Placebo	3	10		10	
Gerris et al., 1991 [74]	Mesterolone 150 mg/d	12	27	NR	26	Negative
	Placebo	12	25	NR	48	

hMG, human menopausal gonadotropin; hCG, human chorionic gonadotropin; IN, intranasally; NR, not reported; NS, no significant change; SC, subcutaneously; WHO, World Health Organization.
[a] Conclusion of authors as to whether drug therapy was more effective than placebo.

are contraindicated in patients with baseline elevations in gonadotropins, and this group may be considered for empiric therapy with gonadotropins.

Gonadotropin-releasing hormone

Pituitary gonadotropin secretion is also increased with the use of the synthetic analogs of GnRH. These agents have been shown to produce better results than hCG and hMG in the treatment of hypogonadotropic hypogonadal men [77], and have been studied in men with idiopathic oligospermia. These drugs have a very short biologic half-life and thus require either frequent administration (intranasally or by subcutaneous injection) or the use of a portable pump for pulsatile subcutaneous infusion.

Schwarzstein and colleagues treated 18 severely oligospermic men with GnRH every other day without observing seminal improvement or a pregnancy [78]. Aparicio et al., using a daily dose of 0.1–0.5 mg GnRH in 21 men with moderate oligospermia, reported improvement in seminal variables in 67% and a pregnancy rate of 24% [79]. However, a controlled study comparing two doses of a long-acting GnRH analog with placebo did not show a significant improvement in seminal variables and yielded no pregnancies (Table 25.2) [69]. A second controlled study did not demonstrate any significant seminal changes, but the pregnancy rates for the treatment and control groups were 36% and 21%, respectively [70]. The pregnancy rates were not significantly different from each other but do demonstrate the wide variation in the treatment-independent fertility potential of the patients being evaluated in these clinical trials, and the absolute necessity of appropriate control groups to assess the efficacy of these treatments.

A prospective trial of a GnRH analog for the treatment of oligoasthenospermia demonstrated a statistically significant improvement in both sperm concentration and motility as compared to results in the group treated with clomiphene citrate [80]. The mean sperm density in the GnRHa group increased from 16.1 million/mL to 26.9 million/mL ($P < 0.05$), while the mean sperm density did not change significantly in the group treated with clomiphene. Similarly, the mean sperm motility increased from 35.9% to 43.9% in the GnRHa group ($P < 0.05$), but did not significantly change in the clomiphene group.

There are still many dosage variables to be evaluated before a definitive judgment can be made on the efficacy of GnRH in the treatment of male infertility. **Because of the enormous expense of GnRH and the lack of specific dosage recommendations, this form of therapy should be used only in clinical trials.**

Androgens

It is well understood that adequate levels of circulating androgens are critical for the maintenance of male sexual and reproductive functions. However, as early as 1939, McCullagh and McGurl noted that administration of testosterone can suppress human testicular function as shown in depression of sperm output [81]. As noted earlier, androgen concentrations within the testis are 50-fold higher than in peripheral serum because of local production [82]. Administration of exogenous androgens results in feedback inhibition of endogenous gonadotropin secretion and reduced concentrations of intratesticular androgens despite apparently normal levels of testosterone in the peripheral serum. Numerous studies of men who abuse anabolic steroids have confirmed these findings [83–86]. Therefore, low doses of exogenous androgens have been employed in the past to avoid significant pituitary feedback suppression. Animal model studies have shown that systemic administration of extraordinarily high doses of androgens can stimulate and maintain spermatogenesis in hypophysectomized rats [87]. In addition, spermatogenesis could be maintained by site-directed intratesticular testosterone administration using testosterone-laden microspheres [88]. These studies suggest that the administration of extremely high doses of testosterone might be effective in the treatment of idiopathic infertility.

There are a variety of synthetic androgens available for oral administration, but they have significant toxicity and their use is not recommended. The most commonly used is mesterolone, in doses ranging from as low as 2 mg/day up to 150 mg/day. Although androgen therapy is thought to improve epididymal function, experimental evidence has not been supportive of this theory. Brown treated 58 men who had isolated asthenospermia and 35 men who had multiple seminal defects with fluoxymesterone, 20 mg/day for six weeks [89]. Improvement of seminal variables was observed in 52% of the first group but in only 11% of the second group. Urry and Cockett noted seminal improvement in 44% of 40 men treated with fluoxymesterone at a much lower dose of 2 mg/day [90]. Aafjes et al., performing a randomized, double-blinded, crossover study of mesterolone (25 mg/day) in 59 men with sperm counts less than 40 million/mL, observed a similar rate of seminal improvement in sperm motility after treatment with mesterolone and placebo; pregnancy rates were the same in both groups as well [71]. The more recent studies on the efficacy of androgen therapy for the management of idiopathic male-factor infertility have used significantly higher doses of mesterolone or testosterone undecanoate. Three randomized prospective controlled studies have been published, and all of them were negative (Table 25.2) [72–74]. Seminal variables were not significantly altered during the course of therapy, and pregnancy rates were either similar to or lower than those of similar patients receiving placebo.

Research attempts at determining a subgroup of responders have been unsuccessful. Although some studies demonstrate improvement in seminal variables after oral androgen therapy, pregnancy rates have been low. Oral androgens are readily metabolized by the liver, and it is doubtful that low doses have any effect on serum androgen levels in eugonadal men. Toxicity, including cholestatic jaundice, peliosis hepatitis, and occasional gynecomastia, appears to outweigh the efficacy of this form of therapy. **It is for these reasons** that oral androgens are not recommended in the treatment of the infertile male or any man desiring of fertility.

Testosterone-rebound therapy

Exogenous testosterone therapy can produce azoospermia or severe oligospermia through the inhibition of gonadotropin secretion. It is for this reason that exogenous testosterone should never be administered in men desiring fertility. "Testosterone-rebound therapy" is based on the theory that after the withdrawal of testosterone therapy, spermatogenesis will resume within four months, and the sperm count may be even higher. Heller *et al.* noted improvement in spermatogenesis in oligospermic men after a course of suppression with testosterone [91]. Subsequent studies demonstrated improvement in seminal variables in 20–67% of men so treated, and pregnancy rates ranging from 14% to 41% [92–95]. Suppression of spermatogenesis has been induced with either testosterone ester injections given weekly (200 mg) or combined testosterone ester injections (200 mg every third week) and high-dose oral androgens (norethandrolone, 20 mg/day). Unfortunately, from 4% to 8% of patients have had lower sperm counts after therapy, and Charny reported that azoospermia persisted in two patients [92]. Interestingly, Charny and Gordon observed an 8% pregnancy rate after testosterone-rebound therapy of 38 patients with azoospermia due to maturation arrest confirmed by testicular biopsy results [93]. This pregnancy rate suggests that testosterone-rebound therapy may be worth trying in select azoospermic patients who have no other therapeutic option. However, the only controlled study of testosterone-rebound therapy was performed in a very small group of patients and did not show any efficacy of this form of treatment (Table 25.2) [15]. **It is for this reason, together with the overwhelming evidence that exogenous testosterone is in fact detrimental to sperm production, that this form of empiric medical therapy has been abandoned by the medical community and has not been the subject of further study in recent years. Exogenous testosterone should therefore not be used in men desiring of fertility.**

Miscellaneous treatments

Numerous non-endocrine treatments aimed at improving the quality of semen have been tested or are currently being evaluated. These treatments are varied, and include those with possible benefit and those without proved effect. Thyroxine, arginine [96],

corticosteroids [97], antibiotics [98], zinc, methylxanthines [15], bromocriptine [99], and vitamins A, E, and C have all been shown to be of little or no benefit in the treatment of subfertile men without evidence of a specific deficiency. **With the exception of patients with a specific vitamin deficiency, the efficacy of any vitamin therapy in normal men is questionable.**

Kallikrein

Kallikrein is a polypeptide enzyme, found in a variety of tissues and serum, that will cleave kininogen to produce kinins, such as bradykinin and kallidin. These polypeptides act locally in the inflammatory response and are closely related to the coagulation and fibrinolysis systems. The kallikrein–kinin system has been shown to play a role in the regulation and stimulation of sperm motility [100,101].

The major source of kallikrein is the pancreas, and pancreatic kallikrein is available in both oral and parenteral forms. Kallikrein therapy has been studied extensively. Schill compared 600 kU/d of kallikrein with placebo in a double-masked fashion over a two-month period in 90 oligospermic men (sperm count < 40 million/mL), and found the rate of improvement in seminal parameters and the pregnancy rate to be significantly better in the kallikrein group (Table 25.3) [102]. However, two more recent studies using the same dose did not observe any significant benefit of kallikrein over placebo [103,104]. Homonnai *et al.*, in an uncontrolled study, noted worsening of sperm counts in a similar group of men treated with kallikrein, and a pregnancy rate of only 17% [107]. Side effects are rare, but epididymal or prostatic inflammation may be exacerbated by kallikrein therapy. **The cumulative results are not very promising, and further study is required to determine any efficacy of this drug.**

Indomethacin

Prostaglandins have been shown to have an inhibitory effect on testicular steroidogenesis [108] and spermatogenesis in vivo [109], and on sperm motility in vitro [110]. These observations suggest that prostaglandins may play a role in both testicular function and sperm maturation. **Although the mechanisms are unclear, most of the evidence demonstrates an inhibitory influence of prostaglandins on reproductive function. Therefore, suppression of prostaglandin synthesis with nonsteroidal anti-inflammatory drugs has been suggested as a form of therapy for subfertile men.**

447

Table 25.3. Results of controlled studies of empiric medical therapy using kallikrein, bromocriptine, indomethacin, ketoprofen, and glutathione

Reference	Dosage	Duration of treatment (months)	No. of patients	Rate of seminal improvement (%)	Pregnancy rate (%)	Results [a]
Kallikrein						
Schill, 1979 [102]	600 KU/d	2	48	Significant	38	Positive
	Placebo	2	42		16	
Glezerman et al., 1993 [103]	600 KU/d	3	55	NS	NR	Negative
	Placebo	3	59		NR	
Keck et al., 1994 [104]	600 KU/d	3	44	NS	9	Negative
	Placebo	3	47		9	
Bromocriptine mesylate						
Hovatta et al., 1979 [99]	5 mg/d	3	20	NS	0	Negative
	Placebo	3	20		0	
Indomethacin						
Barkay et al., 1984 [105]	150 mg/d	2	20	NR	35	Positive
	Placebo	2	25	NR	8	
Ketoprofen						
Barkay et al., 1984 [105]	150 mg/d	2	20	NR	20	Positive
	Placebo	2	25	NR	8	
Glutathione						
Lenzi et al., 1993 [106]	600 mg IM QOD	4	20	Significant	NR	Positive
	Placebo	4	20			

NR, not reported; NS, no significant change; QOD, every other day.
[a] Conclusion of authors as to whether drug therapy was more effective than placebo.

One controlled study by Barkay et al. has suggested an increase in FSH, LH, and testosterone levels in men treated with both indomethacin and ketoprofen (Table 25.3) [105]. They examined the effect of various doses of indomethacin and ketoprofen on both seminal parameters and fertility in 100 oligospermic men. They observed an increase in both FSH and LH with a simultaneous decrease in testosterone in the men receiving either indomethacin or ketoprofen. Prostaglandin levels in the seminal fluid decreased as well. With 75 mg/day of indomethacin, there was a significant increase in both sperm count and motility, and the pregnancy rate was 35%. Other doses of indomethacin and ketoprofen yielded a significant but less dramatic improvement in these variables over placebo. This is an interesting, inexpensive, and relatively nontoxic form of therapy, the only adverse side effect being gastritis. Further study is required to identify the patients best suited for this form of therapy.

Glutathione

Glutathione is a simple, naturally occurring, three-amino-acid compound that is thought to act as an antioxidant and prevent lipid peroxidation. For this reason, glutathione therapy has been used in various pathologic conditions in which reactive oxygen species are thought to play a pathogenic role. In an uncontrolled study, Lenzi et al. used glutathione therapy (600 mg/day IM) for two months in a group of 11 men with a history of genitourinary inflammatory disease and noted significant improvement in sperm motility [111]. These findings were confirmed in a subsequent placebo-controlled, double-masked study performed by Lenzi et al. (Table 25.3) [106]. Forty men were randomized between placebo and intramuscular glutathione therapy using 600 mg every other day for four months. Significant improvement in sperm motility was observed in the glutathione group, but pregnancy rates were not reported. Glutathione is a safe but cumbersome form of empiric medical therapy. Further study is necessary to confirm these early findings by a single investigative team, but this drug should be considered for patients with asthenospermia.

Phosphodiesterase inhibitors

The administration of sildenafil, pentoxifylline, and other methylxanthines has been suggested to potentially increase sperm motility in vitro. Systemic administration of these agents has not demonstrated a significant or reliable response in sperm function and production [112].

Zinc

Semen is normally rich in zinc, as contributed by prostatic secretions. It has been suggested that the administration of exogenous systemic zinc to malnourished men can improve sperm production [113,114].

Although it has been shown to potentially increase the sperm count in both fertile and infertile men, exogenous zinc treatment is probably of little benefit except in the presence of zinc deficiency, and high doses may have a detrimental effect overall on sperm function.

Vitamins C, E, A, and other antioxidants

Reactive oxygen species (ROS) include free radicals, oxygen ions and peroxides and are found at high levels in up to 40% of infertile men [115]. ROS are usually not found in the semen of fertile men. Vitamins such as vitamin C and E, as well as pentoxifylline and allopurinol, are known to have antioxidant activity. It has also been shown that infertile men as well as male smokers have low levels of ascorbic acid in their semen, which can contribute to their infertility [116]. It is for this reason that supplementation with these agents has been proposed to decrease the endogenous oxidative damage to sperm.

It is important to note, however, that low levels of superoxide anion may in fact be important to the acrosome reaction and thereby critically affect ability to fertilize. No randomized, controlled studies have demonstrated a benefit of systemic administration of antioxidant on male infertility. **Administration of high-dose antioxidants has potential beneficial effect on male fertility, but also has theoretical adverse effects. It is for this reason that their use should be limited to low or moderate doses only.**

A variety of different agents, specifically isoflavones (i.e., genistein, daidzein) have recently gained attention as possible treatments for men with abnormal semen parameters. Isoflavones, which are derived from plants, have profound antioxidant capabilities and have already been implicated in the treatment of a variety of different disease states, specifically coronary artery disease and endocrine-secreting tumors. Results on the efficacy of isoflavones are immature, but may suggest the possibility of an interesting future treatment [117].

Summary

An extensive variety of therapeutic agents exists for the treatment of the subfertile male with idiopathic oligospermia, not limited to the agents reported here. Empiric therapy might also include the various assisted reproductive technologies (ART) employed to assist couples with male-factor infertility, specifically intrauterine insemination (IUI), in-vitro fertilization (IVF), and IVF combined with intracytoplasmic sperm injection (ICSI). Couples with severe male-factor infertility should also be counseled about alternatives such as adoption or artificial insemination with donor sperm.

It is essential to rule out any treatable cause of infertility with a thorough evaluation by a male infertility specialist. Potentially correctable causes may include varicocele, antisperm antibodies, endocrinopathy, infection, and obstruction. It is also important to identify any chromosomal abnormality by obtaining a karyotype and Y-chromosome microdeletion test prior to initiating a possibly lengthy and expensive course of empiric treatment. A complete female factor evaluation is also necessary, and may obviate the need for nonspecific therapy in the male partner.

Hopefully, as the understanding of male reproductive physiology broadens, the opportunity to better identify specific problems and develop targeted, specific therapies will grow. It is these new discoveries upon which improved fertility treatments and pregnancy success will depend.

References

[1] Dubin L, Amelar RD. Etiologic factors in 1294 consecutive cases of male infertility. *Fertil Steril* 1971; **22**: 469–74.

[2] Greenberg SH, Lipshultz LI, Wein AJ. Experience with 425 subfertile male patients. *J Urol* 1978; **119**: 507–10.

[3] Collins JA, Wrixon W, Janes LB, Wilson EH. Treatment-independent pregnancy among infertile couples. *N Engl J Med* 1983; **309**: 1201–6.

[4] Read MD, Schnieden H. Variations in sperm count in oligozoospermic or asthenozoospermic patients. *Andrologia* 1978; **10**: 52–5.

[5] Matsumoto AM, Karpas AE, Bremner WJ. Chronic human chorionic gonadotropin administration in normal men: Evidence that follicle-stimulating hormone is necessary for the maintenance of quantitatively normal spermatogenesis in man. *J Clin Endocrinol Metab* 1986; **62**: 1184.

[6] De Kretser DM, Burger HG, Fortune D, *et al.* Hormonal, histological and chromosomal studies in adult males with testicular disorders. *J Clin Endocrinol Metab* 1972; **35**: 392–401.

[7] Schellen TMCM. Clomiphene citrate in male infertility. *Int J Fertil* 1982; **27**: 136–45.

[8] Mellinger RC, Thompson RJ. The effect of clomiphene citrate in male infertility. *Fertil Steril* 1966; **17**: 94–103.

[9] Heller CG, Rowley MJ, Heller GV. Clomiphene citrate: a correlation of its effect on sperm concentration and morphology, total gonadotropins, ICSH, estrogen and testosterone excretion, and testicular cytology in normal men. *J Clin Endocrinol Metab* 1969; **29**: 638–49.

[10] Paulson DF, Hammond CB, de Vere White R, Wiebe RH. Clomiphene citrate: pharmacologic treatment of hypofertile male. *Urology* 1977; **9**: 419–21.

[11] Foss GL, Tindall VR, Birkett JP. The treatment of subfertile men with clomiphene citrate. *J Reprod Fertil* 1973; **32**: 167–70.

[12] Paulson DF. Cortisone acetate versus clomiphene citrate in pre-germinal idiopathic oligospermia. *J Urol* 1979; **121**: 432–4.

[13] Rönnberg L. The effect of clomiphene citrate on different sperm parameters and serum hormone levels in preselected infertile men: a controlled double-blind cross-over study. *Int J Androl* 1980; **3**: 479–86.

[14] Abel BJ, Carswell G, Elton R, *et al.* Randomised trial of clomiphene citrate treatment and vitamin C for male infertility. *Br J Urol* 1982; **54**: 780–4.

[15] Wang C, Chan CW, Wong KK, Yeung KK. Comparison of the effectiveness of placebo, clomiphene citrate, mesterolone, pentoxifylline, and testosterone rebound therapy for the treatment of idiopathic oligospermia. *Fertil Steril* 1983; **40**: 358–65.

[16] Micic S, Dotlic R. Evaluation of sperm parameters in clinical trial with clomiphene citrate of oligospermic men. *J Urol* 1985; **133**: 221–2.

[17] Sokol RZ, Steiner BS, Bustillo M, Petersen G, Swerdloff RS. A controlled comparison of the efficacy of clomiphene citrate in male infertility. *Fertil Steril* 1988; **49**: 865–70.

[18] Check JH, Chase JS, Nowroozi K, Wu CH, Adelson HG. Empirical therapy of the male with clomiphene in couples with unexplained fertility. *Int J Fertil* 1989; **34**: 120–2.

[19] World Health Organization. A double-blind trial of clomiphene citrate for the treatment of idiopathic male infertility. *Int J Androl* 1992; **15**: 299–307.

[20] Wieland RG, Ansari AH, Klein DE, *et al.* Idiopathic oligospermia: control observations and response to cisclomiphene. *Fertil Steril* 1972; **23**: 471–4.

[21] Willis KJ, London DR, Bevis MA, *et al.* Hormonal effects of tamoxifen in oligospermic men. *J Endocrinol* 1977; **73**: 171–8.

[22] Török L. Treatment of oligospermia with tamoxifen (open and controlled studies). *Andrologia* 1985; **17**: 497–501.

[23] AinMelk Y, Belisle S, Carmel M, Jean-Pierre T. Tamoxifen citrate therapy in male infertility. *Fertil Steril* 1987; **48**: 113–17.

[24] Krause W, Holland-Moritz H, Schramm P. Treatment of idiopathic oligozoospermia with tamoxifen – a randomized controlled study. *Int J Androl* 1992; **15**: 14–18.

[25] Clark RV, Sherins RJ. Clinical trial of testolactone for treatment of idiopathic male infertility [abstract]. *J Androl* 1983; **4**: 31.

[26] Clark RV, Sherins RJ. Treatment of men with idiopathic oligozoospermic infertility using the aromatase inhibitor, testolactone: results of a double-blinded, randomized, placebo-controlled trial with crossover. *J Androl* 1989; **10**: 240–7.

[27] Bardin CW, Ross GT, Lipsett MB. Site of action of clomiphene citrate in men: a study of the pituitary–Leydig cell axis. *J Cell Endocrinol* 1967; **27**: 1558–64.

[28] Paulson DF. Clomiphene citrate in the management of male hypofertility: predictors for treatment selection. *Fertil Steril* 1977; **28**: 1226–9.

[29] Shanis B, Check JH, Bollendorf A. Adverse effect of clomiphene citrate on sperm morphology. *Arch Androl* 1991; **27**: 109–11.

[30] Hussein A, Ozgok Y, Ross L, Niederberger C. Clomiphene administration for cases of nonobstructive azoospermia: a multicenter study. *J Androl* 2005; **26**: 787–91.

[31] Lee PA. The occurrence of gynecomastia upon withdrawal of clomiphene citrate treatment for idiopathic oligospermia. *Fertil Steril* 1980; **34**: 285–6.

[32] Nilsson A, Nilsson S. Testicular germ cell tumors after clomiphene therapy for subfertility. *J Urol* 1985; **134**: 560–2.

[33] Chamberlain RA, Cumming DC. Pulmonary embolism during clomiphene therapy for infertility in a male: a case report. *Int J Fertil* 1986; **31**: 198–9.

[34] Akin JW. The use of clomiphene citrate in the treatment of azoospermia secondary to incomplete androgen resistance. *Fertil Steril* 1993; **59**: 223–4.

[35] Comhaire F. Treatment of oligospermia with tamoxifen. *Int J Fertil* 1976; **21**: 232–8.

[36] Bartsch G, Scheiber K. Tamoxifen treatment in oligozoospermia. *Eur Urol* 1981; **7**: 283–7.

[37] Brigante C, Motta G, Fusi F, Coletta MP, Busacca M. Treatment of idiopathic oligozoospermia with tamoxifen. *Acta Eur Fertil* 1985; **16**: 361–4.

[38] Buvat J, Ardaens K, Lemaire A, *et al.* Increased sperm count in 25 cases of idiopathic normogonadotropic oligospermia following treatment with tamoxifen. *Fertil Steril* 1983; **39**: 700–3.

[39] Danner CH, Frick J, Maier F. Results of treatment with tamoxifen in oligozoospermic men. *Andrologia* 1983; **15**: 584–7.

[40] Dony JM, Smals AG, Rolland R, Fauser BC, Thomas CM. Effect of lower versus higher doses of tamoxifen on pituitary-gonadal function and sperm indices in oligozoospermic men. *Andrologia* 1985; **17**: 369–78.

[41] Lewis-Jones DI, Lynch RV, Machin DC, Desmond AD. Improvement in semen quality in infertile males after treatment with tamoxifen. *Andrologia* 1987; **19**: 86–90.

[42] Noci I, Chelo E, Saltarelli O, Donati Cori G, Scarselli G. Tamoxifen and oligospermia. *Arch Androl* 1985; **15**: 83–8.

[43] Schieferstein G, Adam W, Armann J, *et al.* Therapeutic results with tamoxifen in oligozoospermia. I. Remarks on mode of action and metabolism based on clinical findings and laboratory investigations. *Andrologia* 1987; **19**: 113–18.

[44] Schill WB, Landthaler M. Tamoxifen treatment of oligozoospermia. *Andrologia* 1980; **12**: 546–8.

[45] Schill WB, Schillinger R. Selection of oligozoospermic men for tamoxifen treatment by an antiestrogen test. *Andrologia* 1987; **19**: 266–72.

[46] Traub AI, Thompson W. The effect of tamoxifen on spermatogenesis in subfertile men. *Andrologia* 1981; **13**: 486–90.

[47] Vermeulen A, Comhaire F. Hormonal effects of an antiestrogen, tamoxifen, in normal and oligospermic men. *Fertil Steril* 1978; **29**: 320–7.

[48] Adamopoulos DA, Pappa A, Billa E, *et al.* Effectiveness of combined tamoxifen citrate and testosterone undecanoate treatment in men with idiopathic oligozoospermia. *Fertil Steril* 2003; **80**: 914–20.

[49] MacDonald PC, Madden JD, Brenner PF, Wilson JD, Siiteri PK. Origin of estrogen in normal men and in women with testicular feminization. *J Clin Endocrinol Metab* 1979; **49**: 905–16.

[50] Longcope C, Pratt JH, Schneider SH, Fineberg SE. Aromatization of androgens by muscle and adipose tissue in vitro. *J Clin Endocrinol Metab* 1978; **46**: 146–52.

[51] Vigersky RA, Glass AR. Effects of delta1-testolactone on the pituitary–testicular axis in oligospermic men. *J Clin Endocrinol Metab* 1981; **52**: 897–902.

[52] Jarow JP, Kirkland J, Koritnik DR, Cefalu WT. Effect of obesity and fertility status on sex steroid levels in men. *Urology* 1993; **42**: 171–4.

[53] Schlegel PN, Raman JD. Aromatase inhibitors for male infertility. *J Urol* 2002; **167**: 624–9.

[54] Whitcomb RW, Crowley WF. Male hypogonadotropic hypogonadism. *Endocrinol Metab Clin North Am* 1993; **22**: 125–43.

[55] Wang C, Dahl KD, Leung A, Chan SY, Hsueh AJ. Serum bioactive follicle-stimulating hormone in men with idiopathic azoospermia and oligospermia. *J Clin Endocrinol Metab* 1987; **65**: 629–33.

[56] Glass SJ, Holland HM. Treatment of oligospermia with large doses of human chorionic gonadotropin. *Fertil Steril* 1963; **14**: 500–6.

[57] Lytton B, Mroueh A. Treatment of oligospermia with urinary human menopausal gonadotropin: a preliminary report. *Fertil Steril* 1966; **17**: 696–700.

[58] Danezis JM, Batrinos ML. The effect of human postmenopausal gonadotropins on infertile men with severe oligospermia. *Fertil Steril* 1967; **18**: 788–800.

[59] Lunenfeld B, Mor A, Mani M. Treatment of male infertility. I. Human gonadotropins. *Fertil Steril* 1967; **18**: 581–92.

[60] Troen P, Yanihar T, Nankin H, *et al.* Assessment of gonadotropin therapy in infertile males. In: Rosenberg E, Paulsen CA, eds. *The Human Testis*. New York, NY: Plenum Press, 1970.

[61] Mehan DJ, Chehval MJ. Human chorionic gonadotropin in the treatment of the infertile man. *J Urol* 1982; **128**: 60–3.

[62] Sherins RJ. Clinical aspects of treatment of male infertility with gonadotropins: testicular response of some men given HCG with and without Pergonal. In: Mancini RE, Martini L, eds. *Male Fertility and Sterility*. New York, NY: Academic Press, 1974.

[63] Homonnai ZT, Peled M, Paz GF. Changes in semen quality and fertility in response to endocrine treatment of subfertile men. *Gynecol Obstet Invest* 1978; **9**: 244–55.

[64] Dubin L, Amelar RD. Varicocelectomy as therapy in male infertility: a study of 504 cases. *Fertil Steril* 1975; **26**: 217–20.

[65] Acosta AA, Khalifa E, Oehninger S. Pure human follicle stimulating hormone has a role in the treatment of severe male infertility by assisted reproduction: Norfolk's total experience. *Hum Reprod* 1992; **7**: 1067–72.

[66] Ben-Shlomo I, Bider D, Dor J, *et al.* Failure to fertilize in vitro in couples with male factor infertility: what next? *Fertil Steril* 1992; **58**: 187–9.

[67] Molloy D, Harrison K, Breen T, Hennessey J. The predictive value of idiopathic failure to fertilize on the first in vitro fertilization attempt. *Fertil Steril* 1991; **56**: 285–9.

[68] Knuth UA, Hönigl W, Bals-Pratsch M, Schleicher G, Nieschlag E. Treatment of severe oligospermia with human chorionic gonadotropin/human menopausal gonadotropin: A placebo-controlled, double blind trial. *J Clin Endocrinol Metab* 1987; **65**: 1081–7.

[69] Badenoch DF, Waxman J, Boorman L, *et al.* Administration of a gonadotropin releasing hormone analogue in oligozoospermic infertile males. *Acta Endocrinol (Copenh)* 1988; **117**: 265–7.

[70] Crottaz B, Senn A, Reymond MJ, *et al.* Follicle-stimulating hormone bioactivity in idiopathic normogonadotropic oligoasthenozoospermia: Double-blind trial with gonadotropin-releasing hormone. *Fertil Steril* 1992; **57**: 1034–43.

[71] Aafjes JH, van der Vijver JC, Brugman FW, Schenck PE. Double-blind crossover treatment with mesterolone and placebo of subfertile oligozoospermic men: value of testicular biopsy. *Andrologia* 1983; **15**: 531–5.

[72] World Health Organization. Mesterolone and idiopathic male infertility: a double-blind study. *Int J Androl* 1989; **12**: 254–64.

[73] Comhaire F. Treatment of idiopathic testicular failure with high-dose testosterone undecanoate: a double-blind pilot study. *Fertil Steril* 1990; **54**: 689–93.

[74] Gerris J, Comhaire F, Hellemans P, Peeters K, Schoonjans F. Placebo-controlled trial of high-dose mesterolone treatment of idiopathic male infertility. *Fertil Steril* 1991; **55**: 603–7.

[75] Schill WB. Recent progress in pharmacological therapy of male subfertility: a review. *Andrologia* 1979; **11**: 77–107.

[76] Namiki M, Nakamura M, Okuyama A, *et al.* Testicular follicle stimulating hormone receptors and effectiveness of human menopausal gonadotrophin–human chorionic gonadotrophin treatment in infertile men. *Clin Endocrinol (Oxf)* 1986; **25**: 495–500.

[77] Liu L, Chaudhari N, Corle D, Sherins RJ. Comparison of pulsatile subcutaneous gonadotropin-releasing hormone and exogenous gonadotropins in the treatment of men with isolated hypogonadotropic hypogonadism. *Fertil Steril* 1988; **49**: 302–8.

[78] Schwarzstein L, Aparicio NJ, Schally AV. D-tryptophan-6-luteinizing hormone-releasing hormone in the treatment of normogonadotropic oligoasthenozoospermia. *Int J Androl* 1982; **5**: 171–8.

[79] Aparicio NJ, Schwarzstein L, Turner EA, *et al.* Treatment of idiopathic normogonadotropic oligoasthenospermia with synthetic luteinizing hormone-releasing hormone. *Fertil Steril* 1976; **27**: 549–55.

[80] Matsumiya K, Kitamura M, Kishikawa H, *et al.* A prospective comparative trial of a gonadotropin-releasing hormone analogue with clomiphene citrate for the treatment of oligoasthenozoospermia. *Int J Urol* 1998; **5**: 361–3.

[81] McCullagh EP, McGurl FJ. Further observations on the clinical use of testosterone propionate. *J Urol* 1939; **42**: 1265–7.

[82] Turner TT, Jones CE, Howards SS, *et al.* On the androgen microenvironment of maturing spermatozoa. *Endocrinology* 1984; **115**: 1925–32.

[83] Alèn M, Reinilä M, Vihko R. Response of serum hormones to androgen administration in power athletes. *Med Sci Sports Exerc* 1985; **17**: 354–9.

[84] Alèn M, Suominen J. Effect of androgenic and anabolic steroids on spermatogenesis in power athletes. *Int J Sports Med* 1984; **5** (suppl): 189–92.

[85] Clerico A, Ferdeghini M, Palombo C, *et al.* Effect of anabolic treatment on the serum levels of gonadotropins, testosterone, prolactin, thyroid hormones and myoglobin of male athletes under physical training. *J Nucl Med Allied Sci* 1981; **25**: 79–88.

[86] Jarow JP, Lipshultz LI. Anabolic steroid-induced hypogonadotropic hypogonadism. *Am J Sports Med* 1990; **18**: 429–31.

[87] Santulli R, Sprando RL, Awoniyi CA, Ewing LL, Zirkin BR. To what extent can spermatogenesis be maintained in the hypophysectomized adult rat testis with exogenously administered testosterone? *Endocrinology* 1990; **126**: 95–101.

[88] Turner TT, Howards SS, Gleavy JL. On the maintenance of male fertility in the absence of native testosterone secretion: Site-directed hormonal therapy in the rat. *Fertil Steril* 1990; **54**: 149–56.

[89] Brown JS. The effect of orally administered androgens on sperm motility. *Fertil Steril* 1975; **26**: 305–8.

[90] Urry RL, Cockett ATK. Treating the subfertile male patient: improvement in semen characteristics after low dose androgen therapy. *J Urol* 1976; **116**: 54–5.

[91] Heller CG, Nelson WO, Hill IB, *et al.* Improvement in spermatogenesis following depression of the human testis with testosterone. *Fertil Steril* 1950; **1**: 415–22.

[92] Charny CW. The use of androgens for human spermatogenesis. *Fertil Steril* 1959; **10**: 557–70.

[93] Charny CW, Gordon JA. Testosterone rebound therapy: a neglected modality. *Fertil Steril* 1978; **29**: 64–8.

[94] Lamensdorf H, Compere D, Begley G. Testosterone rebound therapy in the treatment of male infertility. *Fertil Steril* 1975; **26**: 469–72.

[95] Rowley MJ, Heller CG. The testosterone rebound phenomenon in the treatment of male infertility. *Fertil Steril* 1972; **23**: 498–504.

[96] Jungling ML, Bunge RG. The treatment of spermatogenic arrest with arginine. *Fertil Steril* 1976; **27**: 282–3.

[97] Uehling DT. Low-dose cortisone for male infertility. *Fertil Steril* 1978; **29**: 220–1.

[98] Hellstrom WJ, Schachter J, Sweet RL, McClure RD. Is there a role for Chlamydia trachomatis and genital mycoplasma in male infertility? *Fertil Steril* 1987; **48**: 337–9.

[99] Hovatta O, Koskimies AI, Ranta T, Stenman UH, Seppälä M. Bromocriptine treatment of oligospermia: a double blind study. *Clin Endocrinol* 1979; **11**: 377–82.

[100] Schill WB. Improvement of sperm motility in patients with asthenozoospermia by kallikrein treatment. *Andrologia* 1975; **20**: 61–3.

[101] Schill WB, Braun-Falco O, Haberland GL. The possible role of kinins in sperm motility. *Int J Fertil* 1974; **19**: 163–7.

[102] Schill WB. Treatment of idiopathic oligozoospermia by kallikrein: results of a double-blind study. *Arch Androl* 1979; **2**: 163–70.

[103] Glezerman M, Lunenfeld E, Potashnik G, et al. Efficacy of kallikrein in the treatment of oligozoospermia and asthenozoospermia: a double-blind trial. *Fertil Steril* 1993; **60**: 1052–6.

[104] Keck C, Behre HM, Jockenhövel F, Nieschlag E. Ineffectiveness of kallikrein in treatment of idiopathic male infertility: a double-blind, randomized, placebo-controlled trial. *Hum Reprod* 1994; **9**: 325–9.

[105] Barkay J, Harpaz-Kerpel S, Ben-Ezra S, Gordon S, Zuckerman H. The prostaglandin inhibitor effect of antiinflammatory drugs in the therapy of male infertility. *Fertil Steril* 1984; **42**: 406–11.

[106] Lenzi A, Culasso F, Gandini L, Lombardo F, Dondero F. Placebo-controlled, double-blind, cross-over trial of glutathione therapy in male infertility. *Hum Reprod* 1993; **8**: 1657–62.

[107] Homonnai ZT, Shilon M, Paz G. Evaluation of semen quality following kallikrein treatment. *Gynecol Obstet Invest* 1978; **9**: 132–8.

[108] Bartke A, Kupfer D, Dalterio S. Prostaglandins inhibit testosterone secretion by mouse testes in vitro. *Steroids* 1976; **28**: 81–8.

[109] Abbatiello ER, Kaminsky M, Weisbroth S. The effect of prostaglandins and prostaglandin inhibitors on spermatogenesis. *Int J Fertil* 1975; **20**: 177–82.

[110] Cohen MS, Colin MJ, Golimbu M, Hotchkiss RS. The effects of prostaglandins on sperm motility. *Fertil Steril* 1977; **28**: 78–85.

[111] Lenzi A, Lombardo F, Gandini L, Culasso F, Dondero F. Glutathione therapy for male infertility. *Arch Androl* 1992; **29**: 65–8.

[112] Burger M, Sikka SC, Bivalacqua TJ, Lamb DJ, Hellstrom WJ. The effect of sildenafil on human sperm motion and function from normal and infertile men. *Int J Impot Res* 2000; **12**: 229–34.

[113] Ebisch IM, Pierik FH, De Jong FH, et al. Does folic acid and zinc sulphate intervention affect endocrine parameters and sperm characteristics in men? *Int J Androl* 2006; **29**: 339–45.

[114] Wong WY, Merkus HM, Thomas CM, et al. Effects of folic acid and zinc sulfate on male factor subfertility: a double-blind, randomized, placebo-controlled trial. *Fertil Steril* 2002; **77**(3): 491–8.

[115] Agarwal A, Sharma RK, Nallella KP, et al. Reactive oxygen species as an independent marker of male factor infertility. *Fertil Steril* 2006; **86**: 878–85.

[116] Mostafa T, Tawadrous G, Roaja MM, et al. Effect of smoking on seminal plasma ascorbic acid in infertile and fertile males. *Andrologia* 2006; **38**: 221–4.

[117] Sierens J, Hartley JA, Campbell MJ, Leathem AJ, Woodside JV. *In vitro* isoflavone supplementation reduces hydrogen peroxide-induced DNA damage in sperm. *Teratog Carcinog Mutagen* 2002; **22**: 227–34.

Chapter 26

Abnormalities of ejaculation

Nancy L. Brackett, Dana A. Ohl, Jens Sønksen, and Charles M. Lynne

Introduction

The purpose of ejaculation is to allow rapid transport of sperm through the urethra into the vagina during intercourse to allow procreation. There are anatomic and neuroanatomic structures essential for ejaculation, and these structures are coordinated in a very exact way to allow normal ejaculation to take place.

The description and management of ejaculatory dysfunction have historically taken a "back seat" to the issues of erectile dysfunction (ED) for a variety of reasons. For example, ED of some degree is widespread, whereas ejaculatory dysfunction is not as widespread, and may occur in only a subset of patients with severe ED. Additionally, ED is often attributed to the latest new medicine prescribed for another disease, or may be part of a more diffuse neurological or anatomic condition. Even when present in conjunction with ED, ejaculatory dysfunction is usually tolerated or ignored as long as the ED can be managed well (which is often the case). Ejaculatory dysfunction obviously becomes more important in the younger male when fatherhood is of concern but, even then, its role in fertility is often looked at only as a problem in transport of sperm.

In men with spinal cord injury (SCI), the relationship of ejaculatory dysfunction to infertility has been studied extensively. In these patients, sperm production has been shown to be essentially normal, yet the semen quality of men with SCI and the function of their sperm are grossly abnormal, indicating more than a simple problem of sperm transport. A special section on male partners with SCI has been included in this chapter.

Anatomy and physiology of ejaculation

The organs involved in the process of ejaculation are the epididymides, vasa deferentia, prostate, seminal vesicles, bladder neck, and bulbourethral glands [1].

Sperm are stored in the cauda epididymidis prior to ejaculation. An elegant animal study by Prins and Zaneveld has shown that during sexual stimulation, fluid is slowly expelled from the cauda epididymidis into the vas deferens. During ejaculation, the sperm are rapidly transported via peristalsis through the vas deferens and into the urethra. Interestingly, residual caudal fluid persisting in the urethra is transported back into the cauda epididymidis, where it is again stored until the next ejaculation [2]. If this storage function is disordered by infrequent ejaculation [2,3] or neurological conditions [4], distal migration down the Wolffian structures can occur, leading to seminal vesicle storage of sperm, and the **seminal vesicles are not a very hospitable environment for the sperm. Sperm stored in the seminal vesicles exhibit very low motility** [4].

From the cauda epididymidis, sperm are transported through the vas deferens, which courses through the external and internal inguinal rings, over the ureter, and turns medially under the prostate. There, the two vasa run medial and parallel to the seminal vesicles, eventually coalescing into the ejaculatory ducts. These ductal systems are completely separate in normal circumstances. The ejaculatory ducts course though the tissue of the prostate and open into the urethra.

Once seminal fluid is expelled through the ejaculatory ducts into the urethra, it still needs to be forced out in the antegrade direction. First, the bladder neck closes, preventing retrograde ejaculation. Then rhythmic contractions of the periurethral muscles cause rhythmic forceful expulsion of semen through the urethra. It has been suggested that expansion of the posterior urethra causes the rhythmic contraction to take place, but in men with absence of seminal emission, who are otherwise neurologically normal, such as testis cancer patients who underwent a radical retroperitoneal lymph node dissection, the rhythmic contraction takes place nevertheless. This observation

Infertility in the Male, 4th edition, ed. Larry I. Lipshultz, Stuart S. Howards, and Craig S. Niederberger. Published by Cambridge University Press. © Cambridge University Press 2009.

suggests that the **periurethral muscle activity is part of the central reflex**, and not due to posterior urethral expansion.

The exact mechanisms that cause this coordinated reflex to occur are not completely clear. However, studies on ejaculation induction procedures in men with spinal cord injury suggest that the event which immediately precedes the ejaculatory reflex threshold is an extremely high-pressure contraction of the external sphincter/periurethral muscles. Men with high-pressure contractions in response to vibratory stimulation always ejaculated, while those without such muscle contraction never ejaculated [5]. **This finding suggests that proprioception within the external sphincter may be important in initiating responses through the neurological pathways described below.**

Neural control of ejaculation

Neural control of ejaculation consists of the ejaculatory reflex, which is mediated at the thoracolumbar level and involves a coordinated interaction of the sympathetic and parasympathetic autonomic nervous systems. Control of the ejaculatory reflex is probably initiated centrally, and it may be inhibited centrally as well via the cortex, thalamus, hypothalamus, midbrain, and pons [6,7]. **Centrally, dopaminergic structures are thought to be excitatory to the ejaculatory reflex while serotonergic receptors are thought to be inhibitory** [8,9].

Additional input directly into the reflex may come from the dorsal nerve of the penis. **Sympathetic outflow via the lumbar sympathetic ganglia and then the hypogastric nerve is responsible for seminal emission and closure of the bladder neck to create a "pressure chamber" phenomenon. Parasympathetic outflow (S2–4) via the pelvic nerve stimulates secretions of the prostate and seminal vesicles while somatic efferents from the same segments are responsible for the contractions of the bulbocavernosal and ischiocavernosal muscles and the pelvic floor resulting in forceful expulsion of the ejaculate.** One may now understand how an abnormality at any point in the system may result in some form of ejaculatory dysfunction (Fig. 26.1).

Abnormalities of ejaculation
Glossary of terms

Although there are a number of specific etiologies for ejaculation disorders, it is important to define the

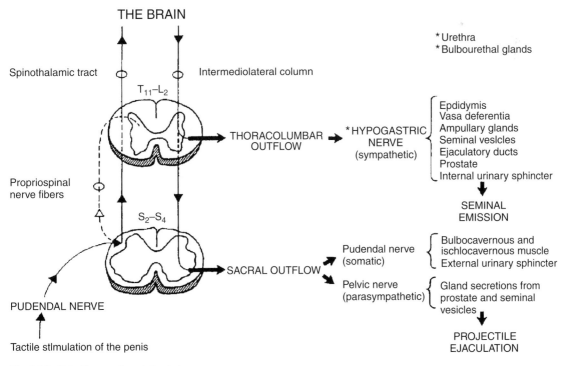

Fig. 26.1. Spinal innervation of ejaculation.

general nature of the dysfunctions. The conditions can be functional or pathological, lifelong or acquired, and exhibit different clinical manifestations, as listed here:

Anemission: Absence of seminal emission, despite climax.

Anejaculation: Absence of seminal emission and projectile ejaculation, although this term is commonly applied to neurologically impaired individuals who lack all aspects of the ejaculatory reflex, including loss of orgasm.

Premature ejaculation (rapid ejaculation): Climax occurring too soon, and before the patient wishes it to occur.

Retarded ejaculation (delayed ejaculation, anorgasmia): Inability to achieve climax, or extreme delay in achieving climax.

Retrograde ejaculation: Passage of semen backwards into the bladder during an ejaculatory reflex, due to failure of bladder neck closure.

Abnormalities of ejaculation: functional

There are abnormalities of ejaculation in which anatomic or neurological problems usually are not seen. These functional issues are perhaps more commonly termed abnormalities of orgasm threshold. Premature ejaculation and delayed ejaculation are the two conditions of importance.

Premature ejaculation

This condition is receiving a great deal more attention than in years past, most likely because of the development of drugs that promise effective on-demand treatment. Premature ejaculation (PE) is defined as reaching climax and ejaculating before the person wishes it. To be considered a dysfunction, it must cause distress. **PE is likely the most common sexual complaint in men, affecting 31% of men between the ages of 18 and 59** [10].

Recent studies on premature ejaculation have focused on the intravaginal ejaculatory latency time (IELT). Studies in men self-reporting whether they suffer from PE have examined the correlation between IELT and perceived dysfunction. Waldinger *et al.* have suggested that those with an IELT of less than one minute have "definite" premature ejaculation, and those with an IELT of 1–1.5 minutes have "probable" premature ejaculation [11].

Treatment for premature ejaculation is aimed at improving sexual performance. Most men with PE do not have ejaculation occurring prior to intromission,

and thus will be able to deposit the semen into the vagina. The rapid-onset, short-acting selective serotonin reuptake inhibitor (SSRI), dapoxetine, has demonstrated promise as an on-demand treatment for men with PE [12].

Delayed ejaculation (retarded ejaculation, primary anejaculation, anorgasmia)

Delayed ejaculation is present when a man is unable to achieve climax. It may be lifelong or acquired. Inability to achieve climax is seen in 8% of men aged 18–59 [10]. This condition can be more common with aging, and recent evidence has suggested that masturbation pattern can affect the ability to climax during sexual activity [13].

Many cases of lifelong anorgasmia are thought to be psychogenic in nature. The characteristics of such cases include the inability of the man to ejaculate during any kind of sexual activity; absence of known neurological conditions; presence of nocturnal emissions, suggesting that the ejaculatory reflex can function normally. Psychogenic cases have historically been thought to be very resistant to psychotherapy. Many times, extreme measures have been necessary to allow men with this condition to initiate a pregnancy, such as rectal probe electroejaculation [14] or surgical sperm retrieval with in-vitro fertilization (IVF).

It is important to remember that some men with apparently functional anorgasmia may have subtle neurological changes indicative of an etiology. Some diagnoses might include occult spina bifida with cord tethering or early multiple sclerosis. The diagnosis of a psychogenic source should be made only after an effort to exclude an organic cause.

Abnormalities of ejaculation: anatomic

Ejaculatory duct obstruction

Ejaculatory duct obstruction (EDO) can be partial or total. Partial EDO is a relatively controversial area, in that some believe previously idiopathic problems with sperm morphology or sperm motility can be explained by partial EDO. Others argue that therapeutic intervention can lead to worsening of fertility, with urine contamination of the ejaculate, possible scarring, and development of complete occlusion of the ducts [15].

Congenital or acquired complete EDO is more clear-cut. This condition is manifest by low semen volume (< 1.0 mL), absence of sperm in the ejaculate, and acidic (prostatic) pH. Patients with complete EDO may complain of testis pain with sexual stimulation. Lifelong EDO is due to either atresia of the very end of the duct or to midline cysts, most likely of utricular origin, that compress the ejaculatory ducts. Men with atresia may have a variant of cystic fibrosis, similar to men with absence of the vas.

Men with EDO can be treated with a transurethral resection to open the ducts, with a high rate of success in increasing semen volume and restoring sperm flow. Urine contamination of the ejaculate and scarring of the urethra, however, can complicate the situation.

Congenital bilateral absence of the vas deferens (CBAVD)

Men with this variation of cystic fibrosis mutations generally appear on physical examination to have nonformation of the entire vas deferens and partial formation of the epididymis. On prostate ultrasound, there is hypoplasia or atresia of one or both seminal vesicles [16]. There may be ejaculatory duct obstruction as well. The clinical presentation is similar to that of men with EDO, and they present with azoospermia and low-volume ejaculate, with normal sensation of orgasm. **The difference between EDO and CBAVD is determined by physical examination.**

CBAVD is a nonreconstructible condition. Initiation of pregnancy is possible with sperm retrieval and IVF.

Bladder neck incompetence

Open bladder neck is occasionally seen as a spontaneous problem due to poor sympathetic outflow, but this is a rare event. More commonly, retrograde ejaculation, due to an incompetent internal sphincter, is a result of medication (see below), diabetic neuropathy, or anatomic causes.

An increasingly uncommon anatomic cause of retrograde ejaculation is previous surgical Y-V plasty revision of the bladder neck [17]. This operation was used in the past to treat boys for a variety of conditions, including urinary infections, dysfunctional voiding, vesicoureteral reflux, and enuresis. It was not effective for these conditions, and has been abandoned.

Reversal of Y-V plasty is difficult and not advisable. These men should be managed with protocols designed for use of retrograde sperm, as discussed later in this chapter.

Abnormalities of ejaculation: neuropathic

Table 26.1 lists the major causes of neurogenic ejaculatory dysfunction.

Table 26.1. Neurogenic causes of ejaculatory dysfunction

Spinal cord injury
Low abdominal/pelvic surgery
Retroperitoneal lymph node dissection
Diabetes and other diseases causing peripheral neuropathy
Myelodysplasia
Multiple sclerosis
Stroke/traumatic brain injury

Spinal cord injury (SCI)

The majority of spinal cord injuries occur to young men. The percentage of men with SCI who retain the ability to ejaculate via sexual activity varies by level of injury. For example, only 4% of men with SCI who have a high complete lesion can ejaculate, versus approximately 18% of those with lower lesions, i.e., injuries that involve only the conus or cauda equina [18]. The former situation presumes an intact ejaculatory reflex mechanism but with few or no central connections remaining. The latter situation presumes an SCI below the cord levels of S2–4 *and* integrity of the respective spinal nerves throughout the cauda equina; a situation unfortunately uncommon. In those men who are able to ejaculate with the assistance of penile vibratory stimulation (PVS, described later in this chapter) some sort of propulsive ejaculation is usually seen. This propulsive feature is an indication that the intact ejaculatory reflex has been recruited. Lack of propulsive ejaculation, and/or appearance of retrograde ejaculation, indicates incomplete and/or uncoordinated stimulation of the spinal cord centers of the ejaculatory reflex.

Low abdominal/pelvic surgery

Putting aside the obvious consequences of radical prostatectomy and radical cystectomy on ejaculatory function, certain operations in the retroperitoneum and pelvis place the sympathetic and parasympathetic nerves at risk for injury. The superior hypogastric plexus is in a midline presacral position just below the aortic bifurcation. Surgery for certain rectal and other less common pelvic tumors may damage this structure, leading to retrograde ejaculation. Extensive dissection of the pelvic splanchnic nerve in the perirectal area can lead to erectile, urinary, and ejaculatory dysfunction [19]. Rates of ejaculatory dysfunction of 36–60% have been reported after radical rectal surgery [19]. Surgery for repair of abdominal aortic aneurysm or aortoiliac bypass grafting may lead to some degree of damage to

457

the lumbar sympathetic ganglia and/or the superior hypogastric plexus, with resultant loss of emission and bladder neck closure.

Retroperitoneal lymph node dissection (RPLND)

The paravertebral sympathetic ganglia at the T2–L3 levels and the convergence of the postganglionic fibers from these ganglia at the superior hypogastric plexus put these structures, which are essential for seminal emission, at risk for damage or removal with the surgical specimen. Templates designed to spare at least a part of these structures on the contralateral side of the tumor have reduced the risk. The highest rates of success in preserving ejaculatory function have been reported with nerve-sparing RPLND. Assuming the surgical anatomy and findings are favorable, ejaculation can be preserved in up to 95% of patients undergoing this procedure, with paternity rates as high as 76% [20]. More recently, laparoscopic RPLND has been reported to be successful in preserving ejaculation in all of the patients in which the procedure was successfully completed [21,22].

Diabetes

Genitourinary autonomic neuropathy is recognized as an important component of the diabetic autonomic neuropathy complex and is seen in one form or another in the majority of type I diabetics. It is the paradigm for the study of peripheral neuropathies affecting the urinary tract. Up to 87% of type I diabetics have physiologic evidence of bladder dysfunction, and erectile dysfunction (ED) is estimated to be present in 35–75% of affected males [23]. Ejaculatory dysfunction is less commonly reported, or is often lumped with ED; **however, ejaculatory failure is said to be present in up to 40% of men with type I diabetes** [24]. The ejaculatory dysfunction may manifest as either retrograde ejaculation or anejaculation (complete failure of emission) depending on the degree of sympathetic autonomic neuropathy involved.

For purposes of conception, any sympathomimetic drug may be administered to mitigate the failure of bladder neck closure in cases of retrograde ejaculation [25], although for assisted conception, sperm retrieval from the bladder is usually satisfactory. Ephedrine sulfate, 50 mg four times a day, pseudoephedrine, 60 mg four times a day, and phenylpropanolamine, 75 mg twice a day, are typically used for this purpose [26,27]. Currently, the most practical drugs administered are pseudoephedrine or phenylpropanolamine, typically compounded with other ingredients as cold remedies.

Because most sympathomimetics will exhibit tachyphylaxis with prolonged use, their administration should be timed to the five or seven days prior to the partner's ovulation. Occasionally these sympathomimetics will reverse anejaculation, but more commonly electroejaculation, or surgical sperm retrieval from the testis, will be necessary to achieve biologic fatherhood.

Myelodysplasia

Spinal dysraphism is a relatively common congenital disorder which involves the lumbar vertebrae in over 90% of cases and the lower thoracic vertebrae in another 5% [28]. As imagined, the majority will have multiple sexual and urologic problems. Decter et al. studied a group of men $\geq$ 18 years of age who were patients at a multidisciplinary clinic [29]. Erections were experienced by 41 men, including 27 who ejaculated with erection. Eleven patients attempted to father children and eight were successful. They concluded that the level of the neurologic lesion was not predictive of erectile or ejaculatory function. However, men with lower and less severe lesions had a greater chance for successful fatherhood. For example, seven of the eight fathers had an L5 or sacral level lesion, were ambulatory, and did not have a ventriculoperitoneal shunt.

Multiple sclerosis (MS)

MS is a demyelinating disease of the nervous system, most common in the spinal cord but sometimes also affecting areas of the brain which have input into the autonomic nervous system. Plaques may affect any white-matter tracts, and some manifestation of autonomic dysfunction is often the first sign of the disease. Voiding dysfunction is reported in up to 97% of the patients, and may be the most disturbing of their symptoms [30]. **Erectile dysfunction may be present in up to 73% of men, and ejaculatory and/or orgasmic dysfunction in about 50%.** Interestingly, reduced libido is reported to occur less frequently, in about 40%. With respect to ejaculatory dysfunction, these men may respond to electroejaculation, but since they are sensate the procedure may have to be performed with conscious sedation or even general anesthesia.

Stroke and traumatic brain injury (TBI)

There is much literature about "sexual disorders" after stroke and TBI. In general, the types and frequencies of sexual disorders are similar for stroke and TBI [19]. The majority of patients report a decline in libido, sexual satisfaction, coital frequency, erection, and orgasmic ability. Psychological and social factors seem to have as much or even more impact on these functions as the resultant physical disability [31]. Ejaculatory dysfunction after stroke and TBI is rarely discussed in the literature.

Further impacting on this subject are the side effects of the various drugs which may be used to treat the underlying causes. These drugs include antihypertensive medicines as well as medications to treat affective disturbances which often accompany stroke and TBI. Nevertheless, based on our ever-expanding knowledge of the role of supraspinal dopaminergic and serotonergic centers on ejaculatory function, it would be reasonable to think that ejaculatory dysfunction in cases of brain injury may have a strong biochemical basis, and that this condition may respond well to appropriate pharmacologic manipulation.

Abnormalities of ejaculation: pharmacologic

Antidepressants

Older antidepressants (e.g., tricyclics), as well as the newer selective serotonin reuptake inhibitors (SSRIs) are powerful inhibitors of climax [32]. This inhibition is via a central effect and is limited to anorgasmia. If orgasm is present, ejaculation is usually noted to be normal in these men. The effect is due to elevation of CNS levels of serotonin (SSRIs) or catecholamines (tricyclics).

Alpha-adrenergic antagonists

Transport of seminal fluid and bladder neck closure are controlled by activation of α-adrenergic nerves. Therefore, α-blockers, given for hypertension or voiding dysfunction from prostatism, can inhibit both seminal emission and bladder neck closure. The result may be a decrease in the amount of semen emitted into the urethra and/or retrograde ejaculation due to inhibition of bladder neck closure [33]. These men present with a normal sensation of orgasm, but a significant decrease or absence of seminal fluid output. Hellstrom and Sikka compared the effects of tamsulosin 0.8 mg daily versus alfuzosin 10 mg daily on ejaculatory function in normal volunteers [33]. A marked decrease in ejaculate volume (not related to retrograde ejaculation) was seen in almost 90% of those taking tamsulosin 0.8 mg daily, with approximately 35% having anejaculation. Twenty-one percent of the alfuzosin group and 12.5% of the placebo group had decreased ejaculatory volume.

Management of abnormalities of ejaculation
Nonsurgical

Pharmacologic management
Alpha-adrenergic agonists

For individuals suffering from a neurogenic source of anemission or retrograde ejaculation, α-agonists may have some value (see *diabetes*, above). The basis for this treatment is to overstimulate pharmacologically those nerves that are ostensibly not being stimulated by endogenous mechanisms. Clearly, if there is a profound and total malfunction of the entire ejaculatory reflex, such as that seen with complete spinal cord injury, pharmacological management will have little effect. However, in other situations, the effect may be beneficial [34].

The types of conditions in which alpha stimulation may be helpful are those in which there is a well-defined peripheral problem that tends to be incomplete. Candidates for this type of therapy have a normal sensation of orgasm, but have either retrograde ejaculation or anemission during climax.

Men with a nerve-sparing RPLND will commonly have some innervation of the ejaculatory organs, and the stimulation afforded by drug therapy may be enough to allow seminal emission or bladder neck closure. Diabetic neuropaths commonly have a progressive decline in adrenergic function, and when either retrograde ejaculation or anemission occurs α-agonist therapy may temporarily "reverse" the effects of the neuropathy for a period of time, until it progresses, making drug therapy ineffective [35].

Selective serotonin reuptake inhibitors (SSRIs) for premature ejaculation

One of the adverse effects of the SSRI drug class is delayed ejaculation, and this adverse effect has been of benefit in delaying ejaculation in men with PE [36]. Pryor *et al.* reported on the short-acting agent dapoxetine for men with PE [12]. IELT increased from a mean of 0.9 minutes to 3.32 minutes at the 60 mg dose. This effect was significantly better than placebo. Adverse events included nausea, headache, diarrhea, and dizziness.

Treatment of refractory retrograde ejaculation

In individuals who suffer from retrograde ejaculation that is unresponsive to medical management, the sperm can be retrieved and utilized for assisted reproductive techniques [37]. **It is essential to optimize the sperm quality prior to use for attempts at pregnancy. Urine is toxic to sperm, and any steps that will improve the sperm quality will improve the chance of success.** There are several steps that can optimize the quality of a retrograde ejaculate. Complete emptying of the bladder immediately prior to ejaculation, and again immediately after, can limit urine contact with the sperm. Administration of bicarbonate to prevent acid formation in the urine may help.

It is controversial whether to fluid load to limit osmolality of the urine, or fluid restrict to prevent urine formation between voids. In patients with very poor semen quality in the retrograde specimen, a catheter should be passed with nonspermicidal lubricant prior to ejaculation, and sperm-friendly buffered media placed in the bladder. After ejaculation, another plastic catheter is used to empty the specimen and the bladder can be rinsed with media for complete collection.

Typically, if sperm production is normal, the above-mentioned maneuvers will be successful in retrieving a specimen suitable for intrauterine insemination (IUI). If, despite the maneuvers, the total motile sperm count after processing is still less than 10 million, in-vitro fertilization, with or without intracytoplasmic sperm injection, may be needed.

Neurostimulation

Neurostimulatory methods may be used to induce ejaculation in men with neurogenic anejaculation. One of the largest and most-studied groups of patients with neurogenic anejaculation includes men with spinal cord injury (SCI) [38]. The most common neurostimulatory methods to induce ejaculation in men with SCI are penile vibratory stimulation (PVS) and electroejaculation (EEJ).

Penile vibratory stimulation

PVS is usually recommended as the first line of treatment for anejaculation in men with SCI [39–41]. PVS involves placing a vibrator on the dorsum or frenulum of the glans penis (Fig. 26.2) [42]. Mechanical stimulation produced by the vibrator recruits the ejaculatory reflex to induce ejaculation [43]. This method is more effective in men with an intact ejaculatory reflex, i.e., men with a level of injury T10 or above (88% success rate) compared to men with a level of injury T11 and below (15% success rate) [44–46].

Unlike the methods of EEJ, surgical sperm retrieval, or prostate massage, the method of PVS may be performed at home by selected couples. Couples should

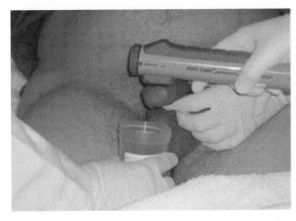

Fig. 26.2. Penile vibratory stimulation is recommended as the first line of treatment for anejaculation in men with SCI.

first be evaluated in a clinic prior to trying PVS at home. The evaluation should include assessment for risk of autonomic dysreflexia, assessment for optimal stimulation parameters to induce safe ejaculation in the given patient, and demonstration that the patient and/or his partner can perform the procedure properly [42].

Autonomic dysreflexia is a risk for any method of sperm retrieval in patients with a level of injury T6 and above [45,47]. Briefly, autonomic dysreflexia is a potentially life-threatening medical complication resulting from an uninhibited sympathetic reflex response to an irritating stimulus below the level of injury. Symptoms of autonomic dysreflexia include hypertension, bradycardia, sweating, chills, and headache. In some cases, autonomic dysreflexia can lead to dangerously high blood pressure levels, and this complication can lead to stroke, seizure, or even death. **Autonomic dysreflexia symptoms can be well managed or prevented by oral administration of nifedipine** [47,48].

PVS may be attempted using any of a number of commercially available devices sold over the counter as wand massagers. One of the most effective commercially available vibrators is the Ferti Care (Multicept, Denmark), engineered specifically for inducing ejaculation in men with SCI (Fig. 26.3). The advantage of this vibrator is its ability to deliver high-amplitude stimulation, i.e., 2.5 mm excursions of the vibrating head, at a frequency of 90–100 Hz. These stimulus parameters were found to be most effective for ejaculatory success in men with SCI [49].

The procedure of PVS has been well described in a number of publications [41,42,50]. Most practitioners

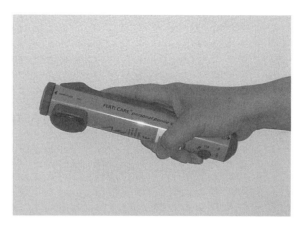

Fig. 26.3. The Ferti Care vibrator, pictured here, was engineered specifically for ejaculation by men with SCI.

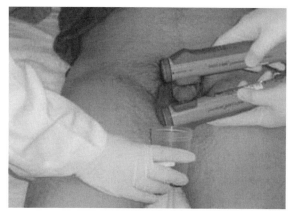

Fig. 26.4. Individuals who cannot respond to PVS with one vibrator may respond to PVS with two vibrators.

follow some form of the following protocol. PVS may be administered to any man with SCI, although in men with certain medical conditions it is relatively contraindicated. Severe inflammation or irritation of the glans penis, which sometimes occurs in patients who wear condom catheters, is a relative contraindication because PVS may lead to further skin breakdown. PVS should not be administered to patients with untreated hypertension or cardiac disease, as it may cause an increase in blood pressure. In patients with a penile prosthesis, PVS must be applied with care, as the pressure of the vibrator may push the glans onto the distal end of the prosthesis. An additional contraindication is the patient's inability to comprehend instructions about the procedure. Additionally, patients recently injured (i.e., < 18 months) may not respond readily to PVS.

Patients with a level of injury T6 or above should be pretreated with nifedipine, which is typically administered sublingually 15 minutes prior to stimulation onset. A dose of 20 mg is usually administered on the first trial of PVS, and adjusted on subsequent trials based on the patient's blood pressure during PVS.

For safety and efficacy, it is advisable to perform PVS after transferring the patient from his wheelchair to an exam table or hospital bed; however, the PVS procedure may be performed with the patient remaining in his wheelchair. The wheelchair site is recommended when transfer is problematic, such as with patients who have high cervical injuries, those with severe pain or extreme obesity, or those wearing spinal cord stabilization devices.

The goal of PVS is to activate the ejaculatory reflex in the thoracolumbar area of the spinal cord. After the

patient has been safely positioned, and pretreated with nifedipine (if necessary), the vibrator is applied to the glans penis (dorsum or frenulum). **This placement stimulates the dorsal penile nerve, which must be intact (S2–4) for ejaculatory success** [51]. Placement of the vibrator on the shaft of the penis or on the perineum is less effective. Placement on the testicles could cause injury. The vibrator is applied for 2–3 minutes or until antegrade ejaculation occurs. If no ejaculation occurs, the stimulation period is followed by a rest period of 1–2 minutes, and stimulation begins again. In patients who are responsive to PVS, the majority (89%) ejaculate within two minutes of stimulation onset [39].

If a patient is unable to ejaculate with a high-amplitude vibrator, then auxiliary methods may be employed to facilitate ejaculation with PVS, such as application of two vibrators (Fig. 26.4) [52], use of abdominal electrical stimulation in addition to PVS (Fig. 26.5) [53], or oral administration of a PDE-5 inhibitor prior to PVS [54].

The definition of PVS failure varies among practitioners. There is a degree of uncertainty about how many trials to administer, how many minutes per trial, or what methods beyond administration of one vibrator should be tried before considering the patient or the trial a PVS failure. **Studies have shown that SCI patients with a bulbocavernosus response (BCR) and a hip flexor response (HR) are more likely to ejaculate with PVS than patients without these responses** [55–57]. The BCR and HR are more useful for predicting ejaculatory success in patients whose injuries are below the cervical level [55]. For example, in men whose injuries were between T1 and T6, ejaculation occurred in

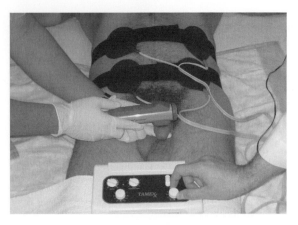

Fig. 26.5. PVS, in combination with abdominal electrical stimulation using a commercially available device, has been shown to be successful in some men who do not respond to PVS alone.

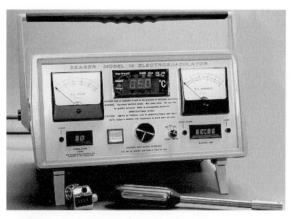

Fig. 26.6. Electroejaculation is a method to retrieve semen when PVS fails.

94% of those who had a positive BCR plus a positive HR, versus 0% with neither response. Similarly, in men whose injuries were between T7 and T12, ejaculation occurred in 67% of men who had both responses, versus 0% with neither response. In contrast, presence of both responses was nearly as predictive as level of injury in men with cervical injuries, with an ejaculation success rate of 78% in men with both responses versus 50% in those with neither response.

In reality, the degree of effort and commitment to PVS will vary based on the skill and experience of the practitioner. Two consecutive failed PVS trials, spaced at least one week apart, typically defines the patient as a PVS failure.

Electroejaculation

Individuals who cannot respond to PVS are often referred for EEJ (Fig. 26.6). Electroejaculation is performed with the patient in the lateral decubitus position (Fig. 26.7). A probe is placed in the rectum, and electrodes on the probe are oriented anteriorly toward the prostate and seminal vesicles. Current delivered through the probe stimulates nerves that lead to emission of semen.

The method of EEJ was first developed in the 1930s for use in veterinary medicine [58] and modified in the 1980s for use in humans [59,60]. Prior to the development of the high-amplitude vibrator in the mid-1990s, EEJ was the most common method of semen retrieval in men with SCI because it had a higher success rate than PVS. Currently, EEJ is recommended for those individuals who fail to achieve semen retrieval via PVS because, compared to PVS, EEJ is more invasive,

preferred less by patients, and results in a lower yield of total motile sperm in the antegrade fraction [61,62].

The technique of EEJ has been described in numerous publications [63–66]. Patients with a level of injury T6 or above are pretreated with nifedipine to manage possible autonomic dysreflexia.

Immediately prior to EEJ, the bladder is catheterized to empty it completely of urine, and to limit the potential retrograde sperm/urine contact. Through this catheter, 10–20 mL of buffering medium (e.g., Ham's F-10 medium) can be instilled into the bladder to optimize the environment for the sperm ejaculated in the retrograde direction. Rectoscopy is performed prior to stimulation to assure that there are no pre-existing lesions and there is no colitis, either of which is a relative contraindication for the procedure.

The EEJ stimulation is delivered in a wave-like pattern with voltage progressively increasing in 1–5 V increments until ejaculation occurs. It has been previously recommended that a low level of electrical baseline (100 mA) be maintained between voltage peaks and during ejaculation, based on the veterinary experience. However, as is discussed below, recent evidence suggests that complete cessation of electrical activity between peaks may be optimal for maximum antegrade ejaculation.

Antegrade ejaculate is released intermittently during the procedure, but it is usually dribbling in nature. The urethra may have to be milked. The voltages and currents that have been reported to produce successful ejaculation range from 5 to 25 V and 100 to 600 mA, respectively. Ten to twenty stimulations are necessary for complete emptying of the system.

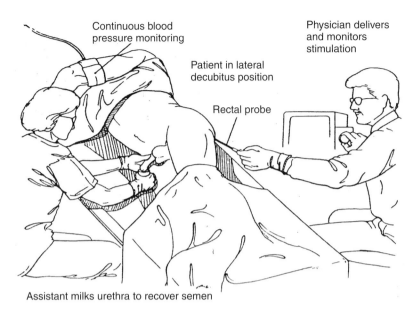

Continuous blood
pressure monitoring

Patient in lateral
decubitus position

Physician delivers
and monitors
stimulation

Rectal probe

Assistant milks urethra to recover semen

Fig. 26.7. Electroejaculation must be performed by a specially trained physician. Electroejaculation is effective in retrieving semen in 95% of men with SCI.

After the procedure, the bladder is catheterized again to empty the retrograde fraction, which may be substantial in some patients. Rectoscopy is performed after the procedure to exclude injury to the rectum.

Patients with complete spinal injuries can undergo EEJ without anesthesia. This is not the case for those with significant sensory sparing or those with other neurological conditions leading to anejaculation. In those with normal sensation, general anesthesia is required for EEJ. It should be noted that EEJ can cause significant discomfort in men with partly preserved sensation, and they may require either general anesthesia or conscious sedation before treatment [67,68].

A study was undertaken to define physiological events surrounding EEJ and PVS in SCI men [5]. **Unsurprisingly, PVS resulted in a stereotypical set of sphincteric events typical of a coordinated ejaculatory reflex.** Extremely high-pressure external sphincter contraction always preceded the reflex. This was followed by relative relaxation of the external sphincter with a rise in pressure of the internal sphincter in conjunction with seminal emission. Rhythmic contractions of the periurethral muscles led to expulsive projectile ejaculation. All these findings were expected.

What was more interesting was the situation observed during EEJ. Application of electricity led to high-pressure contraction of the external sphincter, but after a period of tonic contraction, high-pressure contraction of the *internal* sphincter ensued. If the electrical stimulation was discontinued during this internal

sphincter pressure rise, the course of events continued, and mimicked the events seen following PVS. In other words, **the electrical stimulation was capable of initiating what appeared to be a typical ejaculatory reflex**, with high-pressure internal sphincter contraction coincident with seminal emission, followed by rhythmic contraction of the striated muscle and projectile ejaculation. Again, this pattern was seen to continue, despite discontinuation of the electrical activity.

When the electrical stimulation was continued throughout these events, as was suggested by the "continuous baseline" teaching of the past, the external sphincter pressure always exceeded internal sphincter pressure, favoring retrograde ejaculation. If the stimulus was stopped upon reaching the plateau of external sphincter contraction, the external sphincter pressure dropped below that of the internal sphincter, with the pressure differential favoring antegrade ejaculation. This led to the possibility that stopping the stimulation at peak skeletal muscle contraction would lead to an increased antegrade fraction.

This theory was tested in a "before–after" observational study by Sønksen *et al.* Seven patients who had undergone an average of 5.1 EEJ procedures with the old technique (continuous baseline) were subjected to the new stimulation pattern for an average of 2.7 "new pattern" procedures. The antegrade ejaculate fraction increased from 38.9% to 67.9% [5].

Brackett *et al.* tested this new technique in a randomized study of 12 SCI men. The EEJ trials with interrupted current delivery showed advantages over those with continuous current in several semen parameters. Interruption of the current resulted in increased antegrade semen volume (2.0 mL vs. 0.9 mL), antegrade total sperm count (130 million vs. 79 million) and total antegrade motile sperm count (35 million vs. 25 million) [66].

PVS and EEJ continue to be the most widely used methods of semen collection in men with SCI. PVS has several advantages over EEJ. Although both methods are safe, reliable, and effective [38,69,70], the cost of purchasing PVS equipment is approximately one-twentieth the cost of purchasing EEJ equipment (i.e., approximately $800 versus $16 000 in the year 2007). PVS is preferred by patients, and the semen obtained by PVS is usually of better quality than the semen obtained by EEJ [61,62]. PVS does not require administration by a physician, and selected patients may thus use PVS to attempt home insemination. In contrast, an advantage of EEJ is its effectiveness with PVS failures [40,66,71].

A review was performed on the ejaculatory success rates in a large series of SCI patients [44]. A total of 412 men with SCI underwent 1701 PVS procedures and 845 EEJ procedures. Patients' neurological level of injury ranged between C2 and S4. In patients whose level of injury was T10 or higher, 88% responded to PVS, whereas in patients whose level of injury was T11 or lower, 15% responded to PVS. EEJ was performed only in PVS failures, 95% of whom ejaculated with EEJ. Of the 5% of men who did not ejaculate with EEJ, all were patients with retained pelvic sensation who experienced pain at low voltages (1–4 volts) on their first trial of EEJ, and did not want to continue with further trials of EEJ under sedation or general anesthesia.

Clearly, the ejaculatory success rates obtained with PVS and EEJ merit their continued use as semen retrieval methods in men with SCI.

Prostate massage

"Prostate massage" is a common misnomer, because the intimately located seminal vesicles and ampullae of the vasa are incorporated in the digital mechanical stripping and expulsion of their contents. Prostate massage has been used to collect semen from men with SCI for use in insemination [72–74]. In a recent report, prostatic massage was performed in 69 men with SCI [75]. Sperm were retrieved in 22 patients (31.9%). In these patients, the mean ± SEM sperm concentration was 69.2 ± 15.8 million/mL (range 0.4–325 million/mL), and the sperm motility was 7.3 ± 1.37% (range 0–25%). In the remaining 47 patients, fluid without sperm was obtained in 29 patients. No fluid was obtained in 18 patients. Results for the 22 men from whom sperm were obtained were as follows: IUI was attempted 11 times in six couples, resulting in one live birth (9% success rate per cycle).

It is not clear when prostatic massage should be used in the algorithm of semen retrieval methods in men with SCI. The success rate of ejaculation and the total motile sperm counts obtained with PVS and EEJ are higher than those obtained with prostatic massage. When practitioners lack training or equipment for PVS or EEJ, prostatic massage may be a useful alternative for semen retrieval in men with SCI.

Surgical sperm retrieval

A variety of surgical sperm retrieval methods may be used to retrieve sperm from men with ejaculatory dysfunction (Fig. 26.8), including testicular sperm extraction (TESE), testicular sperm aspiration (TESA), microsurgical epididymal sperm aspiration (MESA), percutaneous epididymal sperm aspiration (PESA), and aspiration of sperm from the vas deferens [76–82]. Unlike the methods discussed previously, surgical sperm retrieval was not developed to treat anejaculation. Instead, these methods were originally developed to retrieve sperm from men who were azoospermic.

Fig. 26.8. Sperm may be surgically removed from men with ejaculatory dysfunction. Use of surgical sperm retrieval in men with SCI is controversial.

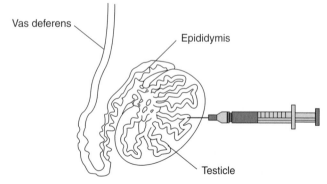

Vas deferens

Epididymis

Testicle

The **application of surgical sperm retrieval to men with SCI is controversial.** A recent survey indicated that some practitioners are using surgical sperm retrieval as the first line of treatment for anejaculation in men with SCI [44]. The primary reasons given by these practitioners for not offering PVS or EEJ were a lack of equipment and/or lack of training in these techniques. It is unclear why practitioners are not being trained in the techniques of PVS and EEJ. One possible reason is that anejaculatory men with SCI represent only a small fraction of the infertile male population, whereas azoospermic men represent a much larger proportion of infertile male patients. Thus, physicians may possess the necessary equipment for, and become adept at, performing the procedures that are appropriate for the majority of their client population. **Ejaculation success rates indicate that PVS and EEJ warrant consideration in centers not currently offering these options for couples with SCI male partners** [44].

Special concerns for male partners with spinal cord injury

Semen quality in men with spinal cord injury

With the advent of PVS and EEJ, data have accumulated on semen quality in men with spinal cord injury. The majority of these men have a distinct semen profile characterized by normal total sperm numbers but abnormally low sperm motility [43,83–85]. This semen profile is uncommon in the general population; therefore, historically, there has been no precedent for understanding the cause of abnormal semen quality in men with SCI. Initial investigations tended to focus on lifestyle factors such as elevated scrotal temperature from sitting in a wheelchair, infrequency of ejaculation, methods of bladder management, and methods of assisted ejaculation as the cause for low sperm motility. Studies showed that such factors could not entirely account for the problem. For example, scrotal temperature was similar in injured and noninjured men [86], frequent ejaculation did not normalize low sperm motility [87–90], and sperm motility remained subnormal despite some improvements by method of bladder management [91] and some improvements by method of assisted ejaculation [61,62].

With lifestyle factors apparently not the cause of abnormal sperm parameters in men with SCI, attention turned to secondary physiological factors as possible

mechanisms for this condition. Again, this line of investigation yielded negative results. For example, there was no correlation between low sperm motility and level of injury, time post-injury, or age of subject [85,92]. Low sperm motility was also not related to endocrine profiles [93,94] or urinary tract infections [91].

Abnormal accessory gland function

Examination of semen from men with SCI shows numerous abnormalities in addition to abnormal sperm parameters. For example, 27% of men with SCI have brown-colored semen which does not become normally colored with repeated ejaculations (Fig. 26.9) [95]. The brown color is not simply hematospermia, but instead indicates a dysfunction of the seminal vesicles [95]. Additional evidence of seminal vesicle dysfunction is the finding that men with SCI show an abnormal pattern of transport and storage of sperm in the seminal vesicles [4].

In addition to dysfunction of the seminal vesicles in men with SCI, there is also evidence of prostate gland

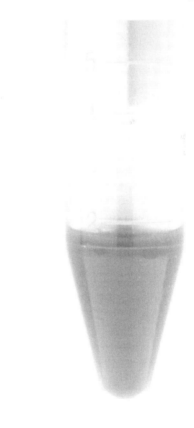

Fig. 26.9. Twenty-seven percent of men with SCI have brown-colored semen. The brown color is not related to semen stasis from infrequency of ejaculation. *See color plate section.*

dysfunction in these men. Prostate-specific antigen (PSA) was higher in the blood, but lower in the semen of men with SCI compared to healthy, age-matched control subjects [96,97]. This pattern of PSA expression indicates an autonomic dysfunction of the prostate gland in men with SCI.

Additional evidence of accessory gland dysfunction in men with SCI is found in studies showing abnormal concentrations of various biochemical substances in the semen of men with SCI compared with semen of control subjects. For example, compared to non-SCI men, men with SCI have higher concentrations of platelet-activating factor acetylhydrolase (PAFah) [98], reactive oxygen species [99–101], and somatostatin (in patients with lesions at or above T6) [102]. Conversely, the semen of men with SCI has lower levels of fructose, albumin, glutamic oxaloacetic transaminase, alkaline phosphatase [103], and TGF-β1 than the semen of able-bodied men [104].

Toxic seminal plasma

Evidence of abnormal accessory gland function in men with SCI led to studies investigating the role of the seminal plasma as a contributing factor to the abnormal sperm parameters found in these men. The studies showed that the seminal plasma of men with SCI is toxic to normal sperm. For example, when seminal plasma of men with SCI was mixed with sperm from normospermic men, a rapid and profound impairment to normal sperm motility occurred [105]. Furthermore, sperm unexposed to the seminal plasma (i.e., aspirated from the vas deferens) had significantly higher motility than sperm in the ejaculate of these men (Fig. 26.10) [106]. These findings introduced the concept of an **abnormal seminal plasma environment as a cause of impaired sperm motility in men with SCI.**

Leukocytospermia

One of the most pronounced semen abnormalities in men with SCI is leukocytospermia [107–109]. Flow cytometric analysis has shown the presence of large numbers of activated T lymphocytes in the semen of these men [107]. Activated T lymphocytes are known to secrete cytotoxic cytokines [110].

Cytokines contribute to low sperm motility

Cytokines play an important role in the function of the immune system [110]. Elevated concentrations of cytokines can be harmful to sperm [111–113]. The seminal plasma of men with SCI contains elevated concentrations of specific cytokines [104]. **When these**

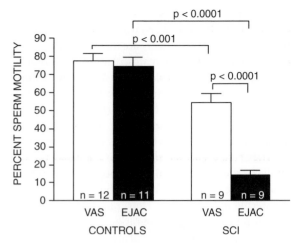

Fig. 26.10. In each of 12 men with SCI, sperm motility was 2–13 times higher when obtained from the vas deferens than from the ejaculate. In contrast, in control subjects, there was little difference in sperm motility between the two sites. This study provided definitive evidence that seminal plasma was a major contributor to low sperm motility in men with SCI. Although the vas-aspirated sperm from these men generally had lower motility than that of controls, suggesting that some epididymal or testicular factor may also have a role in decreasing sperm motility, the major decrease in motility was due to contact with the seminal plasma. (Adapted from Brackett NL *et al.* Sperm motility from the vas deferens of spinal cord injured men is higher than from the ejaculate. *J Urol* 2000; **164**: 712–15, with authors' permission.)

cytokines were neutralized, sperm motility improved [114,115]. **This treatment represented the first intervention that significantly improved sperm motility in men with SCI.**

Reproductive options for couples with SCI male partners

Intravaginal insemination at home

The majority of men with SCI cannot ejaculate during sexual intercourse, and require some form of technical or medical assistance to father a child (Fig. 26.11). The least invasive and least expensive of the assisted reproductive options is intravaginal insemination, sometimes called "in-home insemination." It is advisable for couples to be evaluated in a clinic prior to attempting intravaginal insemination at home. The clinic should evaluate the male partner to determine the optimal method for safe and effective ejaculation at home. This evaluation should assess the male partner with SCI for risk of, and management of, autonomic dysreflexia. The evaluation should also determine the optimal method of inducing ejaculation, such as use of one vibrator [42], two vibrators [52], or oral medications, such as a

PDE-5 inhibitor [116], prior to PVS. The clinic should also evaluate the semen quality of the male partner with SCI. While minimum numbers of total motile sperm have not been established for successful pregnancy using intravaginally inseminated sperm from men with SCI, the clinic should discuss guidelines regarding the number of intravaginal insemination cycles that will be attempted prior to choosing more advanced methods of assisted conception.

The female partner should be evaluated for the absence of any tubal or uterine pathology and for the presence of normal ovulatory cycles. She should also be counseled regarding methods of ovulation prediction at home. Insemination should occur at the time of ovulation. If the male partner with SCI cannot ejaculate during intercourse, the couple may collect his semen by PVS into a clean specimen cup. The semen is then drawn into the barrel of a syringe.

The semen is delivered after inserting the syringe deep into the vagina. Some clinics advise the female to remain recumbent for 15–30 minutes following insemination, to allow gravity to help keep the semen in the vagina. However, there are no data to indicate if this recumbence increases the probability of pregnancy.

There are reports in the literature of the successful use of intravaginal insemination to achieve pregnancy in couples with a male partner with SCI (Table 26.2). In these studies, pregnancy rates were 25–65% per couple.

Intrauterine insemination (IUI)

IUI has been used to achieve pregnancy in couples with an SCI male partner (Table 26.3). In men with SCI, semen to be used in IUI is usually collected by PVS or EEJ. IUI can be performed during unstimulated cycles, where no fertility drugs are prescribed to the woman or during stimulated cycles, where fertility drugs are prescribed to stimulate the production of oocytes and/ or to stimulate ovulation.

The largest recent series of IUI in couples with SCI male partners was reported by Ohl et al. [117]. EEJ was used to obtain sperm from 121 anejaculatory men, 87 of whom had SCI. Assisted reproductive techniques were applied in a stepwise fashion, beginning with IUI and proceeding to IVF in those couples failing at least three cycles of IUI. Thirty-two percent of couples

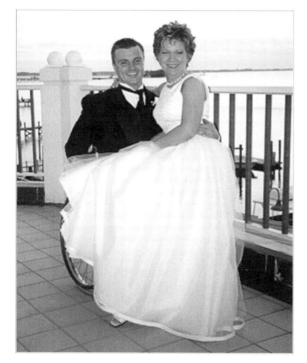

Fig. 26.11. Numerous options are available to assist conception in couples with a male partner with SCI.

Table 26.2. Summary of studies using intravaginal insemination in couples with male partners with SCI

Author, year	Couples (n)	Cycles (n)	Pregnancies (n)
Sønksen et al., 1997	16	ND	4
Löchner-Ernst et al., 1997	22	ND	37
Nehra et al., 1996	8	ND	5
Dahlberg et al., 1995	ND	≤ 48 [a]	12
Elliott et al., 2003	31	ND	14 [a]
Rutkowski et al., 1999	17	45	6
Hultling et al., 1997	19	ND	8

For each study, summarized are the total number of couples, the total number of attempts at pregnancy (cycles), and the total number of pregnancies. ND, no data
[a] Data estimated from information provided in study.

Table 26.3. Summary of studies using intrauterine insemination in couples with male partners with SCI

Author, year	Couples (*n*)	Cycles (*n*)	Pregnancies (*n*)	Medications used in study
Sønksen *et al.*, 1997	4	17	3	CC/hCG
Nehra *et al.*, 1996	13	25	5	None/CC/hMG
Dahlberg *et al.*, 1995	15	≤ 90[a]	9	CC/hMG
Ohl *et al.*, 2001	87	479	41	CC/hMG/hCG/LA
Pryor *et al.*, 2005	10	19	6	CC/hCG
Rutowski *et al.*, 1999	5	10	3	ND
Taylor *et al.*, 1999	14	92	11	ND
Chung *et al.*, 1996	10	50	5	CC/hCG
Heruti *et al.*, 2001	15	33	4	ND

For each study, summarized are the total number of couples, the total number of attempts at pregnancy (cycles), and the total number of pregnancies. Medications used in the study are listed. Some women had multiple cycles with different medications. CC, clomiphene citrate; hCG, human chorionic gonadotropin; hMG, human menopausal gonadotropin; LA, leuprolide acetate; ND, no data.
[a] Data estimated from information provided in study.

Table 26.4. Summary of studies using IVF/ICSI in couples with male partners with SCI

Author, year	Couples (*n*)	Cycles (*n*)	Pregnancies (*n*)	Medications used in study
Hultling *et al.*, 1997	25	52	15	GnRH/hMG/FSH/hCG
Heruti *et al.*, 2001	20	68	18	ND
Sønksen *et al.*, 1997	8	10	3	GnRH/hMG/hCG
Brindten *et al.*, 1997	35	85	18	GnRH/hMG/FSH
Shieh *et al.*, 2003	9	11	9	GnRH/hMG/FSH
Löchner-Ernst *et al.*, 1997	11	ND	13 (2 sets of twins)	ND
Nehra *et al.*, 1996	12	15	6	LA/hMG/FSH/hCG
Dahlberg *et al.*, 1995	9	14	4	CC/hMG
Rutowski *et al.*, 1999	21	42	8	ND
Taylor *et al.*, 1999	15	40	12	ND

For each study, summarized are the total number of couples, the total number of attempts at pregnancy (cycles), and the total number of pregnancies. Medications used in the study are listed. Some women had multiple cycles with different medications. CC, clomiphene citrate; FSH, follicle-stimulating hormone; GnRH, gonadotropin-releasing hormone agonist; hCG, human chorionic gonadotropin; hMG, human menopausal gonadotropin; LA, leuprolide acetate; ND, no data.

became pregnant with IUI alone, with a cycle fecundity of 8.7%. In those failing IUI, the IVF pregnancy rate was 37% per cycle. There was no correlation of any female management factor to IUI pregnancy rate. The only factor related to cycle fecundity was the inseminated total motile sperm count [117].

A cost analysis was performed on the retrospective data. It was found to be cost-effective to perform EEJ on SCI men, and to use the semen specimens for IUI, as long as anesthesia was not required to perform the EEJ. In men who required anesthesia, it was found to be cost-effective to go directly to IVF. Therefore, the current recommendation is to perform sperm

aspiration under local anesthesia coupled with IVF, and not to perform EEJ/IUI in individuals who require anesthesia for the EEJ procedure to be performed.

In-vitro fertilization (IVF)/intracytoplasmic sperm injection (ICSI)

Advanced assisted reproductive technologies are available when fertilization by intravaginal insemination or IUI is not possible or not indicated. In-vitro fertilization (IVF) may be performed with or without intracytoplasmic sperm injection (ICSI). Current IVF protocols develop embryos up to five days in vitro before transfer to the uterus [118]. The highest pregnancy rates are obtained with transfer of high-quality blastocysts compared to transfer of poorly formed blastocysts [119].

IVF and ICSI have been used to achieve pregnancy in couples with SCI male partners. In the studies presented in Table 26.4, pregnancy rates were 19–82% per cycle and 38–100% per couple.

Although definitive studies have not yet been performed, pregnancy outcomes using sperm from men with SCI seem to be similar to those using sperm from nonSCI patients with male-factor infertility [120–122]. Although there are some studies showing impaired sperm function in men with SCI [84,123], these functional impairments apparently do not lower pregnancy rates in couples. These findings may reflect the increasing ability of laboratory-assisted reproductive technologies to overcome all forms of male infertility [124,125] .

Summary

The purpose of ejaculation is to allow rapid transport of sperm through the urethra into the vagina during intercourse to allow procreation. There are anatomic and neuroanatomic structures essential for ejaculation, and these structures are coordinated in a very exact way to allow normal ejaculation to take place. The organs involved in the process of ejaculation are the epididymis, vas deferens, prostate, seminal vesicles, bladder neck, and bulbourethral glands. The process is moderated and coordinated by the brain and certain spinal cord centers. A normal neuromuscular pharmacological milieu must be maintained. In certain situations, the sequelae of the primary condition causing the ejaculatory dysfunction result in sperm dysfunction as well.

Currently, there are numerous options for assisted ejaculation and/or sperm retrieval in affected patients wishing to achieve fatherhood. Regardless of issues of fatherhood, men with ejaculatory dysfunction may seek help to restore normal sexual function. Identification of the point or points of disruption of the processes and structures involved in normal ejaculatory function can allow more precise and efficient management in either situation.

References

[1] Thomas AJ. Ejaculatory dysfunction. *Fertil Steril* 1983; **39**: 445–53.

[2] Prins GS, Zaneveld LJ. Radiographic study of fluid transport in the rabbit vas deferens during sexual rest and after sexual activity. *J Reprod Fertil* 1980; **58**: 311–19.

[3] Jarow JP. Seminal vesicle aspiration of fertile men. *J Urol* 1996; **156**: 1005–7.

[4] Ohl DA, Menge A, Jarow J. Seminal vesicle aspiration in spinal cord injured men: insight into poor semen quality. *J Urol* 1999; 162: 2048–51.

[5] Sønksen J, Ohl DA, Wedemeyer G. Sphincteric events during penile vibratory ejaculation and electroejaculation in men with spinal cord injuries. *J Urol* 2001; **165**: 426–9.

[6] Giuliano F, Clement P. Neuroanatomy and physiology of ejaculation. *Annu Rev Sex Res* 2005; **16**: 190–216.

[7] Coolen LM, Allard J, Truitt WA, McKenna KE. Central regulation of ejaculation. *Physiol Behav* 2004; **83**: 203–15.

[8] Wolters JP, Hellstrom WJ. Current concepts in ejaculatory dysfunction. *Rev Urol* 2006; **8** (Suppl 4): S18–25.

[9] Giuliano F, Clement P. Physiology of ejaculation: emphasis on serotonergic control, *Eur Urol* 2005; **48**: 408–17.

[10] Laumann EO, Paik A, Rosen RC. Sexual dysfunction in the United States: prevalence and predictors. *JAMA* 1999; **281**: 537–44.

[11] Waldinger MD, Zwinderman AH, Olivier B, Schweitzer DH. Proposal for a definition of lifelong premature ejaculation based on epidemiological stopwatch data. *J Sex Med* 2005; **2**: 498–507.

[12] Pryor JL, Althof SE, Steidle C, *et al.* Efficacy and tolerability of dapoxetine in treatment of premature ejaculation: An integrated analysis of two double-blind, randomised controlled trials. *Lancet* 2006; **368**: 929–37.

[13] Perelman MA, Rowland DL. Retarded ejaculation. *World J Urol* 2006; **24**: 645–52.

[14] Stewart DE, Ohl DA. Idiopathic anejaculation treated by electroejaculation. *Int J Psychiatry Med* 1989; **19**: 263–8.

[15] Fisch H, Lambert SM, Goluboff ET. Management of ejaculatory duct obstruction: etiology, diagnosis, and treatment. *World J Urol* 2006; **24**: 604–10.

[16] Samli H, Samli MM, Yilmaz E, Imirzalioglu N. Clinical, andrological and genetic characteristics of patients with congenital bilateral absence of vas deferens (CBAVD). *Arch Androl* 2006; **52**: 471–7.

[17] Ochsner MG, Burns E, Henry HH. Incidence of retrograde ejaculation following bladder neck revision as a child. *J Urol* 1970; **104**: 596–7.

[18] Bors E, Comarr AE. Neurological disturbances of sexual function with special reference to 529 patients with spinal cord injury. *Urol Surv* 1960; **10**: 191–222.

[19] Rees PM, Fowler CJ, Maas CP. Sexual function in men and women with neurological disorders. *Lancet* 2007; **369**: 512–25.

[20] Walsh PC, Retik AB, Vaughan ED, Wein AJ, eds. *Campbell's Urology*, 8th edn. Philadelphia, PA: Saunders, 2002.

[21] Holman E, Kovacs G, Flasko T, *et al.* Hand-assisted laparoscopic retroperitoneal lymph node dissection for nonseminomatous testicular cancer. *J Laparoendosc Adv Surg Tech A* 2007; **17**: 16–20.

[22] Neyer M, Peschel R, Akkad T, *et al.* Long-term results of laparoscopic retroperitoneal lymph-node dissection for clinical stage I nonseminomatous germ-cell testicular cancer. *J Endourol* 2007; **21**: 180–3.

[23] Vinik AI, Maser RE, Mitchell BD, Freeman R. Diabetic autonomic neuropathy. *Diabetes Care* 2003; **26**: 1553–79.

[24] Dunsmuir WD, Holmes SA. The aetiology and management of erectile, ejaculatory, and fertility problems in men with diabetes mellitus. *Diabet Med* 1996; **13**: 700–8.

[25] Lue TF, Giuliano F, Montorsi F, *et al.* Summary of the recommendations on sexual dysfunctions in men. *J Sex Med* 2004; **1**: 6–23.

[26] Proctor KG, Howards SS. The effect of sympathomimetic drugs on post-lymphadenectomy aspermia. *J Urol* 1983; **129**: 837–8.

[27] Thiagarajah S, Vaughan ED, Kitchin JD. Retrograde ejaculation: successful pregnancy following combined sympathomimetic medication and insemination. *Fertil Steril* 1978; **30**: 96–7.

[28] Bauer S, Koff S, Jayanthi V. Voiding dysfunction in children: neurogenic and non-neurogenic. In: Walsh P, Retik A, Vaughn E, Wein A, eds. *Campbell's Urology*, 8th edn. Philadelphia, PA: Saunders, 2002.

[29] Decter RM, Furness PD, Nguyen TA, *et al.* Reproductive understanding, sexual functioning and testosterone levels in men with spina bifida. *J Urol* 1997; **157**: 1466–8.

[30] Haensch CA, Jorg J. Autonomic dysfunction in multiple sclerosis. *J Neurol* 2006; **253** (Suppl 1): I3–9.

[31] Korpelainen JT, Nieminen P, Myllyla VV. Sexual functioning among stroke patients and their spouses. *Stroke* 1999; **30**: 715–9.

[32] Seidman S. Ejaculatory dysfunction and depression: pharmacological and psychobiological interactions. *Int J Impot Res* 2006; **18** (Suppl 1): S33–8.

[33] Hellstrom WJ, Sikka SC. Effects of acute treatment with tamsulosin versus alfuzosin on ejaculatory function in normal volunteers. *J Urol* 2006; **176**: 1529–33.

[34] Kamischke A, Nieschlag E. Update on medical treatment of ejaculatory disorders. *Int J Androl* 2002; **25**: 333–44.

[35] Gilja I, Parazajder J, Radej M, Cvitkovic P, Kovacic M. Retrograde ejaculation and loss of emission: possibilities of conservative treatment. *Eur Urol* 1994; **25**: 226–8.

[36] Riley A, Segraves RT. Treatment of premature ejaculation. *Int J Clin Pract* 2006; **60**: 694–7.

[37] Zhao Y, Garcia J, Jarow JP, Wallach EE. Successful management of infertility due to retrograde ejaculation using assisted reproductive technologies: a report of two cases. *Arch Androl* 2004; **50**: 391–4.

[38] Brown DJ, Hill ST, Baker HW. Male fertility and sexual function after spinal cord injury. *Prog Brain Res* 2006; **152**: 427–39.

[39] Brackett NL, Ferrell SM, Aballa TC, *et al.* An analysis of 653 trials of penile vibratory stimulation on men with spinal cord injury. *J Urol* 1998; **159**: 1931–4.

[40] DeForge D, Blackmer J, Garritty C, *et al.* Fertility following spinal cord injury: a systematic review. *Spinal Cord* 2005; **43**: 693–703.

[41] Sønksen J, Ohl DA. Penile vibratory stimulation and electroejaculation in the treatment of ejaculatory dysfunction. *Int J Androl* 2002; **25**: 324–32.

[42] Brackett NL. Semen retrieval by penile vibratory stimulation in men with spinal cord injury. *Hum Reprod Update* 1999; **5**: 216–22.

[43] Sønksen J, Ohl DA. Penile vibratory stimulation and electroejaculation in the treatment of ejaculatory dysfunction. *Int J Androl* 2002; **25**: 324–32.

[44] Kafetsoulis A, Brackett NL, Ibrahim E, Attia GR, Lynne CM. Current trends in the treatment of infertility in men with spinal cord injury. *Fertil Steril* 2006; **86**: 781–9.

[45] Elliott S, Krassioukov A. Malignant autonomic dysreflexia in spinal cord injured men. *Spinal Cord* 2006; **44**: 386–92.

[46] Sønksen J. Assisted ejaculation and semen characteristics in spinal cord injured males. *Scand J Urol Nephrol Suppl* 2003; 1–31.

[47] Sheel AW, Krassioukov AV, Inglis JT, Elliott SL. Autonomic dysreflexia during sperm retrieval in spinal cord injury: influence of lesion level and sildenafil citrate. *J Appl Physiol* 2005; **99**: 53–8.

[48] Steinberger RE, Ohl DA, Bennett CJ, McCabe M, Wang SC. Nifedipine pretreatment for autonomic dysreflexia during electroejaculation. *Urology* 1990; **36**: 228–31.

[49] Sønksen J, Biering-Sorensen F, Kristensen JK. Ejaculation induced by penile vibratory stimulation in men with spinal cord injuries: the importance of the vibratory amplitude. *Paraplegia* 1994; **32**: 651–60.

[50] Elliott S. Sexual dysfunction and infertility in men with spinal cord disorders. In: Lin V, ed. *Spinal Cord Medicine: Principles and Practice*. New York, NY: Demos Medical Publishing, 2003: 349–65.

[51] Wieder J, Brackett N, Lynne C, Green J, Aballa T. Anesthetic block of the dorsal penile nerve inhibits vibratory-induced ejaculation in men with spinal cord injuries. *Urology* 2000; **55**: 915–17.

[52] Brackett NL, Kafetsoulis A, Ibrahim E, Aballa TC, Lynne CM. Application of 2 vibrators salvages ejaculatory failures to 1 vibrator during penile vibratory stimulation in men with spinal cord injuries. *J Urol* 2007; **177**: 660–3.

[53] Kafetsoulis A, Ibrahim E, Aballa TC, *et al.* Abdominal electrical stimulation rescues failures to penile vibratory stimulation in men with spinal cord injury: a report of two cases. *Urology* 2006; **68**: 204–11.

[54] Giuliano F, Rubio-Aurioles E, Kennelly M, *et al.* Efficacy and safety of vardenafil in men with erectile dysfunction caused by spinal cord injury. *Neurology* 2006; **66**: 210–16.

[55] Bird VG, Brackett NL, Lynne CM, Aballa TC, Ferrell SM. Reflexes and somatic responses as predictors of ejaculation by penile vibratory stimulation in men with spinal cord injury. *Spinal Cord* 2001; **39**: 514–19.

[56] Ohl DA, Sønksen J. Penile vibratory stimulation and electroejaculation. In: Hellstrom WJG, ed. *Male Infertility and Sexual Dysfunction*. New York, NY: Springer-Verlag, 1997: 219–29.

[57] Brindley GS. Reflex ejaculation under vibratory stimulation in paraplegic men. *Paraplegia* 1981; **19**: 299–302.

[58] Gunn RMC. Fertility in sheep: artificial production of seminal ejaculation and the characteristics of the spermatozoa contained therein. *Australian Commonwealth Council of Scientific and Industrial Research* 1936; **94**: 1–5.

[59] Brindley GS. Electroejaculation and the fertility of paraplegic men. *Sexuality Disabil* 1980; **3**: 223–9.

[60] Seager SWJ, Halstead LS, Ohl DA, et al. Electroejaculation: may give hope of fatherhood for some spinal cord injured and other neurologically impaired men. International Andrology Congress 1989.

[61] Brackett NL, Padron OF, Lynne CM. Semen quality of spinal cord injured men is better when obtained by vibratory stimulation versus electroejaculation. *J Urol* 1997; **157**: 151–7.

[62] Ohl DA, Sønksen J, Menge AC, McCabe M, Keller LM. Electroejaculation versus vibratory stimulation in spinal cord injured men: sperm quality and patient preference. *J Urol* 1997; **157**: 2147–9.

[63] Ohl DA. Electroejaculation. *Urol Clin North Am* 1993; **20**: 181–8.

[64] Seager SW, Halstead LS. Fertility options and success after spinal cord injury. *Urol Clin North Am* 1993; **20**: 543–8.

[65] Sønksen J, Ohl DA, Momose H, *et al.* Treatment of infertility. *Spinal Cord* 1999; **37**: 89–95.

[66] Brackett NL, Ead DN, Aballa TC, Ferrell SM, Lynne CM. Semen retrieval in men with spinal cord injury is improved by interrupting current delivery during electroejaculation. *J Urol* 2002; **167**: 201–3.

[67] Perkash I, Martin DE, Warner H, Blank MS, Collins DC. Reproductive biology of paraplegics: results of semen collection, testicular biopsy and serum hormone evaluation. *J Urol* 1985; **134**: 284–8.

[68] Sarkarati M, Rossier AB, Fam BA. Experience in vibratory and electro-ejaculation techniques in spinal cord injury patients: a preliminary report. *J Urol* 1987; **138**: 59–62.

[69] Kolettis PN, Lambert MC, Hammond KR, *et al.* Fertility outcomes after electroejaculation in men with spinal cord injury. *Fertil Steril* 2002; **78**: 429–31.

[70] Utida C, Truzzi JC, Bruschini H, *et al.* Male infertility in spinal cord trauma. *Int Braz J Urol* 2005; **31**: 375–83.

[71] Nehra A, Werner M, Bastuba, Title C, Oates R. Vibratory stimulation and rectal probe electroejaculation as therapy for patients with spinal cord injury: semen parameters and pregnancy rates. *J Urol* 1996; **155**: 554–9.

[72] Taylor Z, Molloy D, Hill V, Harrison K. Contribution of the assisted reproductive technologies to fertility in males suffering spinal cord injury. *Aust N Z J Obstet Gynaecol* 1999; **39**: 84–7.

[73] Engin-Uml SY, Korkmaz C, Duru NK, Baser I. Comparison of three sperm retrieval techniques in spinal cord-injured men: pregnancy outcome. *Gynecol Endocrinol* 2006; **22**: 252–5.

[74] Marina S, Marina F, Alcolea R, *et al.* Triplet pregnancy achieved through intracytoplasmic sperm injection with spermatozoa obtained by prostatic massage of a paraplegic patient: Case report. *Hum Reprod* 1999; **14**: 1546–8.

[75] Arafa MM, Zohdy WA, Shamloul R. Prostatic massage: a simple method of semen retrieval in men with spinal cord injury. *Int J Androl* 2007; **30**: 170–3.

[76] Craft I, Tsirigotis M. Simplified recovery, preparation and cryopreservation of testicular spermatozoa. *Hum Reprod* 1995; **10**: 1623–6.

[77] Tsirigotis M, Pelekanos M, Beski S, *et al.* Cumulative experience of percutaneous epididymal sperm aspiration (PESA) with intracytoplasmic sperm injection. *J Assist Reprod Genet* 1996; **13**: 315–19.

[78] Haberle M, Scheurer P, Muhlebach P, *et al.* Intracytoplasmic sperm injection (ICSI) with testicular sperm extraction (TESE) in non-obstructive azoospermia: two case reports. *Andrologia* 1996; **28** (Suppl 1): 87–8.

[79] Kahraman S, Ozgur S, Alatas C, *et al.* High implantation and pregnancy rates with testicular sperm extraction and intracytoplasmic sperm

injection in obstructive and non-obstructive azoospermia. *Hum Reprod* 1996; **11**: 673–6.

[80] Craft I, Tsirigotis M, Courtauld E, Farrer-Brown G. Testicular needle aspiration as an alternative to biopsy for the assessment of spermatogenesis. *Hum Reprod* 1997; **12**: 1483–7.

[81] Westlander G, Hamberger L, Hanson C, et al. Diagnostic epididymal and testicular sperm recovery and genetic aspects in azoospermic men. *Hum Reprod* 1999; **14**: 118–22.

[82] Chiang H, Liu C, Tzeng C, Wei H. No-scalpel vasal sperm aspiration and in vitro fertilization for the treatment of anejaculation. *Urology* 2000; **55**: 918–21.

[83] Linsenmeyer TA. Male infertility following spinal cord injury. *J Am Paraplegic Soc* 1991; **14**: 116–21.

[84] Denil J, Ohl DA, Menge AC, Keller LM, McCabe M. Functional characteristics of sperm obtained by electroejaculation. *J Urol* 1992; **147**: 69–72.

[85] Brackett NL, Nash MS, Lynne CM. Male fertility following spinal cord injury: facts and fiction. *Phys Ther* 1996; **76**: 1221–31.

[86] Brackett NL, Lynne CM, Weizman MS, Bloch WE, Padron OF. Scrotal and oral temperatures are not related to semen quality or serum gonadotropin levels in spinal cord-injured men. *J Androl* 1994; **15**: 614–19.

[87] Siosteen A, Forssman L, Steen Y, Sullivan L, Wickstrom I. Quality of semen after repeated ejaculation treatment in spinal cord injury men. *Paraplegia* 1990; **28**: 96–104.

[88] Laessoe L, Sønksen J, Bagi P, et al. Effects of ejaculation by penile vibratory stimulation on bladder reflex activity in a spinal cord injured man. *J Urol* 2001; **166**: 627.

[89] Hamid R, Patki P, Bywater H, Shah PJ, Craggs MD. Effects of repeated ejaculations on semen characteristics following spinal cord injury. *Spinal Cord* 2006; **44**: 369–73.

[90] Das S, Dodd S, Soni BM, et al. Does repeated electro-ejaculation improve sperm quality in spinal cord injured men? *Spinal Cord* 2006; **44**: 753–6.

[91] Ohl DA, Denil J, Fitzgerald-Shelton K, et al. Fertility of spinal cord injured males: effect of genitourinary infection and bladder management on results of electroejaculation. *J Am Paraplegic Soc* 1992; **15**: 53–9.

[92] Brackett NL, Ferrell SM, Aballa TC, Amador MJ, Lynne CM. Semen quality in spinal cord injured men: does it progressively decline post-injury? *Arch Phys Med Rehabil* 1998; **79**: 625–8.

[93] Brackett NL, Lynne CM, Weizman MS, Bloch WE, Abae M. Endocrine profiles and semen quality of spinal cord injured men. *J Urol* 1994; **151**: 114–9.

[94] Naderi AR, Safarinejad MR. Endocrine profiles and semen quality in spinal cord injured men. *Clin Endocrinol* 2003; **58**: 177–84.

[95] Wieder JA, Lynne CM, Ferrell SM, Aballa TC, Brackett NL. Brown-colored semen in men with spinal cord injury. *J Androl* 1999; **20**: 594–600.

[96] Lynne CM, Aballa TC, Wang TJ, et al. Serum and seminal plasma prostate specific antigen (PSA) levels are different in young spinal cord injured men compared to normal controls. *J Urol* 1999; **162**: 89–91.

[97] Brasso K, Sønksen J, Sommer P, et al. Seminal plasma PSA in spinal cord injured men: a preliminary report. *Spinal Cord* 1998; **36**: 771–3.

[98] Zhu J, Brackett NL, Aballa TC, et al. High seminal platelet-activating factor acetylhydrolase activity in men with spinal cord injury. *J Androl* 2006; **27**: 429–33.

[99] Padron OF, Brackett NL, Sharma RK, et al. Seminal reactive oxygen species and sperm motility and morphology in men with spinal cord injury. *Fertil Steril* 1997; **67**: 1115–20.

[100] de Lamirande E, Leduc BE, Iwasaki A, Hassouna M, Gagnon C. Increased reactive oxygen species formation in semen of patients with spinal cord injury. *Fertil Steril* 1995; **63**: 637–42.

[101] Rajasekaran M, Hellstrom WJ, Sparks RL, Sikka SC. Sperm-damaging effects of electric current: Possible role of free radicals. *Reproductive Toxicology* 1994; **8**: 427–32.

[102] Odum L, Sønksen J, Biering-Sorensen F. Seminal somatostatin in men with spinal cord injury. *Paraplegia* 1995; **33**: 374–6.

[103] Hirsch IH, Jeyendran RS, Sedor J, Rosecrans RR, Staas WE. Biochemical analysis of electroejaculates in spinal cord injured men: comparison to normal ejaculates. *J Urol* 1991; **145**: 73–6.

[104] Basu S, Aballa TC, Ferrell SM, Lynne CM, Brackett NL. Inflammatory cytokine concentrations are elevated in seminal plasma of men with spinal cord injuries. *J Androl* 2004; **25**: 250–4.

[105] Brackett NL, Davi RC, Padron OF, Lynne CM. Seminal plasma of spinal cord injured men inhibits sperm motility of normal men. *J Urol* 1996; **155**: 1632–5.

[106] Brackett NL, Lynne CM, Aballa TC, Ferrell SM. Sperm motility from the vas deferens of spinal cord injured men is higher than from the ejaculate. *J Urol* 2000; **164**: 712–15.

[107] Basu S, Lynne CM, Ruiz P, et al. Cytofluorographic identification of activated T-cell subpopulations in the semen of men with spinal cord injuries. *J Androl* 2002; **23**: 551–6.

[108] Trabulsi EJ, Shupp-Byrne D, Sedor J, Hirsh IH. Leukocyte subtypes in electroejaculates of spinal cord injured men. *Arch Phys Med Rehabil* 2002; **83**: 31–3.

[109] Aird IA, Vince GS, Bates MD, Johnson PM, Lewis-Jones ID. Leukocytes in semen from men with spinal cord injuries. *Fertil Steril* 1999; **72**: 97–103.

[110] Parham P. *The Immune System*. New York, NY: Garland Science, 2005.

[111] Kocak I, Yenisey C, Dundar M, Okyay P, Serter M. Relationship between seminal plasma interleukin-6 and tumor necrosis factor alpha levels with semen parameters in fertile and infertile men. *Urol Res* 2002; **30**: 263–7.

[112] Eggert-Kruse W, Boit R, Rohr G, *et al*. Relationship of seminal plasma interleukin (IL) -8 and IL-6 with semen quality. *Hum Reprod* 2001; **16**: 517–28.

[113] Sikka SC, Champion HC, Bivalacqua TJ, *et al*. Role of genitourinary inflammation in infertility: Synergistic effect of lipopolysaccharide and interferon-gamma on human spermatozoa. *Int J Androl* 2001; **24**: 136–41.

[114] Cohen DR, Basu S, Randall JM, *et al*. Sperm motility in men with spinal cord injuries is enhanced by inactivating cytokines in the seminal plasma. *J Androl* 2004; **25**: 922–5.

[115] Brackett NL, Cohen DR, Ibrahim E, Aballa TC, Lynne CM. Neutralization of cytokine activity at the receptor level improves sperm motility in men with spinal cord injuries. *J Androl* 2007; **28**: 717–21.

[116] Giuliano F, Rubio-Aurioles E, Kennelly M, *et al*. Efficacy and safety of vardenafil in men with erectile dysfunction caused by spinal cord injury. *Neurology* 2006; **66**: 210–16.

[117] Ohl DA, Wolf LJ, Menge AC, *et al*. Electroejaculation and assisted reproductive technologies in the treatment of anejaculatory infertility. *Fertil Steril* 2001; **76**: 1249–55.

[118] della Ragione T, Verheyen G, Papanikolaou EG, *et al*. Developmental stage on day-5 and fragmentation rate on day-3 can influence the implantation potential of top-quality blastocysts in IVF cycles with single embryo transfer. *Reprod Biol Endocrinol* 2007; **5**: 2.

[119] Balaban B, Urman B, Sertac A, *et al*. Blastocyst quality affects the success of blastocyst-stage embryo transfer. *Fertil Steril* 2000; **74**: 282–7.

[120] Brackett NL, Abae M, Padron OF, Lynne CM. Treatment by assisted conception of severe male factor infertility due to spinal cord injury or other neurological impairment. *J Assist Reprod Genet* 1995; **12**: 210–16.

[121] Shieh JY, Chen SU, Wang YH, *et al*. A protocol of electroejaculation and systematic assisted reproductive technology achieved high efficiency and efficacy for pregnancy for anejaculatory men with spinal cord injury. *Arch Phys Med Rehabil* 2003; **84**: 535–40.

[122] Sønksen J, Sommer P, Biering-Sorensen F, *et al*. Pregnancy after assisted ejaculation procedures in men with spinal cord injury. *Arch Phys Med Rehab* 1997; **78**: 1059–61.

[123] Buch JP, Zorn BH. Evaluation and treatment of infertility in spinal cord injured men through rectal probe electroejaculation. *J Urol* 1993; **149**: 1350–4.

[124] Maduro MR, Lamb DJ. Understanding new genetics of male infertility. *J Urol* 2002; **168**: 2197–205.

[125] Isidori A, Latini M, Romanelli F. Treatment of male infertility. *Contraception* 2005; **72**: 314–18.

Chapter 27

Male contraception and vasectomy

Stanton C. Honig and Jay I. Sandlow

Introduction

Male contraception has traditionally consisted of either barrier methods, such as condoms, or more permanent surgical techniques, such as vasectomy. However, men are now more likely than ever to participate in the choice of contraceptive techniques. Therefore, it has become quite important to develop less invasive, more tolerable, and more reversible methods of male contraception. This chapter will outline some of the more traditional methods of male contraception, as well as describe newer techniques, some of which are currently available, others of which are on the horizon.

Vasectomy
Preoperative considerations

Vasectomy is a safe and effective method of permanent contraception [1]. **In the United States, it is employed by nearly 11% of all married couples and performed on approximately 500 000 men per year, more than any other urologic surgical procedure.** However, fewer vasectomies are performed worldwide than female sterilizations by tubal ligation [2]. This is in spite of the fact that vasectomy is less expensive and associated with much less morbidity and mortality than tubal ligation. Some men fear pain and complications, while others falsely equate vasectomy with castration or loss of masculinity.

About 2–6% of patients undergoing vasectomy later seek reversal. With divorce rates at approximately 50%, insurance for future costly fertility procedures should be addressed by the physician before vasectomy. In the authors' practice, patients are informed that if they are considering sperm cryopreservation, they probably should reconsider having a vasectomy. It makes patients think about the permanent nature of the procedure.

Technical aspects

The procedure should be performed in a warm room and using warm preparation solution to relax the scrotum. Shaving should be performed in the room just prior to prepping, thus reducing the chance of infection. The decision to utilize a single midline incision rather than bilateral incisions is left to the surgeon. However, it is the authors' opinion that bilateral incisions are superior for several reasons. First, there is no chance of dividing the same side twice, as there is with a single midline incision (although this situation can be avoided by gently pulling on the vas and asking the patient to identify which side is being manipulated). Second, it is much easier to divide the vas far from the testis with bilateral incisions. This may help to prevent post-vasectomy congestive pain (see below). Finally, the longer the testicular vasal remnant, the greater the likelihood of a successful vasectomy reversal (if desired) [3]. Although this should not necessarily be a consideration when performing vasectomy, leaving a longer testicular remnant does nothing to lessen the chances of a successful vasectomy outcome.

Local anesthesia

Vasectomy is typically performed as an outpatient procedure using local anesthetics. Some physicians also give sedatives, such as diazepam, orally one hour before the procedure, in order to relax the patient. The choice of local anesthesia is determined by the surgeon, although the authors prefer a mixture of 1% plain lidocaine and 0.5% bupivacaine in a 1 : 1 ratio. The vas deferens is separated from the spermatic cord vessels and manipulated to a superficial position under the scrotal skin. The vas is firmly trapped between the middle finger, the index finger, and the thumb of the left hand. A small superficial skin wheal is raised using a 1.5-inch 25-gauge needle. The needle is then advanced within

Infertility in the Male, 4th edition, ed. Larry I. Lipshultz, Stuart S. Howards, and Craig S. Niederberger. Published by Cambridge University Press. © Cambridge University Press 2009.

the perivasal sheath, and a small amount of local anesthetic is injected around the vas without moving the needle in and out. This produces a vasal nerve block and minimizes edema at the actual vasectomy site [4]. The contralateral vas deferens may be anesthetized at the same time or just before addressing that side. A no-needle device is also available, utilizing a high-pressure jet injection of local anesthesia [5].

Conventional incisional technique

After adequate anesthesia is induced, 1 cm bilateral transverse incisions are carried down through the vasal sheath until bare vas is exposed. The vas is delivered and the deferential artery, veins, and accompanying nerves are dissected free of the vas and spared. A small segment is removed and the ends occluded using one of the techniques described later in this section. Fluff gauze dressings are held in place by a snug-fitting athletic supporter.

No-scalpel vasectomy

This method was developed in China in 1974 [6] and introduced to the United States in 1985 [4]. **This method eliminates the incision, results in fewer hematomas and infections, and leaves a much smaller wound than conventional methods of accessing the vas deferens for vasectomy** [7]. In the original description, a vasal nerve block is performed as described previously. The ring-tipped fixation clamp is grasped with the surgeon's dominant hand and opened while pressing downward, stretching the scrotal skin tightly over the vas and locking the vas within the clamp. The ring clamp is placed in the other hand and the trapped vas is elevated with the index finger of that hand, tightening the scrotal skin over the vas. **A sharp-pointed, curved mosquito hemostat (introduced through the same needle puncture hole used for anesthesia) is used to puncture the scrotal skin, vas sheath, and vas wall with one blade of the clamp. In an alternative method, particularly if the scrotum is thick or tight, following mobilization and anesthetization of the vas, the skin is punctured first with the sharp, curved hemostat and spread until the vertical slit-like opening is just large enough for introduction of the ringed clamp.** The ringed clamp is introduced into the opening, the vas is grasped and brought up to the opening, and the surgeon proceeds as described earlier. The vas is then divided and occlusion is effected using one of the techniques described later in this section. **Many authors advocate closing the fascia over one end of the cut vas (fascial interposition) in order to reduce the likelihood of recanalization** [8,9].

After checking for bleeding, the authors use a small hemostat to tag the vasal ends in order to inspect for any bleeding prior to returning the vas to the scrotum. The contralateral vas is then approached in an identical fashion. **After both vasa are returned to the scrotum, the puncture hole is pinched for a minute and inspected for bleeding.** The puncture hole contracts and is virtually invisible. Antibiotic ointment is applied to the site, and sterile fluff dressings are held in place with a snug-fitting athletic supporter. Studies in the United States and China [4], as well as a large controlled study carried out in Thailand [10], comparing no-scalpel with conventional vasectomy have clearly shown that the no-scalpel technique results in a significantly reduced incidence of hematoma, infection, and pain. In addition, the no-scalpel vasectomy is performed in about 40% less time.

Histological evaluation

Many urologists insist on removal of a segment of vas for pathologic verification, primarily for medicolegal reasons. Even from the legal point of view, a pathologist's report confirming the presence of vas in the vasectomy specimen offers little or no protection from litigation. **Documented counseling, diligent follow-up to obtain at least one azoospermic semen specimen postoperatively, and careful selection of appropriate candidates for vasectomy in the first place provide the best protection from malpractice suits.**

Androlog, an internet-based discussion group for andrologists, addressed this issue and published their findings in the September/October 2006 issue of *Journal of Andrology* [11]. An international discussion relayed information regarding the benefits and drawbacks of sending vasectomy specimens to pathology.

The major benefit of histological confirmation is removal of the appropriate organ. This does not guarantee a successful outcome, however. If a specimen is *not* confirmed as the vas deferens, it signals the surgeon that the operation is clearly not successful. We are sometimes confronted with a structure that we are not 100% sure is the vas deferens, as can happen with patients who have undergone orchidopexy for cryptorchidism. Sometimes the vas is somewhat atretic, and histologic confirmation reassures the surgeon that what he removed was actually the vas deferens.

Pathological confirmation does not confirm postoperative success, however. Success can only be confirmed with postoperative semen analysis. In addition, pathological confirmation of vasa does not assure that a segment was removed from both the left and right vasa, as opposed to two segments from the same vas deferens. In cases of postoperative failure, this gives lawyers more ammunition to confirm poor surgical technique.

The American Urological Association (AUA) has a policy statement regarding the standard of care for sending vasectomy specimens. It reads as follows:

Routine histologic confirmation is unnecessary in performing vasectomy. The American Urological Association, Inc. (AUA) recommends that physicians in practice and that residency training programs no longer require histologic confirmation of the vas deferens as a measurement of vasectomy success. The finding of azoospermia after a bilateral vasectomy is the standard for success. The persistence of sperm in the semen after a bilateral vasectomy is a surgical failure regardless of a pathologic confirmation that two segments of the vas were removed. The lack of clinical value makes the routine histologic evaluation of surgical specimens obtained by a surgeon experienced in performing vasectomies clinically unnecessary. The surgeon should decide whether a histologic evaluation is warranted. The surgeon should document in the patient's record comprehensive preoperative counseling, careful patient selection, meticulous surgical technique, and whether azoospermia was achieved in the postoperative semen – Board of Directors, 1998, reaffirmed 2003.

Therefore, for now, histologic confirmation of vas deferens is *not* considered the standard of care.

Percutaneous vasectomy

The Chinese have performed over 500 000 truly percutaneous vasectomies (and an equal number of vasographies) using chemical occlusion with a combination of cyanoacrylate and phenol [12–14]. After fixation of the vas with the same ring clamp described earlier, the scrotal skin and vas wall are punctured with a 22-gauge needle and the lumen cannulated with a 24-gauge blunt needle. The needle's position within the vas lumen is confirmed by a series of ingenious tests, with final confirmation obtained by injection of Congo red into the abdominal side of the right vas deferens and methylene blue into the left vas. Injection of 20 μL of two parts phenol mixed with one part N-butyl-2-cyanoacrylate mixture through the 24-gauge blunt-tipped needle occludes the lumen. The patient voids at the termination of the procedure. Excretion of red urine means the left side was missed. Blue urine means the right side was missed, and brown urine means both sides were successfully cannulated. Pharmacologic tests of the cyanoacrylate–phenol mixture in China have

demonstrated no toxicity or carcinogenesis. However, these chemicals are not approved by the US Food and Drug Administration for use in the United States. Furthermore, gaining percutaneous access to the 300 μm diameter lumen of the vas is a feat requiring great skill and considerable training.

High-frequency ultrasound

High-frequency ultrasound has been used for percutaneous vasectomy [15] and epididymal occlusion [16] in dogs. Occlusion is unreliable, and skin burns are problematic. To date, it does not appear that this will be a feasible method of vasectomy.

Intra-vas device

The intra-vas device is a flexible, hollow, silicone plug molded from medical grade silicone rubber. This device is placed in both the testicular and abdominal ends of the vas deferens following a hemivasotomy. The vas is either allowed to close spontaneously or is sutured with a small (6–0) stitch. Removal is similar, although the vas defect is typically closed with a small suture [17,18]. The device currently is being investigated in a multicenter trial for both contraceptive efficacy and reversibility.

Methods of vasal occlusion and vasectomy failure

The technique employed for occlusion of the vasal lumina may influence the incidence of recanalization. Suture ligature, still the most common method employed worldwide, may result in necrosis and sloughing of the cut end distal to the ligature. If this occurs on the testicular end of the cut vas, a sperm granuloma will result. If both ends slough, recanalization is more likely to occur. The incidence of vasectomy failure ranges from 1% to 5% when ligatures alone are used for occlusion. When the vasa are sealed with two medium hemoclips on each end, failure rates are reduced to less than 1% [19,20]. The diameter of hemoclips, wider than that of sutures, distributes pressure more evenly on the vasal wall and results in less necrosis and sloughing.

Intraluminal occlusion with needle electrocautery, or battery-driven thermal cautery set at a power sufficient to destroy mucosa but not high enough to cause transmural destruction of the vas, reduces recanalization rates to less than 0.5% [21,22]. At least 1 cm of lumen should be cauterized in each direction. Thermal wires should be rotated to cauterize the entire mucosal surface.

Interposition of fascia between the cut ends, folding back of the vasal ends, and securing one end within the dartos muscle are all techniques that have been advocated with the intent of reducing vasectomy failure rates [8,23]. It appears that fascial interposition may lead to lower rates of recanalization, regardless of the occlusion technique utilized [9].

Standards of successful outcome and postoperative semen testing

No technique of vasal occlusion, short of removing the entire scrotal vas, is 100% effective [24]. **There is no absolute standard of care when it comes to declaring a patient sterile.** Follow-up semen analysis at least 2–3 months post-vasectomy, with the goal of obtaining at least one and preferably two absolutely azoospermic specimens 4–6 weeks apart, is recommended [25].

There are no guidelines in the United States regarding successful outcome except for the recommendation of postoperative azoospermia. Whether the semen sample should be a centrifuged specimen remains unclear, as do the timing and the number of semen analyses. Although many urologists obtain a semen analysis at 6–8 weeks postoperatively, several papers suggest that only 72% and 85% of patients are azoospermic at 3 and 6 months, respectively [26]. Both time and number of ejaculations have been used to determine the optimal time to obtain the initial semen analysis. After 10–20 ejaculations, variable percentages (10–87%) of men will be azoospermic [25]. One publication [27] suggests that 62% and 97% of patients will have no sperm in the ejaculate at 3 and 4 months postoperatively. The researchers also found an 84% compliance rate with one postoperative semen analysis at 3 months compared with only 71% compliance with two specimens at 3 and 4 months. It is rare that once a patient has become azoospermic he will return for further semen analyses [28]. Smucker et al. surveyed patients to determine why they were noncompliant, and concluded that inconvenience was the most common reason, not lack of understanding or forgetfulness [29].

The British Andrology Society recommends that patients should be instructed to have had at least 24 ejaculations and preferably wait at least 16 weeks before submitting a first semen sample for review [30]. In their Guidelines for the Assessment of Post Vasectomy Semen Samples, the Society recommends that a freshly produced sample be examined for the presence of sperm, and if no sperm are seen, the centrifugate should be examined for presence of motile or nonmotile sperm. They advise that clinicians give clearance to discontinue other contraceptive precautions after two consecutive sperm-free ejaculates. The risk of paternity after vasectomy and postoperative azoospermia is estimated to be 1 in 2000 [31]. Smith et al. reported six cases of DNA-confirmed paternity after vasectomy and two consecutive negative semen analyses. This constitutes a late failure, likely from recanalization. Rare complete sperm in a spun semen analysis pellet are found in 10% of semen specimens at a mean of 10 years after vasectomy [32].

Persistence of sperm in the ejaculate

It is relatively clear that patients with motile sperm persistently present in the post-vasectomy ejaculate must be considered failures. This likely is a result of the vas being cut twice on the same side, or of early recanalization. Early failures also include patients who do not use continued protection before having semen analyses that show postoperative azoospermia. When to consider a repeat vasectomy based on persistent presence of motile sperm in the ejaculate is unclear. However, if the counts remain stable, the procedure should be repeated.

Early persistence of nonmotile sperm in the ejaculate is not uncommon, and has been attributed to sperm residing in the vasal ampulla duct or seminal vesicles. This hypothesis has never been proven, however, and the possibility of recanalization certainly exists. A recent study suggests that if rare nonmotile sperm are found, contraception may be cautiously discontinued, as recent evidence demonstrates that these men will ultimately become azoospermic [33].

The British Andrology Society has addressed this problem by creating a category of "special clearance" for patients with persistent nonmotile sperm. The laboratory is asked to confirm viability of sperm with vital staining. If any motile sperm or substantial numbers of nonmotile sperm are present, clinicians are informed promptly, because many surgeons will opt to repeat the vasectomy. Patients with low sperm counts (< 1 million) of persistent nonmotile sperm in their ejaculates (after at least seven months and at least 24 ejaculations) may be given special clearance following appropriate oral counseling and written advice regarding the risk of pregnancy. The literature suggests that the risk of pregnancy with persistent nonmotile sperm in the ejaculate is similar to pregnancy rates associated with postoperative azoospermia [34]. These are British guidelines, and the AUA policy statement states that "the persistence of sperm in the semen after bilateral vasectomy is a surgical failure." However, the AUA is currently developing guidelines for vasectomy that will specifically address this issue.

Complications

Hematoma and infection

Hematoma is the most common complication of vasectomy, with an average incidence of 2% (range 0.09–29%) [35]. Infection is relatively uncommon with the no-scalpel technique, although older series report rates from 12% to 38% [36–38]. The experience of the vasectomist is the single most important factor relating to complications [35]. The hematoma rate was significantly higher among physicians performing 1–10 vasectomies (4.6%) than among those performing 11–50 vasectomies (2.4%) or more than 50 vasectomies (1.6%) per year. A similar relationship was seen for hospitalization rate.

Sperm granuloma

Sperm granulomas form when sperm leak from the testicular end of the vas. Sperm are highly antigenic, and an intense inflammatory reaction occurs when sperm escape outside the reproductive epithelium. Although sperm granulomas are rarely symptomatic, the presence or absence of a sperm granuloma at the vasectomy site seems to be of importance in modulating the local effects of chronic obstruction on the male reproductive tract. The sperm granuloma's complex network of epithelialized channels provides an additional absorptive surface that helps vent the high intraluminal pressure in the obstructed excurrent ducts. Numerous animal studies have correlated the presence or absence of sperm granuloma at the vasectomy site with the degree of epididymal and testicular damage. Species that always develop granulomas after vasectomy have minimal damage to the seminiferous tubules. Some studies of men undergoing vasectomy reversal have revealed somewhat higher success rates in men who have a sperm granuloma at the vasectomy site [39], whereas another large study has not [40]. Although sperm granulomas at the vasectomy site are present microscopically in 10–30% of men undergoing reversal, it is likely that, given enough time, virtually all men develop sperm granulomas at the vasectomy site, the epididymis, or the rete testis.

Long-term effects

Long-term effects of vasectomy in humans may include vasitis nodosa, chronic testicular and/or epididymal pain, alterations in testicular function, chronic epididymal obstruction, and postulated systemic effects [41]. Although vasitis nodosa has been reported in up to 66% of vasectomy specimens in men undergoing vasectomy reversal [42], this entity does not appear to be associated with pain or significant medical sequelae.

In humans, micropuncture studies have revealed that the markedly increased pressures that occur on the testicular side of the vas as well as the epididymis after vasectomy are not transmitted to the seminiferous tubules [43]. Therefore, little disruption of spermatogenesis is expected in humans. Biopsies up to 15 years after vasectomy show the testes to be essentially normal by light microscopy. Electron microscopic studies, however, have revealed thickening of the basal lamina and scattered areas of disrupted spermatogenesis in portions of the biopsy specimens [44]. Chronic orchialgia and/or epididymal pain after vasectomy occurs in perhaps 1 in 1000 patients [45]. In some cases, vasectomy reversal might be considered or, alternatively, an open-ended vasectomy as described previously. The brunt of pressure-induced damage after vasectomy falls on the epididymis and efferent ductules. These structures become markedly distended and then adapt to reabsorb large volumes of testicular fluid and sperm products. When pain and tenderness are localized in the epididymis, very limited published data show that total epididymectomy relieves pain in 95% of men [46]. However, anecdotal experience does not always yield such optimistic results.

Systemic effects of vasectomy have been postulated. Vasectomy results in detectable levels of serum antisperm antibodies in 60–80% of men [47,48]. Some studies suggest that the antibody titers diminish two or more years after vasectomy. Others suggest that these antibody titers persist. However, neither circulating immune complexes nor deposits are increased after vasectomy in humans [49]. Studies in animals and humans have failed to find any association between antisperm antibodies and immune complex-mediated diseases such as lupus erythematosus, scleroderma, rheumatoid arthritis, or myasthenia gravis [50].

Regarding a causal relationship between vasectomy and cardiovascular disease, early studies suggested that vasectomized monkeys had a higher incidence of atherosclerosis [51]. Although one study in cynomolgus monkeys found more frequent and extensive atherosclerosis of the major vessels in previously vasectomized monkeys fed a high-cholesterol diet [52], no evidence of excess cardiovascular disease [53], illness requiring hospitalization [54,55], or biochemical alterations [56] has been found in more than 15 reports (12 employing matched controls) examining thousands of men [57]. An immunologic basis was hypothesized. However, clinical data in humans have not confirmed this relationship, but population size was small and the study was of short duration [58,59]. The recent study by Goldacre *et al.* also showed no association between vasectomy and cardiovascular disease such as myocardial infarction, coronary heart disease, or stroke [58].

Major among the controversies is the possible link between vasectomy and prostate cancer. Studies have found an increased risk of prostate cancer in men who had a vasectomy 20 years previously [60,61]. **But two large-scale cohort studies evaluated men from a wide range of socioeconomic strata and did not find a link between vasectomy and prostate cancer.** Another study of vasectomy sequelae found no increased incidence of cancer or other diseases [57]. However, despite this evidence, many urologists have changed the way they practice and the way they counsel patients, screening vasectomized men earlier [62].

The most likely explanation for the increased diagnosis of prostate cancer in vasectomized men is detection bias. Vasectomized men are more likely to visit a urologist and therefore are more likely to have cancer diagnosed earlier. Furthermore, men who choose to undergo vasectomy may be more likely to seek health care, increasing their opportunity for prostate cancer detection. **A multidisciplinary National Institutes of Health panel concluded that the epidemiologic associations between vasectomy and prostate cancer are weak. It recommended no change in clinical or public health practice and said that screening for prostate cancer should not be any different for vasectomized men** [63]. Possible explanations for this association include an immunologic response (antisperm antibodies), changes in androgen levels, alterations in local growth factors such as epidermal growth factor and transforming growth factor α, and decreased inhibition of factors responsible for prostate cancer [64]. No basic science studies have confirmed any of the postulated explanations.

Significant concerns about the safety of vasectomy and prostate cancer first arose in 1990 when the publication of two case–control (retrospective) studies suggested an increased risk of prostate cancer for men who

had undergone a vasectomy [65,66]. The analysis of a further set of cases and controls from one of these hospital-based surveillance systems found no significant association, suggesting that the earlier conclusion was due to chance [67,68]. Further reviews of these studies by a panel of experts at the World Health Organization concluded that there did not appear to be a relationship between vasectomy and prostate cancer [69]. However, the panel also recommended that additional research should be conducted to examine this link. Controversy was renewed again in 1993 when Giovannucci and colleagues published two large cohort studies (one prospective, one retrospective) showing a significantly increased risk of prostate cancer, especially for men 20 or more years after having a vasectomy [60,61]. The studies evaluated large numbers of health professionals and husbands of nurses through mailed questionnaires. A committee from the American Urological Association reviewed the existing data and literature and concluded that there was not convincing evidence of a link between vasectomy and prostate cancer [69]. This decision was based on data that were subsequently published suggesting no relationship was present [65,70,71]. The committee recommended that men who had had a vasectomy undergo screening for prostate cancer in the same manner as those who had not had a vasectomy, and that they should be advised of a possible link between vasectomy and prostate cancer [69]. Since 1995, subsequent studies from the National Institutes of Health, US academic centers, and international institutions have continued to question the validity of a significant relationship between vasectomy and prostate cancer [68,70–75]. Despite numerous studies reporting inconclusive evidence of a link between prostate cancer and vasectomy, the initial media attention surrounding this controversy continues to have an effect on urologists, who may be inclined to screen vasectomized men earlier for prostate cancer or to discourage vasectomy in men with a strong family history of prostate cancer [62]. A recent study based on long-term follow-up examined the possibility of a relationship between vasectomy and prostate cancer. This cohort study evaluating almost 25 000 patients undergoing vasectomy showed no elevated risk of cancer of the prostate [64]. **Based on the existing data, there is no evidence that vasectomy results in a higher short- or long-term incidence of prostate cancer.**

Historical, conflicting data about the possibility of an elevated risk factor for testicular cancer in men having undergone a vasectomy further complicates the informed discussion between practitioner and patient regarding the safety of vasectomy [74,76–78]. The recent cohort study also showed no higher incidence of testis cancer in patients undergoing vasectomy [64].

Hormonal treatment

The concept of male hormonal manipulation for contraception predated the era of female hormonal contraception by 20 years. In 1939, two investigators independently tested testosterone for suppression of spermatogenesis [79,80]. Since that time, female birth control pills have dominated the contraceptive market. The bar has been set quite high to improve upon safety, efficacy, and reversibility.

In 2007, the 10th Summit Group published their updated recommendations for regulatory approval for hormonal male contraception. This international group was designed to review the status of clinical development projects for male hormonal contraception [81]. Although much has been published regarding the safety and efficacy of different methods of hormonally based male contraception, there has been no clear consensus as to how to measure successful suppression of spermatogenesis, inclusion criteria for studies, reversibility of treatment, length of study to determine safety, and power of study necessary to prove efficacy. The ideal hormonally based male contraceptive would be safe, affordable, 100% effective, reversible, with no short- or long-term side effects. Such a drug does not exist at the present time. There have been several review articles published in the last few years on male contraception [82–88]. The purpose of this section is to review the published data regarding hormonally based male contraceptive treatment options.

An understanding of the endocrinology of male reproduction, specifically the male hypothalamic–pituitary–gonadal axis, and the basic science of spermatogenesis is required to understand the methodologies utilized for male contraception. This is nicely summarized in Chapters 2–5 and will not be repeated in detail here. Briefly, spermatogenesis is regulated by the pulsatile release of gonadotropin-releasing hormone (GnRH), which stimulates the anterior pituitary to episodically release follicle-stimulating hormone (FSH) and luteinizing hormone (LH). LH stimulates the Leydig cells to produce testosterone, which has a local effect on the interstitium and seminiferous tubules and results in sperm production and maturation. FSH acts directly on the Sertoli cells to promote spermatogenesis. The complex interplay between testosterone, FSH,

Table 27.1. Male hormonal contraceptive options

Testosterone
Testosterone propionate
Testosterone enanthate
Testosterone undecanoate
Testosterone buciclate
7α-methyl-19-nortestosterone (MENT)
Testosterone gels
Testosterone–progestin combinations
Medroxyprogesterone acetate (MPA and depoMPA)
Cyproterone acetate (CPA)
Levonorgestrel (LNG)
Desogestrel and etonogestrel
Dienogest (DNG)
Norethisterone (NET, NETA, nestorone gel)
Testosterone with GnRH analogs
GnRH agonists
GnRH antagonists
Selective androgen receptor modulators (SARMs)

and other factors is important for normal spermatogenesis. Inhibin B is released by Sertoli cells and acts as a negative feedback on FSH. Testosterone and estradiol are negative feedback modulators of GnRH.

Endocrinological treatment strategies for male contraception are listed in Table 27.1 [88].

Testosterone alone

In 1939, independent studies on male contraception were performed by Heckel and McCullagh with short-acting testosterone propionate (TP) [79,80]. Subsequent studies revealed reversible azoospermia by 60 days in some patients with daily use of 25 mg IM testosterone propionate [89]. Improved frequency and dosage was achieved with the advent of longer-acting testosterone enanthate (TE), spurring interest in studies with an improved delivery frequency.

The WHO, in conjunction with the Contraceptive Research and Development program (CONRAD), conducted two large multicenter studies on testosterone enanthate. In the initial multicenter study conducted in seven countries, subjects received 200 mg TE IM weekly and used no other contraception for one year once sperm concentrations fell below 3 million/mL [90]. This study revealed that 70% of 271 patients became azoospermic after six months of treatment. The mean time to azoospermia was three months. The azoospermic patients were enrolled in a 12-month efficacy phase, in which one pregnancy occurred. Sperm reappeared in the ejaculate in 11 patients. Once the testosterone was discontinued, the mean time to sperm recovery was 3.7 months. Of note, this international study revealed that 91% of Asian and 60% of Caucasian patients became azoospermic, suggesting an ethnic difference in endocrine response. This difference has been seen in subsequent studies. Possible explanations include differences in levels of 5α-reductase levels in these groups [91], lower baseline testosterone levels, or differing negative feedback responses.

The second WHO testosterone study was performed as a 15-center, 9-country study with 399 volunteers. In 98% of men spermatogenesis was suppressed to below 3 million/mL with weekly 100 mg IM TE after induction phase with 200 mg IM TE [92]. There was a significant difference in pregnancy rates between azoospermic patients (1.4 pregnancies/100 person-years) and patients between 0.1 and 3 million/mL (8.1 pregnancies/100 person-years). Approximately 25% of patients discontinued the study for personal reasons, such as dislike of injections, or for medical reasons. This study confirmed the relative efficacy of treatment, and laid the groundwork for further studies with different longer-acting testosterone regimens.

A phase 2 multicenter study was performed with longer-acting monthly injections of testosterone undecanoate (TU) in 380 Chinese men. In 76% of patients, spermatogenesis was sufficiently suppressed to lead to the initiation phase. If suppression was to azoospermia or less than 3 million/mL, there were no pregnancies. However, there was reappearance of sperm in five patients, with one pregnancy [93].

Studies with testosterone buciclate (TB), another long-acting testosterone derivative, were initially performed by the WHO collaborating center and showed moderate suppression of spermatogenesis at a dose of 1200 mg IM monthly. Minimal side effects were noted, and this set the stage for combining long-acting testosterone with progesterone derivatives [94].

A dose-response trial of 7α-methyl-19-nortestosterone (MENT) was initiated in 35 healthy volunteers to assess effects of serum gonadotropins and sperm production [95]. This synthetic androgen is more potent than testosterone, it is resistant to 5α reduction, and it

has diffusion characteristics that make it well suited for a depot implant. Initial data showed relatively good results, but typical testosterone-related side effects occurred.

Newer delivery systems have been FDA-approved for the treatment of hypogonadism, but it is unclear whether men would tolerate daily gel application of testosterone. Studies combining testosterone gel with other agents are under way.

Use of testosterone alone has side effects, including acne and oily skin, mood changes, increased hemoglobin and hemocrit, weight gain, decrease in testicular volume, sleep apnea, gynecomastia, and possible effects on cholesterol. There are no long-term data on testosterone use in normal males with regard to prostate symptoms, growth, or cancer. In an era of fear of using medications on relatively healthy individuals, acceptability of routine use may be a major concern, given recent data on medical treatment of menopause with estrogen/progestin therapy. In addition, anabolic steroids are a controlled substance, and regulation of this industry is very strict at this time. Abuse of these drugs could easily become prevalent with its widespread use and availability for contraception.

Although data suggest that testosterone therapy will create a milieu of oligospermia and/or azoospermia in most cases, its reliability is clearly uncertain at this point. The efficacy bar has been set very high with "the pill." Greater efficacy, with fewer short- and long-term side effects, will be needed before use of testosterone alone becomes a viable option. In addition, close follow-up with regular semen analyses is necessary since there may be breakthroughs in sperm suppression. However, the use of testosterone with other agents may have more promise.

Combination therapy

Significant side effects and lack of high efficacy with testosterone alone have pushed researchers towards combination therapy. The goal of combination therapy is to effectively create sterility while utilizing a lower dose of testosterone to maintain physiological levels.

Testosterone and progestins

Progestins have been used in multiple small studies for suppression of spermatogenesis and testosterone production in men. Progestins utilized alone result in significant side effects such as loss of libido and erectile dysfunction. The mechanism of action of progestins is thought to be either negative feedback on the pituitary–gonadal axis, inhibition of LH receptor expression, or direct effect on sperm [96,97]. Progestins alone cannot suppress spermatogenesis in dosages safe for administration and without significant side effects. However, combining lower doses of progestins with testosterone supplementation to restore exogenous testosterone may improve safety and efficacy, and lessen side effects.

Medroxyprogesterone acetate (MPA and depot MPA)

The contraceptive efficacy of medroxyprogesterone acetate (MPA) has been studied since the 1970s [84]. Unlike studies on testosterone monotherapy, randomized, multicenter, large-population studies evaluating efficacy of testosterone/progestin preparations are few [98].

A recent review of MPA/testosterone preparations showed that only 67% of patients receiving MPA with different testosterone preparations achieved azoospermia [99]. The 1993 WHO study comparing testosterone alone and 19-nortestosterone with depot MPA showed consistent azoospermia in 95.6% and 97.8%, respectively, in 90 Indonesian males [100]. From these data, it was not clear whether the effect was from testosterone alone or from combination therapy. Subsequent studies [101] in 55 men with testosterone implants plus depot MPA showed suppression to below 1 million/mL in 94% of patients, with no pregnancies in this suppression subgroup. Median time to counts returning to 20 million/mL was five months, but return to baseline numbers took much longer, suggesting an accumulation of drug in adipose tissue. These studies were performed in the Asian population only. Recently, two papers reported on the same group of 38 men with testosterone gel and depot MPA for sperm suppression, and evaluated patient acceptability of this combination [102,103]. Over 90% of patients had sperm suppression to below 1 million/mL, but acceptability was low, with only 45% saying they would use it if commercially available; one-third of patients said it would interfere with their daily routine, and questionnaire data showed mild changes in overall satisfaction with sexual activity and ejaculatory function. Interestingly, a subgroup of patients received GnRH antagonist, but there was no additive effect in terms of sperm suppression. A recent study by the same group looked at factors that might differentiate azoospermic groups from nonazoospermic groups [104]. They showed increased levels of insulin-like factor 3 (INSL3) in the nonazoospermic group, and hypothesized that this may be the target for refining future treatment.

Cyproterone acetate (CPA)

Cyproterone acetate (CPA) is an active antiandrogen with progestin effects. It has been studied as hormone deprivation for prostate cancer. It has profound effects on libido, energy, and decreases in hematocrit. Multiple studies have been performed with combination CPA and TE or TU [105–112]. Doses ranging from 25 to 100 mg/day have suppressed spermatogenesis, but side effects have precluded subsequent studies. It has been postulated that antiandrogens may work well to suppress the effects of residual intratesticular testosterone not suppressed by other means [84].

Levonorgestrel (LNG)

Several small studies [99,113–115] have been performed with levonorgestrel (LNG). This progestin is either an oral or an implant preparation. Unfortunately, the studies performed with a combination of LNG and testosterone resulted in only partial suppression of spermatogenesis even in the Asian population. The concept of a two-implant preparation of progesterone/testosterone is appealing, but data regarding efficacy with this progestin are lacking at the present time.

Desogestrel and etonogestrel

Desogestrel is a potent oral progestin that is converted to the active agent etonogestrel. Initial small studies performed with doses of 75, 150, and 300 µg/day showed variable results. A two-center study in Scotland and China with oral desogestrel 300 µg PO/day and 400 mg depot testosterone SC pellets led to suppression of spermatogenesis with azoospermia in 100% of men [116]. There was noted to be a rise in high-density lipoprotein (HDL) and weight gain. A subsequent study of 21 African men given desogestrel and testosterone pellets showed similar results, but slightly less complete suppression with no negative effects on lipoprotein or hemoglobin [117]. Another study, with 15 patients taking etonogestrel and testosterone pellets at three-month intervals, resulted in azoospermia in all subjects by 28 weeks [118]. A subsequent larger study (n = 130) by the same investigators showed excellent sperm suppression with combination implant when utilized monthly [119]. The combination of this two-drug pellet given every three months is a very palatable option for patients. A multicenter phase 2 trial was initiated in 2003, but terminated in 2006 by Schering-Organon for unclear reasons.

Dienogest (DNG)

Dienogest (DNG) is a progestin with a lower degree of antiandrogenic and estrogenic activity. Preliminary data suggest that it can suppress gonadotropins without adverse side effects [111]. Minimal data are available on the subject of sperm suppression.

Norethisterone (NETE, NETA), nestorone gel

Norethisterone is a depot female contraceptive with similar effects to testosterone undecanoate, making this combination attractive for male contraception. A 1988 study showed suppression with a combination of oral norethisterone and TU [120]. Subsequent studies have shown high efficacy in a small group of Caucasian patients (74 total patients) with either oral or IM norethisterone and testosterone undecanoate [121,122]. Treatment at eight-week intervals resulted in a higher azoospermic rate than 12-week treatment. No short-term changes in the prostate were seen. Longer-term studies are necessary to better evaluate changes in prostate size, prostate-specific antigen (PSA), etc. This combination is very attractive for a depot, since the eight-weekly injection of both testosterone and norethisterone is highly efficacious in a potentially single injection. In addition, a clinical trial is under way evaluating a combination of nestorone gel with testosterone gel.

Testosterone and GnRH analogs (agonists and antagonists)

GnRH is released in a pulsatile fashion that is thought to be responsible for the episodic release of LH and FSH. GnRH agonists work by having paradoxical antigonadotropic effects through the down-regulation of GnRH after an initial GnRH surge. GnRH antagonists cause competitive inhibition of GnRH receptors. They are familiar to clinicians for the regulation of ovulation induction, and in the treatment of advanced prostate cancer and endometriosis.

There have been 12 clinical trials with different GnRH agonists and testosterone, resulting in a combined 23% suppression to azoospermia in a total of 106 patients [123,124]. It appears that the lack of suppression is related to breakthrough of FSH secretion. Therefore, at this point, this combination has not been actively pursued.

However, trials combining TE and GnRH antagonists seem to have better results. Several studies dating back to the early 1990s suggest a rapid onset of suppression of spermatogenesis to azoospermia [125–129]. This group of studies, each with small populations, suggested a good response to this combined therapy. When GnRH was stopped, and

maintenance was performed with testosterone alone, suppression of spermatogenesis was not maintained [130]. Initial trials were performed with short-acting GnRH antagonists, which had local side effects such as significant irritation at the injection site. With the longer-acting GnRH antagonists having fewer local side effects, this therapy may take on a more critical role in the future.

Selective androgen receptor modulators (SARMs)

Selective androgen receptor modulators mimic the central and peripheral androgenic and anabolic effects of testosterone and are being investigated for treatment of prostate disease. In animal models, SARM C6 was found to induce significant suppression of spermatogenesis [131]. This serves as an interesting model for testing in humans as either primary or adjunctive therapy.

In summary, is not completely clear why testosterone, either alone or in combination, does not suppress spermatogenesis completely, or results in evidence of "breakthrough" sperm production. Two theories suggested are incomplete suppression of FSH and persistent or episodic incomplete suppression of intratesticular testosterone that allows for low levels of sperm production [88]. Recent studies have shown increased levels of insulin-like factor 3 (INSL3) in incompletely suppressed patients [104].

Male hormonal contraception is approaching the high bar set by "the pill" and vasectomy. However, much more work is necessary to determine the combination therapy providing the best timing, efficacy, short- and long-term safety before it will reach phase 3 trials. The criteria for studies on treatment modalities from the 10th Summit Meeting on Hormonal Male Contraception (2006) are listed in Table 27.2 [81].

Immunocontraceptives

Along with hormonal manipulation, immunocontraception appears to offer reasonable hope for a nonsurgical contraceptive option in men [132]. It appears to fulfill the criteria necessary for further study, including the ability to synthesize vaccines relatively cheaply, provide effective contraception, have a minimum of side effects, and be reversible. The molecules that have been studied include those that target gamete production (luteinizing hormone-releasing hormone [LHRH]/ GnRH, FSH]), gamete function (sperm antigens and oocyte zona pellucida [ZP]), and gamete outcome

Table 27.2. Criteria for studies on treatment modalities. (From Nieschlag E. 10th Summit Meeting consensus: recommendations for regulatory approval for hormonal male contraception. *Contraception* 2007; **75**: 166–7 [81]. With permission from Elsevier.)

1. Phase 2 studies evaluating efficacy should use WHO sperm concentration parameters and the goal should be suppression ≤ 1 million/mL.

2. After cessation of therapy, patients need to be followed until normal fertility is restored (criterion utilized is 20 million/mL).

3. Inclusion criteria must include men with sperm concentrations > 20 million/mL.

4. Open label, noncomparative contraceptive efficacy studies are acceptable if the primary endpoint is not susceptible to bias, e.g., pregnancy rate.

5. For efficacy, two independent phase 3 trials for 1 year from suppression to < 1 million/mL should include 200 men/couples per trial.

6. For safety, new agents require studies with 300–600 men for 6 months at the intended combination and dose, 100 men exposed for 1 year, and a total of 1500 men in phase 1–3 studies at a minimum.

7. Long-term safety will be monitored by post-marketing surveillance.

8. Laboratory data need to be performed under strict quality control.

(human chorionic gonadotropin [hCG]) [133]. This section will outline some of the more promising immunocontraceptives that have been studied.

Gamete production

In that GnRH stimulates pituitary secretion of gonadotropic hormones, it was logical to predict that immunoneutralization of GnRH would prevent endogenous GnRH from binding to its gonadotropin receptors, and would thereby delay sexual maturation in adolescent animals and cause gonadal atrophy in adults, arrest of gametogenesis, and libido loss. The effects of vaccination using a GnRH vaccine in the dog and the rat were reversible [134]. One obvious drawback to this method in humans is the loss of hormone production.

Human FSH (hFSH) and ovine FSH (oFSH) have also been studied as possible target antigens. Attempts were made to use hFSH linked to cholera toxin and interleukin to produce effective antibodies. The immunization using hFSH caused a 75–100% decease in sperm counts in the ejaculate. The fertility of male monkeys after hFSH immunization was significantly reduced, as well as the ability of spermatozoa to penetrate hamster ova [135]. To date, no studies have been performed on humans.

Gamete function

Development of a vaccine(s) based on sperm antigens represents a promising approach to contraception. The utility of a sperm antigen in immunocontraception is contingent upon its tissue specificity and involvement in fertility, and on raising high antibody titers, especially locally in the genital tract, that are capable of inducing reversible infertility. Several sperm antigens, such as lactate dehydrogenase C4, PH-20, sperm protein (SP)-10, fertilization antigen (FA)-1, FA-2, cleavage signal (CS)-1, NZ-1, and NZ-2 have been proposed as potential candidates for the vaccine development. Sperm–ZP binding is a pivotal issue, a mostly species-specific event in the fertilization process, and the molecules involved in this site constitute the most exciting candidates for immunocontraception [136,137].

Proteins interacting with zona pellucida (ZP)

RSA-1/SP-17 are families of low molecular weight membrane glycoproteins (14, 16, 17, 18 kDa) that function as ZP binding proteins. These autoantigens were immunolocalized on the rabbit sperm surface to the postacrosomal region of the head. Immunization of mice with a synthetic peptide based on an RSA-1 B-cell epitope reduced fertility by 80% compared to controls [138]. SP-17 peptide epitope was used as contraceptive vaccine in an animal model [139].

The fertilization antigen 1 (FA-1) is a glycoprotein first identified on the postacrosomal region, midpiece, and tail of human sperm cell membranes by a monoclonal antibody (MA-24) isolated from mice immunized with human sperm [140]. MA-24 antibody to FA-1 completely prevented human sperm function, and fertilization in vitro in rabbit and mouse [141]. The mechanism is by FA-1 reaction with ZP3 to block sperm–egg interaction. Active immunization of animals with recombinant FA-1 antigen causes a long-lasting reversible inhibition in fertility by raising a sperm-specific immune response. This antigen may also be involved in human immunoinfertility.

The mouse sperm plasma membrane antigen M42 is a relatively diffusible 200/220 kDa doublet glycoprotein found at the posterior region of mouse sperm heads. A mAb directed against this protein, M42 mAb, blocks mouse fertilization in vitro in a concentration-dependent manner; such inhibition depends upon the presence of the ZP. M42 mAb specifically inhibits induction of the acrosome reaction (AR), and does not interfere with sperm–ZP binding or with sperm penetration through the ZP once the AR has been triggered [142].

P95 is a 95 kDa protein that localizes to the anterior region of mouse sperm and contains phosphorylated tyrosine residues. Studies have suggested that P95 is the ligand for ZP3 and possesses tyrosine kinase activity that initiates the AR cascade. The inhibition of kinase activity using tryphostin completely blocked sperm AR and sperm–egg interaction. Studies with the antibody to P95 found a significant reduction of human sperm binding to human ZP and a complete block of ZP penetration in a concentration-dependent manner [143].

β-1,4-galactosyl-transferase (β-GTase) is a receptor in sperm plasma membrane surface for ZP3 binding and involves sperm–egg recognition during fertilization. Antibodies to GTase can inhibit sperm binding to eggs or mZP3. Since GTase is present on both acrosome-intact and acrosome-reacted spermatozoa function, it would not appear to be a good candidate for a contraceptive vaccine as it shows no tissue specificity in its expression [144].

Sperm-specific LDH-C$_4$

The testis-specific isozyme lactate dehydrogenase C$_4$ (LDH-C$_4$) described by Goldberg and colleagues is perhaps the most extensively characterized sperm antigen [145]. LDH-C$_4$ functions in lactate metabolism and glycolysis of developing and mature spermatozoa. Although the somatic lactate dehydrogenases are cytoplasmic, LDH-C$_4$ is localized both intracellularly and extracellularly. Beyler et al. identified LDH-C4 on the surface of human and murine sperm using a solid phase radioimmunoassay with rabbit anti-mouse LDH-C$_4$ antisera [146]. Furthermore, the agglutinating and cytotoxic effects of anti-LDH-C$_4$ antibodies implicated their binding to the sperm surface. The LDH-C subunit is an independent gene product expressed only in spermatogenic cells, and is immunologically distinct from the LDH-A and LDH-B subunits [147]. Identification of this tissue-specificity led to the investigation of LDH-C$_4$'s antigenicity and its potential as an immunocontraceptive. Active immunization with

LDH-C$_4$ suppressed fertility in a variety of mammalian species, including both male and female primates [148]. The observed effects were attributed to multiple immunologic mechanisms. In one study, the immunodominant B-cell epitope of human LDH-C$_4$ was tested as a peptide vaccinogen in female baboons [149]. This LDH-C$_4$ peptide–diphtheria toxoid conjugate was shown to decrease fertility by 75% compared to controls. Furthermore, the contraceptive effect was reversed within one year after the final immunization. Since serum antibody titers did not directly correlate with infertility, the report suggested that cell-mediated immunity rather than humoral immunity might be the critical effector mechanism. In this view, LDH-C$_4$ research can provide useful background information for the development of other types of immunocontraceptive technology.

Acrosomal proteins

Acrosin is a member of the serine protease family that is localized within the acrosome membrane of mammalian sperm. It plays an important role in the AR and sperm–egg binding during fertilization. Antibodies to acrosin have been shown to inhibit fertilization in the human and rabbit, but not in sheep [144].

Herr and colleagues identified the testis/sperm-specific, intra-acrosomal sperm antigen SP-10 (18–34 kDa) using MHS-10, a mAb generated against whole human spermatozoa. MHS-10 was studied for in-vitro fertilization, and the results demonstrated that mAb can inhibit the acrosome reaction, as well as sperm fertilization in human, bovine and mouse [150]. SP-10 is currently under investigation as a model sperm antigen for the development of an oral contraceptive recombinant form of the human SP-10 antigen.

Epididymal proteins

Eppin is a testis/epididymal-specific protein that binds to semenogelin. A report examining the immunization of nonhuman male primates demonstrated reversible infertility in 58% of animals tested. The authors speculated that the antibodies to eppin interfere with the interaction of eppin on the sperm surface to semenogelin, thus preventing fertilization. However, the authors pointed out that high serum titers of the antibody were necessary for contraception [151,152]. Studies are currently under way to further characterize this as a possible immunocontraceptive.

Nonhormonal contraception

Gossypol, nitroimidazole derivatives, Tripterygium wilfordii

The plant product gossypol has been utilized as a reversible contraceptive. It is a natural constituent of cottonseed oil and has been reported in several reviews to have effects on fertility [153,154]. Side effects include nausea and weakness due to hypocalcemia, with severe cases causing paralysis. Experimentally, gossypol has been shown to cause irreversible damage to the germinal cell epithelium, and this has been documented in long-term use in human males as well. Gossypol exists in two isomers, which differ in both their toxicity and fertility-suppressing characteristics. Unfortunately, efforts at separating these two isomers have been unsuccessful, and therefore gossypol does not seem to be an acceptable form of male contraception. Another plant derivative has been utilized. Whereas gossypol acts as a spermatogenic suppressant, *Tripterygium wilfordii* prevents sperm migration. However, this also has toxic side effects that have prevented clinical application [155].

Heat

Heat has been shown to negatively influence spermatogenesis and sperm maturation. Assessment of the contraceptive efficacy of a daily mild increase (1–2°C) in testicular temperature during waking hours was reported in nine couples using two techniques of immobilization of the testes in a suprascrotal position (close to the inguinal canal). In the first technique, immobilization was achieved with specific underwear; there was one undesired pregnancy from a man who stopped the heating for three weeks. With the second technique, immobilization was achieved by adding a supplementary ring to the specific underwear; there were no pregnancies. These methods were found to be both safe and reversible. This study suggested that a daily mild increase in testis temperature could be a potential contraceptive method for men. Although the authors were able to reduce the pregnancy rate, it was not a consistent finding and was associated with a high failure rate [156].

Compounds with antispermatogenic action

These compounds target Sertoli cell–germ cell junctions, preventing maturation and/or increasing germ cell depletion. These drugs cause premature release of the developing sperm into the tubular lumen,

thus leading to infertility [157]. Lonidamine (1-[2,4-dichlorobenzyl]-1H-indazole-3-carboxylic acid) is an anticancer drug. During the course of examining its mechanism of action and toxicity, it was found that lonidamine did not target rapidly dividing cells; rather, it became associated with biological membranes, causing conformational changes that resulted in the disruption of the respiratory process in cells that contained condensed mitochondria, such as tumor cells sensitized by X-irradiation and certain types of germ cells, such as spermatids and spermatocytes. Studies to date have been in rats only, but they have shown no effect on hormonal status, including LH, FSH, and testosterone levels, and results have been completely reversible.

Epididymal factors

Recent animal studies have examined the role of the epididymis in male contraception. Inducing sterility by altering sperm transport through the epididymis has not yet been achieved. The induction of infertility in males of several species is easier to achieve by direct actions of drugs on sperm function (e.g., inhibition of sperm-specific isozymes of the glycolytic pathway by chloro-compounds) than by indirectly reducing amounts of epididymal secretions normally present in high concentration (e.g., α-glucosidase, L-carnitine). Drugs that affect sperm function show clinical promise, since human spermatozoa are susceptible to inhibition. Targeting a specific sperm protein acquired in the testis, but depleted in the epididymis by toxicants that induce rapid infertility, may also lead to the discovery of new contraceptives, but these will require developing new means of organ-specific delivery of contraceptive drugs [158]. This approach is not yet applicable to humans.

Future: nonsurgical male contraception

The role of nonsurgical treatment for male contraception will certainly increase in the future, although vasectomy will likely remain a very popular option. However, as men's participation in the contraceptive process grows, the demand for safer, cheaper, and more easily reversible methods will increase as well.

References

[1] Schwingl PJ, Guess HA. Safety and effectiveness of vasectomy. *Fertil Steril* 2000; **73**: 923–36.
[2] Rowlands S, Hannaford P. The incidence of sterilisation in the UK. *BJOG* 2003; **110**: 819–24.

[3] Witt MA, Heron S, Lipshultz LI. The post-vasectomy length of the testicular vasal remnant: a predictor of surgical outcome in microscopic vasectomy reversal. *J Urol* 1994; **151**: 892–4.

[4] Li S, Goldstein M, Zhu J, Huber D. The no-scalpel vasectomy. *J Urol* 1991; **145**: 341–4.

[5] Weiss RS, Li PS. No-needle jet anesthetic technique for no-scalpel vasectomy. *J Urol* 2005; 173(5): 1677–80.

[6] Li S. Ligation of vas deferens by clamping method under direct vision. *Chin Med J* 1976; **4**: 213–14.

[7] Sokal D, McMullen S, Gates D, Dominik R. The male sterilization investigator team: a comparative study of the no scalpel and standard incision approaches to vasectomy in 5 countries. *J Urol* 1999; **162**: 1621–5.

[8] Sokal D, Irsula B, Hays M, Chen-Mok M, Barone MA, Investigator Study Group. Vasectomy by ligation and excision, with or without fascial interposition: a randomized controlled trial [ISRCTN77781689] *BMC Med* 2004; **2**: 6.

[9] Sokal D, Irsula B, Chen-Mok M, Labrecque M, Barone MA. A comparison of vas occlusion techniques: cautery more effective than ligation and excision with fascial interposition. *BMC Urol* 2004; **4**: 12.

[10] Nirapathpongporn A, Huber DH, Krieger JN. No-scalpel vasectomy at the King's birthday vasectomy festival. *Lancet* 1990; **335**: 894–5.

[11] Makhlouf AA, Niederberger CS. Ensuring vasectomy success: what is the standard? *J Androl* 2006; **27**: 637–40.

[12] Li S. Percutaneous injection of vas deferens. *Chin J Urol* 1980; **1**: 193–8.

[13] Ban SL. Sterility by vas injection method. *Hu Nan Med J* 1980; **5**: 49–50.

[14] Tao T. Vas deferens sterility by injection method. *Qeng Dao Med J* 1980; **5**: 65–8.

[15] Roberts WW, Chan DY, Fried NM, *et al.* High intensity focused ultrasound ablation of the vas deferens in a canine model. *J Urol* 2002; **167**(6): 2613–17.

[16] Roberts WW, Wright EJ, Fried NM, *et al.* High-intensity focused ultrasound ablation of the epididymis in a canine model: A potential alternative to vasectomy. *J Endourol* 2002; **16**: 621–5.

[17] Zaneveld LJ, Burns JW, Beyler S, Depel W, Shapiro S. Development of a potentially reversible vas deferens occlusion device and evaluation in primates. *Fertil Steril* 1988; **49**: 527–33.

[18] Zaneveld LJD, De Castro MP, *et al.* The soft, hollow plug ("SHUG"): a potentially reversible vas deferens occlusive device. In: Rajalakshmi M, Griffin PD, eds. *Male Contraception: Present and Future.* New Delhi: New Age Int, 1999: 293–307.

[19] Moss WM. Sutureless vasectomy, an improved technique: 1300 cases performed without failure. *Fertil Steril* 1974; **27**: 1040–5.

[20] Bennett AH. Vasectomy without complication. *Urology* 1976; **7**: 184–5.

[21] Schmidt SS. Vasectomy. *Urol Clin North Am* 1987; **14**: 149–54.

[22] Barone MA, Irsula B, Chen-Mok M, Sokal DC, Investigator study group. Effectiveness of vasectomy using cautery. *BMC Urol* 2004; **4**: 10.

[23] Esho JO, Cass AS. Recanalization rate following methods of vasectomy using interposition of fascial sheath of vas deferens. *J Urol* 1978; **120**: 178–9.

[24] Maatman TJ, Aldrin L, Carothers GG. Patient noncompliance after vasectomy. *Fertil Steril* 1997; **68**: 552–5.

[25] Barone MA, Nazerali H, Cortes M, *et al.* A prospective study of time and number of ejaculations to azoospermia after vasectomy by ligation and excision. *J Urol* 2003 **170**: 892–6.

[26] Cortes M, Flick A, Barone MA, *et al.* Results of a pilot study of the time to azoospermia after vasectomy in Mexico City. *Contraception* 1997; **56**: 215–22.

[27] Badrakumar C, Gogooi NK, Sundaram SK. Semen analysis after vasectomy: when and how many. *BJU Int* 2000; **86**: 479–81.

[28] Belker AM, Sexter MS, Sweitzer SJ, Raff MJ. The high rate of noncompliance for post-vasectomy semen examination: Medical and legal considerations. *J Urol* 1990; **144**: 284–6.

[29] Smucker DR, Mayhew HE, Nordlund DJ, Hahn WD, Palmer KE. Postvasectomy semen analysis: why patients don't follow-up. *J Am Board Fam Pract* 1991; **4**: 5–9.

[30] Hancock P, McLaughlin E, for the British Andrology Society. British Andrology Society guidelines for the assessment of post vasectomy semen samples (2002). *J Clin Path* 2002; **55**: 812–16.

[31] Smith JC, Cranston D, O'Brien T, *et al.* Fatherhood without apparent spermatozoa after vasectomy. *Lancet* 1994; **344**: 30.

[32] Lemack GE, Goldstein M. Presence of sperm in the pre-vasectomy reversal semen analysis: Incidence and implications. *J Urol* 1996; **155**: 167–9.

[33] Aradhya KW, Best K, Sokal DC. Recent developments in vasectomy. *BMJ* 2005; **330**: 296–9.

[34] Haldar N, Cranston D, Turner E, *et al.* How reliable is vasectomy? Long-term follow-up of vasectomised men. *Lancet* 2000; **356**: 43–4.

[35] Kendrick J, Gonzales B, Huber D, *et al.* Complications of vasectomies in the United States. *J Fam Prac* 1987; **25**: 245–8.

[36] Appell R, Evans P. Vasectomy: etiology of infectious complications. *Fertil Steril* 1980; **33**: 52–3.

[37] Randall PE, Ganguli L, Marcuson RW. Wound infection following vasectomy. *Br J Urol* 1983; **55**: 564–7.

[38] Randall PE, Ganguli LA, Keaney MGL, Marcuson RW. Prevention of wound infection following vasectomy. *Br J Urol* 1985; **57**: 227–9.

[39] Silber SJ. Sperm granuloma and reversibility of vasectomy. *Lancet* 1977; **2**: 588–9.

[40] Belker AM, Thomas AV, Fuchs EEF. Results of 1469 microsurgical vasectomy reversals by Vasovasostomy Study Group. *J Urol* 1991; **145**: 505–11.

[41] Choe JM, Kirkemo AK. Questionnaire-based outcomes study of nononcological post-vasectomy complications. *J Urol* 1996; **155**: 1284–6.

[42] Freund MJ, Weidmann JE, Goldstein M, *et al.* Microrecanalization after vasectomy in man. *J Androl* 1989; **10**: 120–32.

[43] Johnson AL, Howards SS. Intratubular hydrostatic pressure in testis and epididymis before and after vasectomy. *Am J Physiol* 1975; **228**: 556–64.

[44] Jarow JP, Budin RE, Dym M, *et al.* Quantitative pathological changes in the human testis after vasectomy. *N Engl J Med* 1985; **313**: 1252–6.

[45] McConaghy P, Paxton LD, Loughlin V. Chronic testicular pain following vasectomy. *Br J Urol* 1996; **77**: 328.

[46] Selikowitz AM, Schned AR. A late post-vasectomy syndrome. *J Urol* 1985; **134**: 494–7.

[47] Lepow IH, Crozier R. *Vasectomy: Immunologic and Pathophysiologic Effects in Animal and Man*. New York, NY: Academic Press, 1979.

[48] Fuchs EF, Alexander N. Immunologic considerations before and after vasovasostomy. *Fertil Steril* 1983; **40**: 497–9.

[49] Witkin SS, Zelikovsky G, Bongiovanni AM. Sperm-related antigens, antibodies, and circulating immune complexes in sera of recently vasectomized men. *J Clin Invest* 1982; **70**: 33–40.

[50] Massey FJ, Bernstein GS, O'Fallon WM, *et al.* Vasectomy and health: results from a large cohort study. *JAMA* 1984; **252**: 1023–9.

[51] Clarkson TB, Alexander NJ. Long term vasectomy: effects on the occurrence and extent of atherosclerosis in rhesus monkeys. *J Clin Invest* 1980; **65**: 15–25.

[52] Alexander NJ, Clarkson TB. Vasectomy increases the severity of diet-induced atherosclerosis in Macaca fasciculoris. *Science* 1978; **201**: 538–41.

[53] Walker AM, Hunter JR, Watkins RN, *et al.* Vasectomy and non-fatal myocardial infarction. *Lancet* 1981; **1**: 13–15.

[54] Walker AM, Jick H, Hunter JR, Danford A, Rothman KJ. Hospitalization rates in vasectomized men. *JAMA* 1981; **245**: 2315–17.

[55] Petitti DB, Klein R, Kipp H, Friedman GD. Vasectomy and the incidence of hospitalized illness. *J Urol* 1982; **129**: 760–2.

[56] Smith MS, Paulson DF. The physiologic consequences of vas ligation. *Urol Survey* 1980; **30**: 31–3.

[57] Schuman LM, Coulson AH, Mandel JS, Massey FJ, O'Fallon WM. Health status of American men: a study of post-vasectomy sequelae. *J Clin Epidemiol* 1993; **46**: 697–958.

[58] Goldacre MJ, Holford TR, Vessey MP. Cardiovascular disease and vasectomy: findings from two epidemiologic studies. *N Engl J Med* 1983; **308**: 805–8.

[59] Manson JE, Ridker PM, Spelsberg A, *et al.* Vasectomy and subsequent cardiovascular disease in US physicians. *Contraception* 1999; **59**: 181–6.

[60] Giovannucci E, Ascherio A, Rimm EB, *et al.* A prospective cohort study of vasectomy and prostate cancer in US men. *JAMA* 1993; **269**: 873–7.

[61] Giovannucci E, Tosteson TD, Speizer FE, *et al.* A retrospective cohort study of vasectomy and prostate cancer in US men. *JAMA* 1993; **269**: 878–82.

[62] Sandlow JI, Kreder KJ. A change in practice: current urological practice in response to reports concerning vasectomy and prostate cancer. *Fertil Steril* 1996; **66**: 281–4.

[63] Healy B. From the National Institutes of Health. Does vasectomy cause prostate cancer? *JAMA* 1993; **269**: 2620.

[64] Goldacre MJ, Wotton CJ, Seagroatt V, Yeates D. Cancer and cardiovascular disease after vasectomy: an epidemiological database study. *Fertil Steril* 2005; **84**: 1438–43.

[65] Rosenberg L, Palmer JR, Zauber AG, *et al.* Vasectomy and the risk of prostate cancer. *Am J Epidemiol* 1990; **132**: 1051–5.

[66] Mettlin C, Natarajan N, Huben R. Vasectomy and prostate cancer risk. *Am J Epidemiol* 1990; **132**: 1056–61.

[67] Rosenberg L, Palmer JR, Zauber AG, *et al.* The relation of vasectomy to risk of cancer. *Am J Epidemiol* 1994; **140**: 431–8.

[68] Cox B, Sneyd MJ, Paul C, Delahunt B, Skegg DCG. Vasectomy and risk of prostate cancer. *JAMA* 2002; **287**: 3110–15.

[69] Howards SS. Editorial comment on vasectomy and prostate cancer. *J Urol* 1999; **161**: 1852–3.

[70] John EM, Whittemore AS, Wu AH, *et al.* Vasectomy and prostate cancer: results from a multiethnic case–control study. *J Natl Cancer Inst* 1995; **87**: 662–9.

[71] Zhu K, Stanford JL, Daling JR, *et al.* Vasectomy and prostate cancer: a case–control study in a health maintenance organization. *Am J Epidemiol* 1996; **144**: 717–22.

[72] Lesko SM, Louik C, Vezina R, Rosenberg L, Shapiro S. Vasectomy and prostate cancer. *J Urol* 1999; **161**: 1848–53.

[73] Lynge E. Prostate cancer is not increased in men with vasectomy in Denmark. *J Urol* 2002; **168**: 488–90.

[74] Bernal-Delgado E, Latour-Perez J, Pradas-Amal F, Gomez-Lopez LI. The association between vasectomy and prostate cancer: a systematic review of the literature. *Fertil Steril* 1998; **70**: 191–200.

[75] Moller H, Knudsen LB, Lynge E. Risk of testicular cancer after vasectomy: cohort study of over 73,000 men. *BMJ* 1994; **309**: 295–9.

[76] Thornhill JA, Conroy RM, Kelly DG, *et al.* An evaluation of predisposing factors for testis cancer in Ireland. *Eur Urol* 1988; **14**: 429–33.

[77] Cale ARJ, Farouk M, Prescott RJ, Wallace IWJ. Does vasectomy accelerate testicular tumour? Importance of testicular examination before and after vasectomy. *BMJ* 1990; **300**: 370.

[78] Strader CH, Weiss NS, Daling JR. Vasectomy and the incidence of testicular cancer. *Am J Epidemiol* 1988; **128**: 56–63.

[79] Heckel NJ. Production of oligospermia in a man by the use of testosterone propionate. *Proc Soc Exp Biol Med* 1939; **40**: 658–9.

[80] McCullagh EP, McGurl FJ. Further observations on the clinical use of testosterone propionate. *J Urol* 1939; **42**: 1265–7.

[81] Nieschlag E. 10th Summit Meeting consensus: recommendations for regulatory approval for hormonal male contraception. *Contraception* 2007; **75**: 166–7.

[82] Wenk M, Nieschlag E. Male contraception: a realistic option? *Eur J Contraception Reprod Health Care* 2006; **11**: 69–80.

[83] Hoesl CE, Saad F, Poppel M, Altwein JE. Reversible, non barrier male contraception: status and prospects. *Eur Urol* 2005; **48**: 712–13.

[84] Anderson RA, Baird DT. Male contraception. *Endocrine Rev* 2002; **23**: 735–62.

[85] Pasqualotto FF, Lucon AM, Pasqualotto EB, Arap S. Trends in male contraception. *Rev Hosp Clin Fac Med S Paulo* 2003; **58**: 275–83.

[86] Herdiman J, Nakash A, Beedham T. Male contraception: past, present and future. *J Obstet Gynaecol* 2006; **26**: 721–7.

[87] Handelsman DJ. Editorial: hormonal male contraception-lessons from the East when the Western market fails. *J Clin Endocrinol Metab* 2003; **88**: 559–61.

[88] Matthiesson KL, McLacnlan RI. Male hormonal contraception: concept proven, product in sight? *Hum Reprod Update* 2006; **12**: 463–82.

[89] Reddy PR, Rao JM. Reversible antifertility action of testosterone propionate in human males. *Contraception* 1972; **5**: 295–301.

[90] Who Task Force on Methods for the Regulation of Male Fertility. Contraceptive efficacy of testosterone-induced azoospermia in normal men. *Lancet* 1990; **336**: 955–9.

[91] Lookingbill DP, Demers LM, Wang C, *et al.* Clinical and biochemical parameters of androgen action in normal healthy Caucasian versus Chinese subjects. *J Clin Endocrinol Metab* 1991; **72**: 1242–8.

[92] Who Task Force on Methods for the Regulation of Male Fertility. Contraceptive efficacy of testosterone-induced azoospermia and oligozoospermia in normal men. *Fertil Steril* 1996; **65**: 821–9.

[93] Gu YQ, Wang XH, Xu D, *et al.* A multicenter contraceptive efficacy study of injectable testosterone undecanoate in healthy Chinese men. *J Clin Endocrinol Metab* 2003; **88**: 562–8.

[94] Behre HM, Baus S, Kliesch S, *et al.* Potential of testosterone buciclate for male contraception: endocrine differences between responders and non-responders. *J Clin Endocrinol Metab* 1995; **80**: 2394–403.

[95] von Eckardstein S, Noe G, Brache V, *et al.* Clinical trial of 7α-methyl-19-nortestosterone implants for possible use as a long-acting contraceptive in men. *J Clin Endocrinol Metab* 2003; **88**: 5232–9.

[96] El-Hefnawy T, Huhtaniemi I. Progesterone can participate in down-regulation of the luteinizing hormone receptor gene expression and function in cultured murine Leydig cells. *Mol Cell Endocrinol* 1998; **137**: 127–38.

[97] El-Hefnawy T, Manna PR, Luconi M, *et al.* Progesterone action in a murine Leydig tumor cell line (mLTC-1), possibly through a nonclassical receptor type. *Endocrinology* 2000; **141**: 247–55.

[98] Grimes DA, Gallo MF, Grigorieva V, *et al.* Steroid hormones for contraception in men: systematic review of randomized controlled trials. *Contraception* 2005; **71**; 89–94.

[99] Meriggiola MC, Farley TM, Mbizvo MT. A review of androgen-progestin regimens for male contraception. *J Androl* 2003; **24**: 466–83.

[100] Who Task Force on Methods for the Regulation of Male Fertility. Comparision of two androgens plus depot-medroxyporgesterone acetate for suppression to azoospermia in Indonesian men. *Fertil Steril* 1993; **60**: 1062–8.

[101] Turner L, Conway AJ, Jimenez M, *et al.* Contraceptive efficacy of a depot progestin and androgen combination in men. *J Clin Endocrinol Metab* 2003; **88**: 4659–67.

[102] Amory JK, Page ST, Anawalt BD, Matsumoto AM, Bremner WJ. Acceptability of a combination testosterone gel and depomedroxyprogesterone acetate male contraceptive regimen. *Contraception* 2007; **75**: 218–23.

[103] Page ST, Amory JK, Anawalt BD, *et al.* Testosterone gel combined with depomedroxyprogesterone acetate is an effective male hormonal contraceptive regimen and is not enhanced by the addition of a GnRH antagonist. *J Clin Endocrinol Metab* 2006; **91**: 4374–80.

[104] Amory JK, Page ST, Anawalt BD, Matsumoto AM, Bremner WJ. Elevated serum INSL3 is associated with failure to completely suppress spermatogenesis in men receiving male hormonal contraception. *J Androl* 2007; **28** (Suppl 2): 46.

[105] Petry R, Mauss J, Rausch-Stroomann JG, Vermeulen A. Reversible inhibition of spermatogenesis in men. *Horm Metab Res* 1972; **4**: 386–8.

[106] Fredricsson B, Carlstrom K. Effects of low doses of cyproterone acetate on sperm morphology and some other parameters of reproduction in normal men. *Andrologia* 1981; **13**: 369–75.

[107] Roy S, Chatterjee S, Prasad MR, Poddar AK, Pandey DC. Effects of cyproterone acetate on reproductive functions in normal human males. *Contraception* 1976; **14**: 403–20.

[108] Meriggiola MC, Bremner WJ, Paulsen CA, *et al.* A combined regimen of cyproterone acetate and testosterone enanthate as a potentially highly effective male contraceptive. *J Clin Endocrinol Metab* 1996; **81**: 3018–23.

[109] Meriggiola MC, Bremner WJ, Costantino A, *et al.* An oral regimen of cyproterone acetate and testosterone undecanoate for spermatogenic suppression in men. *Fertil Steril* 1997; **68**: 844–50.

[110] Meriggiola MC, Bremner WJ, Costantino A, Di Cintio G, Flamigni C. Low dose of cyproterone acetate and testosterone enanthate for contraception in men. *Hum Reprod* 1998; **13**: 1225–9.

[111] Meriggiola MC, Bremner WJ, Costantino A, *et al.* Twenty-one day administration of dienogest reversibly suppresses gonadotropins and testosterone in normal men. *J Clin Endocrinol Metab* 2002; **87**: 2107–13.

[112] Meriggiola MC, Costantino A, Bremner WJ, Morselli-Labate AM. Higher testosterone dose impairs sperm suppression induced by a combined androgen-progestin regimen. *J Androl* 2002; **23**: 684–90.

[113] Anawalt BD, Bebb RA, Bremner WJ, Matsumoto AM. A lower dosage levonorgestrel and testosterone combination effectively suppresses spermatogenesis and circulating gonadotropin levels with fewer metabolic effects than higher dosage combinations. *J Androl* 1999; **20**: 407–14.

[114] Bebb RA, Anawalt BD, Christensen RB, *et al.* Combined administration of levonorgestrel and testosterone induces more rapid and effective suppression of spermatogenesis than testosterone alone: a promising male contraceptive approach. *J Clin Endocrinol Metab* 1996; **81**: 757–62.

[115] Gui YL, He CH, Amory JK, *et al.* Male hormonal contraception: suppression of spermatogenesis by injectable testosterone undecanoate alone or with levonorgestrel implants in chinese men. *J Androl* 2004; **25**: 720–7.

[116] Kinniburgh D, Zhu H, Cheng L, *et al.* Oral desogestrel with testosterone pellets induces consistent suppression of spermatogenesis to azoospermia in both Caucasian and Chinese men. *Hum Reprod* 2002; **17**: 1490–501.

[117] Anderson RA, van def Spuy ZM, Dada OA, *et al.* Investigation of hormonal male contraception in african men: suppression of spermatogenesis by oral desogestrel with depot testosterone. *Hum Reprod* 2002; **17**: 2869–77.

[118] Brady BM, Walton M, Hollow N, *et al.* Depot testosterone with etonogestrel implants result in induction of azoospermia in all men for long-term contraception. *Hum Reprod* 2004; **19**: 2658–67.

[119] Brady BM, Amory JK, Perheentupa A, *et al.* A multicentre study investigating subcutaneous etonogestrel implants with injectable testosterone decanoate as a potential long-acting male contraceptive. *Hum Reprod* 2006; **21**: 285–94.

[120] Guerin JF, Rollet J. Inhibition of spermatogenesis in men using various combinations of oral progestagens and percutaneous or oral androgens. *Int J Androl* 1988; **11**: 187–99.

[121] Kamischke A, Heuermann T, Kruger K, *et al.* An effective hormonal male contraceptive using testoerone undecanoate with oral or injectable norethisterine preparations. *J Clin Endocrinol Metab* 2002; **87**: 530–9.

[122] Meriggiola MC, Costantino A, Saad F, *et al.* Norethisterone enanthate plus testosterone undecanoate for male contraception: effects of various injection intervals on spermatogenesis, reproductive hormones, testis and prostate. *J Clin Endocrinol Metab* 2005; **90**: 2005–14.

[123] Huhtaniemi I, Nikula H, Ranniko S. Treatment of prostatic cancer with a gonadotropin releasing hormone agonist analog: acute and long term effects on endocrine functions of testis tissue. *J Clin Endocrinol Metab* 1985; **61**: 698–704.

[124] Nieschlag E, Behre HM, Weinbauer GF. Hormonal male contraception: a real chance? In: Nieschlag E, Habenicht UF, eds. *Spermatogenesis-Fertilization-Contraception. Molecular, Cellular and Endocrine Events in Male Reproduction.* Berlin/Heidelberg/New York: Springer, 1992: 477–501.

[125] Pavlou SN, Brewer K, Farley MG, *et al.* Combined administration of a gonadotropin-releasing hormone antagonist and testosterone in men induces reversible azoospermia without loss of libido. *J Clin Endocrinol Metab* 1991; **73**: 1360–9.

[126] Tom L, Bhasin S, Salameh W, *et al.* Induction of azoospermia in normal men with combined Nal-Glu

gonadotropin-releasing hormone antagonist and testosterone enanthate. *J Clin Endocrinol Metab* 1992; **75**: 476–83.

[127] Bastias MC, Kamijo H, Pavlou SN. Sperm motion parameters after suppression of spermatogenesis with a gonadotropin-releasing hormone antagonist plus testosterone supplementation. *Fertil Steril* 1993; **59**: 1261–5.

[128] Bagatell CJ, Matsumoto AM, Christensen RB, Rivier JE, Bremner WJ. Comparison of a gonadotropin releasing-hormone antagonist plus testosterone (T) versus T alone as potential male contraceptive regimens. *J Clin Endocrinol Metab* 1993; **77**: 427–32.

[129] Bagatell CJ, Rivier JE, Bremner WJ. Dose effects of the gonadotropin-releasing hormone antagonist, Nal-Glu, combined with testosterone enanthate on gonadotropin levels in normal men. *Fertil Steril* 1995; **64**: 139–45.

[130] Behre HM, Kliesch S, Lemcke B, von Eckardstein S, Nieschlag E. Suppression of spermatogenesis to azoospermia by combined administration of GnRH antagonist and 19-nortestosterone cannot be maintained by this non-aromatizable androgen alone. *Hum Reprod* 2001; **16**: 2570–7.

[131] Chen J, Hwang DJ, Bohl CE, Miller DD, Dalton JT. A selective androgen receptor modulator for hormonal male contraception. *J Pharmacol Exp Ther* 2005; **312**: 546–53.

[132] Feng HL, Sandlow JI, Sparks AET, Sandra A. Development of Immunocontraceptives: current status. *J Reprod Med* 1999; **44**: 759–65.

[133] Naz RK, Gupta SK, Gupta JC, Vyas HK, Talwar AG. Recent advances in contraceptive vaccine development: A mini-review. *Hum Reprod* 2005; **20**: 3271–83.

[134] Murdoch WJ. Immunoregulation of mammalian fertility. *Life Sci* 1994; **55**: 1871–86.

[135] Moudgal NR, Jeyakumar M, Krishnamurthy HN, Sridhar S, Martin F. Development of male contraceptive vaccine: a perspective. *Hum Reprod Update* 1997; **3**: 335–46.

[136] Naz RK. Vaccine for contraception targeting sperm. *Immunol Rev* 1999; **171**: 193–202.

[137] Naz RK. Fertilization-related sperm antigens and their immunocontraceptive potentials. *Am J Reprod Immunol* 2000; **44**: 41–6.

[138] O'Rand MG, Widgren EE, Fisher SJ. Characterization of the rabbit sperm membrane autoantigen, RSA, as a lectin-like zona binding protein. *Dev Biol* 1988; **129**: 231–40.

[139] Lea IA, O'Rand MG. Immune response to immunization with sperm antigens in the macaque oviduct. *Biol Reprod* 1998; **58**: 794–800.

[140] Naz RK. The fertilization antigen (FA-1): applications in immunocontraception and infertility in humans. *Am J Reprod Immunol Microbiol* 1988; **16**: 21–7.

[141] Naz RK, Wolf DP. Antibodies to sperm-specific human FA-1 inhibit in vitro fertilization in rhesus monkeys: Development of a simian model for testing of anti-FA-1 contraceptive vaccine. *J Reprod Immunol* 1994; **27**: 111–21.

[142] Saling P. Mouse sperm antigens that participate in fertilization. IV. A monoclonal antibody prevents zona penetrating by inhibition of the acrosome reaction. *Dev Biol* 1986; **117**: 511–18.

[143] Bruks DJ, Caballada R, Moore HD, Saling PM. Interaction of a tyrosine kinase from human sperm with the zona pellucida at fertilization. *Science* 1995; **269**: 83–6.

[144] Yee AJ, Silver LM. Contraceptive vaccine formulations with sperm proteins. In: Bronson RA, ed. *Reproductive Immunology*. Boston, MA: Blackwell, 1996: 693–712.

[145] Anderson DJ, Alexander NJ. A new look at antifertility vaccines. *Fertil Steril* 1983; **40**: 557–71.

[146] Beyler SA, Wheat TE, Goldberg E. Binding of antibodies against antigenic domains of murine lactate dehydrogenase-C4 to human and mouse spermatozoa. *Biol Reprod* 1985; **32**: 1201–10.

[147] Goldberg E, Shelton J. Immunosuppression of fertiliy by LDH-C4. In: Talwar GP, ed. *Immunological Approaches to Contraception and Promotion of Fertility*. New York, NY: Plenum, 1986: 219–30.

[148] Goldberg E, VandeBerg JL, Mahony MC, Doncel GF. Immune response of male baboons to testis-specific LDH-C(4). *Contraception* 2001; **64**: 93–8.

[149] O'Hern PA, Goldberg E. Reversible contraception in female baboons immunized with a synthetic epitope of sperm-specific lactate dehydrogenase. *Biol Reprod* 1995; **52**: 331–9.

[150] Diekman AB, Herr JC. Sperm antigens and their use in the development of an immunocontraceptive. *Am J Reprod Immunol* 1997; **37**: 111–17.

[151] O'Rand MG, Widgren EE, Sivashanmugam P, et al. Reversible immunocontraception in male monkeys immunized with eppin. *Science* 2004; **306**: 1189–90.

[152] O'Rand MG, Widgren EE, Wang Z, Richardson RT. 2006 Eppin: an effective target for male contraception. *Mol Cell Endocrinol* 2006; **250**: 157–62.

[153] Prasad MR, Diczfalusy NE. Gossypol. *Int J Androl* 1982; **28** (Suppl): 53–70.

[154] Segal SJ. *Gossypol: A Potential Contraceptive for Men*. New York, NY: Plenum, 1985.

[155] Waites GMH. Male fertility regulation: the challenges for the year 2000. *Br Med Bull* 1993; **49**: 210–21.

[156] Mieusset R, Bujan L. The potential of mild testicular heating as a safe, effective and reversible contraceptive method for men. *Int J Androl* 1994; **17**: 186–91.

[157] Cheng CY, Silvestrini B, Grima J, *et al.* Two new male contraceptives exert their effects by depleting germ cells prematurely from the testis. *Biol Reprod* 2001; **65**: 449–61.

[158] Cooper TG, Yeung CH. Recent biochemical approaches to post-testicular, epididymal contraception. *Hum Reprod Update* 1999; **5**: 141–52.

Chapter 28

Intrauterine insemination from the urologist's perspective

Christine Mullin, James Stelling, and Richard A. Schoor

Introduction

Urologists have been at the forefront in the study of infertility for over 100 years, and have been responsible for some of the greatest success stories in the field of infertility treatment. However, a large percentage of patients cannot achieve success with urologic intervention alone. Thus, advances in assisted reproductive technology (ART) for treatment of infertile couples have played an integral role in achieving fertility in this group of patients. These technologies, such as in-vitro fertilization (IVF), intrauterine insemination (IUI), and intracytoplasmic sperm injection (ICSI), have evolved along with the advances in male reproductive medicine. Despite the rapid technological advances made with ART, urologists still play an integral part in the evaluation and management of infertile couples.

Assisted reproductive technologies (ART) are interventions directed at the female partner, including gonadotropin therapy, IUI, IVF, ICSI, and preimplantation genetic diagnosis (PGD). Artificial insemination – also called intrauterine insemination or IUI – is a relatively "low-tech" form of ART, though it is by far the most frequently used of all ART techniques. While urologists in the United States do not perform IUI, the spouses of many of our patients will ultimately undergo this procedure. Therefore, it is important that urologists have a working knowledge of the indications, technique, side effects, complications, and success rates of IUI, especially as they relate to associated male factors. Such is the goal of the present chapter.

History

Artificial insemination (AI) in its current form owes it origins to animal husbandry research. The earliest accounts of AI experimentation date back more than 300 years. The first successful artificial insemination took place in Italy in 1784. Russian researchers heralded the modern era of AI beginning in the 1890s and pioneered work that started in dogs, rabbits, and poultry, then progressed to horses, sheep, and dairy cattle. The Russians developed innovative techniques to collect semen, such as use of the artificial vagina [1].

In the 1940s, Danish researchers developed two important innovations that dramatically improved the efficacy of AI in animal husbandry: rectocervical fixation and the semen packing straw. Rectocervical fixation enables improved success rates of AI with the use of fewer sperm, and is thus a type of semen extender. The semen packing straw, in various forms, is still used today, even in human AI [1].

In the United States, agricultural research on AI accelerated in the 1940s as well, and tremendous advances were made in sperm collection and processing methods, semen evaluation and selection, and sire selection – the animal equivalent of donor selection. Tests of sperm fertilization potential such as the hypo-osmotic swell test, mucous penetration assay, and even sperm DNA integrity tests, were all developed for the purposes of animal husbandry and adopted later for human usage. Other useful tools in human infertility medicine have their roots in agricultural research and include semen specimen transport, sperm cryopreservation, and gender selection using in-situ hybridization [1]. In the United States today, nearly 100% of dairy cattle and poultry are bred using AI technology.

Indications and technique

IUI is indicated for couples with unexplained infertility, mild to moderate male-factor infertility, or certain female factors, such as antisperm antibodies or a hostile cervical environment. In the United States, IUI is performed by gynecologists or reproductive endocrinologists, not urologists. Women, therefore,

Table 28.1. Female screening tests

HIV
Hepatitis B
Hepatitis C
Trepopnema pallidum
Neisseria gonorrhea
Chlamydia trachomatis
Cytomegalovirus
CBC
Blood type and screen
Day 2 follicle-stimulating hormone
Day 2 estradiol
TSH
Prolactin
Pap Smear
Genetic screening

are evaluated by the gynecologist with histories, physical examination, and laboratory assessments [2]. Tubal patency tests, such as the hysterosalpingogram, saline salpingogram, or diagnostic laparoscopy, are performed as indicated. Indications for tests of tubal patency include prior pelvic inflammatory disease, ectopic pregnancies, or unexplained infertility, among others. The endocrine profile for a woman is similar to a man's, and includes assays for day 2 follicle-stimulating hormone (FSH), luteinizing hormone (LH), and estradiol. For a woman, the only absolute contraindication to IUI is bilateral tubal occlusions. Advanced maternal age and severe elevations in FSH are not contraindications, but are indicators of a poor prognosis. In addition, IUI complications, such as low-birthweight babies and birth defects, are increased in women of advanced maternal age [3,4].

The most common male factor is oligospermia, mild to moderate. **Historically, the presence of 10 million motile sperm was a prerequisite for performing IUI, although now many centers have success with lower cutoff values, such as 5 million motile sperm, or even 1 million motile sperm.** Forward progression on semen analysis is important, though interestingly, centers that use the lower cutoff values often do not make a distinction between the various grades of motility, 1–4. The decision to proceed with IUI in the face of male factors, even severe ones, is complicated by many factors, including the patients' ability to pay

for the more expensive ART procedures such as IVF with ICSI. In addition, whether or not an ART practice refers men with a male factor to the urologist for evaluation is variable from practice to practice, physician to physician, and region to region.

Pre-screening for couples attempting an IUI procedure includes testing for infectious diseases, genetic abnormalities, and general medical problems, such as anemia [5–7]. Women are screened for syphilis, hepatitis B and C, HIV, parvovirus, rubella, and varicella. The total list of female screening tests may be seen in Table 28.1. Men are screened for hepatitis B, hepatitis C, and HIV. Genetic tests routinely performed include testing for cystic fibrosis as well as for those conditions that more commonly affect a particular ethnic group (Table 28.2). For example, there is an Ashkenazi panel for Jewish patients of Eastern European descent [8–10]. **Severely oligospermic men have an increased likelihood of harboring genetic anomalies, such as Y-chromosome microdeletions [11,12]. Couples may benefit from screening and, at the very least, an informed consent discussion prior to proceeding with ART.**

Donor IUI is indicated in cases of severe, insurmountable male-factor infertility in which it is not possible to acquire sperm in sufficient quantities to perform IUI. Factors that lead a patient to choose donor IUI include severe oligospermia, azoospermia, or severe, uncorrectable asthenospermia. In addition, female patients without male partners are able to conceive with donor sperm. Donor IUI is also utilized when there is a high probability of a low sperm retrieval. Donor sperm are commercially available, and recipients can select sperm from donors with a variety of physical traits. In the USA, state and federal laws dictate that donor sperm must be extensively screened for infectious disease and certain genetic diseases [13]. For the complete list, see Table 28.3. Though laws may vary slightly from state to state, in New York at least, anonymous donors cannot claim any parental rights over the offspring [14].

Sperm testing prior to IUI varies from center to center, and can range from a basic semen analysis (volume, concentration, motility) to a complete analysis (the basic plus morphology). Some centers will also perform additional assays for sperm strength and function, such as the "swim-up" test and tests of sperm DNA integrity. Poor sperm DNA integrity has been shown to negatively impact IUI success rates, although the utility of this test in day-to-day practice is limited [15].

Table 28.2. Genetic screening in high-risk groups

Ethnic group	Disorder	Screening test
Ashkenazi Jews	Tay–Sachs disease	Decreased serum hexosaminidase-A, molecular analysis
Ashkenazi Jews	Canavan disease	DNA analysis
Mediterranean	Beta-thalassemia	MCV < 80, Hgb electrophoresis
Southeast Asian and Chinese	Alpha-thalassemia	MCV < 80, Hgb electrophoresis
African-Americans	Sickle cell anemia	Hgb electrophoresis
All ethnic groups	Cystic fibrosis	DNA analysis of 25 *CFTR* mutations

Table 28.3. Sperm donor lab test panel

HIV type 1 and HIV type 2	Cytomegalovirus
Hepatitis B	Hepatitis C
Trepopnema pallidum	*Chlamydia trachomatis*
Neisseria gonorrhea	HTLV-1 and HTLV-II

With the help of the semen analysis results, patients are counseled regarding the likelihood of success with each IUI attempt. The IUI sample is then processed as follows. The man is asked to ejaculate into a sterile specimen cup that is subsequently labeled with a unique identifier, such as an accession number. The specimen will then be allowed to sit at room temperature for 20 minutes, so that it liquefies. A basic semen analysis (volume, concentration, motility) is then performed on an aliquot of the sample. If the specimen's parameters are adequate, 1.5 mL of sperm wash media (SWM) are added to the remainder of the sample, which is then centrifuged at $300 \times g$ for 15 minutes. This step is repeated twice, and the resultant pellet is ultimately resuspended in the SWM (0.5 mL) and transferred to a sterile syringe and packing straw for the actual insemination.

The intrauterine insemination takes place in the physician's office, and must be done on the expected day of ovulation. The female patient lies in a dorsal lithotomy position on a standard gynecological examination table with her feet in stirrups. A speculum is placed in the vagina and the cervix is visualized. Neither local anesthetic nor antibiotic prophylaxis is needed. The sperm specimen is aspirated into a 1.0 mL syringe. The needle is removed and the plastic syringe is attached to a flexible 18 cm polyethylene catheter (a standard intrauterine insemination catheter). All air is removed from the syringe and the catheter is inserted through the endocervical canal; it should extend 5.5 cm in a typical uterus. The sperm are then injected.

Mild cramping may occur. After the injection, the catheter is slowly removed and the patient is instructed to remain lying flat and still for 15 minutes. The woman can resume her normal activities upon leaving the office, and subsequent sexual intercourse has not been shown to impede fertilization, but most physicians recommend abstinence for 24 hours after insemination.

IUI treatment costs

Costs will depend on whether or not the female partner is taking fertility-enhancing medications, the type of medications, necessary monitoring, and the insemination itself. Some estimates of costs of IUI in the United States (not actual costs) are shown in Table 28.4.

The cost per cycle can vary greatly, depending on the center where treatment is undertaken and whether the medication is clomiphene or gonadotropins. For example, a woman taking clomiphene and timing her IUI with an ovulation kit could spend about $750 in one cycle. A woman using gonadotropins with IUI could spend up to $5000, depending on the amount of medication needed and the number of monitoring ultrasounds needed. Some programs monitor blood levels for estrogen along with ultrasounds, particularly for gonadotropin and IUI cycles. Fees for donor sperm vary by sperm bank and are based upon how sperm were prepared (washed versus unwashed) and donor characteristics (i.e., level of education). Typical prices for unwashed sperm are $180–350, and $250–400 for washed sperm. These prices do not include storage, shipment, routine evaluation, blood tests, or physician fees for performing the inseminations.

Success rates

For the purpose of this chapter, IUI success will be defined as clinical pregnancy rates. Success rates for IUI depend upon a variety of factors such as patient age, presence

Table 28.4. Estimates of costs associated with IUI

Clomiphene citrate	$55–165 (depending on dose)
Gonadotropins	$40–75 per ampule (approximately 10–40 ampules/cycle)
Human chorionic gonadotropin (hCG)	$60
Ultrasound monitoring	$300 per test
Estradiol blood test	$85–100 per test
Insemination with sperm preparation	$350

of comorbid conditions, ovulation method, and presence of a male factor. **Age is perhaps the most important factor** [3,16]. Women in the 35- to 39-year range have an approximately 50% reduction in pregnancy rates per natural IUI cycle. These women tend to benefit dramatically from the addition of ovulation inducers – clomiphene citrate or gonadotropins. Pregnancy rates continue to drop off as women advance beyond 50 years of age. It is unclear whether or not the addition of ovulation inducers helps women above the age of 40. The addition of ovulation inducers does seem to help women in the 35- to 39-year range, with gonadotropins having greater efficacy than clomiphene citrate [16].

The presence of a male factor impacts success rates of IUI. Severe oligospermia negatively impacts success rates of IUI [17]. **In general, patients need 5–10 million motile sperm to have a successful IUI. However, there are exceptions, with some centers reporting success with as few as 1 million motile sperm. This emphasizes the importance of the role played by urologists as they evaluate and treat male infertility to improve sperm counts.**

Abnormal sperm morphology has been associated with poorer IUI outcomes both for IUI alone and for IUI with clomiphene or gonadotropin stimulation [18–20]. In addition, abnormal sperm morphology has been associated with higher IUI complication rates such as miscarriage [17]. When a patient is referred to the urologist with a semen analysis consistent with an abnormal morphology, it is imperative for the urologist to identify any underlying condition that may be responsible for this condition, and to treat the cause if possible. The presence of abnormal morphology does not preclude the use of the sperm in IUI.

Varicocele is the most commonly encountered male factor in infertility, present in up to 35% of men in subfertile couples. While surgical correction of varicoceles in subfertile men is accepted and standard, some controversy may exist regarding whether or not to correct a varicocele if the couple needs to resort to

IUI anyway. **Numerous studies have shown that varicocelectomy in such a situation improves success rates for IUI with and without ovulation induction** [21–27]. Correction of varicoceles can improve sperm counts, even in severely oligospermic patients, sufficiently to allow couples to avoid IVF/ICSI and to have a successful IUI. Some men have clinically significant varicoceles and normal semen analyses yet the couple still has unexplained infertility and will ultimately require IUI. Whether or not correcting the varicocele in these patients improves pregnancy rates with IUI beyond those rates achieved when the varicocele remains uncorrected is unknown and has not been specifically studied. Some urologists do recommend varicocelectomy in some of these patients for a variety of reasons, but controlled scientific data on the utility of this approach are currently lacking.

Azoospermia can be due to problems of sperm production or sperm ductal obstruction. Using advanced sperm retrieval techniques, sperm may be harvested from men with both obstructive and nonobstructive azoospermia. In nonobstructive azoospermic men, sperm can be located in small numbers, but neither the quantity of sperm nor their motility is sufficient for IUI. Obstructive azoospermia patients, on the other hand, can be candidates for IUI. Congenital and acquired blockages can be reversed and ejaculatory duct obstruction corrected, often leading to natural, spontaneous pregnancies. Occasionally it is not possible to restore natural fecundity, but it is possible to restore several million motile sperm to the ejaculate. In such a situation, a couple might use IUI rather than IVF/ICSI, and thus save money and avoid unnecessary risk to the woman. On occasion, enough sperm can be retrieved, via an epididymal sperm aspiration, for a successful IUI.

Complications

IUI is safe, though it is not complication-free. IUI complications may be classified into three categories:

medication side effects, pregnancy complications, and laboratory errors. Each will be discussed separately.

Medication side effects

Drug-induced side effects are not dose-related, as they can occur at the 50 mg dose of clomiphene citrate. Uncomplicated ovarian enlargement develops in approximately 14% of women, but true ovarian hyperstimulation syndrome is rare.

Hot flashes are common, occurring in 10–20% of women [28]. They may be due to hypoestrogenism at the hypothalamic level due to clomiphene blockade of estrogen receptors. Problems related to the hyperestrogenic environment induced by clomiphene citrate include abdominal distension (5.5%), nausea and vomiting (2.2%), and breast discomfort (2%). These side effects rapidly abate soon after cessation of therapy.

Visual symptoms, such as blurring, double vision, and/or scotomata develop in 1–2% of women and are usually reversible. Mood swings, depression, and headaches can occur, but are rarely sufficiently serious to require termination of treatment.

The use of fertility drugs has been associated with neoplasia, particularly borderline ovarian tumors, in some, but not all, studies. The apparent association between fertility drug use and epithelial ovarian cancer appears to be related to the fact that these drugs are more likely to be used in infertile women, who are known to be at higher risk of developing ovarian cancer. There does not appear to be an increased risk of breast cancer in women treated with fertility drugs [29]. However, interpretation of the available data is limited by several confounding factors.

Pregnancy complications

Pregnancy complications include multiple gestations, birth defects, low birthweight, and ectopic pregnancies. **The probability of multifetal pregnancy is increased:** twins have been reported in 6.9–9% of pregnancies, triplets in 0.3–0.5%, quadruplets in 0.3%, and quintuplets in 0.13% [30,31]. The risk may be reduced by ultrasound monitoring and withholding hCG, IUI, or intercourse if more than two follicles are greater than 15 mm in diameter. The frequency of congenital malformations and spontaneous abortion does not appear to increase in pregnancies after ovulation induction with IUI. This was illustrated in a report that examined 1034 pregnancies and 935 newborns after clomiphene citrate induction [32]. Spontaneous abortion and visible

congenital malformations occurred in 14.2% and 2.3%, respectively, rates that are comparable to those in mothers who ovulated spontaneously [33]. Rates of ectopic pregnancy are not increased with clomiphene citrate IUI [34]. There is no evidence of developmental delays or learning disabilities in children whose mothers took clomiphene citrate [35]. Several studies found a mildly increased risk of preterm birth in pregnancies (singleton and multiples) after assisted reproduction as compared to natural pregnancies [35]. This effect has not been shown to be specific to clomiphene and is likely due to comorbidities in subfertile women [36]. There is less than a 1% chance of pelvic infection with intrauterine insemination.

Laboratory errors

Chain of custody is a concept that dictates exactly which person or facility has physical control of a laboratory specimen from the time it leaves the patient's body until it arrives at its ultimate destination. In IUI, the initial specimen is the man's ejaculate and the final destination is his designated partner's uterus. Unlike in natural conception – intercourse – the ejaculate in an IUI cycle must pass through many links in the chain prior to reaching this destination. Though uncommon, mix-ups do occur, and from time to time the wrong man's sperm is used for insemination. **From the perspective of those involved, this type of error is a catastrophe that often results in high-profile media coverage and a myriad of legal problems for the provider, the laboratory, the parents, and the child.** Aside from obvious claims of medical negligence, legal ramifications of such an error may include questions of legal custody of the child [14]. Other mechanisms for "mix-ups" exist, including inadvertent – or intentional – use of a pre-used insemination straw. These errors are avoidable with carefully devised protocols for specimen management and chain of custody.

Conclusion

IUI is the most commonly performed ART procedure and can help millions of infertile couples achieve their dream of parenthood. It is important that the urologist have at least a working knowledge of IUI. IUI, in contrast to IVF or ICSI, is relatively "low tech" and straightforward to perform. Success rates vary with maternal age, associated female and male factors, and adjunctive use of clomiphene citrate and gonadotropins. Correction of a male factor, even in a couple that will ultimately require IUI, is indicated and recommended.

Patients who are to undergo IUI, as in any other medical procedure, should be given information regarding the risks of the procedure.

References

[1] Foote RH. *The History of Artificial Insemination: Selected Notes and Notables* American Society of Animal Science, 2002.

[2] Smith S, Pfeifer SM, Collins JA. Diagnosis and management of female infertility. *JAMA* 2003; **290**: 1767–70.

[3] Damario M, Davis OK, Rosenwaks Z. The role of maternal age in the assisted reproductive technologies. *Reprod Med Rev* 1999; **7**: 41–60.

[4] Nuojua-Huttunen S, Gissler M, Martikainen H, Tuomivaara L. Obstetric and perinatal outcome of pregnancies after intrauterine insemination. *Hum Reprod* 1999; **14**: 2110–15.

[5] McKee TA Avery S Majid A Brinsden PR. Risks for transmission of hepatitis C during artificial insemination. *Fertil Steril* 1996; **66**: 161–3.

[6] Hummel WP Talbert LM. Current management of a donor insemination program. *Fertil Steril* 1990; **53**: 382.

[7] Mascola L Guinan ME. Screening to reduce transmission of sexually transmitted diseases in semen used for artificial insemination. *N Engl J Med* 1986; **314**: 1354–9.

[8] Leib JR, Gollust SE, Hull SC, Wilfond BS. Carrier screening panels for Ashkenazi Jews: is more better? *Genet Med* 2005; **7**: 185–90.

[9] Grody WW, Cutting GR, Klinger KW, *et al.*; Subcommittee on Cystic Fibrosis Screening, Accreditation of Genetic Services Committee, American College of Medical Genetics. Laboratory standards and guidelines for population-based cystic fibrosis carrier screening. *Genet Med* 2001; **3**: 149–54.

[10] Practice Committee of the American Society for Reproductive Medicine Information on commonly asked questions about genetic evaluation and counseling for infertile couples. *Fertil Steril* 2004; **82** (Suppl 1): S97–101.

[11] Calleja Macias IE, Martinez Garza SG, Gallegos MC, *et al.* Y chromosome micro-deletion identification in infertile males. *Ginecol Obstet Mex* 2003; **71**: 25–31.

[12] Yao G, Chen G, Pan T. Study of microdeletions in the Y chromosome of infertile men with idiopathic oligo-or azoospermia. *J Assist Reprod Genet* 2001; **18**: 612–16.

[13] Human Rights Campaign. Donor insemination laws: state by state. www.hrc.org/issues/2490.htm. Accessed February 23, 2009.

[14] Fass M. Paternal duties apply to child born of artificial insemination. *New York Law Journal* 2007, January 24.

[15] Duran EH, Morshedi M, Taylor S, Oehninger S.. Sperm DNA quality predicts intrauterine insemination outcome: A prospective cohort study. *Hum Reprod* 2002; **17**: 3122–8.

[16] De Sutter P, Veldeman L, Kok P, *et al.* Comparison of outcome of pregnancy after intra-uterine insemination (IUI) and IVF. *Hum Reprod* 2005; **20**: 1642–6.

[17] Burr RW, Siegberg R, Flaherty SP, Wang XJ, Matthews CD. The influence of sperm morphology and the number of motile sperm inseminated on the outcome of intrauterine insemination combined with mild ovarian stimulation. *Fertil Steril* 1996; **65**: 127–32.

[18] Toner JP, Mossad H, Grow DR, *et al.* Value of sperm morphology assessed by strict criteria for prediction of the outcome of artificial (intrauterine) insemination. *Andrologia* 1995; **27**: 143–8.

[19] Ombelet W, Vandeput H, Van de Putte G, *et al.* Intrauterine insemination after ovarian stimulation with clomiphene citrate: predictive potential of inseminating motile count and sperm morphology. *Hum Reprod* 1997; **12**: 1458–63.

[20] Van Waart J, Kruger TF, Lombard CJ, Ombelet W. Predictive value of normal sperm morphology in intrauterine insemination (IUI): a structured literature review. *Hum Reprod Update* 2001; **7**: 495–500.

[21] Penson DF, Paltiel AD, Krumholz HM, Palter S. The cost-effectiveness of treatment for varicocele related infertility. *J Urol* 2002; **168**: 2490–4.

[22] Marmar JL, Corson SL, Batzer FR, Gocial B. Insemination data on men with varicoceles. *Fertil Steril* 1992; **57**: 1084–90.

[23] Gat Y, Bachar GN, Everaert K, Levinger U, Gornish M. Induction of spermatogenesis in azoospermic men after internal spermatic vein embolization for the treatment of varicocele. *Hum Reprod* 2005; **20**: 1013–17.

[24] Fisher LM, Sandlow J. The role of varicocele treatment in the era of assisted reproductive technologies. *Braz J Urol* 2001; **27**: 19–25.

[25] Hargreave TB. Debate on the pros and cons of varicocele treatment: In favour of varicocele treatment. *Hum Reprod* 1995; **10**: 151–7.

[26] Daitch J, Pasqualotto E, Hendin B, *et al.* Fertility outcome in patients undergoing intrauterine insemination after varicoceletomy. *Fertil Steril* 1999; **72**: 524.

[27] O'Brien JH, Bowles B, Kamal KM, Jarvi K, Zini A. Varicocelectomy for infertile couples with advanced female age: natural history in the era of ART. *J Androl* 2004; **25**: 939–43.

[28] American College of Obstetricians, and Gynecologists. *Management of Infertility Caused by Ovulatory Dysfunction.* ACOG Practice Bulletin #34. Washington, DC: American College of Obstetricians and Gynecologists, 2002.

[29] Venn A, Watson L, Bruinsma F, Giles G, Healy D. Risk of cancer after use of fertility drugs with in-vitro fertilisation. *Lancet* 1999; **354**: 1586–90.

[30] Dickey RP, Holtkamp DE. Development, pharmacology and clinical experience with clomiphene citrate. *Hum Reprod Update* 1996; **2**: 483–506.

[31] Scialli AR. The reproductive toxicity of ovulation induction. *Fertil Steril* 1986; **45**: 315–23.

[32] Kurachi K, Aono T, Minagawa J, Miyake A. Congenital malformations of newborn infants after clomiphene-induced ovulation. *Fertil Steril* 1983; **40**: 187–9.

[33] Dickey RP, Matis R, Olar TT, *et al.* The occurrence of ectopic pregnancy with and without clomiphene citrate use in assisted and nonassisted reproductive technology. *J In Vitro Fert Embryo Transf* 1989; **6**: 294–7.

[34] Hack M, Brish M, Serr DM, *et al.* Outcome of pregnancy after induced ovulation: follow-up of pregnancies and children born after clomiphene therapy. *JAMA* 1972; **220**: 1329–33.

[35] Lambalk CB, van Hooff M. Natural versus induced twinning and pregnancy outcome: a Dutch nationwide survey of primiparous dizygotic twin deliveries. *Fertil Steril* 2001; **75**: 731–6.

[36] Gaudoin M, Dobbie R, Finlayson A, *et al.* Ovulation induction/intrauterine insemination in infertile couples is associated with low-birth-weight infants. *Am J Obstet Gynecol* 2003; **188**: 611–16.

Chapter 29

In-vitro fertilization and micromanipulation for male infertility

Rodrigo L. Pagani, Paulo C. Serafini, and Miguel Srougi

Introduction

A couple is usually considered infertile after one year of unprotected intercourse with adequate exposure in the absence of a pregnancy. Infertility affects around 15% of married couples, with pure male factors and pure female factors each accounting for approximately 30% of these. In the remaining couples, a combination of both factors exists. Therefore, **the male is involved in the childless process half of the time.**

The live birth of Louise Brown in 1978 following in-vitro fertilization (IVF) by Steptoe and Edwards commenced a new era in assisted reproductive technology (ART) [1]. Subsequently, gamete intrafallopian transfer (GIFT) and zygote intrafallopian transfer (ZIFT) were also developed to treat infertility [2,3].

Although IVF was first used with success for couples with male-factor infertility in 1984 [4], it soon became apparent that patients with severe oligospermia or azoospermia were still considered sterile.

To solve this problem, gamete micromanipulation techniques have been applied in couples where conventional IVF could not be used. Initially, the formation of a small hole in the zona pellucida allowing the sperm direct access to the oolemma was elaborated (zona drilling [ZD] and partial zona dissection [PZD]). After that, the microsurgical injection of sperm in the perivitelline space was settled (subzonal insertion of sperm [SUZI]). More recently, the microinjection of sperm directly into the egg itself has resulted in a significant improvement in pregnancy rates (intracytoplasmic sperm injection [ICSI]).

In-vitro fertilization

Initially created for female infertility due to tubal disease, IVF has also rapidly become a treatment for male-factor infertility. Using this technique, fewer sperm are required to achieve oocyte fertilization than with natural intercourse or intrauterine insemination (IUI). This feature of IVF has made it a prominent option in male-factor patients in whom surgical or pharmacologic therapy has not succeeded or is unsuitable.

Controlled ovarian hyperstimulation

Controlled ovarian hyperstimulation (COH) is defined as hormonal manipulation during the ovulatory cycle so that instead of producing one oocyte, the ovary is stimulated to release multiple oocytes. Most patients are down-regulated with a gonadotropin-releasing hormone (GnRH) agonist and then treated with gonadotropins (Fig. 29.1). GnRH antagonists have been introduced in recent years in ovarian stimulation for ART. They exert their pharmacological effect via an immediate and reversible blockade of the pituitary GnRH receptors, and are used to prevent premature LH surges in IVF/ICSI cycles (Fig. 29.2). Follicular growth is monitored by serum estradiol quantification and transvaginal sonographic evaluation of the follicular volume. When lead follicles reach a mean diameter of 17–19 mm, human chorionic gonadotropin (hCG) is given, and about 35 hours later oocytes are collected by ultrasound-guided transvaginal aspiration.

Oocyte preparation and classification

After retrieval, the oocytes are separated from the follicular fluid and classified according to their morphology. Immature oocytes (PI) are still in the prophase of the first meiotic division; they are characterized by the presence of the germinal vesicle. Oocytes in an intermediate degree of maturation (MI) are recognized by the absence of the germinal vesicle and the first polar body. A mature oocyte (MII) contains chromosomes at metaphase II and is characterized by the presence of a first polar body. Postmature oocytes have darkened cytoplasm with a poorly formed corona.

Infertility in the Male, 4th edition, ed. Larry I. Lipshultz, Stuart S. Howards, and Craig S. Niederberger. Published by Cambridge University Press. © Cambridge University Press 2009.

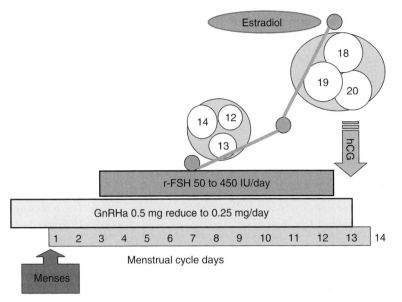

Fig. 29.1. In-vitro fertilization: diagrammatic scheme of a long protocol using a GnRH agonist. GnRHa, gonadotropin-releasing hormone agonist; hCG, human chorionic gonadotropin; r-FSH, recombinant follicle-stimulating hormone.

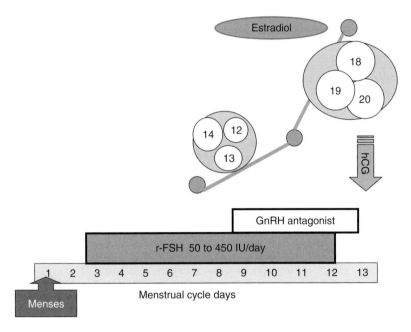

Fig. 29.2. In-vitro fertilization: diagrammatic scheme of a short protocol using a GnRH antagonist. GnRH, gonadotropin-releasing hormone; hCG, human chorionic gonadotropin; r-FSH, recombinant follicle-stimulating hormone.

Semen preparation techniques for IVF

Semen parameters are usually evaluated according to the World Health Organization criteria for sperm concentration, progressive motility, and morphology [5]. Determination of strict criteria for normal morphology is also estimated [6]. Ideally, **sperm preparation should (1) be quick and cost-effective, (2) isolate the highest amount of motile spermatozoa, (3) not cause any harm to sperm, (4) eliminate dead cells, leukocytes, and bacteria, (5) eliminate toxic or bioactive substances, and (6) allow processing of larger volumes of ejaculates.** Unfortunately, there is no such a method available [7].

These techniques are divided into migration, density gradient centrifugation, and filtration techniques. For all migration methods, sperm motility is an essential prerequisite, while for density gradient centrifugation and filtration techniques, both motility and sperm retention at phase borders and adherence to filtration matrices are important. The migration techniques can further be subdivided into swim-up, under-lay, and

501

migration–sedimentation methods. For density gradient centrifugation, separation media such as IxaPrep®, PureSperm®, Isolate®, SilSelect®, and Nicodenz® have recently been introduced to replace Percoll®, due to its risks of contamination of endotoxins. The filtration methods, such as glass wool filtration and use of Sephadex beads and membranes, are alternative techniques [7].

In severe oligoasthenoteratozoospermia, or in sperm aspirated from the epididymis or testicles, Ord *et al.* have developed a mini-Percoll discontinuous gradient layering technique that is associated with fertilization rates that are double or triple those obtained with the swim-up technique [8]. The enhanced fertilization rate obtained by this method is probably due to a sperm fraction with fewer chromatin defects, protection against excessive reactive oxygen species, and healthier sperm due to lower centrifugation spin rates.

Embryo transfer

Mature oocytes are inseminated in a Petri dish and examined 18 hours later for morphologic proof of fertilization. A fertilized zygote contains two pronuclei and two polar bodies in the perivitelline space. Seventy-two hours later, the embryos are at the 4-cell to 8-cell stage and are ready to transfer. Some embryos can benefit from an extended culture to reach the blastocyst stage.

An IVF center's primary concern should be to maximize the live birth rate and minimize the number of multiple gestations. These factors are determined by the number and quality of embryos transferred. The American Society for Reproductive Medicine (ASRM) and the Society for Assisted Reproductive Technology (SART) have developed guidelines to assist ART programs (Table 29.1).

Male-factor outcomes with IVF

No single test or sperm parameter is unquestionable in its prediction of male fertility, as no single sperm feature or function can represent the ability of spermatozoa to accomplish a clinical pregnancy. Therefore, several methods have been created to prevent total failure of fertilization of the eggs following IVF. These methods include the acrosome reaction test, hemizona assay, and the sperm penetration assay.

Sperm concentration and motility are directly connected with fertilization rates. In the normozoospermic patient, 50 000–100 000 motile sperm/mL per oocyte are commonly used for IVF. In the oligospermic patient, however, because of innate dysfunction of the gamete, more sperm are usually inseminated with each oocyte (0.5–1 million motile sperm/mL) [10]. **The introduction of strict morphological criteria in 1986 has been remarkably useful in prognosticating the fertilizing ability of spermatozoa in assisted reproduction** [6]. Oehninger *et al.* studied the correlation between normal sperm morphology and the insemination concentration and discovered that, by increasing the insemination concentration of severely teratozoospermic patients from 100 000 to 500 000 spermatozoa per oocyte, fertilization could be significantly optimized [11].

Fertilization and pregnancy rates in patients undergoing IVF for male factors, however, have been noted to be lower than for patients undergoing IVF for other reasons. A large comparative series from the Center for Reproductive Medicine in Brussels, Belgium, revealed a 68% fertilization rate among 480 couples undergoing IVF for female tubal factors and a 23% fertilization rate after 226 cycles in 175 strictly male-factor couples [12]. In general, very low pregnancy rates resulted from conventional IVF with epididymal or testicular spermatozoa [13,14].

Impaired acrosomal status can be associated with unexplained unsuccessful fertilization. Patients with low spontaneous acrosome loss and high response to A23187 have more than 50% of oocytes fertilized in an IVF cycle [15,16]. Sperm–zona pellucida binding is an essential requisite during human fertilization. This biological step can be measured by hemizona assay. Patients

Table 29.1. Guidelines for the number of embryos transferred [9] (With permission; copyright © 2006 American Society for Reproductive Medicine)

Female age	# Cleavage stage in good prognosis	# Blastocysts in good prognosis	# Cleavage stage in other cases	# Blastocysts in other cases
< 35	1	1	No more than 2	No more than 2
35–37	No more than 2	No more than 2	No more than 3	No more than 2
38–40	No more than 3	No more than 2	No more than 4	No more than 3
> 40	No more than 5	No more than 3	No more than 5	No more than 3

with a hemizona index (HZI) higher than 30% achieved a fertilization rate of approximately 75%, whereas those with HZI lower than 30% had a rate of only 35% [17]. The use of the sperm penetration test (SPA) as a measure of fertility is based on the theory that healthy sperm will penetrate processed hamster ova and result in a significant amount of polyspermia. With the lower limit of normal being five penetrations per egg, couples with a normal SPA have a 95% chance of fertilizing human ova in vitro, as compared with couples with a negative SPA, who have a 50% chance [18].

Gamete and zygote intrafallopian transfer

Gamete intrafallopian transfer (GIFT) is designated for women who have at least one functioning fallopian tube. In GIFT procedures oocytes and sperm are returned to the fallopian tube(s) promptly following oocyte retrieval [2]. Tubal environment may improve oocyte maturation and sperm function, resulting in enhanced fertilization and embryo development and reaching the uterine cavity at an evolutional stage which is concomitant with that of the endometrium [19]. **As it was never demonstrated that GIFT had any advantage over standard IVF, and because it requires laparoscopy, GIFT is now used only in certain instances because of religious beliefs, difficulties in embryo transfer, or as a heroic measure** [20].

Zygote intrafallopian transfer (ZIFT) combines the advantages of the GIFT and IVF procedures, i.e., it enables confirmation of fertilization before transfer, exclusion of polypoid embryos, zygote maturation before entry to the uterine cavity, and greater synchronization

with the uterus [3]. Although retrospective uncontrolled studies comparing ZIFT and IVF demonstrated an increase in implantation and pregnancy rates for ZIFT [21–23], **a recent meta-analysis failed to show any statistically significant difference and concluded that since ZIFT is more expensive and invasive, as it requires laparoscopy, intrauterine transfer of the embryos should be the treatment of choice** [24].

Gamete micromanipulation

Various micromanipulation techniques have been created to increase fertilization rates in cases of severe male infertility. These strategies fall into three basic categories (Fig. 29.3):

(1) manipulation of the zona pellucida to provide an opening in which sperm can gain easier access to the egg – ZD and PZD;
(2) the placement of spermatozoa into the perivitelline space (the space between the zona pellucida and the ovum plasma membrane) – SUZI;
(3) direct injection of a single spermatozoon into the ooplasm – ICSI.

All of these techniques require the use of microinjection tools. Micromanipulation procedures are performed using an inverted phase-contrast microscope, preferably with a heated stage to avoid gamete cooling. Pressure in the holding and injection pipettes is controlled with water or oil-filled high-precision microinjectors. Pipettes are manipulated in three dimensions using sets of hydraulic micromanipulators.

Micromanipulation pipettes are made from 30 μL borosilicate glass tubes. The oocyte-holding pipettes

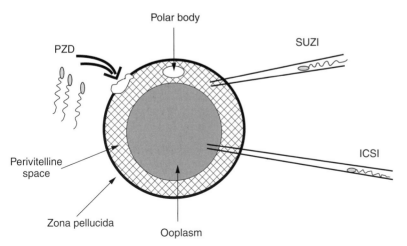

Fig. 29.3. Micromanipulation-assisted fertilization techniques. PZD, partial zona dissection; SUZI, subzonal insertion of sperm; ICSI, intracytoplasmic sperm injection.

are cut and fire-polished on a microforge to obtain the desirable outer and inner diameters (for ICSI, 60 μm and 20 μm, respectively). To make the injection pipettes, the pulled capillary is opened on a microgrinder (for ICSI, to an outer diameter of 7 μm and an inner diameter of 5 μm) with a beveled angle of 45–50°. A sharp spike is made using the microforge to facilitate the injection procedure.

Zona drilling and partial zona dissection

Micromanipulation procedures progressed because of discouraging results with IVF for the male-factor patient. **Although application of acid solutions or enzymes (ZD), and mechanical opening (PZD) of the human zona pellucida have been developed, only PZD has been successful in humans.** One particular problem observed with PZD was the high rate of polyspermia, a lethal condition involving the entrance of more than one sperm into the egg [25].

Subzonal insertion of sperm

This procedure involves the injection of 3–4 sperm per oocyte between the zona pellucida and the plasma membrane of the egg [26]. SUZI represented an advance over PZD, as revealed by pregnancy rates per oocyte retrieval of 10.3% versus 3.8%, respectively [27]. In cases of severe male-factor infertility with fewer than 50 000 motile sperm retrieved, a 57.3% fertilization rate and a 14.5% pregnancy rate were observed, compared with a 4.2% fertilization rate and no pregnancy in a similar population treated with conventional IVF [28]. Unfortunately, high rates of polyspermia still occurred with SUZI.

Intracytoplasmic sperm injection

Technique of ICSI

Originally described in 1988 [29], with the first reported pregnancies documented in 1992, ICSI was created to offer a new treatment option for couples with severe male-factor infertility who could not be helped by conventional IVF [30]. **Polyspermia was finally overcome with ICSI, a procedure which involves the injection of a single sperm into the oocyte.**

Ovarian stimulation, oocyte retrieval, and sperm preparation are performed as for conventional IVF. Oocytes are prepared by removing the surrounding acellular material with enzymes. ICSI is performed on all metaphase II oocytes. Metaphase II oocytes have their diploid complement of chromosome disposed on the metaphase plate near the polar body. The oocyte is stabilized with a holding micropipette and injected under an inverted microscope at 400×. Individual single sperm are aspirated from a prepared semen specimen and injected directly into an oocyte immobilized in a droplet of medium under paraffin oil. The polar body is held at the 12 or 6 o'clock position, and the injection micropipette containing the single sperm is pushed through the zona pellucida and oolemma into the cytoplasm of the oocyte.

Indications for ICSI

In 1995, ICSI was used in nearly 20% of all IVF cycles. By 2004, the percentage of fresh nondonor cycles with ICSI almost tripled. Despite the fact that ICSI was initially developed to treat male-factor infertility, and that the success rates for IVF patients without a diagnosis of male-factor infertility who use ICSI are generally lower than those without a diagnosis of male-factor infertility who use conventional IVF, approximately 50% of ICSI cycles were performed on patients without a male-factor diagnosis (Fig. 29.4) [31]. Furthermore, several prospective controlled randomized trials failed to show that ICSI has any advantage over IVF regarding pregnancy rates in couples with non-male-factor infertility [32–34] or unexplained infertility [35].

Therefore, **ICSI should be used mainly for irreversible or uncorrectable male-factor infertility, except for couples who have had a fertilization failure in a previous IVF cycle or in a condition called "rescue" ICSI, where ICSI is performed on day 2, after the failure of fertilization on the first day utilizing standard IVF** (Table 29.2).

ICSI outcome

The establishment of the Society for Assisted Reproductive Technology (SART) in 1989, and the passage of the Fertility Clinic Success Rate and Certification Act in 1992, allowed consumers to evaluate the success rates of individual centers. This law requires the Centers for Disease Control and Prevention (CDC) to publish pregnancy success rates for ART in fertility clinics in the United States. These data are now readily available, and allow us to assess the true success and impact of IVF and ICSI since 1995 (Table 29.3) [31].

Several factors have been evaluated as predictors of success with IVF/ICSI, but maternal age is the single most important predictor for having a successful outcome in IVF and ICSI. In a report by Oehninger et al., women aged over 40 years were noted to have one-sixth the number of clinical pregnancies of women aged under 34 years [36]. Devroey et al. also

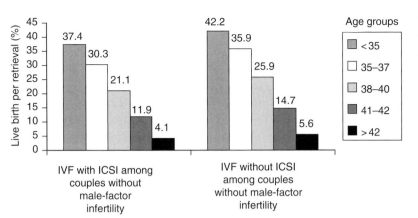

Fig. 29.4. Live births per retrieval among couples without male-factor infertility (Adapted from SART/CDC website) [31].

Table 29.2. Indications for ICSI

Female factor	
Failed previous IVF cycles	
"Rescue" ICSI	
Male factor	
Ejaculated sperm	Severe oligoasthenospermia
	Abnormal sperm morphology
	Immunologic infertility
	Ejaculatory disorders
Epididymal sperm	Obstructive azoospermia
Testicular sperm	Nonobstructive azoospermia
	Necrospermia

found significantly decreased pregnancy and delivery rates in older women (aged ≥ 40 years) after ICSI, and concluded that female age was a predictive factor for embryonic implantation [37].

The effect of paternal age on reproductive outcomes has recently been investigated. Spandorfer *et al.* reported a significant linear decline in semen volume, with no differences in concentration, motility, or morphology of spermatozoa with paternal aging among 821 men undergoing ICSI [38]. Pregnancy outcomes were not influenced by the age of the male partner, although an increase in tripronuclear zygotes was noted with men aged over 50 years. By contrast, in a study by Klonoff-Cohen and Natarajan, sperm number, pregnancy, and live birth delivery were all inversely related to increasing paternal age [39]. Recently, it was stated that "similar to maternal age over 35 years, paternal age over 40 years is a key risk factor in reproduction," as the odds ratio of failure to conceive for paternal age over 40 years was 2.00 (95% CI 1.10–3.61) when the woman

was 35–37 years old, and 5.74 (95% CI 2.16–15.23) for women of 41 years and older [40]. Fathers aged 40 years and over are also associated with higher risks of miscarriage and early fetal death [41–43].

Nagy *et al.* reviewed the effect of spermatozoa factors on results of ICSI in 966 cycles [44]. Despite no normal forms in a semen preparation, virtual azoospermia, or essentially no motile sperm in the ejaculate, pregnancy could still be achieved. **The only time semen parameters had a significantly adverse effect on fertilization and pregnancy rates with ICSI was when there were no motile sperm.** Therefore, sperm viability tests such as the hypo-osmotic swelling test (HOST), the modified HOST (50% mili-Q water/50% culture media), pentoxifylline-enriched media, and the mechanical touch technique have been found to be useful in severe asthenospermia [45–48].

Several studies have demonstrated that fertilization, embryo transfer, and pregnancy are not related to sperm morphology following ICSI [49–51]. Additionally, a study conducted at Baylor College of Medicine has indicated that pregnancy result and newborn status of couples using ICSI with serious teratozoospermia (0% normal morphology) were identical to controls having strict morphology greater than zero [52]. These findings indicate that ICSI success would depend on the evaluation of the single sperm injected. De Vos *et al.* found lower fertilization, pregnancy, and implantation rates, when the individual sperm morphology was observed [53]. The lower success rates applying to morphologically abnormal sperm for ICSI is further supported by evaluating the rate of aneuploidy in these cells. Ryu *et al.* studied the rate of aneuploidy of the sex chromosomes and chromosome 18, using fluorescence in-situ hybridization (FISH) in men undergoing ICSI, and found that morphologically abnormal sperm had a

Table 29.3. Results from the SART/CDC success rates, 2000–2004 [31]

Year	# Cycles	# Cycles with embryo transfer	# Live births	% Live birth ICSI	% Live birth IVF
2000	74 957	60 299	19 042	31.0%	28.6%
2001	80 864	65 363	21 813	30.6%	32.6%
2002	85 826	74 519	24 324	31.9%	34.0%
2003	91 032	74 296	25 775	31.9%	33.4%
2004	94 242	76 533	26 059	30.9%	32.9%
Total	426 921	351 010	117 013	36 625 (31.3%)	37 795 (32.3%)

mean aneuploidy rate of 29%, compared to 1.8–5.5% in the morphologically normal sperm from the same sample [54]. Furthermore, patients with a high frequency of sperm aneuploidy have lower pregnancy rates and higher miscarriage rates than those with normal sperm aneuploidy frequency [55].

Sperm DNA integrity is an essential requirement to achieve pregnancy in natural conception [56] **as well as for IVF outcomes where the natural process of fertilization is circumvented** [57]. A higher degree of sperm DNA damage has been found in couples presenting with unexplained recurrent pregnancy loss [58]. In another study, all male partners of couples who achieved a pregnancy during the first three months attempting to conceive had fewer than 30% sperm with fragmented DNA, whereas 10% of the couples who achieved pregnancy in 4–12 months, and 20% of those who never achieved a pregnancy, had over 30% sperm with fragmented DNA. Moreover, 84% of the men who initiated pregnancy before three months of trying had sperm DNA damage levels below 15% [59]. Bungum et al. reported that for intrauterine insemination there was a significantly higher chance of pregnancy/ delivery in the group with DNA fragmentation index (DFI < 27% and HDS (highly DNA stainable) < 10% [60]. Although no statistical difference between the outcomes of IVF and ICSI was observed in the group with DFI < 27%, ICSI had significantly better results than those of IVF in patients with DFI > 27%.

A meta-analysis reviewed two different types of tests to identify DNA damage and their relationship with ART. It was observed that the DNA fragmentation assessed by the terminal dUTP nick end-labeling (TUNEL) assay significantly decreases the chance of conventional IVF clinical pregnancy, but not that of ICSI clinical pregnancy. When the sperm chromatin structure assay was used, there was no significant effect on the chance of clinical pregnancy after IVF or ICSI treatment [61]. Levels of DFI, as high as 47.9%, are

compatible with ongoing pregnancy and delivery, especially with ICSI [62]. In the largest study to date, including 998 cycles of IVF and ICSI, Bungum et al. concluded that a high DFI does not exclude successful treatment by IVF, but the odds ratio for biochemical pregnancy was three times higher using ICSI than with IVF when the DFI exceeded a level of 30% [63].

Because of these conflicting results, **the Practice Committee of the American Society for Reproductive Medicine recently summarized the current understanding of the impact of abnormal sperm DNA integrity on reproductive outcomes. This committee concluded that current methods for evaluating sperm DNA integrity alone do not predict pregnancy rates achieved with intercourse, IUI, IVF, or ICSI** [64].

Antisperm antibodies may impair the fertilizing ability in vivo and prevent fertilization after IUI or conventional IVF. Only ICSI seems to overcome this problem, and this technique demonstrates comparable fertilization, pregnancy, implantation, and miscarriage rates for males with and without autoantibodies [65].

Aitken et al. reported that men with elevated ROS levels in semen have a sevenfold reduction in conception rates when compared with men who have low ROS [66]. High ROS levels are also associated with decreased pregnancy rate following IVF or ICSI, and arrested embryo growth. Based on a recent meta-analysis, which included all of the available evidence from the literature, our group found that there is a significant correlation between ROS levels in spermatozoa and the fertilization rate after IVF (estimated overall correlation 0.374, 95% CI 0.520–0.205) [67]. Thus, **measuring ROS levels in semen specimens before IVF may be useful in predicting IVF outcome and in counseling selected patients with male-factor or idiopathic infertility.**

Patients with obstructive azoospermia (OA) and nonobstructive azoospermia (NOA) are successfully treated with ICSI using surgically retrieved sperm from the epididymis or testis. In one retrospective review, Aboulghar *et al.* demonstrated that epididymal and testicular sperm from OA patients had fertilization and pregnancy rates comparable to those from patients for whom ejaculated sperm could be used [68]. For patients with OA, only the etiology of the obstruction appears to influence the outcome of ICSI cycles. **A meta-analysis suggested a higher fertilization rate for patients with acquired causes of OA, while patients with congenital bilateral absence of vas deferens (CBAVD) have a higher miscarriage rate** [69].

Testicular sperm from patients with NOA has also been reported to achieve acceptable fertilization and pregnancy rates [70–72]. However, **there was a statistically significant decrease in fertilization and clinical pregnancy rates in the NOA group when compared to patients with OA** [73]. This is possibly due to the use of less mature spermatozoa than in men with normal spermatogenesis. When the NOA patients were further subdivided according to histological categories (tubular sclerosis, germ cell aplasia, and maturations arrest), all of them showed lower fertilization rates than OA patients [74].

In the era of ICSI, cryopreservation has been used to avoid multiple surgical procedures and to have extracted sperm available prior to female ovarian induction. Although the freezing–thawing process may disrupt the quality and especially the motility of the spermatozoa, there is no significant difference in quality between fresh and frozen–thawed epididymal or testicular spermatozoa in patients with OA [75,76].

There is much concern about NOA patients undergoing testicular sperm extraction (TESE), because of the inherently lower number and unsatisfactory quality of sperm that are retrieved using this procedure [77]. There are contradictory reports in the literature about the success of using fresh or frozen sperm from both the epididymis and testis for ICSI [77–81]. The outcomes from a meta-analysis showed an enhanced pregnancy rate when using fresh sperm, but when the data were further subdivided into epididymal and testicular samples separately, no difference in fertilization or pregnancy outcome was noted with testicular samples [73].

Risks of assisted reproductive technology

One of the most significant risks associated with ART is the ovarian hyperstimulation syndrome (OHSS). It occurs in 1–4% of patients undergoing stimulation

and usually occurs 5–7 days after hCG administration. Extensive transudation of fluids rich in albumin leads to intravascular depletion, with subsequent hemoconcentration and hypoalbuminemia. Accumulation of fluid into the peritoneal and thoracic cavity is responsible for symptoms such as abdominal distension and pain, nausea, vomiting, diarrhea, and dyspnea. More serious sequelae can infrequently occur (< 1%) and include hemorrhage, peritonitis, hypercoagulable state, and even death.

The major risk after ART is the occurrence of multiple pregnancies. According to the 2004 SART/CDC data, approximately 29% of all IVF and ICSI cycles resulted in a twin gestation, and an additional 5% of cycles were reported to be triplets or higher order [31]. Recently, efforts have been initiated by fertility centers to reduce the number of embryos transferred. Using the database established by the Human Fertilisation and Embryology Authority in the UK, Templeton and Morris showed that the success rate for three or two embryos transferred were similar, and this reduction essentially eliminated the risk of higher-order multiple pregnancies [82]. In another prospective multicenter trial, women less than 36 years old with at least two good-quality embryos were randomized to either double-embryo transfer (DET) or single-embryo transfer (SET) [83]. This technique reduced the multiple gestations from 33.1% to 0.8%, but unfortunately also diminished the live birth rate from 42.9% to 27.6% for the SET cycle, which may not be cost-effective.

The bypass of natural barriers to fertilization, the possibility of genetic defects in men with severe oligoasthenoteratozoospermia, and the use of severely abnormal sperm for ICSI have aroused doubts about the impact of ICSI on the genetic complement of the offspring. Prenatal testing (chorionic villus sampling or amniocentesis) was used in 1586 ICSI fetuses after fresh embryo transfer. Abnormal fetal karyotypes were found in 47 samples (22 inherited and 25 de novo anomalies). In 17/22 inherited cases the chromosomal structural defect was inherited from the father. A significantly higher percentage of 2.1% de novo anomalies were observed for sperm concentrations below 20 million sperm/mL [84].

In one of the largest retrospective studies, Hansen *et al.* found that children born after IVF and IVF/ICSI had more major and minor birth defects than normally conceived (NC) controls [85]. These authors noticed a greater than twofold risk of birth defects in both conventional IVF (9.0%) and IVF/ICSI (8.6%) children compared to controls (4.2%). There was a higher risk of chromosomal defects, musculoskeletal defects, and multiple major defects in the ICSI cohort than in the NC controls. Another group from Germany prospectively evaluated 3372 ICSI children and compared them to matched controls [86]. A significant increase in major malformations of the heart, gastrointestinal tract, and urinary tract, as well as chromosomal abnormalities, was seen in the ICSI infants as compared to controls. Additionally, there was a significant difference in gestational age, birthweight, body length, head circumference, and Apgar scores in the ICSI children compared to NC controls. Most recently, the International Collaborative Study of ICSI: Child and Family Outcomes (ICSI-CFO) showed a significant increase in pregnancy complications, neonatal unit admissions, and admissions to the hospital greater than seven days for ICSI children compared to controls. Additionally, there was a greater incidence of significant childhood illnesses in ICSI children (74% vs. 57%). ICSI children had a greater likelihood of requiring physiotherapy and speech/language therapy, acquiring upper and lower respiratory tract infections, having dermatological or gastrointestinal problems, or requiring any type of surgery than NC controls [87]. A meta-analysis suggests a statistically significant increased risk of 30–40% of birth defects associated with ART [88].

Two recently published studies provide the first long-term (eight-year) follow-up of children born after IVF with ICSI. Leunens *et al.* showed that ICSI children do not show any delay of cognitive and motor development compared to naturally conceived children [89]. Belva *et al.* performed a thorough neurological examination and found no clinically important differences between ICSI and naturally conceived children, although a major congenital malformation was more frequently found in ICSI children (10% vs. 3.3%) [90].

In cases of male infertility due to severe oligoasthenoteratozoospermia or nonobstructive azoospermia, a peripheral karyotype and a search for AZF deletion on Yq11 should be performed. In men with CBAVD, mutations in the cystic fibrosis transmembrane conductance regulator (*CFTR*) gene should be evaluated. The most common genetic abnormality identified on genetic screening of infertile men is Klinefelter syndrome (47,XXY), which has an occurrence of 1 in 500 live male births and is reported to be present in 13% of cases of azoospermia [91]. Sperm are easily found in testicular biopsies from these patients [92], and fertilization rates greater than 50% using ICSI

have been reported [93]. Structural chromosomal aberrations of autosomes such as Robertsonian and reciprocal translocations are not infrequent in oligospermic males [94].

The overall prevalence of Y-chromosome microdeletions in infertile patients is 8%, and incidence of deletions reported varies among different studies from 1% to 35% [95]. These deletions are extremely rare (0.7%) in patients with sperm concentrations greater than 5 million/mL [96]. Male children conceived after ICSI will carry the same Y microdeletions as their father [97]. It has been reported that up to one-third of patients with Turner's stigmata and sexual ambiguity have associated Y microdeletions [98].

Cystic fibrosis (CF) is the most common autosomal recessive disease in Caucasians, with an incidence of 1 in 2500 and a carrier rate reported as 1 in 25. The *CFTR* identification has allowed the diagnosis of CF mutations in 72% of patients with CBAVD, 30% with CUAVD, and 34% with epididymal obstruction [99]. The obvious implications for reproduction in this population require that the female partners are also screened prior to any attempts at ICSI, and appropriate genetic counseling given.

DNA instability has been studied by examining trinucleotide repeats in the androgen receptor gene (CAG repeats). Normally, fewer than 30 repeats are found in exon 1 of this gene. Significant expansion of these repeats, most likely due to failure of the DNA to repair itself, leads to the development of a severe neurodegenerative syndrome (Kennedy's disease or Kennedy syndrome) [100]. Yoshida *et al.* detected longer than normal CAG nucleotide repeats in normally virilized men with normal genitalia and idiopathic azoospermia [101]. Maduro *et al.* showed an increase in CAG repeat lengths in testicular tissue from infertile men when compared with blood tissue [102]. This suggests that CAG repeat expansion may be the cause of some forms of severe infertility. More importantly, repeat expansion may represent a more global problem with DNA repair. Finally, **while many DNA microsatellites have no functional importance, accelerated expansion of the CAG repeat lengths with ICSI may not place the direct offspring in danger, but may place future generations from such a family at risk of developing Kennedy's disease.**

Beckwith–Wiedemann syndrome (BWS) and Angelman syndrome (AS) are both associated with imprinted gene clusters. Recent reports have implicated a higher rate of BWS and AS in children born after ICSI [103,104]. **There is evidence for an increased risk of imprinting disorders in ICSI children, and that childhood cancers could be associated**, but only a few observations in the literature are available.

Cost-effectiveness

Economic factors play a major role in the consideration of treatment options for male reproduction. **The costs of ART must take numerous factors into consideration, including the evaluation of the patient, the need for expensive fertility drugs to cause the eggs to mature, surgical intervention to retrieve the eggs, fertilizing and incubating the embryos, multiple gestation pregnancies, complications associated with preterm labor, prolonged hospitalization, retrieving and processing the sperm, and, finally, the desire for future children** [105]. Neumann *et al.* reported that the cost was as low as $50 000 per delivery for the first cycle in couples with tubal-factor infertility, while the cost increased to $160 000 for the first cycle in women over 40 years old [106].

Given the relatively high pregnancy rates from ICSI combined with epididymal or testicular sperm, some people have been questioning the need for microsurgical reconstruction of the male reproductive tract after vasectomy. However, in a recent review that compared the costs of vasectomy reversal to ICSI, the average cost per delivery for vasectomy reversal was only $25 475, with a delivery rate of 47%. This is in contrast to the cost of sperm retrieval and ICSI at an average of $72 521, with a delivery rate of 33% [107]. Similar findings were demonstrated by Kolettis and Thomas when they compared the costs of performing vasoepididymostomy to MESA with IVF/ICSI [108]. The average cost for vasoepididymostomy was $31 099, with a delivery rate of 36%, compared to $51 024 and a delivery rate of 29% for MESA with IVF/ICSI. Even a repeat microsurgical reconstruction is more cost-effective than ART [109].

Adjunctive procedures
Assisted hatching

The ability of a blastocyst to hatch, or escape, from the zona pellucida (ZP) that surrounds and protects the embryo during its first few days of development is one of many critical events that must occur for successful reproduction. Assisted hatching (AH) is achieved by zona dissection, drilling, or thinning, making use of acid solutions, proteases, piezon vibrators, and lasers [110].

A systematic review that analyzed data on 2572 women and more than 8036 transferred embryos, reported from all five continents, suggests that AH has no statistically significant impact on the odds of a live birth [111]. The review pooled data from all suitable trials irrespective of the AH method employed, population of women studied, or type of assisted conception procedure.

Assisted hatching may be clinically useful in patients with a poor prognosis, including those with two or more failed IVF cycles, poor embryo quality, and older women ($\geq$ 38 years of age) [112]. However, some reports suggest that it might be associated with higher rates of embryo damage and monozygotic twinning [113].

Preimplantation genetic diagnosis

Preimplantation genetic diagnosis (PGD) was first clinically applied in 1990 for genetic testing of embryos developed through IVF for couples who were at risk of transmitting an X-linked recessive disorder [114]. Nowadays, **it is offered as a method of allowing couples at risk for having children with genetic aberrations an opportunity to transfer only unaffected embryos and to discard embryos with genetic abnormalities.** PGD is tested for the following conditions [115]:

(1) autosomal single-gene disorders such as thalassemia, cystic fibrosis, Tay–Sachs disease, and sickle cell disease;
(2) chromosomal rearrangements (inherited chromosomal abnormalities);
(3) aneuploidy;
(4) X-linked diseases;
(5) nonmedical sex selection;
(6) human leukocyte antigen (HLA) typing.

Initially, single blastomeres were analyzed using multiplex polymerase chain reaction (PCR) to amplify X- and Y-chromosome-specific sequences. Now, FISH technology is routinely used for sex-chromosome assessment [116,117]. For single gene defects, identification of the specific mutations has led to the development of specific PCR probes to identify affected, carrier, and normal embryos [118]. A second strategy in PGD is the use of the first and second polar body, which are extruded during maturation and fertilization of oocytes, for PCR and FISH analysis [119].

Preimplantation genetic screening (PGS) for aneuploidies has been performed in patients with advanced maternal age, unexplained recurrent miscarriage, recurrent implantation failure, nonobstructive and obstructive azoospermia (NOA and OA), and severe sperm morphology anomalies.

As far as male factors are concerned, an increased aneuploidy rate has been observed on both testicular and epididymal spermatozoa from NOA and OA compared with normozoospermic men (19.6% vs. 8.2% vs. 1.6%, respectively) [120]. Increased aneuploidy and mosaicism rates have also been demonstrated on embryos derived from azoospermic men (NOA and OA) compared with embryos derived from fertile men [121,122]. Multiple studies have documented an enlarged frequency of sperm chromosomal anomalies in teratozoospermic spermatozoa [123,124], thereby generating controversy as to whether these patients should undergo ICSI. Although infrequent, macrocephalic spermatozoa have been more extensively studied in the context of PGS, because they seem to be more strongly related to aneuploidy [125].

The current follow-up of children born after PGD indicates, so far, no detrimental effect of the biopsy, as no differences have been reported when compared with children conceived in conventional ICSI cycles [126]. Verlinsky and coworkers have also reported on the follow-up of 754 babies born after 4748 PGD cycles without a significant increase in the prevalence of congenital malformations [116].

Experimental procedures

Round spermatid nucleus injection

Round spermatid nucleus injection (ROSNI) is a method of IVF in which immature sperm are injected directly into the egg. Although some reproductive centers have shown some success with ROSNI [127–130], there is much concern about the health of the offspring conceived through this technique, especially sex-chromosome abnormalities and genomic imprinting [131].

Cytoplasmic transfer

Normal development capability has been returned to eggs with ooplasmic deficiencies by transfer of ooplasm from a normal donor egg. This procedure is prohibited in many countries because of concerns raised over the insertion of third-party mitochondrial DNA, which appears to be maintained in the offspring. To date, there has been no evidence of abnormalities in these children as a result of this foreign DNA [132].

Somatic cell nuclear transfer: cloning

In 1997, the use of a somatic cell nucleus in the sheep culminated in the birth of the famous Dolly. This has been successfully followed in rodents, cats, pigs, cows, sheep, mules, dogs, and horses. The cloning process has great research potential, i.e., a cloned entity could be the source of an inner cell mass for the creation of a stem cell line. It is obvious that a clear distinction needs to be made between nuclear cloning for reproductive purposes and nuclear cloning for therapeutic or investigational purposes [133].

Conclusion

The availability of in-vitro fertilization, further expanded to the use of micromanipulation, has allowed couples with severe male-factor infertility, previously considered sterile, to conceive a child of their own biological background. On the other hand, this technology is followed by great expense together with known and unknown risks to the offspring. Therefore, the urologist should be aware of the limitations of these procedures, and identify the cause of the male's infertility and treat it whenever possible.

References

[1] Steptoe PC, Edwards RG. Birth after the reimplantation of a human embryo. *Lancet* 1978; **2**: 366.

[2] Asch RH, Balmaceda JP, Ellsworth LR, Wong PC. Pregnancy after translaparoscopic gamete intrafallopian transfer. *Lancet* 1984; **2**: 1034–5.

[3] Devroey P, Braeckmans P, Smitz J, *et al.* Pregnancy after translaparoscopic zygote intrafallopian transfer in a patient with sperm antibodies. *Lancet* 1986; **7**: 1329.

[4] Cohen J, Fehilly CB, Fishel SB, *et al.* Male infertility successfully treated by in-vitro fertilisation. *Lancet* 1984; **1**: 1239–40.

[5] World Health Organization. *WHO Laboratory Manual for the Examination of Human Semen and Sperm–Cervical Mucus Interaction*, 4th edn. Cambridge: Cambridge University Press, 1999.

[6] Kruger TF, Menkveld R, Stander FS, *et al.* Sperm morphological features as a prognostic factor in in vitro fertilization. *Fertil Steril* 1986; **46**: 1118–23.

[7] Henkel RR, Schill WB. Sperm preparation for ART. *Reprod Biol Endocrinol* 2003; **1**: 108.

[8] Ord T, Patrizio P, Marello E, Balmaceda JP, Asch RH. Mini-Percoll: a new method of semen preparation for IVF in severe male factor infertility. *Hum Reprod* 1990; **5**: 987–9.

[9] Practice Committee of the Society for Assisted Reproductive Technology; Practice Committee of the American Society for Reproductive Medicine. Guideline on number of embryos transferred. *Fertil Steril* 2006; **86** (Suppl 4): S51–2.

[10] Wolf DP, Byrd W, Dandekar P, Quigley MM. Sperm concentration and the fertilization of human eggs in vitro. *Biol Reprod* 1984; **31**: 837–48.

[11] Oehninger S, Acost, AA, Morshedi M, *et al.* Corrective measures and pregnancy outcome in in vitro fertilization in patients with severe sperm morphology abnormalities. *Fertil Steril* 1988; **50**: 283–7.

[12] Tournaye H, Devroey P, Camus M, *et al.* Comparison of in vitro fertilization in male and tubal infertility: a 3 year survey. *Hum Reprod* 1992; **7**: 218–22.

[13] Hirsh AV, Mills C, Bekir J, *et al.* Factors influencing the outcome of in vitro fertilization with epididymal spermatozoa in irreversible obstructive azoospermia. *Hum Reprod* 1994; **9**: 1710–16.

[14] Tournaye H, Camus C, Bollen N, *et al.* In vitro fertilization techniques with frozen–thawed sperm: a method for preserving the progenitive potential of Hodgkin patients. *Fertil Steril* 1991; **55**: 443–5.

[15] Fénichel P, Donzeau M, Farahifar D, *et al.* Dynamics of human sperm acrosome reaction: Relation with in vitro fertilization. *Fertil Steril* 1991; **55**: 994–9.

[16] Henker R, Müller C, Miska W, Gips H, Schill WB. Determination of the acrosome reaction in human spermatozoa is predictive of fertilization in vitro. *Hum Reprod* 1993; **8**: 2128–32.

[17] Franken DR, Kruger TF, Oehninger S, *et al.* The ability of the hemizona assay to predict human fertilization in different and consecutive in vitro fertilization cycles. *Hum Reprod* 1993; **8**: 1240–4.

[18] Johnson A, Bassham B, Lipshultz LI, Lamb DJ. A quality control system for the optimized sperm penetration assay. *Fertil Steril* 1995; **64**: 832–7.

[19] Tournaye H, Camus M, Ubaldi F, *et al.* Tubal transfer: A forgotten ART? Is there still an important role for tubal transfer procedures? *Hum Reprod* 1996; **11**: 1815–22.

[20] Gamete intrafallopian transfer. *Fertil Steril* 2007; **87** (Suppl 1): S61.

[21] Devroey P, Staessen C, Camus M, *et al.* Zygote intrafallopian transfer as a successful treatment for unexplained infertility. *Fertil Steril* 1989; **52**: 246–9.

[22] Hammitt DG, Syrop CH, Hahn SJ, *et al.* Comparison of concurrent pregnancy rates for in vitro fertilization: embryo transfer, pronuclear stage embryo transfer and gamete intrafallopian transfer. *Hum Reprod* 1990; **5**: 947–54.

[23] Yovich JL, Yovich JM, Edirisinghe WR. The relative chance of pregnancy following tubal or uterine transfer procedures. *Fertil Steril* 1988; **49**: 858–64.

[24] Habana AE, Palter SF. Is tubal transfer of any value? A meta-analysis and comparison with the Society of Assisted Reproductive Technology database. *Fertil Steril* 2001; **76**: 286–93.

[25] Malter HE, Cohen J. Partial zona dissection of the human oocyte: a nontraumatic method using micromanipulation to assist zona pellucida penetration. *Fertil Steril* 1989; **51**: 139–48.

[26] Ng SC, Bongso A, Ratnam SS, *et al.* Pregnancy after transfer of sperm under zona. *Lancet* 1988; **2**: 790.

[27] Tarin JJ. Subzonal insemination, partial zona dissection or intracytoplasmic sperm injection? An easy decision? *Hum Reprod* 1995; **10**: 165–70.

[28] Lippi J, Mortimer D, Jansen PS. Sub-zonal insemination for extreme male factor infertility. *Hum Reprod* 1993; **8**: 908–15.

[29] Lazendorf SE, Malony MK, Veeck LL, *et al.* A preclinical evaluation of pronuclear formation by microinjection of human spermatozoa into human oocytes. *Fertil Steril* 1988; **49**: 835–42.

[30] Palermo G, Joris H. Devroey P, Van Steirteghem AC. Pregnancies after intracytoplasmic injection of single spermatozoon into an oocyte. *Lancet* 1992; **340**: 17–18.

[31] Society for Assisted Reproductive Technology and Centers for Disease Control and Prevention. ART success rates: national summary and fertility clinic reports. 1996–2004. www.cdc.gov/reproductivehealth.

[32] Staessen C, Camus M, Clasen K, De Vos A, Van Steirteghem A. Conventional in-vitro fertilization versus intracytoplasmic sperm injection in sibling oocytes from couples with tubal infertlity and normozoospermic semen. *Hum Reprod* 1999; **14**: 2474–9.

[33] Bhattacharya S, Hamilton MPR, Shaaban M, *et al.* Conventional in-vitro fertilization versus intracytoplasmic sperm injection for the treatment of non-male-factor infertility: a randomized controlled trial. *Lancet* 2001; **357**: 2075–9.

[34] Poehl M, Hollagschwandtner M, Bichler K, *et al.* IVF-patients with nonmale factor "to ICSI" or "not to ICSI" that is the question? *J Assist Reprod Genet* 2001; **18**: 205–8.

[35] Foong SC, Fleetham JA, O'Keane JA, *et al.* A prospective randomized trial of conventional in vitro fertilization versus intracytoplasmic sperm injection in unexplained infertility. *J Assist Reprod Genet* 2006; **23**: 137–40.

[36] Oehninger S, Veeck L, Lanzendorf S, *et al.* Intracytoplasmic sperm injection: Achievement of high pregnancy rates in couples with severe male factor infertility is dependent primarily upon female and not male factors. *Fertil Steril* 1995; **64**: 977–81.

[37] Devroey P, Godoy H, Smitz J, *et al.* Female age predicts embryonic implantation after ICSI: A case controlled study. *Hum Reprod* 1996; **11**: 1324–7.

[38] Spandorfer SD, Avrech OM, Colombero LT, Palermo GD, Rosenwaks Z. Effect of parental age on fertilization and pregnancy characteristics in couples treated by intracytoplasmic sperm injection. *Hum Reprod* 1998; **13**: 334–8.

[39] Klonoff-Cohen HS, Natarajan L. The effect of advancing paternal age on pregnancy and live birth rates in couples undergoing in vitro fertilization or gamete intrafallopian transfer. *Am J Obstet Gynecol* 2004; **191**: 507–14.

[40] de La Rochebrochard E, de Mouzon J, Thépot F, Thonneau P, the French National IVF Registry (FIVNAT) Association. Fathers over 40 and increased failure to conceive: The lessons of in vitro fertilization in France. *Fertil Steril* 2006; **85**: 1420–4.

[41] Nybo Andersen AM, Hansen KD, Andersen PK, Davey Smith G. Advanced paternal age and risk of fetal death: a cohort study. *Am J Epidemiol* 2004; **160**: 1214–22.

[42] de La Rochebrochard E, Thonneau P. Paternal age and maternal age are risk factors for miscarriage; results of a multicentre European study. *Hum Reprod* 2002; **17**: 1649–56.

[43] Slama R, Bouyer J, Windham G, *et al.* Influence of paternal age on the risk of spontaneous abortion. *Am J Epidemiol* 2005; **161**: 816–23.

[44] Nagy Z, Liu J, Cecile J, *et al.* Using ejaculated, fresh, and frozen–thawed epididymal and testicular spermatozoa gives rise to comparable results after intracytoplasmic sperm injection. *Fertil Steril* 1995; **63**: 808–15.

[45] Casper RF, Meriano JS, Jarvi KA, Cowan L, Lucato ML. The hypo-osmotic swelling test for selection of viable sperm for intracytoplasmic sperm injection in men with complete asthenozoospermia. *Fertil Steril* 1996; **65**: 972–6.

[46] Verheyen G, Joris H, Critz K, *et al.* Comparison of different hypo-osmotic solutions to select viable immotile spermatozoa for potential use in intracytoplasmic sperm injection. *Hum Reprod Update* 1997; **3**: 195–203.

[47] Terriou P, Hans E, Giorgetti C, *et al.* Pentoxifylline initiates motility in spontaneously immotile epididymal and testicular spermatozoa and allows normal fertilization, pregnancy and birth after intracytoplasmic sperm injection. *J Assist Reprod Genet* 2000; **17**: 194–9.

[48] de Oliveira NM, Vaca Sanchez R, Rodriguez Fiesta S, *et al.* Pregnancy with frozen–thawed and fresh testicular biopsy after motile and immotile sperm microinjection, using the mechanical touch technique to assess viability. *Hum Reprod* 2004; **19**: 262–5.

[49] Hammadeh ME, Al-Hasani S, Stieber M, *et al.* The effect of chromatin condensation (Aniline Blue staining) and morphology (strict criteria) of human spermatozoa on fertilization, cleavage and pregnancy rates in an intracytoplasmic sperm injection programme. *Hum Reprod* 1996; **11**: 2468–71.

[50] Svalander P, Jakobsson AH, Forsberg AS, Bengtsson AC, Wikland M. The outcome of intracytoplasmic sperm injection is unrelated to "strict criteria" sperm morphology. *Hum Reprod* 1996; **11**: 1019–22.

[51] Gómez E, Pérez-Cano I, Amorocho B, *et al.* Effect of injected spermatozoa morphology on the outcome of intracytoplasmic sperm injection in humans. *Fertil Steril* 2000; **74**: 842–3.

[52] McKenzie LJ, Kovanci E, Amato P, *et al.* Pregnancy outcome of in vitro fertilization/intracytoplasmic sperm injection with profound teratospermia. *Fertil Steril* 2004; **82**: 847–9.

[53] De Vos A, Van De Velde H, Joris H, *et al.* Influence of individual sperm morphology on fertilization, embryo morphology, and pregnancy outcome of intracytoplasmic sperm injection. *Fertil Steril* 2003; **79**: 42–8.

[54] Ryu HM, Lin WW, Lamb DJ, *et al.* Increased chromosome X, Y, and 18 nondisjunction in sperm from infertile patients that were identified as normal by strict morphology: implication for intracytoplasmic sperm injection. *Fertil Steril* 2004; **76**: 879–83.

[55] Burrello N, Vicari E, Shin P, *et al.* Lower sperm aneuploidy frequency is associated with high pregnancy rates in ICSI programmes. *Hum Reprod* 2003; **18**: 1371–6.

[56] Spano M, Bonde JP, Hjollund HI, *et al.* Sperm chromatin damage impairs human fertility. The Danish First Pregnancy Planner Study Team. *Fertil Steril* 2000; **73**: 43–50.

[57] Seli E, Gardner DK, Schoolcraft WB, Moffatt O, Sakkas D. Extent of nuclear DNA damage in ejaculated spermatozoa impacts on blastocyst development after in vitro fertilization. *Fertil Steril* 2004; **82**: 378–83.

[58] Carrell DT, Liu L, Peterson CM, *et al.* Sperm DNA fragmentation is increased in couples with unexplained recurrent pregnancy loss. *Arch Androl* 2003; **49**: 49–55.

[59] Evenson DP, Jost LK, Marshall D, *et al.* Utility of the sperm chromatin structure assay as a diagnostic and prognostic tool in the human fertility clinic. *Hum Reprod* 1999; **14**: 1039–49.

[60] Bungum M, Humaidan P, Spano M, *et al.* The predictive value of sperm chromatin structure assay (SCSA) parameters for the outcome of intrauterine insemination, IVF and ICSI. *Hum Reprod* 2004; **19**: 1401–8.

[61] Li Z, Wang L, Cai J, Huang H. Correlation of sperm DNA damage with IVF and ICSI outcomes: a

systematic review and meta-analysis. *J Assist Reprod Genet* 2006; **23**: 367–76.

[62] Boe-Hansen GB, Fedder J, Ersbøll AK, Christensen P. The sperm chromatin structure assay as a diagnostic tool in the human fertility clinic. *Hum Reprod* 2006; **21**: 1576–82.

[63] Bungum M, Humaidan P, Axmon A, *et al.* Sperm DNA integrity assessment in prediction of assisted reproduction technology outcome. *Hum Reprod* 2007; **22**: 174–9.

[64] The Practice Committee of the American Society for Reproductive Medicine. The clinical utility of sperm DNA integrity testing. *Fertil Steril* 2006; **86** (Suppl 4): S35–7.

[65] Check ML, Check JH, Katsoff D, Summers-Chase D. ICSI as an effective therapy for male factor with antisperm antibodies. *Arch Androl* 2000; **45**: 125–30.

[66] Aitken RJ, Irvine DS, Wu FC. Prospective analysis of sperm–oocyte fusion and reactive oxygen species generation as criteria for the diagnosis of infertility. *Am J Obstet Gynecol* 1991; **164**: 542–51.

[67] Agarwal A, Allamaneni SS, Nallella KP, George AT, Mascha E. Correlation of reactive oxygen species levels with the fertilization rate after in vitro fertilization: a qualified meta-analysis. *Fertil Steril* 2005; **84**: 228–31.

[68] Aboulghar MA, Mansour RT, Serour GI, *et al.* Fertilization and pregnancy rates after intracytoplasmic sperm injection using ejaculated semen and surgically retrieved sperm. *Fertil Steril* 1997; **68**: 109–11.

[69] Nicopoullos JDM, Gilling-Smith C, Ramsay JWA. Does the cause of obstructive azoospermia affect the outcome of intracytoplasmic sperm injection: a meta-analysis. *BJU Int* 2004; **93**: 1282–6.

[70] Devroey P, Liu J, Nagy Z, *et al.* Pregnancies after testicular sperm extraction and intracytoplasmic sperm injection in non-obstructive azoospermia. *Hum Reprod* 1995; **10**: 1457–60.

[71] Schlegel PN, Palermo GD, Goldstein M, *et al.* Testicular sperm extraction with intracytoplasmic sperm injection for non-obstructive azoospermia. *Urology* 1997; **49**: 435–40.

[72] Silber S, Van Steirteghem A, Nagy Z, *et al.* Normal pregnancies resulting from testicular sperm extraction and intracytoplasmic sperm injection for azoospermia due to maturation arrest. *Fertil Steril* 1996; **55**: 110–17.

[73] Nicopoullos JD, Gilling-Smith C, Almeida PA, *et al.* Use of surgical sperm retrieval in azoospermic men: a meta-analysis. *Fertil Steril* 2004; **82**: 691–701.

[74] Vernaeve V, Tournaye H, Osmanagaoglu K, *et al.* Intracytoplasmic sperm injection with testicular spermatozoa is less successful in men with nonobstructive azoospermia than in men with obstructive azoospermia. *Fertil Steril* 2003; **79**: 529–33.

[75] Tournaye H, Merdad T, Silber S, *et al.* No differences in outcome after ICSI with fresh or with frozen–thawed epididymal spermatozoa. *Hum Reprod* 1999; **14**: 90–5.

[76] Griffiths M, Kennedy CR, Rai J, *et al.* Should cryopreserved epididymal or testicular sperm be recovered from obstructive azoospermic men for ICSI? *BJOG* 2004; **111**: 1289–93.

[77] Aoki VW, Wilcox AL, Thorp C, Hamilton BD, Carrell DT. Improved in vitro fertilization embryo quality and pregnancy rates with intracytoplasmic sperm injection of sperm from fresh testicular biopsy samples vs. frozen biopsy samples. *Fertil Steril* 2004; **82**: 1532–5.

[78] Habermann H, Seo R, Cieslak J, *et al.* In vitro fertilization outcomes after intracytoplasmic sperm injection with fresh or frozen–thawed testicular spermatozoa. *Fertil Steril* 2000; **73**: 955–60.

[79] Schlegel PN, Liotta D, Hariprashad J, Veeck LL. Fresh testicular sperm from men with nonobstructive azoospermia works best for ICSI. *Urology* 2004; **64**: 1069–71.

[80] Veheyen G, Vernaeve V, Van Landuyt L, *et al.* Should diagnostic testicular sperm retrieval followed by cryopreservation for later ICSI be the procedure of choice of all patients with non-obstructive azoospermia? *Hum Reprod* 2004; **19**: 2822–30.

[81] Wald M, Ross LS, Prins GS, *et al.* Analysis of outcomes of cryopreserved surgically retrieved sperm for IVF/ICSI. *J Androl* 2006; **27**: 60–5.

[82] Templeton A, Morris IK. Reducing the risk of multiple births by transfer of two embryos after in vitro fertilization. *N Engl J Med* 1998; **339**: 573–7.

[83] Thurin A, Hausken I, Hillensjo T, *et al.* Elective single-embryo transfer versus double-embryo transfer in in vitro fertilization. *N Engl J Med* 2004; **351**: 2392–402.

[84] Bonduelle M, Van Assche E, Joris H, *et al.* Prenatal testing in ICSI pregnancies: incidence of chromosomal anomalies in 1586 karyotypes and relation to sperm parameters. *Hum Reprod* 2002; **17**: 2600–14.

[85] Hansen M, Kurinczuk JJ, Bower C, Webb S. The risk of major birth defects after intracytoplasmic sperm injection and in vitro fertilization. *N Engl J Med* 2002; **346**: 725–30.

[86] Katalinic A, Rosch C, Ludwig M, for the German ICSI Follow-up Study Group. Pregnancy course and outcome after intracytoplasmic sperm injection: a controlled prospective cohort study. *Fertil Steril* 2004; **81**: 1604–16.

[87] Bonduelle M, Wennerholm UB, Loft A, *et al.* A multi-centre cohort study of the physical health of 5-year-old children conceived after intracytoplasmic sperm injection, in vitro fertilization and natural conception. *Hum Reprod* 2005; **20**: 413–19.

[88] Hansen M, Bower C, Milne E, de Klerk N, Kurinczuk JJ. Assisted reproductive technologies and the risk of birth defects – a systematic review. *Hum Reprod* 2005; **20**: 328–38.

[89] Leunens L, Celestin-Westreich S, Bonduelle M, Liebaers I, Ponjaert-Kristoffersen I. Cognitive and motor development of 8-year-old children born after ICSI compared to spontaneously conceived children. *Hum Reprod* 2006; **21**: 2922–9.

[90] Belva F, Henriet S, Liebaers I, *et al*. Medical outcome of 8-year-old singleton ICSI children (born ≥ 32 weeks' gestation) and a spontaneously conceived comparison group. *Hum Reprod* 2007; **22**: 506–15.

[91] Rucker GB, Mielnik A, King P, Goldstein M, Schlegel PN. Preoperative screening for genetic abnormalities in men with nonobstructive azoospermia before testicular sperm extraction. *J Urol* 1998; **160**: 2068–71.

[92] Tournaye H, Staessen C, Liebaers I, *et al*. Testicular sperm recovery in nine 47,XXY Klinefelter patients. *Hum Reprod* 1996; **11**: 1644–9.

[93] Staessen C, Toumaye H, Van Assche E, *et al*. PGD in 47,XXY Klinefelter's syndrome patients. *Hum Reprod Update* 2003; **9**: 319–30.

[94] Yoshida A, Miura K, Shirai M. Cytogenetic survey of 1007 infertile males. *Int J Urol* 1997; **58**: 166–76.

[95] Pagani R, Brugh VM III, Lamb DJ. Y chromosome genes and male infertility. *Urol Clin North Am* 2002; **29**: 745–53.

[96] Krausz C, Forti G, McElreavey K. The Y chromosome and male fertility and infertility. *Int J Androl* 2003; **26**: 70–5.

[97] Silber S, Repping S. Transmission of male infertility to future generations: lessons from the Y chromosome. *Hum Reprod Update* 2002; **8**: 217–29.

[98] Patsalis PC, Sismani C, Quintana-Murci L, *et al*. Effects of transmission of Y chromosome AZFc deletions. *Lancet* 2002; **360**: 1222–4.

[99] Mak V, Zielenski J, Tsui LC, *et al*. Proportion of cystic fibrosis gene mutations not detected by routine testing in men with obstructive azoospermia. *JAMA* 1999; **281**: 2217–24.

[100] Mak V, Jarvi KA. The genetics of male infertility. *J Urol* 1996; **156**: 1245–56.

[101] Yoshida KI, Yano M, Chiba K, Honda M, Kitahara S. CAG repeat length in the androgen receptor gene is enhanced in patients with idiopathic azoospermia. *Urology* 1999; **54**: 1078–81.

[102] Maduro MR, Casella R, Kim E, *et al*. Microsatellite instability and defects in mismatch repair proteins: a new aetiology for Sertoli-cell-only syndrome. *Mol Hum Reprod* 2003; **9**: 61–8.

[103] Cox GF, Burger J, Lip V, *et al*. Intracytoplasmic sperm injection may increase the risk of imprinting defects. *Am J Hum Genet* 2002; **71**: 162–4.

[104] DeBaun MR, Niemitz EL, Feinberg AP. Association of in vitro fertilization with Beckwith–Wiedemann syndrome and epigenetic alteration of LIT1 and H19. *Am J Hum Genet* 2003; **72**: 150–60.

[105] Karpman E, Williams DH, Lipshultz LI. IVF and ICSI in male infertility: update on outcomes risks and costs. *Scientific World Journal* 2005; **5**: 922–32.

[106] Neumann PJ, Gharib SD, Weinstein MC. The cost of a successful delivery with in vitro fertilization. *N Engl J Med* 1994; **331**: 239–43.

[107] Pavlovich CP, Schlegel PN. Fertility options after vasectomy: a cost-effectiveness analysis. *Fertil Steril* 1997; **67**: 133–41.

[108] Kolettis PN, Thomas AJ. Vasoepididymostomy for vasectomy reversal: a critical assessment in the era of intracytoplasmic sperm injection. *J Urol* 1997; **158**: 467–70.

[109] Donovan JF, DiBaise M, Sparks AE, Kessler J, Sandlow JI. Comparison of microscopic epididymal sperm aspiration and intracytoplasmic sperm injection/in vitro fertilization with repeat microscopic reconstruction following vasectomy: is second attempt vas reversal worth the effort? *Hum Reprod* 1998; **13**: 387–93.

[110] Al-Nuaim LA, Jenkins JM. Assisted hatching in assisted reproduction. *BJOG* 2002; **109**: 856–62.

[111] Edi-Osagie E, Hooper L, Seif MW. The impact of assisted hatching on live birth rates and outcomes of assisted conception: a systematic review. *Hum Reprod* 2003; **18**: 1828–35.

[112] Practice Committee of the Society of Assisted Reproductive Technology; Practice Committee of the American Society for Reproductive Medicine. The role of assisted hatching in in vitro fertilization: a review of the literature. A Committee opinion. *Fertil Steril* 2006; **86** (Suppl 4): S124–6.

[113] Hershlag A, Paine T, Cooper GW, *et al*. Monozygotic twinning associated with mechanical assisted hatching. *Fertil Steril* 1999; **71**: 144–6.

[114] Handyside AH, Kontogianni EH, Hardy K, Winston RM. Pregnancies from biopsied human preimplantation embryos sexed by Y-specific DNA amplification. *Nature* 1990; **344**: 768–70.

[115] IFFS Surveillance 07. Chapter 14: Preimplantation genetic diagnosis. *Fertil Steril* 2007; **87** (Suppl 1): S47–9.

[116] Verlinsky Y, Cohen J, Munne S, *et al*. Over a decade of experience with preimplantation genetic diagnosis: a multicenter report. *Fertil Steril* 2004; **82**: 292–4.

[117] Baruch S, Adamson GD, Cohen J, *et al*. Genetic testing of embryos: a critical need for data. *Reprod Biomed Online* 2005; **11**: 667–70.

[118] Kalfoglou A, Scott J, Hudson K. PGD patients' and providers' attitudes about the use and

regulation of PGD. *Reprod Biomed Online* 2005; **11**: 486–96.

[119] Verlinsky Y, Cieslak J, Ivakhnenko V, *et al.* Prepregnancy genetic testing for age-related aneuploidies by polar body analysis. *Genet Test* 1997–1998; **1**: 231–5.

[120] Calogero A, Burello N, De Palma A, *et al.* Sperm aneuploidy in infertile men. *Reprod Biomed Online* 2003; **6**: 310–17.

[121] Silber S, Escudero T, Lenahan K, *et al.* Chromosomal abnormalities in embryos derived from testicular sperm extraction. *Fertil Steril* 2003; **79**: 30–8.

[122] Platteau P, Staessen C, Michiels A, *et al.* Comparison of the aneuploidy frequency in embryos derived from testicular sperm extraction in obstructive and nonobstructive azoospermic men. *Hum Reprod* 2004; **19**: 1570–4.

[123] Bernardini L, Borini A, Preti S, *et al.* Study of aneuploidy in normal and abnormal germ cells from semen of fertile and infertile men. *Hum Reprod* 1998; **13**: 3406–13.

[124] Vicari E, de Palma A, Burello N, *et al.* Absolute polymorphic teratozoospermia in patients with oligo-asthenozoospermia is associated with an elevated sperm aneuploidy rate. *J Androl* 2003; **24**: 598–603.

[125] Viville S, Mollard R, Bach M, *et al.* Do morphological anomalies reflect chromosomal aneuploidies? *Hum Reprod* 2000; **15**: 2563–6.

[126] Sermon KD, Michiels A, Harton G, *et al.* ESHRE PGD Consortium data collection VI: cycles from January to December 2003 with pregnancy follow-up to October 2004. *Hum Reprod* 2007; **22**: 323–36.

[127] Tesarik J, Mendoza C, Testart J. Viable embryos from injection of round spermatids into oocytes. *N Engl J Med* 1995; **333**: 525.

[128] Fishel S, Green S, Bishop M, *et al.* Pregnancy after intracytoplasmic injection of spermatid. *Lancet* 1995; **345**: 641–2.

[129] Gianaroli L, Selman HA, Magli MC, *et al.* Birth of a healthy infant after conception with round spermatids isolated from cyopreserved testicular tissue. *Fertil Steril* **72**: 539–41.

[130] Al-Hasani S, Ludwig M, Palermo I, *et al.* Intracytoplasmic injection of round and elongated spermatid from azoospermic patients: Results and review. *Fertil Steril* 1999; **14** (Suppl 1): 97–107.

[131] Practice Committee of the American Society for Reproductive Medicine; Practice Committee of the Society for Assisted Reproductive Technology. Round spermatid nucleus injection (ROSNI). *Fertil Steril* 2006; **86** (Suppl 4): S184–6.

[132] IFFS Surveillance 07. Chapter 10: Micromanipulation. *Fertil Steril* 2007; **87** (Suppl 1): S37–40.

[133] IFFS Surveillance 07. Chapter 17: Cloning. *Fertil Steril* 2007; **87** (Suppl 1): S59–60.

Chapter 30

Psychological issues of infertility and assisted reproductive technology

Linda D. Applegarth

Introduction

Parenthood has profound meanings for most people. For women, motherhood is often pivotal to identity. Our culture has clearly encouraged women to assume the biologic role of giving birth and nurturing children. For men, fatherhood may mean responsibility, a "relinquishment of a way of life that in the Western world is implanted into the male psyche from birth … On the one hand is the unquantifiable drive and desire to father children, which neither experience of life nor role models seem yet to disillusion us about, whilst on the other hand is the potential fear of loss of freedom and the potential restrictions of fatherhood and responsibilities" [1]. It is this type of ambivalence that may explain why men are sometimes less eager or determined than their partners to pursue parenthood.

Nonetheless, the dream of having children is one that is commonly shared by most couples of reproductive age. **The expectation of having a family not only is shared by the individuals themselves, but also is highly valued by society.** In our culture and others, fertility stands for productivity, growth, and continuity [2]. For most, it is a basic expectation of life – a continuation of the human life cycle. For many, parenthood signifies not only a renewal of life, but also immortality. Anything that threatens to leave this dream unfulfilled can be devastating, and may ultimately threaten self-esteem and status as well as relationships. As a result, when both men and women are faced with uncertainty about if or how they will ever become parents, it can be anticipated that they will experience a number of psychological responses.

The objectives of this chapter are fourfold: (1) to provide an overview of the common psychological and emotional responses to infertility; (2) to review current literature as it pertains to the emotional aspects of male-factor infertility as well as gender differences

in the responses to the infertility condition; (3) to discuss some of the psychological issues associated with male-factor infertility and the assisted reproductive technologies; and (4) to provide an overview of some of the common psychosocial issues and ethical concerns associated with disclosure versus nondisclosure in gamete donation (specifically sperm donation). In fulfilling these objectives, recommendations for ways in which the medical team can be sensitive to or assist patients in managing these issues will also be provided.

Overview: common psychological and emotional responses to infertility

The experience of infertility is often defined as a life crisis. Its impact upon self-image, marital relationships, and relationships with family and friends can be significant. The medical evaluation and treatment, including financial costs, can sometimes be exceedingly difficult to manage emotionally. Such a crisis is generally unanticipated, and many individuals and couples tend to lack sufficient strategies and skills for managing the situation.

As with any crisis, infertility can be defined as a pivotal point in life development that presents an individual with both the opportunity for emotional growth and the danger of increased vulnerability to psychiatric distress. Certainly, the outcome of this crisis depends to some degree on the individual's own personality structure and internal coping mechanisms. The emotional upset that many infertile people feel during this crisis is usually associated with subjective feelings such as anxiety, fear, sadness, guilt, and shame. Additionally, the distress can also be accompanied by feelings of helplessness and ineffectuality in the face of what appears to be an unsolvable problem. What is striking about many of those dealing with infertility

Infertility in the Male, 4th edition, ed. Larry I. Lipshultz, Stuart S. Howards, and Craig S. Niederberger. Published by Cambridge University Press. © Cambridge University Press 2009.

is that they may experience a great deal of anger, anxiety, or depression relative to being unable to predict or control treatment outcomes.

From a professional standpoint, many health and mental health professionals share the same kinds of uncertainty when working with this population. As Malstedt notes,

> Physicians who specialize in reproductive medicine and their staffs are also having to live with the frustrations of not knowing what is going to happen next or how to respond to patients' needs for answers … It appears that all participants in assisted reproductive technology live each day with hope that their medical goals will be achieved, with uncertainty about the duration and ramifications of their treatment decisions, and with the desire to create a happy ending for all involved [3].

For infertile couples who enter treatment using the assisted reproductive technologies, there is a tendency to move forward with both hope and fear.

Unlike many other types of life crises, infertility is particularly noteworthy with respect to its chronicity. This condition seldom resolves itself within a matter of days, weeks, or even months. Often, infertile individuals find that they must endlessly come up with the energy and resources (physical, emotional, and financial) necessary to adapt to the cyclic changes in their bodies, to treatment disappointments, to the newest medical technologies and interventions, to overt as well as covert pressures from family, friends, and society – not to mention to the detrimental effects that the infertility often has on a couple's relationship.

The infertility experience can also become a part of every waking moment for many patients and their partners. It can dictate decisions regarding career development and employment, vacations, and holiday and family get-togethers. It can sometimes make household expenditures nearly impossible. In effect, many patients often describe themselves as feeling "stuck," or as seeing their lives as out of balance and out of control.

As noted, infertility can be a threat to the patient's self-esteem, identity, and self-confidence. When both men and women are faced with uncertainty about if or how they will ever become parents, it can be anticipated that they may have a number of specific psychological responses to this condition. These include depression, guilt, stress and anxiety, and social isolation.

Depression

The inability to conceive a child is fraught with loss, or potential loss. Mahlstedt notes that, in varying degrees, the experience of infertility involves (1) loss of a relationship, (2) loss of health, (3) loss of status or prestige, (4) loss of self-esteem, (5) loss of self-confidence, (6) loss of security, (7) loss of a fantasy or the hope of fulfilling an important fantasy, and (8) loss of something or someone of great symbolic value [3]. She adds that each of these losses in adulthood has been seen as an etiologic factor in depression. The inability to do what many others do so naturally is particularly painful. Some individuals describe themselves as feeling defective and worthless. For those whose self-esteem is significantly dependent on the ability to accomplish goals, the failure to conceive or bear a child becomes easily reinterpreted as failure as a person. Individuals and couples then tend to focus on what they do not have or have not accomplished, and they lose sight of the many positive, productive components of their lives. Depression often results from this style of thinking.

Depression is an understandable response to the emotional pain engendered by infertility. It should be stressed, however, that severe, ongoing depression can develop that results in feelings of hopelessness, inability to function in daily life, severe anxiety or agitation, and suicidal ideation or behavior. This condition requires prompt mental health intervention, and should not be ignored or dismissed as an overreaction to the infertility.

Guilt

Closely associated with the sense of personal failure is guilt. Patients may describe themselves as feeling personally responsible for their infertility. The condition may therefore be seen as punishment for working in stressful jobs, for having had a previous abortion or an affair, or for having postponed parenting decisions because of career demands. It is not uncommon for such guilt to take on an obsessive quality, particularly as patients begin to feel less and less in control of their treatment outcomes and consequently their futures. **Regret and self-blame become common psychological sequelae as the infertility continues.**

Stress and anxiety

Infertility has often been described as an emotional roller-coaster ride, a ride that is fraught with hope one day and despair the next. These ongoing emotional ups and downs can create significant levels of chronic stress and anxiety on a monthly basis. Couples must manage the physical, emotional, and financial concerns related

517

to infertility – concerns that are particularly true for those undergoing the assisted reproductive technologies. Women often have to juggle medical tests and appointments with work responsibilities; financial burdens may mount; and men often worry about their partners' well-being as well as occasional male-factor issues. Couples can never truly be guaranteed that their efforts will be rewarded, and the anxiety goes on and on. **The infertility experience creates significant stress for couples. Although most experts note that there is little evidence that stress causes infertility, most believe that there can be a relationship between the two.**

Social isolation

Another common and difficult aspect of the infertility crisis can be social isolation. **Because few infertile couples have friends or family members who have also confronted infertility, they usually feel different or alone.** With some exceptions, those who have not personally experienced infertility may not truly understand the emotional pain and suffering it brings. Those who choose to talk about their infertility are often subjected to insensitive, rude, or even insulting comments from others. Couples who decide not to share their fertility problems may carry around a painful emotional burden. In either case, there is a tendency to withdraw, to avoid people with children and/or activities that include children. **In so doing, the resulting feeling of isolation can significantly affect self-esteem, and the couple feels prohibited from being part of a larger, childbearing society.**

Review of literature

Lipshultz has pointed out that male infertility is a widespread problem that often continues undiagnosed or untreated [4]. He notes that men are commonly poorly informed about possible treatments, embarrassed about discussing the issue with medical professionals, or "concerned about the stigma of being labeled 'infertile.'" Lipshultz adds that some men's hesitancy to be tested for infertility can confound the worry and frustration of "an already stressed couple." **Clearly, there appear to be a wide range of psychosocial issues that impact and/or result from male-factor infertility.**

Overall, the data pertaining to the psychological components of male-factor infertility are relatively scarce, since it appears that infertile men have been studied with less frequency than women. More research has been done within the context of gender-specific responses to infertility diagnoses. **Such a diagnosis may have profoundly different meanings for each gender.** As Petok notes, "Infertility denies a woman the important function of mothering … At the same time, the loss for a man becomes a failure to create a commodity that will carry on his name and genetic line" [5].

Hjelmstedt *et al.* found that women reacted more strongly to their infertility than men, and significantly more men than women had not confided in anyone about their infertility problem [6]. Of additional interest was the finding that men were more likely to use information seeking as a coping style for managing infertility distress than were women. One small, recent study in Ireland undertook to assess mood profiles in infertile men and to investigate whether etiological factors of infertility have any impact on mood [7]. The study found detectable anxiety levels in 32% of male subjects ($n = 50$), and those with oligospermia described higher levels of anxiety than did other patient subgroups. Notably, and perhaps unlike their female counterparts, there were no cases of depression in the study population. Dhaliwal *et al.* found that anxiety was significantly greater in the partner with the infertility problem [8]; however, whereas men tended to experience anxiety, women were more likely to experience depression. **Several research efforts have also pointed to the tendency for infertile men to understate or "disguise" their levels of emotional distress and upset relative to their infertility** [9,10].

Mason also studied infertile men in the United Kingdom [11]. Her small study group ($n = 22$) described their feelings about not being able to have their own biological children. Common themes for these men were feelings of guilt, shame, anger, isolation, loss, and a sense of personal failure. In addition to discussing their pain, they also commented on how they learned to cope with their condition. Nachtigall and colleagues similarly described reactions of infertile men as being feelings of stigmatization, loss of potency, role failure, and reduced self-esteem [12]. Others have also reported feelings of personal and sexual inadequacy, sexual dysfunction, depression and hopelessness, hostility, and guilt [13,14].

A number of studies have found, too, that men typically adopt coping strategies such as denial, distancing, and avoidance that allow them to manage the potentially painful implications and realities of such a diagnosis. As a result they tend to portray themselves as being especially unstressed [10].

Although women seem to have stronger negative responses to the infertile condition, the emotional power and depth of this experience for both men and women cannot be overstated. The inability to have a child ultimately leaves many couples feeling intensely helpless and vulnerable. Regardless of all their physical efforts and financial costs, there are no guarantees or certainties that they will conceive or give birth to a healthy child. **These feelings of powerlessness and loss of control may be foreign to many who confront infertility. The problem may not be solved, and this relentless fear seems to underscore much of the depression and anxiety that many infertile people experience.**

Recommendations to the medical team

It appears that research on the psychological reactions to specific types of male-factor infertility, as well as to specific female-factor infertility diagnoses, is still limited. Hardy and Makuch note the different ways in which men and women view childbearing, but again stress that women are more likely to respond to the condition with depression and anxiety, regardless of which partner carries the diagnosis [15]. In any case, most infertile patients, at one point or another, feel debilitated by their infertility and also tend to describe themselves as feeling unsupported by healthcare professionals in their efforts to become parents.

As a result, it is important for the medical team to develop an awareness of the emotional impact of infertility. Physicians, nurses, laboratory personnel, receptionists, and other healthcare professionals can often be more effective with infertility patients if they also understand the many ways in which infertility and its treatment disrupt all infertile couples' lives. Recognizing that distress, sadness, and frustration are intrinsic to the experience helps couples also feel that their responses are a normal (albeit painful) part of the process. Patients who feel understood and respected tend to respond with respect, and may also respond more effectively to medical recommendations.

Second, the medical team should encourage both partners to participate in treatment whenever possible. When both partners are present for a medical consultation or procedure, their ability to hear and comprehend the information that is imparted is significantly increased. Patients can not only learn from the physician or nurse, but also ask questions, and learn from each other. Putting information in writing also enables couples to discuss what needs to be done,

review instructions and expectations at home, and make informed choices. When both partners are present for consultations, it can also help to prevent one person from feeling that he or she is the sole cause of the problem or the one responsible for fixing it.

Third, it is ultimately helpful to everyone if the medical team can broaden the definition of successful treatment. Patients who are reluctant to continue infertility treatment, or who are definitely committed to ending it, need not be led to feel that they are quitters or failures. Although pregnancy and childbirth are definitions of success, another is feeling a sense of satisfaction and closure with the ways in which the emotional pain was managed and decisions were made during treatment. **Perhaps "success" can then be measured by patients as truly believing that they did the very best they could with the physical, emotional, and financial resources they had available.**

Psychological issues associated with the assisted reproductive technologies
In-vitro fertilization (IVF) and intracytoplasmic sperm injection (ICSI)

Many couples whose infertility treatment requires in-vitro fertilization (IVF) also need intracytoplasmic sperm injection (ICSI) as a part of the procedure. In many respects ICSI has revolutionized infertility treatment as a whole. **Certainly for men with oligospermia or poor semen quality, the use of ICSI has produced dramatic results in terms of pregnancy rates. Nonetheless, the procedure, although potentially making a male infertility diagnosis obsolete in some cases, is also not without emotional side effects.** A 1998 study hypothesized that male ICSI patients with higher-level male-factor diagnoses would experience more emotional distress than their IVF-only counterparts [16]. Additionally, it was hypothesized that the greatest difference in distress scores would occur during active stages of these procedures, such as when men were required to produce a sperm sample and learn whether or not the oocytes had fertilized. Daily data were obtained, and emotional subscale data were divided into distress and optimism variables. Patients needing ICSI were found to report more distress during the two days prior to active stages of treatment. The researchers concluded that men undergoing ICSI experienced more anticipatory anxiety than those in the IVF group. At the same time, the study concluded that the availability of the ICSI procedure may also help reduce feelings of loss and hopelessness, because it offers a possible solution to the couple's infertility that enables them to have a child who is genetically related to both partners. Both research data and clinical experience have shown that providing a sperm sample during this crucial stage of IVF/ICSI treatment could (and does) increase performance anxiety for both fertile and infertile men. Pook *et al.* [17] and Clarke *et al.* [18] have also studied the role of psychological stress, in general, and found that it has a predictive value for changes in sperm concentration and motility, regardless of whether or not there is a male-factor infertility diagnosis.

The use of donated gametes

The successful use of assisted reproductive technologies over the past 25 years or more has brought with it procedures that allow couples who cannot conceive using their own gametes the alternative of achieving pregnancy through the use of donated oocytes, donated sperm, and even donated embryos. **However, for most couples considering gamete donation of any type, this is a difficult and emotionally painful process.** It creates intense feelings of loss, forces couples to contemplate their biologic mortality, and demands that they reconsider their reasons for wanting to become parents.

Hans Kohut, a renowned personality theorist, posited that a stable and sustainable sense of self is central to human happiness [19]. He noted that the self, the organizing force of the personality that guides how we live our lives, can be disrupted by the disappointment or frustration of a person's innermost hopes and aspirations. When the disruption is severe enough, a perceived deficit of the self can occur, with the concomitant loss of hopefulness about life along with other psychosocial dysfunction. A significant effect of a deficient sense of self is shame. **Thus, couples who must face decisions about the use of donated gametes face one such potentially shame-producing disappointment. The decision to move forward with donor conception also tests the couple's relationship.** Together partners must shift to thinking about how parenting a child who is genetically connected to only one of them may be different from parenting a child who is connected to both of them.

Mahlstedt and Greenfeld note that gamete donation is neither a cure nor a treatment for infertility. They stress,

The time has come for the experts in reproductive technologies (1) to consider the likelihood that assisted reproductive technologies with donor gametes is psychologically different from procedures using the biological gametes of both parents conceiving a child and (2) to stop pretending that once the child is in the couple's arms, they will not give another thought to how it all happened. Conceiving with donor sperm is not the same as conceiving with husband sperm; someone else's eggs are not the same as one's own. Because they have tried for yeas to conceive a child biologically related to them both, couples know this [20].

Understanding the need for emotional preparation in relation to gamete donation is an important part of the process both for patients and for the medical team. Requiring that all patients have a consultation with a trained mental health professional eliminates any suggestion that an individual or couple is being asked to see a fertility counselor because they have a particular problem or lifestyle, and places the focus appropriately on the need for support and information. **It is also within this context that the American Society for Reproductive Medicine (ASRM), in its 2006 Guidelines for Gamete and Embryo Donation recommends that referral for evaluation and counseling be made available to couples before they attempt to conceive through gamete or embryo donation so as to avoid adverse emotional and psychological consequences of the procedure** [21]. The psychological evaluation is also intended to rule out gross psychopathology and depression, potential substance abuse, as well as a history of current or past family violence or abuse. Marital stability is also assessed within the context of the consultation.

In addition, the psychological interview and consultation with the recipient couple allows the mental health professional the opportunity to assess the couple's readiness and gives both partners a chance to voice their thoughts and feelings on the donor gamete issue. It allows each person to process his or her partner's thoughts and feelings as well. **Most certainly, couples must be encouraged to grieve their infertility before using donor gametes.** It has been this author's years of clinical experience that all parties are responsive to having the opportunity to spend time with the mental health professional. It is often the first opportunity each partner has to sort out the many feelings regarding the decision to become parents through gamete or embryo donation, and it provides them with a resource person from whom they can seek assistance as they grapple with some of the more complex issues regarding this decision. **Ultimately, these discussions are protective for both the recipient couple and the** potential offspring, and can have important ethical and psychological implications for these families and possibly for their generations to come.

Microepididymal and testicular sperm retrieval and the use of "donor backup"

There are virtually no data at present regarding the psychological impact on couples for whom it is recommended that they arrange for "donor sperm backup" prior to undergoing a surgical sperm aspiration procedure and IVF. One could certainly expect that reactions to this recommendation are usually intense, in part because many patients are ill-prepared psychologically and emotionally for such a possibility.

Most couples who are dealing with a diagnosis of azoospermia are distressed and anxious, at the very least. The notion that a surgical procedure might allow them the possibility of creating a biological child together can fill them with hope and optimism, even when being given less-than-optimistic chances of success. The stated low statistical chances and realities of retrieving sperm for ICSI and IVF can often be denied by the infertile couple, as is the idea of actually *using* donor sperm with the eggs retrieved. Although couples may understand the practical advantages of having "donor backup" sperm available so that the costly IVF cycle is not lost, their lack of emotional readiness for this possibility can potentially result in a crisis. Not only is the couple confronted with deep feelings of shock, grief, and sadness, but they must also simultaneously accept the real possibility of conceiving a child through donated gametes. Berger *et al.* have indicated that most patients diagnosed with severe male-factor infertility have reported major symptoms such as insomnia, depression, weight loss, and reduced libido in the months following the diagnosis [22]. Seibel has, as a result, pointed out that delaying donor insemination for "at least six months after the diagnosis … seems to increase marital satisfaction and improve self-concept. Patients who do not do so are more likely to experience marital strain, anxiety, and depression" [23]. Therefore, patients who must immediately move to "donor backup" may truly be at risk for increased psychological disruption and difficulties. Understanding and responding to the need for emotional preparation relative to this procedure is imperative.

Known versus anonymous donation

In the case of gamete donation, the terms "known" and "anonymous" can be confusing at best. Historically, most of gamete donation was performed anonymously, and this often continues to be the case, especially for sperm donation. (The ready availability of frozen sperm through donor banks, legal and governmental requirements for HIV testing, and the desire for privacy, tend to encourage the use of anonymous, donated sperm.) **In general, anonymous gamete donation means that recipient couples are provided with non-identifying information about the donor, including physical characteristics, ethnic background, profession, as well as hobbies and interests.** It has been pointed out, however, that anonymity implies "no identity," and there appears to be a growing trend toward more openness in the use of donor gametes, as "anonymous" donors are willing and interested in providing information to recipient families, and families are more secure with having social, educational, and medical histories that they can later share with their children [24].

The use of a "known" donor is applied either to an individual whom the couple knows personally or one with whom they have some degree of a relationship, such as a friend, sibling, or other relative. Therefore the use of the term "identified" donor can perhaps be more useful when referring to a gamete donor who is not personally known to the recipient couple, but is someone the couple has selected through a clinic, sperm bank, or agency, on the basis of photos, family and ethnic background, medical, educational, and work information, and so on. There is an anonymous component to the use of an "identified" donor because the recipient couple may or may not know the full name of the donor, nor does the donor know much, if anything, about the recipient couple. Although the recipients and donor may have had direct contact with one another, there is no expectation of an ongoing relationship between them.

It appears that there is a range of psychological benefits and costs to the use of known, identified, or anonymous gamete and embryo donation. Many couples strongly prefer the use of an anonymous donor. They believe that the anonymity helps to distance them emotionally from the donor and allows them to feel that the resulting offspring is truly their child. Knowing the donor, or seeing a photograph, will only serve to remind them of their feelings of loss, sadness, or inadequacy. The use of a known donor may also raise fears of potential boundary confusion between themselves, the child, and the donor.

On the other hand, there are also a significant number of couples, usually undergoing oocyte donation, who strongly prefer the use of a known or identified donor. In selecting this type of gamete donor, the individual or couple may feel that they are given more control over the process. They believe that it is important to know as much as possible about the donor's personality style, genetic and medical background, ethnicity, and appearance. Similarly, many couples have felt that having a sibling or a relative as a gamete donor was critical to their idea of genetic continuity and connection to the offspring. For some, the idea of using the gametes of a "stranger" is not only unacceptable, but also abhorrent.

Confidentiality, privacy, and secrecy in gamete and embryo donation

Consultations, evaluations, and treatment between infertile individuals and healthcare professionals are covered by the expectation that confidentiality is protected by law, medical ethics, and general medical practice. At the same time, an anonymous gamete donor's confidentiality can be protected through the sharing of only nonidentifying information to the recipient couple.

Privacy is another component of the gamete donation process that primarily involves the recipient couple. It refers to "the couple's right to decide who, outside their relationship, will know about the donor conception: family, friends, and society in general" [3]. **Privacy is usually seen as a positive aspect of a family's efforts to protect its boundaries, and there are certainly some aspects of people's lives that are theirs to keep as private as they wish. Secrecy, however, can potentially have negative implications for a family.** In this case, it has to do with withholding information that can affect a person's life – the life of the offspring created with donor gametes. Secrecy therefore involves a decision not to tell a child about his or her genetic origins, and it may intrude on the child's right to know. It also involves pretending that the child is the genetic offspring of them both. Ultimately, as Mahlstedt notes, "The issue of secrecy is controlled by the recipient couples alone" and does not involve the medical team or the donor, unless the donor is known by the couple [3]. **The impact and implications of privacy versus secrecy will be further discussed in the context of disclosure and nondisclosure in a later section of this chapter.**

Recommendations to the medical team

For couples who undertake IVF and ICSI procedures
Prepare the couple using a "team approach." Often the medical team, physicians, nurses, administrators, and mental health professionals are utilized to help inform, prepare, and support couples before, during, and after the procedure. These health professionals all can play a role in meeting with new patients to discuss medical, financial, emotional, and logistical aspects of the IVF process that may or may not involve the ICSI procedure. **From the initial consultation, the staff must create an environment in which patients feel free to ask questions and express their feelings and concerns, knowing that acceptance and support will be given.**

Preparation for the IVF and ICSI procedures also should include a discussion of the potential emotional stresses involved. This process may be started in consultation with a mental health professional or the nursing team. The goals of this consultation are to normalize the many emotional responses and anxieties that couples experience through these procedures, to help them develop more effective coping strategies for dealing with their anxieties, fears, and potential disappointments. Ultimately, the aim of this consultation can be to broaden the focus of the emotional experience of IVF/ICSI so that couples can succeed in achieving certain goals besides conception.

Regardless of whether or not there is diagnosed male-factor infertility, it is important that the male partner be involved in the ART process. He can give injections, come for blood testing and ultrasounds, and be there for oocyte retrieval and recovery. This type of involvement enhances and personalizes the experience for both partners.

Lastly, the medical team should also plan for follow-up. This planning can begin at the time of the initial consultations. This includes suggestions for coping if there is no pregnancy, discussion about the treatment plan and future IVF cycles, and resources for information and support through infertility consumer organizations such as Resolve, the National Infertility Association (www.resolve.org). Couples who do not achieve a pregnancy when embryo transfer has occurred generally experience grief reactions similar to those of couples experiencing spontaneous abortion; severe disappointment and depression are common responses. They are often isolated from support, and a follow-up call from the physician, nurse, or mental health professional can reassure couples of the appropriateness of their feelings. **This type of caring follow-up can go a long way in soothing the pain of a failed IVF/ICSI cycle.** Even those who do conceive will need continued support, as they often fear that they will lose the pregnancy. Guidance and education about the pregnancy should be given immediately.

For couples using "donor backup" or donated gametes

To assess readiness for gamete donation as well as "donor backup," it is important for mental health professionals, as well as others on the medical team, to explore the individual's and couple's reasons for choosing gamete donation. It is important that both partners understand the implications of this decision and take into account the pros and cons of gamete donation versus adoption or child-free living. **Neither partner should agree to move forward with third-party reproduction just because it has been strongly recommended by a professional or because he or she feels coerced by the other partner, family members, societal pressures, or other factors.** The use of "donor backup" in conjunction with other treatments should be carefully explored and considered prior to surgical treatment, and should not be a decision by default at the last minute. Assessing readiness often involves the exploration of covert and overt pressures, such as the husband who is ashamed and ambivalent about his infertility or the wife who must experience pregnancy and childbirth in order to fulfill her views of motherhood. In summary, it is imperative that the couple be in full agreement about the decision to proceed with gamete donation or "donor backup" and consider it a positive alternative method of family building [25]. **Couple acceptance of the means of conception is also imperative for a positive adjustment for the child** [3].

It is also highly recommended and very important that whenever a known or identified gamete donor is used, a psychosocial evaluation and consultation be performed with all involved parties, including the partner of the potential donor. In the case of known donors, it is important to explore the history of the relationship between the donor and the recipient couple to ensure that there is no coercion or other motivations that could lead to emotionally unhealthy and unhappy outcomes for everyone, especially the potential offspring. Marshall also urges that fertility programs require prospective participants, including recipients, intrafamilial sperm donors, and their partners, undergo psychological counseling by a professional knowledgeable about gamete donation [26]. Counseling would include an examination of emotional risks, possible impact on family relationships, and what information will be disclosed to the offspring. In addition, the potential nature of the relationship and boundaries between the child, his or her parents, and the gamete donor must be addressed, examined, and clearly defined. These evaluations and consultations are intended to avoid any likelihood of future traumatization of the child as well as other family members [27]. **The physician or fertility clinic should not feel obligated to agree to every request for intrafamilial sperm donation, especially where there are indications of coercion, or unhealthy family dynamics** [26], **as should be the case in any form of known gamete donation.**

Psychological issues associated with disclosure and nondisclosure in gamete donation

Historical factors

As an alternative family-building option, donor insemination has been around for at least 100 years [28]. It appears that, historically, this option has been shrouded in secrecy for a number of reasons. First, male infertility, as opposed to female-factor infertility, has generally been a more neglected issue in medical treatment and research [1]. Secondly, male infertility still tends to be associated with a lack of masculinity or virility and sexual functioning. **Thus, these factors have resulted in greater stigmatization and shame than has been noted in female-factor infertility.** Moreover, donor insemination (DI) itself has not only been associated with masturbation, but also conjures up fantasies of the involvement of a second male in an adulterous relationship.

Over the years, donor insemination has thus been viewed with suspicion and seen as morally or religiously unacceptable. **As a result, the procedure was seldom publicly acknowledged, and physicians strongly encouraged secrecy.** Similarly, infertile couples themselves felt compelled to maintain secrecy in order to protect themselves and their child(ren) from stigma and shame. As Daniels notes, "this secrecy has been presented as a natural component of DI" [29]. In his view, secrecy breeds inequality in relationships, since some people have significant information about an individual that the individual him- or herself does not have. Secrecy, therefore, has the potential to damage everyone involved, and can specifically damage the well-being and happiness of the families created through donor insemination [29].

It appears that, although secrecy (and anonymity) has historically surrounded the use of donated sperm, this has not necessarily been the case with ovum donation. Cooper and Glazer point out that one of the primary differences between sperm donation and ovum donation is that known donors are much more frequently used for oocyte donation [30]. They identify two major explanations for this difference: practicality and gender differences. From a practical standpoint, oocytes are more difficult to obtain and cannot yet be easily cryopreserved for future use. The physical invasiveness of the procedure means that most donor oocyte programs do not maintain a large pool of available donors. Historically, because of the lack of available oocytes for donation, recipient couples were encouraged by clinics to "bring a donor" – often a sister, cousin, or friend. Clearly the use of a known oocyte donor has significant implications regarding the notion of secrecy (as it also does in the case of sperm donation).

As noted previously, the desire for secrecy and anonymity in sperm donation has been due, in part, to efforts to protect men from the shame associated with their infertility. Women, in addition to being encouraged to bring a known oocyte donor, are more likely to talk with friends and family about their infertility experience. They may feel more comfortable and accepting of using a known donor; at the same time, they also want and need to feel supported by those with whom they are emotionally closest. Sharing their infertility fears and concerns with significant others can be seen as an important coping strategy [25], as opposed to men, who are likely to employ other forms of coping.

It appears that couples, both donor sperm and donor oocyte recipients, recently have become more open to considering disclosing the means of conception to their offspring. Most infertility physicians have also begun to step back and encourage couples to consider this issue, often with the assistance of an infertility counselor or psychotherapist. In fact, the Ethics Committee of the ASRM now supports disclosure from parents to offspring about the use of donor gametes in their conception, and has made suggestions for policies for fertility programs and sperm banks [31]. The use of a known or anonymous donor, as well as thoughts and feelings about secrecy in the use of donor gametes, most certainly impacts couples' decisions regarding disclosure or nondisclosure to others – and, most importantly, to their potential offspring.

Social and religious factors

As Mahlstedt points out, society places a high value on children and parenthood, but is ambivalent about creating families in nontraditional ways [3]. Most certainly, the ability to do so has been underscored

by the medical and scientific developments in the assisted reproductive technologies. At the same time, some forms of Judaism and Islam, as well as Roman Catholicism, forbid the use of donor gametes in conception. Ironically, the pressure placed upon couples by many religious communities to bear children can be palpable. **For many of these individuals, the effort to balance religious beliefs and teachings with the fervent wish to have a biological or genetic connection to a child can prove to be a difficult and painful process – one that might naturally lead to nondisclosure and secrecy.**

Even in more open communities, in the United States and abroad, the decision to use donor sperm or oocytes can be met with disapproval. A recipient couple must therefore be in agreement with one another about with whom (if anyone) they will share important information about their infertility diagnosis and subsequent use of donor gametes. **Disclosure to others as well as to the child must ultimately be the couple's personal decision, and this also will depend on their religious and cultural practices and environment.**

Disclosure versus nondisclosure

The decision to disclose information about donor conception is exceedingly complex. It involves not only the aforementioned religious and cultural factors, but also legal, ethical, and psychosocial issues. **There are arguments both for and against disclosure, and each couple must ultimately be allowed to decide which choice is best for them and their child(ren) within the context of these issues. Consistent with the ASRM Ethics Committee report, it is noted that many infertility counselors are increasingly supportive of disclosure** [25]. Clinical observations have suggested that donor oocyte recipients appear to be choosing more readily to disclose information to their offspring about how they were conceived [32]. Because women generally have been more forthcoming with friends and family about their infertility condition, they appear to be more likely to discuss the donor option before undertaking the procedure. Because they have been open with others, they also appreciate the need to be open with their child.

A recent study of disclosure decisions among pregnant donor oocyte recipients found that disclosing women voiced the right of the child to know, and perceived social and cultural factors as conducive to disclosure [33]. Nondisclosing and undecided women emphasized a need to protect normal family relationships, perceived a social stigma, and were unable to identify a benefit to disclosing. Schover *et al.* also indicated in an earlier study that recipient couples expressed concern that a child who knows about the donor insemination would feel incomplete and frustrated because they would want to find their genetic parent [34]. Another common concern was the idea that family and society would disapprove of DI, and that this would impact negatively on the identified child.

Most research studies indicate that most couples who use sperm donation do not plan to tell the child about his or her conception [35,36]. With the exception of lesbian couples and single women, this also appears to be the case for many couples who use a known donor, including family members. Greenfeld and Klock supported this finding when they discovered that there were no differences among known or anonymous oocyte donation recipients as to whether or not they would disclose to their child [37].

It appears, however, that the willingness of gamete donors themselves to be identified can also impact recipients' disclosure decisions. Scheib *et al.* followed up with couples using "open identity" sperm donors and found that they were relatively open and positive about their use of DI [38]. The authors also found that disclosure did not have a negative impact on the families. There has been controversy in a number of Scandinavian countries regarding anonymous sperm donation. Sweden and Norway have now abolished sperm donor anonymity. Denmark, however, has argued against this policy, stating that donors themselves are in favor of anonymity and that, more importantly, the abolishment of donor anonymity conveys a clear message that nondisclosure by DI parents is unacceptable [39]. Jorgensen and Hartling posit that a substantive alternative to a policy of non-anonymous donors might be to inform recipient parents about avoiding nondisclosure, and to design educational materials for children that would support parents [40].

The decision to disclose the means of conception to donor offspring is also influenced by parents' uncertainties about when and how to disclose. Rumball and Adair found that couples chose to tell when "it just seemed right," or when they believed that children could understand the information [41]. In their study, there appeared to be an advantage in telling the story to children at a young age when the information was processed in a factual, nonemotional way.

A study by Kirkman also concluded that parents who plan to tell should be encouraged to disclose to their offspring before adolescence [42].

Increasingly, more researchers are focusing their attention on the issue of how gamete donor recipient couples, who wish to do so, can best disclose the use of a third party in the conception of their children [43,44].

Recommendations to the medical team

As Mahlstedt has pointed out, the needs and rights of all those participating in gamete and embryo donation can be respected and accommodated around the issues of disclosure and nondisclosure [3]. The medical team can protect both the recipients' and donors' confidentiality while, at the same time, maintaining neutrality regarding recipients' thoughts, feelings, and decisions about disclosure. The recipient couple can therefore be free to reveal the means of conception to whomever they wish, and they can be prepared, with the assistance and support of health and mental health professionals, if needed, to share this information with their children. **Neutrality and the provision of information and support on the part of physicians and medical staff will ultimately create an open environment for managing the complex issues involving gamete or embryo donation.** De Jonge and Barratt have stated it well:

> The key global issue surrounding gamete donation is not the well-rehearsed known vs. anonymous donation argument but rather one of providing patients with a flexible dual-track system (i.e., ability to know or not to know donor identity), complete with psychosocial support and education that enable them to make well-informed choices that benefit all stakeholders present and future [45].

Conclusion

Infertility is a life crisis: it can impact self-esteem, relationships with others, financial security, and social status within a community. Whatever the infertile individual or couple's specific circumstances may be, it is critical that physicians and other healthcare workers have a thorough understanding of the powerful impact of the infertility experience. **As couples spend months and years trying to achieve parenthood, many also find themselves lacking sufficient coping skills for managing their stress and emotional pain.**

For both men and women, involuntary childlessness often reflects a number of real and potential fears

and losses that may result in depression, anxiety, guilt, and isolation. The assisted reproductive technologies continue to carry great promise for infertile people. Because the need to conceive and bear a child is so compelling, it is not surprising that most couples will go to any length to fulfill their desires and dreams of parenthood. Medical breakthroughs and possibilities have revolutionized treatment options, and provide not only great hope but also great potential for disappointment and despair.

Treatment options and opportunities seem limitless; however, it is also increasingly difficult, but necessary, for patients to feel emotionally and psychologically prepared to handle both the successes and failures of treatment. It can also be increasingly difficult for couples to know when and how to end treatment, should it become necessary.

As the medical technology develops, it seems especially important to consider the ethical and psychological aspects of assisted reproduction and understand its impact on people and society. It can also be important and especially helpful to all participants to reframe and redefine success as we gain an understanding of the psychological aspects of infertility. Success can mean much more than merely giving birth to a genetically related child.

Infertile individuals and couples need the assistance of both health and mental health professionals as they move forward into the newest reproductive technologies. The integration of medical and psychological aspects of infertility underscores the effort to meet the needs of the whole person. It also enables everyone involved to consider seriously the impact of these technologies and treatments on the children who are created. Identifying and understanding the psychological implications of human infertility – both male and female – provide the impetus to prevent difficulties before they exact an emotional toll on patients and offspring, as well as on the medical team.

References

[1] Lee S. *Counseling in Male Infertility*. London: Blackwell, 1996.

[2] Becker G. *Healing the Infertile Family: Strengthening Your Relationship in Search of Parenthood*. New York, NY: Bantam, 1990.

[3] Mahlstedt PP. Psychological issues of infertility and assisted reproductive technology. In: Lipshultz LI, Howards SS, eds. *Infertility in the Male*, 3rd edn. St. Louis, MO: Mosby Year Book, 1997: 462–75.

[4] Lipshultz L. Addressing male reproductive issues: the Reproductive Health Council of the American Foundation for Urologic Disease. *Family Building (Resolve)*, 2003; **3** (1): 21.

[5] Petok WD. The psychology of gender-specific infertility diagnoses. In: Covington SN, Burns LH, eds. *Infertility Counseling: a Comprehensive Handbook for Clinicians*, 2nd edn. Cambridge: Cambridge University Press, 2006: 37–60.

[6] Hjelmstedt A, Andersson L, Skoog-Svanberg A, et al. Gender differences in psychological reactions to infertility among couples seeking IVF and ICSI treatment. *Acta Obstet Gynecol Scand* 1999; **78**: 42–8.

[7] Roopnarinesingh R, El-Hantati, Keane D, Harrison R. An assessment of mood in males attending an infertility clinic. *Ir Med J* 2004; **97**: 310–11.

[8] Dhaliwal LK, Gupta KR, Gopalan S, Kulhara P. Psychological aspects of infertility due to various causes: a prospective study. *Int J Fertil Womens Med* 2004; **49**: 44–8.

[9] Sherrod RA. Male infertility: the element of disguise. *J Psychosoc Nurs Men Health Serv* 2006; **44** (10): 30–7.

[10] Felder H, Meyer F, Osborn W, et al. Psychological aspects in the therapy of the andrological sterility factor with regard to the unfulfilled wish for a child. *Andrologia* 1996; **28** (Suppl 1): 53–6.

[11] Mason MC. *Male Infertility: Men Talking*. London: Routledge, 1993.

[12] Nachtigall R, Becker G, Wozny M. The effects of gender specific diagnosis on men's and women's response to infertility. *Fertil Steril* 1992; **57**: 113–21.

[13] Irvine SCE. Male infertility and its effect on male sexuality. *Sex Marital Ther* 1996; **11**: 273–80.

[14] Kadem P, Mikulincer M, Nathanson YE, Bartoov B. Psychological aspects of male infertility. *Br J Med Psychol* 1990; **63**: 73–80.

[15] Hardy E, Makuch MY. Gender, infertility, and ART. In: Vayena E, Rowe PJ, Griffin PD, eds. *Current Practices and Controversies in Assisted Reproduction*. Geneva: World Health Organization, 2002: 272–80.

[16] Boivin J, Shoog-Svanberg A, Andersson L, et al. Distress level in men undergoing ICSI versus IVF. *Hum Reprod* 1998; **13**: 1403–6.

[17] Pook M, Krause W, Rohrie B. Coping with infertility: distress and changes in sperm quality. *Hum Reprod* 1999; **14**: 1487–92.

[18] Clarke RN, Klock SC, Geoghegan A, Travassos DE. Relationship between psychological stress and semen quality among in-vitro fertilization patients. *Hum Reprod* 1999; **14**: 753–8.

[19] Kohut, H. *The Restoration of Self*. New York, NY: International Universities Press, 1977.

[20] Mahlstedt PP, Greenfeld DA. Assisted reproduction with donor gametes: the need for patient preparation. *Fertil Steril* 1989; **52**: 908–14.

[21] Practice Committee of the American Society for Reproductive Medicine; Practice Committee of the Society for Assisted Reproductive Technology. 2006 Guidelines for Gamete and Embryo Donation. *Fertil Steril* 2006; **86** (Suppl 4): S38–50.

[22] Berger DM, Eisen A, Shuber J Doody KE. Psychological patterns in donor insemination. *Can J Psychiatry* 1986; **31**: 818–23.

[23] Seibel, MM. Therapeutic donor insemination. In: Seibel MM, Crockin SL, eds. *Family Building through Egg and Sperm Donation: Medical, Legal, and Ethical Issues.* Boston, MA: Jones and Bartlett, 1996: 33–45.

[24] Mahlstedt PP, Probasco KA. Sperm donors: their attitude toward providing medical and psychosocial information for recipient families. *Fertil Steril* 1991; **56**: 747–53.

[25] Thorn P. Recipient counseling for donor insemination. In: Covington SN, Burns LH, eds. *Infertility Counseling: a Comprehensive Handbook for Clinicians,* 2nd edn. Cambridge: Cambridge University Press, 2006: 305–18.

[26] Marshall LA. Ethical and legal issues in the use of related donors for therapeutic insemination. *Urol Clin North Am* 2002; **29**: 855–61.

[27] Nikolettos N, Asimakopoulos B, Hatzissabas I. Intrafamilial sperm donation: ethical questions and concerns. *Hum Reprod* 2003; **18**: 933–6.

[28] Gregoire AT, Mayer RC. The impregnators. *Fertil Steril* 1965; **16**: 130–4.

[29] Daniels K. *Building a Family with the Assistance of Donor Insemination.* Palmerston North, New Zealand, Dunmore Press, 2004.

[30] Cooper SL, Glazer ES. *Beyond Infertility: New Paths of Parenthood.* New York, NY: Lexington Books, 1994.

[31] Ethics Committee of the American Society for Reproductive Medicine. Informing offspring of their conception by gamete donation. *Fertil Steril* 2004; **82** (Suppl 1): 212–16.

[32] Applegarth LD. Emotional implications. In Adashi EY, Rock JA, Rosenwaks Z, eds. *Reproductive Endocrinology, Surgery, and Technology.* Philadelphia, PA: Lippincott-Raven, l996: vol. 2, 1954–68.

[33] Hershberger P, Klock SC, Barnes RB. Disclosure decisions among pregnant women who received donor oocytes: a phenomenological study. *Fertil Steril* 2007; **87**: 288–96.

[34] Schover LR, Collins RL, Richards S. Psychological aspects of donor insemination: evaluation and follow-up of recipient couples. *Fertil Steril* 1992; **57**: 583–90.

[35] Klock SC, Jacob MC, Maier D. A prospective study of donor insemination recipients: secrecy, privacy, and disclosure. *Fertil Steril* 1994; **62**: 477–84.

[36] Durna EM, Bebe J, Steigrad SJ, Leader LR. Donor insemination: attitudes of parents towards disclosure. *Med J Aust* 1997; **167**: 256–9.

[37] Greenfeld DA, Klock SC. Disclosure decisions among known and anonymous oocyte donation recipients. *Fertil Steril* 2004; **81**: 1565–71.

[38] Scheib JE, Riordan M, Rubin S. Choosing identity release sperm donation: the parents' perspective 13–18 years later. *Hum Reprod* 2003; **18**: 1115–27.

[39] Ernst E, Ingerslev HJ, Schou O, Stoltenberg H. Attitudes among sperm donors in 1992 and 2002: a Danish questionnaire survey. *Acta Obstet Gynecol Scand* 2007; **86**: 327–33.

[40] Jorgensen HK, Hartling OJ. Anonymity in connection with sperm donation. *Med Law* 2007; **26**: 37–43.

[41] Rumball A, Adair V. Telling the story: parents' scripts for donor offspring. *Hum Reprod* 1999; **14**: 1392–9.

[42] Kirkman M. Parents' contributions to the narrative identity of offspring of donor-assisted conception. *Soc Sci Med* 2003; **57**: 2229–42.

[43] MacDougall K, Becker G, Scheib JE, Nachtigall RD. Strategies for disclosure: how parents approach telling their children that they were conceived with donor gametes. *Fertil Steril* 2007; **87**: 524–33.

[44] Leeb-Lundberg S, Kjellberg S, Sydsjö G. Helping parents to tell their children about the use of donor insemination (DI) and determining their opinions about open-identity sperm donors. *Acta Obstet Gynecol Scand* 2006; **85**: 78–81.

[45] De Jonge C, Barratt CLR. Gamete donation: a question of anonymity. *Fertil Steril* 2006; **85**: 500–1.

Chapter 31

Legal issues in fertility preservation in the male

Susan L. Crockin and Elizabeth M. Bloom

Introduction

Treatment of male infertility predates the advent of in-vitro fertilization (IVF) and other assisted reproductive technology (ART) procedures by decades. Combining older techniques, such as artificial insemination and sperm cryopreservation, with newer technologies and applying them to evolving family constellations have both extended treatment options to more individuals and significantly complicated and expanded the attendant legal issues. The availability and use of cryopreserved sperm, artificial insemination, including donor insemination, and IVF have spawned litigation involving parenthood status between and amongst married (and divorcing) heterosexual couples, same-sex couples, and a child's biological father; inheritance rights for children born from donated sperm; competing claims to gametes and embryos; and provider liability involving sperm banks, medical programs, and insurance carriers as to the patients and families whose fertility they attempt to preserve.

This chapter is intended to identify and discuss these issues and the efforts that legislatures, courts, professional guidelines, programs, and patients have made to resolve them, in the hope of giving professionals some guidance in these evolving areas. **This chapter examines (1) fertility preservation from the perspectives of the various male patients and donors; (2) posthumous reproduction and extraction, including usage of cryopreserved sperm and embryos; (3) the potential responsibilities and liability of providers in the context of preserving their patients' fertility and parentage status; (4) model legislation addressing these issues within the United States; and (5) a brief look into the future in terms of identifying prospective medical advances that will likely impact and potentially alter these currently identified legal issues.**

Adult males and informed consent issues

Preserving male fertility through sperm collection and freezing is the most commonly recognized, and likely most frequently performed, of all fertility preservation measures. **Legal issues raised by this practice center around informed consent for obtaining and using collected semen – most critically, the future circumstances under which the sperm may be used and the legal status of any child or children resulting from such use.** Informed consent issues may also arise over posthumous extraction, as discussed in a subsequent section. It is assumed that the reader is acquainted with the standard elements of informed consent: disclosure, comprehension, voluntariness, competence, and consent [1]. As in other medical contexts, professionals should be well aware of the need to ensure that their patients are fully informed of and understand the risks, benefits, and alternatives to any potential treatment(s) that will impact or protect their current or future fertility; and that the patients are fully competent to choose to consent, or refuse to consent, to certain forms of preservation or usage of their genetic material. Legal liability may also arise over the handling of frozen sperm samples, including mislabeling, misuse, or failure to safely maintain samples in a usable, frozen state. Finally, legal issues may be raised if physicians or other medical professionals do not discuss collection and banking as an option prior to offering or administering medical treatment, such as chemotherapy or radiation, which may impair their patients' fertility. While many of these legal principles apply within any country or legal jurisdiction, readers should be mindful that specific laws can vary both amongst countries and in states within a country. A number of the court cases and legal precedents cited

Infertility in the Male, 4th edition, ed. Larry I. Lipshultz, Stuart S. Howards, and Craig S. Niederberger. Published by Cambridge University Press. © Cambridge University Press 2009.

within this chapter refer to conflicts that arose within the United States.

Frozen sperm has an indefinite "shelf-life," and published reports indicate children have been born from sperm frozen for well over a decade. Legal issues surrounding frozen sperm usage therefore involve multiple future scenarios, and require carefully drawn informed consent documents.

As an initial matter, medical professionals will want to recognize those medical conditions and treatments that may impair fertility, and to inform their patients accordingly. **Failure to explain both the risks of compromised fertility and the available measures to preserve fertility prior to treatment might give rise to a legal claim for negligence or malpractice, depending on the facts and circumstances.** The authors are unaware of any reported cases of this nature to date. A published report from a 2002 study found that of 201 male cancer patients between the ages of 14 and 40 diagnosed with cancer within the previous two years, 60% were warned about infertility and 51% were offered an opportunity to bank their sperm [2]. A more recent study confirmed that 30–40% of male cancer patients report that their physicians fail to raise the issue of fertility or sperm preservation [3]. One consumer organization reports that although 91% of oncologists agree sperm banking should be offered to all male patients at risk of infertility from cancer treatments, only 10% do so; only 57% of patients recall receiving such information from a healthcare provider, and 40–50% do not recall any discussion of infertility before their cancer treatment [4].

Appropriate informed consent documents will obviously need to address adult male patients' future volitional use of their sperm. Less commonly included, but highly recommended, is language that explicitly addresses (1) any approved use following a patient's incapacity or death, as well as (2) a patient's intended relationship to any resulting child. **Professionals should be aware of both of these significant, potential legal issues in order to counsel their patients, provide supplemental documentation, and obtain appropriate informed consent.**

Adult male patients will want to consider the possibility that their present or future partner, or even another family member, may wish to have a child with their sperm at a point in time when they are incapable of giving contemporaneous informed consent to the use of the sperm due to incapacity or death. If a specific medical condition has been diagnosed, such as cancer

or amyotrophic lateral sclerosis (ALS), informed consents may be tailored to explicitly identify such condition and the adult male's consent for specific, delineated future usages. The more specific and comprehensive the consent document, the more likely conflicts will be avoided and partners, physicians, sperm banks, or courts can avoid the need to interpret ambiguous or contested intentions. Within the United States, these issues are discussed in professional guidelines [3,5].

In the alternative, addenda to standard informed consent documents can provide needed specificity and should be considered. Either language can be drafted on behalf of the medical provider, or patients can be referred to knowledgeable legal counsel to draft proposed language (which the program or its own legal counsel can then review and modify as needed). Care should be taken to include language stating that any explicit addendum is intended to supplement and, as necessary, override a more general consent form. In many cases, the situation may be sufficiently unique that the medical program may not have, nor should it be expected to produce, a consent form tailored to the individual patient's condition. **However, failure to recognize and advise of the need for such a documented consent may not only deprive the patient of his reproductive choices but expose the provider to potential litigation involvement, if not actual liability.** It is thus advisable, at a minimum, to refer any such patient and/or his family for a legal consultation. These authors have drafted specific additional consents for posthumous sperm usage following multiple unusual scenarios, including: pre-chemotherapy storage; creation and future dispositions of embryos created with an about-to-be-infertile, unmarried partner; and a patient facing an ALS progression. At the other end of the spectrum, the authors have also advised surviving family members as to limitations on their access to, and use of, their deceased son's and spouse's sperm in the absence of such documentation. The latter scenarios are to be avoided if at all possible.

Male patients and cryopreserved gametes and embryos during lifetime

Because male patients can bank their own sperm, they are likely to have fewer legal issues surrounding cryopreserved material than female patients, who must either create and freeze embryos, and thereby compromise their autonomy, or freeze their eggs under protocols that are still widely considered experimental.

Nonetheless, the reader will want to be aware that cases involving divorce disputes over control and disposition of frozen embryos suggest an important judicial trend toward supporting the contributor who does not wish to procreate. Within the United States, all of these cases have raised the issue of aging and/or declining fertility for the female partner. Only outside the United States have a few recently reported cases involved patients with diseases or disease treatments that resulted in an inability to create additional gametes.

In the United Kingdom, Natalie Evans was denied access to frozen embryos she created with her ex-fiancé in anticipation of cancer treatments, which later rendered her infertile. When their relationship ended and he withdrew his consent, Evans argued that her former fiancé should not be allowed to withdraw his earlier consent to creation, storage, and implantation of the embryos. In ruling against her, the British and European courts cited with approval the Human Fertilisation and Embryology Act (HFEA), which requires consent from both partners at every stage of the IVF process, including implantation [6]. In 2007, after years of legal efforts, Evans lost her final appeal before the Grand Chamber of the European Court of Human Rights. The Grand Chamber rejected Evans' arguments that there were either discrimination or human rights violations under the European Convention of Human Rights, ruling that no violations of law had occurred. The Grand Chamber noted that the rules were clear, and fairly balanced her and her former fiancé's rights. No further avenues of appeal are available [7].

Within the United States, a couple's prior recorded agreement to dispose of the embryos in a way that does not implicate child-bearing has typically been enforced [8], while prior choices to allow one spouse to use the embryos for procreation over a current objection by the other have been rejected with increasing predictability. Thus, in cases in Massachusetts, New Jersey, and Washington [9], courts have been unwilling to enforce a prior agreement to allow (1) a wife to use embryos following the couple's "separation" [10]; (2) a husband to donate the embryos to another couple [11]; and (3) a wife to use embryos created with donor eggs to be implanted in the same gestational carrier who had carried the couple's first child [12].

Typically, courts are extremely reluctant to interfere with procreative or non-procreative decisions and the constitutional rights underlying them. Thus, this trend rests on the stated principle that ordering such usage amounts to "forced procreation," which, in the

words of one court, "is not amenable to judicial enforcement" [13]. Forced sterilization, contraception restrictions, and abortion laws have all been struck down as violative of individual constitutional rights [14]. An additional consideration is that under most states' laws, public policy considerations preclude a parent from waiving parental status and obligations such as child support. Thus, any agreement between spouses enabling one to use frozen embryos and the other to be relieved of parental rights and obligations is likely unenforceable as against public policy in most jurisdictions.

With significant state law variation, there remain many unsettled issues regarding establishing parenthood by intention. With regard to frozen embryos, regardless of whether embryos were created with donor gametes or not, the current trend is to require both partners to re-consent before either can use embryos they created at an earlier time for procreation, regardless of any prior agreement.

Donor gametes have also been involved with legal claims regarding embryo donation, discard, or custody of resulting children. Recent litigation involving donor eggs may shed some light on how courts approach such claims, regardless of whether the donated gametes in question are eggs or sperm. In at least two cases, intended genetic fathers have attempted to rely on the use of donor eggs as a factor in "tipping the scales" toward themselves in determining custody of children created with their former spouse who could not contribute genetic material. In each of those cases, the courts rejected the fathers' arguments [15]. In cases involving sperm donation, similar attempts and results occurred [16]. In a 2003 California case, the husband but not the wife involved in an embryo mix-up case involving a donor egg was granted legal parenthood of a child born to a single woman. His wife was found to have no standing whatsoever to the resulting child, despite the fact that the child was the genetic sibling of the couple's child and they had intended to use their remaining embryos for another child [17]. While these cases suggest there may be additional uncertainty and vulnerability for women who attempt to preserve their ability to parent, if not their fertility, through donor egg and frozen embryos, the applicability to males remains somewhat more attenuated.

Fertility preservation through donor insemination

Use of donor (sperm) insemination to create a family raises additional legal issues for infertile men, their spouses or partners, and the sperm donors involved. With sperm donation, an intended father's interest is both in preserving his legal parentage status despite not having a biological link to the resulting child, and in ensuring that the donor's health history and medical information are provided and do not raise health concerns for any resulting child.

Paternity issues with donor insemination

Within the United States, every state has adopted into law some version of a parentage act, which generally provides for establishing paternity through voluntary acknowledgment or through adjudication, and standards and rules for genetic testing. But with sperm donation long predating many of the developments in ART and IVF, and new statutes being crafted, approximately 42 states currently have laws that address sperm donation [18]. Most (approximately 28) apply to married couples, affirming the legal status of the infertile husband as the father of the child. A minority of the states (at least seven) – Delaware, Texas, Washington, North Dakota, Utah, Oklahoma, and Wyoming, with Nevada, Maine and Illinois recently introducing the 2002 version of the Uniform Parentage Act in their legislatures – are more inclusive, protecting unmarried and married men whose partners use donor insemination with their consent and who intend to father the resulting child. With multiple statutory variations from state to state, and state legislatures updating their ART statutes, it is impossible to generalize as to the currently applicable, specific requirements for any given state law. Some laws require written consent of the intended father; some require physician involvement; some require documentation of any consent by the intended father and/or physician. Following such requirements or practices can significantly reduce any ambiguity as to either proper consents or the resulting legal status of the child. **Careful medical practice would be to document all consents, regardless of whether such is a legal requirement in any given jurisdiction.**

Male patients and their spouses or partners will want to be careful to follow any prescribed steps to ensure their intended child is deemed their legal child. With married couples, and long-standing legal principles that a man is considered the father of any child born to his wife, there should be little reason for concern that a married man whose wife uses donor sperm with his consent will be legally recognized as the father of any resulting child. Less certain parentage outcomes may arise for children born to unmarried heterosexual

couples, to married men claiming lack of knowledge of or consent to any such inseminations, to gay male couples, or from sperm of a single man providing sperm to a female friend or acquaintance. In an example of how variable legal treatment of these arrangements can be, a court in Pennsylvania found a man to be the father of a child his former girlfriend conceived using his banked sperm, despite an agreement that the man would have no paternal obligations. The woman did not publicly acknowledge the donor father, but held out the child as the child of her ex-husband. The court called the woman's deception "despicable" but found her regrettable conduct to be outweighed by the child's right to a father [19]. A Washington court found that the unconsented use of a man's sperm also supported assigning him paternity obligations to the resulting child [20]. Many of these issues are outside the scope of this chapter, but they are noted here to highlight some of the unique and, in many respects, unsettled legal parentage issues involved in collaborative or third-party family-building efforts.

For all nontraditional couples whose family-building efforts do not fit neatly within a state's existing statutory laws, it will be imperative that they take additional steps to understand and, to the extent possible, legally protect their intended parentage. Independent legal consultations with knowledgeable attorneys in the field are strongly recommended. For both unmarried heterosexual or same-sex couples, a nonbiological intended parent might have no legal status regarding the resulting child absent an adoption proceeding or other legal steps that may be possible in a given jurisdiction.

For inseminations involving single women, determining whether from a legal perspective a known male who provides his sperm is a donor or an intended father may prove difficult. As noted above, different state courts have reached different outcomes interpreting their respective artificial insemination statutes and judicial precedent. A recent landmark decision from the Kansas Supreme Court upheld the constitutionality of its donor insemination statute [21]. That law requires a written agreement in order for a man who provides sperm to a woman to be deemed the legal father of any resulting child. Absent such an agreement, any man – known or unknown – is deemed a sperm donor with no parental rights or obligations. The statute was unsuccessfully challenged by a man who claimed that he had expected to be the legal father of any child born from his sperm to an unmarried acquaintance, and that to rule otherwise would unconstitutionally deprive him of his right to fatherhood. The court instead upheld the statute, finding the man had the responsibility of knowing and following the law. Many law professors and other legal observers had submitted "amicus" (friend-of-the-court) legal briefs to offer competing views to the court, and the case was watched with keen interest, given the significance of the ruling.

Donor screening and record keeping

Donor screening is required under a variety of state and federal laws, as well as professional guidelines. At a minimum, current practice dictates obtaining a donor's own and family medical history, FDA-required screening tests [22], and freezing and quarantining sperm samples for a minimum of six months prior to use. Guidelines for donor sperm currently come from individual states' laws, FDA and Centers for Disease Control and Prevention (CDC) regulations, and professional guidelines promulgated by the American Association of Tissue Banks and the American Society for Reproductive Medicine (ASRM). Guidelines recommend different types of testing, including initial donor screening, disease testing, and quality testing. Initial donor screening involves age selection (usually between 18 and 40), a physical examination, and personal interviews with the donor to evaluate his family history and psychological state [23]. Screening for diseases ensures that the donor does not carry harmful diseases such as HIV, hepatitis, or syphilis. Genetic tests are increasingly being performed as well [24]. Lastly, a donor's sperm is tested to confirm sufficient sperm count and sperm motility [25]. **A medical professional's failure to follow these rules will be a potential basis for liability.** Thus, for example, although quite common in the past, few physicians today would agree to use fresh semen for an artificial donor insemination procedure, even if patients offer to waive any future claims. ASRM recommends that only sexually intimate couples use fresh semen, because of the risk of transmission of HIV and other infectious organisms from fresh semen as opposed to frozen and quarantined semen [26].

With respect to record keeping, a number of state laws as well as ASRM guidelines require donor records to be kept for varying lengths of time. Current ASRM guidelines require maintenance of "permanent records about each donor's initial selection process and subsequent follow-up evaluations," as well as requiring that a "mechanism must exist to maintain these records as a future medical resource for any offspring produced" [27]. Although not legally mandated, there is continuing interest in, and efforts to create, donor gamete registries amongst many professional groups, and private registries have begun to spring up as well.

Minor male patients

Minors as patients raise unique informed consent issues in any medical context. Elements of informed consent include not only providing patients with adequate information as to the risks, benefits, and alternatives to any proposed treatment, but also the ability of the particular patient to comprehend and make informed choices. Depending on the age and mental capacity of a minor, he may or may not be able to give informed consent. A "mature minor" is capable of giving consent on his own behalf; a younger child is not. When incapable of giving informed consent for themselves, child patients – like other patients considered incompetent – may have adults do so on their behalf under a legal concept of "substituted judgment," interpretations of which vary from state to state. In theory, such judgment is intended to mean that the designated adult makes the decision he or she feels the patient, if competent, would make for himself. When that standard is impossible to meet, as is typically the case with a very young child, the adult is charged with making the decision he or she feels is in the minor patient's "best interest." Under no circumstances should a substitute decision maker be deciding what he or she wants independently of the minor child and his interests.

Preserving a child's fertility can be both a particularly sensitive issue and one not always recognized by providers or guardians when a child is facing a serious illness. Reports of scientific advances in the field of fertility preservation for children treated for cancer suggest that while the majority can expect to be cured and remain fertile, a significant minority remain at risk for subfertility. One reported estimate is that childhood cancer survivors will represent 1 in 250 adults aged 15–44 by the year 2010 [28]. Another study reports that 15% of child cancer survivors will have compromised reproductive function after their treatment [29]. **Given increasing survival rates for many childhood cancers and other serious illnesses whose treatment may affect future fertility, providers should be cognizant of, and inform their patients of, available options for fertility preservation, as well as the degree to which such options are experimental or of proven efficacy.**

Treatment options range from sperm retrieval to invasive procedures in order to harvest gonadal tissue [30]. The latter procedures have been described as experimental, with some medical professionals calling for "appropriate regulation and ethical scrutiny in order to prevent the exploitation of vulnerable individuals by commercially driven technology" [31]. Providers will want to proceed cautiously in terms of providing sufficient information as to available treatments and appropriate cautions as to the level of experimentation of some of those treatments, particularly in light of the increased vulnerability of child patients. Substituted judgment issues may arise, and jurisdictions (states) vary on the legal requirements for a parent to give consent on behalf of a minor child. **The core principle, however, should remain that the judgment being substituted for the child's is intended to be that which he, if mature and able to reach his own judgment, would make on his own – not another's – behalf.**

As a matter of cautious medical practice, providers will need to ascertain whether any requested or offered sperm preservation is in their patients' best interests or is being requested by a family member for other future potential uses. To the extent that fertility preservation is offered for patients whose life expectancy is anticipated or hoped to extend sufficiently into adulthood to use any cryopreserved sperm, good medical practice will require offering that option to the patients or their representatives. If, however, a minor patient's condition is terminal, any request by parents or other family members to preserve the patient's sperm may raise serious questions as to the appropriateness of honoring such a request, and professionals will want to ensure that they can obtain informed consent from and on behalf of the minor patient. Anecdotal evidence of cases where grieving parents have sought to preserve sperm of adolescent or preadolescent sons suggests that this is an area invoking extreme sensitivity and caution.

Posthumous reproduction and extraction

Posthumous reproduction raises additional legal complexities, including determination of the legal status of any resulting child under applicable law, which varies from jurisdiction to jurisdiction, within the United States as well as internationally. In recent years, a number of US courts have been presented with issues involving children whose biological fathers died before their conception through either artificial insemination or in-vitro fertilization. Most of these cases have arisen in the context of a child's qualification for governmental (Social Security) survivor benefits, which, although a federal entitlement, rests on state law definitions of who is a legal heir, and thus requires courts to interpret and apply state laws to determine whether the child is the legal child of the deceased for purposes of intestate (without a will) inheritance [32]. Most such state laws were drafted prior to, and thus without any thought of, the possibilities of posthumous reproduction.

Over the past decade, there have been at least eight reported cases within the United States involving posthumous parenting, and others reported internationally. Anecdotally, there appear to be many more. Two of the reported cases in the United States and one in the United Kingdom have involved issues of whether or not to release sperm of a deceased man to attempt a pregnancy. Five of the reported decisions by United States state courts or administrative bodies have decided cases involving posthumous parenting in the context of survivor benefits for born children.

The two known United States cases involving whether to release sperm of a deceased man to his former fiancée or girlfriend for her to attempt a pregnancy reached opposite conclusions. A California court, in an unpublished decision, awarded some banked sperm to a deceased's fiancée, ruling that his written intention was clear and that posthumous conception was not against the public policy of that state [33]. In the second case, a Louisiana court affirmed a preliminary injunction against the use of sperm where evidence was conflicting as to the decedent's intentions for posthumous use: his extended family – including his adult son, sister, and mother – all objected, he and his female partner had not been actively undergoing inseminations at the time of his death, and the written "Act of Donation" she attempted to rely upon was drawn up by her law partner rather than a disinterested professional [34].

In Britain, one widow successfully pursued a lengthy court battle to get access to her deceased husband's stored sperm and to have him legally recognized as the father of the two children she conceived after his death [35]. Diane Blood's efforts ultimately resulted in a London High Court judge ruling that the 1998 European Convention on Human Rights overrides inconsistent language in Britain's Human Fertilisation and Embryology Act 1990 and Deceased Fathers Act

2003, which stated that a man is not the father of a child created posthumously with his sperm. Subsequent efforts to amend the Act resulted in its repeal and passage of the Human Fertilisation and Embryology Act 2008, effective April 6, 2009 [36]. The new British law addresses posthumous parentage and requires specific consents be executed prior to death. Under the new law, if proper consents are in place prior to death, a husband or partner may be considered the legal father of a child born from his previously stored sperm or embryos. If donor sperm was used, only if embryos were created prior to the husband's or partner's death can any child be considered his offspring. For any posthumously conceived child using donor sperm, the deceased husband or partner cannot legally be considered a parent.

Decisions in Louisiana, New Jersey, Arizona, Massachusetts, Florida, and New Hampshire have come down regarding the legal parentage of posthumously born children. In Massachusetts, New Jersey, Louisiana, and Arizona, the children were found to be the legal children of the deceased; in Florida and New Hampshire the court rejected parenthood. Each court's decision was based on its interpretations of its own, controlling state law.

Judith Hart, born in Louisiana in 1991, was conceived three months after her father died from cancer, using sperm he had banked for that purpose. Because Louisiana law recognizes parentage only if a child is born during or within several months of the father's lifetime, the Social Security Administration initially denied social security benefits, but later reversed, acknowledging that the case "raises significant policy issues that were not contemplated when the … Act was passed many years ago … recent advances in … the field of reproductive medicine necessitate a careful review of current laws and regulations to ensure that they are equitable in awarding Social Security payments" [37].

Following the ground-breaking *Hart* case, a New Jersey court in *In re Estate of William Kolacy* essentially reversed a federal court's refusal to recognize the paternity of twins born 18 months after their biological father's death and conceived via in-vitro fertilization [38]. The court ruled that "once a child has come into existence … a fundamental policy of the law should be to enhance and enlarge the rights of each human being to the maximum extent possible, consistent with the duty not to intrude unfairly upon the interests of other persons." The court emphasized that while this new technology could be applied in positive ways, it also creates ethical, legal, and social policy problems.

Thus, prospective parents should consider carefully the consequences of using posthumous conception technology, and "the law should certainly be cautious about encouraging parents to move precipitously in this area" [39].

The Massachusetts Supreme Judicial Court became the first highest appellate state court to rule on this issue in *Woodward* v. *Commissioner of Social Security* [32]. In that case, the court found paternity for twins conceived by the decedent's widow after his death, identifying three critical proof requirements for inheritance eligibility: (1) that the children are in fact the genetic children of the deceased; (2) that he affirmatively consented to posthumous reproduction; and (3) that he affirmatively consented to support any resulting children. The court required such "double consent" because the mere act of storing sperm to preserve fertility during life does not necessarily indicate an intention to father children after death. Further, the court advised that parties seeking inheritance rights must establish paternity and consent in court, and must formally notify "every other interested party," including other potential heirs. As the first high state court decision on this issue, the court's opinion may provide guidance to ART programs for creating appropriate consent forms concerning permissible posthumous uses of gametes and embryos.

Arizona law awarded benefits to twins born 10 months after their biological father's death in the case of *Gillett-Netting* v. *Commissioner of Social Security* [40]. In that case, a cancer patient's widow conceived after her husband's death by using his banked sperm, and relying on his prior consent. The Social Security Administration had denied inheritance rights because the twins were not alive or in gestation during the father's lifetime, as required under Arizona's intestate succession law. The Ninth Circuit reversed, finding that the twins were the decedent's legitimate children, since it had been conceded that they were the decedent's biological children. As legitimate children, the twins were "entitled to support and education as if born in lawful wedlock" under Arizona law, thus constructively fulfilling the additional legal inheritance requirement of dependency on an insured wage earner. Consequently, the twins were deemed to be dependent and entitled to benefits based on the decedent's earnings.

In contrast, in *Stephen* v. *Commissioner of Social Security*, a Florida federal district court held that a child conceived from the sperm of an insured individual who died before the transfer of sperm to his widow's body was not entitled to child's survivor benefits [41]. Under Florida law, a child conceived from the sperm of a person who died before the transfer of his sperm to a woman's body is not eligible for a claim against the decedent's estate unless the decedent provided for the child in his will. Here, there was no evidence that the decedent had left a will, and thus the child was found to have no standing to pursue the claim.

Most recently, two state courts within the United States have rejected a deceased man's legal parentage of a child conceived after this death. The Supreme Court of New Hampshire weighed in on this issue in *Khabbaz* v. *Commissioner, Social Security Administration*, holding that a child conceived after her father's death via artificial insemination was not eligible to inherit from her father as his surviving issue under New Hampshire intestacy law [42]. Rejecting a series of arguments made on behalf of the child based on various New Hampshire statutes, the court concluded that the question was governed solely by the intestacy statute, and interpreted the statute's term "surviving issue" to preclude any child not born prior to the decedent's death. Although, like the decedent in *Woodward*, the decedent had affirmatively consented both to posthumous reproduction and to support any resulting children, the court declined to read the statute more broadly or follow the ruling or rationale of *Woodward*. It did, however, emphasize the need for clarifying legislation to address the important public policy considerations at stake. Similarly, the Arkansas Supreme Court rejected a posthumous parentage claim involving a child born from a posthumous frozen embryo transfer created from the deceased husband's sperm [43]. That court refused to either apply its artificial insemination statute (which recognized posthumous parentage) to IVF or to read its 1969 statute more liberally given the advance in reproductive medicine. The court also rejected a novel claim by the widow that the child was "conceived" when the frozen embryo was created, an argument that could have had far-reaching implications for reproductive law and medicine far beyond the issues in dispute.

The war in Iraq has raised additional legal issues related to posthumous reproduction. With sperm banking increasingly common prior to deployment, several children are reported to have been conceived using the sperm of dead military personnel. Posthumous sperm *retrieval*, where sought, may also be complicated due to the protocols involved in releasing a body for the necessary procedures. All of the issues involving posthumous parentage may be compounded, since military families are typically more mobile so that the state of residence may be more fluid, qualification for military benefits may be defined differently than other entitlements, and documents provided by the military in terms of consents at banking may be interpreted differently in different jurisdictions [44].

Posthumous parenthood raises both issues of law and concerns about intentionality. While laws clearly vary from jurisdiction to jurisdiction, courts are also being forced to interpret and extend existing laws. **Thus, patients and providers will want to be aware of, and act consistently with, applicable law in their jurisdiction. It is also advisable to put in writing, as clearly as possible, the intentions of the adult male who is preserving his sperm. It is highly advisable to use consent forms with the sperm bank and physician, and between donors and recipients, to identify explicitly who may use the sperm, and to limit the purposes, time frame, and circumstances for use. Such anticipatory steps may avoid the need to seek court orders by surviving widows, fiancées, and parents, all of which have been pursued with varying outcomes.**

Posthumous extraction of sperm from deceased patients will also raise significant issues of informed consent to both the procedure and future use. Programs presented with such unusual circumstances may wish to seek immediate legal or judicial advice, as without specific informed consent prior to death it is difficult to imagine that there is adequate authorization to use the genetic material. Anecdotal evidence of such extraction and use has been documented; one court reportedly "froze the status quo" by ordering the sperm collected but not used without further investigation and inquiry [45].

The question of whether an adult male intended to father a child after his death has troubled courts and ethicists alike. Even with clearly stated intentions, legal recognition of paternity will depend on both applicable laws and evolving public policy in the relevant country and jurisdiction.

Provider liability issues
Providers of medical and insurance services may be found liable for breaches of duties owed to recipients of their services. As discussed above, provider liability may arise from possible breaches of the informed consent doctrine. Not disclosing or not offering an available treatment that has the potential of improving patients' chances of preserving their fertility, or not disclosing the experimental or unproven nature of

some of such treatments or the legal uncertainty associated with such treatments, may each create liability. Although no known cases have arisen in this context to date, today's experimental procedures, such as testicular sperm extraction and testicular tissue freezing, will continue to be explored and developed [46], and providing patients with this information will likely be within the required duties of providers. Further, genetics research indicates that microdeletions in intervals 5 and 6 on the Y chromosome may be associated with male infertility [47]. Thus, genetics tests may increasingly become available to diagnose and to effectively treat this condition, widening potential liability to a larger group of healthcare providers. **If and when any such procedures become an accepted standard, failure to inform patients of the procedures or to offer them may incur liability.**

In addition, providers may find themselves liable for other possible breaches of duty to their patients or to affected, surviving, or even potentially future family members. Each of those potential sources of liability is discussed briefly.

First, failure to maintain cryopreserved gametes or embryos may be grounds for negligence and/or breach of contract claims. Power failures, mistaken transfers or destruction, and lost or misappropriated embryos or gametes all take on added significance and legal vulnerability if the patients who created and stored the genetic material can no longer recreate and replace it. Thus, although the standards for liability will be the same as in a suit brought by any patient, the measures of damages can be expected to be much greater for patients with compromised future fertility, or for representatives of deceased patients. One example involved a faulty freezer storage tank resulting in lost sperm samples of 28 cancer patients in England, who filed a lawsuit against the hospital where the samples were stored [48]. The hospital later admitted liability [49]. A 2000 case brought against the Medical College of Wisconsin for allegedly lost and damaged sperm of a cancer patient was dismissed for lack of evidence to support claims of negligence and breach of contract [50].

Liability may also arise in the context of donor sperm, although a number of such potential claims are outside the sphere of fertility preservation. Adherence to professional guidelines and any applicable laws will minimize liability. **Providers may be vulnerable for alleged failures to screen properly or failure to collect and/or maintain records which reflect a donor's medical condition, genetic or otherwise.** Inadequate initial screening or inadequate safeguards for collecting and sharing donor information collected from other families or sources are all potential sources of liability. Failure to screen out or disclose a donor or his family's medical conditions can lead to litigation, with parents of an affected child claiming malpractice, negligence or their child's "wrongful birth," "wrongful conception," or other theory of injury. For example, at least two reported cases against a sperm bank and a medical program have arisen in the context of donor gametes and affected offspring [51]. Relying on different theories of law under different controlling state laws, and rejecting some of the theories of law put forth by the parents, both courts nonetheless made clear that programs are responsible for accurately screening sperm and disclosing information in such circumstances. One court cited the professional guidelines promulgated by the 33.

Liability may also arise in the context of surviving relatives attempting to access or block access to cryopreserved gametes or embryos of deceased patients. The popular press reported in 2007 that a Manhattan court barred a New Jersey couple from using their son's semen for grandchildren. The judge ruled that a New York sperm bank must destroy the samples from their son, who died in 1998, because the son had signified that he wanted the samples destroyed in the event of his death [52]. Comprehensive informed consent documents that specifically address future uses or restrictions are recommended in an effort to minimize, if not eliminate, such litigation. Alternatively, providers would do well to have language in their consents that permits them to do nothing and await a court order in the event of any dispute over release of genetic material.

Medical professionals should not be expected to know or convey the status of the law in what are widely acknowledged to be unsettled and nonuniform areas of the law. Consent forms should be drafted carefully not to overstate, or indeed in many cases to state at all, the applicable law. Just as lawyers do not perform surgery, medical professionals will not want to advise patients as to the legal status of their fertility preservation or future family-building efforts. **Consent documents that acknowledge the "unsettled state of the law," where applicable, and that recommend seeking independent, experienced legal counsel, are both appropriate and protective of medical providers and patients alike.** Addenda or supplemental consent forms should be considered in many circumstances. If programs do not have such documents, or the resources to develop them easily (more likely if there are rare circumstances applicable to an individual patient only), they may want to consider referring their patients to independent counsel to draft a proposed addendum or supplemental consent, which the program and its counsel can then review and modify if advisable.

With respect to medical liability claims, there remains at least the theoretical possibility of liability to a child born following treatments to preserve the fertility of his or her genetic parent(s). Informed consent or other defenses to actions brought by adult patients do not preclude lawsuits brought by resulting children who could not have been a party to any agreement, waiver, or consent. One obvious possibility is a child born following intracytoplasmic sperm injection (ICSI) due to a man's subfertility, claiming that his own subfertility is a direct result of his genetic father's condition. Most states have substantially developed law on the subject of "wrongful birth," "wrongful conception," and "wrongful life," with the majority rejecting claims for the latter essentially on the theory that any life has value over no life and therefore damages cannot be calculated. On the other hand, suits by parents for "wrongful birth" and "wrongful conception" have been recognized in some jurisdictions, with damages most frequently assessed for the cost of rearing an affected child [53]. Most of the law in this area predates developments in the fields of ART. **Thus, if efforts to preserve fertility result in children with genetic or other impairments, or impaired fertility, depending on applicable, evolving state law, medical professionals involved in those efforts may find themselves vulnerable to subsequent claims by or on behalf of such children.**

Finally, insurance providers may be found liable for failing to insure fertility preservation procedures that are ancillary to cancer treatments. In one case, a man being treated for cancer sued his insurance carrier for denying his request to insure sperm banking costs, alleging claims of breach of contract and breach of the duty of good faith and fair dealing [54]. As medical advances give patients access to more options, including more proven options, to preserve fertility, insurance providers will need to provide very specific coverage rules and clearly communicate them to their clients.

Model legislation

Within the United States, family law and determinations of parenthood are governed by state law and therefore vary from state to state. Old donor insemination laws apply in some states, while more recently enacted ART legislation or court decisions govern parental relationships in others. **In an effort to update the law, and to encourage consistency, at least two national bodies of lawyers have proposed model legislation for states to adopt that clarify varying state laws and provide standards to address the rights and obligations of those who are involved with and using assisted reproductive technology.** The 2000 Uniform Parentage Act, as amended in 2002, drafted by the National Conference of Commissioners on Uniform State Laws [55] (UPA) and the Proposed Model Act Governing Assisted Reproductive Technology drafted by the American Bar Association Section of Family Law's Committee on Assisted Reproductive Genetic Technologies [56] ("Model Act") will be addressed in this section. Although the existing proposed legislation is broader in scope than the current topic of male fertility, both the UPA and the Model Act attempt to address the rights and obligations of males involved in fertility treatments in the areas of posthumous reproduction, and both attempt to clearly delineate donor and fatherhood status. It should be noted that the sections in the Model Act dealing with parentage are drawn from and identical to the corresponding provisions of the UPA. Accordingly, they will be discussed concurrently.

One of the issues addressed in the proposed legislation is the parent–child relationship of a posthumously conceived child. The proposed language within the UPA and the Model Act states, "if an individual who consented in a record to be a parent by assisted reproduction dies before placement of eggs, sperm or embryos, the deceased individual is not a parent of the resulting child unless the deceased spouse consented in a record that if assisted reproduction were to occur after death, the deceased individual would be a parent of the child" [57]. The Comment to the UPA explains that the section is designed to avoid the problems of intestate succession that might arise if the posthumous use of a person's genetic material led to the deceased being determined to be a parent. Thus, the provision makes clear that consent to posthumous reproduction and posthumous intended parentage must be in writing and explicit. It does not, however, address multiple other significant concerns, including the marital status of the donor and recipient, indefinite or extended time periods, or potential competing claims by other heirs.

Both acts also address the male's status as parent or donor to children born as the result of assisted reproductive technologies. Both the UPA and Model Act state that while "a donor is not a parent of a child conceived by means of assisted reproduction, ... a man who provides sperm for, or consents to, assisted reproduction by a woman ... with the intent to be the parent of her child, is a parent of the resulting child" [58]. Thus, whether a male is considered to be a parent or donor hinges on consent, as a man who intends to be a parent of a child must consent in a record to all forms of assisted reproduction, while the requirement of consent does not apply to a male donor. Both acts go on to clarify that a male who fails to sign a consent can still be determined to be the father if "the woman and the man, during the first two years of the child's life resided together in the same household with the child and openly held out the child as their own" [59].

The effect of dissolution of marriage or withdrawal of consent is also addressed by both the UPA and Model Act. If a former wife proceeds with assisted reproduction after a divorce, the former husband is not the legal parent of the resulting child unless he has previously consented that if assisted reproduction were to occur after a divorce, the former spouse would be a parent of the child. This right is extended to unmarried men also by allowing a man to withdraw his consent to assisted reproduction at any time before it occurs, in which case, "an individual who withdraws consent under this section is not a parent of the resulting child" [60]. The Comment in the UPA points out that a child born through assisted reproduction accomplished after consent has been voided by a divorce or withdrawn in a record will have a genetic father but not a legal father. The section is intended to encourage careful drafting of assisted reproduction agreements to clarify intent.

The growing number of court cases and emerging medical technologies in a country of varying laws and precedent make it clear that legislation is needed. This need is further articulated in the prefatory note to the Model Act, citing a 10-year-old Fourth Circuit Court of Appeals decision, still apt today, that states: "We join the chorus of judicial voices pleading for legislative attention to the increasing number of complex legal issues spawned by recent advances in the field of assisted reproduction. Whatever merit there may be to a fact-driven case-by-case resolution of each new issue, some overall legislative guidelines would allow the participants to make informed choices and the courts to strive for uniformity in their decisions" [61]. **Until and unless uniform or model legislation is widely adopted by a majority of states, courts will need to continue interpreting the varying laws of individual states, and inconsistent rulings are likely to continue in this area.** Until that time, none of the proposed language or paradigms have legal authority, because to give legal effect to any model legislation requires the approval of state legislatures. Even with uniform legislation, uncertainties are likely to arise and need to be resolved.

Conclusion

Predicting the future has never been an easy task for the law, and the law surrounding male fertility preservation is no exception. An increased awareness and interest by patients, families, and offspring is inevitable, given the inquisitiveness of those who use these technologies and their resulting children, and the burgeoning of the field of collaborative reproduction, which continues to invent creative uses of technology, gametes, and embryos, including techniques of posthumous reproduction. If there is one thing that media stories of adolescents finding their "donor sibs" and cases involving posthumous parentage, donor versus dad arguments, donor registries, "yes banks," and freezing gametes and embryos have taught us, it is that the unimaginable of yesterday is the likely reality of tomorrow.

The legal issues surrounding male fertility preservation strongly suggest that professionals should have an increased awareness of both the availability of medical fertility preservation treatments and the degree to which various treatments are experimental or proven, as well as a broader understanding of the concept of fertility preservation as one that includes legal parentage issues. Medical professionals will want to be informed about appropriate and available treatment options, and their risks and benefits. They will need to thoroughly inform and advise their adult and child patients accordingly. Carefully drafted consent documents, including supplemental consents, or separate legal agreements, drawn up in consultation with experienced legal counsel, may be determinative as to patients' wishes being carried out. Both patients and their physicians may benefit from having separate, independent legal counsel advise them on novel issues, such as future use of cryopreserved gametes or embryos and the legal status of any resulting child. Physicians and patients will want to understand the legal aspects of preserving legal fertility or parenthood, beyond biological fertility, and the limitations and vulnerabilities that may surround that aspect of fertility preservation.

This chapter has focused on a general understanding of the legal issues involved in fertility preservation, both biological and legal. With rapid medical advances and variations in laws, definitive guidelines are not possible. It is hoped that this discussion will increase awareness of the relevant legal issues, aid medical professionals in their efforts to provide comprehensive care to their patients, and help protect the families they and their patients hope to create.

Acknowledgments

The authors would like to express their gratitude to Amy Tindell for her insightful research and editing assistance.

References

[1] Meisel A, Loren HR. Towards an informed discussion of informed consent: a review and critique of the empirical studies. *Arizona Law Rev* 1983; **25**: 265–346.

[2] Schover LR, Brey K, Lichtin A, Lipshultz LI, Jeha S. Knowledge and experience regarding cancer, infertility, and sperm banking in younger male survivors. *J Clin Oncol* 2002; **20**: 1880–9.

[3] Ethics Committee of the American Society for Reproductive Medicine. Fertility preservation and reproduction in cancer patients. *Fertil Steril* 2005; **83**: 1622–8.

[4] Fertile Hope. Community statistics. www.fertilehope.org/participate/community-stats.cfm. Accessed March 10, 2009.

[5] Ethics Committee of the American Society for Reproductive Medicine. Posthumous reproduction. *Fertil Steril* 2004; **82**: S260–2.

[6] BBC News. Woman loses frozen embryos fight. 2006, March 7. news.bbc.co.uk/1/hi/health/4779876.stm.

[7] BBC News. Woman "distraught" over embryos. 2007, April 10. news.bbc.co.uk/1/hi/health/6542657.stm.

[8] *Kass* v. *Kass*, 696 N.E.2d 174 (N.Y. 1998).

[9] *A.Z.* v. *B.Z*, 431 Mass. 150, 160, 725 N.E.2d 1051, 1058 (Mass. 2000); *J.B.* v. *M.B*, 170 N.J. 9, 783 A.2d 707 (N.J. 2001); *Litowitz* v. *Litowitz*, 146 Wash.2d 514, 48 P. 3d 261 (Wash. 2002).

[10] *A.Z.* v. *B.Z*, 431 Mass. 150, 725 N.E.2d 1051 (Mass. 2000).

[11] *J.B.* v. *M.B*, 170 N.J. 9, 783 A.2d 707 (N.J. 2001).

[12] *Litowitz* v. *Litowitz*, 146 Wash.2d 514, 48 P. 3d 261 (Wash. 2002).

[13] *A.Z.* v. *B.Z*, 431 Mass. 150, 160, 725 N.E.2d 1051, 1058 (Mass. 2000).

[14] *Skinner* v. *Oklahoma*, 316 U.S.535 (1942); *Eisenstadt* v. *Baird*, 405 U.S. 438 (1972); *Roe* v. *Wade*, 410 U.S. 113 (1973).

[15] *MacDonald* v. *MacDonald*, 608 N.Y. S. 2d 477 (App. Div. 1994); *Ezzone* v. *Ezzone*, No. 96-DR-000359 (Ohio Lake County Ct. C.P. 1996).

[16] *State ex rel. H.* v. *P*, 90 A.D.2d 434, 457 N.Y.S.2d 488 (N.Y.A.D. 1982); *In re Marriage of Phillips*, 274 Kan. 1049, 58 P. 3d 680 (Kan. 2002); *In re Raphael P*, 97 Cal.App. 4th 716, 118 Cal.Rptr.2d 610 (Cal.App. 1 Dist. 2002); *Lane* v. *Lane*, 121 N.M. 414, 912 P. 2d 290 (N.M.App. 1996).

[17] *Robert B.* v. *Susan B*, 109 Cal.App. 4th 1109, 135 Cal. Rptr.2d 785 (Cal.App. 6 Dist. 2003).

[18] Roberts P. Biology and beyond: the case for passage of the new Uniform Parentage Act. Center for Law and Social Policy, 2000. www.clasp.org/publications/biology_and_beyond.pdf. [The District of Columbia, Hawaii, Maine, Pennsylvania, South Dakota, and Vermont do not have laws governing artificial insemination.]

[19] *Ferguson* v. *McKiernan*, 855 A.2d 121 (Pa.Super. 2004), *appeal granted in part by* 868 A.2d 378 (Pa. 2005).

[20] *In re Parentage of J.M.K*, 155 Wash.2d 374, 119 P. 3d 840 (Wash. Sep 15, 2005).

[21] *In the Interest of K.M.H. and K.C.H.*, 169 P. 3d 1025 (Kansas 2007).

[22] American Society for Reproductive Medicine. 2006 Guidelines for gamete and embryo donation. *Fertil Steril* 2006; **86** (5 Suppl): S38–50, § VI(B)(5). [HIV-1 and -2, hepatitis C antibody, hepatitis B surface antigen, hepatitis B core antibody, serologic test for syphilis, HTLV-1 and -2, CMV, *Neisseria gonorrhoeae*, abbreviated retesting every 6 months, tests required by local or state laws.]

[23] 2006 ASRM Guidelines § VI(A).

[24] 2006 ASRM Guidelines § VI(2, 3, 5).

[25] 2006 ASRM Guidelines § VI((1).

[26] 2006 ASRM Guidelines § VI(B)(9).

[27] 2006 ASRM Guidelines § VI(B)(5).

[28] Bleyer WA. The impact of childhood cancer on the United States and the world. *CA Cancer J Clin* 1990; **40**: 355–67.

[29] British Fertility Society. A strategy for fertility services for survivors of childhood cancer. British Fertility Society, 2002. www.britishfertilitysociety.org.uk/practicepolicy/documents/fccpaper.pdf.

[30] Grundy R, Gosden RG, Hewitt M, *et al.* Fertility preservation for children treated for cancer (1): scientific advances and research dilemmas. *Arch Dis Child* 2001; **84**: 355–9.

[31] Grundy R, Larcher V, Gosden RG, *et al.* Fertility preservation for children treated for cancer (2): ethics of consent for gamete storage and experimentation. *Arch Dis Child* 2001; **84**: 360–2.

[32] *Woodward* v. *Commissioner of Soc. Security*, 435 Mass. 536, 760 N.E. 2d 257 (Mass. 2002).

[33] *Johnson* v. *Superior Court*, 101 Cal.App. 4th 869, 882 (Cal.App. 2 Dist. 2002).

[34] *Hall, executrix* v. *Fertility Institute of New Orleans*, 647 So.2d 1348, 1994 La.App.LEXIS 3294 (1994).

[35] Dyer C. Diane Blood law victory gives her sons their "legal" father. *Guardian Unlimited* 2003, Sep. 19. www.guardian.co.uk/science/2003/sep/19/genetics.uknews; News PA. Diane Blood wins paternity rights for children. *Times Online* 2003, Feb. 28.

[36] Human Fertilisation and Embryology Act 2008; www.hfea.gov.uk/en/1784.html. Accessed March 11, 2009.

[37] *Hart* v. *Charter*, No. 94–3944 (E.D. La. dismissed March 18, 1996).

[38] *In re estate of William Kolacy*, 332 NJ Super.593, 753 A.2d 1257 (N.J.Super.Ch. 2000).

[39] *In re estate of William Kolacy*, 332 NJ Super.593, 605, 753 A.2d 1257 (N.J.Super.Ch. 2000).

[40] *Gillett-Netting* v. *Commissioner of Soc. Security*, 371 F.3d 593 (9th Cir. 2004), rev'ing 231 F.Supp. 2d 961 (D.Ariz. 2002).

[41] *Stephen* v. *Commissioner of Social Security*, 386 F.Supp. 2d 1257 (M.D.Fla. 2005).

[42] *Khabbaz* v. *Commissioner, Social Security Administration*, 930 A.2d.1180 (N.H. 2007).

[43] *Finley v. Astrue,* 2008 Ark. LEXIS 2 (1/10/08).

[44] Douncettperry M. To be continued: a look at posthumous reproduction as it relates to today's military. *The Army Lawyer* 27-50-420, May 2008. www.loc.gov/rr/frd/Military_Law/pdf/05-2008.pdf. Accessed March 11, 2009.

[45] Trial court personnel, personal communication to the author.

[46] Fertile Hope. Parenthood options. www.fertilehope.org/learn-more/cancer-and-fertility-info/parenthood-options-men.cfm. Accessed March 10, 2009.

[47] Choi JM, Chung P, Veeck L, *et al.* AZF microdeletions of the Y chromosome and in vitro fertilization outcome. *Fertil Steril* 2004; **81**: 337–41.

[48] Thompson J. Faulty freezer ruins 28 cancer patients' stored sperm. *The Independent* 2003, Jul. 20. news.independent.co.uk/uk/health_medical/article96871.ece; Kaiser Network. British patients whose stored sperm was destroyed when freezer tank failed sue hospital, *Daily Reports* 2003, Aug. 13. www.kaisernetwork.org/daily_reports/rep_index.cfm?DR_ID=19342.

[49] Armstrong R. Cancer patients sue over sperm damage. *Evening News* 2004, Dec. 14. WLNR 13993819.

[50] *Levsen* v. *Medical College of Wisconsin*, 241 Wis.2d 50, 622 N.W.2d 770 (Wis.App. 2000).

[51] *Johnson* v. *Superior Court*, 101 Cal.App. 4th 869, 124 Cal.Rptr.2d 650 (Cal.App. 2 Dist. 2002); *Paretta* v. *Med. Offices for Human Reproduction*, 760 N.Y.S.2d 639 (N.Y.Sup. 2003).

[52] Gregorian D, MacIntosh J. Son is "dead" again: kin denied his sperm. *New York Post* 2006, Nov. 3; United Press International. Use of son's semen for grandchild denied. 2006, Nov. 3. www.newsdaily.com.

[53] *Lloyd* v. *North Broward Hospital District*, 570 So. 2d 984 (Fla. Ct. App. 1990); *Siemieniec* v. *Lutheran General Hospital*, 117 Ill. 2d 230, 512 N.E. 2d 691 (Ill. 1987).

[54] *Lombard* v. *Kyocera Wireless Corp. Employee Health Benefit Plan*, Memorandum of P&A for Opposition to Defendant's Motion to Dismiss the Complaint Without Leave to Amend, 2004 WL 1558969 (S.D.Ca. 2004).

[55] National Conference of Commissioners on Uniform State Laws. *Uniform Parentage Act* (Last Amended or Revised in 2002) § 707, (2002). www.law.upenn.edu/bll/archives/ulc/upa/final2002.htm. Accessed March 10, 2009.

[56] American Bar Association Family Law Section Committee on Assisted Reproductive Technology and Genetics. *Proposed Model Act Governing Assisted Reproductive Technology*, 2007. www.abanet.org/family/committees/artmodelcode_feb2007.pdf. Accessed March 10, 2009.

[57] UPA, § 707; Model Act, § 607.

[58] UPA, §§ 702–3; Model Act, §§ 602–3.

[59] UPA, § 704; Model Act, § 604.

[60] UPA, § 706; Model Act, § 606.

[61] *In re Marriage of Buzzanca*, 61 Cal.App. 4th 1410, 1428–29 (4th Cir. 1998).

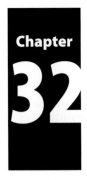

Analyzing male fertility data

Antoine A. Makhlouf and Craig S. Niederberger

The paradox of our times is that we are inundated by information yet starved for knowledge.

William R. Brody

Introduction

Our knowledge of male infertility, its causes and treatments, ultimately derives from raw observational and experimental data. Transforming those data into information depends on statistical analysis. Thus despite most clinicians' understandable reluctance when it comes to mathematical formulae, the male infertility specialist should have some understanding of the fundamentals of statistics, its foundation in the laws of probability, and its application to clinical problems. In this chapter, we will briefly review the basics of probability, statistics, and computer modeling, with special attention to problems relating to male infertility.

A quick review of statistics

Probabilities

Probability can be defined as the chance of a particular event happening. Mathematically, probabilities are represented by a value between 0 (impossibility of the event happening) and 1 (the event is certain to happen). For example, the probability of a random toss of a fair coin coming up tails is intuitively ½ or $P(\text{tails}) = 0.5$. Probabilities have some interesting properties that are relevant to clinicians. If two outcomes are mutually exclusive, the probability of getting one or the other outcome is simply the sum of the individual properties:

$$P(event1 \text{ or } event2) = P(event1) + P(event2)$$

For example, the chance of rolling a 1 or a 2 on a fair die is $1/6 + 1/6 = 2/6$. Since the sum of probabilities of all possible outcomes of an event is 1, the probability of an event *not* occurring can be easily calculated as:

$$P(not\ event1) = 1 - P(event1)$$

Two events are said to be independent if the occurrence of one does not alter the probability of the other happening. In this case, the probability of both events happening is the product of the individual probabilities:

$$P(event1 \text{ and } event2) = P(event1) \times P(event2)$$

Combining the above equations allows solving some problems of clinical relevance. For example, a 25-year-old woman's chance of pregnancy with natural intercourse is about 20% per month [1], and so the cumulative rate of pregnancy for an entire year is:

$$1 - P(\text{no pregnancy per month})^{12}$$
$$= 1 - 0.8^{12} = 0.93 \text{ or } 93\%$$

Thus a normal couple has an approximate chance of 7% of reaching the common clinical definition of infertility (failure to conceive in 12 months of unprotected intercourse) simply due to bad luck.

Similar calculations can be made when counseling couples on the chances of success using alternative strategies such as in-vitro fertilization with intracytoplasmic sperm injection (IVF/ICSI) versus vasectomy reversal [2]. For example, in a couple with a 40-year-old woman, assuming a 70% reversal surgical success rate and a 3% fecundity per month from natural intercourse at age 40, we can estimate the likelihood of conceiving within a year:

$$P(\text{birth in one year}) = P(\text{surgical success})$$
$$\times P(\text{birth from any of 12 cycles})$$
$$= 0.7 \times (1 - 0.97^{12}) = 0.21 \text{ or } 21\%$$

Assuming a 16% live birth rate per IVF cycle with testicular sperm in a 40-year-old female [3], we find that the reversal strategy success rates lie somewhere between one and two cycles of IVF/ICSI:

$P(\text{birth per one cycle}) = 0.16$
$P(\text{birth per two cycle}) = 1 - (0.84 \times 0.84) = 0.29 \text{ or } 29\%$

Infertility in the Male, 4th edition, ed. Larry I. Lipshultz, Stuart S. Howards, and Craig S. Niederberger. Published by Cambridge University Press. © Cambridge University Press 2009.

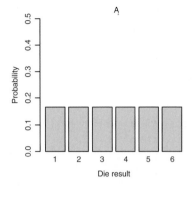

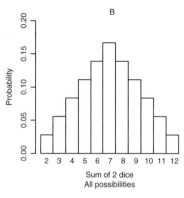

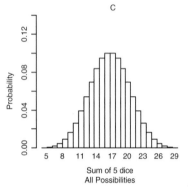

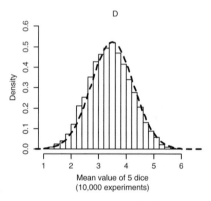

Fig. 32.1. The normal curve and central limit theorem. (A) Plot of probability of obtaining a particular result with the cast of one die, an example of a uniform distribution. Note that the area of all the columns (assuming unit width) sums to one. (B) Plot of probability of obtaining a particular sum with the roll of two dice. (C) Same as B, with five dice. (D) Results of 10 000 computer-simulated experiments in which the mean value of five dice was calculated (calculations and graphs done with the R statistical package). The Gaussian curve with the predicted mean (3.5) and standard deviation equal to predicted standard error of the mean (0.763) is superimposed.

Of course, the above example is highly simplified, and assumes constant conception rates per cycle independent of previous cycle outcomes (which is clearly not the case). For a more in-depth treatment of this problem, the reader is referred to papers dealing with cost-benefit analyses [4–8].

The Gaussian distribution

A probability distribution describes how the probabilities of all possible outcomes of an event are divided or distributed. When the chances of all outcomes are equal, we have a uniform distribution, such as the chance of getting a certain value with a roll of a die (Fig. 32.1A). When we are computing the number of successes or failures in a set of experiments, say the number of heads in a certain number of coin tosses, the binomial distribution is obtained.

In Figure 32.1B and C, we see the distribution of the sums of rolled dice as the roller increases the number of dice. Readers will immediately recognize the shape of the curve obtained after a large number of attempts as the "bell-shaped curve," or the Gaussian distribution. This distribution has a remarkable property. **No matter what distribution we start with, be it uniform, binomial, skewed, etc., if we take enough samples of** **the distribution and average their mean, the distribution of the means will follow the Gaussian curve.** This is illustrated in Figure 32.1D, where 10 000 simulated experiments of rolling five dice and taking their average was done. Most averages lie around 3.5, as predicted (3.5 = (6 + 1)/2 = mean of all possibilities). This is the central-limit theorem that lies at the heart of most statistical analyses. The formula of the curve, discovered by and named after the great mathematician Karl Friedrich Gauss, is:

$$P(x) = \frac{1}{\sigma\sqrt{2\pi}} e^{\frac{-(x-\mu)^2}{2\sigma^2}}$$

This is where μ is the mean and σ is the standard deviation of the population. These two parameters are all that is needed to describe the curve.

The probability that the mean from a certain population lies within a particular range is simply the area under the curve in that range (Fig. 32.2). This area cannot be calculated analytically, and is instead approximated numerically. In Figure 32.2, the area included is within two standard deviations from the mean and covers about 96% of the total surface, and so we expect 96% of experiments to give a result that lies within it. If

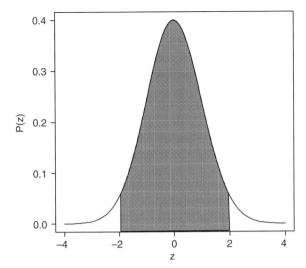

Fig. 32.2. The area under the normal curve determines the chance of obtaining a result within the hashed area.

we perform an experiment and get a result that lies outside that range, then we should be suspicious that the result obtained came from a different population with a different true mean. This forms the basis of inferential statistical tests, as we describe below.

P-value pitfalls

"*P* < 0.05" is the holy grail sought by many investigators. Readers have been conditioned to look for this statement in deciding the value of a treatment, or the importance of a factor. But what is a *P*-value of 0.05? Simply put, it means that whatever one says has a 95% chance of being right, and a 5% chance of being wrong. If the *P*-value is below a certain threshold – by convention 5%, or 0.05 – then the statement can be described as "statistically significant."

What kind of statements can we calculate a *P*-value for? A large number as it turns out. All we have to do is transform the statement into a mathematical statistic that has a known probability distribution (often the normal distribution in Figure 32.2), and then see whether the result falls within the proscribed range. Proper understanding of how the statements are framed, however, is necessary to avoid some pitfalls in interpreting *P*-values.

One of the most common examples in biomedicine is comparing the means in two groups. Let us say we wanted to prove that a certain drug *X* improved sperm counts with 95% confidence (i.e., *P* < 0.05). We would set up an experiment where one group of patients received drug *X* and another got placebo. We would then calculate the mean sperm counts in the two

groups, and determine if the difference was statistically significant. At this stage, many would recognize this as a situation requiring a *t*-test, employ their favorite software, and calculate the *P*-value. If the *P*-value was found to be < 0.05, they would interpret the study as a success, and rush to publication. But what if *P* was 0.06? Do they conclude the reverse and throw away all the work done on researching drug X? And even if *P* was less than the magical 0.05, does it really mean that drug *X* has an effect? To answer these questions, let us break the *t*-test into its components.

The first step is to formulate a mathematically testable hypothesis called the null hypothesis and denoted by H_0:

$$H_0 : \mu_1 = \mu_2$$

In other words, H_0 states that there is no difference between the means and that the drug has no effect and any observed difference is due to chance. The alternative hypothesis (the one we'd like to prove) is denoted as H_1:

$$H_1 : \mu_1 \neq \mu_2$$

To state that the drug had an effect, we have to accept H_1 by proving that H_0 is false with 95% confidence (or *P* < 0.05). While somewhat counterintuitive, this reasoning is at the basis of most inferential statistics. To disprove H_0, we first calculate the *t*-statistic:

$$t = \frac{\mu_1 - \mu_2}{SEM}$$

Where SEM is the standard error of the mean in the observed samples.

For calculation, the reader is referred to standard statistical texts. If H_0 is true, then the calculated *t*-value should lie close to zero. If the observed *t* falls outside an area covering 95% of the *t*-distribution curve around the value 0, then we can be confident that H_0 is unlikely to be true. In that case the *P*-value of the test is less than 0.05, and is in fact the chance of obtaining a *t*-value similar to or more extreme than the one observed. The smaller the *P*-value, the more confident we are in rejecting the null hypothesis and accepting the alternative hypothesis.

Having understood the *t*-test, we can easily answer the questions posed at the beginning of the section. A *P*-value under 0.05 simply indicates that the means of the two groups are different, but *P* < 0.05 does not tell us whether the difference has any clinical meaning.

On the other hand, a *P*-value higher than 0.05 means we could not reject the null hypothesis and that the results observed could be due to chance, and not a true difference between the two means. It does not disprove the alternative hypothesis. Thus with a *P* = 0.06, the investigator should not reject drug X, and should perform further studies. In fact, rejecting the alternative hypothesis when in fact it is true is known as a type II error. The likelihood of avoiding a type II error is known as the power of a study. In practice, many studies have low power because of high variability in the data and a small sample size. While the power of a study can usually be easily calculated, this parameter is seldom reported in most papers. Another pitfall in using *P*-values is the problem of multiple testing. Since a *P*-value is simply an indication of likelihood of getting results due to chance, if an investigator performs enough experiments and comparisons, he or she is eventually bound to reach a significant *P*-value under 0.05. This problem of multiple *P*-value testing is seldom taken into account in biomedical papers.

Diagnostic tests
Diagnostic thresholds and predictive values
Diagnosis (from Greek *dia*, apart; *gignoskein*, recognize or discern) means to separate medical conditions. The purpose of a diagnostic test is therefore to allow the clinician to confirm or predict the presence versus absence of a condition. **Mathematically, the utility of a test can be described by various parameters, the most commonly used being sensitivity, specificity, positive predictive value, and negative predictive value** [9].

Table 32.1 shows the four possible outcomes of a diagnostic test prediction when compared to the true condition. Table 32.2 demonstrates various ways to mathematically describe the performance of a test. An ideal test would have values close to 100% on all parameters. In the real world, however, this is seldom the case, and trade-offs abound. The relative importance of each parameter depends on the way the test is used, and the potential cost of a wrong decision (whether false positive or false negative).

In a screening test, where a positive (abnormal) result prompts further testing, the cost of a false negative (missed diagnosis) is clearly much higher than that of a false positive (additional unnecessary testing). Thus a high sensitivity is desired. The use of the semen analysis to determine if a full male evaluation is indicated is a clear example of its use in screening [10].

Table 32.1. Possible outcomes of a dichotomous test

		Actual state	
		Positive (abnormal)	Negative (normal)
Test result	Positive (abnormal)	True positive (TP)	False positive (FP)
	Negative (normal)	False negative (FN)	True negative (TN)

Table 32.2. Threshold-dependent parameters describing the performance of a test

Metric	Calculation
Classification accuracy	(TP + TN)/total
Sensitivity	TP/(TP + FN)
Specificity	TN/(TN + FP)
Positive predictive value	TP/(TP + FP)
Negative predictive value	TN/(TN + FN)

In contrast, when a test is used to decide whether or not to employ invasive therapy, then a high positive predictive value (PPV) is needed. For example, the diagnosis of ejaculatory duct obstruction must be well established prior to performing resection of the ejaculatory ducts (TURED), as the cost of performing a needless surgery can be very high. One strategy to use in these cases is to employ a sequence of confirmatory tests, so that the cumulative positive predictive value becomes acceptable (e.g., low semen volume combined with azoospermia combined with dilated seminal vesicles on TRUS is much more predictive of ejaculatory duct obstruction than each individually: see Chapter 23 for further details). Mathematically, this is due to the dependence of the PPV on prevalence. A positive preliminary test increases the prevalence of the disease, and therefore the predictive value of the confirmatory test.

Receiver operating characteristic curve
The calculation of sensitivity, specificity, and predictive values presuppose a test with a dichotomous outcome. Most tests in medicine, however, measure numerical values (e.g., sperm count in millions in a semen analysis, or transverse diameter of seminal vesicles in millimeters on a TRUS). Converting these into a dichotomous outcome typically involves choosing a cutoff point (or threshold) which separates normal from abnormal values. Clearly, moving this threshold

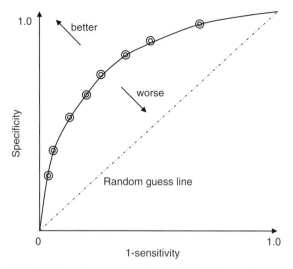

Fig. 32.3. Receiver operating characteristic (ROC) curve. The curve is traced by plotting the specificity versus 1-sensitivity at various thresholds (circles). The diagonal (dashed line) represents a random guess. The further away the curve is from the diagonal, the better the test.

affects the prevalence, sensitivity, and specificity of the test. A more stringent cutoff would give lower sensitivity but higher specificity. **To properly assess the utility and accuracy of a test, we have to come up with a measure that is threshold-independent. Such a measure exists, and can be obtained from the receiver operating characteristic curve of the diagnostic test in question** [11,12].

The roots of the receiver operating characteristic (ROC) curve are based in signal detection theory, and the concept was initially developed for enhancing detection of enemy airplanes on radar signals during World War II (hence the "receiver operating" part of the name). The curve can be obtained by plotting the specificity versus 1 – sensitivity of a test for all possible thresholds (Fig. 32.3). This traces a line with a characteristic appearance. The diagonal on the plot is the tracing of a test in which the outcome is a pure random guess (i.e., a useless test). The further away from the diagonal the curve is, the better the test (i.e., higher sensitivity and specificity). This quality of the test can be quantified by measuring the area under the curve (AUC). A perfect test has an AUC = 1.0, while a worthless test has an area of 0.5. The AUC value can thus be used as a means to globally assess the discriminating ability of a test regardless of thresholds, and allows proper comparison of the power of various diagnostic tests.

A mathematical look at semen analysis

The 20 million/mL cutoff for diagnosing oligospermia is arguably the most notable threshold in the field of andrology. We owe this number to the scientist John MacLeod, who published his studies on the semen quality of fertile and infertile men in the 1950s [13]. In the conclusion to his studies he wrote:

> the striking feature … is that the really significant differences are in the count range between 1 and 20 million/cc, where more than 3 times as many infertile men as fertile men are to be found … if an arbitrary level [for fertile sperm counts] is to be established, it should be set well below the 60 million mark previously accepted.

Let us look at MacLeod's data in light of our previous discussion. Figure 32.4 shows the distribution of sperm concentrations in 1000 fertile men, and in 800 men presenting with infertility (data derived from MacLeod [13]). Inspection of the histograms shows that the distribution in the infertile group is heavily skewed, while that of the fertile group is closer to the normal distribution. This is due to the fact that only 5% of the fertile men had densities below 20 million/mL, compared to 17% of the infertile cohort, a finding emphasized by MacLeod in his conclusions. Thus it seems that the 20 million/mL cutoff is reasonable. But superimposition of smoothed density curves shows a significant degree of overlap between the two groups. In fact, Table 32.3 lists the discriminating metrics of the sperm density test using the 20 million threshold value. **The low sensitivity of 17% makes semen density a poor screening test for infertility.** Can we improve the test by moving the threshold? The answer lies in calculating the area under its ROC. We have previously shown this to be a poor 0.59 [11]. Thus, the test itself and not the threshold is the culprit for the poor accuracy. This has been confirmed by a recent study by Guzick *et al.*, who found that a diagnostic threshold for fertility could not be established based on semen parameters alone [14]. Furthermore, 14% of men over the age of 45 fail to reach the current WHO criterion of 20 million/mL, and age-specific thresholds have been suggested as a remedy [15].

Does all this mean we should discard the semen density as a diagnostic test? Certainly not! However, caution in its interpretation and in counseling patients on its significance is in order. Similar limitations exist with other tests of fertility, including the traditional semen parameters of motility and morphology, as well as more novel tests such as sperm DNA integrity [16]. One indication of the complexity of this problem

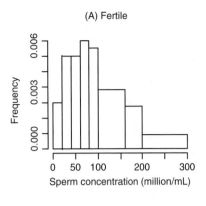

(A) Fertile

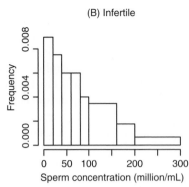

(B) Infertile

Fig. 32.4. (A and B) Frequency histogram of sperm concentration in 1000 fertile and 800 infertile men, from the data in MacLeod [13]. (C) Superimposed smoothed density functions of the same data. Infertile men are in bold dashed line.

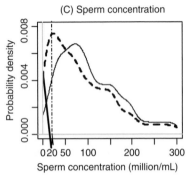

(C) Sperm concentration

Table 32.3. Metrics of semen density as a fertility predictor according to MacLeod's data using a threshold of 20 million/mL [13]. Data from Niederberger [11].

Metric	Value
Classification accuracy	56%
Sensitivity	17%
Specificity	95%
Positive predictive value	77%
Negative predictive value	53%

has been that agreement on new threshold values for the upcoming WHO Manual on Semen Analysis has lagged behind other sections of the manual. We eagerly await newer, more powerful tests of male fertility.

Outcome studies

The regression to the mean problem

Regression to the mean is a statistical phenomenon first described by the nineteenth-century English scientist Francis Galton. In his "Regression towards mediocrity in hereditary stature," he correlated the height of children to the mean of the height of their respective parents [17]. Not surprisingly, he found that there was

a linear correlation between the two variables. He also observed that when parents had a height well above the mean of 68.2 inches (173.2 cm), their children's height was usually lower (i.e., closer to the mean). Conversely, if the parents were shorter than 68.2 inches, say 65 inches (165.1 cm), their children tended to be taller, and again closer to the mean. He called this phenomenon, which is statistical and not genetic, the "regression to mediocrity." We now call it regression to the mean, and we refer to the line describing the relation between two variables as the "regression line."

For the mathematically inclined, this phenomenon can be expected by examining the slope of the regression line [18], which is:

$$slope = \frac{S_y}{S_x} r$$

Where S_x and S_y are the standard deviations of each variable, and r the correlation coefficient. Since r is always less than 1, then for any value of x, the predicted value of y is fewer standard deviation units from its mean compared to the deviation of x.

An intuitive way of thinking of the problem is that if we select "high scoring" cases by a criterion that involves some random element, then one reason those cases scored high is sheer luck, and that luck will not be a factor in a repeat measurement. The next score will therefore be closer to the average. In other words, in any measure with Gaussian distribution, spurious high scores are likely to descend, while low scores are likely to ascend. In male infertility studies, low semen parameters are often used as a selection criterion for study entry. **Because semen parameters exhibit high variability, regression to the mean dictates that an increase will be observed on repeat measurements, regardless of intervention. Thus a strong placebo effect is to be expected, and the use of controls in such studies becomes of the utmost importance.**

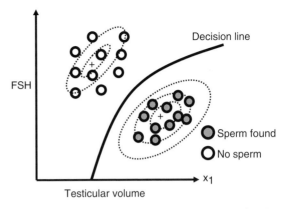

Fig. 32.5. Hypothetical decision space for the problem of predicting the outcome of testicular biopsy based on two variables.

The multivariate problem

Another problem confronting the andrologist is the multifactorial nature of male infertility. In practical terms, this means that it is often difficult to predict response to treatment because the outcome depends on the interplay of multiple factors. This problem is approached mathematically through the use of multivariate models. Understanding how these models are designed is important if one is to properly use the predictive tools derived from them.

A simple bivariate problem is presented in Figure 32.5, which depicts the outcome of testicular biopsy as it varies in patients with different testicular size and follicle-stimulating hormone (FSH). The entire range of possible combinations of variables is referred to as the "decision space." In this (hypothetical) example, a line can be drawn that neatly separates the two groups. The prediction problem then becomes a case of finding the equation of this or a similar line that separates the two outcome groups. There are several methods for obtaining the proper line. These methods are broadly divided into those that are linear and those that are nonlinear.

Linear models

In discriminant function analysis, the observed data are used to create a Gaussian probability distribution centered at the multidimensional mean of each group and with the appropriate standard deviations (represented by the plus sign and dashed contours in Figure 32.5). The value of each distribution at a particular point (x,y) corresponds to the conditional probability of finding a case at that point given a priori that the case belongs to that particular group. By using Bayes' theorem, the posterior probability of belonging to each group can be calculated, and the case classified into the group with

the highest posterior probability. This approach can be used to solve classification problems involving more than two groups.

Logistic regression is another, more popular, approach applicable only to dichotomous outcomes. In this method, each predictor variable is multiplied by a particular weight, and the sum of these products is then used to predict the outcome. The weights are adjusted by an iterative process until the classification errors for the known cases are minimized. **One reason for the popularity of logistic regression is that inferential statistical tests exist to determine if the weights are statistically significant (i.e., not zero). This allows researchers to report the predictive variables, and ignore the others in the predictive model.**

One example of the use of logistic regression is the prediction of sperm retrieval on biopsy. In a study of 100 patients with nonobstructive azoospermia, Tsujimura *et al.* found that serum testosterone, FSH, and inhibin B are predictive of sperm retrieval success according to the following formula [19]:

$$P(sperm\ found) = \frac{1}{1 + e^{(5.201 - 0.048\,FSH - 0.449T - 0.021\,Inhibin)}}$$

Interestingly, they found that age and testicular size were not significant predictors of success. The ROC area for this model was 0.76, a reasonable value.

Nonlinear models

What if the two groups could not be separated by a simple line, such as in Figure 32.6? In this case, the linear models, which can only generate simple lines or curves, cannot be used. Instead, a nonlinear model that allows

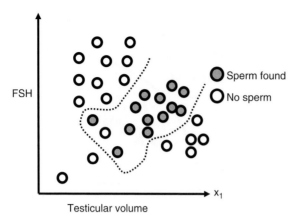

Fig. 32.6. Hypothetical decision space for the nonlinear problem of predicting the outcome of testicular biopsy based on two variables.

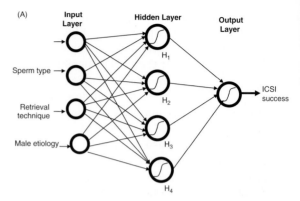

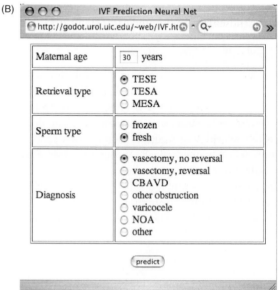

Fig. 32.7. (A) Schematic depiction of an artificial neural network (ANN) to predict IVF/ICSI outcome from surgically derived sperm (based on Wald et al. [20]). (B) Screenshot of computer-based prediction tool.

the generation of separating lines of any arbitrary complexity is used. Artificial neural networks (ANNs) are a prime example of such models. ANNs were initially inspired by the function of biological neurons, but they have acquired solid statistical foundation, and are currently considered but a single aspect of pattern recognition analysis. A typical ANN consists of several layers, each composed of one or more nodes. For example, the ANN in Figure 32.7 has one input layer, one hidden layer, and one output layer. Each node takes a series of inputs, which are summed after multiplication by adjustable weights. The output of the node is modified by the logistic activation function before being passed to the nodes in the next layer. The key parameters of neural networks are the weights, which are adjusted during training by minimizing the error function on known samples.

An example of ANN used in fertility studies is the prediction of IVF/ICSI outcomes with surgically retrieved sperm [20]. By examining 83 known cases, Wald et al. devised a predictive tool that can be easily accessed from any browser-enabled computing device (Fig. 32.7B), and that allows the clinician to counsel patients on the odds of success given various parameters such as female age and method of sperm retrieval. A similar approach has been used to predict the need for vasoepididymostomy at the time of vasectomy reversal [21]. As access to computing devices increases, we expect such tools to gain in utility and popularity.

Conclusion

In this chapter, we have presented a bird's-eye view of the application of statistical and computational methods to the field of male infertility. We have shown how

these applications can lie at the heart of clinical day-to-day decision making, such as in the use of semen analysis cutoff points. Beyond the classical statistical concepts taught in medical school, we have shown how emerging computational models can be used as clinical tools. We hope the reader has gained an appreciation of how data analysis impacts their practice, and that, for the mathematically curious, we have provided a starting point for learning more.

References

[1] Baird DT, Collins J, Egozcue J, et al.; ESHRE Capri Workshop Group. Fertility and ageing. *Hum Reprod Update* 2005; **11**: 261–76.

[2] Niederberger C, Makhlouf AA. Vasectomy reversal in the presence of diminished ovarian reserve: a complex clinical conundrum. *J Androl* 2006; **27**: 3–5.

[3] US Department of Health, and Human Services, Centers for Disease Control, and Prevention. *Assisted Reproductive Technology Success Rates, National Summary and Fertility Clinic Reports.* Atlanta, GA: CDC, 2005. www.cdc.gov/ART/ART2003.

[4] Shin D, Honig SC. Economics of treatments for male infertility. *Urol Clin North Am* 2002; **29**: 841–53.

[5] Kolettis PN, Sabanegh ES, Nalesnik JG, *et al.* Pregnancy outcomes after vasectomy reversal for female partners 35 years old or older. *J Urol* 2003; **169**: 2250–2.

[6] Heidenreich A, Altmann P, Engelmann UH. Microsurgical vasovasostomy versus microsurgical epididymal sperm aspiration/testicular extraction of sperm combined with intracytoplasmic sperm injection: a cost-benefit analysis. *Eur Urol* 2000; **37**: 609–14.

[7] Deck AJ, Berger RE. Should vasectomy reversal be performed in men with older female partners? *J Urol* 2000; **163**: 105–6.

[8] Pavlovich CP, Schlegel PN. Fertility options after vasectomy: a cost-effectiveness analysis. *Fertil Steril* 1997 Jan; **67**: 133–41.

[9] Altman DG, Bland JM. Diagnostic tests 2: predictive values. *BMJ* 1994; **309**: 102.

[10] Jarow JP, Sharlip ID, Belker AM, *et al.* Male Infertility Best Practice Policy Committee of the American Urological Association, Inc. Best practice policies for male infertility. *J Urol* 2002; **167**: 2138–44.

[11] Niederberger CS. Understanding the epidemiology of fertility treatments. *Urol Clin North Am* 2002; **29**: 829–40.

[12] Zweig MH, Campbell G. Receiver-operating characteristic (ROC) plots: a fundamental evaluation tool in clinical medicine. *Clin Chem* 1993; **39**: 561–77.

[13] MacLeod J. Semen quality in 1000 men of known fertility and in 800 cases of infertile marriage. *Fertil Steril* 1951; **2**: 115–39.

[14] Guzick DS, Overstreet JW, Factor-Litvak P, *et al.* Sperm morphology, motility, and concentration in fertile and infertile men. *N Engl J Med* 2001; **345**: 1388–93.

[15] Hellstrom WJ, Overstreet JW, Sikka SC, *et al.* Semen and sperm reference ranges for men 45 years of age and older. *J Androl* 2006; **27**: 421–8.

[16] Makhlouf AA, Niederberger C. DNA integrity tests in clinical practice: it is not a simple matter of black and white (or red and green). *J Androl* 2006; **27**: 316–23.

[17] Galton F. Regression towards mediocrity in hereditary stature. *J Anthropol Inst* 1886; **15**: 246–63.

[18] Bland JM, Altman DG. Regression towards the mean. *BMJ* 1994; **308**: 1499.

[19] Tsujimura A, Matsumiya K, Miyagawa Y, *et al.* Prediction of successful outcome of microdissection testicular sperm extraction in men with idiopathic nonobstructive azoospermia. *J Urol* 2004; **172**: 1944–7.

[20] Wald M, Sparks AET, Sandlow J, *et al.* Computational models for prediction of IVF/ICSI outcomes with surgically retrieved spermatozoa. *Reprod Biomed Online* 2005; **11**: 325–31.

[21] Parekattil SJ, Kuang W, Kolettis PN, *et al.* Multi-institutional validation of vasectomy reversal predictor. *J Urol* 2006; **175**: 247–9.

Chapter 33

Semen analysis

Susan A. Rothmann and Angela A. Reese

Introduction

Semen analysis is an important "gateway test" for evaluating male fertility [1–5]. As a noninvasive and relatively inexpensive test, semen analysis often is the first test ordered when a couple presents for a fertility workup or when a man is interested in permanent contraception [6–10]. The consequences of incorrect semen analysis results can be expensive invasive treatment or inappropriate focus on finding pathology in the wrong partner [11]. The utility of semen analysis in reproductive toxicant exposure assessment makes it an important tool for environmental and occupational health [12–14]. Semen analysis also is vital in monitoring conception control after interventions such as vasectomy [15,16].

Semen analysis does not test for a solitary analyte but is actually a panel of tests that measure many organ and gland functions (Table 33.1), each requiring different technologies and skills [17]. Semen is the composite product of fluids and cells from the testes and the male accessory glands, and contains primarily the following key elements [18–21]:

(1) a minute amount of clear mucoid secretions from the bulbourethral (Cowper's) glands that serve to lubricate the urethra and neutralize any residual acidic urine;

(2) a small amount of acidic secretions from the prostate that contain zinc, citric acid, acid phosphatase, and prostate-specific antigen (PSA);

(3) secretions from the cauda epididymidis and vas deferens that contain spermatozoa;

(4) alkaline secretions from the seminal vesicles that constitute most of the semen volume and contain fructose, prostaglandins, and seminogelin proteins.

Semen analysis is performed primarily in two types of settings: (1) general reference or hospital pathology clinical laboratories, where most of the initial screening is performed, and (2) andrology or fertility laboratories for more intense analysis, usually in a fertility treatment setting. Some post-vasectomy screening is still performed in physicians' offices, but the medico-legal environment, regulatory compliance, and certification costs have made many physicians unwilling to provide laboratory results.

No matter where it is performed, semen analysis is often unreliable [22]. In spite of the importance of semen analysis in fertility diagnosis and treatment, it remains in most clinical laboratories, "the neglected laboratory test" [6]. Some of the factors that make semen analysis results controversial and questionable are:

(1) Semen analysis is practically the last routine manual microscopic test in the laboratory, because of a lack of technology that is reliable, affordable, operator-friendly, and easy to integrate into laboratory workflow.

(2) Many laboratories use procedures that are outmoded or overly complex, or use equipment and supplies not designed for semen analysis. For many laboratories, the semen analysis procedure passes on through the years without any effort to modernize or validate it. **Conflicting opinions among experts about how to perform semen analysis are apparent in publications, notably the World Health Organization (WHO) manuals** [20,23].

(3) **Unlike most of current clinical pathology, semen analysis is not merely a data stream from an instrument, but relies upon and values the professional judgment of the analyst.** Unfortunately, training for semen analysis is often minimal or inadequate. Semen analysis is discussed for a few hours at most in medical technology education and often is not included in clinical training. The testing may not be

Infertility in the Male, 4th edition, ed. Larry I. Lipshultz, Stuart S. Howards, and Craig S. Niederberger. Published by Cambridge University Press. © Cambridge University Press 2009.

Table 33.1. Characteristics measured by semen analysis

Parameter	Characteristic or function
Semen volume	Fluid and protein products of male accessory glands (indirectly)
Coagulation	
Liquefaction	
Consistency (also known as viscosity)	
Sperm count	Spermatogenesis, spermiogenesis
Sperm motility	
Sperm maturity	
Sperm morphology	
Sperm viability	
Leukocyte concentration	Inflammation or infection

performed daily, so competency and speed are difficult to accumulate. In most clinical settings, few funds are available for postgraduate training. Many reference books and manuals on semen analysis give impractical advice for the laboratory that primarily performs screening semen analyses.

(4) Too many laboratories fail to understand principles of laboratory quality management. Many use quality controls (QC) that bear no resemblance to sperm or semen, or do not use any at all. More laboratories (but not all) participate in the many available external quality control or proficiency testing (PT) programs, but in many cases routine QC is overlooked and competency is rarely evaluated outside of a PT challenge. Without the benchmark that appropriate quality measures give, knowing whether a test is performed properly is very difficult.

(5) Although an important part of evaluating the male reproductive system, semen analysis only provides a snapshot of a few fertility markers, at a single point in time. Other, more sophisticated tests of sperm function add to the ability to predict fertility and find pathology. Several semen analyses are needed to provide a consistent picture of a man's seminal health. The results need to be taken in context with the man's history and clinical presentation, as well as his partner's [24]. Unfortunately, many men do not receive appropriate clinical consultation to accompany semen analysis.

Initial evaluation of semen

Semen specimens usually are collected by masturbation into a wide-mouthed polypropylene container from a batch or lot tested for lack of sperm toxicity. Collection of semen into a nonlatex, usually Silastic, condom during coitus appears to yield a higher-quality sample, but this practice is used infrequently [25–27]. Most references suggest that a period of 2–5 days of ejaculatory abstinence should precede semen analysis, but a recent study suggests that an abstinence of 1–2 days yields a specimen with better motility and morphology in men with oligospermia [28]. Declines in all semen parameters, especially sperm morphology, were associated with abstinence prolonged for more than 10 days [28].

Semen should be evaluated 60–90 minutes after collection. Recording both the time the sample was collected and the time the sample analysis was initiated is essential. When samples are transported to a central laboratory, or when patients cannot collect the sample at the laboratory site, the elapsed time can exceed many hours. This practice should be avoided, but, if necessary, should at least be brought to the physician's attention on the analysis report. Sperm motility decreases significantly after three hours, and continues to decline over the next 6–18 hours [29,30]. If delays are inevitable, samples should be kept at room temperature, since exposure to refrigerator or body temperatures accelerates the decline in motility [29,30]. Whenever possible, semen should be collected at the laboratory to permit observation immediately after collection and during liquefaction.

Creating a private and comfortable environment for both collection and sample receipt improves patient experience [31]. **The amount of time the man spends on sample collection is correlated with arousal and better sperm quality** [32]. Most men experience some embarrassment in discussing their semen collection, and all personnel, from the receptionist to the receiving technologist, must put the patient at ease. The patient must understand that honesty about abstinence time and any collection difficulties is an important part of the semen evaluation. At the time of sample receipt, the man should be asked when he last ejaculated, if the sample is complete, and if any portion was lost during collection. When this information is requested in multiple open-ended questions, the patient is more likely to give the true answer [31].

After the sample is received, it must undergo liquefaction before analysis commences. Upon ejaculation, semen immediately coagulates into a semi-solid gel, primarily by the action of seminal vesicle semenogelin proteins [33,34]. The proteolysis of semenogelin by PSA causes semen to liquefy, usually within 5–20 minutes [18], and thus loss or partial secretion of the first prostatic fraction during collection can cause incomplete liquefaction [35,36]. The change from the coagulated to the liquid state should be evaluated at 30 minutes and, if incomplete, at 60 minutes, by swirling the sample. Any residual gelatinous material or particles indicate incomplete liquefaction. Decreased motility can be a consequence, since intact semenogelin can immobilize sperm [33].

As with handling all biological fluids, handling semen samples carries the risk of exposure to infectious pathogens. Laboratory workers must use protective measures, such as gloves, fluid-resistant gowns, and eye protection, and dispose of materials contaminated by semen as biohazardous waste [37]. Many countries have specific laboratory occupational safety regulations that must be followed and documented (e.g., in the USA, Occupational Safety and Health Administration, or OSHA).

After liquefaction, the semen is assessed macroscopically. An obvious, unpleasant odor should be noted, as it may indicate infection or excessive sample age. The normal color is an opalescent off-white. Brown-colored semen is found frequently in assisted ejaculates of men with spinal cord injury, unrelated to red blood cells or heme [38].

Routine measurement of pH is not necessary and provides no useful clinical information if sperm are present [20,39]. Human semen pH measurements vary with technique and time after ejaculation, increasing immediately after ejaculation but decreasing as the specimen ages [40]. In the case of low volume and complete lack of sperm (azoospermia), pH may give some indication whether the problem relates to dysfunction of the accessory glands as opposed to specimen loss during collection, but other tests using biochemical markers or ultrasound examination are more reliable.

Some references recommend weighing the semen sample to get the most accurate volume measurement [41,42]. This practice seems overly stringent, given the variability of ejaculation during semen collection. Clear evidence exists that for many men, the typical practice of collecting a semen sample by masturbation yields less volume than found during coitus [25–27,32]. At best, volume measures are an estimate of the man's natural semen output, and probably are an underestimate.

As noted above, duration of ejaculatory abstinence has a major influence on semen volume, and rarely are sufficient ejaculates from a single man examined to determine his specific optimum. For these reasons, using a 5 mL serological pipette gives a volume measurement that is probably as reliable as possible or necessary with much less effort.

Mixing a semen sample thoroughly is critical for accurate sperm counts, both initially and throughout each step of semen analysis [17,43,44]. The liquefied sample should be pipetted into a conical centrifuge tube and vortexed at a medium speed for 2–3 seconds twice. During pipetting, volume can be measured and consistency (commonly referred to as viscosity) can be evaluated. If the sample leaves the pipette in drops, the consistency is normal; if it exits as a long strand or "thread," the consistency is high or abnormal. Samples with high consistency can be difficult to mix and pipette, and this should be noted to alert the physician that test results may be inaccurate due to unavoidable sample handling errors. Treatment of semen with chymotrypsin usually is effective in reducing the consistency and making the sample easier to process [43–45]. Any chemical alterations should be reported.

Microscopic examination

Next, the semen should be examined microscopically for the presence of bacteria, round cells, debris, agglutination (adherence of motile sperm to other sperm), or aggregation (adherence of sperm to other cells or debris). This can be accomplished by placing a drop or a 10 µL aliquot of the semen on a glass slide and coverslipping it to make a "wet preparation," or it can be performed at the same time as sperm counting if a chamber that does not require dilution is used (see below). Most semen contains a minor amount of debris, generally anucleate material smaller than a sperm head [8]. Moderate to heavy debris should be noted. Bacteria may indicate infection if the concentration exceeds 1000/mL, but can also represent contamination during sample collection, or colonization of the urethra [46]. Sperm agglutination suggests the presence of antisperm antibodies [47]. Enzymatic treatment can reduce agglutination and allow sample analysis [48–49].

Round cells include leukocytes and immature germinal cells, which can be reported as an average number per 10–20 high-power (× 40) fields or can be counted using phase microscopy. A peroxidase test can be used to detect polymorphonuclear neutrophils

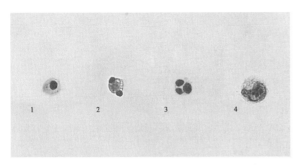

Fig. 33.1. Comparison of leukocytes and sperm precursors: (1) spermatocyte; (2) spermatid; (3) polymorphonuclear leukocyte (PMN) – note nuclear bridges; (4) monocyte – note large U-shaped nucleus, foamy cytoplasm. *See color plate section.*

(PMN), but peroxidase staining will not detect non-PMN leukocytes such as macrophages and monocytes, which can account for half of total leukocytes [50]. In a well-stained semen smear, PMNs can be identified easily by their multilobed nuclei connected by nuclear bridges and cytoplasmic granules not found in sperm precursor cells and other leukocytes (Fig. 33.1). If enumerated as number of leukocytes, or specifically PMNs, per 100 sperm, the absolute number can be calculated from the total sperm count. The common thresholds for leukocytospermia are over 1 million total leukocytes per mL of semen or over 500 000 PMN/mL [42,50]. Using the total leukocyte definition, approximately 10–20% of infertile men have leukocytospermia [51]. Leukocytes are poorly associated with infection, with about 20% of specimens positive microbiologically [51–53], and commonly indicate an inflammatory response in the epididymis or prostate [54,55]. Episodic leukocytospermia secondary to long-distance cycling-induced acute epididymitis has been observed in sperm donors (S. A. Rothmann and D. Houlihan, unpublished observations), and may occur chronically in competitive cyclists due to testicular trauma [56–58]. Leukocytospermia is associated with poor sperm quality due to the production of cytokines, hydrogen peroxide, and reactive oxygen species [50,51,59–61].

Manual sperm counting

The best way to view sperm is with a microscope equipped with a 20× phase-contrast objective. Many clinical laboratories do not use phase-contrast and use a 10× objective, making the procedure much more difficult. Adding phase optics to an existing microscope is a relatively inexpensive way to improve semen analysis.

Optimizing microscope illumination and maintaining the instrument are essential for good optical quality and specimen viewing.

In order to quantify the cellular elements in semen, a counting chamber must be used. Several types are available (Fig. 33.2). For many years, the hemacytometer was the only chamber available for sperm counting. However, the hemacytometer was not designed for semen or sperm counts, and using one generates a great deal of unnecessary labor and time spent, not to mention incorrect results [62,63]. Hemacytometers are associated with the largest variation in proficiency tests [64]. The semen must be diluted, requiring parallel dilutions and duplicate testing of the diluted sample to detect pipetting errors, which commonly occur [65]. The chamber depth of approximately 100 μm is completely inappropriate for a mixture of motile and non-moving cells. Figure 33.3 illustrates the problem. As time elapses, the nonmoving cells settle to the bottom of the chamber. The moving cells continue to swim up and down the depth of the chamber, with the result that all of the sperm are never in the same focal plane, making it impossible to get an accurate count of moving cells. A common mistake is to report no moving cells when in fact they are just above the plane of view, or to estimate that all are moving when the nonmotile cells are lying on the bottom of the chamber below the plane of view.

The hemacytometer chamber and coverslip must be thoroughly cleaned and dried before reusing, leaving no spermicidal residue. Sperm cells have a tendency to adhere to glass, and can contaminate future samples if the chamber is not cleaned adequately. Repeated cleaning will gradually wear down the surface, increasing the depth of the chamber and potentially leading to incorrect sperm count and calculation values. A hemacytometer that is used regularly should be replaced every 1–2 years or when scratched, although many laboratories admit to using their hemacytometer well beyond this time.

The better choice is to **use counting chambers designed specifically for sperm counting.** Sperm counting chambers have two advantages: they do not require dilution, eliminating the need for duplicate counts, and they have a depth appropriate for semen (10–20 μm), which allows viewing of the motile and immotile sperm in the same focal plane [17,66,67]. The Makler counting chamber, introduced in the late 1970s for semen analysis, is reusable but requires extremely careful loading and handling to produce reliable results [68–70]. Using disposable chambers

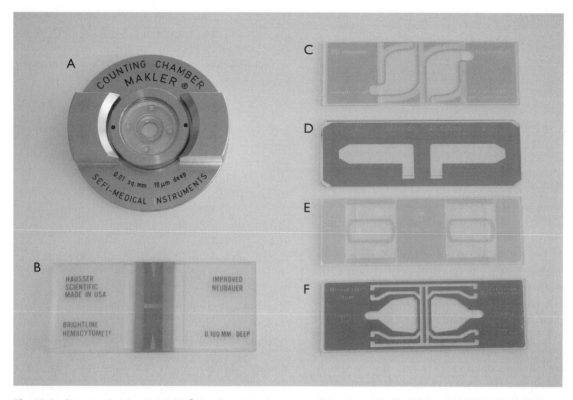

Fig. 33.2. Counting chambers: (A) Makler® chamber; (B) Neubauer hemacytometer; (C) Standard count, Leja slide; (D) Cell Vision®; (E) Cell-Vu®; (F) Microcell™.

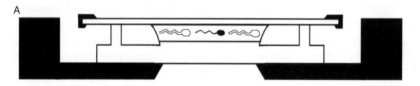

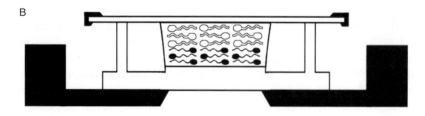

Fig. 33.3. Comparisons of counting chamber depths: (A) 10–20 μm deep sperm counting chamber, sperm in one plane of view; (B) 100 μm deep hemacytometer, sperm in multiple planes of view.

eliminates chamber cleaning, saving labor and inconvenience while at the same time providing a volumetric loading, which appears to increase counting precision. However, the fluid dynamics of particle flow in capillary-loaded chambers can lead to migration of particles or cells into the filling front as the sample flows into the chamber, termed the Segre–Silberberg effect. The effect is very pronounced for spheres, and has been documented with porcine semen [71,72], but the consequences for human semen and sperm have not been reported. The Segre–Silberberg compensation factor for undiluted semen is close to 1.0, which reduces the impact of the effect [73]. Deeper chambers are less prone to the effect.

Comparisons of counting chambers abound in the literature, but the use of different analytic techniques, quality control, and methodology leads to conflicting recommendations [67,74–78]. Failure to take the Segre–Silberberg effect and chamber volume into account may explain some contradictions among chamber comparison reports. All counting chambers have intrinsic strengths and weaknesses, many of which may be masked by semen properties, and laboratories must choose which characteristics are most important.

At least 200 sperm should be counted, which may require either examination of multiple fields in a chamber that uses an eyepiece reticule or multiple loads of chambers that have grids on cover glasses [79]. Once the count of sperm within the chamber is completed, calculations must be performed to obtain the number of sperm per milliliter of semen. Although technically that number is sperm concentration, it has a different connotation for semen analysis than most clinical parameters. Because sperm production is not tightly regulated like blood cell or hormone production, **concentration is not a measure with clinical relevance**, but instead has become a convenient way to compare samples and is often used, erroneously, as a key reference variable. The **total sperm output is a more relevant measure**, and it depends on testicular size, a variable that is almost never known to the laboratory and often not known to the treating physician [20]. Total sperm count is a compromise that has more meaning than concentration, and it is obtained simply by multiplying the concentration of sperm in the semen by the semen volume. Unfortunately, the WHO and many authors perpetuate the use of concentration as a key parameter, and until a major shift in thinking occurs, it probably will continue.

Manual assessment of sperm motility

Sperm motility testing is another area in which many mistakes are made and procedures are overly complicated and more time-consuming than needed. The three methods commonly used are shown in Table 33.2.

The most common method for analyzing sperm motility is estimating the percentage of motile sperm in several microscopic fields and computing the average. Since this is almost completely subjective, the accuracy and precision are poor. A more objective, but still difficult, method requires counting both the motile and the nonmotile sperm, then calculating the percentage that are motile. If the sperm are moving very slowly and the sample has very few sperm, counting them can

be performed without much problem. If the sperm are moving normally and quickly, the method is extraordinarily difficult to perform with any accuracy and precision. Since sperm swim randomly, it is difficult to determine whether a sperm at a given point in a chamber was counted previously before it reached a new location. Very rapidly moving sperm in a concentrated specimen are virtually impossible to count.

An easier, much more objective and reproducible method for motility analysis can be used (Fig. 33.4) [17,80,81]. First, a small (~100 μL) aliquot of the well-mixed, liquefied sample is pipetted into a 1 mL microvial. The vial is incubated in a 56 °C water bath for about five minutes to immobilize the sperm. While this incubation proceeds, the fresh semen sample is loaded into a counting chamber, and only the nonmotile sperm are counted. At the completion of the incubation period, the immobilized sample is loaded into a counting chamber, and the number of sperm is counted (this number is also the total sperm count). The difference between the two, the total number of sperm in the immobilized sample minus the number of nonmotile sperm in the fresh sample, is the number of motile sperm. From these two numbers, calculations can be performed to determine the sperm concentration, total number of sperm in the ejaculate, percentage motility, and total number of motile sperm. Counting nonmoving sperm is easy and reproducible, within and among technologists.

For decades, WHO and other references recommended that semen analysis should include a progressive motility score derived from counting motile sperm in separate progression categories – rapid, slow, and nonprogressive [8,42,82–84]. This difficult and time-consuming task requires discriminating the speed of movement of the sperm cells, either subjectively or more objectively, by counting the number of squares each sperm swims through during a given amount of time. An ability to take into account many variations in the sperm cells' movements is essential, almost impossible for the human eye [20,85]. As a consequence, many technologists simply look at the sample and estimate the progression subjectively. However, the objective motility method described above (Fig. 33.4) also can be used to discern slow and nonprogressive from rapidly progressive sperm, based on the idea that slowly moving sperm can be counted more easily and accurately than rapidly moving sperm. For the fresh semen aliquot, one button of a multi-button tally is used to count nonprogressive and slow-swimming sperm (those sperm that do not move more than one square while counting

Table 33.2. Comparison of sperm motility methods

Method	Procedure	Ease	Accuracy	Precision
Estimate	Estimate percentage of moving sperm	Difficult	Poor	Poor
Semi-objective	Count moving and nonmoving sperm	Difficult	Poor	Poor
Objective	Count nonmoving and immobilized sperm	Easy	Excellent	Excellent

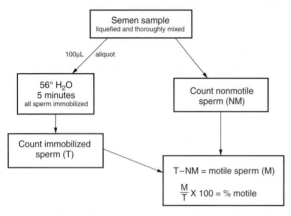

Fig. 33.4. Method for objective determination of sperm motility.

across a row of squares), and the second button is used to count nonmotile sperm. The immobilized aliquot is analyzed as usual. The difference between the nonmotile, slow, and nonprogressive sperm in the fresh sample and the total sperm in the immobilized sample is the number of rapidly progressive sperm.

Several other manual sperm count and motility assessment procedures are not worth the time and effort in most settings. Many facilities try to keep the semen sample at 37 °C throughout the semen analysis, including microscopy. Since short-term percent sperm motility *in semen* is not noticeably affected by changes of temperature between room air and body temperature, this practice is unnecessary [20,29,30]. However, sperm progression and kinematic measures (see *Automation*, below) are temperature-dependent, and are most relevant clinically when analyzed at 37 °C. For clarity, the temperature of the analysis should be noted on the report. Measuring sperm motility at multiple times after collection is a completely time-wasting measure that yields no useful clinical information.

Sperm viability

Sperm viability testing typically uses a nuclear exclusion stain to determine whether nonmotile sperm are alive and not able to move, or actually dead (necrospermia). Viability testing requires a very simple two-

step staining procedure, using eosin Y as the stain and nigrosin as a counterstain [86–88]. The method is quick and easy to evaluate. Sperm that exclude the stain are alive and those that take up the eosin are dead. Both can be visualized well against the blue–black nigrosin counterstain (Fig. 33.5). Smears stained with eosin alone can be evaluated for viability percentage but will be more difficult to analyze [86–88].

In a freshly collected sample, the percentage of motile and viable sperm should be similar, making viability a good check of motility. Since dead sperm do not swim, the number of viable sperm should always be higher than or close to the number of motile sperm. Some accrediting organizations require viability testing when sperm motility is low in order to rule out necrospermia. In practical use, the threshold should be very low (< 10–30% motile), since necrospermia as a clinical condition is rare. Probably the most common cause of low viability is contamination of the sample with lubricants, most of which are spermicidal [89,90].

Sperm morphology

The component of sperm morphology is one of the most predictive measures of fertility potential and therapeutic outcome [1,4,23,91–93]. For an infertile couple, abnormal sperm morphology can suggest the next therapeutic step such as varicocele repair, in-vitro fertilization (IVF), or intracytoplasmic sperm injection (ICSI). Morphology also is an important measure of toxic exposure from environmental and occupational sources [12–14]. Ironically, **sperm morphology is probably the most confusing component of semen analysis to perform and the most difficult part to interpret** [6,20,22,94–98]. There are many different staining methods used, not all suitable for semen, and some technologists even attempt to determine morphology from unstained wet preps, an impossible task. There are many classification systems in use, each with its own criteria for what constitutes a normal cell, and most with poor standardization of morphologic variants. Some systems describe the location of the defects, some the specific types of defects, and some only report the percentage of normal sperm cells.

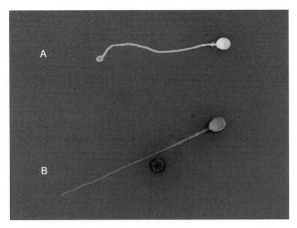

Fig. 33.5. Sperm viability using eosin–nigrosin staining: (A) live (white) cell – excludes the stain; (B) dead (pink) cell – takes up the stain. *See color plate section.*

Morphology methodology

The first step in sperm morphology is to make a good, even semen smear, not too thin and not too thick. Too thin and there will not be enough sperm present for a good evaluation. Too thick and the sperm can be layered and difficult to focus on clearly. Roughly made smears can also separate the sperm heads from the tails as an artifact, leading to an incorrectly high percentage of midpiece abnormalities.

To make the smear, a small drop of semen (approximately 10 µL) should be placed near the labeled end of the slide [80]. Another glass slide is held at a 45° angle to the smear slide and used to pull the semen slowly across the slide. The angle can be increased or decreased to make the smear slightly thicker or thinner, depending on the concentration of the sample. Ideally, the smear should immediately be fixed using a spray cytology fixative to reduce air-drying artifacts, dried thoroughly, and then stored in a dry place until stained.

The best stain for semen smears and sperm is a modified Papanicolaou (Pap) stain [42,82–84,97], providing good clarity and color differentiation among the regions of the cell. Pap-stained smears also are stable over time, allowing later review. The traditional Pap staining method was time-consuming to prepare and perform, but with most of the stains available commercially as ready-to-use solutions, the labor is greatly reduced. Although passing the smears through multiple solutions takes about 20–30 minutes longer than alternative three-step methods, the results are worth the effort [99]. Using limonene-based xylene substitutes eliminates old concerns about the organic solvents

in Pap stain procedures. A three-step quick Pap stain also can be purchased. Because semen analysis often is performed in body fluid sections of hematopathology, stains such as Wright–Giemsa commonly are used. Although rapid and available commercially in one-step and three-step kits, these stains do not provide the same clarity and color variation as the Pap stain. The one-step kits should always be avoided. A particular problem is that semen mucoprotein, which is almost unnoticeable in a Pap-stained smear, stains vivid purple with Wright–Giemsa stains, obscuring much of the fine detail of the sperm morphology. A third option for semen smears is to use pre-stained blood film slides, but the visual quality for sperm cells usually is very poor and the stain is not stable, so that the smears cannot be stored for later review.

After staining, the smear should be coverslipped and examined using a 100× oil objective with a 10× eyepiece. The head, midpiece, and tail of each sperm are separately evaluated (Fig. 33.6). If any of the three major structures is abnormal, the sperm is classified as abnormal [84]. A single-key tally is used in one hand to keep track of the number of sperm analyzed, while a multi-key tally is used with the other hand to tally normal, borderline abnormal, or abnormal [99]. Depending on what information the ordering physician or study needs, the location of the abnormality (head, midpiece, tail) or type of abnormality, such as shape of head, size, etc., can also be determined and tallied [20,91,92,97,99]. At least 200 cells must be evaluated to ensure a statistically valid evaluation of the sample [42,79].

Classification of sperm morphology

Ideally, a classification scheme provides a standardized system that allows many observers to compare results, has clinical relevance, and relates in a meaningful way to fertility [95]. **Consistent classification of sperm cells among individual observers and across time has been difficult to achieve.** Many examples of this can be found in external quality control and proficiency testing programs [96,100–102]. Often participants' results encompass the entire potential result range of 0–100% normal forms, and in spite of extremely large standard deviations generated by the results, about 5% of observations exceed acceptable limits [96].

Why is sperm morphology so difficult to standardize and quantify? Unlike those of many other species, human sperm are extremely pleiomorphic in several respects: many subtle variations of normal exist, and many irregular and abnormal forms are present [12,95].

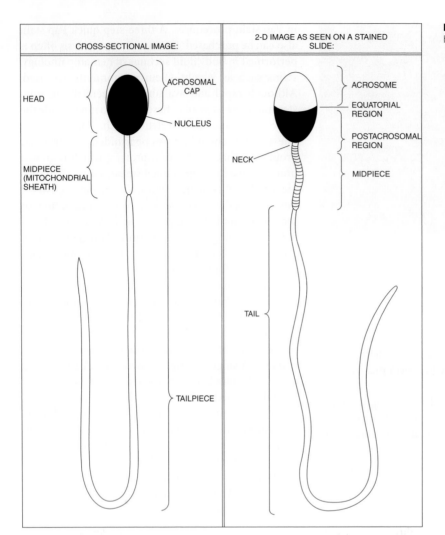

| CROSS-SECTIONAL IMAGE: | 2-D IMAGE AS SEEN ON A STAINED SLIDE: |

HEAD

ACROSOMAL CAP

NUCLEUS

MIDPIECE (MITOCHONDRIAL SHEATH)

TAILPIECE

ACROSOME

EQUATORIAL REGION

POSTACROSOMAL REGION

NECK

MIDPIECE

TAIL

Fig. 33.6. Diagram of normal human sperm.

Agreeing on correct classification of different morphologic forms is difficult when they display continuous variation rather than precise and unique typologies [95,98,103,104]. A discrete form along the morphologic spectrum may be readily identifiable, but intermediate variations can be difficult to differentiate and often may be misclassified. The effect of this problem can be minimized with larger sample sizes of 200–500 cells but can be profound if too few cells are assessed. The use of poor cytological techniques, such as evaluation of unstained preparations, inadequate cell fixation, or unsatisfactory staining, aggravates the effect; however, incorrect classification remains the fundamental problem [22].

Over the last 50 years, five major published classification systems have endured in wide clinical practice:

MacLeod [3,91], WHO Manual 2nd edition [83], WHO Manual 3rd edition [84], ASCP [105], and Strict, described by Menkveld [106,107] and Kruger [93,108] and promoted in the WHO Manual 4th edition [42]. Tables 33.3 and 33.4 summarize the main components of these five schemes in common use. Many other sperm classification schemes exist, usually developed by individual laboratories and adopted as their personal methods. Between 10% and 25% of laboratories use a nonstandard system [96,109]. The practice of such local conventions makes comparison with other systems impossible, and they should not be used.

Most classification schemes defined normal as an idealized sperm cell with an oval head (Fig. 33.6) and were validated by finding the ideal form prominently

Table 33.3. Normal sperm morphology from common sperm classifications

	ASCP	McLeod	WHO 2nd edition	WHO 3rd edition	Strict / WHO 4th edition
Normal reference range	> 80% normal forms	> 60% normal forms	> 50% normal forms	> 30% normal forms	> 14% normal forms
Head					
Shape	Oval	Oval	Oval	Oval	Oval Smooth border
Acrosome	1/2–2/3 of head surface		> 1/3 of head surface	40–70% of head surface	40–70% of head surface
Size	4–5 μm long 2–3 μm wide		3–5 μm long 2–3 μm wide (width = 1/2–2/3 length)	4–5.5 μm long 2.5–3.5 μm wide (length/width = 1.5–1.75)	3–5 μm long 2–3 μm wide
Vacuoles	Not clear	Not stated		< 20% of head area	Up to 4
Midpiece					
Shape		Not considered	Straight, regular outline Axially attached	Straight, regular outline Axially attached	Slender, straight, regular outline Axially attached
Size	1 μm wide 5 μm long		< 1/3 head width, 7–8 μm long	< 1/3 head width, 7–8 μm long	< 1 μm wide length = 1.5 × head length
Cytoplasmic drople (CD)		Considered to be immature sperm		< 1/3 head area	< 1/2 head area
Tail					
Shape		Not considered	Slender, uncoiled, regular outline	Slender, uncoiled, regular outline	Uniform size, uncoiled
Width	1 μm at base 0.1 μm at tip				Thinner than midpiece
Length	50–55 μm long		> 45 μm long	> 45 μm long	10 × head length

in ejaculates of men with proven fertility and relatively infrequently in those of infertile men [1,4,5]. Others attempted to find a consensus definition of normal sperm shape by surveying multiple experts [95]. A newer approach defined normal based on a reference population of sperm found in cervical mucus [106,107]. Examples of basic sperm morphology are shown in Figure 33.7. Much of the classification difficulty and controversy arises over just how perfect a sperm must be to be considered normal. In actual practice, smearing, fixation, air-drying, and staining can induce artifacts that must be identified and distinguished from the sperm cell's natural morphology.

Compounding the problem, individual observers or laboratories often develop variations on a scheme, and frequently do not identify the classification method used, making comparison of results obtained in different laboratories impossible. Surveys show that 25–50% of PT participants do not know what classification they use, how it was derived, or how to reference it [96,101,102]. In a recent unpublished survey by the authors, one-third of the proficiency challenge participants and one-fifth of the attendees in a morphology training class were using the wrong atlas for their system, leading to incorrect classification (Table 33.5). One atlas is available that compares classification schemes and lists appropriate references [97].

The classification systems most commonly used in fertility laboratories, the WHO 3rd edition scheme and the strict criteria (adopted in the WHO 4th edition), rarely are used in general hospital and reference laboratories and are not taught in most medical technology or pathology programs. This dichotomy creates problems of appropriate referral, since there are many more initial semen analyses performed in general laboratories than in fertility centers. However, **little consensus about what a normal sperm looks like**

Table 33.4. Abnormal sperm morphology from common sperm classifications

	ASCP	McLeod	WHO 2nd edition	WHO 3rd edition	Strict / WHO 4th edition
Head	Acrosomal abnormality Postacrosomal abnormality Bicephalic Paired Large head Small head Vacuolated	Megaloform Small form Tapering Amorphous Double	Large Small Tapering Amorphous Double Pyriform Pin Round	Large Small Tapering Amorphous Double Pyriform Pin Round Vacuolated	Borderline abnormal: slight deviation from oval Abnormal: acrosome < 40% or > 70% of head area round head small head tapered head double head large head diadem defect (vacuoles)
Midpiece	Abnormal size Thickened Bent tail Missing tail CD present		Abnormal size Thickened Bent tail Missing tail Cd present	Abnormal size Thickened Bent tail Missing tail Cd present	Borderline abnormal: slightly thick Abnormal: abnormal length very thick bent tail missing tail CD present
Tail	Coiled tail Curled tail Multi-tailed Variation in length Terminal droplet		Multiple tails Short tail Broken tail Hairpin Coiled tail Irregular width Terminal droplet	Multiple tails Short tail Broken tail Hairpin Coiled tail Irregular width Terminal droplet	Abnormal: all tail defects

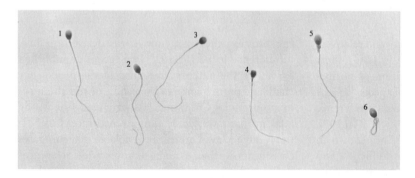

Fig. 33.7. Examples of normal and abnormal sperm: (1) normal sperm; (2) normal sperm; (3) borderline abnormal head (normal for WHO 3rd, abnormal for strict/WHO 4th); (4) abnormal head (small, small acrosome, irregular), normal midpiece and tail; (5) abnormal midpiece (thick), normal head and tail; (5) abnormal tail (coiled), normal head and midpiece. *See color plate section.*

is evident even among sperm morphology experts, judging from the results of the American Association of Bioanalysis Proficiency Testing Service (AAB-PTS), in which the majority of participants were fertility laboratories [101].

The evolution of the major classification systems begins with John MacLeod. In the 1950s, he organized the descriptions of previous observers into a method and nomenclature for classifying sperm based on head shapes [91,92]. Normal was defined as an oval head, and abnormal forms were classified into five categories by their geometric shape. MacLeod correlated morphologic findings with fertility of many men [4]. The MacLeod system was widely promulgated and remains the basis for sperm morphology classification in most general pathology laboratories. Its utility is limited by several conventions: only head defects are categorized, which can result in classification of sperm as normal in

Table 33.5. Classification system and atlas discordance: results from a survey of participants in a proficiency challenge and a morphology training class

Group	Inappropriate atlas	No reference atlas
Proficiency test	32%	6%
Morphology class	19%	28%

spite of significant defects of midpiece or tail; only one defect is assigned per sperm, which can mask the presence of other significant abnormalities; and normal is defined very generously at 60–80%.

The World Health Organization (WHO) published four editions of a manual on semen analysis in 1980, 1987, 1992, and 1999. Each edition of the WHO manual has discussed guidelines for morphology categorization and provided some photographs illustrating various sperm shapes. In the 1st and 2nd editions [82,83], classification was described in a manner very similar to MacLeod's, where each sperm was assigned a single defect. Midpiece and tail defects also were added as category possibilities in a hierarchical way, with head abnormalities taking precedence over midpiece over tail defects.

In the 3rd edition [84], the approach to classification changed. Instead of assigning each sperm a single defect, the manual recommended tallying defects in each of the three main regions of the sperm, head, midpiece, and tail, and calculating the total number of defects as a percentage of abnormal, giving a more comprehensive description of abnormalities present. However, the manual is contradictory about how complete the abnormality description should be, in one section recommending the specific defects listed in previous editions and in another suggesting that abnormalities simply be grouped by region of the sperm as unspecified defects of head, midpiece, or tail.

The inability of the expert editorial panel to agree on how to classify normal sperm is obvious upon reading the manual text. The manual states that the assignment of normal should be strict, but does not state how "strictness" should be determined. The percent normal expected in a fertile individual is listed as greater than 30%, a decrease of 20% from the previous edition, but how the value was derived is unclear. Panel members candidly acknowledge that consensus was difficult to reach, and the compromise was ambiguity [23].

The 4th edition of the WHO manual [42] attempted to resolve these problems by declaring that the Strict classification developed by Menkveld and Kruger should be used (see below). Many clinicians believe that this recommendation is not appropriate, and that such strict interpretation of the image is not justified except in the setting of IVF, where investigators have shown predictive value [93,110]. In fact, the 4th edition of the WHO manual does not cite any references showing that the Strict system has value outside of IVF treatments. As in previous editions, the few images in the text give insufficient information or rationale to learn classification. The manual introduces a slight variation on the typical Strict classification, which reports percent normal only, by stating that defects in the functional regions (head, midpiece, and tail) should be categorized generally, and prevalent defects should be noted. However, unless the technologist identifies all defects as the analysis progresses, it is impossible to know if a defect is truly prevalent.

In 1989, the American Society of Clinical Pathologists (ASCP) published an atlas authored by Adelman and Cahill [105]. Unlike most other schemes, the ASCP classifies head defects not by geometric shape, but by the anatomic location of the defect, a rational and useful classification method. For example, a sperm that has no acrosome is classified as an acrosomal defect, where other schemes would call it round. It is unfortunate that this useful method of classifying sperm defects is rarely used. However, when surveyed, many technologists think they are using this scheme when in fact they are using the MacLeod system [96], probably because so many have ASCP Board certification. The major problem of the ASCP scheme is the definition of normal at 80–90%, which limits adequate discrimination from abnormal.

Leading a group of South African investigators, Roelof Menkveld approached classification in a different way from previous observers [106,107]. Reasoning that most sperm present in upper endocervical canal mucus after coitus were biologically selected for normality, they found a remarkably homogeneous population of oval-headed sperm in postcoital mucus. Using this very specific and morphologically similar group of sperm as a reference population, they defined normal very critically and strictly. Rather than identify specific abnormalities, they classified sperm as normal or abnormal. A third typology, borderline normal, was added as an intermediate class but eliminated later. The WHO 3rd-edition system classifies borderline as normal. Biological relevance and normal values were determined by comparison with oocyte fertilization in

561

vitro [93]. For this reason, many IVF clinics and fertility specialists use the Strict classification scheme, although the predictive value for non-IVF fertility treatments is not clear [111,112]. Even Menkveld and coworkers recently reported that the best discriminator between fertile and infertile men was the WHO 3rd-edition classification [113].

The Strict classification system has been criticized for several problems:

(1) a failure to recognize that the appearance of "normal" sperm in the semen may in fact be different from the strict reference population in the cervical mucus, or that these biological secretions may impact the appearance on a stained slide;

(2) the fact that the lower limit of normal nearly always includes zero;

(3) its dependence on detecting very subtle morphologic differences, many of which are detectable only in enlarged photographs of the sperm;

(4) the tendency to become "stricter" in classification as time goes on until no men have a normal analysis [M. Gerrity, personal correspondence; 114];

(5) the semantic implication that "strict" is "better" than other methods; and

(6) how "strict" to be.

In a College of American Pathologists proficiency testing survey, 37 laboratories using Strict classification reported values ranging from 10% to 95% normal on one smear, and for another, 35 laboratories reported values ranging from 3% to 100% normal [10]. Recent studies recommend that the lower reference limit for Strict normal should be only 3% [113]. About the same time, the Kruger group published a lower reference value of 5% [115]. It is difficult to accept that a normal fertile man would have only 4–8% normal forms, or that normal shapes in fertile men would decrease from 14% to 3% in 10 years. In a recently published atlas, Kruger recommends 14% as the lower reference limit for Strict normal, with the range from 5% to 14% normal forms designated as abnormal but a "good prognosis" range [108], similar to recommendations in earlier publications [93].

A criticism of older, "non-strict" classifications is the tendency to overrate normal as 70–100% of the sperm population. The Strict classification carries the opposite risk of overrating abnormal. In a typical 200-cell analysis, just one or two sperm can make a difference between normal or abnormal. Neither extreme seems clinically valuable for most settings.

Fertility specialists are in widespread agreement that the WHO 3rd and the Strict/WHO 4th classifications

Table 33.6. Simple distinctions between WHO 3rd and strict/WHO 4th sperm classification methods

	WHO 3rd	Strict/WHO 4th
Reference value for normal	Over 30% normal forms	Over 14% normal forms
Classification of borderline abnormal	Normal	Abnormal
Utility of classification	Screening Fertility treatment	Fertility treatment

are the most appropriate systems currently in common practice; however, experts disagree about which of the two is the best to use. Unfortunately, there are so many variations of the two schemes that learning either one or comparing the results is very difficult [96]. Judging from their individual atlases [107,108], the two main proponents of the Strict classification do not agree about what is a normal sperm. Confusion about how to classify sperm can be reduced by education and discussion [94,114,116], but until a universal standard is available, ambiguity will exist [95].

A summary of the major distinctions between the WHO 3rd edition and the Strict/WHO 4th edition is shown in Table 33.6. **As a general recommendation, laboratories that primarily perform routine semen analysis for non-fertility specialists, as an initial screening, should use the more liberal WHO 3rd edition, where normal includes borderline forms and has a reference value of greater than 30%. Laboratories that perform analysis as part of a specialty fertility practice should use either the WHO 3rd or the Strict/WHO 4th classification, or both.**

MacLeod wrote in 1951, "There are as many different interpretations of morphology as there are authors, without general agreement as to the various cell types which constitute abnormal forms … a cell considered 'abnormal' by one is not always classified as such by another" [4]. Almost 60 years later this statement is still true.

Automation

Several types of automated semen analyzers are commercially available. In general, however, automation of semen analysis has failed to answer the needs of the clinical laboratory. Current technology is either too expensive and difficult to use in a sophisticated andrology laboratory or busy hematology laboratory, where most semen analysis is performed, or is not sufficiently robust to be useful.

The oldest, most reliable technology is computer-assisted semen analysis (CASA), which has been extensively investigated over the last 25 years [104,117–120] and recently reviewed [121].

CASA instruments digitize the video image of some portion of the sperm, usually the head or its outline, and track its movement over many video frames. Proprietary algorithms analyze the tracks and calculate motile and nonmotile sperm, and many sperm kinematic functions such as straight-line and curvilinear velocity. Kinematic measures have value in treatment outcome prediction [118,122]. Several automated programs for sperm morphology have been developed by CASA manufacturers, and these have the potential to reduce analytic variability by standardizing instruments to a set of images, if an expert panel could agree on the classifications [121]. At the present time, the analysis time and reliability of CASA morphology is not acceptable for routine laboratory use [124].

Unfortunately, the purchase price and steep operational learning curve of CASA instruments make them impractical and cost-prohibitive in most clinical laboratory settings. Reviewers estimate that less than 2% of clinical laboratories and less than 20% of andrology laboratories use CASA [64,121]. However, CASA has proven valuable in toxicology, primarily by increasing the sensitivity of detecting changes in sperm kinematics or sperm morphometry associated with potential toxicants [12,124–129].

Instrumentation based on optical density is in the marketplace as well. The family of SQA instruments use signal processing to measure sperm concentration and motility indirectly using photoelectric detection of light absorption and optical density fluctuations caused by motility. Semen is loaded into a proprietary testing capillary for analysis. To measure concentration, the instrument compares the difference between the amount of light absorbed by sperm and the amount absorbed by seminal plasma. Motility is measured by disturbances or interruptions in light [130]. Various algorithms convert the signals either to a sperm motility index of general semen quality or, in newer versions, into traditional sperm measures. Although slightly less expensive than CASA instruments, the cost of supplies, especially quality control, increases operating expense to a very high level.

Only a few reports exist that compare the technology to manual methods [131,132], suggesting that unpublished anecdotal reports of the technology's lack of reliability in both accuracy and operation may represent the wider experience. If this technology were widely adopted and validated, one would expect to see the andrology field flooded with publications, just as it was in the early CASA years.

Several operational factors limit the value of the SQA technology. The use of optical density to measure concentration of sperm poses several technical problems. Spectrophotometry best measures color in solutions, not opacity from cell suspensions [76]. It also requires a relatively large volume (~1 mL) for sample loading into a proprietary testing capillary [130]. Low-volume or high-consistency samples cannot be used, and in settings of insemination or IVF therapy too much semen will be used for analysis to make the technology usable in this application. The high volume requirement also greatly increases the cost of QC to a prohibitive level. The technology requires motile sperm to generate a result, so that settings and channels for quality control and patient samples are different. Although the instrument can detect beads in the QC channel without difficulty, it cannot measure them in the patient sample channel, suggesting that the channels use different optical density settings. This is also suggested by the appearance of a new service parameter used to calibrate the instrument to read latex beads accurately, which apparently amplifies the optical density. The fact that measurement of stabilized sperm QC is nonlinear with the factory settings could present a problem in analyzing proficiency test samples, since all programs are based on stabilized sperm. Sperm morphology is calculated from a look-up reference table that assumes the sperm motility and morphology are correlated, an assumption that is neither functionally correct [133] nor valid [134]. As a consequence, as the number of motile sperm declines in the sample over time, the instrument falsely underreports the number of morphologically normal sperm. Thus morphology studies should still be performed manually, reducing the cost–benefit ratio even further. Because no specific defects are described, utility for toxicology is limited. A visualization screen allows viewing of samples or smears, albeit poorly, but the instrument cannot analyze smears directly or accept video feed, limiting the ability to analyze existing QC or PT for these parameters.

Automation would solve many problems of standardization. Since few semen analyses are performed in most settings, manufacturers of laboratory equipment have not been convinced that sales will justify development expense and have not been motivated to solve the problem of automation. Keeping in mind that semen

Table 33.7. Reference values established by the World Health Organization

Volume (mL)	Concentration (million/mL)	Total sperm count	% Motility	% Normal forms	Edition, year	Reference
N/A	20	N/A	60	48	1st, 1980	[82]
2	20	40	50	50	2nd, 1987	[83]
2	20	40	50	30	3rd, 1992	[84]
2	20	40	50	15	4th, 1999	[42]

analysis is a set of very different tests, it is difficult to create technology that can satisfy all parameters. At this time, **semen analysis remains predominately a manual test.**

Reference ranges for semen parameters

The value of semen analysis as a predictor of male fertility has been debated [77,135]. In part, this is due to an unrealistic expectation that traditional semen analysis describes absolute criteria for fertility, when in fact many functional variables exist that are not measured by the test (e.g., capacitation, egg penetration). Furthermore, large fertility trials that can be performed in animals, where semen from a single animal can be used to inseminate many females, are not possible in humans [136,137]. Thus, **the influence of the female partner in human fertility plays a huge confounding role in both defining fertility and interpreting the association of specific semen analysis measures with fertility** [138,139]. An additional problem is the lack of quality control benchmarks in many studies, as well as the ambiguity of methodology, especially for sperm motility and morphology.

About the best that can be expected is an emergence of predictive patterns from large studies associating specific sperm factors with probability of fertility. From these, reference ranges can be calculated, but they will suffer the same limitations described above. The earliest comprehensive and well-controlled studies that identified and controlled many variables were described in the early 1950s by John MacLeod and statistician Ruth Gold [4,140–149]. Their series of publications still forms the basis for clinical reference values in semen analysis. The papers described a data analysis problem confirmed over the years, that semen variables are distributed in a non-Gaussian manner, because of marked right skewing [150,151]. The lower 95% confidence limits usually give biologically meaningless negative values,

the mean is very different from the median, and this makes distinction between group means very difficult [151]. Furthermore, varying definitions of fertility as well as subject age considerations confound comparison of studies [152]. As a consequence of all these factors, the **reference values for semen analysis are not as clear as needed.**

MacLeod's research found the greatest difference between the fertile and infertile populations of 1800 men at the lowest concentration of 20 million sperm per milliliter or the lowest total sperm count of 50 million [141]. Unfortunately, he and most authors subsequently ignored the total sperm count number, and concentration became the unit of measurement most often cited. The lower limit of normal remains 20 million sperm/mL in most laboratories and in the latest WHO manual [42,102]. Values currently cited by the WHO are shown in Table 33.7. It cannot be overemphasized that although this "cutoff" implies a lower threshold concept for male fertility, it merely indicates a level below which probability of pregnancy is less [153]. Many men father children without therapy in spite of having sperm counts, morphology, or motility well below lower reference limits.

Reference ranges for hematology and clinical chemistry are commonly set with upper and lower limits for a 95% confidence interval, so that the lower limit is the 2.5th percentile and the upper limit, the 97.5th percentile [154]. However, since pathology has not been linked to good sperm quality, upper limits for parameters such as sperm count, motility, viability, or morphology are probably unnecessary. As shown in Table 33.8, many studies define a lower reference limit anywhere from the 2.5 to the15th percentile, but limits described by MacLeod and Gold continue to be validated [2,4,113,115,155–162].

In spite of the data available, a wide variety of reference ranges are used by laboratories that perform semen analysis, many of them far outside of the limits generally accepted as valid [102].

Table 33.8. Lower reference limits for semen parameters based on surveys of fertile, infertile, or healthy populations

Test Population	n	Method	Percentile	Volume (mL)	Total sperm count (million)	Concentration (million/mL)	% Motility	% Normal forms	Classification	Publication year	Study location	Ref
Fertile men	99	Manual	2.5	1.2	15.4	9.1	29	2	Strict	2006	Norway	[159]
Fertile men	49	Manual	NR	1.5	30[a]	20	20	40	WHO 2nd	1988	UK	[155]
Fertile men	315	CASA	5	NR	56	16	14	NR	NR	2002	Denmark	[156]
Fertile men	99	Manual	5	1.7	22.3	10.6	33	3	Strict	2006	Norway	[159]
Fertile men	287	Manual	5	1	15.3	7	18	4	Strict	1997	Belgium	[161]
Fertile men	1081	Manual	5	2	70	20	50	10	Strict	2002	Europe	[162]
Fertile men	99	Manual	10	2.1	54.3	16.9	43	4	Strict	2006	Norway	[159]
Fertile men	210	Manual	10	NR	NR	20	30	24	WHO 3rd	2001	Netherlands	[113]
Fertile men	210	Manual	10	NR	NR	20	30	2	Strict	2001	Netherlands	[113]
Fertile men	1081	Manual	10	1.3	29.6	14.3	28	5	Strict	1997	Belgium	[161]
Fertile men	243	Manual	25	1.3	30[a]	23	46	12	WHO 3rd	1998	Singapore	[1579]
Fertile men	696	Manual	NR	NR	NR	48	63	12	Strict	2001	USA	[1]
Fertile men	1958	Manual	NR	NR	NR	20	40	60	MacLeod	1951	USA	[4,142,143]
Healthy men	1191	Manual	5	2.3	154	65	67	39	WHO 3rd	2007	China	[158]
Healthy men	562	Manual	15	1.5	50	30	45	68	WHO 3rd	2002	China	[160]
Healthy men	162	Manual	15	3.2	131[a]	41	52	12	MacLeod/Eliasson	2001	Turkey	[115]
Infertile men	765	Manual	NR	NR	NR	13.5	32	9	Strict	2001	USA	[1]

NR, Not reported.
[a] Calculated from data in manuscript (volume × concentration).

Benchmarks for semen analysis: training, quality control, proficiency, and competency testing

Formal semen analysis training is rare, and without adequate education it is very difficult to feel confident about clinical test results [22]. Training is especially critical for semen analysis when technical skill and judgment are not assisted by automation. Training can improve analytic skill, as demonstrated in a series of courses offered by ESHRE–SIGA between 1994 and 1999 when notable improvement in testing ability was evident by the end of the course [163]. Other studies have also documented improved performance after a standardized training course, demonstrating the value of such training [164–166]. Some professional societies offer instruction, but many laboratories do not have budgets for training, especially when travel is involved. However, self-paced training courses [17,99] and video [80] are available for the laboratory that wants to improve the technical skills of its staff.

The use of quality control (QC) is a requirement for any good laboratory assay. To ensure its use, many countries and states have specific regulations for QC in semen analysis. In the USA, semen analysis is categorized as a high-complexity test requiring two levels of quality controls on each day of patient testing [167,168]. This not only documents the ability to perform the test correctly, but also gives the technologist confidence in the results of the test [165,166,169]. Without the benchmark that QC provides, knowing whether a test has been performed properly is very difficult [170]. Properly designed QC demonstrates both accuracy (obtaining the correct result) and precision (obtaining the same result multiple times). In a 2002 survey, 67% of laboratories did not perform any QC for semen analysis [102].

A quality control for sperm count is like that for any other test, one that can be analyzed in any counting chamber or semen analyzer in the same way as a patient sample. **In order to truly mimic a clinical test material, the quality control must resemble the sample being analyzed. No surrogate materials come close to looking as complex as sperm cells in semen** (Fig. 33.8). Sperm are oval and have tails that often overlap or coil around the head, changing the appearance and making them harder to differentiate from nonsperm cells. Semen contains debris, immature germ cells, leukocytes, and other non-sperm cells, some of which can be confused with sperm. Although latex beads have been promoted

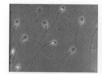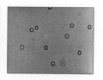

Fig. 33.8. Human sperm QC suspension vs. beads: (a) human sperm patient sample; (b) stabilized human sperm QC; (c) latex beads.

as a control for sperm count [171], beads are really not a valid control [76,172]. Sphere suspensions are a different shape and easy to count since there are no tails or other particles present to cause visual confusion. A suspension of human sperm is the only valid quality control for sperm count. Beads do have a role in calibration of counting chambers as long as the Segre–Silberberg effect on particle distribution is taken into account [71,173].

Sperm motility quality controls are available in two formats: frozen aliquots of semen or video recordings on CD-ROM, tape, or digital file. The frozen aliquots allow the controls to be analyzed in a counting chamber, but due to the variation in sperm cell death during thawing, the motility of frozen–thawed sperm is highly variable [174]. The fact that these controls must be stored in liquid nitrogen greatly adds both to the expense of the product and to the necessity for increased safety practices for dealing with the ultra-low-temperature materials.

Video recordings, although they lack the direct handling aspects of a semen sample, are easy to use, inexpensive, and reproducible. Generally, the only equipment needed is a computer and a tally counter. When images of both fresh and immobilized aliquots of a sample are provided, video-based quality controls can be used as a surrogate for any manual method of motility analysis. Many CASA instruments can accept video feed but may require certain formats [175].

Semen smears stained with the appropriate stain can be used for sperm viability or sperm morphology quality controls. QC smears for sperm morphology must be assayed for the classification system being used. Most of the morphology quality controls commercially available are assayed for WHO 3rd and Strict/WHO 4th classifications. QC for the Strict/WHO 4th scheme is especially important, as viewers tend to get stricter with time, often until no normal sperm can be identified [M. Gerrity, personal correspondence; 114]. Assayed ranges for the older classification systems, such as ASCP, McLeod, and WHO 2nd edition, are not provided with any commercial controls. Facilities that use these classification systems must establish control ranges by analyzing the control smears at least 20 times [176,177]. Switching to a modern system probably is more cost-effective and makes more sense, as it allows results to be compared with known standards. Morphology quality control smears are usually stained, but unstained smears from an assayed lot can be obtained from some manufacturers to stain using the laboratory's individual procedures.

External quality control, or proficiency testing (PT) as it is called in the USA, is an important way for a laboratory to see how its results compare with those of a peer group of other laboratories. Unlike QC supplies, PT uses materials with unknown assay values. Laboratory results are stratified by method (type of counting chamber, stain, classification scheme, etc.) and the mean of each group calculated. Results outside of 95% confidence limits (two standard deviations) or in some programs a fixed interval, are considered unacceptable. Note that the peer group results determine the mean, not the reference value as with internal QC. In the USA, laboratories must participate in PT twice a year [167,168], and a number of providers offer appropriate PT materials. Laboratories that use automated analysis for any part of semen analysis must be able to analyze PT materials on the same equipment. If PT materials can only be analyzed manually, the patient testing must also be performed manually or referenced daily to manual results of known QC.

PT for semen analysis identifies many of the analytic problems discussed earlier. For example, morphology PT results often show a range of normal from 0–100% [96]. Early semen analysis PT showed a high level of disagreement among participants, with reported sperm concentrations ranging from 3×10^6 mL to 492×10^6/mL from one sample, and 2×10^6/mL to 147×10^6/mL from another [101]. Ranges of results appear to be narrowing as laboratories use the data to identify their need to improve testing.

PT can be valuable for indicating areas where more training is needed, or where procedures should be updated and improved [100]. At its best, PT serves an important educational purpose, by providing interpretation of data and resources for improving procedures [178], for example, newly available virtual PT challenges for motility and morphology.

Annual competency testing of technologists should be part of a laboratory quality program and is required in the USA by Clinical Laboratory Improvement Amendments (CLIA) [168]. PT participation can be used as part of competency testing, to show how a technologist performs compared to peers. Additional competency testing must include direct observation of test performance by a technical supervisor and review of intermediate test results, QC records, proficiency testing results, and preventive maintenance records, as well as assessment of problem-solving skills, usually by written examination or quizzes on important aspects of semen analysis. Some training programs include cognitive testing [80]. Commercial products are available for documenting training and competency [17,33,99].

Acknowledgments

The authors thank Anna Bort, Jeremy Paul, and Paul Weis for their contributions to the manuscript.

Disclosure

Both authors are employees of Fertility Solutions Inc., a company that manufactures and distributes semen analysis quality controls, reagents, and training materials.

References

[1] Guzick DS, Overstreet JW, Factor-Litvak P, et al. Sperm morphology, motility, and concentration in fertile and infertile men. N Engl J Med 2001; 345: 1388–93.

[2] Jouannet P, Czyglik F, David G, et al. Study of a group of 484 fertile men. Part 1: distribution of semen characteristics. Int J Androl 1981; 4: 440–9.

[3] MacLeod J. The semen examination. Clin Obstet Gyn 1965; 8: 115–27.

[4] MacLeod J, Gold RZ. The male factor in fertility and infertility. IV. Sperm morphology in fertile and infertile marriage. Fertil Steril 1951; 2: 394–414.

[5] Rehan NE, Sobrero AJ, Fertig JW. The semen of fertile men: statistical analysis of 1,300 men. Fertil Steril 1974; 26: 408–13.

[6] Chong AP, Walters CA, Weinrieb SA. The neglected laboratory test: the semen analysis. J Androl 1983; 4: 280–2.

[7] Lipshultz LI, Howards SS, eds. Infertility in the Male, 2nd edn. St. Louis, MO: Mosby Year Book, 1991.

[8] Mortimer D. Practical Laboratory Andrology. New York, NY: Oxford University Press, 1994.

[9] Rothmann SA. Semen analysis: a practical guide to performance and interpretation. In: Seibel MM, ed. Infertility: a Comprehensive Text. Stamford, CT: Appleton and Lange, 1997: 45–58.

[10] Rothmann SA, Morgan BW. Laboratory diagnosis in andrology. Cleveland Clinic J Med 1989; 56: 805–10.

[11] McLachlan RI, Baker HW, Clarke GN, *et al.* Semen analysis: its place in modern reproductive medical practice. *Pathology* 2003; **35**: 25–33.

[12] Katz DF. Human sperm as biomarkers of toxic risk and reproductive health. *J NIH Res* 1991; **3**: 63–7.

[13] Schrader SM, Ratcliffe JM, Turner TW, Hornung RW. The use of new field methods of semen analysis in the study of occupational hazards to reproduction: the example of ethylene dibromide. *J Occup Med* 1987; **29**: 963–6.

[14] Schrader SM, Chapin RE, Clegg ED, *et al.* Laboratory methods for assessing human semen in epidemiologic studies: a consensus report. *Repro Toxicol* 1992; **6**: 275–9.

[15] Meacham RB. Criteria for determining that a vasectomy has succeeded. *J Androl* 2003; **24**: 494–5.

[16] Nazerali H, Thapa S, Hays M, *et al.* Vasectomy effectiveness in Nepal: a retrospective study. *Contraception* 2003; **67**: 397–401.

[17] Kinzer DR, Rothmann SA. *The Andrology Trainer*, 2nd edn. Cleveland, OH: Fertility Solutions Inc., 2003.

[18] Amelar RD. Coagulation, liquefaction and viscosity of human semen. *J Urol* 1962; **87**: 187–90.

[19] Chughtai B, Sawas A, O'Malley RL, *et al.* A neglected gland: a review of Cowper's gland. *Int J Androl* 2005; **28**: 74–7.

[20] Eliasson R. Basic semen analysis. In: *Current Topics in Andrology*. Perth: Ladybrook Publishing, 2003.

[21] Jeyendran RS. *Interpretation of Semen Analysis Results: a Practical Guide*. Cambridge: Cambridge University Press, 2000.

[22] Baker DJ, Paterson MA, Klaassen JM, Wyrick-Glatzel J. Semen evaluations in the clinical laboratory: how well are they being performed? *Lab Med* 1994; **25**: 509–14.

[23] Mortimer D, Menkveld R. Sperm morphology assessment: historical perspectives and current opinions. *J Androl* 2001; **22**: 192–205.

[24] American Urological Association and American Society for Reproductive Medicine. *Report on Optimal Evaluation of the Infertile Male*, 2001.

[25] Gerris J. Methods of semen collection not based on masturbation or surgical sperm retrieval. *Hum Reprod Update* 1999; **5**: 211–15.

[26] Zavos PM. Seminal parameters of ejaculates collected from oligospermic and normospermic patients via masturbation and at intercourse with the use of a seminal fluid collection device. *Fertil Steril* 1985; **44**: 517–20.

[27] Zavos PM, Goodpasture JC. Clinical improvements of specific seminal deficiencies via intercourse with a seminal collection device versus masturbation. *Fertil Steril* 1989; **51**: 190–3.

[28] Levitas E, Lunenfeld E, Weiss N, *et al.* Relationship between the duration of sexual abstinence and semen quality: analysis of 9,489 semen samples. *Fert Steril* 2005; **83**: 1680–6.

[29] Appell RA, Evans PR. The effect of temperature on sperm motility and viability. *Fertil Steril* 1977; **28**: 1329–32.

[30] Appell RA, Evans PR, Blandy JP. The effect of temperature on the motility and viability of sperm. *Br J Urol* 1977; **49**: 751–6.

[31] Clarke RN, Klock SC, Geoghegan A, Travassos DE. Relationship between psychological stress and semen quality among in-vitro fertilization patients. *Hum Reprod* 1999; **14**: 753–8.

[32] Pound N, Javed MH, Ruberto C, Shaikh MA, Del Valle AP. Duration of sexual arousal predicts semen parameters for masturbatory ejaculates. *Physiol Behav* 2002; **76**: 685–9.

[33] Robert M, Gagnon C. Purification and characterization of the active precursor of a human sperm motility inhibitor secreted by the seminal vesicles: identity with semenogelin. *Biol Reprod* 1996; **55**: 813–21.

[34] Robert M, Gagnon C. Semenogelin I: a coagulum forming, multifunctional seminal vesicle protein. *CMLS Cell Mol Life Sci* 1999; **55**: 944–60.

[35] Lee C, Keefer M, Zhao ZW, *et al.* Demonstration of the role of prostate-specific antigen in semen liquefaction by two-dimensional electrophoresis. *J Androl* 1989; **10**: 432–8.

[36] Mikhailichenko VV, Esipov AS. Peculiarities of semen coagulation and liquefaction in males from infertile couples. *Fertil Steril* 2005; **84**: 256–8.

[37] Schrader SM. Safety guidelines for the andrology laboratory. *Fertil Steril* 1989; **51**: 387–9.

[38] Wieder JA, Lynne CM, Ferrell SM, Aballa TC, Brackett NL. Brown-colored semen in men with spinal cord injury. *J Androl* 1999; **20**: 594–600.

[39] Meacham R. Perspectives and editorials: from Androlog. *J Androl* 2002; **23**: 330–1.

[40] Owen DH, Katz DF. A review of the physical and chemical properties of human semen and the formulation of a semen simulant. *J Androl* 2005; **26**: 459–69.

[41] Cooper TG, Brazil C, Swan SH, Overstreet JW. Ejaculate volume is seriously underestimated when semen is pipetted or decanted into cylinders from the collection vessel. *J Androl* 2007; **28**: 1–4.

[42] World Health Organization. *WHO Laboratory Manual for the Examination of Human Semen and Sperm–Cervical Mucus Interactions*, 4th edn. Cambridge: Cambridge University Press, 1999.

[43] Chen F, Lu J, Xu H, Huang Y, Lu N. Chymotrypsin effects on the determination of sperm parameters and seminal biochemistry markers. *Clin Chem Lab Med* 2006; **44**: 1335–9.

[44] Zavos PM, Correa JR, Zarmakoupis-Zavos PN. Effect of treatment of seminal viscosity difficulties with a-chymotrypsin on the recovery of spermatozoa for assisted reproductive technologies: comparisons between the SpermPrepT filtration and Percoll gradient centrifugation methods. *Middle East Fert Soc J* 1997; **2**: 223–9.

[45] Adler A, Lu L, Macanas E. Chymotrypsin increases the number of sperm isolated from viscous male factor specimens. *Fertil Steril Suppl* 1997; **1**: S107.

[46] Keck C, Gerber-Schafer C, Clad A, Wilhelm C, Breckwoldt M. Seminal tract infections: impact on male fertility and treatment options. *Hum Reprod Update* 1998; **4**: 891–903.

[47] Shibahara H, Shiraishi Y, Hirano Y, *et al.* Diversity of the inhibitory effects on fertilization by anti-sperm antibodies bound to the surface of ejaculated human sperm. *Hum Reprod* 2003; **18**: 1469–73.

[48] Pattinson HA, Mortimer D, Curtis EF, Leader A, Taylor PJ. Treatment of spermagglutination with proteolytic enzymes. I. Sperm motility, vitality, longevity and successful disagglutination. *Hum Reprod* 1990; **5**: 167–73.

[49] Pattinson HA, Mortimer D, Taylor PJ. Treatment of spermagglutination with proteolytic enzymes. II. Sperm function after enzymatic disagglutination. *Hum Reprod* 1990; **5**: 174–8.

[50] Anderson DJ, Politch JA. White blood cells in semen and their impact on fertility. In: Centola G, Ginsberg K, eds. *Evaluation and Treatment of the Infertile Male.* Cambridge: Cambridge University Press, 1996: 263–76.

[51] Wolff H. The biologic significance of white blood cells in semen. *Fertil Steril* 1995; **63**: 1143–57.

[52] Wolff H, Politch JA, Martinez A, *et al.* Leukocytospermia is associated with poor semen quality. *Fertil Steril* 1990; **53**: 528–36.

[53] Barratt CL, Robinson A, Spencer RC, *et al.* Seminal peroxidase positive cells are not an adequate indicator of asymptomatic urethral genital infection. *Int J Androl* 1990; **13**: 361–8.

[54] Schaeffer AJ. Chronic prostatitis and the chronic pelvic pain syndrome. *N Engl J Med* 2006; **355**: 1690–8.

[55] Motrich RD, Maccioni M, Ponce AA, *et al.* Pathogenic consequences in semen quality of an autoimmune response against the prostate gland: from animal models to human disease. *J Immunol* 2006; **177**: 957–67.

[56] Frauscher F, Klauser A, Stenzl A, *et al.* US findings in the scrotum of extreme mountain bikers. *Radiology* 2001; **219**: 427–31.

[57] Leibovitch I, Mor Y. The vicious cycling: bicycling related urogenital disorders. *Eur Urol* 2005; **47**: 277–86.

[58] Southorn T. Great balls of fire and the vicious cycle: a study of the effects of cycling on male fertility. *J Fam Plan Reprod Health Care* 2002; **28**: 211–13.

[59] Aitken RJ. Free radicals, lipid peroxidation and sperm function. *Reprod Fertil Dev* 1995; **7**: 659–68.

[60] Agarwal A, Saleh RA, Bedaiwy MA. Role of reactive oxygen species in the pathophysiology of human reproduction. *Fertil Steril* 2003; **79**: 829–43.

[61] Fraczek M, Kurpisz M. Inflammatory mediators exert toxic effects of oxidative stress on human spermatozoa. *J Androl* 2007; **28**: 325–33.

[62] Cooper TG, Neuwinger J, Bahrs S, Nieschlag E. Internal quality control of semen analysis. *Fertil Steril* 1992; **58**: 172–8.

[63] Freund M, Carol B. Factors affecting haemocytometer counts of sperm concentration in human semen. *J Reprod Fert* 1964; **8**: 149–55.

[64] Keel BA, Vanderslice WE. Comparison of sperm counting chambers used by participants in a national andrology proficiency testing program. *Fertil Steril* 2004; **82**: S329–30.

[65] Niederberger C. Semen analysis: are 2 counts truly better than 1? *J Androl* 2004; **25**: 19–21.

[66] Ginsburg KA, Armant DR. The influence of chamber characteristics on the reliability of sperm concentration and movement measurements obtained by manual and videomicrographic analysis. *Fertil Steril* 1990; **53**: 882–7.

[67] Johnson JE, Boone WR, Blackhurst DW. Manual versus computer-automated semen analyses. Part I. Comparison of counting chambers. *Fertil Steril* 1996; **65**: 150–5.

[68] Makler A. The improved ten-micrometer chamber for rapid sperm count and motility evaluation. *Fertil Steril* 1980; **33**: 337–8.

[69] Bailey E, Fenning N, Chamberlain S, *et al.* Validation of sperm counting methods using Limits of Agreement. *J Androl* 2007; **28**: 364–73.

[70] Yanagida K, Hoshi K, Sato A, Burkman L. Automated semen analysis shows an increase in sperm concentration and motility with time in Makler chambers having excess sample volume. *Hum Reprod* 1990; **5**: 193–6.

[71] Douglas-Hamilton DH, Smith NG, Kuster CE, Vermeiden JP, Althouse GC. Particle distribution in low-volume capillary-loaded chambers. *J Androl* 2005; **26**: 107–14.

[72] Douglas-Hamilton DH, Smith NG, Kuster CE, Vermeiden JP, Althouse GC. Capillary-loaded particle fluid dynamics: effect on estimation of sperm concentration. *J Androl* 2005; **26**: 115–22.

[73] Leja Products BV. *Manual for the Assessment of Sperm Counts.* Nieuw-Vennep, The Netherlands.

[74] Johnson JE, Boone WR, Blackhurst DW. Manual versus computer-automated semen analyses. Part III. Comparison of old versus new design MicroCell Chambers. *Fertil Steril* 1996; **65**: 446–7.

[75] Seaman EK, Goluboff E, BarChama N, Fisch H. Accuracy of semen counting chambers as determined by the use of latex beads. *Fertil Steril* 1996; **66**: 662–5.

[76] Prathalingam NS, Holt WW, Revell SG, Jones S, Watson PF. The precision and accuracy of six different methods to determine sperm concentration. *J Androl* 2006; **27**: 257–62.

[77] Tomlinson MJ, Kessopoulou E, Barratt CL. The diagnostic and prognostic value of traditional semen parameters. *J Androl* 1993; **20**: 588–93.

[78] Tomlinson M, Turner J, Powell G, Sakkas D. One-step disposable chambers for sperm concentration and motility assessment: how do they compare with the World Health Organization's recommended methods? *Hum Reprod* 2001; **16**: 121–4.

[79] ESHRE (European Society of Human Reproduction, and Embryology). *Manual on Basic Semen Analysis. ESHRE Monographs.* Oxford: Oxford University Press, 2002.

[80] Muller CH, Rothmann SA, Reese AA, Orkand AR, Astion ML. *Semen Analysis Video Training Reference.* Seattle, WA: University of Washington, 2002.

[81] Keel A. The semen analysis. In: Keel BA, Webster BW, eds. *CRC Handbook of the Laboratory Diagnosis and Treatment of Infertility.* Boca Raton, FL: CRC Press, 1990: 27–69.

[82] World Health Organization. *Laboratory Manual for the Examination of Human Semen and Sperm–Cervical Mucus Interactions.* Singapore, Press Concern, 1980.

[83] World Health Organization. *Laboratory Manual for the Examination of Human Semen and Sperm–Cervical Mucus Interactions,* 2nd edn. Cambridge: Cambridge University Press, 1987.

[84] World Health Organization. *WHO Laboratory Manual for the Examination of Human Semen and Sperm–Cervical Mucus Interactions,* 3rd edn. Cambridge, UK, Cambridge University Press, 1992.

[85] Yeung CH, Cooper TG, Nieschlag E. A technique for standardization and quality control of subjective motility assessments in semen analysis. *Fertil Steril* 1997; **67**: 1156–8.

[86] Blom E. A one minute live–dead sperm stain by means of eosin–nigrosin. *Fertil Steril* 1950; **1**: 176–7.

[87] Dougherty KS, Emilson LB, Cockett AT, Urry RL. A comparison of subjective measurements of human sperm motility and viability with two live–dead staining techniques. *Fertil Steril* 1975; **26**: 700–2.

[88] Eliasson R. Supravital staining of human spermatozoa. *Fertil Steril* 1977; **28**: 1257.

[89] Davis NS, Rothmann SA, Tan M, Thomas AJ. Effect of catheter composition on sperm quality. *J Androl* 1993; **14**: 66–9.

[90] Kaye MC, Schroeder-Jenkins M, Rothmann SA. Impairment of sperm motility by water soluble lubricants as assessed by computer-assissted sperm analysis. *J Androl* 1991; **12**: P52.

[91] MacLeod J. A possible factor in the etiology of human male infertility: preliminary report. *Fertil Steril* 1962; **13**: 29–33.

[92] MacLeod J. Human seminal cytology as a sensitive indicator of the germinal epithelium. *Int J Fertil* 1964; **9**: 281–95.

[93] Kruger TF, Acosta AA, Simmons KF, *et al.* Predictive value of abnormal sperm morphology in in vitro fertilization. *Fertil Steril* 1988; **49**: 112–17.

[94] Davis RO, Gravance CG. Consistency of sperm morphology classification methods. *J Androl* 1994; **15**: 83–91.

[95] Freund M. Standards for the rating of human sperm morphology: a cooperative study. *Int J Fertil* 1966; **11**: 97–180.

[96] Kinzer DR, Caruso C, Quigley J, Rothmann SA. Sperm morphology analysis: problems as demonstrated by proficiency testing. *J Androl* 1998; **19** (Suppl): 54.

[97] Rothmann SA, ed. *Sperm Confirm: Human Sperm Morphology and Semen Cytology Atlas.* Cleveland, OH: Fertility Solutions Inc., 1997.

[98] Souchier C, Czyba J, Grantham R. Difficulties in morphologic classification of human spermatozoa. *J Reprod Med* 1978; **21**: 244–8.

[99] Rothmann SA, Reese AA. *Sperm Wizard Sperm Morphology Training Program. Master Curriculum.* Cleveland, OH: Fertility Solutions Inc., 2002.

[100] Cooper TG, Atkinson AD, Nieschlag E. Experience with external quality control in spermatology. *Hum Reprod* 1999; **14**: 765–9.

[101] Keel BA, Quinn P, Schmidt CF, *et al.* Results of the American Association of Bioanalysts national proficiency testing programme in andrology. *Hum Reprod* 2000; **15**: 680–6.

[102] Keel BA, Stembridge TW, Pineda G, Serafy NT. Lack of standardization in performance of the semen analysis among laboratories in the United States. *Fertil Steril* 2002; **78**: 603–8.

[103] Bedford JM, Bent MJ, Calvin H. Variations in the structural character and stability of the nuclear chromatin in morphologically normal human spermatozoa. *J Reprod Fertil* 1973; **33**: 19–29.

[104] Katz DF, Overstreet JW, Samuels SJ, *et al.* Morphometric analysis of spermatozoa in the assessment of human male fertility. *J Androl* 1986; 7: 203–10.

[105] Adelman MM, Cahill EM, eds. *Atlas of Sperm Morphology*. Chicago, IL: ASCP Press, 1989.

[106] Menkveld R, Stander FSH, Kotze TJ, Kruger TF, van Zyl JA. The evaluation of morphological characteristics of human spermatozoa according to stricter criteria. *Hum Reprod* 1990; **5**: 586–92.

[107] Menkveld R, Oettle EE, Kruger TF, *et al*. *Atlas of Human Sperm Morphology*. Baltimore, MD: Williams and Wilkins, 1991.

[108] Kruger TF, Franken DR. *Atlas of Human Sperm Morphology Evaluation*. London: Taylor & Francis, 2004.

[109] College of American Pathologists. *Semen Analysis Survey SEM-B*. Northfield, IL, 1999.

[110] Chow V, Cheung AP. Male infertility. *J Reprod Med* 2006; **51**: 149–56.

[111] Check JH, Adelson HG, Schubert BR, Bollendorf A. Evaluation of sperm morphology using Kruger's strict criteria. *Arch Androl* 1992; **28**: 15–17.

[112] Karabinus DS, Gelety TJ. The impact of sperm morphology evaluated by strict criteria on intrauterine insemination success. *Fertil Steril* 1997; **67**: 536–41.

[113] Menkveld R, Wong WY, Lombard CJ, *et al*. Semen parameters, including WHO and strict criteria morphology, in a fertile and subfertile population: an effort towards standardization of in-vivo thresholds. *Hum Reprod* 2001; **16**: 1165–71.

[114] Franken DR, Barendsen R, Kruger TF. A continuous quality control program for strict sperm morphology. *Fertil Steril* 2000; **74**: 721–4.

[115] Gunalp S, Onculoglu C, Gurgan T, Kruger TF, Lombard CJ. A study of semen parameters with emphasis on sperm morphology in a fertile population: an attempt to develop clinical thresholds. *Hum Reprod* 2001; **16**: 110–14.

[116] Davis RO, Gravance CG, Overstreet JW. A standardized test for visual analysis of human sperm morphology. *Fertil Steril* 1995; **63**: 1058–63.

[117] Boyers SP, Davis RO, Katz DF. Automated semen analysis. *Curr Prob Obstet Gynecol Fertil* 1989; **12**: 165–200.

[118] Garrett C, Baker HWG. A new fully automated system for the morphometric analysis of human sperm heads. *Fertil Steril* 1995; **63**: 1306–17.

[119] Moruzzi JF, Wyrobek AJ, Mayall BH, Gledhill BL. Quantification and classification of human sperm morphology by computer-assisted image analysis. *Fertil Steril* 1988; **50**: 142–52.

[120] Davis RO, Katz DF. Operational standards for CASA instruments. *J Androl* 1993; **14**: 385–94.

[121] Amann RP, Katz DF. Reflections on CASA after 25 years. *J Androl* 2004; **25**: 317–25.

[122] Hirano Y, Shibahara H, Obara H, *et al*. Relationships between sperm motility characteristics assessed by the computer-aided sperm analysis (CASA) and fertilization rates in vitro. *J Assist Reprod Genet* 2001; **18**: 213–18.

[123] Graves JE, Higdon HL, Boone WR, Blackhurst DW. Developing techniques for determining sperm morphology in today's andrology laboratory. *J Assist Reprod Genet* 2005; **22**: 219–25.

[124] Boyle CA, Khoury MJ, Katz DF, *et al*. The relation of computer-based measures of sperm morphology and motility to male infertility. *Epidemiology* 1992; **3**: 239–46.

[125] Eskenazi B, Wyrobek AJ, Fenster L, *et al*. A study of the effect of perchloroethylene exposure on semen quality in dry cleaning workers. *Am J Indust Med* 1991; **20**: 575–91.

[126] Perreault SD, Cancel AM. Significance of incorporating measures of sperm production and function into rat toxicology studies. *Reproduction* 2001; **121**: 207–16.

[127] Moline JM, Golden AL, Bar-Chama N, *et al*. Exposure to hazardous substances and male reproductive health: A research framework. *Environ Health Perspect* 2000; **108**: 803–13.

[128] Slott VL, Suarez JD, Poss PM, *et al*. Optimization of the Hamilton-Thorn computerized sperm motility analysis system for use with rat spermatozoa in toxicological studies. Fundam Appl Toxicol 1993; **21**: 298–307.

[129] Toth GP, Wang SR, McCarthy H, Tocco DR, Smith MK. Effects of three male reproductive toxicants on rat cauda epididymal sperm motion. *Reprod Toxicol* **6**: 507–15.

[130] Medical Electronic Systems, Inc. *Spermalite™ SQA-V User Guide*. Version 245, 2005.

[131] Agarwal A, Sharma RK. Automation is the key to standardized semen analysis using the automated SQA-V sperm quality analyzer. *Fertil Steril* 2007; **87**: 156–62.

[132] Akashi T, Mizuno I, Okumura A, Fuse H. Usefulness of sperm quality analyzer-V (SQA-V) for the assessment of sperm quality in infertile men. *Arch Androl* 2005; **51**: 437–42.

[133] Royster MO, Lobdell DT, Mendola P, *et al*. Evaluation of a container for collection and shipment of semen with potential uses in population-based, clinical, and occupational settings. *J Androl* 2000; **21**: 478–84.

[134] Martinez C, Mar C, Azcarate M, *et al*. Sperm motility index: a quick screening parameter from sperm quality analyser-IIB to rule out oligo- and asthenozoospermia in male fertility study. *Hum Reprod* 2000; **15**: 1727–33.

[135] McDonough PG. Has traditional semen analysis lost its clinical relevance. *Fertil Steril* 1997; **67**: 586–7.

[136] Amman RP. Can the fertility potential of a seminal sample be predicted accurately? *J Androl* 1989; **10**: 89–98.

[137] Amman RP, Hammerstedt RH. In vitro evaluation of sperm quality: an opinion. *J Androl* 1992; **14**: 397–406.

[138] Eliasson R. Sperm count and fertility: facts and myths. In: Frajese G, *et al.*, eds. *Oligozoospermia: Recent Progress in Andrology*. New York, NY: Raven Press, 1981; 1–8.

[139] MacLeod J, Wang C. Male fertility potential in terms of semen quality. *Fertil Steril* 1979; **31**: 103–16.

[140] MacLeod J. The male factor in fertility and infertility: an analysis of the ejaculate volume in 800 fertile men and in 600 men in infertile marriage. *Fertil Steril* 1950; **1**: 347–61.

[141] MacLeod J. Semen quality in 1000 men of known fertility and in 800 cases of infertile marriage. *Fertil Steril* 1951; **2**: 115–39.

[142] MacLeod J, Gold RZ. The male factor in fertility and infertility. II. Spermatozoon counts in 1000 men of known fertility and in 1000 cases of infertile marriage. *J Urol* 1951; **66**: 436–49.

[143] MacLeod J, Gold RZ. The male factor in fertility and infertility. III. An analysis of motile activity in the spermatozoa of 1000 fertile men and 1000 men in infertile marriage. *Fertil Steril* 1951; **2**: 187–204.

[144] MacLeod J, Gold RZ. The male factor in fertility and infertility. V. Effect of continence on semen quality. *Fertil Steril* 1952; **3**: 297–315.

[145] MacLeod J, Gold RZ. The male factor in fertility and infertility. VI. Semen quality and certain other factors in relation to ease of conception. *Fertil Steril* 1953; **4**: 10–33.

[146] MacLeod J, Gold RZ. The male factor in fertility and infertility. VII. Semen quality in relation to age and sexual activity. *Fertil Steril* 1953; **4**: 194–209.

[147] MacLeod J, Gold RZ. The male factor in fertility and infertility. VIII. A study of variation in semen quality. *Fertil Steril* 1956; **7**: 387–410.

[148] MacLeod J, Gold RZ. The male factor in fertility and infertility. IX. Semen quality in relation to accidents of pregnancy. *Fertil Steril* 1957; **8**: 36–49.

[149] MacLeod J, Gold RZ, McLane CM. Correlation of the male and female factors in human infertility. *Fertil Steril* 1955; **6**: 112–43.

[150] Berman NG, Wang C, Paulsen CA. Methodological issues in the analysis of human sperm concentration. *J Androl* 1996; **17**: 68–73.

[151] Handelsman DJ. Optimal power transformations for analysis of sperm concentration and other semen variables. *J Androl* 2002; **23**: 629–34.

[152] Hellstrom WJ, Overstreet JW, Sikka SC, *et al.* Semen and sperm reference ranges for men 45 years of age and older. *J Androl* 2006; **27**: 421–8.

[153] Silber S. Controversial problems involving male infertility. www.infertile.com/pdf_files/inthenew/sci/keye.pdf

[154] Sasse EA. Objective evaluation of data in screening for disease. *Clin Chim Acta* 2002; **315**: 17–30.

[155] Barratt CL, Dunphy BC, Thomas EJ, Cooke ID. Semen characteristics of 49 fertile males. *Andrologia* 1988; **20**: 264–9.

[156] Andersen AG, Ziebe S, Jorgensen N, *et al.* Time to pregnancy in relation to semen quality assessed by CASA before and after sperm separation. *Hum Reprod* 2002; **17**: 173–7.

[157] Chia SE, Tay SK, Lim ST. What constitutes a normal seminal analysis? Semen parameters of 243 fertile men. *Hum Reprod* 1998; **13**: 3394–8.

[158] Gao J, Gao ES, Yang Q, *et al.* Semen quality in a residential, geographic and age representative sample of healthy Chinese men. *Hum Reprod* 2007; **22**: 477–84.

[159] Haugen TB, Egeland T, Magnus O. Semen parameters in Norwegian fertile men. *J Androl* 2006; **27**: 66–71.

[160] Junqing W, Qiuying Y, Jianguo T, *et al.* Reference value of semen quality in Chinese young men. *Contraception* **65**: 2002; 365–8.

[161] Ombelet W, Bosmans E, Janssen M, *et al.* Semen parameters in a fertile versus subfertile population: A need for change in the interpretation of semen testing. *Hum Reprod* 1997; **12**: 987–93.

[162] Slama R, Eustache F, Ducot B, *et al.* Time to pregnancy and semen parameters: A subfertile population: A need for change in the interpretation of semen testing. *Hum Reprod* 2002; **17**: 503–15.

[163] Björndahl L, Barratt CLR, Fraser L, Kvist U, Mortimer D. ESHRE basic semen analysis courses 1995–1999: Immediate beneficial effects of standardized training. *Hum Reprod* 2002; **17**: 1299–305.

[164] Auger J, Eustache F, Ducot B, *et al.* Intra- and inter-individual variability in human sperm concentration, motility and vitality assessment during a workshop involving ten laboratories. *Hum Reprod* 2000; **15**: 2360–8.

[165] Franken DR, Smith M, Menkveld R, *et al.* The development of a continuous quality control programme for strict sperm morphology among sub-Saharan African laboratories. *Hum Reprod* 2000; **15**: 667–71.

[166] Toft G, Rignell-Hydbom A, Tyrkiel E, Shvets M, Giwercman A. Quality control workshops in standardization of sperm concentration and motility assessment in multicentre studies. *Int J Androl* 2005; **28**: 144–9.

[167] Department of Health, and Human Services, Health Care Financing Administration. Clinical Laboratory Improvement Amendments of 1988, Final Rule [42 CFR 493] *Federal Register* 1992 (Friday, February 28); **57**: 7002–86.

[168] Department of Health, and Human Services, Center for Medicare, and Medicaid Services. Chapter IV, Part

493 Clinical Laboratory Improvement. In: *42 Code of Federal Regulations* (October 1, 2004, edn). Washington, DC: Government Printing Office, 2004: 967–1087.

[169] Dunphy BC, Kay R, Barratt CLR, Cooke ID. Quality control during the conventional analysis of semen, an essential exercise. *J Androl* **10**: 378–85.

[170] Bjorndahl L, Tomlinson M, Barratt CLR. Raising standards in semen analysis: professional and personal responsibility. *J Androl* 2004; **25**: 862–3.

[171] Peters AJ, Zaneveld LJ, Jeyendran RS. Quality assurance for sperm concentration using latex beads. *Fertil Steril* 1993; **60**: 702–5.

[172] Mahmoud AMA, Depoorter B, Piens N, Comhaire FH. The performance of 10 different methods for the estimation of sperm concentration. *Fertil Steril* 1997; **68**: 340–5.

[173] Shiran E, Stoller J, Blumenfeld Z, Feigin PD, Makler A. Evaluating the accuracy of different sperm counting chambers by performing strict counts of photographed beads. *J Assist Reprod Genet* 1995; **12**: 434–42.

[174] Clements S, Cooke ID, Barratt CLR. Implementing comprehensive quality control in the andrology laboratory. *Hum Reprod* 1995; **10**: 2096–106.

[175] Davis RO, Rothmann SA, Overstreet JW. Accuracy and precision of computer-aided sperm analysis in multicenter studies. *Fertil Steril* 1992; **57**: 648–53.

[176] Cembrowski GS, Carey RN. *Laboratory Quality Management*. Chicago, IL: American Society of Clinical Pathologists Press, 1989.

[177] Westgard JO. *Basic QC Practices*, 2nd edn. Madison, WI: Westgard QC, 2002.

[178] Hassemer DJ. Interlaboratory surveys to assess performance: more than proficiency testing. *MLO Med Lab Observer* 2006; **38**: 20–5.

Chapter 34

Strict criteria for sperm morphology

Grace M. Centola and Rajasingam S. Jeyendran

Introduction

Traditionally, a sperm is defined as "normal" by its overall shape and size relative to those of the other spermatozoa in the ejaculate. Such an evaluation is in large part due to the human eye's appreciation of uniformity and symmetry.

Despite this convention, however, the majority of sperm in an ejaculate are neither uniform nor symmetrical, instead displaying tremendous variation in shape and size to the point of being classified as "abnormal." To further complicate matters, sperm take on many transitional shapes and sizes, making the identification of "normal" sperm morphology difficult. The inability to prove definitely that the fertilization potential of such transitional types is impaired exacerbates the confusion.

Determination of the structure of the sperm is an important part of the routine semen analysis. Sperm morphology has been proven to be the single most important seminal parameter with regard to predicting fertilization rate and pregnancy outcome in assisted reproduction [1–3]. **The percentage of sperm with normal structure of the head and tail can assist the physician in determining a treatment regimen for the infertile couple.** Normal sperm morphology by strict criteria has also been shown to be positively correlated with the sperm zona-induced acrosome reaction [4], tight sperm–zona pellucida binding [5], and ability to penetrate cervical mucus [6], and to be negatively correlated with leukocytospermia [7]. Guzick et al. demonstrated that the percentage of normal sperm had greater power to discriminate between fertile and infertile men than did sperm concentration and motility [8]. They suggest that threshold values for morphology, concentration, and motility can be used to classify men as subfertile, indeterminate, or fertile, but none is diagnostic of infertility. On the other hand, Nallella et al. reported that sperm motility and concentration provide more accurate information than sperm morphology, since half of the *fertile* men that were examined had abnormal morphology [9].

Sperm morphology classification schemes range from the traditional methods of McLeod and Eliasson [10–14] to the American Society for Clinical Pathology method (ASCP) [15] and guidelines from earlier editions from the World Health Organization (WHO) [16,17]. The strict criteria methods include those described in the most recent edition of the WHO manual [18], and the Tygerberg (or Kruger) Strict method [1,19]. In a recent survey of 536 laboratories enrolled in the American Association of Bioanalysts Andrology Proficiency Testing Program, more than 20 different criteria were reported as being used, with the strict method the most common (30% of laboratories), followed by the WHO method (23%) and the ASCP method (10%) [20]. Interestingly, this survey also showed that at least 28% of respondents did not indicate the morphology criteria used in their labs, and only 60% indicated the method on the semen analysis report. Furthermore, the cutoff for the normal range varied widely, from > 5% to > 80% [21]. The cutoff value for normal in each of the methods was also decidedly different: 60%, 30%, and 14% respectively for ASCP, WHO, and strict methods.

Regardless of the method a laboratory might choose for determining sperm morphology, it is essential that the method be standardized within the laboratory, and that strict quality control measures be employed [14], including proficiency testing (PT) [20,21]. Lack of adherence to accepted standards and widely different interpretations of sperm structure are prevalent and have led to the inability of physicians to compare results between different laboratories [20–24]. With continued participation in PT programs, it is hoped that there will be decreased interlaboratory variation and a marked improvement in overall laboratory analysis of sperm morphology [21].

Infertility in the Male, 4th edition, ed. Larry I. Lipshultz, Stuart S. Howards, and Craig S. Niederberger. Published by Cambridge University Press. © Cambridge University Press 2009.

Preparation of morphology slides

In theory, preparation of slides for morphology analysis is quite simple. In practice, however, the lack of performance standardization makes it difficult if not impossible to compare sperm morphologies within and between laboratories [20,21]. **One way to control for some variation is a consistent and standardized protocol for slide preparation.**

Slides are simply prepared by applying 5–20 μL of raw semen or washed sperm to a pre-cleaned glass slide. Pre-cleaning the slide with an ethanol wipe insures that the smear will adhere to the slide. The semen drop can be smeared onto the slide using a second slide or coverslip. It is important to make a thin smear of semen to allow easy visualization of individual spermatozoa. Following air-drying, the slide can be stained using various cell stains. A previous WHO method allowed examination of unstained smears using phase-contrast optics [17], but this was corrected in a later approach [18]. **Sperm morphology should never be assessed using an unstained or wet-prep slide. It is difficult, if not impossible, to determine accurate sperm morphology on an unstained preparation.**

There are several types of cell stains available for easy visualization of the sperm head, midpiece, and tail structures. The most commonly used stains are the Papanicolaou stain, modified for semen cytology by Eliasson [11], DiffQuick (Allegiance Healthcare, McGraw Park, IL, USA), and Stat III (MidAtlantic Diagnostics, Mt. Laurel, NJ, USA). The duration of the staining process and the quality of cell staining varies with each staining method. For example, a Papanicolaou stain may take hours, whereas a DiffQuick stain takes only a few minutes at most.

Following slide fixation in methanol or formalin or CytoPrep (Fisher Scientific, Pittsburg, PA, USA), the slide is immediately stained using the method of choice. When a Wright–Giemsa stain is employed, the fixative must be removed by soaking in ethanol for 20 minutes prior to staining [22]. Finally, the slide is washed in distilled water and air-dried.

For proper assessment of sperm morphology, it is important that slides be prepared using a standardized protocol. Smears should be air-dried and fixed within a set amount of time, usually within a few hours of the semen analysis. Following staining and drying of the slide, it is important to assess the stained sperm microscopically within 24 hours of slide preparation. **With increasing time from staining to observation, the cells will shrink, and thus accurate determination of head and midpiece dimensions will be compromised.** Generally, two slides are prepared for staining, with one slide proceeding through the staining process. An unstained slide can be stored and stained at a later date should the need arise to compare with subsequent semen analyses, or verify the stained sperm morphology.

Assessment of sperm morphology

A minimum of 100–200 spermatozoa are counted on the stained slide using 100× oil-immersion magnification. This allows clear visualization of the individual sperm structure. An eyepiece reticule is recommended for measuring the sperm head size (length and width) as well as the length of the sperm tail. However, with experience, an eyepiece reticule may not be necessary. Depending on the custom of the referring physicians, the andrology laboratory provides percent normal and percent abnormal, and may classify the abnormalities into the types of structural defects. With the strict classification method for assessing sperm morphology, a percent normal and abnormal is determined. Using other methods, such as WHO 2nd, 3rd, 4th edition [16–18] the percent abnormal may be further divided into head, tail, and midpiece defects. If one particular defect is more prevalent, a comment to that effect can be made in the report.

When a stained slide is assessed, only sperm with a recognizable tail are counted in the morphology tally. Tail-less sperm are not counted in the morphology assessment, since removal of the tail most likely occurred during slide preparation. Immature sperm forms, such as spermatocytes and spermatids, are not counted as part of the total percent abnormal. However, if increased numbers of round cells are seen, the trained technician can quantify the immature forms as compared with other round cells, such as lymphocytes, and other white blood cells [14]. This can provide useful information to the physician. Furthermore, it is important to insure that the presence of coiled tails is not due to hypo-osmotic stress. If increased numbers of coiled tails are seen, a wet-mount smear should be observed under phase-contrast microscopy.

Strict criteria for morphology assessment

Table 34.1 compares the strict and WHO classification methods. In most instances, an abnormal spermatozoon is obvious. It is the borderline structural variations, such as head or tail size and acrosome size, that

Table 34.1. Comparison of WHO and strict criteria for assessment of sperm morphology.

	WHO (2nd edition) [16]	WHO (3rd edition) [17]	Strict criteria [1,13,18,23]
Head	Regular oval Length 3–5 μm, width 2–3 μm Acrosome > 1/3 size of head	Smooth oval Length 4–5 μm, width 2.5–3.5 μm Acrosome 40–70% of head	Smooth and perfect oval 4–6 μm × 2.4–3.5 μm Well-defined acrosome (40–70% of sperm head)
Midpiece	Straight, regular Width < 1 μm, length 5–7 μm	Slender, regular Width < 1 μm, length 1.5 × head size	No midpiece defects Slender, regular Width < 1 μm, length 1.5 × head size
Tail	Slender, uncoiled 45 μm long	Slender, uncoiled 45 μm long	No tail defects Uniform size, 10 × head length, 45 μm long
Cytoplasmic droplets	< ½ the head size	< ½ size of the head	No cytoplasmic droplets > ½ size of the head
Vacuoles	Not stated	< 20% of head	Up to 4
General	If in doubt = normal	Borderline = abnormal	Borderline = abnormal

can stump the andrologist. Utilizing the strict method, a spermatozoon that might be considered "borderline" would be classified as abnormal [18,23], whereas with other methods, particularly the WHO [16,17] and Eliasson methods [11–14], the "borderline" spermatozoa would be classified as normal. **Utilizing strict criteria, a sperm is defined as _normal_ if its conformation agrees exactly with four strict criteria. Normal spermatozoa are identified as those with no recognizable defects that might affect their function; an ideal spermatozoon is expected to have a normal function [14,23]. All sperm not conforming to the strict criteria are classified as _abnormal_ [14].**

When strict criteria are used, a normal spermatozoon is characterized by a smooth oval head, 4.0–6.0 μm in length and 2.4–3.5 μm in width (Table 34.1) [1,13,14,18]. The acrosome must be well defined, covering 40–70% of the sperm head. There must be no midpiece or tail defects. Lastly, there should be no cytoplasmic droplets greater than half the size of the sperm head. **With these criteria, it is obvious that a well fixed and stained slide is essential for accurate determination of normal sperm.**

Attempt at a differential evaluation

Clear-cut distinctions between "normal" and "abnormal" sperm morphology have not been established, and since the majority of sperm in an ejaculate have been found to be abnormal, attempts initially were made to identify the cause for the abnormality [24–27]. Researchers probably hoped that once the etiology was identified, therapies could be implemented.

For example, a high percentage of abnormal sperm may be associated with varicocele, whereby allergic reactions may cause an increase in amorphous forms and sperm precursors. Any debilitating illness, or exposure to certain drugs that affect spermatogenesis (e.g., nitrofurans), may also produce an increase in the number of abnormal sperm [28]. The percentage of abnormal sperm forms has also been observed to increase under physical or psychological stress, as in chronic hashish users [29] and men exposed to heat [30]. The presence of a high number of sperm with cytoplasmic droplets may indicate that inadequate sperm maturation has occurred, thereby suggesting a type of epididymal pathology.

The diagnosis of a particular pathologic condition through the evaluation of specific sperm abnormalities is only possible, however, when such abnormalities occur frequently and in relatively high concentration. But as interest in male infertility and the use of advanced diagnostic techniques increased, the differential evaluation of sperm morphology lost its usefulness.

The link between sperm morphology and fertility

As sperm morphology assays were discarded, however, other facts suggested that normal morphology is essential for sperm to reach the fertilization site. Specifically, homogeneous sperm populations with normal morphology are found in the endocervical mucus, in contrast to heterogeneous sperm populations found in the ejaculate and in the lower part of the endocervical

Table 34.2. Prognostic value of strict morphology analysis [1,19]

< 4 % Normal	Severely impaired sperm
4 % – 14 % Normal	Questionably impaired sperm
> 14 % Normal	Potentially normal sperm

canal [31]. However, the percentage of abnormal sperm found in the cervical mucus is high enough to invalidate this thinking [14]. **A higher percentage of morphologically normal than abnormal spermatozoa are found bound to the zona pellucida [32–35].**

The creation of "strict criteria" to describe an ideal "normal" was therefore based on the morphology of postcoital spermatozoa found in the endocervical mucus [23]. This criterion was founded on the logic that **if normal sperm morphology is necessary for sperm to reach the fertilization site, then normal sperm morphology is de facto essential for fertilization.** Thus, by defining normal sperm morphology with very strict criteria, a number of publications seem to suggest an association between normal sperm morphology and fertility, but this association remains controversial.

Sperm morphology and IVF

The clinical value of strict morphology as a prognostic tool in IVF was initially reported by Kruger *et al.* [1]. As a way to predict fertility, Kruger *et al.* subsequently defined the range of normal sperm morphology (Table 34.2) [19]. A number of publications have confirmed the positive predictive value of strict criteria [36–47], but a number of others contradict these findings [14,23,48–50].

Sperm morphology and ICSI

Sperm morphology assessed by strict criteria, along with other male-factor analyses, was reported to be a good predictor of fertilization [51]. More specifically, researchers reported that in selecting sperm for use in ICSI, the head and midpiece must be positioned closely together in order for successful fertilization to occur [52]. Researchers also discovered, however, that no significant differences were apparent between the good and poor prognosis groups regarding their respective rates of fertilization, pregnancy, and implantation – indicating that strict morphology scores are not related to ICSI outcome [53].

Sperm morphology and IUI

Not surprisingly, the predictive power of strict morphology in IUI is also contested. A morphological evaluation based on the strict criteria was discovered to be the best predictor of pregnancy, with higher rates of success in men with 14% or higher normal morphology compared to a lower score [54]. **Strict morphology was also reported to be a good predictor of IUI success [55–60]. Strict morphology was also reported to affect pregnancy rates when IUI was used [61–64].**

Clinical relevance

The usefulness of sperm morphology

Although strict criteria for sperm morphology have been widely accepted, their usefulness remains an issue of contention. For example, the strict criteria of identifying sperm morphology as "normal" if the postcoital sperm in the endocervical mucus is normal may be imperfect: the cervical mucus is not a barrier for abnormal sperm, because ejaculates containing only sperm with no acrosomes are able to penetrate and migrate into the cervical mucus [65]. In addition, sperm morphology was not a reliable predictor in selecting sperm without chromosomal aberrations [66], while normal morphology was not a good indicator of genetically normal sperm [67].

Given this lack of objectivity and consensus in strict morphology, and also considering the large range of sperm defects as equally problematic, this type of analysis may not be appropriate in diagnosing infertility, and can detract from determining which defects are more significant than others [68,69]. Guzick *et al.* have also determined the existence of significant overlap between men considered to be fertile and men considered to be infertile, and neither sperm morphology, sperm concentration, nor motility was a powerful discriminator between the two groups [8]. Establishing high quality control standards in evaluating morphology may improve the clinical utility of morphology, especially after continuous technologist training and refresher courses [70].

The meaning of abnormal sperm cells

Improved sperm morphology observed following surgical correction of varicocele [71,72], is probably the result of influencing spermatogenesis. The ultrastructure of irregular sperm heads often shows acrosomal abnormalities [73] that appear to originate at the early spermatid stage [74,75]. Spermatozoa with no acrosome have a low concentration of phosphorus, a high content of zinc, and a variable amount of lysine, suggesting an immature nucleus [76]. The levels of FSH, LH, inhibin

B, and testosterone – the primary controllers of spermatogenesis – were related to lower levels of normal sperm morphology [77]. Similarly, low levels of nitrous oxide and testosterone in seminal plasma were related to defective sperm morphology, indicating their role in spermatogenesis [78]. **Therefore, it appears that the presence of a high number of abnormal sperm cells probably indicates a testicular and/or epididymal abnormality – but not necessarily fertility problems, since good fertilization rates can still occur** [19].

Sperm morphology tends to vary less than sperm count and sperm motility in the same male [79]. Morphology, count, and motility may be likened to a fingerprint, except when some acute process (e.g., viral infection or a heat experiment) produces a temporary change, and morphology may therefore be an indicator of the health of the germinal epithelium [80]. If so, the presence of a high number of abnormal sperm in an ejaculate is an indicator of yet unknown factor(s) that negatively influence the integrity of spermatogenesis without altering sperm production.

Normal sperm morphology and fertilization potential

It is important to re-emphasize that in no study was normal sperm morphology found to be the only predictive semen parameter with regard to fertilization and pregnancy outcome. Considering the complex biological sequences leading to these reproductive events, the lack of any provable relationship should be entirely expected. **In the absence of other male or female factors, a very high percentage of spermatozoa need to be abnormal before strict criteria can provide a definitive assessment of infertility.** Specifically, more than 96% of the sperm in an ejaculate must be abnormal for the prediction of poor fertilization potential, suggesting that morphology appears to reflect spermatogenetic quality. If so, then more steps should be taken to determine how each defect might lead to infertility before blind acceptance that all abnormal forms imply abnormal function.

Conclusions

We must accept the fact that, despite the tests applied to the ejaculate, a conclusive determination of fertilization potential may remain impossible. However, the determination of a couple's definitive inability to conceive (e.g., when almost no spermatozoa are ejaculated or when almost all spermatozoa are immotile and show severe morphological abnormalities) is

possible. In accord with this concept, presently available assays should be based on prescribed limits below which there exists a 95% certainty that fertilization cannot occur.

As a consequence, any test result that falls above this "infertility cutoff" is of little or no diagnostic use at the present time – whether or not it falls in the "normal" or "abnormal" morphological range. Although talk about "relative" fertilization capacity is tempting when such abnormal sperm assay values are obtained, such an approach is fraught with error, because fertility depends on numerous factors, including those related to the woman. Only after a sufficient number and variety of sperm tests have been developed and validated can large-scale studies be performed to determine if a combination of all these tests (coupled with multifactorial analyses) will be able to indicate the fertilization potential of an ejaculate. At the present time, such studies are premature.

We hope that the explanation provided here will dispel some of the myths surrounding the clinical significance and application of sperm morphology results. **A better understanding of exactly what a sperm morphology assessment is measuring should eliminate the apparent confusion between "normal" sperm forms and actual fertilization potential.**

References

[1] Kruger TF, Menkveld R, Stander FSH, et al. Sperm morphologic features as a prognostic factor in in vitro fertilization. Fertil Steril 1986; **46**: 1118–23.

[2] Donnelly ET, Lewis SEM, McNally JA, Thompson W. In vitro fertilization and pregnancy rates: the influence of sperm motility and morphology on IVF outcome. Fertil Steril 1998; **70**: 305–14.

[3] Sallam HN, Ezzeldin F, Sallam A, Agameya AF, Farrag A. Sperm velocity and morphology, female characteristics and the hypo-osmotic swelling test as predictors of fertilization potential: experience from the IVF model. Int J Fertil Women's Med 2003; **48**: 88–95.

[4] Bastian HS, Windt ML, Menkveld R, et al. Relationship between zona pellucida-induced acrosome reaction, sperm morphology, sperm–zona pellucida binding and in vitro fertilization. Fertil Steril 2003; **79**: 49–55.

[5] Rafaelli RJ, Spaine DMG, Cedenho AP, Srougi M. The relationship between morphology of human spermatozoa and hemizona assay. Braz J Urol 2001; **27**: 255–61.

[6] Eggert-Kruse W, Reimann-Anderson J, Rohr G, et al. Clinical relevance of sperm morphology assessment using strict criteria and relationship with sperm–mucus interaction in vivo and in vitro. Fertil Steril 1995; **63**: 612–24.

[7] Aziz N, Agarwal A, Lewis-Jones I, Sharma RK, Thomas AJ. Novel associations between specific sperm morphological defects and leukocytospermia. *Fertil Steril* 2004; **82**: 621–7.

[8] Guzick DS, Overstreet JW, Factor-Litvak P, *et al.* Sperm morphology, motility, and concentration in fertile and infertile men. *N Engl J Med* 2001; **345**: 1388–93.

[9] Nallella KP, Sharma RK, Aziz N, Agarwal A. Significance of sperm characteristics in the evaluation of male infertility. *Fertil Steril* 2006; **85**: 629–34.

[10] McLeod J. A testicular response during and following a severe allergic reaction. *Fertil Steril* 1962; **13**: 531–41.

[11] Eliasson R. Standards for investigation of human semen. *Andrologia* 1971; **3**: 49–64.

[12] Eliasson R. Analysis of semen. In: Behrman SJ, Kistner RW, eds. *Progress in Infertility, II*. Boston, MA: Little Brown, 1975: 691–713.

[13] Eliasson R. Analysis of semen. In: Burger H, DeKretser D, eds. *The Testis*. New York, NY: Raven Press, 1981: 381–99.

[14] Eliasson R. Basic semen analysis. In: Matson P, ed. *Current Topics in Andrology*. Perth: Ladybrook, 2003: 35–89.

[15] Adelman MM, Cahill EM, eds. *Atlas of Sperm Morphology*. Chicago, IL: ASCP Press, 1989.

[16] World Health Organization. *WHO Laboratory Manual for the Examination of Human Semen and Semen–Cervical Mucus Interaction, 2nd edn*. Cambridge: Cambridge University Press, 1987.

[17] World Health Organization. *WHO Laboratory Manual for the Examination of Human Semen and Sperm–Cervical Mucus Interaction, 3rd edn*. Cambridge: Cambridge University Press, 1992.

[18] World Health Organization. *WHO Laboratory Manual for the Examination of Human Semen and Sperm–Cervical Mucus Interactions, 4th edn*. Cambridge: Cambridge University Press, 1999.

[19] Kruger TF, Acosta AA, Simmons KF, *et al.* Predictive value of abnormal sperm morphology in *in vitro* fertilization. *Fertil Steril* 1988; **49**: 112–17.

[20] Keel BA, Stembridge TW, Pineda G, Serafy NT. Lack of standardization in performance of the semen analysis among laboratories in the United States. *Fertil Steril* 2002; **78**: 603–8.

[21] Keel BA. How reliable are results from the semen analysis? *Fertil Steril* 2004; **82**: 41–4.

[22] Keel BA, Quinn P, Schmidt CF, *et al.* Results of the American Association of Bioanalysts national proficiency testing programme in andrology. *Hum Reprod* 2000; **15**: 680–6.

[23] Mortimer D, Menkveld R. Sperm morphology assessment: historical perspectives and current opinions. *J Androl* 2001; **22**: 192–205.

[24] Ombelet W, Pollet H, Bosmans E, Vereecken A. Results of a questionnaire on sperm morphology assessment. *Hum Reprod* 1997; **12**: 1015–20.

[25] MacLeod J, Gold RZ. The male factor in fertility and infertility. IV. Sperm morphology in fertile and infertile marriage. *Fertil Steril* 1951; **2**: 394–414.

[26] MacLeod J. The basis and clinical significance of deviations in human cytology. In: Moghissi KS, Hafez ESE, eds. *Biology of Mammalian Fertilization and Implantation*. Springfield, IL: Charles C. Thomas, 1972: 139–52.

[27] Hellinga G. *Clinical Andrology*. London: Heinemann, 1976.

[28] Jeyendran RS, Zaneveld LJD. Semen analysis: the method and interpretation. In: Sciarra JJ, ed. *Gynecology and Obstetrics*. Philadelphia, PA: Lippincott, 1993; **5**: 1–15.

[29] Issidorides MR. Observations in chronic hashish users: nuclear aberrations in blood and sperm and abnormal acrosomes in spermatozoa. *Adv Biosci* 1978; **22–23**: 377–88.

[30] Brun B, Clavert A. Morphologic acrosomal malformation in man exposed to heat. *J Gynecol Obstet Biol Reprod (Paris)* 1977; **6**: 907–11.

[31] Menkveld R, Stander FSH, Kotze TJ, Kruger TF, van Zyl JA. The evaluation of morphological characteristics of human spermatozoa according to stricter criteria. *Hum Reprod* 1990; **5**: 586–92.

[32] Menkveld R, Franken D, Kruger TF, Oehninger S, Hodgen GD. Sperm selection capacity of the human zona pellucida. *Mol Reprod Devel* 1991; **30**: 346–52.

[33] Liu, DY, Baker, HWG Morphology of spermatozoa bound to the zona pellucida of human oocytes that failed to fertilize *in vitro*. *J Reprod Fertil* 1992; **94**: 71–84.

[34] Liu DY, Baker HWG. Acrosome status and morphology of human spermatozoa bound to the zona pellucida and oolemma determined using oocytes that failed to fertilize *in vitro*. *Hum Reprod* 1994; **9**: 673–9.

[35] Garrett C, Liu DY, Baker HWG. Selectivity of the human sperm–zona pellucida binding process to sperm head morphometry. *Fertil Steril* 1997; **67**: 362–71.

[36] Oehninger S, Acosta AA, Morshedi M, *et al.* Corrective measures and pregnancy outcome in in-vitro fertilization in patients with severe sperm morphology abnormalities. *Fertil Steril* 1988; **50**: 283–7.

[37] Van Zyl JA, Kotze TJ, Menkveld R. Predictive value of spermatozoa morphology in natural fertilization. In: Acosta AA, Swanson RJ, Ackerman SB, *et al.*, eds. *Human Spermatozoa in Assisted Reproduction*. Baltimore, MD: Williams & Wilkins, 1990.

[38] Enginsu ME, Dumoulin JCM, Pieters MHEC, *et al*. Evaluation of human sperm morphology using strict criteria after Diff-Quik staining: correlation of morphology with fertilization *in vitro*. *Hum Reprod* 1991; **6**: 854–8.

[39] Enginsu ME, Dumoulin JCM, Pieters MHEC, Evers JLH, Geraedts JPM. Predictive value of morphologically normal sperm concentration in the medium for *in vitro* fertilization. *Int J Androl* 1993; **16**: 113–20.

[40] Enginsu ME, Pieters MHEC, Dumoulin JCM, Evers JLH, Geraedts JPM. Male factor as determinant of *in vitro* fertilization outcome *Hum Reprod* 1992; **7**: 1136–40.

[41] Grow DR, Oehninger S, Seltman HJ, *et al*. Sperm morphology as diagnosed by strict criteria: probing the impact of teratozoospermia on fertilization rate and pregnancy outcome in a large *in vitro* fertilization population *Fertil Steril* 1994; **62**: 559–67.

[42] Ombelet W, Fourie FL, Vandeput H, *et al*. Teratozoospermia and in-vitro fertilization: a randomized prospective study. *Hum Reprod* 1994; **9**: 1479–84.

[43] Yang YS, Chen SU, Ho HN, *et al*. Correlation between sperm morphology using strict criteria in original semen and swim-up inseminate and human *in vitro* fertilization. *Arch Androl* 1995; **34**: 105–13.

[44] Vawda AI, Gunby J, Youglai EV. Semen parameters as predictors of in-vitro fertilization: The importance of strict criteria sperm morphology. *Hum Reprod* 1996; **11**: 1445–50.

[45] Oehninger S, Kruger TF, Simon T, *et al*. A comparative analysis of embryo implantation potential in patients with severe teratozoospermia undergoing in-vitro fertilization with a high insemination concentration or intracytoplasmic sperm injection. *Hum Reprod* 1996; **11**: 1086–9.

[46] Coetzee K, Kruger TF, Lombard CJ. Predictive value of normal sperm morphology: a structured literature review. *Hum Reprod Update* 1998; **4**: 73–82.

[47] Salumets A, Suikkari AM, Mols T, Soderstrom-Anttila V, Tuuri T. Influence of oocytes and spermatozoa on early embryonic development. *Fertil Steril 2002*; **78**: 1082–7.

[48] Morgentaler A, Fung MY, Harris DH, Powers RD, Alper MM. Sperm morphology and *in vitro* fertilization outcome: a direct comparison of World Health Organization and strict criteria methodologies. *Fertil Steril* 1995; **64**: 1177–82.

[49] Lundin K, Soderlund B, Hamberger L. The relationship between sperm morphology and rates of fertilization, pregnancy and spontaneous abortion in an in-vitro fertilization/intracytoplasmic sperm injection programme. *Hum Reprod* 1997; **12**: 2676–81.

[50] Host E, Ernst E, Lindenberg S, Smidt-Jensen S. Morphology of spermatozoa used in IVF and ICSI from oligozoospermic men. *Reprod Biomed Online* 2001; **3**: 212–15.

[51] Mahutte NG, Arici A. Failed fertilization: is it predictable? *Curr Opin Obstet Gynecol* 2003; **15**: 211–18.

[52] Emery BR, Thorp C, Malo JW, Carrell DT. Pregnancy from intracytoplasmic sperm injection of a sperm head and detached tail. *Fertil Steril* 2004; **81**: 686–8.

[53] Svalander P, Jakobsson AH, Forsberg AS, Bengtsson AC, Wikland M. The outcome of intracytoplasmic sperm injection in unrelated to "strict criteria" sperm morphology. *Hum Reprod* 1996; **11**: 1019–22.

[54] Toner JP, Mossad H, Grow DR, *et al*. Value of sperm morphology assessed by strict criteria for prediction of the outcome of artificial (intrauterine) insemination. *Andrologia* 1995; **27**: 143–8.

[55] Ombelet W, Deblaere K, Bosmans E, *et al*. Semen quality and intrauterine insemination. *Reprod Biomed Online* 2003; **7**: 485–92.

[56] Lindheim SR, Barad DH, Zinger M, *et al*. Abnormal sperm morphology is highly predictive of pregnancy outcome during controlled ovarian hyperstimulation and intrauterine insemination. *J Assist Reprod Genet* 1996; **13**: 569–72.

[57] Hauser R, Yogev L, Botchan A, *et al*. Intrauterine insemination in male factor subfertility: Significance of sperm motility and morphology assessed by strict criteria. *Andrologia* 2001; **33**: 13–17.

[58] Van Waart J, Kruger TF, Lombard CJ, Ombelet W. Predictive value of normal sperm morphology in intrauterine insemination (IUI): a structured literature review. *Hum Reprod Update* 2001; **7**: 495–500.

[59] Lee RK, Hou JW, Ho HY, *et al*. Sperm morphology analysis using strict criteria as a prognostic factor in intrauterine insemination. *Int J Androl* 2002; **5**: 277–80.

[60] Spiessens C, Vanderschueren D, Meuleman C, D'Hooghe T. Isolated teratozoospermia and intrauterine insemination. *Fertil Steril* 2003; **80**: 1185–9.

[61] Check JH, Adelson HG, Schubert BR, Bollendorf A. Evaluation of sperm morphology using Kruger's strict criteria. *Arch Androl* 1992; **28**: 15–17.

[62] Matorras R, Corcostegui B, Perez C, *et al*. Sperm morphology analysis (strict criteria) in male infertility is not a prognostic factor in intrauterine insemination with husband's sperm. *Fertil Steril* 1995; **63**: 608–11.

[63] Karabinus DS, Gelety TJ. The impact of sperm morphology evaluated by strict criteria on intrauterine insemination success. *Fertil Steril* 1997; **67**: 536–41.

[64] Check ML, Bollendorf A, Check JH, Katsoff D. Reevaluation of the clinical importance of evaluation

sperm morphology using strict criteria. *Arch Androl* 2002; **48**: 1–3.

[65] Jeyendran RS, Van der Ven HH, Kennedy WP, *et al.* Acrosomeless sperm: a cause of primary male infertility. *Andrologia* 1985; **17**: 31–6.

[66] Celik-Ozencil C, Jakab A, Kovacs T, *et al.* Sperm selection for ICSI: shape properties do not predict the absence or presence of numerical chromosomal aberrations. *Hum Reprod* 2004; **19**: 2052–9.

[67] Ryu HM, Lin WW, Lamb DJ, *et al.* Increased chromosome X Y 18 nondisjunction in sperm from infertile patients that were identified as normal by strict morphology: implication for intracytoplasmic sperm injection. *Fertil Steril* 2001; **76**: 879–83.

[68] Niederberger C. Responses to semen analysis CART report. *J Androl* 2003; **24**: 329–31.

[69] Kruger TF, Coetzee K. The role of sperm morphology in assisted reproduction. *Hum Reprod Update* 1999; **2**: 172–8.

[70] Franken DR, Kruger TF. Lessons learned from a sperm morphology quality control programme. *Andrologia* 2006; **38**: 225–9.

[71] Bouchot O, Prunet D, Gaschignard N, Buzelin JM. Surgery of varicocele: results concerning sperm motility and morphology. *Prog Urol* 1999; **9**: 703–6.

[72] Kibar Y, Seckin B, Erduran D. The effects of subinguinal varicocelectomy on Kruger morphology and semen parameters. *J Urol* 2002; **168**: 1071–4.

[73] Bisson JP, David G, Magnin C. Ultrastructural study of anomalies of the acrosome in spermatozoa with irregular heads. *Bull Assoc Anat* 1975; **59**: 345–56.

[74] Camatini M, Franchi E, Faleri M. Ultraobstructive azoospermia. *Arch Androl* 1978; **1**: 203–9.

[75] Soderstrom KO. An acrosomal abnormality in spermatids from infertile men. *Arch Androl* 1981; **7**: 275–8.

[76] Baccetti B, Renieri T, Rosati F, Selmi MG, Casanova S. Further observations on the morphogenesis of the round headed human spermatozoa. *Andrologia* 1977; **9**: 255–64.

[77] Meeker JD, Godfrey-Bailey L, Hauser R. Relationships between serum hormone levels and semen quality among men from an infertility clinic. *J Androl* 2007; **28**: 397–406.

[78] Huang I, Jones J, Khorram O. Human seminal plasma nitric oxide: correlation with sperm morphology and testosterone. *Med Sci Monit* 2006; **12**: 103–6.

[79] Schrader SM, Turner TW, Breitenstein MJ, Simon SD. Longitudinal study of semen quality of unexposed workers. I. Study overview. *Reprod Toxicol* 1988; **2**: 183–90.

[80] MacLeod J. Human seminal cytology as a sensitive indicator of the germinal epithelium. *Int J Fertil* 1964; **9**: 281–95.

Chapter 35

Sperm processing techniques

Grace M. Centola and Rajasingam S. Jeyendran

Introduction

Following thorough evaluation of both the male and female partners, the physician may employ assisted reproductive technologies (ART) to increase the chances of a successful pregnancy. **One rationale is to enhance the probability of fertilization by bringing the spermatozoa closer to the oocyte, and thus increasing the chance of successful gamete interaction.** The most appropriate choice of ART technique is usually based upon the quality of the spermatozoa, the source of the gametes, and the fertility status of the female partner. Intrauterine insemination (IUI) is often a first-line therapy, especially when the female has a documented normal evaluation, and the male presents with deficits in sperm concentration and/or motility. In-vitro fertilization (IVF) and/or intracytoplasmic sperm injection (ICSI) is most commonly utilized when there are severe deficits in sperm parameters, including questionable sperm fertility potential or long-standing, unexplained infertility of either male or female origin, or both.

The purpose of this chapter is to discuss methods of preparation of spermatozoa for IUI as well as other ART techniques. In addition, a brief discussion of preparation of frozen–thawed semen, surgically retrieved spermatozoa, and retrograde ejaculates will be included, although the reader is directed to specific chapters on semen cryopreservation (Chapter 36) and surgical sperm retrieval (Chapter 22) for details on those topics.

Sperm transport in the female reproductive tract

When mature sperm leave the epididymis and vas deferens, a process called *emission*, they are mixed with glandular secretions and form the ejaculate. These accessory gland secretions provide a vehicle for

transport and survival of the spermatozoa during early stages of transport in the female reproductive tract [1,2]. These secretions protect the spermatozoa from the acidic hostile environment of the vagina, and aid in access of the spermatozoa to the cervix and cervical mucus.

If spermatozoa are deposited in the cervical mucus at or around the time of ovulation, when *periovulatory* cervical mucus is receptive to the sperm, the motile spermatozoa migrate into the mucus and form a reservoir of sperm. These motile sperm are thought to be released into the uterine cavity in pulsatile fashion, with the sole purpose of entering the oviduct and migrating to the ampulla of the Fallopian tube, which is the site of fertilization. **Of an estimated 100 million motile sperm deposited at the cervix, only a few hundred to a thousand sperm actually enter the oviduct.** Only 0.1% of sperm placed in the upper vagina can be found in the cervical canal after one hour [3]. Some investigators have demonstrated a reduction of 5–6 orders of magnitude along the reproductive tract [4].

The periovulatory cervical mucus not only provides a vehicle for sperm entrance into the female reproductive tract but also acts as a biological filter. The mucus acts as a barrier to leukocytes, bacteria, and other contaminating agents present in the seminal fluid [5]. Prostaglandins and decapacitating agents also present in the seminal fluid are prevented from entering the uterine cavity as well.

Freshly ejaculated sperm are incapable of fertilization and must undergo a series of changes in structure and chemical function, termed *capacitation*, which end in the ability of the sperm to successfully interact with and fertilize the oocyte [1,2]. **Capacitation is a series of sperm events characterized by sperm hyperactive motility, which allows the sperm to penetrate through the cumulus cells surrounding the oocyte. The spermatozoa then gain the capability to**

Infertility in the Male, 4th edition, ed. Larry I. Lipshultz, Stuart S. Howards, and Craig S. Niederberger. Published by Cambridge University Press. © Cambridge University Press 2009.

acrosome-react and bind to the zona pellucida of the oocyte through a series of biochemical and molecular events [1,2,6,7]. In order to penetrate the oolemma, spermatozoa must have completed the capacitation process by undergoing the acrosome reaction. Whereas acrosome-reacted spermatozoa can bind to the zona pellucida and penetrate the oolemma, acrosome-intact spermatozoa cannot penetrate the zona pellucida and bind to the oolemma.

In summary, **transport of spermatozoa from the male to the site of fertilization in the female involves both active and passive transport processes from the seminiferous tubules through the epididymis and vas deferens, ejaculation into the vagina, and contact with the cervix in the female.** Upon deposition in the female reproductive tract, the spermatozoa make contact with the cervical mucus, and the motile, most normal sperm penetrate the mucus and enter the uterine cavity. Nonmotile, nonfunctional sperm, as well as contaminating cells and debris, are filtered away from the motile sperm and prevented from entering the uterine cavity. **Following a series of events, the spermatozoa undergo capacitation and the acrosome reaction, quickly penetrate through the oocyte vestments (cumulus cells), and bind to receptors in the zona pellucida.** One capacitated, acrosome-reacted sperm will then bind to the oolemma and enter the cytoplasm of the oocyte [6].

Insemination of processed sperm

The ability of spermatozoa to penetrate the cervical mucus and finally bind to the oocyte can be affected by a number of factors. These include inability of the spermatozoa to penetrate the cumulus oophorus, as well as the inability to acrosome-react and bind to the zona pellucida. In order to correct such presumed deficits, ART techniques such as ICSI can be employed. **The inability of spermatozoa to successfully transport to the site of fertilization can be a result of decreased sperm concentration (oligospermia), decreased sperm motility (asthenospermia), increased abnormal sperm forms (teratozoospermia), inability to penetrate the cervical mucus, and of female factors, including hostile cervical mucus and anatomical defects in the female tract. These factors can be circumvented by use of artificial insemination, particularly intrauterine insemination, by which the spermatozoa can be deposited directly into the uterus, closer to the site of fertilization.** The intent is to give the sperm a "head start" in the race to the site of

fertilization, and thus increase the chances of successful sperm–egg interaction.

Under normal circumstances, when the ejaculate is deposited at the cervical os, the periovulatory cervical mucus acts as a filter, allowing only motile sperm to penetrate the cervix and enter the uterine lumen. The cervical mucus filters away contaminating cells, leukocytes, debris, and bacteria, and muscle stimulants such as prostaglandins, present in the semen [8–10]. Furthermore, decapacitating factors present in the seminal fluid are removed from contact with the spermatozoa as they pass through the cervical mucus [1,2].

In order to circumvent hostile cervical mucus, oligospermia, and asthenospermia, as well as many of the other factors hindering successful sperm–egg interaction, the spermatozoa can be placed directly into the uterus. However, this cannot be done with freshly ejaculated sperm, because normally all contents of the ejaculate do not enter the uterus because of the filtering capacity of the cervical mucus. Early studies utilized unwashed semen, centrifuged into a small volume, for an IUI. In early reports, patients complained of severe cramping, and only 1 of 29 patients conceived [11]. **The semen must first be processed to remove all contaminants and to concentrate the motile spermatozoa into a small volume that can easily be placed directly into the uterus.** If done at the periovulatory period, a reasonable chance of pregnancy can be achieved.

Rationale for sperm processing

In order to place the motile sperm directly into the uterus, and thus perform an intrauterine insemination, the spermatozoa must be separated from the seminal fluid. **Some form of sperm processing, or "sperm washing" is required to isolate sperm from the seminal plasma, to initiate capacitation, and to concentrate the motile population of sperm into a small volume that can easily be accommodated by the uterus** [10,12]. The motile sperm, concentrated in a small volume of nutrient medium that is supportive of sperm motility and longevity, can be placed through the cervical opening into the uterus by using a small catheter.

No separation techniques, however, guarantee the removal of all cells and pathogens, including the hepatitis and HIV viruses [10]. Nutrient media used for processing may contain antibiotics, which will help to remove bacterial contamination [13,14], but not viruses. It is therefore prudent that the physician counsel the recipient of IUI as to the possible risks of transmitting communicable disease using untested partner's sperm.

Sperm processing techniques for IUI and for ART (IVF and ICSI) are similar. **The ultimate goal for either type of insemination is the acquisition of a concentrated fraction of motile sperm.** IUI, however, requires a higher concentration of motile sperm for deposition into the uterus, since there is significant loss of sperm during transport through the female reproductive tract. For IVF and ICSI, direct insemination of the oocyte can be achieved with very few sperm (50 000 – 100 000 sperm) in a culture dish, with a single spermatozoon injected directly into each retrieved oocyte [2].

The source of the spermatozoa to be processed for IUI is generally the entire ejaculate or frozen semen specimen, whereas the source of the spermatozoa used for IVF and/or ICSI can be from the ejaculate, from a testicular or epididymal aspirate, or extracted from testicular biopsy tissue. Spermatozoa can also be separated from neutralized urine in cases of retrograde ejaculation [15]. The urine is usually alkalinized by catheterization of the bladder and instillation of nutrient media or buffer prior to attempted ejaculation [12].

Epididymal or testicular aspiration (MESA, TESA) results in very small volumes of fluid that might contain sperm. These sperm are not motile and can be cultured overnight, with or without stimulants, prior to selection for ICSI, with the intent that some spastic or shaking movement might be induced and thus signal a viable sperm for pick-up and injection into the oocyte. Testicular biopsy tissue can be acquired by percutaneous aspiration from the testicles or open biopsy (TESE). The tissue must then be minced or digested to release individual spermatozoa, which can then be treated as for the aspirates. Individual sperm can then be removed from the tissue or contaminating fluid, picked up with a micropipette and used for ICSI. Both cell and tissue fractions can also be cryopreserved and used at a later date. Cryopreservation of epididymal and testicular aspirates and tissue in multiple vials also allows several attempts at ART and possible pregnancy.

Methods for processing semen

Sperm separation techniques have evolved from very simple wash-centrifugation procedures [16–18] to

filtration using glass wool columns[19–21], Sephadex columns [22,23], membrane filtration [24,25], albumin gradients [26,27], magnetic cell sorting [28], migration tubes [29,30], migration methods including swim-up [17,31,32], swim-down [33], and migration through sodium hyaluronate [34,35]. **The use of density gradient centrifugation procedures [28,36–43] for separation of the fraction containing the most normal and motile sperm has most recently been the method of choice [44].**

The physical characteristics of some semen samples may interfere with the efficiency of the separation procedure, e.g., seminal viscosity, incomplete liquefaction, and excessive numbers of cells other than spermatozoa (epithelial cells, leukocytes, and immature spermatogenic cells). A semen specimen should be allowed to liquefy for at least 30 minutes before processing. Extremely viscous semen samples may be gently mixed with culture medium and allowed more time before processing, or passed gently through 18- or 19-gauge needles using a syringe, although this can damage sperm. Alternately, brief treatment of the specimen with chymotrypsin has been shown to help reduce viscosity [10]. Semen that has not completed liquefaction may be gently mixed with culture medium to allow the nonliquefied coagulum to settle to the bottom of a test tube. The supernatant containing the sperm can then be drawn off and processed as desired. Semen that has excessive numbers of nonreproductive cells (e.g., "round" or epithelial cells) may be processed by first diluting the semen with buffered culture medium and increasing the number of tubes for processing.

Whenever possible, methods of sperm preparation should be used that not only enrich the motile population of cells but also increase the opportunities for subsequent fertilization by sperm that are more functional, with respect to sperm membrane and nuclear integrity. Most of the semen processing methods yield enriched populations of motile sperm, but these techniques vary in their ability to produce a finished product with the highest proportion of morphologically normal motile sperm [17,44].

Equipment, media, and supplies

Simple laboratory equipment is needed for processing semen [10]. Equipment includes a compound microscope for assessing sperm count and motility, a dry incubator for warming nutrient media and maintaining the washed preparation, a table-top centrifuge, and a storage refrigerator. Additional supplies include sterile transfer pipettes, sterile 15 mL centrifuge tubes, sterile specimen containers, test-tube racks, and nutrient medium. A standard refrigerator is used to store the medium prior to use. The refrigerator and incubator temperatures must be checked and recorded daily as part of the overall laboratory quality control program. All media must be warmed to 37 °C prior to use. This can be done in the dry incubator, in a water bath, or in a block heater on a slide warming plate.

A small table-top centrifuge is sufficient for physician office laboratories. Various types and models of centrifuges are available, including those with variable and those with fixed speeds. The centrifuge tubes containing the semen and media are centrifuged at $300 \times g$ at room temperature. A standard compound microscope is needed to assess the semen prior to washing, and to determine the sperm count and motility following processing. A counting chamber such as Makler chamber, disposable counting slide, or hemacytometer is needed to determine sperm concentration [45]. Finally, general lab supplies include sterile graduated pipettes for measuring semen volume, nutrient medium and gradients (if used), and sterile disposable transfer pipettes for removing the semen–medium fraction or removal of the pellet to a clean centrifuge tube. Sterile polystyrene centrifuge tubes for semen centrifugation, and sterile specimen containers for collection of the ejaculate, are also standard lab supplies [10].

There are many different commercially available media, such as Ham's F-10 or Tyrode's buffer, that can be used for sperm processing [10,45]. **However, the most commonly used medium for sperm processing is the commercially available synthetic human tubal fluid (HTF), which mimics the uterotubal fluids** [10]. Culture media must be tested for osmolality, pH, lack of endotoxin contamination, and biocompatibility, and must have FDA approval for human use [46]. Two buffering systems are used with gamete culture. The first is HEPES (N-2-hydroxyethylpiperazine-N'-2-ethanesulfonic acid), which has a working pH of 6.8–8.2. HEPES-buffered media is designed for use with room air. The second most common is bicarbonate-buffered medium, which relies on carbonic acid/bicarbonate equilibrium for maintaining pH. If medium is supplemented with bicarbonate buffer, a CO_2 incubator is needed, and the caps of the centrifuge tubes must be kept slightly ajar for gas exchange to maintain the pH of the medium. **Processing sperm for IUI may be done with HEPES-buffered medium, allowing capacitation to proceed in vivo (after the**

insemination). This allows the laboratory to work without the need for CO_2 incubators. Most media used in the andrology laboratory also contain a pH indicator such as phenol red, which gives the medium a light orange to pink color at neutral pH. Keeping an eye on the color of the medium can head off any problems. It is important to remember to keep HEPES-buffered media in room air, or with caps tightly closed, and bicarbonate-buffered media in a 5% CO_2 incubator with caps slightly ajar.

Sperm processing medium is supplemented with a protein source, such as human serum albumin (HSA) or synthetic serum substitute (SSS), which is essential for sperm survival and initiation of sperm capacitation. Most commonly, albumin is added by the manufacturer to the synthetic medium at 3–5 mg/mL. With regard to sperm, capacitation occurs by removal or efflux of cholesterol from the sperm membrane and is promoted by albumin [46,47]. The nutrient medium is also supplemented with antibiotics, such as penicillin/streptomycin or gentamicin, to reduce the possibility of pelvic infection. However, earlier reports suggested that the technique of processing the sperm by any of these methods reduces bacterial content [13,14,48]. Gentamicin is the antibiotic of choice, since the lab cannot always be sure if the female recipient of washed sperm is allergic to penicillin.

Nutrient media are available from several commercial suppliers in various volumes (from 10 mL for single-specimen processing up to 100–500 mL for high-volume laboratories). If purchased in large volumes, the medium should be divided among smaller vials or tubes and stored in the refrigerator. Then only the volume needed for a specimen, or for use in a particular day, can be removed and warmed prior to use.

All nutrient media are stored in the refrigerator until use. Prior to use, all nutrient media are warmed to 37 °C by incubation in an incubator, water bath, or heating block.

Simple centrifugation wash method

A simple dilution and centrifugation wash procedure was first reported by Hanson and Rock [16]. It has been the simplest and most commonly utilized procedure for preparing sperm for IUI, especially in a physician's office laboratory. This technique is especially useful for preparing frozen–thawed semen for IUI, as well as for concentration of low-sperm-count specimens [10,12]. The procedure involves 2–3 times dilution of the liquefied semen with nutrient medium, followed by centrifugation at approximately 280–300 × g for 10 minutes. The supernatant is removed, and the pellet resuspended in fresh nutrient medium, followed by a second centrifugation step. An aliquot is removed to determine the sperm concentration and motility, information which is provided to the physician performing the insemination. The final pellet is resuspended in 0.3–0.5 mL of fresh medium, and this fraction is used for the insemination.

The main disadvantage of the simple wash procedure is that not only motile sperm but nonmotile sperm, debris, contaminating cells, and bacteria are brought down into the pellet. Centrifugation of all of these cellular materials, particularly leukocytes, generates the production of oxygen radicals (reactive oxygen species, ROS) which can induce irreversible damage to the spermatozoa [10,12,45,49–51].

The simple wash procedure is recommended for semen specimens with low sperm count and motility. However, these should also be "clean," that is, with little if any debris or cells. Centrifugation of an oligoasthenospermic ejaculate with contaminating cells and debris will have significant deficits due to generation of ROS. A simple wash procedure can be used for specimens that have normal sperm parameters, with no contaminating cells and debris, and when the laboratory is not equipped to perform other preferred methods. However, the density gradient procedure for sperm preparation for IUI and IVF is still the preferred method (see below).

Simple wash for cryopreserved semen specimens

A simple wash procedure is recommended also for frozen–thawed semen [12]. **Spermatozoa that have been cryopreserved and thawed can be damaged by the freezing and thawing process. It is therefore important not to "over-process" thawed semen to prepare for an IUI.** The thawed semen–cryopreservative mix is removed to a sterile centrifuge tube. The semen–cryopreservative is diluted with twice the thawed volume using nutrient medium. This is done slowly and drop-wise so as to not subject the sperm to osmotic shock with the addition of medium with normal osmolarity. After dilution with medium, the specimen is centrifuged at 280–300 × g for five minutes, the supernatant removed and the pellet gently resuspended in fresh medium. An aliquot can be taken for determination of sperm count and motility prior to the insemination. The mean percentage of motile sperm

recovery following simple wash or even swim-up of thawed sperm is approximately 5% [12]. One study compared simple wash, density gradient centrifugation, and Sephadex column filtration, and showed no statistical differences in pregnancy rates, although density gradient centrifugation was associated with a lower pregnancy rate than the other methods [52].

Simple wash procedure for retrograde ejaculates

Retrograde ejaculation occurs when semen is forced into the bladder rather than outward through the urethra. This may be the result of various medical conditions, such as diabetes, or therapeutic medications, as well as spinal cord injury. If semen enters the bladder, the normally acidic urine renders the spermatozoa nonmotile or dead [10,53].

Laboratories that do not specialize in ART are less likely to be capable of processing urine specimens to recover retrograde ejaculates. Recovery of spermatozoa from the urine is a relatively simple procedure but necessitates strict cooperation between laboratory, urologist, and gynecologist so that sperm recovery can be timed during the periovulatory period.

Sperm can be recovered following retrograde ejaculation and used for inseminations or for other ART techniques. However, preparatory steps should be taken prior to ejaculation to neutralize or alkalinize the urine. It is important to neutralize the urine in order to minimize damage to the spermatozoa. Alkalinization of the urine is accomplished by treatment of the patient with oral bicarbonate or by catheterization of the bladder and instillation of a buffer such as phosphate-buffered saline. The patient is asked to produce a semen sample into a sterile plastic container, then to void the bladder immediately after ejaculation into a separate container. The antegrade ejaculate, if present, is processed according to routine procedures. The urine/buffer sample is examined for sperm, diluted further with nutrient medium, and placed in multiple tubes for concentration. The concentrates are collected and washed again, and then post-wash count and motility are determined. The potentially acidic and hyperosmotic nature of the urine is detrimental to the sperm cells, and reduced motility is often observed, so it is important to process the retrograde sample as soon as possible.

It is important to note that this simple centrifugation wash concentrates not only retrograde sperm, but all other contaminating debris present in the urine at the time of ejaculation. Additional

wash steps may be prudent, especially with nutrient medium supplemented with antibiotics. If motility is not greatly compromised, the sperm may be processed further by swim-up, glass wool filtration, density gradient separation, or other methods to isolate as many motile sperm as possible from the urinary proteins, cells, and other debris.

The choice of processing methods should be based on the concentration of motile sperm present in the urine, and the progressive motility of the sperm, as well as the presence of contaminating debris and dead cells.

Swim-up, swim-down migration methods

Sperm migration methods are based on the natural process of sperm migration through the cervical mucus [54], where viable sperm are filtered from nonviable, nonmotile sperm and other cellular elements. The earliest reports of sperm rise [55] and the swim-up technique [31] relied on the natural ability of motile sperm to migrate from one medium into another, i.e., from semen into nutrient medium or from one layer of nutrient medium into a "cleaner" or cell-free layer. These migration methods involve either the swim-up of motile sperm directly from semen into nutrient medium, the swim-up of motile sperm from a washed pellet of sperm, or the swim-down of motile sperm from semen into nutrient medium [10,12,45].

In the swim-up from semen method, the semen is divided equally into sterile centrifuge tubes, with approximately 1.0 mL of semen per tube. An equal volume of nutrient medium supplemented with protein and antibiotics is gently layered over the semen, and the tube capped and placed in a 37 °C incubator for approximately 1–1.5 hours. Others have suggested an incubation time of 30–45 minutes [54]. Often, the centrifuge tube is tipped on a 45° angle to provide a larger surface area for the medium to interface with the semen [54]. After the incubation, the supernatant containing the motile sperm fraction is removed, and diluted equally with fresh nutrient medium. The motile sperm fraction is then centrifuged for 5–10 minutes at 280–300 × g, and the pellet is resuspended in 0.3–0.5 mL of fresh nutrient medium for the insemination. An aliquot is taken for determination of sperm count and motility. The swim-up from semen method is thought to be the simplest way to obtain a good population of motile sperm, and, depending on the yield required, it can be a rapid procedure with normal semen specimens [32]. Abnormal specimens may

benefit from gradient centrifugation, with an excellent yield of motile sperm [32].

The second migration method involves an initial wash-centrifugation step, followed by layering of nutrient medium on the sperm pellet. After a one-hour incubation, the supernatant containing the motile sperm is removed, diluted with medium, and centrifuged. The final pellet is once again resuspended for the insemination. This procedure of swim-up from a washed pellet is useful for semen specimens with normal to high sperm concentration, normal motility, and a clean, cell-free seminal fluid. As mentioned above, centrifugation of the raw semen into a packed cell pellet may induce the formation of oxygen radicals that can irreversibly damage the viable sperm [45,49,50], especially when there is an increase in cells, particularly leukocytes. It has also been suggested that migration of sperm against the gravitational force results in a lower percentage of motile sperm recovery [12,31].

The swim-down technique involves layering the raw semen directly over nutrient medium in a centrifuge tube [12,33,45,54]. Using gravitational force, motile sperm can swim into the nutrient medium. Following incubation, the semen is removed, and the resulting swim-down fraction can be diluted with fresh medium and centrifuged, and the motile sperm pellet can be resuspended in medium for the insemination. An additional wash step can be included to remove any residual seminal fluid.

Both the swim-up and swim-down procedures have been used to isolate a clean motile population of sperm, leaving behind the nonmotile sperm, cells, and debris [56].

In terms of the efficiency of motile sperm recovery, swim-up methods rely most on quality (speed) of motility, the quantity of motile sperm in the original specimen, and the skill of the clinician/technician with pipettes [10,46,54]. The swim-up procedure is preferable for semen specimens that are relatively free of contaminating cells and debris, and with a high sperm concentration [10], since recovery of numbers of motile sperm is low [10,12,45]. Regarding temperature, swim-up procedures are more efficient if performed at 37 °C rather than room temperature.

Density gradient centrifugation

In 1977, a modified colloidal silica material was developed for gradient separation of cells [36]. Density gradient separation of sperm is based on the sperm size, motility, and density [54]. The gradient should

587

have no or minimal osmotic effect, low viscosity, and high specific gravity [54]. The first type of medium used for density gradient centrifugation of sperm was Percoll (Pharmacia AB, Uppsala, Sweden), which is polyvinylpyrrolidone-coated silica. In the mid-1990s, Percoll was removed from the market for human use and was replaced by silane-coated colloidal silica, available under several trade names. The density gradient centrifugation procedure uses centrifugal force to propel the cellular fraction of the seminal fluid into contact with the gradient material [46].

This method (also called discontinuous gradient separation) is perhaps one of the more popular, utilizing centrifugal force to propel sperm and seminal debris downward and into contact with the fluid interface between the semen and the gradient material. Motile sperm pass through the fluid interface more easily, leaving nonmotile sperm, epithelial cells, and other debris trapped at the interface. If more than one density layer is used, the sperm (and any other cellular or seminal debris) that pass through the first interface are placed in contact with the next fluid interface, and again the motile sperm are better able to pass into the next layer of gradient material. Thus, the multiple-layer gradient method effectively "cleans" the semen sample and concentrates the motile sperm at the bottom of the test tube [10,46].

For density gradient processing, a 45% gradient solution is gently layered over a 90% gradient, and the semen is layered over the top. The tube is then centrifuged at $300 \times g$ for 20 minutes. The resultant pellet is usually removed using a thin-tipped transfer pipette and placed into a clean centrifuge tube. Removal of the pellet first is more advantageous than removing the supernatant (remaining seminal fluid and gradient layers), since the pellet can be removed without contaminating the motile fraction with semen and debris. If the gradient and semen are first removed, the debris and seminal fluid wash down the sides of the tube and can be resuspended with the pellet. The pellet is resuspended in at least 2 mL fresh nutrient medium (more or less depending on the size of the pellet, i.e., sperm concentration) and centrifuged for 5–10 minutes at $300 \times g$. The final pellet is resuspended in 0.3–0.5 mL for the insemination.

Most recently, a single gradient layer has been used for sperm separation. A single interface may be utilized for routine processing of semen (for example, a gradient material of 80% or 90% concentration layered below the semen). Multiple interfaces, using more than one density gradient (for example, two interfaces – semen, 40% gradient, 80% gradient – and three interfaces – semen, 40%, 60%, 80%) are used for either routine semen samples or samples with lower numbers of motile sperm [10,46,54]. Usually a concentration of 80% or 90% gradient is advantageous for the majority of routine semen specimens. A poor specimen, such as one with low concentration, low motility, or low progression, may not penetrate the higher-concentration gradients. In these instances, a 45–60% gradient may be used, or a single gradient of 45% or 60% individually. Some have even recommended a three-layer gradient of 45%, 70%, and 90% [54], and others have recommended a combination of magnetic cell sorting and gradient centrifugation [28]. **However, a single 80% gradient is sufficient for processing almost all specimens for routine IUI, is most cost-effective, and results in recovery of adequate numbers of motile sperm [10].**

The density gradient method for sperm processing is not recommended for specimens with low sperm count and motility, or for frozen–thawed specimens. These specimens should be processed using a simple wash or swim-up procedure. Furthermore, highly viscous ejaculates are difficult to process by any of the standard wash procedures. To reduce viscosity prior to washing, an ejaculate may be pushed through a syringe fitted with an 18- to 20-gauge needle, diluted and mixed with nutrient medium prior to layering on a gradient, or incubated for a swim-up from semen method. Finally, chymotrypsin digestion of viscous samples has been favorable [10,54].

Preparation of semen specimens for IVF and ICSI

Preparation of semen specimens for ART – IVF and/or ICSI – involves the same processing as for IUI, except that a significantly lower concentration of motile sperm is required for IVF/ICSI [57]. Generally, a simple wash procedure is not recommended, once again because of the damage to sperm by oxygen radicals from exposure of sperm to leukocytes and dead cells. **The preferred methods for processing of sperm for IVF are the density gradient centrifugation procedure and the swim-up from semen procedure, with the goal being recovery of motile sperm in a concentration suitable for the desired procedure [46,57].** A combination of these procedures can also be used [46,58,59]. Following a density gradient centrifugation of a specimen with good semen parameters, but increased debris and cells, the pellet can be overlayered with fresh nutrient medium for a swim-up. Following incubation, the supernatant containing the motile fraction of sperm, usually 90–100% motile sperm, can be used directly for IVF. For IVF, 50 000–100 000 sperm are added per dish or per droplet containing the oocytes. The intent therefore is to utilize a fraction with the highest motility possible.

For ICSI, depending on the sperm concentration and the origin of the specimen, gradient centrifugation can be used, as well as swim-up from semen. Individual sperm with normal morphology are injected directly into the oocyte. **Therefore, recovery of numbers of sperm is not necessarily a concern, nor is the need for progressive motility.** Individual sperm with some evidence of viability (i.e., twitching movement) can be picked up by the ICSI pipette. In cases of totally non-motile sperm, the sperm can be diluted with hypo-osmotic buffer (as for the hypo-osmotic swelling test, HOS test), and the swelling (and hence viable) sperm used for ICSI.

In severely oligospermic specimens, more than one ejaculate can be obtained on the day of oocyte retrieval in order to increase the chances of finding motile sperm for ICSI [46]. Additionally, ejaculates can be collected the day before the oocyte retrieval and stored in refrigeration medium, or washed and incubated overnight [60,61].

Epididymal and testicular sperm

Epididymal aspiration and testicular biopsy yield very few motile sperm relative to ejaculated semen [62]. When retrieved from the testicle, spermatozoa are inherently immature, have limited motility, and are incapable of capacitation and penetration of the zona pellucida [46,52]. Epididymal sperm, on the other hand, might exhibit vigorous motility, variable sperm maturation, and a reduced ability to capacitate. **Regardless of the source of the sperm – i.e., epididymal aspiration or testicular biopsy – the lower numbers of mature, motile sperm mandate that ICSI be used to fertilize oocytes.** Processing epididymal aspirates involves the same procedures as those used to process specimens with low sperm count and/or motility, as long as the aspirate demonstrates some forward progressive motility [46]. Red blood cells can be eliminated by addition of hypotonic lysing buffer, which causes the red blood cells to lyse and release pigment into the nutrient medium. The specimen can then be

centrifuged and the pellet containing the spermatozoa retrieved and further washed.

Testicular biopsy tissue is processed by dissection of the tissue with needles, scalpel blades, small-bore pipettes, mortar and pestle, or tissue homogenizers. Tissue can also be macerated between two sterile glass slides in order to release spermatozoa from the seminiferous tubules. Following tissue mincing, nutrient medium is added, and the suspension placed into sterile centrifuge tubes. The larger pieces of tissue are allowed to settle, and are removed. The supernatant can be washed with fresh nutrient medium and examined for the presence of sperm. Usually, the spermatozoa are surrounded by large amounts of debris, cells, and tissue fragments. Spermatozoa are embedded in clumps of cells or debris, and usually show no progressive motility, or may show tail twitching. The preparation can be incubated as a thin smear or microdrop of medium overnight at 37 °C. Motile or twitching sperm may then be found along the periphery of the droplet in which the tissue was incubated, picked up with the micropipette, and then used for ICSI. If sufficient numbers of motile sperm are present, multiple-layer density gradient centrifugation can be used to recover a clean preparation of spermatozoa for use with ICSI [46].

Surgical sperm recovery from the testicle or epididymis can be scheduled to coincide with oocyte retrieval. However, it may be advantageous to schedule the sperm retrieval prior to oocyte retrieval and then cryopreserve small tissue pieces or aspirates in multiple vials. This provides enough specimen for multiple attempts at ICSI, but also allows for a contingency plan (such as use of donor sperm) should no sperm be found that would be suitable for ICSI. The tissue or aspirate is frozen utilizing the same methodology as for semen cryopreservation.

Summary and conclusions

It is relatively simple to set up a sperm preparation laboratory and perform sperm preparation for IUI. Special expertise, however, is necessary for processing of epididymal and testicular specimens for ART procedures. It is clear that with unusual, nonroutine specimens, referral to an andrology or ART laboratory would be prudent. Specimens exhibiting severe oligospermia or hyperviscosity, and retrograde ejaculates, may require more intensive laboratory manipulations to recover sufficient numbers of motile sperm.

It is difficult to identify a technique that should be used for all specimen processing procedures. **It is** important that the method of choice for processing be determined on an individual basis, dependent on sperm concentration and motility, morphology, and semen volume. Not only results of previous semen analyses but also the quality of the specimen presented on the day of the processing must be considered. A trial of sperm processing (by gradient, migration, or simple wash) is often recommended prior to initiating any ART cycle. No single separation technique is always superior. The technique that yields the most normal motile sperm should be used [63]. This is where technical andrology laboratory experience clearly provides an advantage.

References

[1] Wolf DP. Sperm–egg interaction. In: Centola GM, Ginsburg KA, eds. *Evaluation and Treatment of the Infertile Male*. Cambridge: Cambridge University Press, 1996: 6–18.

[2] Battaglia DE. Intracytoplasmic sperm injection: the process, the outcomes and the controversies. In: Patton PE, Battaglia DE, eds. *Office Andrology*. Totowa, NJ: Humana Press, 2005: 241–54.

[3] Settlage DSF, Motoshima M, Tredway DR. Sperm transport from the external os to the fallopian tubes in women: a time and quantitation study. *Fertil Steril* 1973; **24**: 655–61.

[4] Mortimer D, Templeton AA. Sperm transport in the human female reproductive tract in relation to semen analysis characteristics and time of ovulation. *J Reprod Fertil* 1982; **64**: 401–8.

[5] Jeyendran RS, Zhang XJ. Sperm processing methods. In: Jeyendran RS, ed. *Sperm Collection and Processing Methods*. Cambridge: Cambridge University Press, 2003: 107–10.

[6] Fraser LR. Sperm capacitation and the acrosome reaction. *Hum Reprod* 1998; **13** (Suppl 1): 9–19.

[7] Kupker W, Diedrich K, Edwards RG. Principles of mammalian fertilization. *Hum Reprod* 1998; **13** (Suppl 1): 20–32.

[8] Sahmay S, Atasu T, Karacan I. The effect of intrauterine insemination on uterine activity. *Int J Fertil* 1990; **35**: 310–14.

[9] Stone SC, de la Maza LM, Peterson EM. Recovery of microorganisms from the pelvic cavity after intracervical or intrauterine artificial insemination. *Fertil Steril* 1986; **46**: 61–5.

[10] Centola GM. Sperm preparation for insemination. In: Patton PE, Battaglia DE, eds. *Office Andrology*. Totowa, NJ: Humana Press, 2005: 39–52.

[11] Mastroianni L Jr, Laberge JL, Rock J. Appraisal of the efficacy of artificial insemination with husband's sperm and evaluation of insemination techniques. *Fertil Steril* 1957; **8**: 260–6.

[12] Byrd W. Processing human semen for insemination: comparison of methods. In: Centola GM, Ginsburg KA, eds. *Evaluation and Treatment of the Infertile Male*. Cambridge: Cambridge University Press, 1996: 6–18.

[13] Sun L, Gastaldi C, Peterson EM, de la Maza LM, Stone SC. Comparison of techniques for the selection of bacteria-free sperm preparations. *Fertil Steril* 1987; **48**: 659–63.

[14] Wong PC, Balmaceda JP, Blanco JD. Sperm washing and swim-up technique using antibiotics removes microbes from human semen. *Fertil Steril* 1986; **45**: 97–100.

[15] Zavos PM, Wilson EA. Retrograde ejaculation: etiology and treatment via the use of a new noninvasive method. *Fertil Steril* 1984; **42**: 627–32.

[16] Hanson FM, Rock J. Artificial insemination with husband's sperm. *Fertil Steril* 1951; **2**: 162–74.

[17] Dodson WC, Moessner J, Miller J, Legro RS, Gnatuk CL. A randomized comparison of the methods of sperm preparation for intrauterine insemination. *Fertil Steril* 1998; **70**: 574–5.

[18] Depypere H, Milingos S, Comhaire F. Intrauterine insemination in male subfertility: a comparative study of sperm preparation using commercial percoll kit and conventional sperm wash. *Eur J Ob Gyn Reprod Biol* 1995; **62**: 225–9.

[19] Paulson JD, Polakoski K, Leto S. Further characterization of glass wool column filtration of human semen. *Fertil Steril* 1979; **32**: 125–6.

[20] Jeyendran RS, Perez-Pelaez M, Crabo BG. Concentration of viable spermatozoa for artificial insemination. *Fertil Steril* **45**: 132–4.

[21] Johnson DE, Confino E, Jeyendran RS. Glass wool column filtration versus mini-percoll gradient for processing poor quality semen samples. *Fertil Steril* 1996; **66**: 459–62.

[22] Drobnis EZ, Zhong CQ, Overstreet JW. Separation of cryopreserved human semen using Sephadex columns, washing or Percoll gradients. *J Androl* 1991; **12**: 201–8.

[23] Zavos PM, Centola GM. Selection of sperm from oligozoospermic men for ARTA: comparisons between swim-up and Spermprep filtration. *ARTA* 1991; **1**: 338–45.

[24] Agarwal A, Manglona A, Loughlin KR. Filtration of spermatozoa through L membrane: a new method. *Fertil Steril* 1991; **56**: 1162–7.

[25] Agarwal A, Manglona A, Loughlin KR. Improvement in semen quality and sperm fertilizing ability after filtration through the L4 membrane: comparison of results with swim-up technique. *J Urol* 1992; **147**: 1539–41.

[26] Ericsson RJ, Langevin CN, Nishino M. Isolation of fraction rich in human Y sperm. *Nature* 1973; **246**: 421–4.

[27] Glass RH, Ericsson RJ. Intrauterine insemination of isolated motile sperm. *Fertil Steril* 1978; **29**: 535–9.

[28] Said TM, Grunewald S, Paasch U, *et al.* Advantage of combining magnetic cell separation with sperm preparation techniques. *RBM Online* 2005; **10**: 740–6.

[29] Wang FN, Lin CT, Hong CY, *et al.* Modification of the Wang tube to improve in vitro semen manipulation. *Arch Androl* 1992; **29**: 267–9.

[30] Colakoglu M, Kodama H, Fukuda J, Tanaka T. A new variation of swim-up technique in the preparation for intrauterine insemination. *Jap J Fertil Steril* 1995; **40**: 291–5.

[31] Lopata A, Patullo MJ, Chang A, James B. A method for collecting motile spermatozoa from human semen. *Fertil Steril* 1976; **27**: 677–84.

[32] Mortimer D, Mortimer ST. Methods of sperm preparation for assisted reproduction. *Ann Acad Med Sing* 1992; **21**: 517–24.

[33] Gonzales FG, Pella RE. Swim down: a rapid and easy method to select motile spermatozoa. *Arch Androl* 1993; **30**: 29–34.

[34] Wikland M, Wik O, Steen Y, *et al.* A self-migration method for preparation of sperm for in-vitro fertilization. *Hum Reprod* 1987; **3**: 191–5.

[35] Zimmerman ER, Robertson KR, Kim HR, Drobnis EZ, Nakajima ST. Semen preparation with the sperm select system versus a washing technique. *Fertil Steril* 1994; **61**: 269–75.

[36] Pertoft HC, Laurent TC. Isopycnic separation of cells and cell organelles on centrifugation in modified colloidal silica gradients. In: Catsimpoolas N, ed. *Methods of Cell Separation*, Volume 1. New York, NY: Plenum Press, 1977: 25–32.

[37] Gorus FK, Pipeleers DG. A rapid method for the fractionation of human spermatozoa according to their progressive motility. *Fertil Steril* 1981; **35**: 662–5.

[38] Morshedi M, Duran HE, Taylor S, Oehninger S. Efficacy and pregnancy outcome of two methods of semen preparation for intrauterine insemination: a prospective randomized study. *Fertil Steril* 2003; **79** (Suppl 3): 1625–32.

[39] Esteves SC, Sharma RK, Thomas AJ, Agarwal A. Effect of swim-up sperm washing and subsequent capacitation on acrosome status and functional membrane integrity of normal sperm. Int *J Fertil Women's Med* 2000; **45**: 335–41.

[40] Sharma RK, Seifarth K, Garlak D, Agarwal A. Comparison of three sperm preparation media. *Int J Fertil Women's Med* 1999; **44**: 163–7.

[41] Centola GM, Herko R, Andolina E, Weisensel S. Comparison of sperm separation methods: Effect on recovery, motility, motion parameters and hyperactivation. *Fertil Steril* 1998; **70**: 1173–5.

[42] Prakash P, Leykin L, Chen Z, *et al.* Preparation by differential gradient centrifugation is better than swim-up in selecting sperm with normal morphology (strict criteria). *Fertil Steril* 1998; **69**: 722–6.

[43] Moohan JM, Lindsay KS. Spermatozoa selected by a discontinuous percoll density gradient exhibit better motion characteristics, more hyperactivation and longer survival than direct swim-up. *Fertil Steril* 1995; **64**: 160–5.

[44] Carrell DT, Kuneck PH, Peterson CM, *et al.* A randomized, prospective analysis of five sperm preparation techniques before intrauterine insemination of husband sperm. *Fertil Steril* 1998; **69**: 122–6.

[45] Mortimer D. *Practical Laboratory Andrology*. New York, NY: Oxford University Press, 1994.

[46] Gliedt D, Reed ML. Preparation of gametes for assisted reproductive technologies. In: *Andrology and Embryology Review Course Manual*. Chicago, IL: American Association of Bioanalysts, 2003: 8.1–8.58.

[47] Cross NL. Role of cholesterol in sperm capacitation. *Biol Reprod* 1998; **59**: 7–11.

[48] Nicholson CM, Abramsson L, Holm DE, Bjurulf E. Bacterial contamination and sperm recovery after semen preparation by density gradient centrifugation using silane-coated silica particles at different g forces. *Hum Reprod* 2000; **15**: 662–6.

[49] Shekarriz M, DeWire DM, Thomas AJ, Agarwal A. A method of human semen centrifugation to minimize the iatrogenic sperm injuries caused by reactive oxygen species. *Eur Urol* 1995; **28**: 31–5.

[50] Jeyendran RS, Ruiz A, Zhang XJ. General procedures: sperm washing, sperm treatment and cryopreservation. In: Jeyendran RS, ed. *Sperm Collection and Processing Methods*. Cambridge: Cambridge University Press, 2003: 111–22.

[51] Aitken RJ, Gordon E, Harkiss D, *et al.* Relative impact of oxidative stress on the functional competence and genomic integrity of human spermatozoa. *Biol Reprod* 1998; **59**: 1037–46.

[52] Byrd W, Drobnis EZ, Kutteh WH, Marshburn P, Carr BR. Intrauterine insemination with frozen donor sperm: a prospective randomized trial comparing three different sperm preparation techniques. *Fertil Steril* 1994; **62**: 850–6.

[53] Olmstead SS, Dubin NH, Cone RA, Moench TR. The rate at which human sperm are immobilized and killed by mild acidity. *Fertil Steril* 2000; **73**: 687–93.

[54] Ruiz A, Jeyendran RS. Sperm processing procedure for intrauterine insemination. In: Jeyendran RS, ed. *Sperm Collection and Processing Methods*. Cambridge: Cambridge University Press, 2003: 123–40.

[55] Drevius LO. The "sperm-rise" test. *J Reprod Fertil* 1971; **24**: 427–9.

[56] Ing RM, Li DQ, Harding AM, Jones WR. A comparison of swim-down and swim-up methods for the extraction of high motility sperm. *Fertil Steril* 1991; **55**: 817–19.

[57] Phipps WR. Assisted reproductive technology for male factor infertility. In: Centola GM, Ginsburg KA, eds. *Evaluation and Treatment of the Infertile Male.* Cambridge: Cambridge University Press, 1996: 130–54.

[58] Ng FLH, Liu DY, Baker HWG. Comparison of percoll, mini-percoll and swim-up methods for sperm preparation from abnormal semen samples. *Hum Reprod* 1992; **7**: 261–6.

[59] Baker HWG, Ng FLH, Liu DY. Preparation and analysis of semen for IVF/GIFT. In: Trounson A, Gardner DK, eds. *Handbook of In Vitro Fertilization.* Boca Raton, FL: CRC Press, 1993: 33–56.

[60] Veeck L. TES and Tris (TEST)-yolk buffer systems, sperm function testing and *in vitro* fertilization. *Fertil Steril* 1992; **58**: 484–6.

[61] Paulson RJ, Sauer MV, Francis MM, Macaso TM, Lobo RA. A prospective controlled evaluation of TEST-yolk buffer in the preparation of sperm for human in vitro fertilization in suspected cases of male infertility. *Fertil Steril* 1992; **58**: 551–5.

[62] Silber SJ. Testis biopsy and the infertile male. In: Patton PE, Battaglia DE, eds. *Office Andrology.* Totowa, NJ: Humana Press, 2005: 215–40.

[63] Smith S, Hosid S, Scott L. Use of post separation sperm parameters to determine the method of choice for sperm preparation for assisted reproductive technology. *Fertil Steril* 1995; **63**: 591–7.

Chapter 36

Sperm banking: indications and techniques

Moshe Wald and Gail S. Prins

Introduction

Sperm can be obtained for banking purposes from various sources, depending on the clinical circumstances. Possible sources include appropriately collected ejaculated semen, postejaculate urine, and surgically retrieved testicular tissue. This chapter will discuss the various aspects of banking sperm from these sources, focusing on cryopreservation principles, techniques, and applications.

Principles
Basic principles of cryopreservation

Successful cooling and freezing of a cell from physiological to subzero temperatures, with subsequent thawing and achievement of cellular viability and functionality, requires a thorough understanding of the biological ramifications of these processes, which vary both among species and among cell types within a particular species. Thus, cryopreservation protocols should be adjusted to each species and cell type, to assure optimal outcomes [1].

The introduction of permeable cryoprotective agents (CPA), such as glycerol and dimethyl sulfoxide, allowed for the development of many cryopreservation protocols for various cells and tissues. An adequate intracellular concentration of these agents protects from potentially damaging intracellular ice formation and osmotic shock during the freezing phase. **The most widely used cell suspension cryopreservation protocols were based on the use of molar concentrations of CPAs** [1]. As most cell membranes are permeable to water and CPAs, a coupled flow of both is expected to occur at various stages of the process, including the time of CPA addition and removal, as well as during freezing and thawing. The characteristics of this coupled flow dictate cell volume and intracellular osmotic concentrations

throughout the process. As extreme changes might cause unwanted membrane stretching and even rupture [2], impermeable solutes, such as sugars, are often added to the media to prevent osmotic cellular swelling during post-thaw CPA removal [3].

Typically, there is a critical cooling rate for maximal survival, which can vary greatly among different cell types. In general, and for most cells, a high survival rate requires that the cooling rate be sufficiently slow to avoid intracellular ice formation [1,4]. On the other hand, freezing at slow rates over a long period can cause extreme concentration of extracellular solutes, which, in turn, can decrease cell survival through direct effects of the solutes on the cellular membranes or through osmotic dehydration [1,5].

The warming rate also influences cell survival, and the significance of this factor varies among different cell types. The effect of warming rate also depends on the prior cooling rate. For example, a freezing rate is generally associated with cellular accumulation of small, irregular, and thermodynamically unstable ice crystals. Cells in which such ice crystals have formed may still survive if matched with a sufficiently rapid thawing rate. However, if the warming rate is too slow, the small irregular crystals can grow into very large crystals by a process called migratory recrystallization, which can cause fatal damage to the internal cell structure [6].

In general, an inverse correlation exists between successful cryopreservation and the complexity of the biological system being frozen [1,5]. Sperm cell suspensions are considered two-compartment systems, with water shifting from the intracellular compartment to the medium outside upon extracellular ice formation. However, when tissues are cryopreserved, water must cross several layers of cells before reaching the outside medium. This process can cause damaging chemical and thermodynamic gradients [1,7].

Infertility in the Male, 4th edition, ed. Larry I. Lipshultz, Stuart S. Howards, and Craig S. Niederberger. Published by Cambridge University Press. © Cambridge University Press 2009.

Cryopreservation of spermatozoa

Human spermatozoa have a very broad response curve, with little difference in survival observed following a wide range of cooling rates [1,8–11]. Various studies on sperm cryopreservation have been conducted in an attempt to identify the optimal protocol for CPA addition and removal, and cooling and warming rates, as well as to characterize the effect of semen extenders on the sperm membrane, osmotic tolerance, and CPA permeability [1,9,12–14]. These studies suggested that the cryobiological properties of spermatozoa vary among different species [1].

The most successful methods for cryopreservation of human spermatozoa use slow initial cooling to 5 °C (–0.5 °C/min), followed by a faster freezing rate (–20 °C/min) to –80 °C and a very rapid plunge to –196°C (–200 °C/min) in the presence of glycerol buffered with a TRIS–TES egg yolk–citrate medium [9]. When these optimized freezing conditions are achieved, volume and storage container do not seem to be major factors in human sperm cryosurvival, thus permitting each user to choose between straws or vials holding between 0.1 and 1.0 mL. While satisfactory success rates have been achieved with cryopreserved sperm through either intrauterine insemination (IUI) or in-vitro fertilization (IVF), an associated decrease in post-thaw sperm viability has been reported that can be potentially significant in cases of oligospermic samples [1].

Cryopreservation procedures have been reported to cause generation of reactive oxygen species (ROS), which have been shown to have a negative effect on sperm function [15]. The levels of the peroxidative protectant enzyme superoxide dismutase (SOD) have been observed to be consistently lower in thawed cryopreserved sperm than in corresponding fresh samples [16]. Thus it has been hypothesized that inclusion of free radical scavengers (for example, α-tocopherol) in the freezing media may prevent oxidative damage during cryopreservation [15]. However, Alvarez and Storey have shown that lipid peroxidation inhibitors have no detectable effect in preventing loss of sperm viability, and that polyols are essential as cryoprotectants [16]. This suggests that while direct peroxidative contribution to sublethal cryodamage during freeze–thaw is minimal, membrane stress contribution is substantial [16]. A study by Prins and colleagues showed that the addition of dithiothritol, which prevents oxidation damage of sulfhydrol groups, was able to significantly improve post-thaw motility in poor-quality human semen, and motility was further enhanced by cryoseeding the specimen prior to final freeze [11]. While human spermatozoa are known to tolerate manipulation, appropriate sperm handling to minimize mechanical stresses (such as those involved in pipetting, mixing, and centrifugation) was also suggested as one of the determining factors for survival [15].

Cryopreservation of testicular tissue

Advanced-stage germ cells, namely spermatids and spermatozoa, can be retrieved successfully from cryopreserved testicular tissue using mechanical extraction or enzymatic digestion [1,17,18] and used subsequently for IVF with intracytoplasmic sperm injection (ICSI). Live births have been reported using spermatozoa extracted from cryopreserved testicular tissue [19,20]. Interestingly, harvesting of germ cells at earlier stages of development for cryopreservation and subsequent transplantation with further in-vivo maturation in an animal model has been reported [21]. Accumulating evidence suggests that immature male germ cells can be successfully cryopreserved if frozen following appropriate isolation methods [1,21–23].

The possible use of cryopreserved testicular tissue for grafting in an attempt to restore endocrine and reproductive testicular functions following iatrogenic or disease-induced damage has been the subject of extensive research [1]. However, successful cryopreservation of testicular tissue for this purpose is challenging, given the variation of cell types, with different cryobiological properties, and the need to protect intercellular interactions to maintain post-thaw functionality [1,24,25]. Other important considerations include the varying sizes of testicular tissue samples that are harvested, which may have an effect on CPA permeation and removal, as well as the tendency of the seminiferous tubules to trap water, which potentially can lead to ice formation and subsequent damage of the blood–testis barrier and tubule structure [1]. In fact, studies of testicular tissue following cryopreservation utilizing animal models have demonstrated significant tubular damage [26,27], suggesting the need for further experiments to identify protocols that would allow the clinical use of cryopreserved testicular tissue for subsequent transplantation [1].

Techniques
Methods for sperm collection

Donor or patient semen samples that are to be cryopreserved are collected in the same manner that is used for semen analysis at a fertility clinic or physician's office

[28]. **Sexual abstinence for 2–4 days is recommended to obtain an ideal sperm count**; however, when time is of the essence, such as with patients undergoing chemotherapy, specimens can be collected with 24 hours of abstinence on sequential days. **The recommended technique for sample production is masturbation (without lubricants) within a private room associated with the laboratory or physician's office.** This assures that the sample is processed efficiently, a factor that may be critical for poor-quality samples. The sample must be collected in a sterile, nonspermatotoxic container supplied by the laboratory. If the man cannot masturbate, for religious or psychological reasons, the sample can be produced in a condom during intercourse and transferred to a sterile container. Since it is imperative that the condom does not contain spermicides, a Milex sheath or device provided by the laboratory should be used. Coitus interruptus is not acceptable, because of contamination of the specimen.

Several sperm banks offer collection kits that can be used at home, with the sample shipped overnight to the sperm bank using an express carrier. This allows patients who cannot travel to the laboratory because of distance or illness the opportunity to bank their sperm specimens. Typically, the kits contain a sterile collection container and fresh sperm buffer that is to be mixed with the sample following collection. While this buffer preserves sperm viability for more than 24 hours, it should be noted that approximately 10% of the sperm may die during this extended period prior to cryopreservation. While this may not matter for patients with normal sperm counts, it may be less than ideal for patients with oligospermic or asthenospermic specimens.

Methods for testicular sperm retrieval

There are several surgical approaches for retrieval of epididymal and testicular sperm from patients with obstructive or nonobstructive azoospermia. In patients with obvious obstructive azoospermia (e.g., congenital absence of vas deferens, failed vasectomy reversal, etc.) sufficient numbers of sperm can be obtained by simple testicular sperm aspiration or extraction procedures (TESA and TESE, respectively), as well as by microscopic or percutaneous epididymal sperm aspiration (MESA and PESA, respectively). Other procedures, such as microdissection TESE and testis fine-needle aspiration mapping, have been developed for sperm retrieval in cases of nonobstructive azoospermia, in which the limited spermatogenesis is associated with

lower rates of successful retrieval. These methods are discussed in detail in other chapters of this book.

For collected testicular tissue, the specimens are placed in a sterile tube containing 2–4 mL of 37 °C buffered medium such as human tubal fluid (HTF) containing HEPES to maintain pH. If micro-TESE is performed, separate tubes are labeled for the left and right testes tissue. The specimens should be transported to the laboratory in a timely manner.

All procedures in the laboratory are performed under a laminar flow hood using sterile technique. The biopsy specimens are placed in a 35 mm Petri dish with HTF–HEPES supplemented with 0.3% bovine serum albumin (BSA) at 37 °C. Under a dissecting microscope, the seminiferous tubules are gently teased apart using 21-gauge needles, and the contents are gently squeezed into the surrounding media [29]. The tubules are transferred to a 15 mL conical tube containing 1 mL of fresh medium, and the cell suspension is transferred to a separate centrifuge tube. Both tubes are incubated at 37 °C for 15–30 minutes, and the supernatant of the first tube (containing tubules) is combined with the cell suspension in the second tube. The suspension is next centrifuged at $500 \times g$ for 5 minutes, and the pellet is resuspended in 1 mL Ham's F-10 with 0.3% BSA. A cell count is performed with a counting chamber, and the sperm suspension is diluted or concentrated to $0.5–1.0 \times 10^6$ sperm/mL. If the count is very low, the cells should be suspended in 200 μL media. Prior to freezing, an aliquot should be removed to assess sperm quality. The sperm count and motility can be determined manually and a morphology smear made using the feathering technique followed by staining and classification using the WHO third edition criteria [30] or the strict criteria (WHO, fourth edition) [31]. A drop of sperm cells is also stained for cell viability using 0.5% eosin Y vital stain and live : dead ratios determined [31]. This information can prove valuable to the clinician and laboratory at the time of IVF/ICSI.

Medium and specimen preparation

As discussed above, there are several ingredients of sperm cryoprotective buffers that are essential for the successful freeze–thaw of spermatozoa, and those pertinent to humans will be discussed. Successful cryomedia require the cryoprotectant glycerol [32]. However, it should be noted that glycerol itself can be detrimental to survival of human spermatozoa. **Thus it is essential that final concentrations of glycerol in the sperm mixture not exceed 7.5%; that, once added, the** cooling/freezing process commences immediately; and that, post-thaw, the mixture is removed from the sperm cells by immediate washing. Additional use of buffering components such as the zwitterion buffers TES and TRIS [33] and sodium citrate [10] has been shown to aid in the dehydration process. Use of purified egg yolk in the cryomedium has been shown to improve post-thaw recovery of the sperm cells due to protection of sperm membrane fluidity during the freeze–thaw process [10]. A direct comparison of eight different cryoprotective buffer systems for human spermatozoa included glycerol alone, citrate–egg yolk–glycerol, TES–TRIS–citrate–egg yolk–glycerol, TES–TRIS–citrate–egg yolk (no glycerol), HEPES–KOH–glycerol, and human sperm preservation medium (HSPM, a modified Tyrode's with glycerol). The highest post-thaw viability, motility, and penetration capacity was found with the TES–TRIS–citrate–yolk–glycerol mixture named TEST-CII [9,10]. This mixture is now sold commercially by Irvine Scientific (Santa Ana, CA, USA). While widely used in the sperm banking industry, TEST–yolk buffer must be removed from the sperm cells prior to in-vivo or in-vitro applications. Another cryoprotective medium that contains HEPES-buffered human tubal fluid with 1% human serum albumin, 4% sucrose, and 6% glycerol has been introduced that is claimed to be IUI-ready [34]. However, this medium does contain 6% glycerol, which can be toxic to sperm if not removed in a timely manner.

Once the semen specimen has liquefied, a sperm count, motility, and morphology assessment is made and noted in the chart for subsequent use. If the sperm concentration is $> 100 \times 10^6$ sperm/mL, the specimen can be diluted to $< 100 \times 10^6$/mL using a buffered medium such as Ham's F-10. Similarly, if the sperm count is < 20–40×10^6 sperm/mL, the specimen can be concentrated by centrifugation and resuspension to approximately 20–40×10^6 sperm/mL. These steps permit an optimized number of sperm per vial for subsequent use in pregnancy attempts using IUI. In the case of TESE, cells should be appropriately diluted or concentrated to allow for the freezing of multiple aliquots in separate cryovials. This can vary from as low as a few hundred sperm in 200 μL final volume to as many as 1–2×10^6 cells per 0.8 mL final volume.

The cryoprotectant medium is added slowly in a drop-by-drop fashion over a 10- to 15-minute period, with gentle mixing between additions in order to minimize osmotic shock to the cells. In general, a 1 : 1 dilution of sperm suspension and cryobuffer is used. It is ideal to slow-cool the specimens to 4 °C to minimize cold shock. This can be achieved by placing the tubes containing the sperm mixtures in a beaker containing 250 mL room-temperature water and placing this in a 4 °C refrigerator for 1.5–2 hours. The specimens are then transferred in 0.5–1.0 mL volumes (with exceptions noted for low sperm counts) to prelabeled cryovials or cryostraws and immediately processed for freezing. If good cryoprotectants and procedures are used, there is little difference with regard to post-thaw sperm quality when vials are compared to straws [7]. Labeling on the storage container and holding canes must include the patient's name, record number, and date. If an adequate number of sperm are available, a 100 μL aliquot should be separately frozen and thawed within 1–3 days to obtain post-thaw recovery counts and motility information, which can be invaluable during subsequent use.

Specimen freezing, storage, and thawing

Since sperm are the smallest human cells, they possess the highest surface-to-volume ratio of all cells, making them ideally suited for cryosurvival. Consequently, relatively easy methods of sperm freezing and thawing can be utilized, and routine use of programmable freezers is not required. The most common and easiest method for freezing of cryovials is to place them in the vapor phase of liquefied nitrogen for 15–30 minutes [35]. This results in a rapid freeze at the rate of approximately –20 °C per minute to the temperature of –80 °C. This can be accomplished by loading the cryovials on cryocanes and placing them in a nitrogen vapor tank used for sperm shipping, or by suspending the cryovials in the nitrogen vapor phase above the liquid phase in a nitrogen storage tank. Holders for suspending the specimens in the nitrogen vapor are available from several commercial vendors. For cryostraws, the straws can be placed on a rack that is held 10 cm above the liquid phase of nitrogen, which also rapidly freezes the sperm cells. After 15–30 minutes in nitrogen vapor, the sperm containers can be plunged into liquid nitrogen, where they can be held indefinitely at –196 °C. It is critical that the samples remain below the liquid surface until they are removed for thawing. When subsequently checked for specimen identification and location, it is imperative that the canes not be taken into room temperature, even momentarily, and plunged back into liquid nitrogen. Even though a change is not visible to the naked eye, this could result in raising and lowering the core temperature of the frozen specimen, leading to cryodamage to the cells. Specimen identification should instead be done in the mouth of the cryocontainer (–80 °C) or in a Styrofoam box containing liquid nitrogen.

Studies have been performed using programmable freezers for human spermatozoa, with marginally improved results over conventional methods [36]. Use of these systems may be desirable in high-volume facilities or when samples with poor quality and low recovery potential are being frozen. Automated systems typically use a cooling rate of –0.5 °C per minute from room temperature to –0.5 °C, seeding and freezing at –10 °C per minute to –80 °C, followed by rapid plunge to –196 °C. While these rates are similar to what is attainable with the conventional methods described above, the programmable system may provide tighter and more consistent freezing rates.

As a rule of thumb in cryobiology, thaw rates should match the freezing rates. Thus, since human sperm are frozen at rapid freezing rates, the thawing protocols should include rapid thaw rates. This can be best accomplished by placing the cryovials or straws in a 37 °C water bath for five minutes. However, when good protocols are in place, thawing at room temperature can produce equivalent results [10]. Once thawed, the sperm should be processed immediately to remove the cryoprotectants and avoid glycerol toxicity. This can be accomplished by dilution in buffered medium with 0.3% serum albumin, followed by centrifugation and a second wash. Alternatively, the specimens can be passed through glass wool columns or particulate gradients such as Percoll.

Equipment requirements and regulatory agencies

The equipment necessary for sperm cryopreservation in the laboratory includes the following: light microscope, counting chambers, calibrated pipettes, low-speed centrifuge, liquid nitrogen storage tank, nitrogen vapor holding chamber or rack, and nitrogen vapor shipping tanks. These are available from a number of commercial suppliers. Supplies will include routine delivery of liquid nitrogen, freezing medium, freezing vials or straws, canes, disposable tubes, and other standard andrology laboratory supplies. The total cost for this equipment and supplies (beyond those routinely available in an andrology laboratory) will vary between US$10 000 and US$20 000, depending upon size and current availability of a microscope.

In the United States, federal regulations now require that all facilities that freeze and bank human sperm be registered with the Federal Drug Administration, and that they follow the guidelines outlined by the Centers for Disease Control and Prevention, which have been adopted from the American Society for Reproductive Medicine (ASRM) and the American Association of Tissue Banks (AATB). The andrology laboratory performing these procedures must be CLIA-approved as a high complexity laboratory and inspected and certified by an appropriate governmentally approved certifying body.

Applications
Donor semen and screening for HIV and other known sexually transmitted diseases

Cryobanking of donor sperm is a major application for sperm cryopreservation. This use allows for the utilization of carefully screened donor semen for assisted reproductive technologies (ART) in various clinical and personal situations, mainly for couples with an irreversibly infertile male partner. Semen samples obtained from healthy donors can be used for IUI as well as for IVF when indicated by the reproductive status of the female partner. **The option of sperm cryopreservation has contributed to an increase in the availability of donor specimens, since the presence of the donor is not required at the time of the insemination. As cryobanking allows the storage of sperm for longer than six months, donors can be screened before and six months after collection for the human immunodeficiency virus (HIV) and other known sexually transmitted diseases, making the donor pool safer** [37,38].

The ASRM has provided detailed guidelines for sperm donation [39]. These guidelines have been adopted and slightly modified by the FDA, which now mandates specific requirements for all sperm banks. According to these guidelines, donors should be of legal age but younger than 40 years of age, to minimize the potential hazards related to aging. Selecting donors who have established fertility is desirable but not an absolute requirement. While anonymous donors have traditionally been used, directed (nonanonymous or known) donation is acceptable if all parties agree. **While there are no agreed-upon standards, minimal semen parameters recommended for donors include sperm motility of 50%, sperm concentration of at least 50×10^6 motile sperm/mL, sperm morphology** within the normal range and post-thaw sperm motility at > 50% of initial motility. Recommended donor screening and evaluation include a detailed medical history and a complete physical examination, as well as testing for certain genetic and infectious diseases. The latter includes serologic tests for syphilis, serum testing for HIV, active CMV infection, hepatitis B antigen (HBsAg), and hepatitis C antibody, semen or urethral tests for *Neisseria gonorrhoeae*, and urethral or urinary testing for *Chlamydia trachomatis*, to be obtained initially and repeated at six-month intervals. Potential donors who are found to be positive for these infectious agents must be excluded, with the exception of those testing positive for *Neisseria gonorrhoeae* or *Chlamydia trachomatis*, who may be reconsidered after being treated and retested [39]. **Once a donor passes the screening process, samples may be collected, frozen, and stored for a six-month quarantine period. After the donor is retested for the infectious diseases and found to be negative, quarantined samples can be released for usage.** The above criteria are applicable to all anonymous and directed sperm donors. The single exception is intimate partners who do not require the above screens and quarantine period.

Al-Inany *et al.* have studied the fertility potential of individual sperm donors, using progressively motile sperm density (PMSD) as an indicator for semen quality [40]. Semen samples with PMSD between 8 and 12×10^6/mL were considered suboptimal, while samples with PMSD higher than 12×10^6/mL were considered optimal. Interestingly, donor semen samples with suboptimal quality were found to yield pregnancy rates identical to those achieved with semen samples of optimal quality, suggesting that high-fecundability sperm donors cannot be identified on the basis of their semen analysis results.

Collection of sperm from partner for future insemination prior to vasectomy or planned gonadotoxic treatments for cancer

It is estimated that each year 76 600 American men and women treated for cancer are at risk for subsequent infertility [41]. Certain malignant diseases, such as leukemias, lymphomas, and testicular cancer, strike teenagers and young men during their reproductive years. In fact, testicular cancer is the most common malignancy in men of reproductive age [42]. Furthermore, cancers that are common in young men, such as testicular cancer and Hodgkin's lymphoma, are

some of the most treatable, creating a pool of young men who survive their malignancies and go on to potentially desire children.

Treatment methods for these malignancies include chemotherapy, surgery, and irradiation of the abdomen and pelvis, which can negatively impact fertility through direct damage to spermatogenesis or interruption of the neuronal pathways that regulate erection and ejaculation. Men who are treated with combination chemotherapy for nonseminomatous germ cell tumors of the testis were reported to have an approximately 50% risk of permanent azoospermia [41]. The probability of permanent infertility increases with the cumulative dose of the chemotherapy agents [43]. Radiotherapy for testicular seminoma could also cause permanent impairment of spermatogenesis, but most men treated with this modality were reported to recover their fertility in the months after treatment [44]. A recent study has investigated the trends in sperm parameters following chemotherapy and radiotherapy for testicular cancer [45]. A statistically significant decrease in sperm parameters was observed after these treatments, which was most significant three months after the end of chemotherapy and six months after the end of radiotherapy. Two years after therapy, 3% of the patients who received chemotherapy and 6% of those who were treated with radiotherapy remained azoospermic. Moreover, the recovery of spermatogenesis after chemotherapy or radiotherapy in this study of testicular cancer patients was not a function of pretreatment sperm parameter quality, thus providing further support for sperm cryopreservation before the initiation of such therapy.

Use of sperm cryopreservation prior to cancer therapy might be limited by the reduction in sperm parameters observed in some malignant conditions that are caused by the disease process itself. Interestingly, 30–60% of men with testicular cancer already have impaired spermatogenesis prior to any treatment, perhaps because testicular tissue abnormalities contribute to cancer risk [46]. While men with testicular cancer are the most likely to have reduced sperm parameters at the time of diagnosis, patients with other malignancies, particularly Hodgkin's disease, may also have reduced fertility even before cancer treatment begins [47]. The stage of cancer in patients with testicular cancer and Hodgkin's disease shows no relationship to their semen quality. **However, the availability of IVF/ICSI, requiring only a single sperm of good quality to achieve a pregnancy, makes it worthwhile for young men to bank cryopreserved semen prior to cancer** treatment even if their sperm counts and motility are impaired at the time of cancer diagnosis. Even one semen sample can be divided into small aliquots and frozen, to provide sufficient material for several subsequent cycles of IVF/ICSI [48]. A study of IVF procedures performed with cryopreserved semen specimens obtained from men with malignant diseases demonstrated a fertilization rate of 60% and a 40% pregnancy rate. Patients with cancers of the lymphatic system had the best results, while those with testicular neoplasm had the poorest outcome [49]. A more recent study of 10 cancer patients who used cryopreserved semen specimens for assisted reproductive treatments found that the pregnancy rate per cycle of IVF/ICSI was 36% [50], which is not unusual in competent IVF/ICSI programs when the female partner is under age 35 [47,48]. When the sperm parameters at the time of cancer diagnosis are normal or only mildly impaired, cryopreserving more than one semen sample may allow for the use of less complex ART techniques such as IUI, without or with ovarian stimulation [47,48].

Utilization of surgically retrieved sperm for IVF/ICSI in cases of complete azoospermia

The introduction of ICSI, requiring limited sperm numbers for achieving fertilization, has revolutionized the treatment of male infertility [51]. This technique, coupled with IVF, enables men whose infertility was previously considered as uncorrectable to father a biological offspring.

Cryopreserved surgically retrieved sperm can be used for IVF/ICSI in cases of both obstructive and nonobstructive azoospermia (NOA). In patients with clear-cut obstructive azoospermia (OA), such as congenital absence of vas deferens or failed vasectomy reversal, a simple open testis biopsy will yield sufficient numbers of sperm for ART. Couples in whom the male partner had a previous vasectomy and the female partner is older or has known reproductive problems could also benefit from a simple surgical sperm retrieval procedure combined with IVF/ICSI. However, as spermatogenesis is impaired in men with NOA, sperm retrieval rates have been reported to be only 36–64% if a standard testicular sperm extraction (TESE) procedure is performed [27,52,53]. Several microsurgical methods have been suggested to address this problem [54,55]. Microdissection TESE has been reported to provide better sperm retrieval through smaller volumes of testicular tissue removed, as compared to

standard biopsies, with the additional advantage of identification and preservation of the subtunical vessels, potentially lowering the risk of the testicular function impairment observed in larger-volume standard testicular biopsies [54,56].

The possible superiority of cryopreserved surgically retrieved sperm versus fresh sperm (obtained surgically on the day of the actual IVF procedure) in terms of IVF/ICSI outcomes has been subject to much debate in the recent years [57]. In early studies, fertilization and/or pregnancy rates were reported to be lower with frozen–thawed sperm than with fresh [58,59], and associated with higher spontaneous abortions and a lower live birth rate as compared with fresh testicular sperm [60]. **However, evidence is now accumulating to support the use of frozen–thawed sperm, which has multiple benefits.** Cryopreserved TESE sperm from both obstructive and nonobstructive azoospermic patients was shown to maintain adequate viability post thaw and to achieve excellent fertilization and pregnancy rates with IVF/ICSI [27]. A larger follow-up study comparing fresh versus frozen TESE sperm at a single clinic, sometimes on the same patients, with first attempt using fresh and second attempt using frozen, revealed no difference between fresh and frozen–thawed TESE sperm with regard to fertilization rates, embryo cleavage rates, pregnancy rates, delivery rates, and spontaneous abortion rates [61]. Furthermore, there was no difference between patients with OA and those with NOA. Studies at other centers have also demonstrated that in men with OA and NOA, cryopreserved sperm can yield IVF/ICSI outcomes similar to those provided by fresh TESE sperm [51,61,62]. A more recent study has retrospectively compared IVF/ICSI outcomes using fresh and cryopreserved surgically retrieved sperm in a large dataset derived from a total of 318 IVF/ICSI treatment cycles with 3280 ova obtained from 188 women [63]. Interestingly, the fertilization rates for surgically derived sperm were found to be higher for cryopreserved sperm than for freshly retrieved sperm (59.9% vs. 53.6%, respectively; chi-square $P_{-a} < 0.02$, Cramer's phi 0.04). However, the authors estimated that based on the time required to obtain data on 3280 ova, full numerical resolution of the issue of whether cryopreserved sperm are superior or similar to fresh sperm will not be available until approximately 2010. Nonetheless, these results, along with similar pregnancy rates with both types of sperm in this study, clearly indicate that cryopreserved sperm are not inferior to fresh sperm.

Routine consideration of sperm cryopreservation for possible future IVF/ICSI procedures at the time of diagnostic testicular biopsy or reconstructive surgery has been recommended, because of a number of advantages that cryopreservation provides [64]. Advanced attempts to freeze surgically retrieved testicular sperm can avoid a costly ovarian stimulation cycle for the partner if no sperm are retrieved during the TESE procedure. Freezing the specimen at the time of diagnostic biopsy minimizes testicular damage from repeated biopsies, since cryopreservation of TESE specimens allows for storage of multiple vials, which can be used for several cycles of IVF/ICSI [57]. Furthermore, surgical sperm retrieval and cryopreservation in advance may be more convenient to the couple undergoing IVF/ICSI treatment, as this approach obviates the need to perform surgical procedures on both partners on the same day [57].

Summary

The ability to successfully preserve and store male germ cells and testicular tissue offers an important contribution to the advancement of assisted reproductive technologies and reproductive medicine. Depending on its source (i.e., semen, postejaculate urine, or surgically retrieved testicular tissue), quantity, and quality, cryopreserved sperm can be used for either IUI or IVF, with or without ICSI, in various clinical settings. Donor sperm can be used in cases of uncorrectable male infertility, and the partner's semen can be collected and banked prior to vasectomy or planned gonadotoxic treatment, for future insemination. Cryopreserved surgically retrieved sperm can be used for IVF/ICSI in cases of complete azoospermia. While the availability of advanced assisted reproductive technologies (specifically, IVF and ICSI) and the development of new techniques for surgical sperm retrieval allow men whose infertility was previously considered to be uncorrectable to father a biological offspring, sperm and testicular tissue cryopreservation offers an additional advantage, negating the need for synchronization of sperm retrieval and ovulation.

The combination of theoretical techniques, derived from basic scientific principles, with extensive empirical research has resulted in improvements in various aspects of the sperm cryopreservation process, including identification of effective cryoprotectants and optimization of their use, development of appropriate cooling and warming protocols, and avoidance of damaging ice formation, solidifying the role of sperm

banking as an essential tool for state-of-the-art treatment of male-factor infertility.

References

[1] Woods EJ, Benson JD, Agca Y, Critser JK. Fundamental cryobiology of reproductive cells and tissues. *Cryobiology* 2004; **48**: 146–56.

[2] Mazur P, Schneider U. Osmotic responses of pre-implantation mouse and bovine embryos and their cryobiological implications. *Cell Biophys* 1986; **8**: 259–85.

[3] Leibo SP. A one step method for direct non-surgical transfer of frozen thawed bovine embryos. *Theriogenology* 1984; **21**: 767–90.

[4] Leibo SP, McGrath JJ, Cravalho EG. Microscopic observation of intracellular ice formation in unfertilized mouse ova as a function of cooling rate. *Cryobiology* 1978; **15**: 257–71.

[5] Critser JK, Agca Y, Woods EJ. Cryopreservation of mature and immature gametes. In: DeJonge CJ, Barratt CLR, eds. *Assisted Reproductive Technology.* Cambridge: Cambridge University Press, 2002: 144–66.

[6] Leibo SP, Mazur P, Jackowski SC. Factors affecting survival of mouse embryos during freezing and thawing. *Exp Cell Res* 1974; **89**: 79–88.

[7] Mazur P. Freezing of living cells: mechanisms and implications. *Am J Physiol* 1984; **247**: C125–42.

[8] Henry MA, Noiles EE, Gao D, Mazur P, Critser JK. Cryopreservation of human spermatozoa. IV. The effects of cooling rates and warming rate on the maintenance of motility, plasma membrane integrity, and mitochondrial function. *Fertil Steril* 1993; **60**: 911–18.

[9] Prins GS, Weidel L. A comparative study of buffer systems as cryoprotectants for human spermatozoa. *Fertil Steril* 1986; **46**: 147–9.

[10] Weidel L, Prins GS. Cryosurvival of human spermatozoa frozen in eight different buffer systems. *J Androl* 1987; **8**: 41–7.

[11] Sawetawan C, Bruns E, Prins GS. Improvement of post-thaw motility in poor quality human semen. *Fertil Steril* 1993; **60**: 706–10.

[12] Gilmore JA, Liu J, Critser JK. Osmotic tolerance limits of murine spermatozoa in the presence of extender media. *Cryobiology* 1999; **39**: 353–4.

[13] Gilmore JA, Liu J, Woods EJ, Peter AT, Critser JK. Cryoprotective agent and temperature effects on human sperm membrane permeabilities: convergence of theoretical and empirical approaches for optimal cryopreservation methods. *Hum Reprod* 2000; **15**: 335–43.

[14] Gilmore JA, Liu J, Gao DY, Critser JK. Determination of optimal cryoprotectants and procedures for their

addition and removal from human spermatozoa. *Hum Reprod* 1997; **12**: 112–18.

[15] Agca Y, Critser JK. Cryopreservation of spermatozoa in assisted reproduction. *Semin Reprod Med* 2002; **20**: 15–23.

[16] Alvarez JG, Storey BT. Evidence for increased lipid peroxidase damage and loss of superoxide dismutase activity as a mode of sublethal cryodamage to human sperm during cryopreservation. *J Androl* 1992; **13**: 232–41.

[17] Bahadur G, Chatterjee R, Ralph D. Testicular tissue cryopreservation in boys: ethical and legal issues. *Hum Reprod* 2000; **15**: 1416–20.

[18] Res U, Res P, Kastelic D, Stanovnik M, Kmetec A, Merlo A. Birth after treatment of a male with seminoma and azoospermia with cryopreserved–thawed testicular tissue. *Hum Reprod* 2000; **15**: 861–4.

[19] Borini A, Sereni E, Bonu C, Flamigni C. Freezing a few testicular spermatozoa retrieved by TESA. *Mol Cell Endocrinol* 2000; **169**: 27–32.

[20] Salzbrunn A, Benson DM, Holstein AF, Schulze W. A new concept for the extraction of testicular spermatozoa as a tool for assisted fertilization (ICSI). *Hum Reprod* 1996; **11**: 752–75.

[21] Avarbock MR, Brinster CJ, Brinster RL. Reconstituition of spermatogenesis from frozen spermatogonial stem cells. *Nat Med* 1996; **2**: 693–6.

[22] Crabbe E, Verheyen G, Tournaye H, Van Steirteghem A. Freezing of testicular tissue as a minced suspension preserves sperm quality better than whole-biopsy freezing when glycerol is used as a cryoprotectant. *Int J Androl* 1999; **22**: 43–8.

[23] Ogura A, Matsuda J, Asano T, Suzuki O, Yanagimachi R. Mouse oocytes injected with cryopreserved round spermatids can develop into normal offspring. *J Assist Reprod Genet* 1996; **13**: 431–4.

[24] Karlsson JO, Toner M. Long-term storage of tissues by cryopreservation: critical issues. *Biomaterials* 1996; **17**: 243–56.

[25] Paynter S, Cooper A, Thomas N, Fuller B. Cryopreservation of multicellular embryos and reproductive tissues. In: Karow AM, Critser JK, eds. *Reproductive Tissue Banking: Scientific Principles*. New York, NY: Academic Press, 1997: 359–97.

[26] Jezek D, Schulze W, Kalanj-Bognar S, et al. Effects of various cryopreservation media and freezing–thawing on the morphology of rat testicular biopsies. *Andrologia* 2001; **33**: 368–78.

[27] Yin H, Wang X, Kim SS, et al. Transplantation of intact rat gonads using vascular anastomosis: Effects of cryopreservation, ischemia and genotype. *Hum Reprod* 2003; **18**: 1165–72.

[28] Prins GS. Semen analysis. In: Centola G, Lamb DJ, eds. *Andrology and Embryology Review Course*. St. Louis, MO: American Association of Bioanalysts, 2003: 5.1–5.16.

[29] Prins GS, Dolgina R, Studney P, et al. Quality of cryopreserved testicular sperm in patients with obstructive and nonobstructive azoospermia. *J Urol* 1999; **161**: 1504–8.

[30] World Health Organization. *WHO Laboratory Manual for the Examination of Human Sperm and Sperm–Cervical Mucus Interaction*, 3rd edn. Cambridge, Cambridge University Press, 1992.

[31] World Health Organization. *WHO Laboratory Manual for the Examination of Human Sperm and Sperm–Cervical Mucus Interaction*, 4th edn. Cambridge: Cambridge University Press, 1999.

[32] Polge G, Smith AU, Parkes AS. Revival of spermatozoa after vitrification and dehydration at low temperatures. *Nature* 1949; **164**: 666–9.

[33] Graham EF, Crabo B, Brown K. Effects of some zwitter ion buffers on the freezing and storage of spermatozoa. *J Dairy Sci* 1972; **55**: 372–8.

[34] Larson JM, McKinney K, Mixon B, Burry B, Wolf DP. An intrauterine insemination-ready cryopreservation method compared with sperm recovery after conventional freezing and post-thaw processing. *Fertil Steril* 1998; **67**: 81–7.

[35] Sherman JK. Improved methods of preservation of human spematozoa by freezing and freeze-drying. *Fertil Steril* 1963; **14**: 49–54.

[36] Critser JK, Huse-Benda A, Aaker D, Arneson B, Ball G. Cryopreservation of human spermatozoa. I. Effects on holding procedure and seeding on motility, fertilizability and acrosome reaction. *Fertil Steril* 1987; **47**: 656–63.

[37] Witt MA. Sperm banking. In: Lipshultz LI, Howards SS, eds. *Infertility in the Male*, 3rd edn. St. Louis, MO: Mosby Year Book, 1997: 501.

[38] Stewart GJ, Tyler JP, Cunningham AL, Barr JA, Driscoll GL, Gold J, Lamont BJ. Transmission of human T-cell lymphotrophic virus type III (HTLV-III) by artificial insemination by donor. *Lancet* 1985; **2**: 581–5.

[39] American Society for Reproductive Medicine. Guidelines for sperm donation. *Fertil Steril* 2004; **82**: S9–12.

[40] Al-Inany HG, Dunselman GAJ, Dumoulin JCM, Maas JWM, Evers JLH. Fertility potential of individual sperm donors. *Gynecol Obstet Invest* 1999; **47**: 147–50.

[41] Meistrich ML, Vassilopoulou-Sellin R, Lipshultz LI. Gonadal dysfunction. In: Devita VT, Hellman S, Rosenberg SA, eds. *Cancer: Principles and Practice of Oncology*, 5th edn. Philadelphia, PA: Lippincott-Raven, 1997: 2758–73.

[42] Huyghe E, Matsuda T, Thonneau P. Increasing incidence of testicular cancer worldwide: a review. *J Urol* 2003; **170**: 5–11.

[43] Howell SJ, Shalet SM. Pharmacological protection of the gonads. *Med Pediatr Oncol* 1999; **33**: 41–5.

[44] Gordon W, Siegmund K, Stanisic TH, *et al.* A study of reproductive function in patients with seminoma treated with radiotherapy and orchidectomy (SWOG-8711). Southwest Oncology Group. *Int J Radiat Oncol Biol Phys* 1997; **38**: 83–94.

[45] Gandini L, Sgro P, Lombardo F, *et al.* Effect of chemo- or radiotherapy on sperm parameters of testicular cancer patients. *Hum Reprod* 2006; **21**: 2882–9.

[46] Petersen PM, Giwercman A, Skakkebaek N, Rorth M. Gonadal function in men with testicular cancer. *Semin Oncol* 1998; **25**: 224–33.

[47] Naysmith TE, Blake DA, Harvey VJ, Johnson NP. Do men undergoing sterilizing cancer treatments have a fertile future? *Hum Reprod* 1998; **13**: 3250–5.

[48] Opsahl MS, Fugger EF, Sherins RJ, Schulman JD. Preservation of reproductive function before therapy for cancer: new options involving sperm and ovary cryopreservation. *Cancer J Sci Am* 1997; **3**: 189–91.

[49] Khalifa E, Oehninger S, Acosta AA, *et al.* Successful fertilization and pregnancy outcome in in-vitro fertilization using cryopreserved/thawed spermatozoa from patients with malignant diseases. *Hum Reprod* 1992; **7**: 105–8.

[50] Hallak J, Hendin B, Thomas AJ, Agarwal A. Investigation of fertilizing capacity of cryopreserved spermatozoa from patients with cancer. *J Urol* 1998; **159**: 1217–20.

[51] Palermo G, Joris H, Devroey P, Van Steirtghem AC. Pregnancies after intracytoplasmic injection of single spermatozoon into an oocyte. *Lancet* 1992; **340**: 17–18.

[52] Palermo GD, Schlegel PN, Hariprashad JJ, *et al.* Fertilization and pregnancy outcome with intracytoplasmic sperm injection for azoospermic men. *Hum Reprod* 1999; **14**: 741–8.

[53] Schlegel PN, Palermo GD, Goldstein M, *et al.* Testicular sperm extraction with intracytoplasmic sperm injection for nonobstructive azoospermia. *Urology* 1997; **49**: 435–40.

[54] Schlegel PN. Testicular sperm extraction: microdissection improves sperm yield with minimal tissue excision. *Hum Reprod* 1999; **14**: 131–5.

[55] Turek PJ, Ljung BM, Cha I, Conaghan J. Diagnostic findings from testis fine needle aspiration mapping in obstructed and nonobstructed azoospermic men. *J Urol* 2000; **163**: 1709–16.

[56] Manning M, Junemann KP, Alken P. Decrease in testosterone blood concentrations after testicular sperm extraction for intracytoplasmic sperm injection in azoospermic men. *Lancet* 1998; **352**: 37.

[57] Wald M, Niederberger CS, Ross LS. Surgical sperm retrieval for assisted reproduction. *Minerva Ginecol* 2004; **56**: 217–22.

[58] Romero J, Remohi J, Minguez Y, *et al.* Fertilization after intracytoplasmic sperm injection with cryopreserved testicular spermatozoa. *Fertil Steril* 1996; **65**: 877–9.

[59] Verheyen G, Nagy Z, Joris H, *et al.* Quality of frozen–thawed testicular sperm and its preclinical use for intracytoplasmic sperm injection into *in vitro*-matured germinal-vesicle stage oocytes. *Fertil Steril* 1997; **67**: 74–80.

[60] Belker AM. Bioethics and law forum. *J Androl* 1999; **20**: 331.

[61] Friedler S, Raziel A, Soffer Y, *et al.* Intracytoplasmic injection of fresh and cryopreserved testicular spermatozoa in patients with nonobstructive azoospermia – a comparative study. Fertil Steril 1997; **68**: 892–7.

[62] Gil-Salom M, Romero J, Minguez Y, *et al.* Pregnancies after intracytoplasmic sperm injection with cryopreserved testicular spermatozoa. *Hum Reprod* 1996; **11**: 1309–13.

[63] Wald M, Ross LS, Prins GS, Cieslak-Janzen J, Wolf G. Analysis of outcomes of cryopreserved surgically retrieved sperm for IVF/ICSI. *J Androl* 2006; **27**: 60–5.

[64] Habermann H, Seo R, Cieslak J, *et al. In vitro* fertilization outcomes after intracytoplasmic sperm injection with fresh or frozen–thawed testicular spermatozoa. *Fertil Steril* 2000; **73**: 955–60.

Chapter 37

Tests for antisperm antibodies

Suresh C. Sikka and Wayne J. G. Hellstrom

Introduction

Immunologic infertility has long been an important area of investigation in fertility clinics and reproductive research. The concept that immunological factors play a significant role in infertility has been reported in the scientific literature since the early twentieth century [1–3]. **Major advances in this field of study have resulted from the understanding that specific antibodies within the reproductive tract secretions, and especially those that are attached to the sperm surface, are clinically significant** [4]. There is considerable evidence that sperm antibodies impair fertility by blocking penetration of cervical mucus by spermatozoa, by interfering in the fertilization process [5], or possibly by exerting an embryotoxic effect [6–8]. The extent to which some of these effects are expressed is related to the antibody level, immunoglobulin class, and regional specificity of these antibodies.

Immunologic infertility is the most common medically treatable cause of male infertility, but the projected results of current treatments at this time are less than optimal. As many as 60% of candidates for vasectomy reversal may have circulating antisperm antibodies [9]. It is also known that men with primary infertility have a higher incidence of antisperm antibodies in their serum and semen than do age-matched fertile controls [10,11]. Under some circumstances, such as testicular trauma or vasectomy, the "blood–testis barrier" may be broken, thereby allowing the immune system to be exposed to a large number of sperm, facilitating the production of antisperm antibodies [12]. In addition, **the lack of reliable, standardized testing protocols for antisperm antibodies has contributed to uncertainty among fertility specialists concerning the magnitude of such immunologic phenomena in human reproductive failure** [4].

Clinical relevance

Immunologic phenomena are reported in association with infertility in 10–30% of unexplained cases [1,3,7,13]. **Before any treatment of unexplained infertility is initiated, the possible presence of antisperm antibodies should be investigated** under the following clinical scenarios:

(1) in couples with repeated abnormal postcoital tests [14];
(2) when persistent infertility exists after vasovasostomy in association with normal sperm counts and motility [15];
(3) when semen analysis is characterized by excessive agglutination of sperm (mainly tail-to-tail agglutination);
(4) in cases of testicular trauma, torsion, maldescent and persistent pyospermia, or testicular biopsy [12];
(5) when there is a genetic predisposition [16];
(6) in cases of repeated genital infections [17].

All such couples with idiopathic infertility should be adequately screened for antisperm antibodies.

Diagnostic tests

A wide variety of tests (historical and current) are available for screening for antisperm antibodies as a cause of immunologic infertility.

Sperm immobilization tests (Isojima)

These tests **measure complement-dependent cytotoxicity** and are highly specific for immunoglobulins. Therefore, false positive results are rare, while false negative results may occur. Single IgA antibodies may interfere with fertilization [18].

Infertility in the Male, 4th edition, ed. Larry I. Lipshultz, Stuart S. Howards, and Craig S. Niederberger. Published by Cambridge University Press. © Cambridge University Press 2009.

Sperm agglutination tests (Franklin–Dukes, Kibrick, tray agglutination test)

These tests depend on cross-linking of spermatozoa by multivalent antibodies. **Non-immunoglobulin-mediated agglutination may lead to false positive results.** The number of sites for antigen binding varies with immunoglobulin class, so that large multivalent molecules such as IgM are more likely to give a strongly positive reaction [19–21].

Mixed agglutination reaction (MAR)

This test uses a second antibody (e.g., rabbit antibody) that is directed against a human immunoglobulin class [22]. The agglutination response is amplified by including human red blood cells that are also coated with human immunoglobulin. Thus the positive response involves the mixed agglutination of blood cells and sperm cells by the second antibody. **The large size of the agglutinate limits the ability of the assay to determine the region of the sperm to which the antibody is bound**, and restricts its utility in evaluating the percentage of antibody-bound sperm.

Indirect immunofluorescence

In this test, the second antibody is conjugated with a fluorescent label, and the number of antibody-bound sperm can be observed directly with a fluorescence microscope, along with the location of the bound antibody on the sperm surface [23]. If the test is carried out after the sperm are air-dried, exposure of internal sperm antigens as well as surface antigens will occur. **Exposure of internal antigens may lead to false positive results because these antigens may cross-react with antibodies to bacterial antigens that are not related to infertility.**

Enzyme-linked immunosorbent assay (ELISA)

In these tests, the second antibody is linked to an enzyme that has reacted with its substrate to produce a color that can be measured photometrically. Either whole sperm or membrane extracts are fixed to microtiter wells, the second antibody is added, and the color reaction is developed. **Preparation of the sperm cells may lead to exposure of internal antigens or loss of antigens, resulting in false positive and false negative results**, respectively [24].

Radiolabeled antiglobulin assay

In this assay, the second antibody is labeled with a radioisotope, usually [^{125}I]-protein G, as the radioligand, and the result is determined from the radioactivity (bound antibody) remaining in the washed sperm cells. This method allows objective and specific questions to be asked concerning IgG class antibodies [25]. However, if both living and dead cells are assayed together, false positive results may occur because of exposure of internal antigens. **A varying degree of false negative results is possible. Moreover, regional specificity of the antisperm antibody cannot be determined with this method.**

Immunobead rosette test (IBT)

This immunobead test (IBT) is a technically simple assay that evaluates immunologic infertility by identifying the classes of antisperm antibodies and their binding sites on the sperm surface [13,26,27]. The test uses polyacrylamide beads coated with antibodies against human immunoglobulins (Igs) to bind to antibody-coated sperm. This test is one of the most informative and specific of all the assays currently available to detect antisperm antibodies [4,28]. The test makes use of widely available, inexpensive reagents. The immunobeads are microscopic polyacrylamide spheres which carry covalently bound rabbit antibodies directed against human immunoglobulins. Immunobeads are commercially available, and are directed against whole human immunoglobulin (Ig) or against individual immunoglobulin classes (IgG, IgA, IgM). The second antibody is linked to polyacrylamide beads that are smaller in size (approximately 2–10 μm) than the sperm cell. Sperm and beads are mixed, and the suspension is observed microscopically for agglutination of sperm and beads (Fig. 37.1). By using beads coated with Ig-class-specific second antibodies, one can identify the different antibody classes involved (IgG, IgA, IgM) [29]. The capability to determine immunoglobulin class may be particularly useful in assessing fertility in males, since **IgAs are considered to be more detrimental than IgGs to sperm function. The immunobead test also identifies the location on the sperm cell (head, midpiece, tail) to which the antibody is bound. The rate of false positives is low with the immunobead test, but false negatives may occur** [30].

There are **two ways to perform** the immunobead test:

(1) **The direct method.** This IBT can be performed directly to assess native antibodies on sperm by

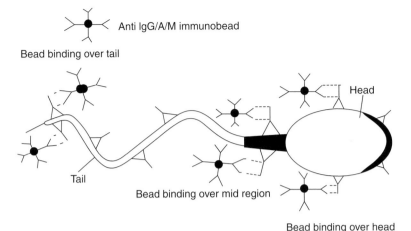

Anti IgG/A/M immunobead

Bead binding over tail

Head

Tail

Bead binding over mid region

Bead binding over head

Fig. 37.1. A diagrammatic cartoon showing sperm with location of immunobead (IgA, IgG, or IgM) binding.

binding immunobeads to the target sperm surface [31]. **This is the method of choice for assessing men who have adequate numbers of motile sperm** in their semen.

(2) **The indirect method.** This is **performed after passive transfer of antibody** from a body fluid (blood, serum, seminal plasma, cervical mucus, or follicular fluid) to donor sperm [32,33]. **Donor sperm that have been found to be negative for antisperm antibodies by testing previously by the direct method are used for the passive transfer method.** Body fluids from both men and women can be evaluated in this manner [4,18,27]. Because only a small sample of the fluid is needed for testing, the remaining aliquot may be stored for retesting or for comparison with another sample obtained at a later date.

Detailed test procedures
SpermMar (SPMAR) test
SPMAR is used only for direct assays employing sperm from washed or unwashed ejaculates [22]. It can be easily incorporated into routine semen analysis as a screening test, but **positive results should be confirmed by IBT (especially of class IgG and IgA).** Ortho Diagnostic Systems (Ortho, Raritran, NJ, USA) introduced a SPMAR kit that relies on an antiserum against the Fc component of human IgG to induce mixed agglutination between antibody-coated sperm and latex beads conjugated with human IgG [34].

Unwashed semen or washed sperm suspension (7–10 µL) is mixed with 10 µL of SPMAR latex particles and 10 µL of the antiserum against the Fc component

of human IgG on a clean microscope slide. After placement of a coverslip, the mixture is observed for agglutination under a phase-contrast objective after 2–3 minutes and after 10 minutes. The majority of 10-minute readings on unwashed semen are unreadable because of excessive clumping and adherence of sperm and beads to debris. However, the **10-minute reading used for analysis of the washed sperm of the patient or the donor provides better results** [34].

Mixed agglutination reaction (MAR) test
This test for evaluation of antisperm antibodies in semen was initially introduced in 1978 [18]. However, widespread application of this test is limited in part by the inconvenience associated with procuring and preparing human IgG-sensitized erythrocytes as target cells for Ig-mediated mixed agglutination with sperm cells. Some reports have suggested that the SPMAR kit, which uses latex beads coated with IgG, may circumvent the use of erythrocytes [22,34]. When the kit is used to screen unwashed semen, it is better to evaluate agglutination within 2–3 minutes of mixing. **SPMAR is more sensitive in identifying sperm with antibodies of the IgG class on their surface. The MAR test, on the other hand, does not require a sperm-washing step and should, therefore, be both time- and cost-effective.**

The data suggest that when 10% or more of the sperm are agglutinated to beads in the SPMAR or MAR test, additional investigation of the semen and/ or serum for the presence of antisperm antibodies is probably indicated [34]. Because clinical experience with SPMAR or MAR currently is limited, all positive results **should be confirmed by the better-established IBT**, as discussed below.

IBT assay

Materials

(1) immunobead reagents (rabbit anti-human IgG, IgA, and IgM) – (Irvine Scientific, Santa Ana, CA, USA);

(2) positive and negative controls – frozen serum aliquots;

(3) antisperm antibody-negative normal donor semen sample (fresh ejaculate);

(4) sperm washing medium (Cat. # 9983, Irvine Scientific, Santa Ana, CA, USA);

(5) spermfuge – Adams Compact II centrifuge (Cat. # 0235, Beckton Dickinson, Sparks, MD, USA) – a fixed-speed centrifuge for sperm processing;

(6) various pipettors, clean glass slides, coverslips;

(7) self-standing conical dispo-beakers (3.0 mL capacity);

(8) phase-contrast microscope with 20× and 40× objectives.

Protocol

Direct immunobead test

In our laboratory, the test is performed by mixing $10\,\mu L$ of washed sperm suspension (approximately 5×10^6 motile sperm/mL) with $10\,\mu L$ of the appropriate immunobead reagent (6 mg/mL of IgG, IgA, or IgM) on a slide covered with a standard (22×22 mm) coverslip. The slide is incubated in a moist chamber at room temperature for 10 minutes before evaluation using phase-contrast optics (200× to 400× magnification). **A test is positive if more than 20% of the motile sperm have two or more attached beads** [34]. **The percentage of motile sperm bound to beads is recorded, along with the pattern of binding, i.e., head (H), midpiece (M), tail endpiece (T), or entire sperm (E)** [26,30].

An indirect IBT (see below) **is performed on seminal plasma if there are not enough motile sperm to perform a direct test.** Seminal plasma is prepared by filtering the semen through a $0.45\,\mu m$ or $0.8\,\mu m$ Millipore filter (disposable) or by centrifugation. Semen with increased viscosity and clumps should be passed through a 21G needle before filtering. Seminal plasma can be tested without heat inactivation of the complement [32].

Indirect immunobead test

In our laboratory, an antibody-positive and a negative serum suspension are simultaneously tested as controls. Specifically, the unknown test serum, previously stored at $-20\,°C$, is heated at $56\,°C$ for 30 minutes along with the control sera aliquots to inhibit the complement. **Freshly obtained semen sample from a normal donor (with negative antisperm antibodies) is processed to collect motile spermatozoa** by either swim-up or swim-down technique using warm sperm wash media. Sperm suspension is washed by centrifugation ($300 \times g$ for 6–8 minutes), and the number of motile spermatozoa is determined using a phase-contrast microscope at 200× magnification. **An aliquot (0.1 mL) of washed sperm suspension ($8–10 \times 10^6$ motile sperm) is mixed with a 0.1 mL aliquot of the test serum (and the controls) and diluted to 1.0 mL with medium in a conical dispo-beaker (≥ 3.0 mL capacity).** Following 60 minutes of incubation at $37\,°C$, the sperm are washed with 2–3 mL medium for three successive washings as described above. A final suspension is prepared using $20–80\,\mu L$ volume of medium (depending upon size of sperm pellet) for IBT testing. Anti-IgA, IgG, and IgM immunobeads are suspended individually (6 mg/mL media) and washed once.

The test is performed by mixing $10\,\mu L$ of washed donor sperm suspension prepared as above with $10\,\mu L$ of the appropriate immunobead reagent (IgA, IgG, or IgM) on a clean glass slide, and covered with a standard (22×22 mm) coverslip. The slide is incubated at temperature ($25–37\,°C$) in a moist chamber for 10 minutes before being read under the phase-contrast optics (200× or 400× magnification). **The number of motile sperm bound to beads is recorded, along with the number of beads and their location, i.e., sperm head (H), midpiece (M), tail endpiece (T), or entire sperm (E). It is important that the normal ranges are determined in each laboratory.**

A common practice is to do a one-step preliminary screening using a mixture of immunobeads (IgA, IgG, and IgM) prepared as described above, followed by secondary testing of positives by these individual immunobeads. Our experience over the last few years suggests such preliminary screening for IgG and IgA-class antibodies only. **Sera are rarely positive for IgM-class antibodies alone, and it is believed that, compared to IgA and IgG, the IgM-class antibodies are not clinically significant for evaluation of immunologic infertility** [34].

Data interpretation

Lab results

The **endpoint in these tests is to determine the percentage of motile sperm that bind to immunobeads.**

The test is considered positive if ≥ 20% of the motile sperm have ≥ 2 attached beads. We consider a binding of 15–20% with a minimum of two beads attached to a motile sperm as "gray area," and the test is repeated. It is not known exactly what degree of sperm immuno-bead binding may indicate a clinically significant level of antisperm antibodies. Some centers consider bead binding of 50% or more of the sperm population as clinically significant [7,35], while others have considered that if 20% or more sperm bind to beads, the antibody levels should be considered positive [13,14,26,36]. **Our own experience with the assay suggests that no single numerical value for bead binding can be considered clinically significant at this time; this is especially true when the results are compared from one laboratory to another.**

Depending on the region of the sperm to which the antibody is attached, different sperm functions may be affected [26]. For example, antibodies attached to the sperm tail may hinder sperm motility and transport, and **those attached to the head region could interfere with sperm binding to the zona pellucida** or block entry of the sperm into the ooplasm itself [3,5,36]. In the presence of antisperm antibodies of the IgG and IgM classes, complement-mediated cell damage may reduce the longevity of these spermatozoa and thus reduce the sperm numbers that are available for upward migration to the site of fertilization. **Antisperm antibodies could interfere with ion pumps or channels that regulate intracellular ion concentrations.** It is possible that antisperm antibodies could also induce a premature and inappropriate acrosome reaction by promoting clustering of intramembranous particles or through sublethal complement-mediated damage to sperm-head membranes.

Clinical significance

The **region of bead binding** is an important factor in determining clinical significance [33]. The **immunoglobulin type** must also be considered when results are interpreted, as **IgA may be more detrimental than IgG**. Thus, the prevalence of IgA in primary immunologic male infertility patients may explain the poor prognosis for such cases. In comparison, immunologic infertility secondary to vasectomy shows predominance of IgG [31]. Nevertheless, **the information provided by the IBT on the location of antibody binding and class of antibody can be used in conjunction with the clinical history and other relevant studies to provide the clinician with important data for the management of infertile couples with potential** immunologic infertility [37]. Initial clinical reports from in-vitro fertilization programs confirm that head-directed antibodies, particularly of the IgA class, can interfere with fertilization, likely through interference with sperm–zona interaction [38].

In a fertility clinic practice, the assessment of circulating antisperm antibodies by passive transfer to donor sperm (indirect assay) is necessary in:

(1) **the workup of the female**;
(2) **evaluation of men prior to vasectomy reversal**; and
(3) **assessing the progress of therapy in men and women with immunologic infertility**.

The female partner should initially be tested by circulating antisperm antibodies in serum. Unlike low to moderate levels of sperm surface-bound antibodies, high levels of circulating antibodies may indicate severely reduced chances of successful treatment by IVF or donor insemination [39]. Regarding the relevance of sperm antibodies to infertility, it can be clinically argued that "if a patient with positive sperm antibody results achieved a pregnancy, then sperm antibodies must be irrelevant" [40]. However, in such cases the possibility of "false positive" results cannot be ruled out, **especially due to lack of standardization of antisperm antibody testing**. There are many factors (e.g., **testing insufficiently diluted serum or using serum without inhibiting the complement) that can lead to such false positive results.** Many laboratories test undiluted or quarter-diluted serum. **A dilution of 1/10 should be the minimum serum dilution used, in order to minimize nonspecific binding factors. However, this criterion alone is not sufficient to conclude that a patient has "immunoinfertility" or "sperm autoimmunity."** It is important to reserve these terms for cases in which either IgA or IgG sperm antibodies have been unequivocally detected and there is evidence of poor cervical mucus penetration by spermatozoa and/or repeated negative postcoital test, indicating functional impairment consistent with infertility or subfertility.

What course should be followed if the female partner has sperm antibodies?

If the patient has a positive indirect IBT for IgA-class antibodies in cervical mucus, associated with poor cervical mucus penetration results, but relatively low titer (< 1/100) of circulating antibodies in serum, then the patient has a reasonable chance of conceiving by intrauterine insemination of her partner's semen or washed spermatozoa (assuming essentially normal semen quality). **High-titer antibodies (> 1/1000) give a generally poor prognosis** [39,40].

Advantages and limitations of IBT

Advantages

The **test offers a number of advantages in both clinical and research studies**:

(1) This method has demonstrated the ability to identify the class of immunoglobulin (IgG, IgA, IgM) that can be associated with the sperm.

(2) The anatomical location of the immunoglobulin on the sperm surface (head, midpiece, tail, or entire surface) can be determined.

(3) **The method requires no specialized equipment, makes use of widely available reagents, and is simple and very informative**.

(4) **An IBT titer can be very useful for monitoring a patient's response to corticosteroid treatment.** For example, tail-tip antibodies do not significantly affect cervical mucus penetration or fertilization and often occur in fertile individuals [38]. There is also evidence that antibody titer is correlated directly with the severity of sperm functional impairment and inversely with fecundability [37].

Limitations

(1) **The subjective nature of the assessment** requires substantial decision making by the observer in selecting sperm for counting and in deciding when and where beads have attached to sperm.

(2) The **reproducibility of this method has never been rigorously studied in a standardized manner**.

(3) The **inherent technical and biological variability** in the test could complicate the transfer of standards from one laboratory to another.

(4) **Strict quality control**, including the repetitive testing of a pooled or single positive serum source, is therefore essential for the clinical application of the test.

Quality control management

Variability

There is always some variability of the test even in the hands of an experienced technician. Studies have indicated that bead binding to the sperm tail is occasionally higher with SPMAR than with IBT, while the

reverse may be true with bead binding to the head. Immunoglobulin of the IgA class may have additional prognostic significance if present on sperm. Because SPMAR does not detect IgA, assays for IgA should be carried out by IBT when SPMAR tests are positive [31]. It is unlikely that many IgA-positive specimens will be missed when semen is screened for antisperm antibodies using SPMAR, because sperm-surface IgA is almost always found in association with IgG [36]. In managing quality control, especially for indirect IBT, besides preference for employing single sperm donor, **the use of positive and negative serum controls is very important for each assay.** Some additional factors that should be looked into while **managing variability and quality control** are listed below.

(1) If different sperm donors are used for indirect assay, **an arc sine variance stabilizing transformation** can be applied to the portions of sperm with each binding pattern before further analysis is done [26]. The goal of the analysis should be to quantify the relative contribution of between-man difference to the total variability in the proportions of sperm in each binding category. Therefore, a **variance components analysis** could be carried out. The variance between these long-term means from different men in the donor population is called the "**between-man**" variance. The computer program in SAS can estimate such a variance. The reasons for these differences are unclear. **There are no data on large-scale clinical studies that relate pregnancy outcome to either IBT or SPMAR results** [34]. Therefore, neither test can be considered a "gold standard." A positive result in either test should raise a suspicion of an immunological factor; the higher the level of bead binding, the greater the suspicion [39]. The fact that **the component of variance between different sperm donors for the indirect assay may be relatively low might suggest that technical variables in the assay are more influential than biological variability.** Many biological factors may induce variation from ejaculate to ejaculate, both within and among donors, including variability in antigen masking by epididymal and seminal plasma components.

(2) The competition among antibodies of different classes from nearby binding sites could result in **masking effects**.

Table 37.1. Hypothetical situation in which percentage of men with antisperm antibodies in serum (predicted positives) can be expected to have antibodies on the sperm surface (true positives). Results will vary for each testing laboratory

Sensitivity (Sn) of IBT test on serum (%)	Specificity (Sp) of IBT test on serum (%)	Prevalence of patients with antisperm antibodies on sperm surface (SS) (%)	Predicted positive (PP) (%) [a]
100	75	20	50
100	75	15	41
100	65	20	42
100	65	15	34
95	75	20	49
95	75	15	40
95	65	20	40
95	65	15	32

[a] $PP = \dfrac{Sn \times SS}{Sn \times SS + (1 - Sp)(1 - SS)}$

Thus, the lower the specificity of IBT in a testing lab, the lower the predicted value of true positives. Sensitivity of IBT plays a minor role. (Adapted from Parslow JM *et al*. The effects of sperm antibodies on fertility after vasectomy reversal. *Am J Reprod Immunol* 1983; **3**: 28–34.)

(3) Our experience also supports the observation by others that **circulating antisperm antibodies in women can most accurately be assessed using their partner's own sperm for antibody transfer** [26].

(4) Studies involving passive antibody transfer **for evaluating multiple serum sources should utilize a single sperm donor in order to minimize the sources of variability** in the experiments. Similar precautions are appropriate for assessing longitudinal changes in antibody levels associated with therapy.

(5) Substantially **more data on the relationship of the test results to fertility will be required before absolute values for "abnormal or "clinically significant" results are established** [31]. In the meantime, the test results cannot be used quantitatively without regard to the clinical history and results of other laboratory tests. These data may be important to the clinician in assessing the role of immunologic phenomena in the evaluation of infertility of a couple.

Proficiency testing

Such **variability can be monitored by frequent evaluation of positive control data, and any shift or drift in these results should be evaluated with appropriate corrective actions.** Fertility labs should participate in proficiency testing with unknown samples that are shipped to various participating labs at regular intervals as part of a proficiency challenge testing for quality assurance purposes.

Pitfalls and recommendations

It is **important to determine the sensitivity, specificity, and predictive value** of a serum screening protocol in identifying a man as having clinically significant amounts of antisperm antibodies on the spermatozoa. Under the worst (but realistic) conditions of test sensitivity of 95%, specificity of 65%, and prevalence of true positives in semen of 15%, only about 32% of patient semen samples would be positive in spite of a "positive" value in the sera (Table 37.1). Even with 100% test sensitivity, the percentage of antibody-positive serum samples that would lead to a positive test in semen would not exceed 50%. These calculations underscore the necessity of testing the semen directly for antibodies whenever a "positive" serum value is obtained [39].

The key question remains, **what is the appropriate course of action after sperm antibodies have been detected in either male or female, or both?** If the antibody test was initially performed on the patient's serum using an indirect assay, then the following steps should be followed:

(1) repeat the indirect IBT on serum, including 1/100 and 1/1000 serum dilutions;

(2) perform an IBT on semen and/or cervical mucus;

(3) if not already done, test for sperm cervical mucus penetration.

It appears that a screening protocol for evaluation of circulating antisperm antibodies of the IgG class can be nearly 100% sensitive for predicting sperm-surface IgG antibodies. However, the data are inadequate to support strong conclusions regarding the sensitivity of serum IgA in predicting seminal IgA [14]. The true positive predictive rate for antisperm antibodies on the sperm surface using circulating antisperm antibodies as a screening assay was estimated to be as low as 35%. **A positive screen dictates that a direct assay on sperm should be performed** [36].

Future directions: what is next?

Since mature sperm first form at puberty, long after recognition of self has occurred, they have antigenic determinants that are capable of stimulating an immune response. In fact the sperm are usually blocked from eliciting an immune response by the blood–testis barrier and the male genital tract. However, **certain events that compromise these biological barriers (e.g., vasectomy, trauma during sexual activity, torsion, infection or obstruction, testicular biopsy, and genetic predisposition, etc.) may lead to the development of antisperm antibodies**.

The presence of circulating antibodies indicates a humoral immune response to sperm cell antigens. It is known that **the presence of circulating antibodies does not necessarily imply their presence within reproductive tract secretions**, and in the case of semen the antibodies in seminal plasma may not be representative of those on the sperm surface. However, there may be valid clinical or logistical reasons to test for antisperm antibodies in blood serum.

The IBT is a sensitive and specific test for detection of sperm antibodies in serum or reproductive tract secretions. So far there is a complete lack of correlation between a commercially available ELISA kit and the IBT. Preliminary experiments have also demonstrated poor correlation between standard Western blotting procedures and IBT. However, it is still safer to use live sperm assays (e.g., direct IBT) for diagnostic screening purposes. Titration using a tenfold dilution series gives a valuable indication of antibody levels in serum or other body fluids, but it lacks sensitivity for patient monitoring.

It is generally acknowledged that **the direct IBT method (rather than the indirect IBT) for measuring antibodies on the surface of the patient's sperm is the preferred approach for workup of the infertile male.** However, the IBT is currently available only in a limited number of clinical laboratories. It may be difficult to schedule a great number of patients from remote locations to give semen specimens. **Logistically, it is easier to send a serum sample by mail, store the samples in a freezer, and at a convenient time perform a number of assays concurrently.** In this way, a test may be repeated or samples may be compared in the same assay with specimens obtained later in the patient's diagnostic workup or therapy. However, the value and limitations of screening men for antisperm antibodies by tests on blood sera are not currently known. **New standardized tests for quantitative antisperm antibody testing are needed**, and are in development [41].

The IBT provides information on immunoglobulin class, and on the anatomical location of sperm-surface antibodies, that is not provided by other classical tests. This information may have clinical value for cases of immunologic infertility in assessing the prognosis for fertility and in choosing the therapeutic approach. **The relationship of these characteristics of circulating antibodies to those of the sperm-surface antibodies is also unknown, and is of scientific and clinical interest.**

Particularly, we assume that only those **antibodies which are bound to the sperm surface are clinically significant** and have the ability to interfere with the sperm transport or fertilization [3]. Fertilization, embryo development, and pregnancy rates after intracytoplasmic sperm injection (ICSI) have not been found to be influenced significantly by the proportion of antisperm antibody-bound spermatozoa, nor by the type or location of the antisperm antibodies, suggesting that **ICSI should be the primary choice for patients who have very high (> 80%) antisperm antibody binding in their semen.**

Conclusions

In conclusion, **a positive test for antibodies, particularly of the IgA class, in sera and on the sperm surface appear to imply a poorer prognosis for male fertility.** Assays that have measured sperm-surface antibody binding have included the radiolabeled antiglobulin test, indirect immunofluorescence, mixed agglutination reaction (MAR) using human red blood cells coated with human immunoglobulin, and the immunobead rosette test (IBT). **The IBT is a simple, sensitive, and specific test for routine sperm antibody screening of semen, cervical mucus, serum, or follicular fluid.** Immunofluorescence assays do not distinguish antibody attachment to living sperm and thus may lead to false positive results when antibodies directed against internal sperm antigens are detected.

The IBT has been widely accepted as a reliable screening test for sperm antibodies. **The role of antisperm antibodies in infertility often may be more relative than absolute.** Improvements in antisperm antibody assays enable us to: (1) quantify the number of sperm-carrying antibodies, (2) identify the class of immunoglobulin involved, and (3) identify the location of antibody binding to the sperm. At best, our treatments employing immunosuppression and sperm washing have been marginally effective. ICSI is currently the "gold standard" for men with high antisperm antibody binding levels (> 80%), and for those who fail simpler, less costly, and less invasive reproductive therapies for immunologic infertility. **Additional emphasis on research with new approaches and the development of new biomedical technologies will give promise** to this area of investigation.

References

[1] Rumke P, Hellinga G. Autoantibodies against spermatozoa in sterile men. *Am J Clin Path* 1959; **32**: 357–62.

[2] Boettcher B. Antigens of the male tract. *J Reprod Fertil* 1973; **18**: 77–80.

[3] Bronson R, Cooper G, Rosenfeld D. Sperm antibodies: their role in infertility. *Fertil Steril* 1984; **42**: 171–5.

[4] Bronson R, Cooper G. Rosenfeld A. Membrane-bound sperm-specific antibodies: their role in infertility. In: Vogel H, Jagiello G, eds. *Bioregulators of Reproduction*. New York, NY: Academic Press, 1981: 521–9.

[5] Bronson RA, Cooper GW, Rosenfeld DL. Autoimmunity to spermatozoa: effect on sperm penetration of cervical mucus as reflected by postcoital testing. *Fertil Steril* 1984; **41**: 609–12.

[6] Menge AC, Medley NE, Mangione CM, Dietrich JM. The incidence and influence of antisperm antibodies in infertile human couples on sperm–cervical mucus interactions and subsequent fertility. *Fertil Steril* 1982; **38**: 439–43.

[7] Ayvaliotis B, Bronson R, Rosenfeld D, Cooper G. Conception rates in couples where autoimmunity to sperm is detected. *Fertil Steril* 1985; **43**: 739–43.

[8] Witkin SS, David SS. Effect of sperm antibodies on pregnancy outcome in a subfertile population. *Am J Obstet Gynecol* 1988; **158**: 59–63.

[9] Parslow JM, Royle MG, Kingscott MMB, Wallace DMA, Hendry WF. The effects of sperm antibodies on fertility after vasectomy reversal. *Am J Reprod Immunol* 1983; **3**: 28–31.

[10] Linnet L, Hjort T, Fogh-Anderson P. Association between failure to impregnate after vasovasostomy and sperm agglutinins in semen. *Lancet* 1981; **117**: 119–21.

[11] Hass GG. Evaluation of sperm antibodies and autoimmunity in the infertile male. In: Santen RJ, Swerdloff RS, eds. *Male Reproductive Dysfunction*. New York, NY: Academic Press, 1985: 147–52.

[12] Rumke P. The origin of immunoglobulins in semen. *Clin Exp Immunol* 1974; **17**: 287–9.

[13] Clarke GN, Stojanoff A, Cauchi MN, *et al.* Detection of sperm antibodies in semen using the immunobead test: a survey of 813 consecutive patients. *Am J Reprod Immunol Microbiol* 1985; **7**: 118–21.

[14] Clarke GN, Stojanoff A, Cauchi MN, *et al.* Detection of antispermatozoal antibodies of IgA class in cervical mucus. *Am J Reprod Immunol* 1984; **5**: 61–6.

[15] Fuchs EF, Alexander NJ. Immunologic considerations before and after vasovasostomy. *Fertil Steril* 1983; **40**: 497–502.

[16] Turek P, Lipshultz LI. Immunologic infertility. *Urol Clin North Am* 1994; **21**: 447–51.

[17] Quesada EM, Dukes CD, Deen GH, Franklin RR. Genital infection and sperm agglutinating antibodies in infertile men. *J Urol* 1968; **99**: 106–8.

[18] Jager S, Kremer J, van Slochteren-Draaisma T. A simple method of screening for antisperm antibodies in the human male: detection of spermatozoal surface IgG with the direct mixed antiglobulin reaction carried out on untreated fresh human semen. *Int J Fertil* 1978; **23**: 12–21.

[19] Kibrick S, Belding DL, Merrill B. Methods for the detection of antibodies against mammalian spermatozoa. II. A gelatin agglutination test. *Fertil Steril* 1952; **3**: 430–4.

[20] Franklin RR, Dukes CD. Antispermatozoal antibody and unexplained infertility. *Am J Obstet Gynecol* 1964; **89**: 6–11.

[21] Fruberg J. A simple and sensitive micro-method for demonstration of sperm-agglutinating activity in serum from infertile men and women. *Acta Obstet Gynecol Scand (Suppl)* 1974; **36**: 21–6.

[22] Ackerman S, McGuire G, Fulgham DL, Alexander NJ. An evaluation of a commercially available assay for the detection of antisperm antibodies. *Fertil Steril* 1988; **49**: 732–6.

[23] Hjort T, Hansen RB. Immunofluorescent studies on human spermatozoa. I. The detection of different spermatozoal antibodies and their occurrence in normal and infertile women. *Clin Exp Immunol* 1971; **8**: 9–14.

[24] Shai S, Bar-Yoseph N, Peer E, Naot Y. A reverse (antibody capture) enzyme-linked immunosorbent assay for detection of antisperm antibodies in sera and genital tract secretions. *Fertil Steril* 1990; **54**: 894–901.

[25] Hass GG, Schreiber AD, Blasco L. The incidence of sperm-associated immunoglobulin and C3, the third component of complement, in infertile men. *Fertil Steril* 1983; **39**: 542–4.

[26] Hellstrom WJG, Overstreet JW, Moore SM, *et al.* Antisperm antibodies bind with different patterns to sperm of different men. *J Urol* 1987; **138**: 895–8.

[27] Clarke GN. An improved immunobead test procedure for detecting sperm antibodies in serum. *Am J Reprod Immunol Microbiol* 1987; **13**: 1–5.

[28] Hellstrom WJG, Overstreet JW, Samuels SJ, Lewis EL. The relationship of circulating antisperm antibodies to sperm surface antibodies in infertile men. *J Urol* 1988; **140**: 1039–44.

[29] Pattinson HA, Mortimer D. Prevalence of sperm surface antibodies in the male partners of infertile couples as determined by immunobead screening. *Fertil Steril* 1987; **48**: 466–71.

[30] Junk SM, Matson PL, O'Halloran F, Yovich JL. Use of immunobeads to detect antispermatozoal antibodies. *Reprod Fertil* 1986; **4**: 199–203.

[31] Parslow JM, Poulton TA, Besser GM, Hendry WF. The clinical relevance of classes of immunoglobulins on spermatozoa from infertile and vasovasostomized males. *Fertil Steril* 1985; **43**: 621–7

[32] Uehling DT. Secretory IgA in seminal fluid. *Fertil Steril* 1971; **22**: 769–73.

[33] Clarke GN. Immunoglobulin class and regional specificity of antispermatozoal antibodies blocking cervical mucus penetration by human spermatozoa. *Am J Reprod Immunol Microbiol* 1988; **16**: 135–43.

[34] Hellstrom WJG, Samuels SJ, Waits AB, Overstreet JW. A comparison of the usefulness of SpermMar and immunobeads tests for the detection of antisperm antibodies. *Fertil Steril* 1989; **52**: 1027–31.

[35] Bronson RA, Cooper GW, Rosenfeld DL. Correlation between regional specificity of antisperm antibodies to the spermatozoan surface and complement-mediated sperm immobilization. *Am J Reprod Immunol Microbiol* 1982; **2**: 222–8.

[36] Shulman S. Immunologic barriers to fertility. *Obstet Gynecol Surv* 1972; **27**: 553–60.

[37] Collins JA, Burrows EA, Yeo J, Younglai EV. Frequency and predictive value of antisperm antibodies among infertile couples. *Hum Reprod* 1992; **8**: 592–8.

[38] Hammitt DG, Muench MM, Williamson RA. Antibody binding to greater than 50% of sperm at the tail tip does not impair male fertility. *Fertil Steril* 1988; **49**: 174–8.

[39] Parslow JM, Royle MG, Kingscott MMB, Wallace DMA, Hendry WF. The effects of sperm antibodies on fertility after vasectomy reversal. *Am J Reprod Immunol* 1983; **3**: 28–34.

[40] Clarke GN. Detection of antisperm antibodies using immunobeads. In: Keel BA, Webster BW, eds. *Handbook of the Laboratory Diagnosis and Treatment of Infertility*. Boca Raton, FL: CRC Press, 1990: 177–92.

[41] Carlsson L, Milsson BO, Ronquist G, Lundquist M, Larsson A. A new test for immunological infertility: an ELISA based on prostasomes. *Int J Androl* 2004; **27**: 130–3.

Chapter

38

Semen white blood cell assay

Joseph A. Politch and Deborah J. Anderson

Introduction

Elevated concentrations of white blood cells (WBCs) in semen have been associated with genital tract infections [1,2] and poor semen quality, including decrements in sperm concentration, motility, morphology, and DNA integrity [3–14]. The World Health Organization (WHO) defines leukocytospermia as seminal WBC concentrations greater than 10^6/mL [15,16]. Elucidating the interaction between leukocytospermia and genital tract infections, and its potential role in infertility, depends on accurate assessment of WBCs in semen. **Numerous techniques have been used in both research and clinical settings to detect seminal WBCs, and a summary and evaluation of several of the various methods are presented in this chapter.**

Round cell counts

The nonspermatozoal cells in the ejaculate comprise primarily either immature germ cells or WBCs [17] and are collectively known as "round cells." Direct counting of round cells in wet mounts, visualized by phase-contrast microscopy, has been widely practiced. **However, because WBCs cannot be distinguished from immature germ cells using this method, total round cell counts are of no value for approximating WBCs in semen [18,19].**

Bryan–Leishman or Papanicolaou stains

The Bryan–Leishman [15,16,20] and Papanicolaou [15,16] **stains, performed on semen smears, are intended to distinguish WBCs from immature germ cells.** In particular, granulocytes can be differentiated from spermatids, and lymphocytes/monocytes from secondary spermatocytes. **However, these techniques involve a lengthy laboratory preparation and**

numerous steps, require a highly trained technician to ensure proper assessment of seminal round cells, and do not permit precise quantification of WBC [15,16,21-23].

Dipstick tests

Wolff *et al.* surveyed a number of commonly used methods for the detection of male genital tract inflammation [23,24]. **Leukocyte esterase urine dipstick tests, used in some infertility units to screen inflammation in semen, were found to be inexpensive as well as quick and easy to perform.** However, the specific dipstick that was tested (Cytur-Test, Boehringer, Mannheim, Germany) had a sensitivity of 57% and a specificity of 31% compared to the Endtz peroxidase method. **Therefore, it was concluded that such dipstick tests were not appropriate for clinical andrological use.**

Peroxidase tests

In 1974, Endtz described a simple peroxidase test for enumerating WBCs in semen [25]. This method is now widely used, and a similar technique [26] has been recommended by the WHO [15,16]. Tests of peroxidase are easy to perform on wet mounts, and are quick, inexpensive, and reliable. These assays detect the peroxidase enzyme present in granulocytes, which are the predominant WBC in semen, and are important indicators of acute infection and inflammation (Fig. 38.1). Peroxidase tests do not detect other WBCs, but because granulocytes represent 50–60% of all WBCs in semen [27,28], peroxidase-positive cell concentrations correlate with total WBC counts as detected by the more technologically sophisticated immunohistology or flow cytometry tests [18]. **For all the reasons stated above, the peroxidase assay has been determined to be the best method for the clinical detection of WBCs in semen at the present time [18,23].**

Infertility in the Male, 4th edition, ed. Larry I. Lipshultz, Stuart S. Howards, and Craig S. Niederberger. Published by Cambridge University Press. © Cambridge University Press 2009.

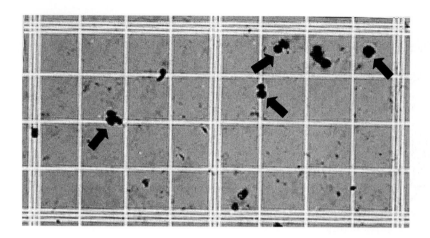

Fig. 38.1. Detection of peroxidase-positive granulocytes in semen using a hemocytometer and the method of Endtz [25] (× 200).

Granulocyte elastase test

Granulocyte elastase, an enzyme specific to granulocytes, is released from activated leukocytes. It has been quantified in human seminal plasma by an enzyme-linked immunosorbent assay (ELISA). Wolff and Anderson demonstrated good correlation ($r = 0.70$) of granulocyte elastase with total WBC concentrations in semen determined by immunohistology [29]. Granulocyte elastase levels above 1000 ng/mL were shown to be diagnostic for leukocytospermia, and high levels reportedly indicate male adnexitis [29,30]. The granulocyte elastase ELISA has the advantage of being quantitative, and is suited for batch testing of frozen specimens. This assay measures the level of granulocyte activation in an ejaculate. **Most studies have correlated WBC or granulocyte numbers with semen parameters; if granulocyte activation is an important factor in male infertility, the elastase test could prove to be a better indicator of WBC-induced male infertility than conventional seminal WBC counts** [21]. **One drawback to this method is that it is relatively expensive compared to peroxidase tests.**

Immunohistology

In addition to granulocytes, other WBC types are also present in semen and may affect fertility. Specifically, macrophages represent 20–30% of all WBCs in semen, whereas T lymphocytes only 2–5%. Plasma cells and B lymphocytes are rarely detected in semen [27,28]. **Immunohistology enables quantitation of total WBC in semen** [27,28,31]. Individual subtypes can be enumerated by detecting WBC phenotypic antigens with specific monoclonal antibodies (Fig. 38.2). **This approach is considered the "gold standard" of semen WBC assessment techniques; however, it requires training, and is time-consuming and expensive** [22,23,27,28,31].

Flow cytometry

The use of automated instrumentation in the andrology laboratory, such as computer-assisted semen analysis, has increased considerably over the past 20 years. **Thus, flow cytometry holds promise for quick, accurate, and relatively inexpensive measurement of WBC in semen.** Flow cytometry is a method frequently used in the field of cellular immunology, and can accurately analyze thousands of cells in a few seconds. Recent studies have raised the possibility of utilizing flow cytometry for a number of andrological measures, including assessing seminal WBC [32–42]. Ricci *et al.* compared the peroxidase and granulocyte elastase assays with a flow cytometry method in combination with pan-leukocyte monoclonal antibodies [41]. They found that the two conventional tests displayed good specificity, but only moderate sensitivity compared to the flow cytometry method. Interestingly, they found a significant correlation between WBC detected by the peroxidase assay and CD45+ cells from flow cytometry, in agreement with a previous paper that showed a similar correlation when the same monoclonal antibody was used in an immunocytochemistry technique [18]. **Thus, as flow cytometry becomes readily available to andrology laboratories, its efficient and economic use for seminal WBC counting and characterization becomes a possibility.**

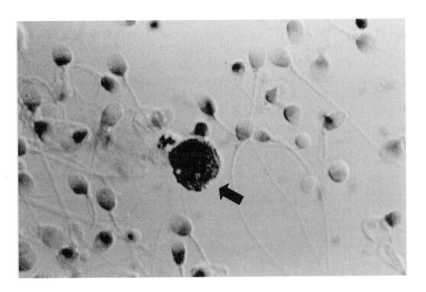

Fig. 38.2. Detection of CD4+ lymphocyte in semen using the immunohistological method of Wolff and Anderson [28] (× 1000).

Conclusion

While there are numerous methods available for detecting WBCs in semen, many of these techniques have disadvantages for clinical or research application. New technologies such as flow cytometry hold great promise for quick, precise and inexpensive assessment of WBCs in semen. **However, at the present time, the peroxidase test is the method of choice for clinical assessment of leukocytospermia.**

Protocol for peroxidase test [18,25]

Materials

Stock solution

> 50 mL distilled water
> 50 mL 100% ethanol
> 100 mg benzidine (Sigma)

Dissolve benzidine in ethanol before adding distilled water. Store in the dark (use dark bottle or wrap container in aluminum foil) at 4 °C. This stock solution is stable for at least six months.

Working solution

> 4 mL stock solution
> 5 µL 30% hydrogen peroxide

Store in dark container at room temperature. The working solution is stable for at least one month.

Diluent

> Normal sterile saline (0.151 M sodium chloride)

Test procedure

The ejaculate is collected by masturbation into a sterile specimen cup after a minimum of 48 hours of abstinence and liquefied for 30 minutes. Twenty microliters of peroxidase test working solution are mixed with 20 µL of liquefied ejaculate and incubated for five minutes at room temperature. Twenty microliters of this solution are then added to 20 µL of saline immediately before counting. Ten microliters of the diluted specimen are loaded into a hemocytometer, and peroxidase-positive (i.e., intensely brown-stained round cells the size of granulocytes, Fig. 38.1), as well as peroxidase-negative (unstained) round cells, are differentially counted at 400× magnification on a microscope.

Of note, benzidine is a carcinogen. Benzidine powder and concentrated solutions should be handled with extreme caution. The concentration of benzidine in the final diluted sample is below that considered to constitute a health risk by the Occupational Safety and Health Administration.

References

[1] Bar-Chama N, Fisch H. Infection and pyospermia in male infertility. *World J Urol* 1993; **11**: 76–81.

[2] Hosseinzadeh S, Eley A, Pacey AA. Semen quality of men with asymptomatic chlamydial infection. *J Androl* 2004; **25**: 104–9.

[3] Alvarez JG, Sharma RK, Ollero M, *et al.* Increased DNA damage in sperm from leukocytospermic semen samples as determined by the sperm chromatin structure assay. *Fertil Steril* 2002; **78**: 319–29.

[4] Arata de Bellabarba G, Tortolero I, Villarroel V, *et al*. Nonsperm cells in human semen and their relationship with semen parameters. *Arch Androl* 2000; **45**: 131–6.

[5] Aziz N, Agarwal A, Lewis-Jones I, Sharma RK, Thomas AJ. Novel associations between specific sperm morphological defects and leukocytospermia. *Fertil Steril* 2004; **82**: 621–7.

[6] Bezold G, Politch JA, Kiviat NB, *et al*. Prevalence of sexually transmissible pathogens in semen from asymptomatic male infertility patients with and without leukocytospermia. *Fertil Steril* 2007; **87**: 1087–97.

[7] Erenpreiss JS, Hlevicka J, Zalkalns J, Erenpreisa J. Effect of leukocytospermia on sperm DNA integrity: a negative effect in abnormal semen samples. *J Androl* 2002; **23**: 717–23.

[8] Gambera L, Serafini F, Morgante G, *et al*. Sperm quality and pregnancy rate after COX-2 inhibitor therapy of infertile males with abacterial leukocytospermia. *Hum Reprod* 2007; **22**: 1047–51.

[9] Lackner JE, Herwig R, Schmidbauer J, *et al*. Correlation of leukocytospermia with clinical infection and the positive effect of antiinflammatory treatment on semen quality. *Fertil Steril* 2006; **86**: 601–5.

[10] Moskovtsev SI, Willis J, White J, Mullen JB. Leukocytospermia: relationship to sperm deoxyribonucleic acid integrity in patients evaluated for male factor infertility. *Fertil Steril* 2007; **88**: 737–40.

[11] Omu AE, Al-Qattan F, Al-Abdul-Hadi FM, Fatinikun MT, Fernandes S. Seminal immune response in infertile men with leukocytospermia: effect on antioxidant activity. *Eur J Obstet Gynecol Reprod Biol* 1999; **86**: 195–202.

[12] Saleh RA, Agarwal A, Kandirali E, *et al*. Leukocytospermia is associated with increased reactive oxygen species production by human spermatozoa. *Fertil Steril* 2002; **78**: 1215–24.

[13] Thomas J, Fishel SB, Hall JA, *et al*. Increased polymorphonuclear granulocytes in seminal plasma in relation to sperm morphology. *Hum Reprod* 1997; **12**: 2418–21.

[14] Wolff H, Politch JA, Martinez A, *et al*. Leukocytospermia is associated with poor semen quality. *Fertil Steril* 1990; **53**: 528–36.

[15] World Health Organization. *WHO Laboratory Manual for the Examination of Human Semen and Sperm–Cervical Mucus Interaction*, 4th edn. Cambridge: Cambridge University Press, 1999.

[16] World Health Organization. *WHO Laboratory Manual for the Examination of Human Semen and Sperm–Cervical Mucus Interaction*, 3rd edn. Cambridge: Cambridge University Press, 1992.

[17] Smith DC, Barratt CL, Williams MA. The characterisation of non-sperm cells in the ejaculates of fertile men using transmission electron microscopy. *Andrologia* 1989; **21**: 319–33.

[18] Politch JA, Wolff H, Hill JA, Anderson DJ. Comparison of methods to enumerate white blood cells in semen. *Fertil Steril* 1993; **60**: 372–5.

[19] Sigman M, Lopes L. The correlation between round cells and white blood cells in the semen. *J Urol* 1993; **149**: 1338–40.

[20] Couture M, Ulstein M, Leonard J, Paulsen CA. Improved staining method for differentiating immature germ cells from white blood cells in human seminal fluid. *Andrologia* 1976; **8**: 61–6.

[21] Anderson DJ, Politch JA. White blood cells in semen and their impact on fertility. In: Centola GM, Ginsburg KA, eds. *Evaluation and Treatment of the Infertile Male*. Cambridge: Cambridge University Press, 1996: 263–76.

[22] Wolff H. The biologic significance of white blood cells in semen. *Fertil Steril* 1995; **63**: 1143–57.

[23] Wolff H. Methods for the detection of male genital tract inflammation. *Andrologia* 1998; **30**(Suppl 1): 35–9.

[24] Wolff H, Panhans A, Zebhauser M, Meurer M. Comparison of three methods to detect white blood cells in semen: leukocyte esterase dipstick test, granulocyte elastase enzyme immunoassay, and peroxidase cytochemistry. *Fertil Steril* 1992; **58**: 1260–2.

[25] Endtz AW. A rapid staining method for differentiating granulocytes from "germinal cells" in Papanicolaou-stained semen. *Acta Cytol* 1974; **18**: 2–7.

[26] Nahoum CR, Cardozo D. Staining for volumetric count of leukocytes in semen and prostate–vesicular fluid. *Fertil Steril* 1980; **34**: 68–9.

[27] Tomlinson MJ, White A, Barratt CL, Bolton AE, Cooke ID. The removal of morphologically abnormal sperm forms by phagocytes: a positive role for seminal leukocytes? *Hum Reprod* 1992; **7**: 517–22.

[28] Wolff H, Anderson DJ. Immunohistologic characterization and quantitation of leukocyte subpopulations in human semen. *Fertil Steril* 1988; **49**: 497–504.

[29] Wolff H, Anderson DJ. Evaluation of granulocyte elastase as a seminal plasma marker for leukocytospermia. *Fertil Steril* 1988; **50**: 129–32.

[30] Jochum M, Pabst W, Schill WB. Granulocyte elastase as a sensitive diagnostic parameter of silent male genital tract inflammation. *Andrologia* 1986; **18**: 413–19.

[31] el-Demiry MI, Young H, Elton RA, *et al*. Leucocytes in the ejaculate from fertile and infertile men. *Br J Urol* 1986; **58**: 715–20.

[32] Ferrara F, Daverio R, Mazzini G, Bonini P, Banfi G. Automation of human sperm cell analysis by flow cytometry. *Clin Chem* 1997; **43**: 801–7.

[33] Gandini L, Lenzi A, Lombardo F, Pacifici R, Dondero F. Immature germ cell separation using a modified discontinuous Percoll gradient technique in human semen. *Hum Reprod* 1999; **14**: 1022–7.

[34] Haas GG, Cunningham ME. Identification of antibody-laden sperm by cytofluorometry. *Fertil Steril* 1984; **42**: 606–13.

[35] Ke RW, Dockter ME, Majumdar G, Buster JE, Carson SA. Flow cytometry provides rapid and highly accurate detection of antisperm antibodies. *Fertil Steril* 1995; **63**: 902–6.

[36] Moilanen JM, Carpen O, Hovatta O. Flow cytometric analysis of semen preparation, and assessment of acrosome reaction, reactive oxygen species production and leucocyte contamination in subfertile men. *Andrologia* 1999; **31**: 269–76.

[37] Moilanen JM, Carpen O, Hovatta O. Flow cytometric light scattering analysis, acrosome reaction, reactive oxygen species production and leukocyte contamination of semen preparation in prediction of fertilization rate in vitro. *Hum Reprod* 1998; **13**: 2568–74.

[38] Pasteur X, Metezeau P, Maubon I, Sabido O, Kiefer H. Identification of two human sperm populations using flow and image cytometry. *Mol Reprod Dev* 1994; **38**: 303–9.

[39] Perticarari S, Ricci G, Granzotto M, *et al.* A new multiparameter flow cytometric method for human semen analysis. *Hum Reprod* 2007; **22**: 485–94.

[40] Rasanen ML, Hovatta OL, Penttila IM, Agrawal YP. Detection and quantitation of sperm-bound antibodies by flow cytometry of human semen. *J Androl* 1992; **13**: 55–64.

[41] Ricci G, Presani G, Guaschino S, Simeone R, Perticarari S. Leukocyte detection in human semen using flow cytometry. *Hum Reprod* 2000; **15**: 1329–37.

[42] Spano M, Evenson DP. Flow cytometric analysis for reproductive biology. *Biol Cell* 1993; **78**: 53–62.

Chapter 39

Determination of seminal oxidants (reactive oxygen species)

Ashok Agarwal and Fnu Deepinder

Introduction

Determination of seminal oxidants is fast emerging as a significant diagnostic and prognostic tool in infertility clinics, andrology, and assisted reproduction laboratories. This is because reactive oxygen species (ROS) play an important role in the pathophysiology of damage to human spermatozoa [1,2]. ROS are highly reactive oxidizing agents belonging to the class of free radicals [3]. A free radical is defined as "any atom or molecule that possesses one or more unpaired electrons" [4]. **Spermatozoa generate ROS in physiological amounts, which play a role in such processes as sperm capacitation, acrosome reaction, and oocyte fusion** [5]. **However, uncontrolled and excessive production of ROS, when it overwhelms the limited antioxidant defenses in semen, results in seminal oxidative stress** [6].

Reports have indicated that high levels of ROS are detected in semen samples of 25–40% of infertile men [7,8]. The production of abnormal levels of ROS is thought to be involved in many aspects of male infertility in which spermatozoa are rendered dysfunctional by altered plasma membrane due to lipid peroxidation, DNA damage, and impaired metabolism, morphology, motility, and fertility [9]. Spermatozoa are highly susceptible to damage induced by ROS because of the high content of polyunsaturated fatty acids within their plasma membranes and a low concentration of scavenging enzymes within the cytoplasm [10,11]. However, "high ROS" is still an unclear concept, because pathological levels of ROS in infertile semen samples have not been defined accurately.

An oxidative stress (OS) test may accurately discriminate between fertile and infertile men and identify those with a clinical diagnosis of male-factor infertility who are likely to initiate a pregnancy if they are followed over a period of time. In addition,
such a test can help select subgroups of patients with infertility in which oxidative stress is a significant factor, and those who may benefit from antioxidant supplementation. In the absence of a standard protocol to assess seminal oxidants, there is no consensus concerning the inclusion of OS analysis as part of the routine diagnostic workup of an infertile male. This chapter will therefore discuss the available techniques which can be used to measure OS in semen.

Types of seminal oxidants

Seminal oxidants represent two broad categories of molecules, the first being oxygen-derived radicals and nonradicals called **reactive oxygen species (ROS)**, e.g., the hydroxyl radical (OH), superoxide anion (O_2^-), hydrogen peroxide (H_2O_2), and the hypochlorite radical ($OHCl^-$). The second category is nitrogen-derived free radicals called **reactive nitrogen species (RNS)**, e.g., nitric oxide (NO) and nitrous oxide (N_2O). These nitrogen-derived radicals are sometimes considered a subclass of ROS [12].

Source and mechanism of generation of ROS

Human semen consists of different types of cells such as mature and immature spermatozoa, round cells at different stages of spermatogenesis, leukocytes, and epithelial cells. **Leukocytes and immature spermatozoa are the two main sources of ROS** [13–15]. Polymorphonuclear neutrophils generate ROS in response to a variety of chemical and bacterial stimuli and overwhelm a spermatozoon's ability to repair or compensate for damage [16,17]. Potent chemoattractants such as formyl methionyl leucyl phenylalanine (FMLP) and phorbol myristate acetate (PMA) stimulate the leukocyte system to generate ROS via discrete

Infertility in the Male, 4th edition, ed. Larry I. Lipshultz, Stuart S. Howards, and Craig S. Niederberger. Published by Cambridge University Press. © Cambridge University Press 2009.

pathways [18–20]. ROS produced by leukocytes forms the first line of defense in any infectious process and is significantly and positively correlated with pro-inflammatory cytokines [21]. **In human sperm, ROS are generated by two major systems: nicotinamide adenine dinucleotide phosphate (NADPH) oxidase at the level of sperm plasma membrane and the nicotinamide adenine dinucleotide (NADH)-dependent oxidoreductase (diphorase) system at the mitochondrial level** [22]. Studies suggest that defects in spermiogenesis that result in retention of cytoplasmic droplets lead to ROS formation [23]. A strong positive correlation exists between immature spermatozoa and ROS production, which in turn is negatively correlated with sperm quality [1,2].

Currently available tests for detecting seminal oxidants

The various methods used for measuring seminal oxidants are described below (Fig. 39.1).

Direct measurement of ROS

Chemiluminescence
Chemiluminescence assay is the most commonly used method for measuring the concentration of ROS within seminal fluid or sperm cell suspension [6,24].

Method
Oxidative end products produced by an in-vitro reaction between ROS and certain reagents produce a light signal that is converted to an electrical signal (photon), which is measured with a luminometer. Two major reagents or probes are used to assess ROS generated by spermatozoa: luminol (5-amino-2,3-dihydro-,1,4-phthalazinedione; also, 3-aminophthalic hydrazide) and lucigenin (N,N'-dimethyl-9,9'-biacridinium dinitrate) [25].

Luminol is a sensitive chemiluminescent probe that provides robust assay results that are highly correlated with sperm function. It is the most intensively investigated and the most frequently used

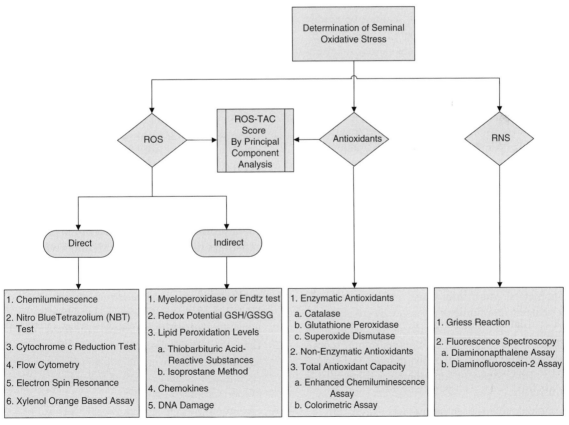

Fig. 39.1. Flowchart demonstrating various methods available to measure seminal oxidative stress. GSH, reduced glutathione; GSSG, oxidized glutathione; RNS, reactive nitrogen species; ROS, reactive oxygen species; TAC, total antioxidant capacity.

dye in clinical chemical ROS measurements. **Being uncharged, it is a membrane-permeable molecule that can react with a variety of free radicals, both intracellularly and extracellularly, like the superoxide anion and the hydrogen peroxide and hydroxyl radicals.** Therefore, it is unable to differentiate between various types of ROS and between intra- and extracellular ROS. Luminol has a very short half-life, thereby allowing for rapid measurement of ROS. The quantum yield of luminol is about 2%, among the highest known. Fundamentally, it measures redox activity, which is characterized by the cellular generation of oxidizing species. Superoxide (O_2^-) is an essential intermediate in the creation of luminol-dependent chemiluminescence. Hence any univalent oxidant that has the potential to generate O_2^- can produce chemiluminescence in the presence of luminol, including ferricyanide, xanthine oxidase, persulfate, hypochlorite, and peroxynitrite [25,26].

Lucigenin, being positively charged, is relatively membrane-impermeable and responds particularly to the superoxide anion in the extracellular space [25,27]. However, the chemiluminescence created by cellular generation of O_2^- cannot be readily distinguished from redox cycling of lucigenin [26]. Therefore, lucigenin is not reliable as a probe for evaluating superoxide production, although it does have value as a nonspecific redox marker for enhanced electron transfer activity associated with defective sperm function [28].

Examples of chemiluminescent probes that do not create a redox cycle, and hence can be used for quantification of superoxide anion, include cypridina luciferin analog2-methyl-6-phenyl-3,7-dihydroimidazo[1,2-a]pyrazin-3-one [29] and coelenterazine [30].

Applications

A variety of luminometers can be used to measure the light intensity resulting from the chemiluminescence reaction. Current luminometer models use two different processing designs. The photon-counting luminometers count individual photons, whereas direct-current luminometers measure electric current, which is proportional to the photon flux. Results are expressed either as counted photons per minute (cpm), as relative light units (rlu), or as millivolts per second (mV/s). Three types of luminometers are available commercially:

(1) Single/double-tube luminometers – these can measure only 1–2 samples at a time and are suitable for small research laboratories.

(2) Multiple-tube luminometers – these are expensive and are more suited for centers that regularly engage in research.

(3) Plate luminometers – these can analyze multiple samples on a single disposable plate and are suitable for commercial entities and core research laboratories.

When luminometers are compared, the coefficient of variation (percent change over a set of readings) and lower limit of detection (minimum sample quantity required for the instrument to generate response) should be considered [31].

Multiple factors may affect and confound the chemiluminescent reaction. The person who operates these instruments should be familiar with all these factors in order to achieve consistently accurate results. Some of these factors are as follows:

(1) Leukocyte contamination – as discussed earlier, leukocytes are a major source of ROS. Thus there is a strong possibility that the responses represent leukocyte contamination rather than abnormal redox activity of spermatozoa [32,33]. In light of these findings, leukocyte removal strategies based on the use of CD45-coated magnetic beads [34] to remove leukocytes selectively from sperm suspensions can be used in conjunction with leukocyte-specific agonists such as FMLP [35] or opsonized zymosan to assess the redox activity of human sperm suspensions.

(2) Analysis time – **the assay is best conducted within one hour of sperm isolation from the seminal plasma** [24], **because the chemiluminescent activity of seminal oxidants declines with time** [36].

(3) **Samples with poor liquefaction give poor chemiluminescent signals, as seminal plasma constituents may interfere with underlying free radical chemistry of the spermatozoa** [28].

(4) **Repeated centrifugation stimulates ROS production because of mechanical shearing forces** [37]. Therefore, centrifugation regimes used in preparation of spermatozoa need to be standardized.

(5) Bovine serum albumin, which is used to supplement culture media, can generate spurious chemiluminescence signals in the presence of human seminal plasma [38].

(6) Chemiluminescent signals, especially those generated by the probe luminol, are sensitive to changes in the pH of the medium [28].

Limitations

The chemiluminescence assay is a nonspecific test, because it measures the total ROS activity in semen. It does not provide any information on the differential contribution of spermatozoa and leukocytes to ROS production [39].

Nitro blue tetrazolium (NBT) test

Method

Nitro blue tetrazolium (NBT) is a yellow, water-soluble, nitro-substituted aromatic tetrazolium compound. It reacts with cellular superoxide ions to form a formazan derivative that can be monitored spectrophotometrically [40,41]. The oxidase system in the cytoplasm transfers electrons from cytoplasmic NADPH (generated by hexose monophosphate shunt) to NBT, thereby reducing it to formazan. **NBT can be used to stain individual cells (spermatozoa and leukocytes), and formazan precipitates can be measured to see NBT reduction.** Thus NBT reaction reflects the ROS generating activity in the cytoplasm of cells, and therefore it can help determine the cellular origin of ROS in semen [42].

Applications

NBT reduction is a readily available, easily performed, inexpensive, and highly sensitive test. **This test can be used for assessing the differential contribution of spermatozoa and leukocytes to ROS production in semen** [42].

Limitations

NBT can also be reduced by many cellular reductases, and changes in the cellular content of various oxidoreductases might alter the rates of NBT reduction [43].

Cytochrome c reduction test

Method

Superoxide formed by the electron transfer from a donor to molecular oxygen can be quenched by the reagent ferricytochrome c, which is reduced to ferrocytochrome c. The reduction of ferricytochrome c to ferrocytochrome c is used to measure superoxide formation. Detection of superoxide is confirmed when addition of enzyme superoxide dismutase completely ceases the production of ferrocytochrome c from ferricytochrome c.

$$Fe^{3+} \text{ cyt c} + O_2^- \rightarrow Fe^{2+} \text{ cyt c} + O_2$$

The rate constant has been estimated at $\sim 1.5 \times 10^5$ M/s at pH 8.5 and room temperature. The spectrophotometric reaction is measured at 550 nm. The extinction coefficient for ferricytochrome c is 0.89×10^4 M/cm, and for ferrocytochrome is 2.99×10^4 M/cm. Emission, $E_{m\,550nm} = 2.1 \times 10^4$ M/cm [44,45].

Applications

This is the gold standard test for detecting extracellularly released superoxide in in-vitro assays [46].

Limitations

(1) The assay is not absolutely specific for superoxide. Various enzymatic and nonenzymatic reductants present in in-vivo conditions are capable of cytochrome c reduction. **This limits the application of the assay for in-vivo detection of the superoxide radical.** It is therefore important that detection of superoxide be confirmed by complete annihilation of cyt-c reduction with externally added superoxide dismutase [47]. Cyt-c can also be acetylated to enhance its specificity for superoxide [48].

(2) The rate of superoxide formation can be underestimated, as the reduced cyt-c can be reoxidized by various oxidants such as hydrogen peroxide and peroxynitrite and enzymes such as cytochrome oxidases. To avoid this event, scavengers of oxidants (100 U/mL catalase for H_2O_2, 10 mM urate for peroxynitrite) or enzyme inhibitors (10 μM cyanide for cytochrome oxidase) can be added [47].

(3) **Cyt-c has limitations in measuring superoxide formation within intact cells as opposed to cellular or tissue extracts because of its restricted intracellular access** [47].

Flow cytometry

Method

Flow cytometry can be used to detect ROS with the use of fluorescent probes: 2,7-dichlorodihydrofluorescein diacetate (DCFH-DA), dihydroethidine (DHE), and dihydrorhodamine 123. These compounds diffuse into the living cells. When oxidized by ROS, which is generated within the cell, they develop fluorescence, the intensity of which can be measured by a flow cytometer. The quantification of fluorescence reflects the rate and quantity of the ROS produced intracellularly [49].

The percentage of cells with a high mitochondrial membrane potential (MMP) can also be estimated using flow cytometry, with mitochondrial probes. **Furthermore, flow cytometry can distinguish between viable and nonviable sperm populations using dyes such as propidium iodide (PI) and Yopro-1, which can enter dead or apoptotic cells only** [50,51].

Applications

Flow cytometry analysis can be used to identify sperm populations that may be dysfunctional because of intracellular ROS. **The assay has an added advantage over the most commonly used method of chemiluminescence as it can measure intracellular ROS exclusively in the viable portion of the sperm population.** Unlike flow cytometry, ROS measured by other methods may only be present extracellularly or in a small proportion of primarily nonviable sperm [51]. **Moreover, specific probes can be used to detect specific intracellular free radicals, e.g., DFCH-DA for hydrogen peroxide and DHE for superoxide detection.**

Limitations

The technique involves the use of a flow cytometer and software for data analysis, which are expensive, not easily available, and require technical expertise. Although our laboratory has standardized this assay in human spermatozoa to measure both hydrogen peroxide and superoxide using DCFH-DA and DHE by single flow cytometry test, no studies are available in the literature regarding the use of this technique to detect ROS in human sperm.

Electron spin resonance (ESR) or electron paramagnetic resonance

Method

ESR uses the magnetic properties of unpaired electrons to detect free radicals directly. When an external magnetic field is applied, the unpaired or the paramagnetic electrons present in the free radicals can exist in two different orientations, either parallel or antiparallel with respect to the applied field. These paramagnetic species absorb electromagnetic radiation and provide absorption spectra utilizing the energy of the electron spin state [52,53].

Applications

ESR spectroscopy is the most direct and least ambiguous method for detecting free radicals of interest without artifacts from added chemicals [52]. Efforts are under way to develop this technique

for the in-vivo evaluation of radical generation and redox status.

Limitations

It is an expensive and cumbersome technique. Moreover, ESR cannot detect oxidants such as superoxide, NO, hydroxyl, alkoxyl, cysteinyl, or glutathiyl radicals, either because their concentration is below the detection limit of the present-generation ESR spectrophotometers ($\sim 10^{-8}$ M) or because their spin relaxation times are very short [54].

However, these problems could be overcome by adding spin-trap molecules such as nitroso and nitrone derivatives to the unstable free radicals, thereby converting them to more stable secondary radicals [54]. The absorption spectrum could then be obtained by applying external magnetic field to these spin-trapped free radicals. Nitroso compounds, such as 2–methyl-2-nitrosopropane (MNP), provide more information than nitrones, as the trapped radical adds directly to the nitroso nitrogen, whereas with the nitrones the trapped radical adds to a carbon adjacent to the nitrogen. However, nitrones are the spin traps of choice for oxygen-centered radicals, as oxygen-centered radical adducts of MNP are quite unstable. To measure ROS in vivo, aromatic traps such as salicylate and phenylalanine can be used, as they are suitable for human consumption [55,56].

Xylenol orange-based assay

Method

This is a new colorimetric automated assay proposed by Ozcan Erel [57]. It is based on the principle that oxidants in sample oxidize the ferrous ion–o-dianisidine complex to ferric ion. The ferric ion makes a colored complex with xylenol orange in an acidic medium, the color intensity of which can be measured by a spectrophotometer. The assay is calibrated with hydrogen peroxide, and the results are expressed in terms of micromolar hydrogen peroxide equivalent per liter (μmol H_2O_2 equiv/L). The assay is performed by an automated analyzer and requires about 35 μL of semen sample.

Applications

It is claimed to be a rapid, easy, stable, reliable, sensitive, inexpensive, and fully automated assay [57].

Limitations

It is a relatively new technique. Hence further research is needed to verify the diagnostic ability and practicality of the assay claimed by the inventors.

Indirect indicators of seminal oxidative stress

Myeloperoxidase or the Endtz test

Method

The myeloperoxidase or Endtz test stains polymorphonuclear granulocytes, thus differentiating these cells from germinal cells. These peroxidase-positive leukocytes are the major source of ROS generation in semen [58].

Applications

It can be used as an indirect indicator of excessive ROS formation in semen.

Limitations

It does not provide any indication of ROS levels produced by spermatozoa.

Redox potential GSH/GSSG

Method

Reduced glutathione (GSH) is one of the most important nonenzymatic oxidant defenses within the body. It detoxifies peroxides and maintains several physiologically important antioxidants such as α-tocopherol and ascorbic acid in their reduced forms. NADPH-dependent oxido-reductase continuously regenerates GSH from GSSG (oxidized form). The balance of GSH and GSSG provides a dynamic indicator of OS in vivo. GSH and GSSG may be determined biochemically or by high-performance liquid chromatography (HPLC) according to the Jones method [59].

Applications

The method can be used to determine generalized OS both in vivo and in vitro.

Limitations

Glutathione-degrading enzymes may lead to artifactual overestimation or underestimation of GSH and GSSG levels. Moreover, the test has not yet been standardized for determination of oxidative stress in semen.

Measurement of lipid peroxidation levels

Lipid peroxidation is one of the most widely used indicators of OS.

Thiobarbituric acid-reactive substances (TBARS)

Method

ROS-induced lipid peroxidation leads to the formation of various aldehydes including propanedial, i.e., malonaldehyde (MDA) [60]. The thiobarbituric acid–propanedial complex can be detected by HPLC, spectrophotometry, or spectrofluorescence [61].

Applications

TBARS is the most widely employed assay for screening and monitoring lipid peroxidation.

Limitations

The assay is not specific, because a variety of TBA-reactive materials such as carbohydrates, bile acids, nucleic acids, and amino acids are not related to lipid peroxidation [62].

Isoprostane (IsoP) method

Method

Nonenzymatic, free radical-induced lipid peroxidation generates oxidized lipid products termed F_2-isoprostanes (IsoP). These substances increase in vivo in response to the known OS generators, and their production can be manipulated by antioxidant supplementation [63].

Applications

Measurement of IsoP is a reliable and attractive marker for measuring OS in vivo, as these are stable compounds and are not produced by enzymatic pathways using arachidonic acid, i.e., cyclooxygenase or lipoxygenase pathways. In addition, IsoP levels are not altered by lipid content in the diet [64].

Limitations

Detection of IsoP requires mass spectrometry, which is an expensive and time-consuming method and requires bioinformatics expertise. Although several commercial immunoassay ELISA kits are available to quantify different IsoPs, considerable interference exists with other substances present in semen, thus necessitating partial purification of samples before analysis [64].

Chemokines

Method

Spermatozoa produce ROS in response to chemo-attractant agents that also stimulate free radical generation by leukocytes [65]. Increased OS amplifies the production of certain cytokines, specifically IL-1α, IL-1β, IL-8, and TNF-α, which in turn results in recruitment of additional neutrophils and increased generation of ROS [66,67]. **Measuring these cytokines in seminal plasma using specific enzyme immunoassay (EIA) kits for each individual cytokine, or by**

623

using cytometric bead array (CBA) flow cytometry for simultaneous cytokines assessment, might provide indirect assessment of OS in semen [6].

Applications

Further research is needed before measurement of cytokines is routinely used as a marker of OS in semen.

Limitations

Determination of a combination of various cytokines is expensive.

DNA damage

Method

ROS has been implicated as one of the important factors leading to sperm DNA damage. This damage can be detected and quantified, providing an indirect measure of OS [68–70]. Some of the currently available tests that are used to evaluate the integrity of sperm DNA include terminal deoxynucleotidyl transferase-mediated deoxyuridine triphosphate nick end-labeling (TUNEL assay), sperm chromatin structure assay (SCSA), comet assay, in-situ nick translation, and DNA breakage detection–fluorescence in-situ hybridization assay (DBD–FISH) [71]. Detailed descriptions of these tests are beyond the scope of this chapter.

Applications

Sperm DNA damage assessment is an objective marker of sperm apoptosis [72].

Limitations

OS is only one of the three main mechanisms behind sperm chromatin damage (defective chromatin packaging and apoptosis being the other two mechanisms) [73,74]. **Hence DNA damage does not necessarily indicate the presence of OS.**

Determination of reactive nitrogen species

Griess reaction

Method

This is an indirect method for determining NO, and it involves the spectrophotometric measurement of its stable decomposition products NO_3^- and NO_2^-. With this method, a two-step diazotization reaction occurs in which the NO-derived nitrosating agent such as N_2O_3 reacts with sulfanilic acid to produce a diazonium ion that is then coupled to N-(1-naphthyl)ethylenediamine to form a chromophoric azo product that absorbs strongly at 543 nm [75,76].

To quantify NO_3^- and NO_2^-, enzymatic reduction of NO_3^- to NO_2^- is achieved by a commercially available preparation of nitrate reductase . NO_2^- is then determined by the Griess reaction [77]. Aspergillus nitrate reductase is used because of its efficiency at reducing very small amounts of NO_3^- to NO_2^- [77].

Applications

It is a simple, rapid, and inexpensive assay for NO_3^- and NO_2^-.

Limitations

It has a practical sensitivity limit of only 2–3 μM [77].

Fluorescence spectroscopy

Fluorescence spectroscopy is a type of electromagnetic spectroscopy which analyzes fluorescence from a sample. It involves using a beam of light, usually ultraviolet, that excites electrons in the molecules and causes them to emit light photons of lower energy. This technique was utilized to measure NO or NO_2^- by exploiting the ability of NO to produce N-nitrosating agents.

Diaminonaphthalene assay

Method

A relatively nonfluorescent aromatic diamino compound, 2,3-diaminonaphthalene, reacts rapidly with the NO-derived N-nitrosating agent (N_2O_3) to form highly fluorescent 2,3-naphthotriazole (NAT) [78].

Applications

This assay is sensitive, specific, and versatile. **It is capable of detecting as little as 10–30 nM NAT, and may also be used to quantify NO generated under physiological conditions with minimal interference by nitrite decomposition [78].**

Limitations

Caution should be taken while using powerful light sources such as lasers, which can result in photochemistry and lead to false positive results.

Diaminofluoroscein 2 assay

Method

Diaminofluoroscein 2 (DAF-2) reacts with the nitrosating agent to form a nitrosamine, which forms a fluorescent triazole through an internal rearrangement [79].

Applications

The adva ntage of DAF-2 is that the wavelength associated with fluorescein can be used, so that equipment currently used for other bioassays can easily be adapted to detect NO in vivo and in vitro [80,81].

Limitations

Nitroxyl (HNO) also reacts with DAF-2, generating triazoles. **Thus there is a possibility that some of the NO detected by DAF-2 is in fact HNO** [79]. As with the above assay, caution should be exercised with powerful light sources such as lasers.

Determination of seminal antioxidants

Various enzymatic and nonenzymatic factors protect cells from harmful effects of free radicals [82]. Measuring the levels of these antioxidants provides an indirect assessment of the level of seminal OS.

Enzymatic antioxidants

Three natural enzyme systems are known to protect spermatozoa against oxygen toxicity: catalase, glutathione peroxidase, and superoxide dismutase [83].

Catalase

Catalase (CAT) is involved in the detoxification of hydrogen peroxide (H_2O_2), which is a toxic product of both normal aerobic metabolism and pathogenic ROS production. This enzyme catalyzes the conversion of two molecules of H_2O_2 to molecular oxygen and two molecules of water [84]:

$$2H_2O_2 \xrightarrow{\text{Catalase}} 2H_2O + O_2$$

CAT also demonstrates peroxidatic activity, in which low molecular weight alcohols can serve as electron donors. While the aliphatic alcohols serve as specific substrates for CAT, other enzymes with peroxidatic activity do not utilize these substrates. CAT activity can be determined spectrophotometrically by utilizing its peroxidative function [85].

Glutathione peroxidase

Glutathione peroxidase (GPx) catalyzes the reduction of hydroperoxides, including hydrogen peroxides, by reduced glutathione, and functions to protect the cell from oxidative damage. The enzyme uses glutathione as the ultimate electron donor. Oxidized glutathione (GSSG), produced upon reduction of an organic hydroperoxide by GPx, is recycled to its reduced state by glutathione reductase (GRD) and NADPH [86]:

$$GSSG + NADPH + H^+ \xrightarrow{\text{GRD}} GSH + NADP^+$$
$$2GSH + R(OOH)COOH \xrightarrow{\text{GPx}} GSSG$$
$$+ R(OH)COOH + H_2O$$

The oxidation of NADPH to $NADP^+$ is accompanied by a decrease in absorbance at 340 nm. The rate of this decrease is directly proportional to the GPx activity in the semen sample [85].

Superoxide dismutase

Superoxide dismutase (SOD) catalyzes the dismutation of superoxide into hydrogen peroxide and oxygen [87]:

$$2O_2^- + 2H^+ \xrightarrow{\text{SOD}} H_2O_2 + O_2$$

It plays a major role in maintaining sperm viability. The SOD levels in spermatozoa are positively correlated with the duration of sperm motility [88]. SOD activity is assessed by measuring the dismutation of superoxide radicals generated by xanthine oxidase and hypoxanthine [85].

Applications

Decreased activity of the above enzymes has been found in seminal plasma of infertile males who have high ROS activity [89].

Limitations

Determination of enzymatic antioxidants does not provide the entire picture of antioxidant defenses in the semen.

Nonenzymatic antioxidants

Besides the enzymatic defenses, other compounds present in human semen such as albumin, α-tocopherol, β-carotene, lycopene, urate, and ascorbic acid play an important role in the protection of spermatozoa against free radical attack [90–92].

Applications

Levels of these antioxidants correlate negatively with the generation of ROS, and their measurement in seminal plasma by high-performance liquid chromatography can provide an indirect assessment of the level of OS in semen [6,91].

Limitations

Determination of individual nonenzymatic antioxidants does not provide complete information about the total seminal antioxidant capacity.

Measurement of total antioxidant capacity (TAC)

Total antioxidant capacity provides biological information more relevant than that obtained by the measurement of individual components because it considers the cumulative effect of all antioxidants present in semen. Several methods have been developed to measure TAC in biological fluids, such as the oxygen radical absorbance capacity (ORAC) [93], the ferric reducing ability of plasma (FRAP) [94], and the phycoerythrin fluorescence-based assay [95]. The following are commonly used methods for measuring TAC in seminal fluid.

Enhanced chemiluminescence assay

Method

A chemiluminescent substrate luminol along with para-iodophenol (an enhancer giving more intense, prolonged, and stable light emission) is mixed with horseradish peroxidase (HRP)-linked immunoglobulin to produce ROS, which in turn is mixed with a substrate, hydrogen peroxidase (H_2O_2). The ability of the antioxidants in the seminal plasma to reduce the chemiluminescence of the signal reagent is compared with that of Trolox (6-hydroxyl-2,5,7,8-tetramethylchroman-2-carboxylic acid), a water-soluble tocopherol analog, and is measured as molar Trolox equivalents [96,97].

Applications

It is an accurate method for measuring total antioxidant capacity in seminal plasma.

Limitations

It is a time-consuming, expensive, and cumbersome method, because fresh signaling reagent solution must be prepared each time the assay is performed and then standardized with Trolox. Moreover, the signal reagent may reduce in intensity within a short time, adding another technical problem [98].

Colorimetric assay

Method

ABTS® (2,2'-azinobis-[3-ethyl-benzothiazoline-6-sulfonic acid]) forms a relatively stable radical cation ABTS$^+$ when it is incubated with a peroxidase (such as met-myoglobin) and H_2O_2 which starts the reaction. The formation of ABTS$^+$ on interaction with ferryl myoglobin produces a relatively stable blue-green color, which can be monitored at 750 nm with a spectrophotometer. Antioxidants present in the semen sample suppress this color production to a degree that is proportional to their concentrations [50,99].

$$HX - Fe^{III} + H_2O_2 \rightarrow X - [Fe^{IV} = 0] + H_2O$$
$$ABTS + X - [Fe^{IV} = 0] \rightarrow ABTS + HX - Fe^{III}$$
$$HX - Fe^{III} = metmyoglobin; \ X - [Fe^{IV} = 0]$$
$$= ferrylmyoglobin$$

Applications

Colorimetric assay is a simple, rapid, relatively inexpensive, and reliable method for measuring seminal TAC. It is less expensive and less time-consuming than the traditional enhanced chemiluminescence assay [98].

Limitations

The sensitivity depends upon the color intensity of the endpoint reaction.

ROS–TAC score

Since neither ROS nor TAC alone can adequately quantify seminal OS, our laboratory introduced a new index called the ROS–TAC score, which combines both variables [96].

Method

The ROS–TAC score is a statistical formula derived from levels of ROS in washed sperm suspensions and TAC in seminal plasma using principal component analysis [96]. A composite ROS–TAC score may be more strongly correlated with OS than ROS or TAC alone.

Levels of ROS are measured in the semen sample by the chemiluminescence assay, and TAC is determined by either colorimetric or enhanced chemiluminescence assay. The ROS–TAC score is calculated using this underlying formula:

$$ROS - TAC = 50 + (principal\ component \times 10.629)$$
$$Principal\ component = (-0.707 \times standardized\ ROS)$$
$$+ (0.707 \times standardized\ TAC)$$
$$Standardized\ ROS = [log\,(ROS + 1) - 1.3885]\,/\,0.7271$$
$$Standardized\ TAC = (TAC - 1650.93)\,/\,532.22$$

Applications

ROS–TAC score may serve as a predictive measure in identifying clinically infertile males who are likely to initiate a pregnancy over a period of time [100]. It appears that individuals with ROS–TAC scores below 30 are at particular risk for prolonged inability to initiate pregnancy [96].

Limitations

There is not enough literature available to validate the clinical usefulness of this assay. **Moreover, this assay was based on the assumption that female factors were absent.**

Protocols of commonly used techniques

Protocols of the techniques used most commonly to measure seminal OS are described below.

ROS measurement by chemiluminescence

A total of 400 µL aliquots of liquefied semen containing sperm and leukocytes and phosphate-buffered saline (PBS) are used to assess basal ROS levels. Eight microliters of horseradish peroxidase (HRP) are added to the cell suspension. The addition of HRP greatly accentuates the sensitivity of luminol to extracellular hydrogen peroxide. Ten microliters of luminol, prepared as 5 mM stock in dimethyl sulfoxide (DMSO), are added to the mixture. Normal ROS levels in neat semen range from 0.02 to 0.2×10^6 cpm per 20×10^6 sperm. A variety of factors such as impurities in the reagents and surrounding equipment can deleteriously affect the results. Therefore, a negative control (10 µL of 5 mM

luminol + 400 µL of PBS) and a blank (400 µL of PBS) aliquot should also be assessed with the test sample. The blank reading provides the background luminescence of the instrument while the control value shows the background luminescence plus the luminescence caused by the presence of impurities in the reagent. Subtract the control reading from the test reading to calculate the true reading of the sample. With pure reagents, the control reading is expected to be equal to that of the blank [24,100]. The control and the samples should be run in duplicate, taking the average of the two readings. It is also advisable to repeat the run if the mean control reading is above 1×10^6 (Fig. 39.2).

ROS can also be measured in a washed semen sample, but there is a significant difference between ROS

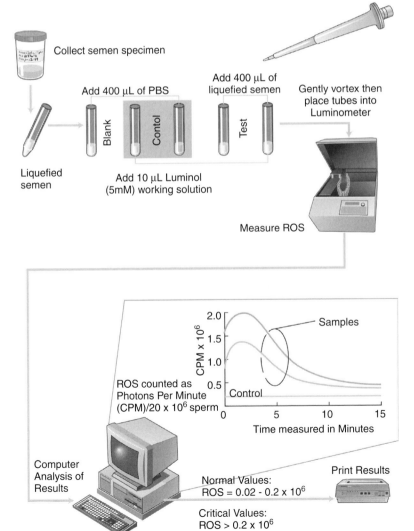

Fig. 39.2. Measurement of ROS in neat semen by chemiluminescence assay.

levels measured in neat semen and those measured in washed spermatozoa. **In fact, ROS levels in neat semen after liquefaction in the presence of seminal antioxidant protection more accurately represent the true in-vivo OS status of an individual than those in washed samples [101]. Therefore, this test can be used as an alternative to an ROS–TAC score for accurate and reliable assessment of seminal OS in the andrology laboratory [100].**

TAC measurement by colorimetric assay

Add 20 μL of diluted seminal plasma to 1 mL of the reconstituted chromogen, ABTS-metmyoglobin (10 mL vial with 10 mL of PBS). Twenty microliters of deionized water is used as a blank and 20 μL of Trolox (6-hydroxy-2,5,7,8-tetramethylchroman-2-carboxylic acid) at a concentration of 1.73 mmol/L is used as a standard. Add 1 mL of chromogen to the standard, the blank, and the sample. Measure the initial absorbance (A_1) with the spectrophotometer adjusted at a wavelength of 600 nm at a temperature of 37 °C.

Add 200 μL of H_2O_2 (250 μmol/L) to the sample, standard, and blank tubes, and measure the absorbance (A_2) after exactly 3 minutes. Calculate the difference (ΔA) between A_2 and A_1. The TAC of the sample in terms of the Trolox equivalents is calculated by the following formula, and the results are expressed as μM of Trolox equivalents:

$$TAC = \text{Concentration of the standard} \times (\Delta A \text{ Blank} - \Delta A \text{ Sample}) / (\Delta A \text{ Blank} - \Delta A \text{ Standard}) \text{ [98]}$$

Commonly used commercially available kits for measuring TAC are Cayman chemical antioxidant kit (Cayman Chemical Company, Ann Arbor, MI, USA) and Randox total antioxidant status kit (Randox Laboratories, San Francisco, CA, USA).

Future research

The discovery of biomarkers is gaining a great deal of interest worldwide, as alterations of these metabolites are involved in many reproductive disorders. Identification of key OS markers has potential for greater diagnostic and therapeutic interventions. With this in mind, a new scientific discipline has been conceived known as metabolomics. Metabolomics is the systematic study of the inventory of metabolites, as small molecule biomarkers that represent the functional phenotype in a cell, tissue, or organism [102,103]. **Recent research suggests that biomarkers of OS (–CH, –NH, –SH, C=C, and –OH) can be** quantified in semen using this technology platform based on various forms of analytical, biochemical, and spectral analysis. It has also been revealed that different levels of OS biomarkers are uniquely associated with normal semen plasma compared to different forms of male-factor infertility [104]. Therefore, in the future, metabolomic profiling of semen using near-infrared spectroscopy and proprietary chemometrics and bioinformatics may provide a rapid, noninvasive, and cost-effective diagnostic method of analyzing semen for abnormalities related to ROS damage and oxidative stress.

Conclusion

The role of oxidative stress (OS) in the pathogenesis of male infertility has been well established. The diagnostic and prognostic capabilities of the seminal OS are beyond those of the conventional sperm quality tests. There is a growing consensus concerning the clinical utility of seminal OS testing in an infertility clinic. As of today, ROS measurement by chemiluminescence and TAC measurement by colorimetric assay are the two most well-described laboratory techniques used for assessing OS in semen. Extensive research in this field has shown tremendous utility of advanced techniques such as flow cytometry and ESR in determining seminal oxidants. Further research is needed, however, before these can be put into clinical practice.

Acknowledments

The authors are grateful to Andrew C. Novick, MD, Chairman, Glickman Urological and Kidney Institute, Cleveland Clinic, for his support and encouragement.

References

[1] Aitken RJ, Clarkson JS, Fishel S. Generation of reactive oxygen species, lipid peroxidation, and human sperm function. *Biol Reprod* 1989; **41**: 183–97.

[2] Agarwal A, Ikemoto I, Loughlin KR. Relationship of sperm parameters with levels of reactive oxygen species in semen specimens. *J Urol* 1994; **152**: 107–10.

[3] Aitken RJ. A free radical theory of male infertility. *Reprod Fertil Dev* 1994; **6**: 19–23.

[4] Warren JS, Johnson KJ, Ward PA. Oxygen radicals in cell injury and cell death. *Pathol Immunopathol Res* 1987; **6**: 301–15.

[5] de Lamirande E, Gagnon C. Human sperm hyperactivation and capacitation as parts of an oxidative process. *Free Radic Biol Med* 1993; **14**: 157–66.

[6] Sharma RK, Agarwal A. Role of reactive oxygen species in male infertility. *Urology* 1996; **48**: 835–50.

[7] Padron OF, Brackett NL, Sharma RK, *et al.* Seminal reactive oxygen species and sperm motility and morphology in men with spinal cord injury. *Fertil Steril* 1997; **67**: 1115–20.

[8] de Lamirande E, Gagnon C. Impact of reactive oxygen species on spermatozoa: a balancing act between beneficial and detrimental effects. *Hum Reprod* 1995; **10** (Suppl 1): 15–21.

[9] Cummins JM, Jequier AM, Kan R. Molecular biology of human male infertility: links with aging, mitochondrial genetics, and oxidative stress? *Mol Reprod Dev* 1994; **37**: 345–62.

[10] Jones R, Mann T, Sherins R. Peroxidative breakdown of phospholipids in human spermatozoa, spermicidal properties of fatty acid peroxides, and protective action of seminal plasma. *Fertil Steril* 1979; **31**: 531–7.

[11] Aitken J, Fisher H. Reactive oxygen species generation and human spermatozoa: the balance of benefit and risk. *Bioessays* 1994; **16**: 259–67.

[12] Darley-Usmar V, Wiseman H, Halliwell B. Nitric oxide and oxygen radicals: a question of balance. *FEBS Lett* 1995; **369**: 131–5.

[13] Sharma RK, Pasqualotto AE, Nelson DR, Thomas AJ, Agarwal A. Relationship between seminal white blood cell counts and oxidative stress in men treated at an infertility clinic. *J Androl* 2001; **22**: 575–83.

[14] Saleh RA, Agarwal A, Kandirali E, *et al.* Leukocytospermia is associated with increased reactive oxygen species production by human spermatozoa. *Fertil Steril* 2002; **78**: 1215–24.

[15] Gil-Guzman E, Ollero M, Lopez MC, *et al.* Differential production of reactive oxygen species by subsets of human spermatozoa at different stages of maturation. *Hum Reprod* 2001; **16**: 1922–30.

[16] Ryan TC, Weil GJ, Newburger PE, Haugland R, Simons ER. Measurement of superoxide release in the phagovacuoles of immune complex-stimulated human neutrophils. *J Immunol Methods* 1990; **130**: 223–33.

[17] Allen RC. Phagocytic leukocyte oxygenation activities and chemiluminescence: a kinetic approach to analysis. *Methods Enzymol* 1986; **133**: 449–93.

[18] Wolfson M, McPhail LC, Nasrallah VN, Snyderman R. Phorbol myristate acetate mediates redistribution of protein kinase C in human neutrophils: Potential role in the activation of the respiratory burst enzyme. *J Immunol* 1985; **135**: 2057–62.

[19] Rossi F. The O2-forming NADPH oxidase of the phagocytes: nature, mechanisms of activation and function. *Biochim Biophys Acta* 1986; **853**: 65–89.

[20] DeChatelet LR, Shirley PS, Johnston RB. Effect of phorbol myristate acetate on the oxidative metabolism of human polymorphonuclear leukocytes. *Blood* 1976; **47**: 545–54.

[21] Nallella KP, Allamaneni SS, Pasqualotto FF, *et al.* Relationship of interleukin-6 with semen

characteristics and oxidative stress in patients with varicocele. *Urology* 2004; **64**: 1010–13.

[22] Gavella M, Lipovac V. NADH-dependent oxidoreductase (diaphorase) activity and isozyme pattern of sperm in infertile men. *Arch Androl* 1992; **28**: 135–41.

[23] Gomez E, Buckingham DW, Brindle J, *et al.* Development of an image analysis system to monitor the retention of residual cytoplasm by human spermatozoa: correlation with biochemical markers of the cytoplasmic space, oxidative stress, and sperm function. *J Androl* 1996; **17**: 276–87.

[24] Kobayashi H, Gil-Guzman E, Mahran AM, *et al.* Quality control of reactive oxygen species measurement by luminol-dependent chemiluminescence assay. *J Androl* 2001; **22**: 568–74.

[25] Aitken RJ, Buckingham DW, West KM. Reactive oxygen species and human spermatozoa: Analysis of the cellular mechanisms involved in luminol- and lucigenin-dependent chemiluminescence. *J Cell Physiol* 1992; **151**: 466–77.

[26] Faulkner K, Fridovich I. Luminol and lucigenin as detectors for O2. *Free Radic Biol Med* 1993; **15**: 447–51.

[27] McKinney KA, Lewis SE, Thompson W. Reactive oxygen species generation in human sperm: luminol and lucigenin chemiluminescence probes. *Arch Androl* 1996; **36**: 119–25.

[28] Aitken RJ, Baker MA, O'Bryan M. Shedding light on chemiluminescence: the application of chemiluminescence in diagnostic andrology. *J Androl* 2004; **25**: 455–65.

[29] de Lamirande E, Gagnon C. Capacitation-associated production of superoxide anion by human spermatozoa. *Free Radic Biol Med* 1995; **18**: 487–95.

[30] Tarpey MM, White CR, Suarez E, *et al.* Chemiluminescent detection of oxidants in vascular tissue: lucigenin but not coelenterazine enhances superoxide formation. *Circ Res* 1999; **84**: 1203–11.

[31] Agarwal A, Allamaneni SS, Said TM. Chemiluminescence technique for measuring reactive oxygen species. *Reprod Biomed Online* 2004; **9**: 466–8.

[32] Whittington K, Ford WC. Relative contribution of leukocytes and of spermatozoa to reactive oxygen species production in human sperm suspensions. *Int J Androl* 1999; **22**: 229–35.

[33] Aitken RJ, West KM. Analysis of the relationship between reactive oxygen species production and leucocyte infiltration in fractions of human semen separated on Percoll gradients. *Int J Androl* 1990; **13**: 433–51.

[34] Aitken RJ, Buckingham DW, West K, Brindle J. On the use of paramagnetic beads and ferrofluids to assess and eliminate the leukocytic contribution to oxygen

radical generation by human sperm suspensions. *Am J Reprod Immunol* 1996; **35**: 541–51.

[35] Krausz C, Mills C, Rogers S, Tan SL, Aitken RJ. Stimulation of oxidant generation by human sperm suspensions using phorbol esters and formyl peptides: relationships with motility and fertilization *in vitro*. *Fertil Steril* 1994; **62**: 599–605.

[36] Aitken RJ, Clarkson JS. Cellular basis of defective sperm function and its association with the genesis of reactive oxygen species by human spermatozoa. *J Reprod Fertil* 1987; **81**: 459–69.

[37] Aitken RJ, Clarkson JS. Significance of reactive oxygen species and antioxidants in defining the efficacy of sperm preparation techniques. *J Androl* 1988; **9**: 367–76.

[38] Quinn P, Whittingham DG, Stanger JD. Interaction of semen with ova *in vitro*. *Arch Androl* 1982; **8**: 189–98.

[39] Fridovich I. Editorial commentary on Zhao H, *et al.* Superoxide reacts with hydroethidine but forms a fluorescent product that is distinctly different from ethidium: potential implications in intracellular fluorescence detection of superoxide. *Free Radic Biol Med* 2003; **34**: 1357–8.

[40] Baehner RL, Boxer LA, Davis J. The biochemical basis of nitroblue tetrazolium reduction in normal human and chronic granulomatous disease polymorphonuclear leukocytes. *Blood* 1976; **48**: 309–13.

[41] Armstrong JS, Bivalacqua TJ, Chamulitrat W, Sikka S, Hellstrom WJ. A comparison of the NADPH oxidase in human sperm and white blood cells. *Int J Androl* 2002; **25**: 223–9.

[42] Esfandiari N, Sharma RK, Saleh RA, Thomas AJ, Agarwal A. Utility of the nitroblue tetrazolium reduction test for assessment of reactive oxygen species production by seminal leukocytes and spermatozoa. *J Androl* 2003; **24**: 862–70.

[43] Fridovich I. Superoxide anion radical (O2–.), superoxide dismutases, and related matters. *J Biol Chem* 1997; **272**: 18515–17.

[44] Massey V. The microestimation of succinate and the extinction coefficient of cytochrome c. *Biochim Biophys Acta* 1959; **34**: 255–6.

[45] Land EJ, Swallow AJ. One-electron reactions in biochemical systems as studied by pulse radiolysis. V. Cytochrome c. *Arch Biochem Biophys* 1971; **145**: 365–72.

[46] Elferink JG. Measurement of the metabolic burst in human neutrophils: a comparison between cytochrome c and NBT reduction. *Res Commun Chem Pathol Pharmacol* 1984; **43**: 339–42.

[47] Fridovich I. Cytochrome c. In: Greenwald RA, ed. *CRC Handbook of Methods for Oxygen Radical Research*. Boca Raton, FL: CRC, 1985: 121–2.

[48] O'Brien PJ. Superoxide production. *Methods Enzymol* 1984; **105**: 370–8.

[49] Bass DA, Parce JW, Dechatelet LR, *et al.* Flow cytometric studies of oxidative product formation by neutrophils: a graded response to membrane stimulation. *J Immunol* 1983; **130**: 1910–17.

[50] Miller NJ, Rice-Evans C, Davies MJ, Gopinathan V, Milner A. A novel method for measuring antioxidant capacity and its application to monitoring the antioxidant status in premature neonates. *Clin Sci (Lond)* 1993; **84**: 407–12.

[51] Guthrie HD, Welch GR. Determination of intracellular reactive oxygen species and high mitochondrial membrane potential in Percoll-treated viable boar sperm using fluorescence-activated flow cytometry. *J Anim Sci* 2006; **84**: 2089–100.

[52] Weber GF. The measurement of oxygen-derived free radicals and related substances in medicine. *J Clin Chem Clin Biochem* 1990; **28**: 569–603.

[53] Bray RC, Pettersson R. Electron-spin-resonance measurements. *Biochem J* 1961; **81**: 194–5.

[54] Buettner GR. Spin trapping: ESR parameters of spin adducts. *Free Radic Biol Med* 1987; **3**: 259–303.

[55] Halliwell B, Kaur H. Hydroxylation of salicylate and phenylalanine as assays for hydroxyl radicals: A cautionary note visited for the third time. *Free Radic Res* 1997; **27**: 239–44.

[56] Coudray C, Favier A. Determination of salicylate hydroxylation products as an in vivo oxidative stress marker. *Free Radic Biol Med* 2000; **29**: 1064–70.

[57] Erel O. A new automated colorimetric method for measuring total oxidant status. *Clin Biochem* 2005; **38**: 1103–11.

[58] Shekarriz M, Sharma RK, Thomas AJ, Agarwal A. Positive myeloperoxidase staining (Endtz test) as an indicator of excessive reactive oxygen species formation in semen. *J Assist Reprod Genet* 1995; **12**: 70–4.

[59] Jones DP. Redox potential of GSH/GSSG couple: assay and biological significance. *Methods Enzymol* 2002; **348**: 93–112.

[60] Pryor WA, Stanley JP, Blair E. Autoxidation of polyunsaturated fatty acids: II. A suggested mechanism for the formation of TBA-reactive materials from prostaglandin-like endoperoxides. *Lipids* 1976; **11**: 370–9.

[61] Yagi K. Simple assay for the level of total lipid peroxides in serum or plasma. *Methods Mol Biol* 1998; **108**: 101–6.

[62] Tarpey MM, Wink DA, Grisham MB. Methods for detection of reactive metabolites of oxygen and nitrogen: *in vitro* and in vivo considerations. *Am J Physiol Regul Integr Comp Physiol* 2004; **286**: R431–44.

[63] Morrow JD, Hill KE, Burk RF, Nammour TM, Badr KF, Roberts LJ. A series of prostaglandin F2-like compounds are produced in vivo in humans by a non-cyclooxygenase, free radical-catalyzed mechanism. *Proc Natl Acad Sci U S A* 1990; **87**: 9383–7.

[64] Roberts LJ, Morrow JD. Measurement of F(2)-isoprostanes as an index of oxidative stress in vivo. *Free Radic Biol Med* 2000; **28**: 505–13.

[65] Weese DL, Peaster ML, Hernandez RD, *et al.* Chemoattractant agents and nerve growth factor stimulate human spermatozoal reactive oxygen species generation. *Fertil Steril* 1993; **59**: 869–75.

[66] Rajasekaran M, Hellstrom WJ, Naz RK, Sikka SC. Oxidative stress and interleukins in seminal plasma during leukocytospermia. *Fertil Steril* 1995; **64**: 166–71.

[67] Buch JP, Kolon TF, Maulik N, Kreutzer DL, Das DK. Cytokines stimulate lipid membrane peroxidation of human sperm. *Fertil Steril* 1994; **62**: 186–8.

[68] Loft S, Kold-Jensen T, Hjollund NH, *et al.* Oxidative DNA damage in human sperm influences time to pregnancy. *Hum Reprod* 2003; **18**: 1265–71.

[69] Aitken RJ, Baker MA, Sawyer D. Oxidative stress in the male germ line and its role in the aetiology of male infertility and genetic disease. *Reprod Biomed Online* 2003; **7**: 65–70.

[70] Aitken RJ, Baker MA. Oxidative stress and male reproductive biology. *Reprod Fertil Dev* 2004; **16**: 581–8.

[71] Evenson DP, Wixon R. Clinical aspects of sperm DNA fragmentation detection and male infertility. *Theriogenology* 2006; **65**: 979–91.

[72] Agarwal A, Allamaneni SS. Sperm DNA damage assessment: a test whose time has come. *Fertil Steril* 2005; **84**: 850–3.

[73] Shen H, Ong C. Detection of oxidative DNA damage in human sperm and its association with sperm function and male infertility. *Free Radic Biol Med* 2000; **28**: 529–36.

[74] Sakkas D, Mariethoz E, Manicardi G, *et al.* Origin of DNA damage in ejaculated human spermatozoa. *Rev Reprod* 1999; **4**: 31–7.

[75] Guevara I, Iwanejko J, Dembinska-Kiec A, *et al.* Determination of nitrite/nitrate in human biological material by the simple Griess reaction. *Clin Chim Acta* 1998; **274**: 177–8.

[76] Granger DL, Taintor RR, Boockvar KS, Hibbs JB. Measurement of nitrate and nitrite in biological samples using nitrate reductase and Griess reaction. *Methods Enzymol* 1996; **268**: 142–51.

[77] Grisham MB, Johnson GG, Lancaster JR. Quantitation of nitrate and nitrite in extracellular fluids. *Methods Enzymol* 1996; **268**: 237–46.

[78] Miles AM, Wink DA, Cook JC, Grisham MB. Determination of nitric oxide using fluorescence spectroscopy. *Methods Enzymol* 1996; **268**: 105–20.

[79] Espey MG, Thomas DD, Miranda KM, Wink DA. Focusing of nitric oxide mediated nitrosation and oxidative nitrosylation as a consequence of reaction with superoxide. *Proc Natl Acad Sci U S A* 2002; **99**: 11127–32.

[80] Espey MG, Miranda KM, Thomas DD, Wink DA. Ingress and reactive chemistry of nitroxyl-derived species within human cells. *Free Radic Biol Med* 2002; **33**: 827–34.

[81] Espey MG, Miranda KM, Thomas DD, Wink DA. Distinction between nitrosating mechanisms within human cells and aqueous solution. *J Biol Chem* 2001; **276**: 30085–91.

[82] Lewis SE, Boyle PM, McKinney KA, Young IS, Thompson W. Total antioxidant capacity of seminal plasma is different in fertile and infertile men. *Fertil Steril* 1995; **64**: 868–70.

[83] Baker HW, Brindle J, Irvine DS, Aitken RJ. Protective effect of antioxidants on the impairment of sperm motility by activated polymorphonuclear leukocytes. *Fertil Steril* 1996; **65**: 411–19.

[84] Jeulin C, Soufir JC, Weber P, Laval-Martin D, Calvayrac R. Catalase activity in human spermatozoa and seminal plasma. *Gamete Res* 1989; **24**: 185–96.

[85] Wheeler CR, Salzman JA, Elsayed NM, Omaye ST, Korte DW. Automated assays for superoxide dismutase, catalase, glutathione peroxidase, and glutathione reductase activity. *Anal Biochem* 1990; **184**: 193–9.

[86] Paglia DE, Valentine WN. Studies on the quantitative and qualitative characterization of erythrocyte glutathione peroxidase. *J Lab Clin Med* 1967; **70**: 158–69.

[87] Peeker R, Abramsson L, Marklund SL. Superoxide dismutase isoenzymes in human seminal plasma and spermatozoa. *Mol Hum Reprod* 1997; **3**: 1061–6.

[88] Alvarez JG, Touchstone JC, Blasco L, Storey BT. Spontaneous lipid peroxidation and production of hydrogen peroxide and superoxide in human spermatozoa: superoxide dismutase as major enzyme protectant against oxygen toxicity. *J Androl* 1987; **8**: 338–48.

[89] Alkan I, Simsek F, Haklar G, *et al.* Reactive oxygen species production by the spermatozoa of patients with idiopathic infertility: Relationship to seminal plasma antioxidants. *J Urol* 1997; **157**: 140–3.

[90] Thiele JJ, Friesleben HJ, Fuchs J, Ochsendorf FR. Ascorbic acid and urate in human seminal plasma: Determination and interrelationships with chemiluminescence in washed semen. *Hum Reprod* 1995; **10**: 110–15.

[91] Palan P, Naz R. Changes in various antioxidant levels in human seminal plasma related to immunoinfertility. *Arch Androl* 1996; **36**: 139–43.

[92] Fraga CG, Motchnik PA, Shigenaga MK, *et al.* Ascorbic acid protects against endogenous oxidative DNA damage in human sperm. *Proc Natl Acad Sci U S A* 1991; **88**: 11003–6.

[93] Cao G, Prior RL. Comparison of different analytical methods for assessing total antioxidant capacity of human serum. *Clin Chem* 1998; **44**: 1309–15.

[94] Benzie IF, Strain JJ. The ferric reducing ability of plasma (FRAP) as a measure of "antioxidant power": the FRAP assay. *Anal Biochem* 1996; **239**: 70–6.

[95] Glazer AN. Phycoerythrin fluorescence-based assay for reactive oxygen species. *Methods Enzymol* 1990; **186**: 161–8.

[96] Sharma RK, Pasqualotto FF, Nelson DR, Thomas AJ, Agarwal A. The reactive oxygen species–total antioxidant capacity score is a new measure of oxidative stress to predict male infertility. *Hum Reprod* 1999; **14**: 2801–7.

[97] Kolettis PN, Sharma RK, Pasqualotto FF, *et al.* Effect of seminal oxidative stress on fertility after vasectomy reversal. *Fertil Steril* 1999; **71**: 249–55.

[98] Said TM, Kattal N, Sharma RK, *et al.* Enhanced chemiluminescence assay vs colorimetric assay for measurement of the total antioxidant capacity of human seminal plasma. *J Androl* 2003; **24**: 676–80.

[99] Miller NJ, Rice-Evans CA. Factors influencing the antioxidant activity determined by the ABTS.+ radical cation assay. *Free Radic Res* 1997; **26**: 195–9.

[100] Saleh RA, Agarwal A. Oxidative stress and male infertility: from research bench to clinical practice. *J Androl* 2002; **23**: 737–52.

[101] Allamaneni SS, Agarwal A, Nallella KP, *et al.* Characterization of oxidative stress status by evaluation of reactive oxygen species levels in whole semen and isolated spermatozoa. *Fertil Steril* 2005; **83**: 800–3.

[102] Rochfort S. Metabolomics reviewed: a new "omics" platform technology for systems biology and implications for natural products research. *J Nat Prod* 2005; **68**: 1813–20.

[103] Hollywood K, Brison DR, Goodacre R. Metabolomics: current technologies and future trends. *Proteomics* 2006; **6**: 4716–23.

[104] Agarwal A, Sharma RK, Prabakaran SA, *et al.* Assessment of oxidative stress levels in semen using spectroscopy-based metabolomic profiling: implications in male infertility. *American Society for Reproductive Medicine* 2006; **P-131**: S180.

Chapter 40

Measurement of DNA fragmentation in human spermatozoa

Denny Sakkas

Introduction

In 1980 Evenson *et al.* published a pioneering paper in *Science* entitled "Relation of mammalian sperm chromatin heterogeneity to fertility," in which they used flow cytometry measurements of heated sperm nuclei to reveal a significant decrease in resistance to in-situ denaturation of spermatozoal DNA in samples from bulls, mice, and humans of low or questionable fertility when compared with others of high fertility [1]. **They postulated that since thermal denaturation of DNA in situ depends on chromatin structure then there were assumed changes in sperm chromatin conformation that may be related to the diminished fertility. They then went on to suggest that flow cytometry of heated sperm nuclei could provide a new and independent determinant of male fertility.**

It was not anticipated by Evenson and colleagues that 12 years later the humans of low or questionable fertility would have the ideal treatment option in intracytoplasmic sperm injection (ICSI) [2]. Moving further forward, we have now become more adept at measuring the abnormalities in the sperm nucleus, and the use of ICSI to treat humans with severe fertility problems is routine. There are, however, valid concerns about the use of ICSI in these low-fertility patients [3], even though large follow-up studies do not show any major differences between ICSI, in-vitro fertilization (IVF), and normal conceptions [4]. **The testing of sperm DNA fragmentation and concerns about ICSI have therefore become further interconnected, because patients with faulty nuclear DNAs are among those most likely to turn to ICSI.** This chapter will therefore examine the main aspects of testing sperm DNA fragmentation, and the impact of these tests on predicting the fertility status of males.

Sperm DNA fragmentation tests

Sperm DNA fragmentation can be measured by a number of different means. In addition to the flow cytometry-based technology initially described by Evenson *et al.* [1], a number of other techniques have since been reported that also provide a measure of sperm nuclear DNA status. These included the TUNEL assay [6], in-situ nick translation [7], and the comet assay [8,9]. Furthermore, numerous other techniques exist that measure the integrity of the sperm nucleus, among them chromomycin A_3 [10,11], the DNA breakage detection–fluorescence in-situ hybridization (DBD–FISH) technique, and the sperm chromatin dispersion (SCD) analysis [12–14]. A number of other "surrogate" markers of sperm integrity have also been reported. Included in these are apoptotic marker proteins [15–17], which, when present, imply that the spermatozoa have been programmed to undergo cell death and degrade the nucleus through apoptosis.

Testing spermatozoal DNA integrity

Two tests have been most commonly reported in recent years as indicators of sperm nuclear integrity. The test most commonly used to detect DNA strand breaks is TUNEL (terminal deoxynucleotidyl transferase-mediated dUTP nick end-labeling). The TUNEL technique labels single- or double-stranded DNA breaks, but does not quantify DNA strand breaks in a given cell. The most widely adapted and therefore most closely scrutinized test that evaluates spermatozoal DNA integrity is, however, the sperm chromatin structure assay (SCSA).

The sperm chromatin structure assay (SCSA)
The SCSA is a flow-cytometric test that measures the susceptibility of sperm nuclear DNA to acid-induced

Infertility in the Male, 4th edition, ed. Larry I. Lipshultz, Stuart S. Howards, and Craig S. Niederberger. Published by Cambridge University Press. © Cambridge University Press 2009.

DNA denaturation in situ, followed by staining with acridine orange [18–20]. Acridine orange is a metachromatic dye that fluoresces red when associated with denatured (fragmented) DNA and green when bound to double-stranded (normal) DNA. Therefore an increase in the percentage of cells with a high ratio of red to green fluorescence indicates an overall increase in DNA fragmentation in the spermatozoa from that ejaculate. Because the SCSA is quantitative (on a continuous scale), as opposed to a qualitative measurement, it has the potential to better define thresholds associated with reproductive outcome [19]. SCSA parameters correlate with DNA strand breaks detected using the TUNEL technique [21,22].

The SCSA, now adapted clinically as a service, measures a number of parameters, which include the DFI (DNA fragmentation index, i.e., the sperm fraction with detectable denaturable single-stranded DNA, mainly due to DNA breaks) [20] **and the HDS** (highly DNA stainable cells, the sperm fraction showing increased double-stranded DNA accessibility to acridine orange, mainly because of defects in the histone-to-protamine transition process). As these parameters are not correlated to each other, they represent independent aberrations of the human mature male gamete in the ejaculate. DFI has been postulated to influence a normally initiated pregnancy [23,24]. Indeed, Evenson et al. showed that increasing levels of DFI (> 30%), independently of WHO standard semen parameters, were associated with a decreased probability of fathering a child [23]. Since the initial studies clinically examining the SCSA test, many studies have been set up also to challenge the SCSA prediction power in the context of assisted reproductive technologies (ART). In some initial small (24 men) pilot studies it was shown that when DFI was above 27%, no pregnancies were achieved after IVF/ICSI [25]. Two other studies reinforced this finding. Larson-Cook et al. examined 89 couples undergoing IVF/ICSI [19]. The endpoint was clinical pregnancy 14 days after embryo transfer as assessed by positive serum hCG and ultrasound detection for a fetal sac. They showed that all patients who achieved a pregnancy had a DFI below 27%. (On the other hand, HDS was not correlated to pregnancy.) Saleh et al. considered 19 couples undergoing intrauterine insemination (IUI), 10 couples undergoing IVF, and four couples undergoing ICSI [26]. In this study, levels of DFI (but not of HDS) were negatively correlated with biochemical pregnancy. The highest DFI value in biological fathers was 28%. Even

though findings were quite consistent, some discrepancies arose from these two studies: (1) sperm concentration, percentage motility, and percentage morphology were significantly lower in patients who failed to initiate a clinical pregnancy in the Saleh et al. study [26] but not in that of Larson-Cook et al. [19]; (2) the fertilization rate was related to DFI in the Saleh et al. study but not in the Larson-Cook et al. study.

The interest generated by the original Evenson and Spano studies [23,24], **on the existence of an upper DNA fragmentation threshold above which no pregnancy can be obtained after ART, has lessened as more investigations have been published.** First, Gandini et al., in a study involving 34 couples (12 IVF and 22 ICSI) did not note any difference between patients who did and did not initiate pregnancies, and, above all, they reported healthy full-term pregnancies even with high levels of DFI (up to 66.3%) [27]. Pregnancy rates were 25% for IVF and 40.9% for ICSI. HDS was not correlated with either pregnancy or delivery. No association was found between the SCSA parameters and the fertility rate. Second, Bungum et al. in two studies have investigated ART treatment cycles and the predictive value of the SCSA test [28,29]. In the initial study they reported results from 131 IUI, 109 IVF, and 66 ICSI cycles, taking into account biochemical pregnancy (positive plasma hCG), clinical pregnancy (intrauterine gestational sac with a heartbeat three weeks after a positive hCG test), and delivery [28]. Delivery rate was 15.3% after IUI, 28.4% after IVF, and 37.9% after ICSI. They reported that, for IUI, the chance of pregnancy/delivery was significantly higher in the group with DFI < 27% (and HDS < 10%): only one delivery was obtained in the 23 males having a DFI > 27%. The combination of DFI and HDS gave a higher predictive value regarding the outcome of IUI. On the other hand, no statistically significant difference in the outcome after IVF/ICSI was noted by dividing patients according to the DFI level above or below 27%. However, the results of ICSI were significantly better than those of IVF. For example, as far as the group with DFI > 27% was concerned, comparing ICSI and IVF performances, the authors reported higher clinical pregnancy (52.9% vs. 22.2%), implantation (37.5% vs. 19.4%), and delivery (47.1% vs. 22.2%) rates. In addition, when the analysis was restricted to IVF patients only, the low DFI level (< 27%) group consistently showed better clinical pregnancy (36.6% vs. 22.2%), implantation (33.3% vs. 19.4%), and delivery (29.7% vs. 22.2%) rates than the group of men with DFI > 27%. In the second, larger study, the IUI results were substantiated, and no statistical difference was seen between the outcomes of ICSI and IVF in the group with DFI ≤ 30% [29]. In the group with DFI > 30%, the results of ICSI were indeed significantly higher than those of IVF. They still recommended that SCSA should be used as a testing method to identify patients being overtreated by IUI and move them more quickly into IVF or ICSI treatment. Finally, Virro et al. studied 249 couples undergoing IVF/ICSI and noted that men with DFI < 33% had a significantly greater chance of initiating a clinical pregnancy (positive hCG), a lower rate of spontaneous abortions, and an increase in ongoing pregnancies at 12 weeks (47% vs. 28%) [30]. HDS and standard WHO parameters were not related to pregnancy outcomes.

More recently, Payne et al. also failed to find a strong correlation between SCSA and ART pregnancy prediction [31]. They concluded that the SCSA failed to identify elevated DFI thresholds for negative pregnancy outcome after ART. Patients with a low DFI (≤ 9%) were least likely to become pregnant, a finding contradictory to SCSA marketing, which states that DFIs of ≤ 15% have excellent fertility potential. On the other hand, patients with HDS ≥ 17% had low pregnancy rates, indicating decreased fertility potential.

The increasing number of publications in this field indicates that the clinical relevance of the SCSA tests is definitely not completely black and white [32]. When the test is correlated to natural fertility and IUI, it seems more appropriate. However, when tested in an IVF or ICSI setting, the results are inconclusive, most probably because of the way spermatozoa are prepared for IVF and ICSI [33,34]. Finally, an advantage of SCSA, compared to other, more specific techniques to detect sperm DNA breaks, resides in its capability to identify two different types of aberrant sperm populations, those mirrored by the DFI (sperm with DNA breaks) and the HDS fraction (sperm with chromatin derailments in the protamination process). The interplay between these two parameters should be tested in more detail in future ART studies.

The TUNEL (terminal deoxynucleotidyl transferase-mediated dUTP nick end-labeling) assay

The TUNEL assay has been adopted as a measure of sperm DNA integrity for two reasons. First, the ease with which available TUNEL kits measure DNA fragmentation allows for a simple assessment of sperm to be made on the basis of whether DNA strand breaks are present. Second, the assumption has been made in numerous studies that TUNEL measurement of sperm is indicative of apoptosis. Whether the presence of DNA strand breaks, as measured by TUNEL, is indicative of apoptosis remains a major question [35,36].

The technique can be used either with flow cytometry, allowing a greater number of spermatozoa to be assessed, or by staining cells on a slide and examining them individually under a fluorescent microscope.

Clinically the TUNEL technique has been placed under far less scrutiny than the SCSA diagnosis. In a study by Benchaib et al., sperm DNA fragmentation was measured with the TUNEL technique [37]. Similar to many other investigators [5,12,38–40], they found that there was a negative statistical correlation between the rate of fragmentation and the semen characteristics. The study examined 322 couples, divided into 88 cycles of IVF or 234 cycles of ICSI. A statistically significant negative relationship was found for sperm DNA fragmentation and fertilization when ICSI and IVF were compared. With ICSI, a statistically significant negative relationship was found between fertilization rate and percentage of sperm DNA fragmentation (DFI). The risk of a failed transfer due to blocked embryo development increased when the DFI exceeded 15% (18.2% for ICSI vs. 4.2% for IVF) with an odds ratio of 5.05. The miscarriage risk increased fourfold when the DFI exceeded 15% (37.5% for ICSI vs. 8.8% for IVF). The study has been corroborated by a more recent study by Borini et al., who also used the TUNEL assay to evaluate DNA fragmentation [41]. They examined 132 men undergoing an ART cycle (82 IVF and 50 ICSI) and correlated outcome with sperm parameters and ART outcome. They also found a highly significant negative correlation between DNA fragmentation and sperm parameters and a close relationship between DNA fragmentation and post-implantation development in ICSI patients: the clinical pregnancy and pregnancy loss rates differed significantly between patients with high and low sperm DNA fragmentation ($P = 0.007$ and $P = 0.009$, respectively). These two TUNEL studies found that sperm DNA fragmentation was a prognostic indicator of the fertilization, pregnancy, and miscarriage rates, and of the pregnancy outcome. Interestingly, both studies performed their TUNEL assays on sperm suspensions after density gradient separation, and not on semen samples such as those utilized by most SCSA studies.

Current clinical relevance regarding tests of sperm DNA integrity

From the ever-increasing wealth of data collected so far about the SCSA and TUNEL techniques, the following has been concluded by meta-analysis of published papers.

Evenson and Wixon reported that couples with no known infertility problems were 7.0 times (CI 3.17–17.7) more likely to achieve a pregnancy/delivery if the DNA fragmentation index (DFI) was < 30% ($n = 362$, $P = 0.0001$) using in-vivo fertilization [42]. Infertile couples using IUI were 7.3 times (CI 2.88–18.3) more likely to achieve a pregnancy/delivery if their DFI was < 30% ($n = 518$, $P = 0.0001$). With routine IVF, infertile couples were approximately 2.0 times (CI 1.02–2.84) more likely to become pregnant if their DFI was < 30% ($n = 381$, $P = 0.03$). For ICSI and/or routine IVF, the results failed to show significance. Their meta-analyses showed that the SCSA infertility test was predictive for reduced pregnancy success using in vivo and IUI but less so for routine IVF, and to a lesser extent ICSI fertilization. A further meta-analysis by Li et al. examined eight studies, five of which used the TUNEL assay and three of which used the SCSA [43]. For studies using the TUNEL assay, the pooled results of IVF outcomes indicated that the clinical pregnancy rate (RR 0.68, 95% CI 0.54–0.85, $P = 0.006$), but not the fertilization rate (RR 0.79, 95% CI 0.54–1.16, $P = 0.23$), decreased significantly for patients with a high degree of sperm DNA damage compared with those with a low degree of sperm DNA damage. For the SCSA papers, the pooled results showed no significant effects of sperm DNA damage on the clinical pregnancy rate after IVF (RR 0.58, 95% CI 0.25–1.31, $P = 0.19$) or ICSI (RR 1.18, 95% CI 0.81–1.74, $P = 0.38$). Their meta-analysis indicated that sperm DNA damage, as assessed by the TUNEL assay, significantly decreased only the chance of IVF clinical pregnancy, but not that of either IVF fertilization or ICSI fertilization, or ICSI clinical pregnancy. In addition, their results revealed that sperm DNA damage, when assessed by the SCSA, had no significant effect on the chance of clinical pregnancy after IVF or ICSI treatment.

Two main conclusions can be drawn, about the impact of DNA damage and about the predictive power of SCSA and TUNEL:

(1) An increased fraction of sperm showing DNA damage is certainly a negative trait that reduces the chances to father a child.

(2) The predictive powers of these tests, and in particular SCSA, seem to be reduced as more rigorous technologies are used to treat infertility. SCSA definitely remains predictive of natural conception and IUI, but once IVF or ICSI treatment is adopted then SCSA loses its predictive power.

Improving sperm nuclear DNA integrity tests

A technical aspect of numerous studies utilizing SCSA is that the commercial application measures values in the semen. This is because the inventors believe that the semen is representing the "tip of the iceberg" of the problem seen in the spermatozoa in general [23]. The decreased predictive power of the SCSA analysis in IVF and ICSI may be due to the fact that a selected sperm population (by swim-up or discontinuous gradient centrifugation) is used in these techniques. It is clear that sperm quality is improved by density gradient centrifugation techniques. Spano and colleagues tried to measure DFI and HDS on both the raw and prepared semen aliquots [44]. They found that enriched cell suspensions to be used in ART contained sperm with better motility, morphology, HDS, and DFI. Interestingly, they also observed that ICSI full-term pregnancies could be also obtained with high-DFI-value semen as assessed in the PureSperm fraction (range was 1.7–60.4%). In addition, we had also previously shown that when sperm samples from different men were prepared using density gradient techniques for ART and then stained using the chromomycin A_3 (CMA_3) fluorochrome, which indirectly demonstrates a decreased presence of protamine, and in-situ nick translation, which examines for the presence of endogenous DNA nicks, a significant ($P < 0.001$) decrease in both CMA_3 positivity and DNA strand breakage occurred [45–47]. As SCSA is performed in the raw semen sample prior to processing, a selective elimination of spermatozoa with DNA fragmentation during sperm preparation for ART cannot be excluded, and additional studies are needed to clarify this point. To further ascertain the relevance of some of the DNA sperm tests to IVF and ICSI outcome, clinical trials should examine predictability when the analysis is performed on the same prepared sample used to inseminate the oocytes or perform ICSI. In a previous small study, when we performed this type of analysis on prepared sperm using TUNEL, we were able to identify differences in blastocyst development between

Table 40.1. Examples of sperm DNA fragmentation tests and their mode of action

Mode of action	Test	References
Direct integration of marked nucleotides into sperm nuclear DNA breaks	Terminal deoxynucleotidyl transferase-mediated dUTP nick end-labeling (TUNEL) In-situ nick translation	[6,7]
Binding of a marker onto DNA after alteration in sperm chromatin conformation	Sperm chromatin structure assay (SCSA) DNA breakage detection–fluorescence in-situ hybridization (DBD–FISH) Sperm chromatin dispersion (SCD) Comet assay	[1,8,12–14,23,24,50]
Integration of a marker into a sperm nucleus representative of abnormal protamine content	Chromomycin A_3 (CMA_3) Aniline blue Toludine blue	[10,11,51,52]
Apoptotic markers	Fas Annexin V Bcl protein family members Caspases	[15,16,17,53,54]

high and low TUNEL patients but failed to observe differences in pregnancy rates [48].

A second major difference between many of the tests is in the steps preparatory to measurement. These can be separated into either (1) an invasive denaturation step of heating, acid exposure, etc., which acts to unwind the chromatin in susceptible areas so that markers such as acridine orange can have greater accessibility, or (2) an in-situ diagnosis whereby the sperm are not pretreated and are either fixed or labeled immediately so that the chromatin is in a more "natural" state. Generally, when different sperm DNA measurement techniques are compared, they do show a strong correlation even though the outcome results may shift in intensity of the DNA fragmentation. For example, Chohan *et al.* found that the TUNEL and SCD assays showed a strong relationship with the SCSA ($r > 0.866$; $P < 0.001$) for sperm DNA fragmentation, both in infertile men and in donors of known fertility [12]. Even different fixation techniques will shift the level of intensity [49]. **The general deduction is that SCSA, TUNEL, and SCD show similar predictive values for DNA fragmentation.**

Numerous tests now exist to measure sperm DNA fragmentation. Ironically, it could be argued that technically they are all measuring similar aberrations in sperm chromatin and DNA structure, with only a slight variation in the way they access the DNA (Table 40.1) [1,6–8,10–17,23,24,50,52–54]. The tests such as the SCSA and TUNEL have been discussed above. **Other tests include the comet assay [8], DNA breakage detection (DBD)–FISH [55], SCD [13,56], and its commercial form the HaloSperm kit [50]. All have shown a strong correlation to sperm quality in examination** **of fertile versus nonfertile males.** Their clinical effectiveness in correlating to pregnancy outcome is still to be determined, as none have come under the same scrutiny as SCSA or even TUNEL. Of all the current tests the comet assay has the added advantage that it can be examined for the presence of both single- and double-stranded breaks, depending on the conditions under which it is run [8]. These tests give an accurate assessment of sperm DNA integrity, but all involve a challenge to the susceptibility of DNA integrity and may give higher than expected values.

Other means exist for surrogate examination of the DNA integrity of spermatozoa. One means is to examine the protamine constituency of the spermatozoa. It is believed that the lower the protamine-to-histone ratio the more likely the chance that the sperm are abnormal and that the DNA integrity may be faulty [57]. Aoki *et al.* measured variations in protamine 1 (P1) and protamine 2 (P2) content between individual sperm cells of fertile and infertile men and correlated them with DNA integrity [58,59]. They found that TUNEL and SCSA positivity correlated with abnormal protamine levels in sperm cells. Chromomycin A_3 measurements are also thought to be representative of protamine levels in spermatozoa [60]. A number of clinical studies subsequently have shown a positive relationship between CMA_3 and sperm DNA integrity [47,61,62].

A final set of interesting surrogate markers include those that examine apoptotic pathway-related markers. In 1999 we showed that abnormal spermatozoa were more likely to possess Fas on their membranes [15]. Subsequently, numerous studies have shown that a number of apoptotic marker proteins correlate with DNA integrity in sperm [16,17,53,54]. Whether these markers reflect apoptotic sperm is still not clearly understood [36]. Unfortunately, because spermatozoa possess a high level of protamines we are unable to perform the classic DNA analysis of apoptosis showing DNA laddering of the histone-complexed DNA.

Interestingly, some of the apoptotic markers are already being used in innovative ways to help select spermatozoa with better DNA integrity [17] and to test whether novel sperm selection techniques provide a better yield of spermatozoa [63,64]. Further scrutiny of all the markers described will provide answers as to how informative they will be in a clinical setting.

The origin of DNA damage

There are two main theories explaining the origin of sperm DNA damage. **First, it is thought that abnormalities in spermatogenesis and/or spermiogenesis lead to the production of sperm with these inherent DNA anomalies.** A breakdown in three key cell system regulators, apoptosis, DNA repair, and chromatin remodeling, are thought to be responsible (reviewed in [5,35,65]). **A second line of thought is that exposure to increased radical oxygen species or failure of antioxidant defense systems during transport through the male reproductive tract is also responsible.** This argument is best illustrated in an excellent commentary by Alvarez [66] and in a review by Aitken and Sawyer [67]. It is also supported by studies demonstrating that DNA fragmentation is higher in epididymal [68] and ejaculated [69,70] spermatozoa than in testicular sperm. It is my belief, however, that a failure in the first system is predominantly responsible, as it will lead to the production of spermatozoa that are more susceptible to ROS in the reproductive tract.

Conclusion

The numerous tests now available to examine deficiencies in spermatozoa provide a significant improvement to the standard concentration, motility, and morphology assessment. In one respect they provide a second level of scrutiny; in a number of studies even normozoospermic men have been shown to possess anomalies in sperm DNA integrity [10,30,71]. **In relation to their clinical relevance, it is unmistakable that a higher level of abnormality in sperm DNA integrity is certainly a negative trait that reduces the chances to father a child.** The mainstream application of this technology, however, still requires further research and improvement. Finally, the armory of techniques now available for measurement of sperm DNA integrity and certain molecular characteristics of ejaculated spermatozoa hopefully will allow us to pinpoint more accurately the origin of these anomalies in spermatozoa, and will lead to better clinical treatment options prior to the use of ICSI.

References

[1] Evenson DP, Darzynkiewicz Z, Melamed MR. Relation of mammalian sperm chromatin heterogeneity to fertility. *Science* 1980; **210**: 1131–3.

[2] Palermo G, Joris H, Devroey P, Van Steirteghem AC. Pregnancies after intracytoplasmic injection of single spermatozoon into an oocyte. *Lancet* 1992; **340**: 17–18.

[3] Devroey P, Van Steirteghem A. A review of ten years experience of ICSI. *Hum Reprod Update* 2004; **10**: 19–28.

[4] Ponjaert-Kristoffersen I, Bonduelle M, Barnes J, *et al.* International collaborative study of intracytoplasmic sperm injection-conceived, in vitro fertilization-conceived, and naturally conceived 5-year-old child outcomes: cognitive and motor assessments. *Pediatrics* 2005; **115**: e283–9.

[5] Seli E, Sakkas D. Spermatozoal nuclear determinants of reproductive outcome: implications for ART. *Hum Reprod Update* 2005; **11**: 337–49.

[6] Gorczyca W, Traganos F, Jesionowska H, Darzynkiewicz Z. Presence of DNA strand breaks and increased sensitivity of DNA in situ to denaturation in abnormal human sperm cells: analogy to apoptosis of somatic cells. *Exp Cell Res* 1993; **207**: 202–5.

[7] Bianchi PG, Manicardi GC, Bizzaro D, Bianchi U, Sakkas D. Effect of deoxyribonucleic acid protamination on fluorochrome staining and in situ nick-translation of murine and human mature spermatozoa. *Biol Reprod* 1993; **49**: 1083–8.

[8] Singh NP, Danner DB, Tice RR, *et al.* Abundant alkali-sensitive sites in DNA of human and mouse sperm. *Exp Cell Res* 1989; **184**: 461–70.

[9] Hughes CM, Lewis SE, McKelvey-Martin VJ, Thompson W. A comparison of baseline and induced DNA damage in human spermatozoa from fertile and infertile men, using a modified comet assay. *Mol Hum Reprod* 1996; **2**: 613–19.

[10] Bianchi PG, Manicardi GC, Urner F, Campana A, Sakkas D. Chromatin packaging and morphology in ejaculated human spermatozoa: evidence of hidden anomalies in normal spermatozoa. *Mol Hum Reprod* 1996; **2**: 139–44.

[11] Bianchi PG, Manicardi G, Bizzaro D, *et al.* Use of the guanine-cytosine (GC) specific fluorochrome,

chromomycin A3, as an indicator of poor sperm morphology. *J Assist Reprod Genet* 1996; **13**: 246–50.

[12] Chohan KR, Griffin JT, Lafromboise M, De Jonge CJ, Carrell DT. Comparison of chromatin assays for DNA fragmentation evaluation in human sperm. *J Androl* 2006; **27**: 53–9.

[13] Fernandez JL, Muriel L, Rivero MT, *et al*. The sperm chromatin dispersion test: a simple method for the determination of sperm DNA fragmentation. *J Androl* 2003; **24**: 59–66.

[14] Muriel L, Meseguer M, Fernandez JL, *et al*. Value of the sperm chromatin dispersion test in predicting pregnancy outcome in intrauterine insemination: A blind prospective study. *Hum Reprod* 2006; **21**: 738–44.

[15] Sakkas D, Mariethoz E, St John JC. Abnormal sperm parameters in humans are indicative of an abortive apoptotic mechanism linked to the Fas-mediated pathway. *Exp Cell Res* 1999; **251**: 350–5.

[16] Oehninger S, Morshedi M, Weng SL, *et al*. Presence and significance of somatic cell apoptosis markers in human ejaculated spermatozoa. *Reprod Biomed Online* 2003; **7**: 469–76.

[17] Said T, Agarwal A, Grunewald S, *et al*. Selection of nonapoptotic spermatozoa as a new tool for enhancing assisted reproduction outcomes: an in vitro model. *Biol Reprod* 2006; **74**: 530–7.

[18] Evenson D, Jost L. Sperm chromatin structure assay is useful for fertility assessment. *Methods Cell Sci* 2000; **22**: 169–89.

[19] Larson-Cook KL, Brannian JD, Hansen KA, *et al*. Relationship between the outcomes of assisted reproductive techniques and sperm DNA fragmentation as measured by the sperm chromatin structure assay. *Fertil Steril* 2003; **80**: 895–902.

[20] Evenson DP, Larson KL, Jost LK. Sperm chromatin structure assay: its clinical use for detecting sperm DNA fragmentation in male infertility and comparisons with other techniques. *J Androl* 2002; **23**: 25–43.

[21] Sailer BL, Jost LK, Evenson DP. Mammalian sperm DNA susceptibility to in situ denaturation associated with the presence of DNA strand breaks as measured by the terminal deoxynucleotidyl transferase assay. *J Androl* 1995; **16**: 80–7.

[22] Aravindan GR, Bjordahl J, Jost LK, Evenson DP. Susceptibility of human sperm to in situ DNA denaturation is strongly correlated with DNA strand breaks identified by single-cell electrophoresis. *Exp Cell Res* 1997; **236**: 231–7.

[23] Evenson DP, Jost LK, Marshall D, *et al*. Utility of the sperm chromatin structure assay as a diagnostic and prognostic tool in the human fertility clinic. *Human Reprod* 1999; **14**: 1039–49.

[24] Spano M, Bonde JP, Hjøllund HI, *et al*. Sperm chromatin damage impairs human fertility. The Danish First Pregnancy Planner Study Team. *Fertil Steril* 2000; **73**: 43–50.

[25] Larson KL, DeJonge CJ, Barnes AM, Jost LK, Evenson DP. Sperm chromatin structure assay parameters as predictors of failed pregnancy following assisted reproductive techniques. *Hum Reprod* 2000; **15**: 1717–22.

[26] Saleh RA, Agarwal A, Nada EA, *et al*. Negative effects of increased sperm DNA damage in relation to seminal oxidative stress in men with idiopathic and male factor infertility. *Fertil Steril* 2003; **79**: 1597–605.

[27] Gandini L, Lombardo F, Paoli D, *et al*. Full-term pregnancies achieved with ICSI despite high levels of sperm chromatin damage. *Hum Reprod* 2004; **19**: 1409–17.

[28] Bungum M, Humaidan P, Spano M, *et al*. The predictive value of sperm chromatin structure assay (SCSA) parameters for the outcome of intrauterine insemination, IVF and ICSI. *Hum Reprod* 2004; **19**: 1401–8.

[29] Bungum M, Humaidan P, Axmon A, *et al*. Sperm DNA integrity assessment in prediction of assisted reproduction technology outcome. *Hum Reprod* 2007; **22**: 174–9.

[30] Virro MR, Larson-Cook KL, Evenson DP. Sperm chromatin structure assay (SCSA) parameters are related to fertilization, blastocyst development, and ongoing pregnancy in in vitro fertilization and intracytoplasmic sperm injection cycles. *Fertil Steril* 2004; **81**: 1289–95.

[31] Payne JF, Raburn DJ, Couchman GM, *et al*. Redefining the relationship between sperm deoxyribonucleic acid fragmentation as measured by the sperm chromatin structure assay and outcomes of assisted reproductive techniques. *Fertil Steril* 2005; **84**: 356–64.

[32] Makhlouf AA, Niederberger C. DNA integrity tests in clinical practice: it is not a simple matter of black and white (or red and green). *J Androl* 2006; **27**: 316–23.

[33] Zini A, Finelli A, Phang D, Jarvi K. Influence of semen processing technique on human sperm DNA integrity. *Urology* 2000; **56**: 1081–4.

[34] Zini A, Mak V, Phang D, Jarvi K. Potential adverse effect of semen processing on human sperm deoxyribonucleic acid integrity. *Fertil Steril* 1999; **72**: 496–9.

[35] Sakkas D, Mariethoz E, Manicardi G, *et al*. Origin of DNA damage in ejaculated human spermatozoa. *Rev Reprod* 1999; **4**: 31–7.

[36] Sakkas D, Seli E, Manicardi GC, *et al*. The presence of abnormal spermatozoa in the ejaculate: did apoptosis fail? *Hum Fertil (Camb)* 2004; **7**: 99–103.

[37] Benchaib M, Lornage J, Mazoyer C, *et al.* Sperm deoxyribonucleic acid fragmentation as a prognostic indicator of assisted reproductive technology outcome. *Fertil Steril* 2007; **87**: 93–100.

[38] Perreault SD, Aitken RJ, Baker HW, *et al.* Integrating new tests of sperm genetic integrity into semen analysis: Breakout group discussion. *Adv Exp Med Biol* 2003; **518**: 253–68.

[39] Spano M, Seli E, Bizzaro D, Manicardi GC, Sakkas D. The significance of sperm nuclear DNA strand breaks on reproductive outcome. *Curr Opin Obstet Gynecol* 2005; **17**: 255–60.

[40] Tarozzi N, Bizzaro D, Flamigni C, Borini A. Clinical relevance of sperm DNA damage in assisted reproduction. *Reprod Biomed Online* 2007; **14**: 746–57.

[41] Borini A, Tarozzi N, Bizzaro D, *et al.* Sperm DNA fragmentation: paternal effect on early post-implantation embryo development in ART. *Hum Reprod* 2006; **21**: 2876–81.

[42] Evenson D, Wixon R. Meta-analysis of sperm DNA fragmentation using the sperm chromatin structure assay. *Reprod Biomed Online* 2006; **12**: 466–72.

[43] Li Z, Wang L, Cai J, Huang H. Correlation of sperm DNA damage with IVF and ICSI outcomes: a systematic review and meta-analysis. *J Assist Reprod Genet* 2006; **23**: 367–76.

[44] Spano M, Cordelli E, Leter G, *et al.* Nuclear chromatin variations in human spermatozoa undergoing swim-up and cryopreservation evaluated by the flow cytometric sperm chromatin structure assay. *Mol Hum Reprod* 1999; **5**: 29–37.

[45] Morrell JM, Moffatt O, Sakkas D, *et al.* Reduced senescence and retained nuclear DNA integrity in human spermatozoa prepared by density gradient centrifugation. *J Assist Reprod Gen* 2004; **21**: 217–22.

[46] Sakkas D, Manicardi GC, Tomlinson M, *et al.* The use of two density gradient centrifugation techniques and the swim-up method to separate spermatozoa with chromatin and nuclear DNA anomalies. *Hum Reprod* 2000; **15**: 1112–16.

[47] Tomlinson MJ, Moffatt O, Manicardi GC, *et al.* Interrelationships between seminal parameters and sperm nuclear DNA damage before and after density gradient centrifugation: Implications for assisted conception. *Hum Reprod* 2001; **16**: 2160–5.

[48] Seli E, Gardner DK, Schoolcraft WB, Moffatt O, Sakkas D. Extent of nuclear DNA damage in ejaculated spermatozoa impacts on blastocyst development after in vitro fertilization. *Fertil Steril* 2004; **82**: 378–83.

[49] Manicardi GC, Tombacco A, Bizzaro D, *et al.* DNA strand breaks in ejaculated human spermatozoa: comparison of susceptibility to the nick translation and terminal transferase assays. *Histochem J* 1998; **30**: 33–9.

[50] Fernandez JL, Muriel L, Goyanes V, *et al.* Halosperm is an easy, available, and cost-effective alternative for determining sperm DNA fragmentation. *Fertil Steril* 2005; **84**: 860.

[51] Erenpreiss J, Bars J, Lipatnikova V, Erenpreisa J, Zalkalns J. Comparative study of cytochemical tests for sperm chromatin integrity. *J Androl* 2001; **22**: 45–53.

[52] Franken DR, Franken CJ, de la Guerre H, de Villiers A. Normal sperm morphology and chromatin packaging: comparison between aniline blue and chromomycin A3 staining. *Andrologia* 1999; **31**: 361–6.

[53] Cayli S, Sakkas D, Vigue L, Demir R, Huszar G. Cellular maturity and apoptosis in human sperm: creatine kinase, caspase-3 and Bcl-XL levels in mature and diminished maturity sperm. *Mol Hum Reprod* 2004; **10**: 365–72.

[54] Cayli S, Jakab A, Ovari L, *et al.* Biochemical markers of sperm function: male fertility and sperm selection for ICSI. *Reprod Biomed Online* 2003; **7**: 462–8.

[55] Fernandez JL, Vazquez-Gundin F, Delgado A, *et al.* DNA breakage detection-FISH (DBD-FISH) in human spermatozoa: Technical variants evidence different structural features. *Mutat Res* 2000; **453**: 77–82.

[56] Fernandez JL, Muriel L, Goyanes V, *et al.* Simple determination of human sperm DNA fragmentation with an improved sperm chromatin dispersion test. *Fertil Steril* 2005; **84**: 833–42.

[57] De Yebra L, Ballesca JL, Vanrell JA, *et al.* Detection of P2 precursors in the sperm cells of infertile patients who have reduced protamine P2 levels. *Fertil Steril* 1998; **69**: 755–9.

[58] Aoki VW, Moskovtsev SI, Willis J, *et al.* DNA integrity is compromised in protamine-deficient human sperm. *J Androl* 2005; **26**: 741–8.

[59] Aoki VW, Emery BR, Liu L, Carrell DT. Protamine levels vary between individual sperm cells of infertile human males and correlate with viability and DNA integrity. *J Androl* 2006; **27**: 890–8.

[60] Bizzaro D, Manicardi GC, Bianch PG, *et al.* In-situ competition between protamine and fluorochromes for sperm DNA. *Mol Hum Reprod* 1998; **4**: 127–32.

[61] Sakkas D, Manicardi G, Bianchi PG, Bizzaro D, Bianchi U. Relationship between the presence of endogenous nicks and sperm chromatin packaging in maturing and fertilizing mouse spermatozoa. *Biol Reprod* 1995; **52**: 1149–55.

[62] Esterhuizen AD, Franken DR, Lourens JG, *et al.* Chromatin packaging as an indicator of human sperm dysfunction. *J Assist Reprod Genet* 2000; **17**: 508–14.

[63] Jakab A, Sakkas D, Delpiano E, *et al.* Intracytoplasmic sperm injection: a novel selection method for sperm

with normal frequency of chromosomal aneuploidies. *Fertil Steril* 2005; **84**: 1665–73.

[64] Ainsworth C, Nixon B, Aitken RJ. Development of a novel electrophoretic system for the isolation of human spermatozoa. *Hum Reprod* 2005; **20**: 2261–70.

[65] Sakkas D, Seli E, Bizzaro D, Tarozzi N, Manicardi GC. Abnormal spermatozoa in the ejaculate: abortive apoptosis and faulty nuclear remodelling during spermatogenesis. *Reprod Biomed Online* 2003; **7**: 428–32.

[66] Alvarez JG. The predictive value of sperm chromatin structure assay. *Hum Reprod* 2005; **20**: 2365–7.

[67] Aitken RJ, Sawyer D. The human spermatozoon: not waving but drowning. *Adv Exp Med Biol* 2003; **518**: 85–98.

[68] Steele EK, McClure N, Maxwell RJ, Lewis SE. A comparison of DNA damage in testicular and proximal epididymal spermatozoa in obstructive azoospermia. *Mol Hum Reprod* 1999; **5**: 831–5.

[69] Ollero M, Gil-Guzman E, Lopez MC, *et al.* Characterization of subsets of human spermatozoa at different stages of maturation: implications in the diagnosis and treatment of male infertility. *Hum Reprod* 2001; **16**: 1912–21.

[70] Greco E, Scarselli F, Iacobelli M, *et al.* Efficient treatment of infertility due to sperm DNA damage by ICSI with testicular spermatozoa. *Hum Reprod* 2005; **20**: 226–30.

[71] Saleh RA, Agarwal A, Nelson DR, *et al.* Increased sperm nuclear DNA damage in normozoospermic infertile men: a prospective study. *Fertil Steril* 2002; **78**: 313–18.

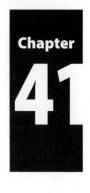

Chapter 41

A look towards the future: advances in andrology expected to revolutionize the diagnosis and treatment of the infertile male

Dolores J. Lamb

Introduction

Diagnoses in male infertility tend to be descriptive. For example, azoospermia is a condition in which there are no sperm in the ejaculate; this derives from the fact that in the overwhelming majority of cases the underlying basis of the patient's infertility is unknown. As molecular medicine enters the clinical arena for many specialties, the diagnosis and treatment of male infertility remains, for the most part, stagnant. Semen analyses, whole blood karyotypes, Y-chromosome microdeletion assays, and endocrine profiles are key laboratory diagnostic tests used to evaluate the infertile male (as discussed in Chapter 15); however, the results of these tests often are uninformative.

Consequently, ongoing investigations in translational research seek to improve the diagnosis and treatment of patients through the development of new and novel molecular approaches for identifying previously unrecognized causes of male infertility. These approaches include state-of-the-art genetics, genomics, proteomics, and metabolomics.

Couples face overwhelming financial and emotional costs related to their infertility, and given the present diagnostic uncertainties they also face difficult choices. The technological advances achieved today ultimately will improve our understanding of the mechanisms regulating all aspects of male reproductive development and function. Approaches to diagnosis will radically change over the next decades with the application of our growing understanding of the etiologies of infertility. Today, treatments available for male infertility are limited; yet as a result of a mechanistic understanding of infertility, new therapies will be

developed to allow for targeted treatment of patients. This will be in stark contrast to the current predominant clinical strategy, which uses defective gametes to overcome sterility with intracytoplasmic sperm injection in almost all cases. For patients, knowledge of the cause of their infertility and the potential consequences for their offspring will allow infertile couples to make informed decisions regarding their options for assisted reproduction. This chapter will explore the advances and technologies currently under development that are likely to advance our ability to diagnose and treat male infertility in the future.

The molecular medicine revolution reveals new etiologies of male infertility

The molecular time line of genetic diagnosis

Diagnosis of genetic defects evolved from simple assessment of the presence or absence of chromosome pairs (numerical alterations in chromosomes) to more complex diagnosis of structural chromosomal abnormality. Our ability to diagnose chromosomal defects in infertile males has improved markedly with each technological advance. This progress began with the simple realization that the sex chromosomes exist. It is noteworthy to realize that this was first postulated by McClung in 1901, and that the exact number of human chromosomes was not discovered until 1956 by Tjio and Levan [1]. It was soon discovered that aneuploidy of the sex chromosomes is associated with infertility (such as Klinefelter syndrome, Turner syndrome), and, as cytogenetic methodology improved, chromosome

Infertility in the Male, 4th edition, ed. Larry I. Lipshultz, Stuart S. Howards, and Craig S. Niederberger. Published by Cambridge University Press. © Cambridge University Press 2009.

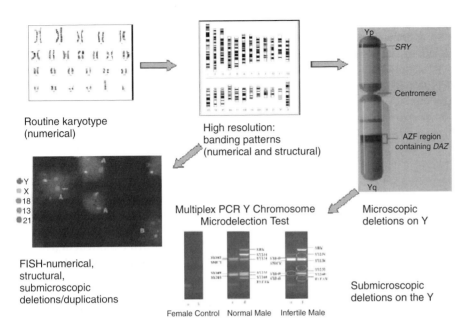

Routine karyotype
(numerical)

High resolution:
banding patterns
(numerical and structural)

FISH-numerical,
structural,
submicroscopic
deletions/duplications

Multiplex PCR Y Chromosome
Microdeletion Test

Female Control   Normal Male   Infertile Male

Microscopic
deletions on Y

Submicroscopic
deletions on the Y

Fig. 41.1. Genetic advances and the diagnosis of male infertility. The routine karyotype first provided information concerning numerical defects of chromosomes, and later technological advances allowed large translocations, insertions, and deletions to be observed as well. The development of polymerase chain reaction (PCR), the sequencing of the human genome, and fluorescence in-situ hybridization (FISH) has permitted previously unrecognized genetic causes of male infertility to be realized. With each new technological advance our ability to diagnose genetic causes of male infertility has improved. *See color plate section.*

translocations and deletions were observed in infertile men. Interestingly, although two cytogeneticists had postulated the presence of genes required for spermatogenesis on the Y chromosome in 1976 using routine cytogenetics [2], this knowledge was not translated to the infertility clinic for another 20 years with the identification of Y-chromosome microdeletions utilizing polymerase chain reaction (PCR) analysis [3]. Importantly, the Y-chromosome microdeletions identified in some men with azoospermia or severe oligospermia represent a genomic disorder not usually found by a routine karyotype; it could be diagnosed only when technology advanced sufficiently to permit the detection of this deletion by PCR. Further refinement by direct sequence analysis permits an even higher level of detection, allowing the definition of mutations in single genes causing male infertility.

The recent molecular revolution in genetics provides the cytogeneticist with an array of approaches to diagnose structural chromosomal defects. These include (1) fluorescence in-situ hybridization (FISH), (2) whole chromosome painting, and (3) comparative genomic hybridization, along with (4) PCR and (5) direct DNA sequencing to define chromosomal or genomic abnormalities (Fig. 41.1). As our ability to identify subtle defects in chromosome structure and gene sequence has improved, so has our ability to diagnose genetic defects in infertile men. **With each new technological advance, previously unrecognized genetic causes of male infertility have been defined.** This chapter will explore these novel approaches and focus on their potential clinical application in the future.

New technologies improve detection of numerical and structural chromosomal abnormalities

Meiotic recombination during gametogenesis involves the exchange of segments of DNA between pairs of homologous chromosomes and guarantees the continual evolution of the species by ensuring genetic diversity in the offspring. Defects in this critical reproductive process result in offspring with numerical or structural chromosomal abnormalities that may result in embryonic or fetal lethality, mental retardation, and birth defects. Importantly, these types of chromosomal aberrations are a significant cause of infertility in both males and females (see Chapter 15). Currently, a routine karyotype analysis provides evidence of numerical and structural defects in about 6% (some estimates are higher) of all infertile men, and thus provides important diagnostic information [4,5].

Technological advances continually improve our ability to define previously unrecognized causes of male infertility. The karyotype remains the gold standard of chromosomal analysis. In recent years, methods were developed to complement, or in some cases improve upon, the diagnostic capability of the karyotype. While some of these diagnostic approaches are used in a few state-of-the-art laboratories, the routine application of these technologies to the diagnosis of the infertile male is rare. They are expected to become commonplace as the genetic basis of male infertility becomes more widely appreciated by clinicians.

Fluorescence in-situ hybridization (FISH)

FISH uses molecular probes specific to regions of chromosomes, and can be designed to detect relatively small chromosome gains or losses. More commonly, it is used to define aneuploidy (gain or loss of chromosome, a deviation from the normal chromosomal complement), as well as the incidence of mosaicism. A powerful use of this technique is to define the incidence of sperm aneuploidy in infertile men [6] (see Chapter 15).

Significant limitations exist to the application of FISH in the routine evaluation of the infertile male. These include the cost of the probes required, the significant technical skills necessary, and the time required for three independent readers to evaluate each slide and count the fluorescent dots on each cell or sperm. Large numbers of sperm or cells are normally analyzed to reach a statistically valid result. Equipment for automated FISH analyses is commercially available, featuring an automated microscope with a multi-slide motorized stage, bright-field and fluorescent illumination, a sensitive 3-CCD color camera, and a sophisticated computer system for image capture and analysis. A stage micro-locator allows the investigator to return to an archived slide and immediately view the cell of interest in real time. This type of approach provides a method for the rapid detection of sperm chromosome disomy. Fertilization with sperm that has a chromosome disomy can lead to pregnancy loss, as well as syndromes compatible with a viable offspring: trisomy 13 (Patau syndrome), 18 (Edwards syndrome), 21 (Down syndrome), and sex chromosome abnormalities (Klinefelter [XXY–XXXXY] and Turner [monosomy X] syndromes).

Chromosome painting

Chromosome painting relies on the use of chromosome-specific fluorescent probes that stain each chromosome a different color. Complex chromosome rearrangements become immediately apparent. It is more commonly used for analysis of cancer cells, because of the cost of the probes and equipment

required, but it is applicable to the assessment of chromosome structures in infertile men and would be used in combination with a karyotype analysis.

Comparative genomic hybridization (CGH)

CGH initially used metaphase chromosomes to analyze chromosomal imbalances. The technique relies on the staining of control (normal) and patient DNA with green and red fluorescent dyes, respectively. Addition of equivalent concentrations of the green control and red patient DNA to metaphase chromosomes under conditions that allow hybridization of the added DNA to each chromosome permits geneticists to analyze structural chromosome defects. If chromosomes are normal in both the patient and the control, target chromosomes will stain yellow (the color yellow results when there is equivalent fluorescence of green and red dyes). A duplication of a chromosome region in the patient would lead to an area of red fluorescence on the target metaphase chromosome, and conversely a loss of a portion of chromosome (such as a Y-chromosome deletion) would stain green. This technology is limited by the resolution of detection of chromosome gains and losses, and was largely replaced with oligonucleotide fragments encoding human DNA sequences hybridized to glass slides (described below). CGH microarrays can be constructed spanning the entire human genome, with 32 433 overlapping fragments of oligonucleotide probe [7]. In essence, this represents a molecular karyotype and is known as a chromosome microarray [8].

Chromosome microarray (CMA)

The CMA method designed in the Kleberg Cytogenetics Laboratory at Baylor College of Medicine was developed for the clinical diagnosis of known chromosomal disorders using oligonucleotides as targets for comparative genomic hybridization. The genomic targets arrayed on the chip specifically focus on known clinical syndromes resulting from a loss or gain of specific chromosomal regions. It has been validated to detect small chromosomal deletions, duplications, and triplications. In general, there are 3–10 oligonucleotide fragments for each disease region, and each fragment hybridizes to only one chromosomal location.

CMA spans all chromosomes to identify imbalances that cannot be detected by current karyotype methods. An example of the type of imbalance detected is a Y-chromosome microdeletion (Fig. 41.2) [9]. In addition to providing the information normally obtained

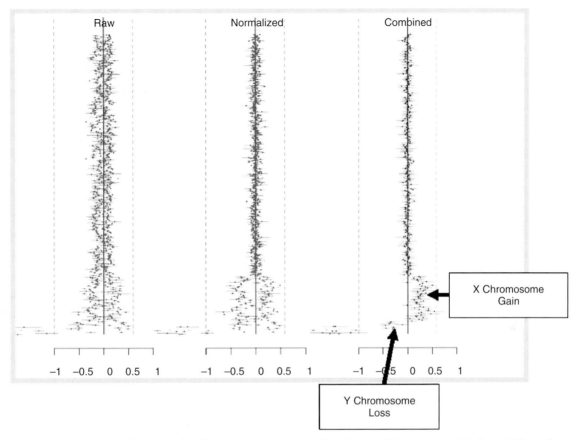

Fig. 41.2. Demonstration of the principles of chromosome microarray analysis. A region of chromosome gain is shown in blue and a loss in red, with the normal regions shown in green. Depicted is a schematic diagram of the data showing that female DNA stained red and male DNA stained green was competitively hybridized to a DNA assay of oligonucleotides spanning specific regions of each human chromosome, including the Y chromosome. The figure shows that the female DNA lacked the Y chromosome (as expected) but had a duplication of the X chromosome, as it should because the DNA is from a female. *See color plate section.*

by karyotype or FISH, CMA can define the extent of an imbalance, since there are multiple array points per telomere and disease region. While CMA's weakness is that it will not detect a balanced translocation or inversion that could be readily defined on a karyotype, CMA's strength is its ability to define imbalances that are undetected by routine cytogenetics. Cheung *et al.* used CMA both to detect previously identified abnormalities and to identify additional cryptic microdeletions and/or duplications in patients with various chromosomal abnormalities and microdeletions [9]. Of interest, CMA was used to rule out Klinefelter syndrome in a patient who was a phenotypic male with a karyotype of 46, X, der(X)t(X;Y)p22.33; p11.2. In a second child with developmental delay and dysmorphic features, CMA demonstrated that he was a 47,XXY Klinefelter male [9].

Advances in our understanding of the molecular defects causing male infertility
Y-chromosome microdeletions and duplications

Y-chromosome microdeletions were first observed over 30 years ago by two cytogeneticists studying men with azoospermia [2]. Subsequently, with the advances realized by the human genome project, Y-chromosome microdeletions were identified as a fairly common cause of nonobstructive azoospermia, being present in about 8–12% of men with nonobstructive azoospermia and a lesser percentage of men with oligospermia [10]. The deleted in azoospermia gene (*DAZ*) was the first putative spermatogenesis gene identified in the distal portion of the Y-chromosome coding region [3], and a number of spermatogenesis genes and types of microdeletions have been identified (reviewed in [10]). This is discussed more fully in Chapter 15. Of note, researchers have found that duplications in regions of the Y chromosome may occur as well and in some instances may be associated with male infertility [11], such as occurs with AZFc duplications in the Han Chinese. The role of duplications of regions of the Y chromosome remains an area of active research.

Gene mutations and male infertility

Studies of genetic causes of male infertility have profoundly altered the urologist's concept of its etiology. As evidence continues to accumulate, investigators speculate that as much as 80% of all male infertility may have a genetic basis. With advances in the field of genetics and technology, it is expected that patients will not just undergo a history and physical examination, but will have a lifelong record of their genetic information (perhaps even obtained through advanced prenatal diagnosis) that will provide prospective information concerning their risk of disease development. The studies described below will set the stage for new and novel approaches to diagnosis of the infertile male in the future.

What have we learned from animal models of male infertility?

As of today, over 300 null mutations and 50 conditional targeted deletions of genes have produced mouse models of male infertility. These mouse models confirmed and extended our understanding of the role of infertility-related genes involved in sex determination/ differentiation, steroidogenesis, steroid metabolism, growth factor, peptide, and steroid receptors, peptide hormones and growth factors, signal transduction pathways, DNA replication and repair, homologous recombination, mitosis, meiosis and differentiation (reviewed in [12]). Study of these mouse models has revealed proteins essential for novel structures vital to normal reproduction, such as the intercellular bridge, intermitochondrial cement and the chromatoid body, and the fibrous sheath [13–18]. Despite such major advances in understanding the importance of these genes in mouse reproductive function, translation of these findings to human male infertility has been slow. Nevertheless, scientists consistently define a high level of conservation of reproductive genes that occurs throughout evolution. Indeed, the ever-expanding

collection of organisms that have undergone complete DNA sequencing, from *Drosophila* to zebrafish to mice to humans, consistently shows large numbers of conserved genes. Thus there is a high likelihood that many of the infertility genes identified in animal models will have relevance to human male infertility.

Examples abound of translation of molecular findings in lower organisms that are applicable to humans

Scientists and the lay public alike marvel at the similarities of gene nucleotide sequences in diverse organisms, and these similarities support the concept of evolution. A few examples illustrate this principle. The *Drosophila* (fruit fly) gene *Boule* is homologous to the human Y-chromosome gene, deleted in azoospermia (*DAZ*) [19], and as in the human this gene product is involved in spermatogenesis [19,20]. The mammalian adenine nucleotide translocase 4 (*Ant4*) gene is highly conserved in both mammals and nonmammalian species, and when it is deleted male infertility results [21]. The *RBMX* gene, essential for brain development in zebrafish is homologous to *RBMY*, a spermatogenesis gene on the Y chromosome [22]. A yeast post-replication repair gene, *RAD18*, is highly homologous to *mRAD19Sc*, a mouse gene expressed in the primary pachytene spermatocyte that binds to single-stranded DNA and interacts with the ubiquitin-conjugating enzyme, RAD6. These are common pathways in both organisms. Indeed, *RAD18*-homologous genes are found in other species such as *Aspergillus nidulans* and *Neurospora crassa* as well [23]. Similarly, the long-sought gene that underlies the juvenile spermatogonial depletion mutation in the mouse was shown to be the mouse homolog of the *Saccharomyces cerviasiae* gene *UTP14*, expressed predominantly in the zygotene through round spermatids [24]. **The literature is replete with examples of fertility-related genes such as those mentioned above that are highly conserved throughout evolution. Thus, evidence of gene defects causing infertility in mouse models raises significant concern about the causes of infertility in humans.**

Gene mutations in human male infertility

With the advent of the human genome project, large numbers of genes implicated in human male infertility have become known. Despite these advances in our understanding of the molecular basis for male infertility, the overall frequency of any individual mutation is generally low, and, with the exception of analysis of the cystic fibrosis transmembrane conductance regulator gene (*CFTR*) variants in couples when the man has bilateral absence of the vas deferens [25,26], DNA sequence analysis is rarely employed in the evaluation of the infertile male. That said, the definition of the nucleotide sequence for the human genome has facilitated the identification of human infertility-related genes, resulting in a virtual explosion of publications over the past few years.

Modulation of gene expression and its association with male infertility

Not surprisingly, the highest rate of RNA synthesis/gene expression in the body is in the testis – specifically during spermatogenesis. Genetic modification of DNA affecting even noncoding regions of the DNA such as the promotor or the 3' untranslated regions can alter RNA expression, as can changes in the transcriptional machinery. During the processing of the mRNA that occurs after transcription, many unique forms of RNAs commonly expressed in other tissues are produced in the testis as a result of alternative splicing. Defects in all of these processes have been associated with male infertility (as well as other systemic defects, in some cases) [12].

Epigenetics and non-Mendelian modifiers of gene expression

One regulator of gene expression is methylation. **Imprinting of genes by methylation is an epigenetic phenomenon that differs from gene mutation but nevertheless carries the possibility of transmitting a phenotypic alternation from parents to offspring through multiple generations.** Imprinting occurs at specific gene loci during gametogenesis with a gender-defined pattern of methylation of certain genes. At fertilization, the union of the male and female gametes brings one gene copy with a male pattern of methylation and one copy of a female pattern of methylation, and these methylation patterns are maintained in the offspring. **When there is a failure of imprinting during gametogenesis, at fertilization two male or two female-patterned methylations may be present, and these are associated with specific disease syndromes.**

Studies in animals suggested that exposure to agents thought to be involved in endocrine disruption (hormone mimics, i.e., agents such as detergents, pesticides, fungicides, plasticizers, herbicides, and insecticides) may affect reproductive development and function through their actions as weak receptor agonists or antagonists. Because estrogens can influence gene methylation, investigators have asked whether fetal exposure to these agents (thought to be steroid hormone agonists or antagonists) can result in adult disease – in this case alterations in the methylation patterns of genes known to be differentially imprinted during gametogenesis, with associated functional deficiencies in male reproductive health [27]. These studies are of importance not only because they raise the possibility that environmental exposures can have long-term consequences for fertility, but also because there are a number of genetic syndromes that result from abnormal gene imprinting. Several rare diseases, such as Beckwith–Wiedemann, Angelman, and Prader–Willi syndromes, appear to occur with increased frequency in the offspring of infertile couples conceived by ICSI [28–30].

Modulation of RNA translation to proteins and its association with infertility

MicroRNA and PIWI RNA are key players in the regulation of gametogenesis

Previously unrecognized infertility pathways regulating translation are under investigation. Noncoding RNAs and their regulation of specific cellular pathways were first revealed in Caenorhabditis *elegans* in 2001 [31]. More recently, the number of noncoding regulatory RNAs, termed microRNAs or miRNAs (about 21 nucleotides in length), as well as the slightly larger PIWI-interacting RNAs (also called P-element induced wimpy testis in *Drosophila*, or piRNAs, about 26–31 nucleotides in length), have increased to ~500 sequences in mice and humans [32], with over 50 000 piRNAs [33]. These small fragments of piRNA derived from long precursor RNAs were first believed to be testis-specific, but are now known to be present in more diverse tissues. There are human homologs, and PIWI is highly expressed in the spermatogenic cells. The number of miRNAs is less for reasons that are not clearly understood, and this remains an area of intense investigation. In females, the ribonuclease Dicer, involved in RNA interference, plays a key role in the female germline, although the role in the male is less clearly understood. Dicer plays a role in the biosynthesis of the miRNAs, which are about 21 nucleotides long. **These unique gene classes, *PIWI* and *MIWI*, are required for spermatogenesis and male fertility [34–36], again** pointing to the importance of this newly identified regulatory pathway in fertility. Obviously, research in this area is rapidly advancing.

Improvements in diagnosis of RNA transcription changes

Expression microarrays define transcriptional changes in male infertility

Molecular techniques progressed from the simple analysis of the level of a single mRNA with techniques such as a Northern blot to define gene expression to the analysis of huge numbers of genes simultaneously with the use of expression microarrays. The basic concept remains the same, and relies upon the principle of hybridization of complementary nucleotide sequences. However, the strategy used for these arrays differs from the CMA described above (which analyzes DNA duplications and deletions) because the assay requires that mRNA be transcribed into cDNA, again with a linked red or green fluorescent dye competitively binding the green control and red experimental cDNAs to the oligonucleotides on the array. While the principles of data analysis are similar to the CMA, and huge amounts of data are generated, the information reflects the complex regulation of expression of thousands of different genes within a tissue of interest. Some arrays focus only on targeted genes, for example those involved in cell cycle control or DNA repair pathways or other signal transduction pathways, while others encompass virtually all known genes. Investigators worked to define tissue signatures representing either specific tissues, cell types, or tumor stages. With regard to the testis, Griswold and colleagues have amassed a large body of data representing testis gene expression in the mouse at various times of development [37]. Turek's group has presented microarray data characterizing gene expression in human testis representing not only normal testis, but also the pathologic histologies of Sertoli-cell-only, hypospermatogenesis, and maturation arrest [38]. Interpretation, however, is challenging because the testis represents a heterogeneous mixture of cell types, and accordingly findings often reflect cell-type-specific changes rather than direct regulator defects. Laser capture microdissection of a single cell within a tissue overcomes these caveats but can be technically challenging. Nevertheless, the gene expression microarray is an important technology that provides a broad view of gene expression.

Genetic analysis of residual RNA in sperm

The precise contribution of an individual locus to an observed phenotype can be challenging in complex disorders. Because infertility results in the absence or paucity of offspring, a simple linkage analysis is nearly impossible to undertake to identify gene defects associated with infertility. This fact presents challenges to the detection of single gene defects in male infertility. The candidate gene approach (targeted gene deletion in mouse models, or gene knockdown) has provided many new insights into previously unrecognized genes required for fertility. However, translation of these findings to the human situation has been slow, although certain advances have been realized. Because oligospermic and normospermic infertile men are not candidates for a testis biopsy, genetic studies of human infertility to date have relied on somatic DNA analysis, an approach that provides no insight into the possibility of germline mutations or splicing variants/mutations. Sperm are transcriptionally inactive because of the condensation of the nucleus and tightly packaged chromatin. However, prior to that time, during meiosis, micro-RNAs are expressed that remain stable up through fertilization in the human (discussed previously) [39–45]. Indeed, the presence of long-lived mRNA in sperm was noted many years ago by Monesi and colleagues [46]. The gene expression microarray studies of Krawetz and colleagues suggested that RNA associated with sperm reflect testicular gene expression, specifically meiotically expressed genes [42]. Matzuk and colleagues used the RNA isolated from human spermatozoa to develop a novel diagnostic strategy [47]. Interestingly, multiple full-length spermatozoal mRNAs encoding candidate fertility-related genes were screened for mutations by reverse transcriptase–polymerase chain reaction (RT–PCR), and over 90% of the haploid-expressed genes tested could be analyzed, even in severely oligospermic samples. The human homolog of the *Drosophila* kelch gene was investigated, because targeted deletion in the mouse results in severe oligospermia due to reduction in elongating spermatids. When this residual sperm RNA analysis approach was used, germ-cell-expressed *hKLHL10* mutations resulting in deficient protein function were identified in 1.3% of patients with oligospermia, demonstrating the utility of this approach [47]. Certainly, this approach holds promise for noninvasive genetic diagnosis of meiotic-expressed gene defects.

Proteomics of human semen and testis

Although many investigations focus on analysis of RNA to assess gene expression, it is imperative to analyze the resulting proteins, because not all RNAs are translated. The technique involves high-resolution, two-dimensional electrophoresis with robotically performed dissection of individual protein spots followed by amino acid analysis for protein identification. Proteomics allows a large-scale investigation into the qualitative and quantitative comparison of proteomes under different conditions to further unravel biological processes. Proteomics is the study of the complete complement of proteins in an organism using both protein profiling and functional assessments. The word proteome comes from PROTEin complement to a genOME. These studies are really in their infancy. Proteomic analysis of semen has provided potentially new markers of prostate cancer [48,49]. Others have attempted to use proteomics to describe protein differences in the sperm of men that fail to penetrate the ova [50]. Elsewhere, the Herr laboratory has focused its proteomic investigations of sperm to identify potential contraceptive targets in sperm [51,52]. The field is developing rapidly.

Therapeutic advances of the future
Stem cells

Stem cells have the potential to differentiate into different functional cell types in the body, and their discovery has given rise to the fields of regenerative medicine and cloning (reviewed in [53]). Investigators have sought to develop methods to use stem cells to correct or restore fertility. Embryonic stem cells have the potential to differentiate into nearly every cell type found in the body. As the cells differentiate, they are thought to lose this plasticity to develop into different tissues; yet specific tissues (gastrointestinal, integumentary, spermatogenic, and hematopoietic systems) maintain their regenerative capacity. In fact, adult stem cells have been functionally identified in a wide range of tissues. The adult stem cells are thought to hold great promise for tissue generation. We focus here solely on the therapeutic potential of stem cells for rejuvenation of male fertility.

Embryonic stem cells

Embryonic stem cells are obtained from embryos, such as those generated during a routine in-vitro fertilization (IVF) cycle. After fertilization and through embryogenesis until about the eight-cell stage, the blastomeres are totipotent, meaning they have the capacity to differentiate into any cell type in the body. Immediately thereafter, the embryonic stem cells derived from the inner cell mass of a blastocyte become pluripotent, meaning they can differentiate into all cell types in the body (tissues derived from all three germ layers) with the exception of the placenta. These cells can be cultured under stringent conditions and expanded, yet maintain their regenerative capacity. Stem cell differentiation is controlled by both intrinsic genetic signals, and extrinsic signals such as growth factors, cell contacts, and the microenvironment or niche. Depending upon the culture conditions in vitro and/or their transplantation to a specific niche in vivo, the cells can be directed to differentiate into different cell lineages. Transplantation of undifferentiated embryonic stem cells results in teratoma formation, and indeed the first observation of stem-cell-like activity occurred during studies of embryonal carcinoma cells. Scientists are beginning to dissect the pattern of gene expression and extrinsic modulator that regulates each step of embryonic germ cell development, and eventually will be able to direct embryonic stem cell differentiation efficiently down different paths to eventually become virtually any tissue in the body [54]. This is the promise of embryonic stem cells.

Embryonic stem cells have the capacity to differentiate directly into either male or female gametes [55–58]. Varying culture conditions have resulted in the presence of some haploid gene expression, although complete spermatogenesis has been difficult if not impossible to achieve in vitro [59]. Using cell culture in combination with transplantation to the testis, male gametes were derived directly from embryonic germ cells [58]. Functional ova have not been as definitively achieved, although follicle-like structures have been generated in vitro [55,56].

Spermatogonial stem cells

Although the existence of spermatogonial stem cells was postulated almost 40 years ago on the basis of morphological studies [60–62] and observations of spermatogenic damage following toxic exposures, it was not until the pioneering work of Brinster and colleagues that their existence was proven [63,64]. Using testicular homogenates of transgenic mice expressing the *LacZ* gene (to provide a marker of cell fate), these investigators transplanted these cells into the

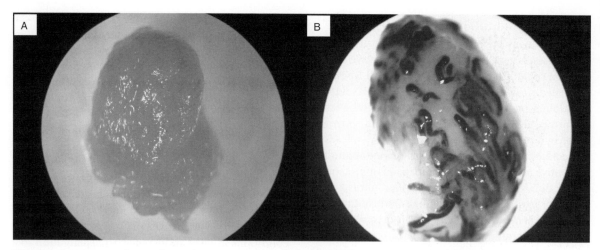

Fig. 41.3. Spermatogonial stem cell transplantation into Sertoli-cell-only histology mouse recipient testis. Spermatogonial stem cells from cryptorchid Rosa26 mouse testis expressing the *LacZ* transgene were enriched based upon exclusion of rhodamine dye and flow cytometry to select the cells that excluded the rhodamine dye. These cells were transplanted by microinjection via the efferent ducts and backwashing the testis of a TAF4b-deficient mouse with a Sertoli-cell-only histology. The cells engrafted, colonized the seminiferous tubules, and spermatogenesis was restored. (A) a noninjected control TAF4b-deficient testis; (B) a TAF4b testis four months after transplantation of the Rosa26 spermatogonial stem cells. The cell fate of the transplanted cells within the recipient seminiferous tubules is evident by the blue staining demonstrating the presence of the *LacZ* transgene [68]. *See color plate section.*

seminiferous tubules of otherwise sterile mice with a Sertoli-cell-only pathology. After three months, the transplanted spermatogonial stem cells had engrafted and colonized the seminiferous tubules. Spermatogenesis was restored (Fig. 41.3). The clinical implications of this work are enormous. It suggests that isolation, enrichment, and cryopreservation of spermatogonial stem cells prior to chemotherapy or radiation therapy, with later autologous transplantation, may offer the potential of subsequent restoration of fertility. This will be especially important for survivors of childhood cancer. Adult patients can bank sperm prior to cryopreservation. However, most couples would prefer a naturally conceived child. Work has progressed in many laboratories to partially enrich the spermatogonial stem cells of species ranging from mice to primates. Many urologists today bank a testicular biopsy from patients about to undergo chemotherapy, with the expectation that the technology will advance rapidly over the next 10 years and allow transplantation in the future.

Guan *et al.* isolated spermatogonial stem cells from immature mice and, after a selection procedure and culture, injected them into blastocysts and showed that they differentiated into all three germlines (endoderm, mesoderm, ectoderm) and differentiated into various organs and tissues [65]. There was germline transmission of the marker protein, showing that these rare cells

had embryonic stem cell activity or could revert down the pathway of differentiation back to a primordial germ-cell-like cell. These studies could have significant implications for the future application of these cells to regenerative medicine without the potential ethical concerns raised by the use of human embryos to derive embryonic stem cells.

Lentiviral transduction of spermatogonial stem cells has permitted germline gene therapy. Using a rat model, Ryu *et al.* transduced germ cells with a fluorescent marker protein, and about 40% of the offspring expressed this transgene [66]. This approach would potentially offer the hope of correction of gene defects through transgenesis.

Leydig stem cell/progenitors

Lo *et al.* enriched Leydig cell progenitors using a combination of castration, flow cytometry based upon differential efflux of Hoechst 33342 dye, and intratesticular transplantation into the interstitial space, to demonstrate both the existence of adult Leydig stem cells in the testis and their potential to increase testosterone production (Fig. 41.4) [67,68]. When an LH-receptor-deficient mouse model was used, transplantation of healthy wild-type Leydig cell progenitors expressing the *LacZ* gene to track cell fate resulted in engraftment and colonization of the interstitial space. Measurable levels of testosterone became apparent in the serum

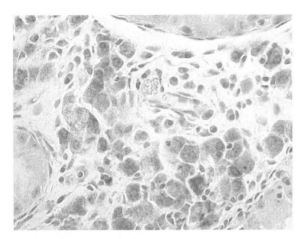

Fig. 41.4. Successful engraftment and colonization of transplanted Leydig cell progenitors into the interstitial space. Adult Leydig stem cell progenitors from the testis of Rosa26 male mice expressing the *LacZ* transgene were enriched by flow cytometry based upon exclusion of Hoechst 33342 dye and transplanted into a Wv mouse testis. The testicular section is stained to show the expression of the β-galactosidase transgene (blue) and counterstained with hematoxylin and eosin (pink) as described by Lo *et al.* [67]. *See color plate section.*

over time after transplantation, and spermatogenesis was restored in these otherwise hypogonadal, infertile mice. The method not only offers the potential to restore and rejuvenate androgen secretion, but also provides a model to study the regulation of Leydig cell differentiation and development.

Conclusions

There is no doubt that technical and scientific advances such as those described in this chapter will drive the development of new and innovative approaches to the diagnosis and treatment of the infertile male by the urologist. As our understanding of the basic mechanisms of mitosis, meiosis, and sperm differentiation grows, along with our knowledge of the processes of sperm maturation and transit through the genital tracts of the male and female, and of the events of fertilization and early embryonic development, the diagnostic, medical, and surgical approaches to the treatment of infertility will coordinately advance and ultimately improve patient care. Thus, in our quest to enhance our knowledge of these basic cellular processes that have gone awry, medical advances will be realized and continually improve our ability to diagnose and treat. To *cure* these infertile patients, rather than *assist* their fertility with assisted reproductive technology (ART) procedures, will require the continued

application of basic research to define these control mechanisms. We look toward the future with excitement – where we will find that a patient's genetic, genomic, and proteomic information provides a view not only of his or her current physical state but a prediction of the likelihood of future illnesses or syndromes. For the urologist, such information will become as important as the patient history in the course of the workup of the infertile male. Couples face overwhelming financial and emotional costs related to their infertility. For these patients, knowledge of the cause of their infertility that will be gained as a result of these new technologies, and of the potential consequences of that infertility for the offspring, will allow them to make informed decisions regarding their options for assisted reproduction. It is hoped that the advanced techniques and research findings discussed will provide not only new treatment options but also insights into the safety and long-term consequences of the predominant current clinical strategy, which largely relies upon the use of defective or deficient sperm for fertilization rather than treating the cause of the infertility.

Acknowledgments

Supported in part by Grants No. 2P01 HD 36289 and the National Institutes of Health Cooperative Centers Program in Reproductive Research (U54 HD07495) from the National Institutes of Health.

References

[1] Tjio HJ, Levan A. The chromosome numbers of men. *Hereditas* 1956; **42**: 1–6.

[2] Tiepolo L, Zuffardi O. Localization of factors controlling spermatogenesis in the nonfluorescent portion of the human Y chromosome long arm. *Hum Genet* 1976; **34**: 119–24.

[3] Reijo R, Alagappan RK, Patrizio P, Page DC. Severe oligozoospermia resulting from deletions of azoospermia factor gene on Y chromosome. *Lancet* 1996; **347**: 1290–3.

[4] Yoshida A, Miura K, Shirai M. Cytogenetic survey of 1,007 infertile males. *Urol Int* 1997; **58**: 166–76.

[5] Nakamura Y, Kitamura M, Nishimura K, *et al.* Chromosomal variants among 1790 infertile men. *Int J Urol* 2001; **8**: 49–52.

[6] Egozcue J, Sarrate Z, Codina-Pascual M, *et al.* Meiotic abnormalities in infertile males. *Cytogenet Genome Res* 2005; **111**: 337–42.

[7] Ishkanian AS, Malloff CA, Watson SK, *et al.* A tiling resolution DNA microarray with complete coverage of the human genome. *Nat Genet* 2004; **36**: 299–303.

[8] Cheung SW, Shaw CA, Scott DA, *et al*. Microarray-based CGH detects chromosomal mosaicism not revealed by conventional cytogenetics. *Am J Med Genet A* 2007; **143**: 1679–86.

[9] Cheung SW, Shaw CA, Yu W, *et al*. Development and validation of a CGH microarray for clinical cytogenetic diagnosis. *Genet Med* 2005; **7**: 422–32.

[10] McElreavey K, Krausz C, Patrat C, Fellous M. Male infertility and microdeletions of the Y chromosome. *Gynecol Obstet Fertil* 2002; **30**: 405–12.

[11] Lin YW, Hsu LC, Kuo PL, *et al*. Partial duplication at AZFc on the Y chromosome is a risk factor for impaired spermatogenesis in Han Chinese in Taiwan. *Hum Mutat* 2007; **28**: 486–94.

[12] Matzuk MM, Lamb DJ. Genetic dissection of mammalian fertility pathways. *Nat Cell Biol* 2002; **4** (Suppl): s41–9.

[13] Parvinen M. The chromatoid body in spermatogenesis. *Int J Androl* 2005; **28**: 189–201.

[14] Greenbaum MP, Ma L, Matzuk MM. Conversion of midbodies into germ cell intercellular bridges. *Dev Biol* 2007; **305**: 389–96.

[15] Roy A, Lin YN, Agno JE, DeMayo FJ, Matzuk MM. Absence of tektin 4 causes asthenozoospermia and subfertility in male mice. *FASEB J* 2007; **21**: 1013–25.

[16] Luk JM, Lee NP, Shum CK, *et al*. Acrosome-specific gene AEP1: Identification, characterization and roles in spermatogenesis. *J Cell Physiol* 2006; **209**: 755–66.

[17] Greenbaum MP, Yan W, Wu MH, *et al*. TEX14 is essential for intercellular bridges and fertility in male mice. *Proc Natl Acad Sci U S A* 2006; **103**: 4982–7.

[18] Escalier D. Knockout mouse models of sperm flagellum anomalies. *Hum Reprod Update* 2006; **12**: 449–61.

[19] Eberhart CG, Maines JZ, Wasserman SA. Meiotic cell cycle requirement for a fly homologue of human Deleted in Azoospermia. *Nature* 1996; **381**: 783–5.

[20] Shan Z, Hirschmann P, Seebacher T, *et al*. A SPGY copy homologous to the mouse gene Dazla and the Drosophila gene boule is autosomal and expressed only in the human male gonad. *Hum Mol Genet* 1996; **5**: 2005–11.

[21] Brower JV, Rodic N, Seki T, *et al*. Evolutionarily conserved mammalian adenine nucleotide translocase 4 is essential for spermatogenesis. *J Biol Chem* 2007; **282**: 29658–66.

[22] Tsend-Ayush E, O'Sullivan LA, Grutzner FS, *et al*. RBMX gene is essential for brain development in zebrafish. *Dev Dyn* 2005; **234**: 682–8.

[23] van der LR, Roest HP, Hoogerbrugge JW, *et al*. Characterization of mRAD18Sc, a mouse homolog of the yeast postreplication repair gene RAD18. *Genomics* 2000; **69**: 86–94.

[24] Rohozinski J, Bishop CE. The mouse juvenile spermatogonial depletion (jsd) phenotype is due to a mutation in the X-derived retrogene, mUtp14b. *Proc Natl Acad Sci U S A* 2004; **101**: 11695–700.

[25] De BM, Ferec C. Mutations in the cystic fibrosis gene in men with congenital bilateral absence of the vas deferens. *Mol Hum Reprod* 1996; **2**: 669–77.

[26] Anguiano A, Oates RD, Amos JA, *et al*. Congenital bilateral absence of the vas deferens: a primarily genital form of cystic fibrosis. *JAMA* 1992; **267**: 1794–7.

[27] Anway MD, Cupp AS, Uzumcu M, Skinner MK. Epigenetic transgenerational actions of endocrine disruptors and male fertility. *Science* 2005; **308**: 1466–9.

[28] Allen C, Reardon W. Assisted reproduction technology and defects of genomic imprinting. *BJOG* 2005; **112**: 1589–94.

[29] Chang AS, Moley KH, Wangler M, Feinberg AP, Debaun MR. Association between Beckwith–Wiedemann syndrome and assisted reproductive technology: a case series of 19 patients. *Fertil Steril* 2005; **83**: 349–54.

[30] Olivennes F, Mannaerts B, Struijs M, Bonduelle M, Devroey P. Perinatal outcome of pregnancy after GnRH antagonist (ganirelix) treatment during ovarian stimulation for conventional IVF or ICSI: a preliminary report. *Hum Reprod* 2001; **16**: 1588–91.

[31] Lau NC, Lim LP, Weinstein EG, Bartel DP. An abundant class of tiny RNAs with probable regulatory roles in Caenorhabditis elegans. *Science* 2001; **294**: 858–62.

[32] Saito K, Nishida KM, Mori T, Kawamura Y, Miyoshi K, Nagami T, *et al*. Specific association of Piwi with rasiRNAs derived from retrotransposon and heterochromatic regions in the Drosophila genome. *Genes Dev* 2006; **20**: 2214–22.

[33] Ro S, Park C, Jin J, Sanders KM, Yan W. A PCR-based method for detection and quantification of small RNAs. *Biochem Biophys Res Commun* 2006; **351**: 756–63.

[34] Kuramochi-Miyagawa S, Kimura T, Ijiri TW, *et al*. Mili, a mammalian member of piwi family gene, is essential for spermatogenesis. *Development* 2004; **131**: 839–49.

[35] Deng W, Lin H. Miwi, a murine homolog of piwi, encodes a cytoplasmic protein essential for spermatogenesis. *Dev Cell* 2002; **2**: 819–30.

[36] Kuramochi-Miyagawa S, Kimura T, Yomogida K, *et al*. Two mouse piwi-related genes: Miwi and mili. *Mech Dev* 2001; **108**: 121–33.

[37] Small CL, Shima JE, Uzumcu M, Skinner MK, Griswold MD. Profiling gene expression during the differentiation and development of the murine embryonic gonad. *Biol Reprod* 2005; **72**: 492–501.

[38] Fox MS, Ares VX, Turek PJ, Haqq C, Reijo Pera RA. Feasibility of global gene expression analysis in testicular biopsies from infertile men. *Mol Reprod Dev* 2003; **66**: 403–21.

[39] Kumar G, Patel D, Naz RK. c-MYC mRNA is present in human sperm cells. *Cell Mol Biol Res* 1993; **39**: 111–17.

[40] Wykes SM, Visscher DW, Krawetz SA. Haploid transcripts persist in mature human spermatozoa. *Mol Hum Reprod* 1997; **3**: 15–19.

[41] Ostermeier GC, Miller D, Huntriss JD, Diamond MP, Krawetz SA. Reproductive biology: delivering spermatozoan RNA to the oocyte. *Nature* 2004; **429**: 154.

[42] Ostermeier GC, Dix DJ, Miller D, Khatri P, Krawetz SA. Spermatozoal RNA profiles of normal fertile men. *Lancet* 2002; **360**: 772–7.

[43] Miller D, Briggs D, Snowden H, *et al.* A complex population of RNAs exists in human ejaculate spermatozoa: Implications for understanding molecular aspects of spermiogenesis. *Gene* 1999; **237**: 385–92.

[44] Ostermeier GC, Goodrich RJ, Diamond MP, Dix DJ, Krawetz SA. Toward using stable spermatozoal RNAs for prognostic assessment of male factor fertility. *Fertil Steril* 2005; **83**: 1687–94.

[45] Ostermeier GC, Goodrich RJ, Moldenhauer JS, Diamond MP, Krawetz SA. A suite of novel human spermatozoal RNAs. *J Androl* 2005; **26**: 70–4.

[46] Monesi V. Ribonucleic acid and protein synthesis during differentiation of male germ cells in the mouse. *Arch Anat Microsc Morphol Exp* 1967; **56**: 61–74.

[47] Yatsenko AN, Roy A, Chen R, *et al.* Non-invasive genetic diagnosis of male infertility using spermatozoal RNA: KLHL10 mutations in oligozoospermic patients impair homodimerization. *Hum Mol Genet* 2006; **15**: 3411–19.

[48] Pilch B, Mann M. Large-scale and high-confidence proteomic analysis of human seminal plasma. *Genome Biol* 2006; **7**: R40.

[49] Banez LL, Srivastava S, Moul JW. Proteomics in prostate cancer. *Curr Opin Urol* 2005; **15**: 151–6.

[50] Pixton KL, Deeks ED, Flesch FM, *et al.* Sperm proteome mapping of a patient who experienced failed fertilization at IVF reveals altered expression of at least 20 proteins compared with fertile donors: case report. *Hum Reprod* 2004; **19**: 1438–47.

[51] Shetty J, Diekman AB, Jayes FC, *et al.* Differential extraction and enrichment of human sperm surface proteins in a proteome: identification of immunocontraceptive candidates. *Electrophoresis* 2001; **22**: 3053–66.

[52] Shetty J, Naaby-Hansen S, Shibahara H, *et al.* Human sperm proteome: immunodominant sperm surface antigens identified with sera from infertile men and women. *Biol Reprod* 1999; **61**: 61–9.

[53] Vieyra DS, Jackson KA, Goodell MA. Plasticity and tissue regenerative potential of bone marrow-derived cells. *Stem Cell Rev* 2005; **1**: 65–9.

[54] Donovan PJ, de Miguel MP. Turning germ cells into stem cells. *Curr Opin Genet Dev* 2003; **13**: 463–71.

[55] Hubner K, Fuhrmann G, Christenson LK, *et al.* Derivation of oocytes from mouse embryonic stem cells. *Science* 2003; **300**: 1251–6.

[56] Toyooka Y, Tsunekawa N, Akasu R, Noce T. Embryonic stem cells can form germ cells in vitro. *Proc Natl Acad Sci U S A* 2003; **100**: 11457–62.

[57] West JA, Park IH, Daley GQ, Geijsen N. In vitro generation of germ cells from murine embryonic stem cells. *Nat Protoc* 2006; **1**: 2026–36.

[58] Geijsen N, Horoschak M, Kim K, *et al.* Derivation of embryonic germ cells and male gametes from embryonic stem cells. *Nature* 2004; **427**: 148–54.

[59] Lee JH, Kim HJ, Kim H, Lee SJ, Gye MC. In vitro spermatogenesis by three-dimensional culture of rat testicular cells in collagen gel matrix. *Biomaterials* 2006; **27**: 2845–53.

[60] Huckins C. The spermatogonial stem cell population in adult rats. 3. Evidence for a long-cycling population. *Cell Tissue Kinet* 1971; **4**: 335–49.

[61] Huckins C. The spermatogonial stem cell population in adult rats. II. A radioautographic analysis of their cell cycle properties. *Cell Tissue Kinet* 1971; **4**: 313–34.

[62] Huckins C. The spermatogonial stem cell population in adult rats. I. Their morphology, proliferation and maturation. *Anat Rec* 1971; **169**: 533–57.

[63] Brinster RL, Avarbock MR. Germline transmission of donor haplotype following spermatogonial transplantation. *Proc Natl Acad Sci U S A* 1994; **91**: 11303–7.

[64] Brinster RL, Zimmermann JW. Spermatogenesis following male germ-cell transplantation. *Proc Natl Acad Sci U S A* 1994; **91**: 11298–302.

[65] Guan K, Nayernia K, Maier LS, *et al.* Pluripotency of spermatogonial stem cells from adult mouse testis. *Nature* 2006; **440**: 1199–203.

[66] Ryu BY, Orwig KE, Oatley JM, *et al.* Efficient generation of transgenic rats through the male germline using lentiviral transduction and transplantation of spermatogonial stem cells. *J Androl* 2007; **28**: 353–60.

[67] Lo KC, Lei Z, Rao C, Beck J, Lamb DJ. De novo testosterone production in luteinizing hormone receptor knockout mice after transplantation of leydig stem cells. *Endocrinology* 2004; **145**: 4011–15.

[68] Falender AE, Freiman RN, Geles KG, *et al.* Maintenance of spermatogenesis requires TAF4b, a gonad-specific subunit of TFIID. *Genes Dev* 2005; **19**: 794–803.

Index

Note: page numbers in *italics* refer to figures and tables